Neuroscience of Nicotine
Mechanisms and Treatment

烟碱神经科学

作用机制与治疗

（英）维克托 R. 普里迪（Victor R. Preedy） 主编

胡清源
侯宏卫 主译
付亚宁

化学工业出版社
·北京·

内容简介

本书汇总了63篇有关烟草神经科学领域的新进展，整合了关于烟碱使用的药理学、细胞学和分子学方面的尖端研究，以及它对神经生物学功能的影响，内容涵盖了烟碱研究、治疗、政策和预防的各个方面，为学生、早期职业研究人员和各级调查人员提供了烟碱滥用各个方面的基本介绍，可以帮助读者快速了解烟草行业发展现状、烟碱的神经生物学机制和毒理学效应、烟碱成瘾的治疗等内容。

Neuroscience of Nicotine: Mechanisms and Treatment, 1st edition
Victor R. Preedy
ISBN: 9780128130353
Copyright © 2019 Elsevier Inc. All rights reserved.
Authorized Chinese translation published by Chemical Industry Press Co. Ltd.

《烟碱神经科学：作用机制与治疗》（胡清源，侯宏卫，付亚宁 主译）
ISBN: 978-7-122-42919-3
Copyright © 2019 Elsevier Inc. and Chemical Industry Press Co. Ltd. All rights reserved.

No part of this publication may be reproduced or transmitted in any form or by any means, electronic or mechanical, including photocopying, recording, or any information storage and retrieval system, without permission in writing from Elsevier (Singapore) Pte Ltd. Details on how to seek permission, further information about the Elsevier's permissions policies and arrangements with organizations such as the Copyright Clearance Center and the Copyright Licensing Agency, can be found at our website: www.elsevier.com/permissions.

This book and the individual contributions contained in it are protected under copyright by Elsevier Inc. and Chemical Industry Press Co. Ltd. (other than as may be noted herein).

This edition of Neuroscience of Nicotine: Mechanisms and Treatment is published by Chemical Industry Press Co.Ltd. under arrangement with ELSEVIER Inc.
This edition is authorized for sale in China only, excluding Hong Kong, Macau and Taiwan. Unauthorized export of this edition is a violation of the Copyright Act. Violation of this Law is subject to Civil and Criminal Penalties.

本版由Elsevier Inc. 授权化学工业出版社有限公司在中国大陆地区（不包括香港、澳门以及台湾地区）出版发行。
本版仅限在中国大陆地区（不包括香港、澳门以及台湾地区）出版及标价销售。未经许可之出口，视为违反著作权法，将受民事及刑事法律之制裁。
本书封底贴有Elsevier防伪标签，无标签者不得销售。

注 意

本书涉及领域的知识和实践标准在不断变化。新的研究和经验拓展我们的理解，因此须对研究方法、专业实践或医疗方法作出调整。从业者和研究人员必须始终依靠自身经验和知识来评估和使用本书中提到的所有信息、方法、化合物或本书中描述的实验。在使用这些信息或方法时，他们应注意自身和他人的安全，包括注意他们负有专业责任的当事人的安全。在法律允许的最大范围内，爱思唯尔、译文的原文作者、原文编辑及原文内容提供者均不对因产品责任、疏忽或其他人身或财产伤害及/或损失承担责任，亦不对由于使用或操作文中提到的方法、产品、说明或思想而导致的人身或财产伤害及/或损失承担责任。

北京市版权局著作权合同登记号：01-2023-0286

图书在版编目（CIP）数据

烟碱神经科学：作用机制与治疗/（英）维克托 R. 普里迪（Victor R. Preedy）主编；胡清源，侯宏卫，付亚宁主译. —北京：化学工业出版社，2023.7

书名原文：Neuroscience of Nicotine: Mechanisms and Treatment
ISBN 978-7-122-42919-3

Ⅰ.①烟… Ⅱ.①维…②胡…③侯…④付… Ⅲ.①烟碱-神经生物学-研究 Ⅳ.①R338

中国国家版本馆CIP数据核字（2023）第023579号

责任编辑：李晓红		文字编辑：林 丹　骆倩文	
责任校对：王 静		装帧设计：王晓宇	

出版发行：化学工业出版社（北京市东城区青年湖南街13号　邮政编码100011）
印　　装：北京虎彩文化传播有限公司
787mm×1092mm　1/16　印张35¾　字数894千字　2023年6月北京第1版第1次印刷

购书咨询：010-64518888　　　　　　　　售后服务：010-64518899
网　　址：http://www.cip.com.cn
凡购买本书，如有缺损质量问题，本社销售中心负责调换。

定　　价：298.00元　　　　　　　　　　　　　　　　　　　　版权所有　违者必究

译者人员名单

主 译：胡清源　侯宏卫　付亚宁

译 者：胡清源　侯宏卫　付亚宁　王红娟　田雨闪　陈　欢
　　　　韩书磊　刘　彤　李凯欣　秦雨涵　刘明达　张　浩
　　　　高铭遥　韩鹏飞　李倩楠　程浩平

前言 PREFACE

烟草使用（吸烟）的历史起源是在美洲，大约400年前烟草就开始了商业规模的种植，现在在世界范围内广泛使用。据估计，全球有10亿人被归类为烟草使用者，每年大约有700万人因吸烟而死亡。美国约有4000万成年人吸烟，其中3/4属于日常吸烟者。每年大约有50万美国人死于吸烟的影响。

烟碱能改变多种神经生物学过程：从分子和细胞生物学到大脑的功能改变。详细了解烟碱及其广泛影响对于为治疗方案奠定基础是必要的。然而"戒烟"是非常困难的，因为吸烟者经历了大量的戒断症状。烟碱戒断在行为层面是明显的，但这也有分子和细胞基础。另一方面，一些报告认为烟碱可以增强认知能力。事实上，与烟碱有关的科学资料非常丰富，在不同学科之间的相互关联，可在不同的资源中发现。因此，在单一的来源中找到可以导致对烟碱的神经科学的更好深入理解的信息迄今为止是很困难的。这在《烟碱神经科学：作用机制与治疗》中得到了解决。全文共分为以下七个部分：

（1）绪论——场景设置部分；
（2）神经科学；
（3）心理、行为、渴求和戒断；
（4）药理学、神经活性物质、分子和细胞生物学；
（5）烟碱和其他成瘾；
（6）生物标志物和筛查；
（7）治疗、策略和资源。

由于许多章节可以被分成两个或更多的章节，所以很难将特定章节归为书的不同部分。尽管如此，与烟碱相关的章节、领域和关键方面的导航都在书末列出了出色的索引。

《烟碱神经科学：作用机制与治疗》超越了多学科和智力的划分，每一章都有以下内容：
- 一组关键事实
- 术语解释
- 一组要点总结

《烟碱神经科学：作用机制与治疗》是为研究和教学目的而设计的，读者对象包括神经学家、卫生科学家、公共卫生助教、工人、医生、药理学家和研究型科学家，以及各级烟草研究和服务项目的主管。另外，领导治疗和预防烟碱滥用的医生也可能感兴趣。它是有价值的个人参考书，也为学术图书馆提供涵盖神经学、健康科学或成瘾领域的书籍。本书作者来自国内外知名专家，包括世界知名机构。本书适用于本科生、研究生、讲师和学术教授。

Victor R. Preedy
伦敦国王学院
英国伦敦

编辑顾问 Editorial Advisors

Dr. Vinood Patel. PhD, FRSC

Reader, Department of Biomedical Sciences, University of Westminister, London, United Kingdom

Dr. Rajkumar Rajendram AKC BSc (Hons) MBBS (Dist) EDIC FRCP (Edin)

Consultant, Department of Internal Medicine, King Abdulaziz Medical City, Riyadh, Saudi Arabia

Chairman, Medication Utilisation & Process Evaluation Subcommittee, Medication Safety Program, Ministry of the National Guard Health Affairs, King Abdulaziz Medical City, Riyadh, Saudi Arabia

Lecturer, Department of Nutrition, Faculty of Life Sciences and Medicine, King's College, London, United Kingdom

1	了解不同国家的烟草使用情况 Fabrizio Ferretti	001
2	孕妇吸烟和胎儿大脑的结果：机制和可能的解决方案 Hui Chen, Yik Lung Chan, Brian G. Oliver, Carol A. Pollock, Sonia Saad	009
3	烟碱对青少年的影响 Sari Izenwasser	019
4	传统卷烟和电子烟对大脑的影响 Ewelina Wawryk-Gawda, Marta Lis-Sochocka, Patrycja Chylińska-Wrzos, Beata Budzyńska, Barbara Jodłowska-Jędrych	027
5	减少烟草中的烟碱及其影响 Yael Abreu-Villaça, Alex Christian Manhães, Anderson Ribeiro-Carvalho	036
6	产前烟碱暴露和神经前体细胞 Tursun Alkam, Toshitaka Nabeshima	044
7	烟碱依赖性神经元中突触定位的烟碱乙酰胆碱受体亚基 Kristi A. Kohlmeier	053
8	在不同模型中，可替宁作为一种可能的烟碱效应的变构调节剂 Oné R. Pagán	063
9	烟碱、神经可塑性和烟碱的治疗潜力 Russell W. Brown, W. Drew Gill	071
10	缰状突触和烟碱 Jessica L. Ables, Beatriz Antolin-Fontes, Ines Ibañez-Tallon	078
11	烟碱对大脑神经元的神经保护：烟碱成瘾的另一面 Dzejla Bajrektarevic, Silvia Corsini, Andrea Nistri, Maria Tortora	087
12	将烟碱、薄荷醇和大脑变化联系起来 Brandon J. Henderson	096
13	吸烟与烟碱：对多发性硬化症的影响 Insa Backhaus, Alice Mannocci, Giuseppe La Torre, Aldo Liccardi	106
14	多巴胺能系统的烟草和正电子发射断层扫描（PET）：人类研究综述 Chidera C. Chukwueke, Bernard Le Foll	116
15	静止状态功能连接成像和烟碱依赖 Victor M. Vergara, Vince D. Calhoun	127
16	急性烟碱效应的功能磁共振成像 Christiane M. Thiel	136
17	精神分裂症中的烟碱依赖：烟碱乙酰胆碱受体的贡献 Robert D. Cole, Vinay Parikh	144

18	注意偏向和吸烟 David J. Drobes, Jason A. Oliver, John B. Correa, David E. Evans	154
19	烟碱对人体抑制控制的影响 Ulrich Ettinger, Veena Kumari	162
20	烟碱、促肾上腺皮质激素释放因子和焦虑样行为 Adriaan W. Bruijnzeel	171
21	6-羟基-L-烟碱和记忆障碍 Lucian Hritcu, Marius Mihasan	178
22	可替宁与记忆：为忘而忆 Valentina Echeverria, Ross Zeitlin	187
23	烟碱在异常学习和皮质纹状体可塑性中的作用 Jessica L. Koranda, Jeff A. Beeler	197
24	产前烟碱暴露及其对后代行为的影响 Tursun Alkam, Toshitaka Nabeshima	206
25	以吸烟为重点的物质使用渴望障碍 Stephen J. Wilson, Michael A. Sayette	214
26	运动对渴望和戒断症状的急性影响 Wuyou Sui, Scott Rollo, Harry Prapavessis	220
27	CRF2 受体激动剂和烟碱戒断 Zsolt Bagosi	229
28	精神错乱和烟碱戒断 Kataria Dinesh, Goel Ankit, Tiwari Sucheta, Kukreti Prerna	237
29	术后烟碱戒断 Paul Zammit	245
30	烟碱和 α3β2 神经烟碱乙酰胆碱受体 Doris Clark Jackson, Sterling N. Sudweeks	251
31	烟碱成瘾和 α4β2* 烟碱乙酰胆碱受体 John J. Maurer, Heath D. Schmidt	260
32	α3β4 烟碱乙酰胆碱受体和 P 物质在烟碱致敏中的作用 Branden Eggan, Sarah McCallum	269
33	靶向烟碱型乙酰胆碱受体治疗疼痛 Deniz Bagdas, S.Lauren Kyte, Wisam Toma, M.Sibel Gurun, M.Imad Damaj	278
34	肌肉型烟碱受体的药理作用 Armando Alberola-Die, Raúl Cobo, Isabel Ivorra, Andrés Morales	287
35	阿片类药物受体参与烟碱相关的强化和愉悦 Ari P. Kirshenbaum	298
36	烟碱诱导的诱发效应：年龄、性别、抗氧化剂预防的影响 Danielle Macedo, Adriano José Maia Chaves Filho, Patrícia Xavier Lima Gomes, Lia Lira Olivier Sanders, David Freitas de Lucena	308

37	烟碱奖励和戒烟：CB1 受体的作用	
	S. Tannous, S. Caille	318
38	烟碱和其他烟碱乙酰胆碱受体激动剂的认知增强作用的治疗潜力	
	Britta Hahn	327
39	烟碱和多巴胺 DA_1 受体药理学	
	Agnieszka Michalak, Barbara Budzyńska	335
40	烟碱奖励背景下的大脑基因表达：对胆碱能基因的关注	
	Mark D. Namba, Gregory L. Powell, Armani P. Del Franco, Julianna G. Goenaga, Cassandra D. Gipson	344
41	HIV 感染者与吸烟：关注烟碱对大脑的影响	
	Manuel Delgado-Vélez, José A. Lasalde-Dominicci	352
42	肾素 – 血管紧张素系统基因与烟碱依赖	
	Sergej Nadalin, Hrvoje Jakovac	362
43	烟碱依赖与 *CHRNA5/CHRNA3/CHRNB4* 烟碱受体调节组	
	Sung-Ha Lee, Elizabeth S. Barrie, Wolfgang Sadee, Ryan M. Smith	372
44	大脑、Nrf2 和烟草：吸烟氧化应激介导的脑血管效应的机制和反馈机制	
	Shikha Prasad, Taylor Liles, Luca Cucullo	380
45	烟碱和组蛋白脱乙酰酶抑制剂对大脑的影响	
	Maria Paula Faillace, Ramon O. Bernabeu	390
46	L 型钙离子通道与烟碱	
	Yudan Liu, Meghan Harding	400
47	烟碱与其他物质使用和成瘾的并存：风险、机制、后果和对实践的影响，以年轻人为重点	
	Linda Richter	412
48	吸烟与赌博并存障碍：潜在机制及未来探索	
	Emma V. Ritchie, David C. Hodgins, Daniel S. McGrath	420
49	烟草和强效可卡因使用的神经科学：新陈代谢、效果和症状学	
	Antonio Gomes de Castro-Neto, Rossana Carla Rameh-de-Albuquerque, Pollyanna Fausta Pimentel de Medeiros, Roberta Uchôa, Beate Saegesser Santos	429
50	唾液可替宁测定	
	M. Inês G.S. Almeida, Luisa Barreiros, Spas D. Kolev, Marcela A. Segundo	438
51	关于吸烟状态分类的可替宁截止值的概述	
	Sungroul Kim	447
52	戒烟预期问卷	
	Lorra Garey, Fiammetta Cosci, Michael J. Zvolensky	459
53	由药剂师主导的戒烟服务：当前和未来的展望	
	Chee Fai Sui, Long Chiau Ming	467
54	青少年的烟碱使用和体重控制：预防和早期干预的意义	
	Adrian B. Kelly, Rebekah Thomas, Gary C. K. Chan	476
55	锻炼是一种戒烟的辅助手段	
	Scott Rollo, Wuyou Sui, Harry Prapavessis	485

56 伐伦克林：治疗吸烟成瘾和精神分裂症
Do-Un Jung, Sung-Jin Kim ··· 494

57 烟碱疫苗：过去、现在和未来
Yun Hu, Zongmin Zhao, Kyle Saylor, Chenming Zhang ··· 503

58 在精神病医院治疗烟碱依赖
Emily A. Stockings ··· 512

59 口服 18- 甲氧基冠醚（18-MC）降低大鼠烟碱自给药
Amir H. Rezvani, Stanley D. Glick, Edward D. Levin ·· 521

60 药物遗传学与戒烟
Taraneh Taghavi, Rachel F. Tyndale ·· 526

61 促食欲素系统与烟碱成瘾：临床前观察
Shaun Yon-Seng Khoo, Gavan P. McNally, Kelly J. Clemens ·· 536

62 烟草控制政策和吸烟者的反应
Philip DeCicca, Erik Nesson ··· 546

63 烟碱神经科学资源
Rajkumar Rajendram, Victor R. Preedy ·· 554

1
了解不同国家的烟草使用情况

Fabrizio Ferretti

School of Social Sciences, Department of Communication and Economics (DCE), University of Modena and Reggio Emilia (UNIMORE), Reggio Emilia, Italy

缩略语

CDC	美国疾病控制和预防中心	**WHO**	世界卫生组织
NIH	美国国立卫生研究院	**GBD**	全球疾病负担
OECD	经济合作与发展组织	**IARC**	国际癌症研究机构
WBG	世界银行集团		

1.1 引言

有多种烟草制品可供世界各地的人们根据当地的喜好和习俗以多种不同的形式消费烟草。例如，烟草产品可以燃烧（如卷烟和比迪烟）、加热（如水烟），甚至口服或鼻咽（如鼻烟、槟榔和咀嚼烟草）。每个民族都有自己的文化传统，例如，印度的比迪烟、中东和南亚国家的水烟和鼻烟（Hammond, 2009, p3）。

然而，随着工业化、城市化和全球化的发展，人造卷烟的消费量在20世纪急剧增长，几乎遍及所有国家。因此，如今卷烟已成为全球烟草使用的主要形式，约占全球烟草产品总销售额的92%。着眼于当前在公共卫生领域的挑战，这就是为什么在烟草流行病学中，"烟草使用"和"吸烟"两个术语经常被作为同义词使用（NIH, 2016, 第2章）。

1.2 烟草流行病学的基本概念

对于每个人来说，烟草消费的规模和模式都是由各种个人和集体影响相互作用的结果（Warner, MacKay, 2006）。如图1.1所示，采用流行病学"三角模型"来描述和概念化这些复杂的关系（Penn State, 2016; Slade, 1993, 第1章），例如，以吸烟的形式存在的烟草起到了媒介的作用（即疾病发生所需的"必要"因素，尽管它可能不是一定会导致疾病。所有习惯性吸烟者都是宿主，至少有可能由于吸烟而患上一种或多种与烟草有关的疾病（通常导致残疾和死亡）。烟草公司通过生产和推广卷烟的使用来扩大市场规模（即吸烟者人数和每个吸烟者所消费的卷烟数量），发挥媒介（即向易感个体运输和传播）的作用。最后，宿主和病媒在由心理、文化、法律和经济等广泛因素相互作用所决定的社会环境中运作和互动（Giovino, 2002）。

鉴于烟草作为几种慢性非传染性疾病（如心血管和呼吸系统疾病以及多种癌症）的主要风险因素的突出作用，衡量全球烟草使用的分布和强度对于①更好地了解吸烟行为的决定因素，②制

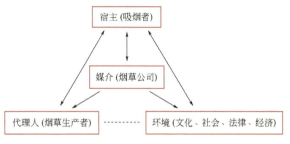

图1.1 烟草流行中代理人、宿主、媒介和环境的相互作用

来自：Penn State. (2016). Epidemiologic Triad. Department of Statistics. Pennsylvania State University. Available at: https://onlinecourses.science.psu.edu/stat507/node/25. Originally adapted from Egger, G.; Swinburn, B.; Rossner, S. (2003). Dusting off the epidemiological triad: could it work with obesity? Obesity Reviews 4(2), 115-119.

订有效的公共卫生计划，③监测各国的进展至关重要（GBD，2015）。总的来说，为了研究烟草使用的模式并模拟烟草控制政策在特定人群中的影响，流行病学家现今依赖于总体（即分区）和个体（即主体）的综合和复杂的模型（CDC，2014，第15章）。然而，国家一级和长期监测烟草使用的"基本原则"仍然包括通过使用直接和间接方法或两者同时使用来测量（或更好地估计）两个关键的卫生政策变量——吸烟流行率和吸烟强度（IARC，2008，第3章）。

在某一特定人群中，吸烟流行率通常采用直接的方法来评估，即通过询问具有代表性的受试者的吸烟状况和行为来评估（Bonnie, Stratton, Wallace, 2007）。调查提供了关于吸烟者身份的信息（例如，年龄、性别、种族、教育程度和收入水平），以及每个吸烟者的习惯和态度。具体来说，根据受访者自我报告的信息，将受访者分为三个主要类别（如图1.2所示）：从不吸烟者、目前吸烟者和曾经吸烟者（CDC，2014，第15章）。每一组的人数是一个存量变量（即在给定时间点测量的量）。随着时间的推移，对被研究人群进行监测，可以得到开始、停止和复发吸烟的人数。这些是流量变量（即在一段时间内测量的数量），表示在给定的时间间隔内（例如，一年）每个库存的变化量。

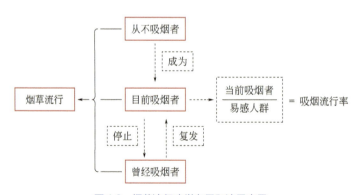

图1.2 烟草流行病学存量和流量变量

如果将某一特定类别的病例数（例如，吸烟者人数）除以处于危险中的人口的相应人数（从不吸烟、目前吸烟和曾经吸烟的人数的总和），关于存量和流量变量的数据转换成比率就更有意义，其中分子和分母可能指研究中的整个样本（通常由15岁及以上的人口组成）或按性别、年龄等分类的特定子集（Bonita, Beaglehole, Kjellstrom, 2006，第2章）。先进的统计技术通常用于从对给定人口的不同调查中收集结果，以获得国家级别的吸烟流行的估计。在这一框架中，一般人口中吸烟的流行率提供了关于某一国家目前吸烟人数比例的信息。最后，对这些国家简单（粗

比率进行年龄标准化，以便在人口年龄结构不同的国家之间进行公平比较（WHO, 2015）。

烟草使用调查还记录了每个吸烟者每天消费卷烟数量的自我报告数据。这些数字再加上流行率数据，就得出了研究对象在一段特定时间（通常是一年）内吸烟总人数的估计值。在一个特定的经济体中，美国的卷烟消费是衡量烟草市场规模的基本指标。总消费量除以该国烟民人数就得到了每个烟民平均消费的卷烟数量。这是一个常用的衡量吸烟强度的国家标准，通常用日均消费来表示，即"平均吸烟者"每天消费的卷烟数量（Guindon, Boisclair, 2003）。然而，使用一种间接的方法也在国家一级评估了卷烟的总消费量和平均消费量。间接估计主要基于国家商品资产负债表的统计数字。事实上，卷烟生产、净出口（即进口减去出口）和库存的变化提供了一种表观烟草消费的衡量标准，即理论上可用于国内消费的卷烟数量。在发达国家，这些估计数字通常与烟草税收统计数据结合在一起。年总表观消费量与15岁或15岁以上人口的比率衡量了该国的人均卷烟消费量（WHO, 2017）。

总的来说，直接法和间接法各有优缺点。间接法是一种相对容易的方法，可以产生基本统计数据，从而概述不同国家的烟草消费情况，而直接法虽然更具挑战性，但提供关于吸烟者身份（例如性别、年龄）的信息，并区分吸烟流行率和吸烟的强度。允许对国家内部和国家之间烟草使用的模式和演变进行深入的流行病学调查（Lopez, Neil, Tapani, 1994）。

1.3 对烟草制品的需求：简要介绍

在市场经济中，卷烟和其他与烟草有关的产品，就像任何制造产品一样，通常对当前和潜在的消费者以一定的价格出售。然而，价格只是影响消费者购买意愿的众多变量之一。消费者的收入和品味、相关商品（补充品和替代品，如酒精和电子卷烟）的价格和烟草控制政策是影响消费者在特定市场和时间段内购买多少卷烟（或烟草相关产品）的主要因素（Gallus, Schiaffino, LaVecchia, Townsend, Fernandez, 2006）。影响需求的相关因素很多，需要对不同国家烟草消费的决定因素进行抽象理解。在经济学中，解决这个问题的方法主要是首先分析价格变化对需求量的影响，保持所有其他可能影响购买的因素不变，然后检查除价格之外任何变量（例如可支配收入或强制性健康警告）的变化对消费的影响，每次只考虑一个（Mankiw, 2012, 第4章）。

这一"思维实验"的结果是经济学分析中的一个基本思维工具：需求曲线模型。广义上讲，需求曲线描述了消费者愿意购买的商品数量与商品价格之间的关系，并保持其他影响消费者购买意愿的因素不变。这种关系可以写成一个方程，如 $Q = D(P; Z)$，其中 Q、P 分别表示数量和价格；Z 是一个矢量（即变量列表）用于解释除价格以外影响需求的所有因素；而 $D(\ )$ 是表示括号中的变量如何决定需求量的函数（Allen et al. 2005, 第3章）。这种关系也可以用图形来描述，如图1.3（a）所示，它展示了一个简化的卷烟需求曲线模型。

具体地说，在图1.3（a）中，横轴衡量的是特定时期内市场对卷烟的需求量 Q，纵轴衡量的是该国卷烟的平均价格 P。标为 D_1 的蓝色曲线显示了不同价格下的需求量，假设在 Z 中列出的任何其他因素没有变化也可能影响 Q。例如，如果价格为 P_1，那么需求量将等于 Q_1。将研究市场所消费的卷烟总数除以相应的有危险人口（即15岁或以上的人口）或根据估计的吸烟者人数，我们获得了1.2节所述的两个主要国家级别的吸烟强度指标，即人均卷烟消费量或每个吸烟者的平均卷烟消费量。

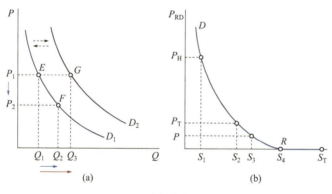

图1.3 卷烟的市场需求

P—市场价格；Q—需求量；P_{RD}—保留价格；P_T—市价加税（t）；P_H—市场价格加税（t）和医疗费用（H）。

1.3.1 价格弹性与需求量变化

大量研究表明，卷烟的需求总体上呈下降趋势，即遵循需求规律（Perucic, 2015）。换句话说，较低的价格往往会鼓励现在已经在购买卷烟的烟民大量购买，也可能会让那些以前买不起卷烟的潜在烟民开始吸烟。这意味着，在其他条件相同的情况下，较低的价格[例如图1.3（a）中的P_2]会导致吸烟强度或吸烟流行率或两者都增加（消费从Q_1到Q_2增加）。需求曲线的形状和位置反映了卷烟价格的变化对吸烟者数量和每个吸烟者消费的卷烟数量的影响程度。为了衡量需求量对价格变化的反应性，经济学家通常计算需求的价格弹性，即需求量变化百分比与价格变化百分比之比（Allen et al. 2005，第3章）。

例如，如果在其他条件相同的情况下，卷烟的数量要求减少6%，以应对增加的平均市场价格为8%，则需求的价格弹性是（-6%）/（8%）= -0.75。对卷烟的需求通常是相对无弹性的，也就是说，价格的上涨会导致需求量的下降。根据最近的估计，卷烟的平均价格弹性范围为-0.5～-0.3，因此价格上涨10%会使需求量减少4%（Chaloupka, Warner, 2000）。

1.3.2 需求和收入弹性的变化

在其他条件不变的情况下，价格的变化会导致需求量的变化，也就是说，沿着给定的需求曲线移动[例如，图1.3（a）中从F点到E点]。相反，除价格以外的任何因素的变化都会引起需求的变化，即整个需求曲线的移动[例如，如图1.3（a）所示，需求从D_1向右移动到D_2]。后者是市场状况的变化。新的需求曲线D_2（用红色表示）表明，在任何给定价格下，消费者对卷烟的需求都更大。

为了更好地理解烟草控制政策对卷烟消费的影响，区分需求曲线的移动（由于价格变化）和需求曲线的偏移（由于收入和口味等任何其他变量的变化）也是至关重要的。例如，卷烟税通过提高市场价格，抑制了卷烟消费，但只影响了需求的数量，而关于吸烟有害健康影响的更好教育可结构性减少卷烟的需求，从而减少消费[如图1.3（a）所示，需求曲线从D_2向左移动到D_1]。烟草公司的降价策略可能会完全抵消卷烟税的影响，但不会完全抵消教育计划的影响，因为如果成功，该计划将降低在任何给定价格下的需求量。

除了味道、规则、相关商品的价格，人群的吸烟习惯和行为主要受消费者收入水平和分布的影响。随着除价格以外的任何因素的变化,可支配收入的变化通过改变需求曲线而影响消费。然而,人均收入的增加可能会使需求曲线向左或向右平移[即人均收入的增加会使需求曲线向左或向右平移,如图1.3(a)所示],从而增加或减少卷烟的消费量。

需求的收入弹性用需求量变化百分比与收入变化百分比的比率来计算,是衡量其他因素相同的情况下,如何以及在多大程度上响应消费者收入的变化。这个系数在确定国家间卷烟消费的差异时很重要。如果收入弹性为正,则卷烟是一种正常商品(例如当收入增加时,需求量增加的商品)。在这种情况下,经济发展往往会增加吸烟者数量和每个吸烟者的消费,从而加剧与烟草健康有关的问题的发生。否则,负的收入弹性表明卷烟是次品(例如一种商品,其需求量随着收入的增加而减少)。在过去几十年里,在大多数发达国家,卷烟已经从一种普通商品(收入弹性低于 $0.5\sim1$)变成了一种次等商品。然而,在许多发展中国家,与传统的烟草消费形式相反,制造卷烟仍然具有积极和巨大的收入弹性(Wilkins, Yurekli, Hu, 2007,第3章)。

1.3.3 利用需求模型了解吸烟流行情况

考虑到烟草消费的其他具体特征,可以进一步发展基本需求模型(Phillips, 2016)。为了达到这个目的,在图1.3(b)中,x 轴测量实际和潜在吸烟者的数量,y 轴测量保留价格 P_{RD}(即每位消费者愿意支付的最高价格)。沿着向下倾斜的需求曲线(D 曲线,用蓝色表示),消费者被按照他们的支付意愿降序排列。换句话说,D 曲线上每个点的高度表示给定消费者的保留价格。这条卷烟需求曲线与 x 轴上的 R 点相交,超过 R 点就变成了水平曲线。S_T(处于风险中的人群)和 S_4 之间的差值给出了保留价格为零的消费者的数量(即那些即使有免费卷烟也不愿意吸烟的人)。相反,其余消费者(S_4 左边)的行为是"吸烟总成本"的函数:卷烟的自由市场价格、税收和与吸烟有关的健康成本之和。

如果没有关于吸烟的健康风险的信息(或教育),并且政府没有采取任何烟草控制政策,吸烟的总成本就是 P,即卷烟的自由市场价格。在这样一个社会中,所有的消费者,其支付意愿大于(或等于)P 的都会选择吸烟[图1.3(b)中的 S_3]。在某一国家和时间吸烟人数与风险人数的比率(在本例中为 S_3/S_T)表示吸烟的流行率(简称吸烟率)(如1.2节所述)。由于消费税(t)而导致的卷烟价格上涨(至 $P_T = P+t$)导致吸烟者人数减少到 S_2,从而导致流行率降低。然而,自由市场价格和税收之和只代表了吸烟总成本的一小部分。吸烟率的急剧下降主要是由于人们普遍认识到吸烟对健康的严重影响。如图1.3(b)所示,直到 S_1,当消费者考虑到吸烟的全部成本时,吸烟者人数下降,$P_H = P+t+H$(H 为健康相关成本)。

尽管吸烟的有害影响是众所周知的,但吸烟的积极和显著的流行率(这里用 S_1/S_T 的比率来衡量)强调了吸烟的主要特征之一:上瘾。从经济学的观点来看,烟瘾和其他药物上瘾很相似,都基于三个关键方面:耐受性、克制力和戒断。因此,容忍意味着一种渐进的适应,也就是说,随着过去的累计消费的增加,当前的消费倾向于变得不那么令人满意。强化反映了吸烟习惯在当前吸烟者行为中的关键作用,而戒断则意味着烟草消费具有一定程度的不可逆性(即戒烟通常不是件容易的事,也不便宜)。因此,当期消费成为过去消费选择的函数。

在基本模型中捕捉上瘾的一种方法是将需求曲线方程写成 $Q = D(P; Q^*, Z)$,其中 Q^* 为前几个时期累计消费卷烟的总和。成瘾的概念可能有助于解释卷烟需求的某些特定属性,例如,①长期吸烟者的付费意愿不可降低;②长期需求对价格和收入变化的反应性更强(即消费者改变与健康相关的习惯的时间越长，价格和收入弹性就越高；③各种替代烟草产品的兴起，如电子烟（IARC, 2011, 第4章）。

最后，鉴于烟草使用给个人和社会带来的有形（医疗支出）和无形（生活质量的损失和生命的损失）成本很高，即使是相当于S_1的吸烟者数量也可能导致市场失灵（即当个人对自身利益的追求给整个社会带来不好的结果时，就会出现一种无效率的情况）。事实上，烟草市场的低效率有两个主要来源：①关于吸烟的健康风险和烟草消费的成瘾性质的信息不全；②吸烟给非吸烟者和卫生系统带来成本。因此，烟草控制措施（除税收外）的目的不仅是减少需求数量，而且最重要的是减少对卷烟的需求（即向左移动D曲线的度量）是有经济依据的。例如在公共场所禁烟、包装上的强制性健康警告以及禁止卷烟广告（Nguyen, Rosenqvist, Pekurinen, 2012）。

1.4 不同国家烟草使用概况

根据最近的综合估计和预测数据来看（Ng et al. 2014; NIH, 2016, 第2章）在撰写本书时，全球大约有11.1亿吸烟者（15岁或15岁以上）。其中一半人生活在西太平洋和东南亚地区，特别是中国、印度和印度尼西亚这三个国家，这三个国家的烟民总数占全球烟民总数的45%。性别在决定吸烟习惯方面起着关键作用。大约85%（9.38亿）的吸烟者是生活在发展中国家的男性。相反，女性烟民为1.75亿，其中约46%是经济合作与发展组织高收入国家的居民。

在过去十年中，吸烟者总数保持相当稳定，但预计到2025年将增加到11.5亿。这一增长主要是由于发展中国家预计将出现人口增长。相比之下，世界大部分地区的吸烟流行率正在下降，除了东地中海和非洲世界卫生组织区域的男性人口（流行率分别约为36%和26%，在未来10年预计将达到45%和34%）。在全球范围内，17年前吸烟率约为26%；2015年逐渐下降至20%左右。俄罗斯、中国和几个欧洲国家的吸烟率仍远高于世界平均水平。例如，在东欧和俄罗斯，近1/3的成年人口（两性加起来）目前吸烟（Ng et al. 2014; NIH, 2016, 第2章）。

对卷烟消费数量的估计表明，2014年全球约有5.8万亿支卷烟。卷烟消费总量前六个国家（即中国、俄罗斯、印度、美国、印度尼西亚和日本）约占世界总消费量的60%。自2000年以来，全球卷烟消费量有所增加，主要是由于几个西太平洋和东地中海国家的消费量增加。在过去10年中，全球范围内的吸烟强度以成年人（15岁及以上的人）的年人均卷烟消费量衡量，从每人每年约1200支卷烟下降到1000支卷烟。这一烟草成瘾的基本指标在经济合作与发展组织国家尤其下降，这些国家的平均消费量远高于2000年的世界平均水平（人均约2200支卷烟），2015年急剧下降至约1400支。在一些巴尔干和东欧国家，例如克罗地亚（2771）、白俄罗斯（2896）和俄罗斯联邦（2838），人均卷烟年消费量超过2500支。此外，不仅在地中海小国（希腊、黎巴嫩和塞浦路斯），而且在人口众多的国家（如沙特阿拉伯、韩国、尤其是中国），人均卷烟消费量约为2000支（Eriksen, Mackay, Schluger, Gomeshtapeh, Drope, 2016; Ferretti, 2015; Ng et al. 2014; NIH, 2016, 第2章）。

最后，卷烟消费的一个关键驱动因素是可承受性，通常用一包卷烟的价格与每日平均可支配收入的比率来衡量（两者都用相同的货币来表示，以考虑到各国生活成本的差异），它抓住了该国平均消费者必须放弃吸烟的资源（金钱或劳动时间）的数量。最近的证据表明，与发达国家相比，发展中国家的卷烟价格越来越便宜，这主要是由于新兴经济体的人均收入迅速增长，以及几乎所有高收入国家对卷烟价格征收的消费税负担日益加重（Blecher, van Walbeek, 2008）。

| 术 语 解 释 | ■ 卷烟负担能力：是衡量资源数量的一个指标。买一包卷烟所需的金钱或时间。
■ 卷烟需求曲线：消费者需求数量与卷烟价格之间的关系，保持其他影响购买的因素不变，如消费者的收入和品味、相关商品的价格和政府管制。
■ 正常（劣质）商品：当收入增加时，需求量增加（减少）的商品。
■ 卷烟的价格弹性：在其他条件不变的情况下，卷烟价格变化1%所产生的需求量的百分比变化。
■ 吸烟强度：特定国家和年份的吸烟总人数与吸烟者人数的比率。
■ 吸烟（流行）率：特定国家和时间吸烟人数与风险人数的比率。 |

| 烟草使用的关键事实 | ■ 烟草可能消耗的不同形式。然而，如今人造卷烟占世界烟草产品总销量的90%以上。
■ 全世界约有11.1亿吸烟者。他们中大约有一半生活在西太平洋和东南亚地区，尤其是三个国家：中国、印度和印度尼西亚。由于发展中国家人口的增长，吸烟者总数正在缓慢增加。
■ 全球吸烟习惯中的性别问题。世界上大约4/5的吸烟者是男性，他们主要生活在发展中国家。相反，女性吸烟者约为1.75亿人，其中40%以上是发达国家居民。
■ 全球吸烟率约为21%，其在过去十年一直在下降，特别是在高度发达的经济合作与发展组织成员国。然而，未来几年，非洲和地中海东部国家的吸烟率预计将上升。吸烟率在俄罗斯联邦、中国和几个东欧国家特别高（平均超过25%）。
■ 近年来，由于消费税的原因，发达经济体的卷烟价格已经大大降低，而新兴经济体的卷烟价格普遍更为低廉，吸烟者的收入增长超过了卷烟的平均价格。
■ 自2000年以来，吸烟强度稳步下降。经合组织国家的人均卷烟消费量大幅下降（从2000年的2240支下降至2013年的1450支）。然而，在一些巴尔干和东欧国家，如克罗地亚（2271）、白俄罗斯（2896）和俄罗斯联邦（2838），人均卷烟年消费量超过2500支。 |

| 要 点 总 结 | ■ 本章简要介绍了烟草经济学和流行病学的一些基本概念。
■ 用代理人（烟草生产者）、宿主（吸烟者）、媒介（烟草公司）的"三角模型"和社会环境组成的"三角模型"来描述给定人群中吸烟决定因素之间的相互作用。
■ 在一个特定的国家，有两个基本的烟草使用指标：吸烟率和吸烟强度。
■ 例如，消费税引起的卷烟价格变化导致需求量的变化（即沿着给定的需求曲线的变化），而消费者收入和口味的变化或烟草监管政策的变化导致需求的变化（即整个需求曲线的变化）。
■ 卷烟需求对价格的变化往往相对缺乏弹性，特别是在短期内。卷烟在发达国家常被视为次品，在发展中国家则被视为正常商品。 |

参考文献

Allen, W. B.; Doherty, N.; Weigelt, K.; Mansfield, E. (2005). Managerial economics. Theory, applications, and cases (6th ed.). New York: W.W. Norton, Company.

Blecher, E.; van Walbeek, C. (2008). An analysis of cigarette affordability (pp. 4-14). Paris: International Union Against Tuberculosis and Lung Disease.

Bonita, R.; Beaglehole, R.; Kjellstrom, T. (2006). Basic epidemiology. Geneva: WHO.

Bonnie, R. J.; Stratton, K.; Wallace, R. B. (Eds.), (2007). Ending the tobacco problem: A blueprint for the nation. Washington, DC: The National Academies Press.

CDC. (2014). The health consequences of smoking—50 years of progress: A report of the surgeon general. Atlanta, GA: Centers for Disease Control and Prevention [Appendix 15.1].

Chaloupka, F.; Warner, K. (2000). The economics of smoking. In A. J. Culyer, J. P. Newhouse (Eds.), Handbook of health economics (pp. 1539-1627). Amsterdam: Elsevier.

Eriksen, M.; Mackay, J.; Schluger, N.; Gomeshtapeh, F. I.; Drope, J. (2016). The tobacco atlas (4th ed.). Atlanta, GA: American Cancer Society. 7 REFERENCES.

Ferretti, F. (2015). Unhealthy behaviours: an international comparison. PLoS ONE, 10(10), e0141834.

Gallus, S.; Schiaffino, A.; LaVecchia, C.; Townsend, J.; Fernandez, E. (2006). Price and cigarette consumption in Europe. Tobacco Control, 15(2), 114-119.

GBD Tobacco Collaborators. (2015). Smoking prevalence and attributable disease burden in 195 countries and territories, 1990-2015: a systematic analysis from the Global Burden of Disease Study 2015. Lancet, 389(10082), 1885-1906.

Giovino, G. A. (2002). Epidemiology of tobacco use in the United States. Oncogene, 21(48), 7326-7340.

Guindon, G. E.; Boisclair, D. (2003). Past, current and future trends in tobacco use. Discussion paper, February, no. 3 Washington DC: WB.

Hammond, K. S. (2009). Global patterns of nicotine and tobacco consumption. Nicotine Psychopharmacology (pp. 3-28). In J. E. Henningfield, E. D. London, S. Pogure (Eds.). Handbook of Experimental Pharmacology (pp. 2-28).

Berlin, Heidelberg: Springer-Verlag. IARC. (2008). Methods for evaluating tobacco control policies. Lyon: International Agency for Research on Cancer and WHO.

IARC. (2011). Effectiveness of tax and price policies for tobacco control. Lyon: International Agency for Research on Cancer and WHO.

Lopez, A. D.; Neil, E. C.; Tapani, P. (1994). A descriptive model of the cigarette epidemic in developed countries. Tobacco Control, 3(3), 242-247.

Mankiw, N. G. (2012). Principles of microeconomics (6th ed.). Mason, OH: South-Western Cengage Learning.

Ng, M.; Freeman, M. K.; Fleming, T. D.; Robinson, M.; Dwyer-Lindgren, L.; Thomson, B. et al. (2014). Smoking prevalence and cigarette consumption in 187 countries, 1980-2012. Journal of the American Medical Association, 311(2), 183-192.

Nguyen, L.; Rosenqvist, G.; Pekurinen, M. (2012). Demand for tobacco in Europe. Report no. 6 Helsinki: National Institute for Health and Welfare.

NIH. (2016). The economics of tobacco and tobacco control. National Cancer Institute, tobacco control monograph, series no 21. Bethesda, MD: NIH and WHO.

Penn State. (2016). Epidemiologic triad. Department of Statistics, Pennsylvania State University. Available at: https://onlinecourses.science.psu.edu/stat507/node/25.

Perucic, A. M. (2015). The demand for cigarettes and other tobacco products. In Tobacco control economics tobacco free initiative. Geneva: WHO.

Phillips, C. V. (2016). Understanding the basic economics of tobacco harm reduction.Discussion paper no. 72 London: The Institute of Economic Affairs.

Slade, J. (1993). Nicotine delivery systems. In C. T. Orleans, J. Slade (Eds.), Nicotine addiction: Principles and management. Oxford: Oxford University Press.

Warner, K. E.; MacKay, J. (2006). The global tobacco disease pandemic: nature, causes, and cures. Global Public Health, 1(1), 65-86.

WHO. (2015). Global report on trends in prevalence of tobacco smoking. Geneva: WHO.

WHO. (2017). Report on the global tobacco epidemic: Monitoring tobacco use and prevention policies. Geneva: WHO [Appendix X]. Wilkins, N.; Yurekli, A.; Hu, T. (2007). Economic analysis of tobacco demand . In A . Yurekli, J. deBeyer (Eds.), Economics of tobacco toolkit. Washington, DC: WB.

2
孕妇吸烟和胎儿大脑的结果：机制和可能的解决方案

Hui Chen[1], Yik Lung Chan[2], Brian G. Oliver[1,2], Carol A. Pollock[3], Sonia Saad[3]

1. School of Life Sciences, Faculty of Science, University of Technology Sydney, Sydney, NSW, Australia
2. Respiratory Cellular and Molecular Biology, Woolcock Institute of Medical Research, The University of Sydney, Glebe, NSW, Australia
3. Renal Group, Department of Medicine, Kolling Institute, Royal North Shore Hospital, St Leonards, NSW, Australia

缩略语

Drp	动力相关蛋白	OXPHOS	氧化磷酸化
Fis	裂变蛋白	Pink	PTEN诱导的假定激酶
HI	缺氧缺血	ROS	活性氧物种
LC	微管相关蛋白轻链	SE	卷烟烟雾暴露
MnSOD	锰超氧化物歧化酶	TLR	Toll样受体
NO	一氧化氮	TOM	线粒体外膜转位酶
Opa-1	视神经萎缩1蛋白		

2.1 引言

在了解胎儿成年后的疾病规划方面，已取得了迅速的进展。某些出生时基因表达的改变可以持续至成年期，大大增加了某些疾病的易感性。报告强调了理想宫内环境对优化胎儿健康结果的关键作用。孕妇吸烟会干扰子宫内环境的稳定性，导致子代的脑炎症反应和氧化应激。这可能导致新生儿缺氧缺血性（HI）损伤和成年期认知改变，如抑郁和焦虑。

2.2 孕妇吸烟和胎儿大脑发育

尽管对怀孕期间吸烟的风险进行了普及教育，但据估计，在一些国家仍有20%～45%的妇女在怀孕期间吸烟，而在某些土著社区，这一比例甚至更高。此外，世界上至少有82%的人无法避免二手烟，其中包括孕妇。

孕妇吸烟/卷烟烟雾暴露（SE）是导致宫内生长受限、低出生体重、围产期发病率和死亡率以及后代长期后果（包括行为问题）的主要因素（Chen, Morris, 2007）。烟碱的血管收缩作用使胎盘血流减少，导致宫内营养和氧气不足，限制胎儿生长，进而永久性改变生理功能。

尽管大脑获得了优先的营养供给，但怀孕期间吸烟与较小的脑重量、额叶和小脑体积密切相关（图2.1）。孕妇单独服用烟碱似乎并不会改变后代的大脑容量（Grove et al. 2001），而孕妇SE会降低新生儿出生时大脑的容量（Chan, Saad, Pollock et al. 2016）。显然，卷烟烟雾中的其他化学物质在胎儿大脑发育不良中起着重要作用。由于烟草烟雾中有超过5000种化学物质的复杂性质，

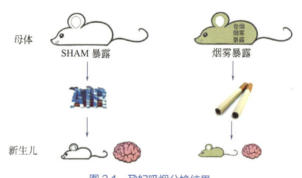

图 2.1　孕妇吸烟分娩结果

孕妇吸烟会降低新生儿的出生重和大脑容量。

单一成分不太可能引起疾病。

2.3　孕妇吸烟与胎儿神经认知结果

孕妇吸烟对胎儿大脑的结构和功能发育造成长期不良影响，从而导致认知障碍（Bublitz, Stroud, 2012）。脑容量小与智商低显著相关（Haier et al. 2004），而语言能力与脑容量呈正相关（Witelson et al. 2006）。与不吸烟者相比，吸烟孕妇的 13～16 岁孩子的语言和视觉记忆能力较低（Fried et al. 2003）。怀孕期间大量吸烟（>20 支/天）会增加幼儿产生恐惧和焦虑等内化行为的风险（Moylan et al. 2015）。此外，孕妇吸烟以剂量依赖的方式增加了患注意缺陷多动障碍的风险（Altink et al. 2009）。因此，怀孕期间吸烟是一个重大的公共健康问题。

然而，一些混杂因素，如父母的社会经济地位、饮酒和父亲吸烟等，可能会导致人类研究中出现不一致的结果（Moylan et al. 2015）。因此，动物模型在消除这些混杂因素以单独确定孕妇吸烟的影响方面具有优势。关于 SE 的直接影响的研究数量有限，而大多数研究采用了烟碱，限制了数据的解释。本章将重点介绍直接 SE 的动物模型。

2.4　孕妇吸烟与新生儿 HI 脑病

出生前后的缺氧可导致新生儿 HI 脑损伤（Johnston, Hoon Jr., 2006）。烟碱会减少流向胎盘的血流量。吸烟还会增加碳氧血红蛋白水平，从而降低胎儿和母体红细胞的携氧能力。因此，动物研究表明，孕妇吸烟会导致胎儿缺氧（Socol et al. 1982）。HI 本身可以导致儿童脑瘫和相关残疾（Johnston, Hoon Jr., 2006），而孕妇每天吸烟量达 10 支以上已被证明会增加脑瘫风险（Streja et al. 2013）。

在 HI 脑病期间，血氧饱和度和血流量降低，中断胎儿大脑的正常发育（Li et al. 2012）。小胶质细胞对缺氧反应迅速并在受损组织中积聚，在受损组织中产生过量的炎性细胞因子，如 TNF-α 和 IL-1β 以及活性氧（ROS），导致炎症和氧化应激。在小鼠中，即使没有损伤，SE 母鼠的后代也已经存在大脑炎症和氧化应激的增加（Chan et al. 2016）。因此，当这些后代患有 HI 脑病时，会有更多的细胞死亡（Chan et al. 2017）。大脑皮层、海马体和脑室下区是最易受 HI 损伤的区域。患有 HI 脑病的雄性幼崽的梗死面积增大，而雌性幼崽的梗死面积没有增大（Li, Xiao et al. 2012），说明存在性别差异，雄性幼崽受影响更严重。

2.5 潜在机制

2.5.1 脑炎性反应

卷烟过滤嘴无法去除烟草燃烧产生的ROS，从而导致多种骨髓细胞和淋巴细胞中炎性通路的激活（Qiu et al. 2017）。ROS还可以激活巨噬细胞，从而进一步产生更多的ROS（Rahman, Adcock, 2006）。妊娠吸烟者长时间的全身炎症也会影响后代。在SE母亲的成年雄性后代中，脑促炎细胞因子IL-6、IL-1α细胞凋亡受体和Toll样受体（TLR）4的表达增加（图2.2）（Chan et al. 2016）。TLRs的激活刺激了单核细胞中IL-1β和IL-6的产生（图2.2），进而通过正反馈回路增强TLR的表达。雌性后代在断奶到成年期间也有类似的变化（Chan, Saad, Al-odat et al. 2016）。

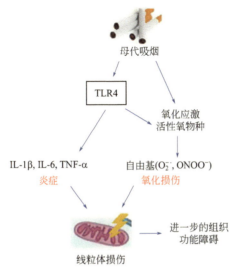

图2.2　母代吸烟诱发子代脑功能障碍的机制

母代吸烟会增加子代大脑的炎症和氧化应激，而这两者都会导致线粒体损伤和神经功能障碍。

神经炎症在神经退行性病变的发展中起着至关重要的作用。TLR4和IL-1水平的升高都会导致β-淀粉样蛋白的升高，这与阿尔茨海默病的发展有关。脑IL-6水平的升高也与焦虑、类似自闭症的行为以及神经衰弱疾病的进展有关（Wei et al. 2012）。事实上，吸烟的母亲血液中炎症细胞因子水平较高，其子女患精神分裂症或自闭症的严重程度也有所增加（Ashwood et al. 2011; Potvin et al. 2008）。

2.5.2 大脑氧化应激

2.5.2.1 ROS

当细胞产生的氧化分子压倒内源性抗氧化防御系统时，就会发生氧化应激。脑组织特别容易受到ROS的损伤，因为它是转运氧气的主要器官（占身体消耗的20%）。ROS的增加与线粒体膜通透性的增加以及最终细胞死亡有关（Popa-Wagner et al. 2013）。

长期的SE本身会增加母亲大脑的氧化应激和细胞损伤（Chan, Saad, Pollock et al. 2016）。母乳富含的抗氧化剂可以暂时保护新生儿。然而，一旦幼崽从母乳喂养中逐渐断奶，雄性幼崽的大脑氧化应激就会持续增加，直到成年，成年后的大脑会出现严重的细胞损伤（Chan, Saad, Pollock et al. 2016）。卷烟烟雾中的某些有毒化学物质可能诱发母亲和后代的氧化应激，因为母亲补充抗氧化剂可以逆转这种影响（Chan et al. 2017）。有趣的是，雌性后代似乎可以避免母亲吸烟的这种不利影响（Chan, Saad, Al-odat et al. 2016）。潜在的机制将在2.6节中讨论。

2.5.2.2　抗氧化防御系统

有一个复杂的抗氧化防御系统清除多余的ROS在大脑中尤为重要，因为神经元容易受到氧化应激的影响。大脑中最重要的抗氧化剂是锰超氧化物歧化酶（MnSOD），它在线粒体中的浓度高于其他细胞内成分。线粒体氧化磷酸化（OXPHOS）复合物Ⅰ和Ⅲ在正常能量代谢过程中产生ROS；因此，线粒体MnSOD对于清除过量ROS非常重要。有趣的是，MnSOD在妊娠后期和新生儿期间出现激增，随后在小鼠出生4天后下降（Khan, Black, 2003）。多项研究表明，MnSOD对神经保护至关重要，它通过防止线粒体功能障碍来防止神经元凋亡并减少缺血性脑损伤（Keller et al. 1998）。

在食管和肺等外周组织中MnSOD水平升高，以清除长期吸烟产生的过量ROS。迄今为止，只有两项研究报告了母亲SE对大脑MnSOD的影响（Chan, Saad, Al-odat et al. 2016; Chan, Saad, Pollock et al. 2016）。在母亲和成年雄性后代的大脑中，MnSOD水平都降低了（Chan, Saad, Pollock et al. 2016）。长远来看，由于ROS过量产生，MnSOD的耗尽会导致线粒体和DNA损伤（Chan et al. 2017）。

2.5.3　线粒体功能与完整性

线粒体是ATP产生的主要场所。在大脑中，由于其高代谢和能量需求，神经元中有高密度的线粒体。线粒体功能障碍被发现存在于许多神经系统疾病如肌萎缩性脊髓侧索硬化症和阿尔茨海默病中，这表明健康的线粒体对维持神经健康至关重要（Jiang et al. 2015）。

2.5.3.1　线粒体膜功能单位

ATP是通过OXPHOS复合物Ⅰ～Ⅴ促进线粒体嵴产生的（图2.3）。复合物Ⅰ和Ⅱ分别作为电子在呼吸链中的第一个和第二个入口点。复合物Ⅲ促进电子转移到复合体Ⅳ，这是ATP生产的一个关键调节剂。复合物Ⅰ、Ⅲ和Ⅳ中的质子驱动ADP转化为ATP。所有5种OXPHOS复合物的大脑水平均因长期SE而增加，表明能源供应的需求增加（Chan, Saad, Pollock et al. 2016）。事实上，大脑ATP酶的活性会因SE而降低（Vani, Anbarasi, Shyamaladevi, 2015）。虽然断奶时脑复合体Ⅰ和Ⅴ水平降低，但成年后所有的Ⅰ～Ⅴ复合体会因母体SE增加，与母亲相似，这表明线粒体功能可能遗传自母亲（Chan, Saad, Al-odat et al. 2016; Chan, Saad, Pollock et al. 2016）。

在OXPHOS过程中，90%的ROS作为复合物Ⅰ和Ⅲ的副产物生成（图2.3）。ROS可与一氧化氮（NO）形成过氧硝酸盐，后者进一步导致蛋白质酪氨酸硝化形成3-硝基酪氨酸，从而破坏线粒体（Beal, 1998）。MnSOD和NO竞争与超氧化物反应，防止生成过氧硝酸盐和3-硝基酪氨酸。硝化本身也能使MnSOD失活（Surmeli, Litterman, Miller, Groves, 2010）。当MnSOD水平降低且硝基酪氨酸水平升高时，线粒体对氧化应激的保护较少，例如在吸烟和孕妇SE期间（Chan, Saad, Pollock et al. 2016）。

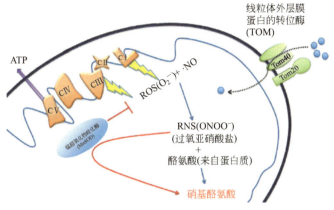

图2.3 线粒体能量代谢单位

活性氧（ROS）是由氧化磷酸化（OXPHOS）复合物（CⅠ～CⅤ）产生的。这些蛋白质通过Tom20和Tom40进入线粒体。ROS与一氧化氮（NO）结合形成过氧亚硝酸盐（RNS），后者与硝酸盐相互作用形成硝基酪氨酸。MnSOD抑制这一过程。

线粒体外膜蛋白复合物转位酶（TOM）是大多数在细胞质中合成的线粒体蛋白前体的主要入口。Tom40在运输过程中在脂质双膜中形成离子通道（Rapaport, Neupert, Lill, 1997）。Tom20（Tom40复合物的外周亚基）通过促进蛋白质插入到线粒体外膜来识别和导入蛋白质前体。Tom20可在氧化应激下降解。虽然SE对雄性后代的脑Tom20没有影响，但在断奶时，由于母体吸烟，其水平降低，成年后升高（Chan, Saad, Pollock et al. 2016）。

2.5.3.2 线粒体的完整性

线粒体结构是高度动态的，通过"线粒体自噬"维持。自噬是指"自食"，即降解细胞成分以维持细胞间稳态。"线粒体自噬"是指通过自噬去除线粒体。

在自噬过程中，微管相关蛋白轻链（LC）形成自噬体吞噬细胞内成分。LC3A/B-Ⅰ向LC3A/B-Ⅱ的转化被用作自噬活性的指标，而LC3A/B-Ⅱ水平与自噬体形成相关。母体SE降低了断奶和成年雄性后代的脑LC3A/B-Ⅱ水平，而增加了同年龄雌性后代的脑LC3A/B-Ⅱ水平（Chan et al. 2017）。这表明雄性后代的自噬能力较雌性后代低。

裂变和融合促进线粒体自噬（分别为图2.4中的步骤1和步骤2）。裂变将受损的线粒体部分从健康片段中分离出来，而融合将两个健康片段结合在一起形成一个新的线粒体。这两个过程是平衡的，以维持线粒体的整体形态。高融合裂变比导致线粒体较少，形状细长且相互关联；低融合裂变比导致线粒体呈小球体状和短棒状，通常被称为"线粒体碎片"。如果不能在大脑中触发线粒体自噬，则会导致神经退行性疾病（Cheung, Ip, 2009）。

（1）裂变机制

动力相关蛋白（Drp-1）存在于线粒体分裂位点，以分离受损的线粒体片段（图2.4，步骤①）。裂变蛋白1（Fis-1）锚定在线粒体外膜上，作为适应Drp-1的平台。分离后，PTEN诱导的假定激酶（Pink-1）积聚在受损线粒体的外膜上，导致Parkin的募集（图2.4，步骤③）。

线粒体Drp-1在出生后第1天增加，但在成年雄性后代中由于孕妇吸烟而减少（Chan et al. 2017）。线粒体Fis-1在出生20天后（断奶年龄）才会增加，成年雄性后代的线粒体Fis-1也会减少，这表明孕妇吸烟降低了裂变能力。这可能与神经细胞凋亡增加导致的脑线粒体密度降低有关。相反，Drp-1在出生后第1天降低，但在成年雌性后代中增加（Chan et al. 2017）。在产后第1

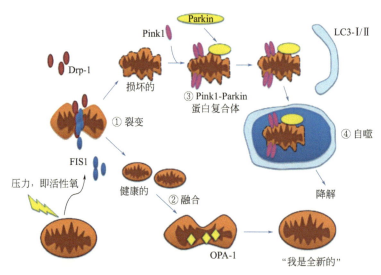

图 2.4 线粒体自噬和自噬机制

线粒体自噬和自噬。受损的线粒体片段在动力相关蛋白（Drp-1）和裂变蛋白（Fis-1）的促进下与健康部分分离。受损的线粒体吸引 PTEN 诱导的假定激酶（Pink-1）和 Parkin。该复合物随后被微管相关蛋白轻链（LC3）A/B-Ⅰ/Ⅱ 吞噬，形成自噬体进行降解。线粒体的健康部分可以通过视神经萎缩 1 蛋白（Opa-1）与另一个线粒体的健康部分结合。

天和第 20 天，雌性后代的 Parkin 也降低了，但成年雌性后代的 Pink-1 有所增加。这种增加与线粒体 MnSOD 的增加和凋亡标志物水平的降低有关。这表明，裂变活动的增加可以防止孕妇吸烟引起的雌性后代大脑细胞凋亡的增加。

（2）融合机制

视神经萎缩 1 蛋白（Opa-1）调节融合过程（图 2.4，步骤②）。Opa-1 基因敲除小鼠在胚胎发育第 9 天死亡；因此，Opa-1 对胚胎发育至关重要（Rahn et al. 2013）。线粒体融合似乎可以保护细胞免于凋亡和延长寿命，但其机制尚不清楚。

由于孕妇吸烟，成年雄性后代的脑 Opa-1 显著减少，脑细胞凋亡增加，表明可循环利用的健康线粒体片段较少（Chan et al. 2017）。在阿尔茨海默病中观察到脑线粒体融合减少（Zhang et al. 2016）。虽然吸烟本身与阿尔茨海默病和痴呆密切相关已经得到充分的研究证实（Anstey et al. 2007），但是这种风险在后代身上的研究还没有在人类身上进行。另一方面，雌性后代的 Opa-1 水平在出生后第 1 天增加，但在成年后没有变化（Chan et al. 2017）。这表明，未知的机制促进了线粒体融合机制，以防止雌性后代过度的脑凋亡。在年轻女性中也发现了类似的线粒体保护观察结果（Azarashvili et al. 2010）。

2.6 孕妇吸烟反应的性别差异

尽管男性和女性的大脑结构相似，但他们对特定神经疾病的敏感性不同。男性更容易患精神疾病，如自闭症、注意力缺陷和多动症（Davies, 2014）。当女性遭受这些脑部疾病时，她们的发病年龄比男性大（Zagni et al. 2016）。

与雌性后代相比，雄性后代更容易受到孕妇吸烟引起的炎症反应、氧化应激、线粒体损伤和大脑凋亡的影响。推测这种性别差异是由雌激素引起的，雌激素被认为具有神经保护和抗炎作用，从而保护了女性的大脑（Brann et al. 2007）。雌激素的另一个作用是作为抗氧化剂，防止脂质过氧化、蛋白质氧化和DNA损伤（Escalante et al. 2017）。雌激素也被证明在线粒体毒素暴露期间维持线粒体膜电位（Wang et al. 2001）。

在男性和女性的大脑中，神经胶质细胞对环境损害的反应是不同的。星形胶质细胞是最丰富的神经胶质细胞，它支持营养稳态和电脉冲的神经传递。从男性获得的星形胶质细胞表达较高水平的IL-1βmRNA，这可能导致神经元损伤后更糟糕的结果（Santos-Galindo et al. 2011）。雌性的星形胶质细胞比雄性的星形胶质细胞更能抵抗应激源，如氧化诱导的细胞死亡（Liu et al. 2008）。卷烟烟雾中发现的脂多糖（Hasday et al. 1999）可增加男性星形胶质细胞中IL-6、TNF-α和IL1mRNA的表达（Santos-Galindo et al. 2011）。同样，母体吸烟SE会增加成年雄性后代的脑IL-6，而不增加雌性后代的脑IL-6（Chan, Saad, Al-Odat et al. 2016; Chan, Saad, Pollock et al. 2016）。2.5.3节中描述了孕妇吸烟对线粒体吞噬反应的性别差异，并在表2.1中进行了总结。

表2.1　孕妇SE对后代脑自噬的影响

性别	雄性后代	雌性后代
线粒体自噬-裂变	↓	↑
线粒体自噬-融合	↓	↑
自噬	没有变化	↑

注：孕妇吸烟减少了雄性后代大脑中的线粒体裂变和融合活动，但对自噬活动没有影响；然而，它增加了裂变、融合和自噬。

2.7　左旋肉碱作为治疗策略

左旋肉碱是一种内源性的天然季铵盐化合物，广泛存在于各种哺乳动物体内。它是线粒体脂肪酸氧化的重要成分（Gülçin, 2006）。左旋肉碱作为线粒体内膜中的能量载体，控制乙酰辅酶A的供应并支持OXPHOS复合体的活性（Virmani, Binienda, 2004）。左旋肉碱充当ROS清除剂，保护MnSOD免受氧化损伤，这表明它可能有助于改善线粒体功能（Gülçin, 2006）。

左旋肉碱也具有保护神经的作用。在线粒体毒素暴露前用左旋肉碱预处理可增加内源性ROS清除剂的活性，以防止机体抗氧化应激（Virmani, Binienda, 2004）。在SE小鼠母亲中，妊娠期和哺乳期补充左旋肉碱可增加新生雄性后代大脑MnSOD和Tom20水平，导致成年期线粒体自噬标志物显著改善（总结于表2.2）（Chan et al. 2017）。细胞凋亡和细胞DNA损伤也减少了，这表明左旋肉碱对孕妇吸烟有持续的神经保护作用。在雌性后代的大脑中也观察到类似的大脑自噬标记的改善。因此，补充左旋肉碱可能是减轻吸烟者后代氧化应激引起的线粒体功能障碍的一个很好的选择。

表2.2　孕妇补充左旋肉碱对后代线粒体自噬的影响

性别	雄性后代	雌性后代
线粒体自噬-裂变	↑	没有变化
线粒体自噬-融合	↑	没有变化
自噬	没有变化	↓

2.8 结论

妊娠期和哺乳期孕妇吸烟可引起雄性后代大脑明显的炎症反应和氧化应激，损害线粒体的完整性，导致细胞死亡。孕妇吸烟似乎可以保护雌性后代免受这种影响。孕妇补充左旋肉碱已在吸烟孕妇的后代中显示出了良好的神经保护作用。

术语解释	
	■ 乙酰辅酶A：由糖酵解产生，是一种代谢中间产物，可转化为碳水化合物、蛋白质和脂肪。
	■ 细胞凋亡：细胞在应激状态下的程序性死亡，如暴露于环境污染和吸烟。
	■ 自噬：意味着"自食"，这是一种细胞通过自我消化去除受损蛋白质的策略。
	■ 脑病：脑疾病或脑障碍。
	■ 缺氧缺血：由于缺氧和血液供应不足引起的一种状况，通常发生在动脉阻塞时。
	■ 线粒体：是细胞的"发电站"，能量物质ATP是由能量底物乙酰辅酶A和氧气产生的。
	■ 线粒体自噬：受损的线粒体的自我吞噬或自我更新过程，以维持体内健康的线粒体种群。
	■ 氧化磷酸化：当柠檬酸循环产生的电子沉积在线粒体内膜的电子传递链中时，它们被酶捕获产生ATP。
	■ 氧化应激：主要是在ATP合成过程中产生的自由基超过了内源性抗氧化剂清除自由基的能力。
	■ 活性氧：含有额外氧分子的化学活性化学物质，可以氧化其他细胞成分。

孕妇吸烟的关键事实	
	■ 吸烟孕妇的后代大脑发育不全，导致学习和记忆功能受损。
	■ 吸烟孕妇的后代更有可能因缺氧和血液短缺而导致脑损伤。
	■ 吸烟孕妇的男性后代比女性后代有更多的脑细胞死亡。
	■ 孕妇吸烟会损害脑细胞线粒体功能。
	■ 与男性后代相比，女性后代的大脑更能免受孕妇吸烟的影响。

要点总结	
	■ 孕妇吸烟使后代大脑发育延迟。
	■ 孕妇吸烟损害后代的认知功能。
	■ 孕妇吸烟与缺氧缺血性脑病的高风险相关。
	■ 孕妇吸烟增加男性后代的大脑细胞凋亡。
	■ 孕妇吸烟增加氧化应激和损害男性后代的大脑线粒体功能。
	■ 与男性后代相比，女性后代的大脑更能免受孕妇吸烟的不利影响。

参考文献

Altink, M. E.; Slaats-Willemse, D. I. E.; Rommelse, N. N. J.; Buschgens, C.J. M.; Fliers, E. A.; Arias-Vásquez, A. et al. (2009). Effects of maternal and paternal smoking on attentional control in children with and without ADHD. European Child, Adolescent Psychiatry, 18(8), 465-475.

Anstey, K. J.; von Sanden, C.; Salim, A.; O'Kearney, R. (2007). Smoking as a risk factor for dementia and cognitive decline: a metaanalysis of prospective studies. American Journal of Epidemiology, 166(4), 367-378.

Ashwood, P.; Krakowiak, P.; Hertz-Picciotto, I.; Hansen, R.; Pessah, I.; Van de Water, J. (2011). Elevated plasma cytokines in autism spectrum disorders provide evidence of immune dysfunction and areassociated with impaired behavioral outcome. Brain, Behavior, and Immunity, 25(1),

40-45.

Azarashvili, T.; Stricker, R.; Reiser, G. (2010). The mitochondria permeability transition pore complex in the brain with interacting proteins - promising targets for protection in neurodegenerativediseases. Biological Chemistry, 391(6), 619-629.

Beal, M. F. (1998). Mitochondrial dysfunction in neurodegenerative diseases. Biochimica et Biophysica Acta (BBA): Bioenergetics, 1366(1-2), 211-223.

Brann, D. W.; Dhandapani, K.; Wakade, C.; Mahesh, V. B.; Khan, M.M. (2007). Neurotrophic and neuroprotective actions of estrogen:basic mechanisms and clinical implications. Steroids, 72(5), 381-405.

Bublitz, M. H.; Stroud, L. R. (2012). Maternal smoking during pregnancy and offspring brain structure and function: review and agenda for future research. Nicotine, Tobacco Research, 14(4), 388-397.

Chan, Y. L.; Saad, S.; Al-Odat, I.; Oliver, B. G.; Pollock, C.; Jones, N. M. et al. (2017). Maternal L-carnitine supplementation improves brain health in offspring from cigarette smoke exposed mothers. Frontiers in Molecular Neuroscience, 10(33).

Chan, Y. L.; Saad, S.; Al-Odat, I.; Zaky, A. A.; Oliver, B.; Pollock, C. et al. (2016). Impact of maternal cigarette smoke exposure on brain and kidney health outcomes in female offspring. Clinical and Experimental Pharmacology, Physiology, 43(12), 1168-1176.

Chan, Y. L.; Saad, S.; Pollock, C.; Oliver, B.; Al-Odat, I.; Zaky, A. A. et al. (2016). Impact of maternal cigarette smoke exposure on brain inflammation and oxidative stress in male mice offspring. ScientificReports, 6, 25881.

Chen, H.; Morris, M. J. (2007). Maternal smoking—a contributor to the obesity epidemic? Obesity Research, Clinical Practice, 1, 155-163.

Cheung, Z. H.; Ip, N. Y. (2009). The emerging role of autophagy in Parkinson's disease. Molecular Brain, 2, 29.Davies, W. (2014). Sex differences in attention deficit hyperactivity disorder: candidate genetic and endocrine mechanisms. Frontiers in Neuroendocrinology, 35(3), 331-346.

Davies, W. (2014). Sex differences in attention deficit hyperactivity disorder: candidate genetic and endocrine mechanisms. Frontiers in Neuroendo-Crinology, 35(3), 331-346.

Escalante, C. G.; Mora, S. Q.; Bolaños, L. N. (2017). Hormone replacement therapy reduces lipid oxidation directly at the arterial wall: a possible link to estrogens' cardioprotective effect through atherosclerosis prevention. Journal of Mid-Life Health, 8(1), 11-16.

Fried, P. A.; Watkinson, B.; Gray, R. (2003). Differential effects on cognitive functioning in 13- to 16-year-olds prenatally exposed to cigarettes and marihuana. Neurotoxicology and Teratology, 25(4), 427-436.

Grove, K. L.; Sekhon, H. S.; Brogan, R. S.; Keller, J. A.; Smith, M. S.; Spindel, E. R. (2001). Chronic maternal nicotine exposure alters neuronal systems in the arcuate nucleus that regulate feeding behavior in the newborn rhesus macaque. The Journal of Clinical Endocrinology, Metabolism, 86(11), 5420-5426. PMID:11701716.

Gül çin I. (2006). Antioxidant and antiradical activities of l-carnitine. Life Sciences, 78(8), 803-811.

Haier, R. J.; Jung, R. E.; Yeo, R. A.; Head, K.; Alkire, M. T. (2004). Structural brain variation and general intelligence. NeuroImage, 23(1), 425-433.

Hasday, J. D.; Bascom, R.; Costa, J. J.; Fitzgerald, T.; Dubin, W. (1999). Bacterial endotoxin is an active component of cigarette smoke. Chest, 115(3), 829-835.

Jiang, Z.; Wang, W.; Perry, G.; Zhu, X.; Wang, X. (2015). Mitochondrial dynamic abnormalities in amyotrophic lateral sclerosis. Translational Neurodegeneration, 4, 14.

Johnston, M. V.; Hoon, A. H.; Jr. (2006). Cerebral palsy. Neuromolecular Medicine, 8(4), 435-450.

Keller, J. N.; Kindy, M. S.; Holtsberg, F. W.; St. Clair, D. K.; Yen, H.-C.; Germeyer, A. et al. (1998). Mitochondrial manganese superoxide dismutase prevents neural apoptosis and reduces ischemic brain injury: suppression of peroxynitrite production, lipid peroxidation, 15 REFERENCES and mitochondrial dysfunction. The Journal of Neuroscience, 18(2), 687-697.

Khan, J. Y.; Black, S. M. (2003). Developmental changes in murine brain antioxidant enzymes. Pediatric Research, 54(1), 77-82.

Li, Y.; Gonzalez, P.; Zhang, L. (2012). Fetal stress and programming of hypoxic/ischemic-sensitive phenotype in the neonatal brain: mechanisms and possible interventions. Progress in Neurobiology, 98(2), 145-165.

Li, Y.; Xiao, D.; Dasgupta, C.; Xiong, F.; Tong, W.; Yang, S. et al. (2012). Perinatal nicotine exposure increases vulnerability of hypoxicischemic brain injury in neonatal rats: role of angiotensin II receptors.Stroke 43(9), 2483-2490.

Liu, M.; Oyarzabal, E. A.; Yang, R.; Murphy, S. J.; Hurn, P. D. (2008). A novel method for assessing sex-specific and genotype-specific response to injury in astrocyte culture. Journal of Neuroscience Methods, 171(2), 214-217.

Moylan, S.; Gustavson, K.; Øverland, S.; Karevold, E. B.; Jacka, F. N.; Pasco, J. A. et al. (2015). The impact of maternal smoking during pregnancy on depressive and anxiety behaviors in children: the Norwegian mother and child cohort study. BMC Medicine, 13(1), 24.

Popa-Wagner, A.; Mitran, S.; Sivanesan, S.; Chang, E.; Buga, A. M. (2013). ROS and brain diseases: the good, the bad, and the ugly. Oxidative Medicine and Cellular Longevity, 2013, 963520.

Potvin, S.; Stip, E.; Sepehry, A. A.; Gendron, A.; Bah, R.; Kouassi, E. (2008). Inflammatory cytokine alterations in schizophrenia: a systematic quantitative review. Biological Psychiatry, 63(8), 801-808.

Qiu, F.; Liang, C.-L.; Liu, H.; Zeng, Y.-Q.; Hou, S.; Huang, S. et al. (2017). Impacts of cigarette smoking on immune responsiveness: up and down or upside down? Oncotarget, 8(1), 268-284.

Rahman, I.; Adcock, I. M. (2006). Oxidative stress and redox regulation of lung inflammation in COPD. The European Respiratory Journal, 28(1), 219-242.

Rahn, J. J.; Stackley, K. D.; Chan, S. S. (2013). Opa1 is required for proper mitochondrial metabolism in early development. PLoS ONE, 8(3)e59218.

Rapaport, D.; Neupert, W.; Lill, R. (1997). Mitochondrial protein import. Tom40 plays a major role in targeting and translocation of preproteins by forming a specific binding site for the presequence. The Journal of Biological Chemistry, 272(30), 18725-18731.

Santos-Galindo, M.; Acaz-Fonseca, E.; Bellini, M. J.; Garcia-Segura, L. M. (2011). Sex differences in the inflammatory response of primary astrocytes to lipopolysaccharide. Biology of Sex Differences, 2, 7.

Socol, M. L.; Manning, F. A.; Murata, Y.; Druzin, M. L. (1982). Maternal smoking causes fetal hypoxia: experimental evidence. American Journal of Obstetrics and Gynecology, 142(2), 214-218.

Streja, E.; Miller, J. E.; Bech, B. H.; Greene, N.; Pedersen, L. H.; Yeargin-Allsopp, M. et al. (2013). Congenital cerebral palsy and prenatal exposure to self-reported maternal infections, fever, or smoking. American Journal of Obstetrics and Gynecology, 209(4), 332.e1-332.e10.

Surmeli, N. B.; Litterman, N. K.; Miller, A. F.; Groves, J. T. (2010). Peroxynitrite mediates active site tyrosine nitration in manganese superoxide dismutase. Evidence of a role for the carbonate radical anion. Journal of the American Chemical Society, 132(48), 17174-17185.

Vani, G.; Anbarasi, K.; Shyamaladevi, C. S. (2015). Bacoside A: role in cigarette smoking induced changes in brain. Evidence-based Complementary and Alternative Medicine: eCAM, 2015, 286137.

Virmani, A.; Binienda, Z. (2004). Role of carnitine esters in brain neuropathology. Molecular Aspects of Medicine, 25(5-6), 533-549.

Wang, J.; Green, P. S.; Simpkins, J. W. (2001). Estradiol protects against ATP depletion, mitochondrial membrane potential decline and the generation of reactive oxygen species induced by 3-nitroproprionic acid in SK-N-SH human neuroblastoma cells. Journal of Neurochemistry, 77(3), 804-811.

Wei, H.; Chadman, K. K.; McCloskey, D. P.; Sheikh, A. M.; Malik, M.; Brown, W. T. et al. (2012). Brain IL-6 elevation causes neuronal circuitry imbalances and mediates autism-like behaviors. Biochimica et Biophysica Acta (BBA): Molecular Basis of Disease, 1822(6), 831-842.

Witelson, S. F.; Beresh, H.; Kigar, D. L. (2006). Intelligence and brain size in 100 postmortem brains: sex, lateralization and age factors. Brain, 129(2), 386-398.

Zagni, E.; Simoni, L.; Colombo, D. (2016). Sex and gender differences in central nervous system-related disorders. Neuroscience Journal, 2016, 2827090.

Zhang, L.; Trushin, S.; Christensen, T. A.; Bachmeier, B. V.; Gateno, B.; Schroeder, A. et al. (2016). Altered brain energetics induces mitochondrial fission arrest in Alzheimer's disease. Scientific Reports, 6, 18725.

# 3
烟碱对青少年的影响

Sari Izenwasser

Department of Psychiatry, Behavioral Sciences, University of Miami Miller School of Medicine, Miami, FL, United States

缩略语

5-HT	血清素	nAChR	烟碱乙酰胆碱受体
AD	成人	NC	没有变化
Adol	青少年	Nic	烟碱
CB recs	大麻素受体	S-A	自给药
CPP	条件位置偏好	Sens	敏化作用
DA	多巴胺	SERT	5-羟色胺转运体
DAT	多巴胺转运体	STR	纹状体

多年来，对烟碱的临床前研究仅针对成年人，主要针对成年男性。在过去的15～20年中，有更多的研究研究了烟碱对青少年的影响。迄今为止，关于男性的研究更多；然而，许多针对男性和女性的研究表明，与成年人的数据相比，不同性别和不同年龄的人有不同的影响。本章将在可能的情况下着重于烟碱在青春期对男性和女性的影响。此外，还将尝试包括青少年和成人两方面的研究，试图确定青少年是否是独特的。然而，如上所述，许多研究仍然只报道了男性的数据，而且往往不包括与成年人的直接比较。因此，比较不同实验室的结果通常是必要的。由于篇幅和参考文献的限制，这不是一篇详尽的文献综述；然而，我们将尝试包括显示该领域的广度的研究。

烟碱使用的平均年龄发生在青少年时期，90%的使用者在18岁之前就开始尝试吸烟（Centers for Disease Control and Prevention, 2017）。尽管在2011—2016年中学生吸烟人数有所下降，但电子烟和水烟的使用却有所增加。据报道，大约10%的高中生和3%的中学生在过去30天内使用过两种或两种以上的烟草产品，高中生一生中使用多种烟草制品的比例略高于30%。总体而言，在高中生和中学生中男生使用水烟的比例高于女生，尽管高中女生使用水烟的比例略高于男生。

3.1 烟碱对青少年和成年男性与女性的影响

临床前实验室研究经常表明，与成人相比，青少年通常对烟碱表现出独特的反应（见表3.1）。一般来说，青少年对烟碱的反应比成年人更敏感，尽管男性和女性的反应往往不同。大多数研究表明，烟碱会刺激身体运动活动，而青春期男性对这种影响并不敏感（Collins, Izenwasser, 2004; Collins, Montano, Izenwasser, 2004; Cruz, Delucia, Planeta, 2005; Faraday, Elliott, Grunberg, 2001; Schochet, Kelley, Landry, 2004）。相反，许多研究表明，致敏作用确实发生在成年男性

（Bracken, Chambers, Berg, Rodd, McBride, 2011; Collins, Izenwasser, 2004; Collins, Montano et al. 2004; Cruz et al. 2005）以及成年和青春期的女性中（Collins, Izenwasser, 2004）。青春期男性的致敏发生在每日给药期间（Collins, Izenwasser, 2004; Collins, Montano et al. 2004），如果在烟碱疗法结束3天后攻击动物，这种敏感症状仍然明显（Cruz et al. 2005）。青春期男性缺乏致敏性的一个潜在原因是烟碱对这一群体的活动的急性影响比成年男性、成年女性或青春期女性要大得多。由于对烟碱的初始反应如此之高，活性的显著增加可能很难发生。通过渗透性微型泵持续给予烟碱也会对烟碱的运动效应产生敏感性；然而，这在青春期和成年男性身上均有发生（Faraday, Elliott, Phillips, Grunberg, 2003）

当第一次接触烟碱是在青春期时，雄性和雌性大鼠自给药的烟碱量明显高于成年大鼠。雌性青春期大鼠自给药的烟碱量约为成年雌性大鼠的两倍（Levin, Rezvani, Montoya, Rose, Swartzwelder, 2003），而青春期的雄性自给药的烟碱量是成年雄性的三倍（Levin et al. 2007）。一旦在青春期建立，这些增加的给药率就会持续到成年期。在青春期（而非成年期）向雄性大鼠重复给予烟碱后，成年后其烟碱自给药(S-A)显著增加（Adriani et al. 2003）。

烟碱条件位置偏好（CPP）在青少年和成年男性与女性中很明显。在两个年龄段，更低的剂量下雄性大鼠在比雌性大鼠表现出更显著的CPP，表明烟碱作为奖励在雄性大鼠中比在雌性大鼠中更有效（Lenoir et al. 2015）。有趣的是，对于其他精神兴奋剂药物，如可卡因和苯丙胺，通常观察到相反的情况（例如，Dow-Edwards, 2010; Festa et al. 2004; Hu, Becker, 2003; Lynch, Carroll, 1999; Russo et al. 2003; Zakharova, Wade, Izenwasser, 2009）。总体而言，青少年比成年人更敏感，尽管其表现方式因性别而异。在男性中，与成年人相比，青少年的剂量反应曲线向左移动。与成年人相比，青春期女性的曲线向上移动，表明青少年的奖励效果比成年人更高（Lenoir et al. 2015）。一项针对男性的早期研究表明，烟碱CPP仅在青春期早期出现，而在青春期后期或成年期则不明显（Belluzzi, Lee, Oliff, Leslie, 2004）。在青春期或成年期反复给予烟碱一个月后，雄性大鼠的烟碱CPP增加（de la Pena et al. 2015）。然而，暴露于卷烟烟雾只会在青春期暴露时导致烟碱CPP增加。这些发现表明，青春期早期可能是特别容易受到烟碱影响的时期。

表3.1 烟碱对青春期和成年期的雄性和雌性的行为影响

给药方式	活动类型	行为变化	参考文献
烟碱7天；注射PND 28, 60；1天或30天后测试	自发活动	Adol: 雄性无感，雌性有感；AD: 雄性和雌性均有感	Collins and Izenwasser (2004); Collins, Montano et al. (2004)
烟碱7天；注射PND 28-34, 90-96；3天后测试	自发活动	雄性Adol无感，AD有感	Cruz et al. (2005)
烟碱10天；PND 28, 70；只有雄性	自发活动，提示条件反射	Adol: 无感，只有条件反射；AD: 两者都有	Schochet et al. (2004)
烟碱PND 31-42；7天后测试；只有雄性	自发活性	成年期疯狂和刻板的敏感度	Bracken et al. (2011)
连续烟碱21天；PND 30, 60	自发活动	Adol, AD: 雄性和雌性在测试期间无感	Faraday et al. (2011)
烟碱持续12天；PND 25, 55；只有雄性	自发活动	Adol, AD: 在测试期间有感	Fara et al. (2003)
日常烟碱；PND 49, 69；只有雌性	8字形迷宫中自发活动	雌性Adol: 无影响；AD: 活力降低	Levin et al. (2003)

续表

给药方式	活动类型	行为变化	参考文献
持续烟碱，PND 30-47	梳理	Adol：雌性无影响，雄性减少；AD：无影响	Trauth, Seidler, Slotkin (2000)
高烟碱	社交焦虑	烟碱在青春期雄性和青春期雌性中产生焦虑；对雌性更有效	Cheeta, Irvine, Tucci, Sandhu, File (2001); Elliott, Faraday, Phillips, Grunberg (2004); Slawecki, Gilder, Roth, Ehlers (2003)
烟碱5天；PND 25-30, 55-60	高架迷宫	Adol：雄性焦虑上升，雌性焦虑下降；AD：雌性、雄性焦虑均下降	Cheeta et al. (2001); Elliott et al. (2004); Slawecki et al. (2003)
烟碱6天；PND 31-36	AD的露天测试	雄性焦虑上升（中心时间减少）	Cheeta et al. (2001); Elliott et al. (2004); Slawecki et al. (2003)
烟碱PND 34-43,60-69；5周后测试	烟碱自给药	Adol：雄性在测试期间后增加	Adriani et al. (2003)
开始烟碱暴露，PND 32, 64	烟碱自给药	雌性Adol：两倍AD摄入量；雄性Adol：三倍AD摄入量	Levin et al. (2003, 2007)
烟碱 PND 28, 38, 90	烟碱CPP	雄性CPP只出现在PND 28中	Belluzzi et al. (2004)
烟碱 PND 28, 28；测试PND 40, 70	烟碱CPP	CPP只出现在Adol，不出现在AD中	Vastola, Douglas, Varlinskaya, Spear (2002)
烟碱CPP PND 34-38, 66-70	烟碱CPP	CPP Adol比AD更敏感。在Adol/AD，烟碱在雄性中更有效	Lenoir et al. (2015)
烟碱或卷烟烟雾 PND 28-41, 63-76；28天后测试	烟碱CPP，自给药	烟碱或吸烟后CPP增加，吸烟后烟碱自给药增加	de la Pena et al. (2015)

注：AD表示成年人，Adol表示青少年。

3.2 青春期的烟碱增加了随后给药的影响

许多研究表明，青春期的男性更容易受到其他药物的交叉敏（例如，在青春期接触烟碱后对另一种药物的反应增加），引发烟碱可能是导致其他药物滥用的"门户"药物的想法（见表3.2）。青春期反复暴露于烟碱会导致雄性大鼠对可卡因（Collins, Izenwasser, 2004）和苯丙胺（Collins, Montano et al. 2004）的运动刺激效应敏感，这些效应会持续到成年期（Collins, Izenwasser, 2004; Collins, Montano et al. 2004）。这种交叉致敏作用在雌性和成年大鼠中都不明显。

在成年后期的测试中，青春期的烟碱暴露会增加大鼠的可卡因条件位置偏好（CPP）（McMillen, Davis, Williams, Soderstrom, 2005）。然而，对小鼠的研究表明，它是下降的（Kelley, Middaugh, 1999;Kelley, Rowan, 2004）。目前尚不清楚是什么导致了这种物种差异。相比之下，Pomfrey等（Pomfrey, Bostwick, Wetzell, Riley, 2015）报道了在青春期烟碱对可卡因CPP或自给药没有影响。虽然在这项研究中测试了多种剂量的可卡因，但数据是以一种不同寻常的方式呈现的，即所有剂量都被压缩成一个单一的柱状图。因此，很难确定是否存在剂量反应或曲线位移，也很难得出关于为什么这个实验室发现的结果与其他实验室不同的结论。

青春期烟碱自给药导致青春期男性乙醇静脉注射自给药增加，而女性或任何性别的成年人则没有增加（Larraga, Belluzzi, Leslie, 2017）。同样，从青春期到成年期，暴露在卷烟烟雾中3周会导致雄性小鼠口服更多的乙醇（Burns, Proctor, 2013）。同样，在雄性大鼠中，在青春期注射烟碱导致甲基苯丙胺的自给药增加（Pipkin et al. 2014）。重复使用烟碱也增加了男性对芬太尼的自给药，而女性则没有变化（Klein, 2001）。暴露于烟碱下的雄性青春期老鼠也会增加可卡因的自给药，而烟碱对成年期雄性老鼠的可卡因的自给药没有显著影响（Reed, Izenwasser, 2017）。

表3.2 青春期烟碱给药对成年期雄性和雌性动物使用其他药物的影响

给药方式	活动类型	行为变化	参考文献
烟碱7天 PND 28, 60; 1天或30天后测试	自发活动——可卡因	Adol: 雄性对可卡因敏感，雌性没有变化; AD: 雄性/雌性没有变化	Collins and Izenwasser (2004)
烟碱7天 PND 28, 60; 1天或30天后测试	自发活动——苯丙胺	Adol: 雄性对苯丙胺敏感，雌性没有变化; AD: 雄性/雌性没有变化	Collins, Montano et al. (2004)
烟碱 PND 35-50；自给药开始 PND 51；只有雄性	甲基苯丙胺自给药	Adol预处理后的甲基苯丙胺自给药↑	Pikin et al. (2014)
烟碱 PND 42-60	芬太尼自给药	雄性↑自给药↑，雌性无变化	Klein (2001)
烟碱 PND 25-60(老鼠)；12天或28天后测试	可卡因CPP	雄性↓条件位置偏好	Kelley and Middaugh (1999); Kelley and Rowan (2004)
烟碱 PND 35-44；测试 PND 80	可卡因CPP	雄性↑CPP	McMillen et al. (2005)
烟碱CPP 28-42；测试 PND 66；只有雄性	可卡因CPP, 自给药	没有变化	—
卷烟烟雾 PND 35-66；只有雄性；老鼠	饮用乙醇	乙醇↑	Burns and Proctor (2013)
日常烟碱 PND 28-34, 60-66; 30天后测试；只有雄性	可卡因自给药	仅经预处理后的Adol可卡因自给药↑	Reed and Izenwasser (2017)
烟碱自给药开始 PND 32	乙醇静脉注射自给药	Adol 雄性: 乙醇↑; 雌性/成年期: 没有变化	Larraga et al. (2017)
烟碱 PND 45-59，每3天测试一次；测试成年的	饮用乙醇	烟碱与手术室配对时致敏	Zipori et al. (2017)

注：↑表示观察到增加，↓表示观察到减少。除非另有说明，所有研究均使用大鼠。

3.3 烟碱对青少年神经化学的影响

在行为研究方面，已经有大量的研究对青春期和成年期大鼠在给予烟碱后的多种受体和大脑通路进行了研究（见表3.3）。我们实验室的研究表明，每天注射烟碱会增加成年雄性大鼠尾壳核和伏隔核中的烟碱乙酰胆碱受体（nAChR）密度，而青春期雄性大鼠则不会（Collins, Wade, Ledon, Izenwasser, 2004）。在经烟碱预处理的成年大鼠中，多巴胺转运体、多巴胺D_1或D_2受体及血清素转运体密度均无变化。在青春期大鼠中，反复给予烟碱后多巴胺转运体密度增加，血清素转运体密度降低。这些数据与行为数据一致，表明青少年在服用烟碱后对可卡因和苯丙胺的运动刺激作用敏感，但对烟碱不敏感，而成年人则相反（Collins, Izenwasser, 2004; Collins,

Montano et al. 2004）。除了 nAChR 密度增加之外，还有证据表明在反复注射烟碱后，几个烟碱受体亚基（例如，α5、α6 和 β2）的基因表达增加（Adriani et al. 2003）。在连续输注烟碱 14 天后，α4 和 β2 受体显著增加，但在青少年和成年人（男性和女性）中 α5 受体没有变化（Hoegberg, Lomazzo, Lee, Perry, 2015）。因此，重复给药与连续输注烟碱的效果可能存在差异。其他研究表明，使用不同的烟碱给药方案会改变大脑多个区域的 nAChRs。例如，通过微型泵持续给药烟碱导致海马区、大脑皮层和中脑 nAChR 密度增加（Abreu-Villaca et al. 2003; Trauth, Seidler, McCook, Slotkin, 1999）。持续给药烟碱也会导致雌性大鼠血清素转运体结合的增加，其速度比雄性大鼠快得多。在雌性中，这种增长是在青春期观察到的，而在雄性中直到成年后才会出现（Xu, Seidler, Ali, Slikker, Slotkin, 2001）。相反，雄性大鼠血清素 $5HT_2$ 的结合增加，而雌性大鼠则没有（Xu, Seidler, Cousins, Slikker, Slotkin, 2002）。

表 3.3　烟碱治疗对青春期与成年期雄性和雌性神经化学的影响

给药方式	行为变化	参考文献
从 PND 28-34, 60-66 每天注射烟碱	Adol: DAT↑, SERT↓, nAChR NC↓; AD: nAChR↑, DAT↑, SERT NC↑	Collins and Izenwasser (2002)
从 PND 34-43, 60-69 每天注射烟碱，仅限雄性	Adol: α5、α6、β2↑; AD: NC	Adriani et al. (2003)
持续烟碱，PND 28-42, 70-84	Adol/AD: 雄性/雌性 α4、β2↑; α5 NC	Hoegberg et al. (2015)
烟碱 2 周，仅 PND 30 Adol	雄性 STR 的初始 AD 转换↑，雄性和雌性的 PND 50-60 AD 转换↑	Trauth, Seidler, Ali, Slotkin (2001)
从 PND 30-47 或 30-37 连续烟碱	Adol、AD: nAChR 在测试期间↑；有些在雄性中持续 30 天，而不是雌性	Abreu-Villaca et al. (2003); Abreu-Villaca, Seidler, Tate, Cousins, Slotkin (2004); Trauth et al. (1999)
持续烟碱，PND 30-47.5，仅限 Adol	雄性/雌性：SERT PND 75↑; $5HT_2$ PND 45、60↑	Xu et al. (2001)
持续烟碱，PND 30-47 然后 90-107；测试 PND 180	雄性：5HT 转换率↑；雌性：更小且延迟的效果	Slotkin et al. (2014)
持续烟碱，PND 30-47 然后 90-107；测试 PND 180	雄性长期 5HT 受体↑，雌性 5HT 受体↓	Slotkin and Seidler (2009)
烟碱 PND 30-47.5，只有 Adol。雄性和雌性一起分析	Adol: M2 毒蕈碱↓，基础和 FSK- 刺激的 AC↑	Chow et al. (2000)
烟碱 PND 30, 70。仅限男性	基线弧和 c-fos: Adol>AD; >↑ Adol 患者 PFC 中的弧比烟碱处理后的 AD 更高	Schochet, Kelley, Landry (2005)
烟碱 4 天，PND 31, 41, 56。雄性和雌性一起分析	烟碱在 Adol 中没有明显的 DA↑; AD 可耐受 DA↑	Badanich, Kirstein (2004)
从 PND 34-43 每天注射烟碱 1 天或 30 天后测试	第 1 天: NC; 30 天: 雄性/雌性比例，STR 中 CB 受体↓，在河马↑，在 STR 和河马中 Mu 型阿片肽↓	Marco et al. (2007)
烟碱 7 天，注射 PND 28-34, 90-96。3 天后测试，仅限雄性	AD: 对皮质酮升高耐受; Adol: NC	Cruz et al. (2005)

注：↑表示观察到增加，↓表示观察到减少。缩写：5-HT 血清素；CB 大麻素；DA 多巴胺；DAT 多巴胺转运蛋白；nAChR 烟碱乙酰胆碱受体；NC 无变化；SERT 血清素转运体；STR 纹状体。

Slotkin 和他的同事已经做了大量的研究来检测烟碱与大脑血清素系统的相互作用（例如，Slotkin et al. 2007; Slotkin, Card, Seidler, 2014; Slotkin, Seidler, 2007, 2009）。他们已经证明，在青春期烟碱对血清素有很大的影响，这种影响会持续到成年期，而且还存在年龄和性别差异。例如，青春期烟碱的暴露大大增加了烟碱对成年人血清素转换的急性影响，导致血清素的显著消耗（Slotkin et al. 2014）。此外，雌性在青春期接触烟碱，减弱了成年人戒断烟碱后血清素转换率的峰值，而这在男性中则没有观察到（Slotkin et al. 2014）。

尽管人们对 nAChR、多巴胺和血清素的研究非常关注，但烟碱对其他受体系统也有影响，例如，在青春期重复给药后 M2 毒蕈碱受体（Chow, Seidler, McCook, Slotkin, 2000）、大麻素受体（Marco et al. 2006）和鸦片类受体（Marco et al. 2006）减少。

3.4 结论

总之，烟碱对行为影响的临床前研究表明，青春期男性对该药物的作用非常敏感。与青春期女性或成年人相比，烟碱作为青春期男性的奖励和行为兴奋剂更有效，这种长期影响在男性青少年中比在其他群体中更为明显。青少年时期接触烟碱增加了其他滥用药物的奖励和重新适应特性，包括刺激剂（可卡因、苯丙胺和甲基苯丙胺）、阿片类药物（芬太尼）和乙醇（见表3.2）。因此，这些调查结果表明，青少年可能特别容易受到烟碱的影响，并在接触烟碱之后容易受到其他药物滥用的风险，此外，男性青少年可能表现出最大的脆弱性。这些研究还表明，在得出有关烟碱和其他药物的影响的结论之前，研究不同的发育阶段和性别是很重要的。大多数研究的结果表明，不同年龄和性别的人对反复使用烟碱有明显的差异和持久的适应。

术语解释
- 条件位置偏好：用于研究药物奖励的方法。
- 自给药：用于研究药物强化的方法，受试者通过执行操作任务来管理药物。
- 敏化作用：增加了药物暴露于某种刺激（如另一种药物）后的效果。

青少年受烟碱影响的关键事实
- 大多数吸烟者在18岁之前开始吸烟；因此，研究这一发展期是很重要的。
- 自给药是实验室使用的一种模式，受试者通过执行一项任务（如压力杠杆机）自行给药。这模仿了人类自发滥用药物的情况。
- 条件位置偏好是一种实验室模型，用于确定使用某一药物是否是有益的。
- 致敏作用表明，药物在反复接触后的效果甚至比第一次接触时的效果更大。

要点总结
- 开始使用烟碱的平均年龄发生在青春期，90%的使用者在18岁之前开始尝试吸烟。
- 临床前实验室研究经常表明与成年人相比，青少年对烟碱往往表现出独特的反应。
- 与成年女性不同，青春期的男性对烟碱的影响特别敏感。
- 青春期摄入烟碱通常会增加其他滥用药物的后续使用。
- 在得出有关烟碱和其他药物影响的结论之前，研究不同的发育阶段和性别是很重要的。

参考文献

Abreu-Villaca, Y.; Seidler, F. J.; Qiao, D.; Tate, C. A.; Cousins, M. M.; Thillai, I. et al. (2003). Short-term adolescent nicotine exposure has immediate and persistent effects on cholinergic systems: critical periods, patterns of exposure, dose thresholds. Neuropsychopharmacology, 28, 1935-1949.

Abreu-Villaca, Y.; Seidler, F. J.; Tate, C. A.; Cousins, M. M.; Slotkin, T. A. (2004). Prenatal nicotine exposure alters the response to nicotine administration in adolescence: effects on cholinergic systems during exposure and withdrawal. Neuropsychopharmacology, 29, 879-890.

Adriani, W.; Spijker, S.; Deroche-Gammonet, V.; Laviola, G.; Le Moal, M.; Smit, A. B. et al. (2003). Evidence for enhanced neurobehavioral vulnerability to nicotine during periadolescence in rats. The Journal of Neuroscience, 23, 4712-4716.

Badanich, K. A.; Kirstein, C. L. (2004). Nicotine administration significantly alters accumbal dopamine in the adult but not in the adolescent rat. Annals of the New York Academy of Sciences, 1021, 410-417.

Belluzzi, J. D.; Lee, A. G.; Oliff, H. S.; Leslie, F. M. (2004). Agedependent effects of nicotine on locomotor activity and conditioned place preference in rats. Psychopharmacology, 174, 389-395.

Bracken, A. L.; Chambers, R. A.; Berg, S. A.; Rodd, Z. A.; McBride, W. J. (2011). Nicotine exposure during adolescence enhances behavioral sensitivity to nicotine during adulthood in Wistar rats. Pharmacology, Biochemistry, and Behavior, 99, 87-93.

Burns, B. E.; Proctor, W. R. (2013). Cigarette smoke exposure greatly increases alcohol consumption in adolescent C57BL/6 mice. Alcoholism, Clinical and Experimental Research, 37(Suppl. 1), E364-E372.

Centers for Disease Control and Prevention. (2017). Tobacco use among middle and high school students—United States, 2011-2016. Morbidity and Mortality Weekly Report.

Cheeta, S.; Irvine, E. E.; Tucci, S.; Sandhu, J.; File, S. E. (2001). In adolescence, female rats are more sensitive to the anxiolytic effect of nicotine than are male rats. Neuropsychopharmacology, 25, 601-607.

Chow, F. A.; Seidler, F. J.; McCook, E. C.; Slotkin, T. A. (2000). Adolescent nicotine exposure alters cardiac autonomic responsiveness: b-adrenergic and m2-muscarinic receptors and their linkage to adenylyl cyclase. Brain Research, 878, 119-126.

Collins, S. L.; Izenwasser, S. (2002). Cocaine differentially alters behavior and neurochemistry in periadolescent versus adult rats. Developmental Brain Research, 138, 27-34.

Collins, S. L.; Izenwasser, S. (2004). Chronic nicotine differentially alters cocaine-induced locomotor activity in adolescent vs. adult male and female rats. Neuropharmacology, 46, 349-362.

Collins, S. L.; Montano, R.; Izenwasser, S. (2004). Nicotine treatment produces persistent increases in amphetamine-stimulated locomotor activity in periadolescent male but not female or adult male rats. Developmental Brain Research, 153, 175-187.

Collins, S. L.; Wade, D.; Ledon, J.; Izenwasser, S. (2004). Neurochemical alterations produced by daily nicotine exposure in periadolescent vs. adult male rats. European Journal of Pharmacology, 502, 75-85.

Cruz, F. C.; Delucia, R.; Planeta, C. S. (2005). Differential behavioral and neuroendocrine effects of repeated nicotine in adolescent and adult rats. Pharmacology, Biochemistry, and Behavior, 80, 411-417.

de la Pena, J. B.; Ahsan, H. M.; Tampus, R.; Botanas, C. J.; de la Pena, I. J.; Kim, H. J. et al. (2015). Cigarette smoke exposure during adolescence enhances sensitivity to the rewarding effects of nicotine in adulthood, even after a long period of abstinence. Neuropharmacology, 99, 9-14.

Dow-Edwards, D. (2010). Sex differences in the effects of cocaine abuse across the life span. Physiology, Behavior, 100, 208-215.

Elliott, B. M.; Faraday, M. M.; Phillips, J. M.; Grunberg, N. E. (2004). Effects of nicotine on elevated plus maze and locomotor activity in male and female adolescent and adult rats. Pharmacology, Biochemistry, and Behavior, 77, 21-28.

Faraday, M. M.; Elliott, B. M.; Grunberg, N. E. (2001). Adult vs. adolescent rats differ in biobehavioral responses to chronic nicotine administration. Pharmacology, Biochemistry, and Behavior, 70, 475-489.

Faraday, M. M.; Elliott, B. M.; Phillips, J. M.; Grunberg, N. E. (2003). Adolescent and adult male rats differ in sensitivity to nicotine's activity effects. Pharmacology, Biochemistry, and Behavior, 74, 917-931.

Festa, E. D.; Russo, S. J.; Gazi, F. M.; Niyomchai, T.; Kemen, L. M.; Lin, S. N. et al. (2004). Sex differences in cocaine-induced behavioral responses, pharmacokinetics, and monoamine levels. Neuropharmacology, 46, 672-687.

Hoegberg, B. G.; Lomazzo, E.; Lee, N. H.; Perry, D. C. (2015). Regulation of alpha4beta2alpha5 nicotinic acetylcholinergic receptors in rat cerebral cortex in early and late adolescence: sex differences in response to chronic nicotine. Neuropharmacology, 99, 347-355.

Hu, M.; Becker, J. B. (2003). Effects of sex and estrogen on behavioral sensitization to cocaine in rats. The Journal of Neuroscience, 23, 693-699.

Kelley, B. M.; Middaugh, L. D. (1999). Periadolescent nicotine exposure reduces cocaine reward in adult mice. Journal of Addictive Diseases, 18, 27-39.

Kelley, B. M.; Rowan, J. D. (2004). Long-term, low-level adolescent nicotine exposure produces dose-dependent changes in cocaine sensitivity and reward in mice. International Journal of Developmental Neuroscience, 22, 339-348.

Klein, L. C. (2001). Effects of adolescent nicotine exposure on opioid consumption and neuroendocrine responses in adult male and female rats. Experimental and Clinical Psychopharmacology, 9, 251-261.

Larraga, A.; Belluzzi, J. D.; Leslie, F. M. (2017). Nicotine increases alcohol intake in adolescent male rats. Frontiersin Behavioral Neuroscience, 11, 25.

Lenoir, M.; Starosciak, A. K.; Ledon, J.; Booth, C.; Zakharova, E.; Wade, D. et al. (2015). Sex differences in conditioned nicotine reward are age-specific. Pharmacology, Biochemistry, and Behavior, 132, 56-62.

Levin, E. D.; Lawrence, S. S.; Petro, A.; Horton, K.; Rezvani, A. H.; Seidler, F. J. et al. (2007). Adolescent vs. adult-onset nicotine selfadministration in male rats: duration of effect and differential nicotinic receptor correlates. Neurotoxicology and Teratology, 29, 458-465.

Levin, E. D.; Rezvani, A. H.; Montoya, D.; Rose, J. E.; Swartzwelder, H. S. (2003). Adolescent-onset nicotine self-administration modeled in female rats. Psychopharmacology, 169, 141-149.

Lynch, W.; Carroll, M. (1999). Sex differences in the acquisition of intravenously self-administered cocaine and heroin in rats. Pyschopharmacology, 144, 77-82.

Marco, E. M.; Granstrem, O.; Moreno, E.; Llorente, R.; Adriani, W.; Laviola, G. et al. (2007). Subchronic nicotine exposure in adolescence induces long-term effects on hippocampal and striatal cannabinoidCB1 and mu-opioid receptors in rats. European Journal of Pharmacology, 557, 37-43.

Marco, E. M.; Llorente, R.; Moreno, E.; Biscaia, J. M.; Guaza, C.; Viveros, M. P. (2006). Adolescent exposure to nicotine modifies acute functional responses to cannabinoid agonists in rats. Behavioural Brain Research, 172, 46-53.

McMillen, B. A.; Davis, B. J.; Williams, H. L.; Soderstrom, K. (2005). Periadolescent nicotine exposure causes heterologous sensitization to cocaine reinforcement. European Journal of Pharmacology, 509, 161-164.

Pipkin, J. A.; Kaplan, G. J.; Plant, C. P.; Eaton, S. E.; Gil, S. M.; Zavala, A. R. et al. (2014). Nicotine exposure beginning in adolescence enhances the acquisition of methamphetamine self-administration, but not methamphetamine-primed reinstatement in male rats. Drug and Alcohol Dependence, 142, 341-344.

Pomfrey, R. L.; Bostwick, T. A.; Wetzell, B. B.; Riley, A. L. (2015). Adolescent nicotine exposure fails to impact cocaine reward, aversion and self-administration in adult male rats. Pharmacology, Biochemistry, and Behavior, 137, 30-37.

Reed, S. C.; Izenwasser, S. (2017). Nicotine produces long-term increases in cocaine reinforcement in adolescent but not adult rats. Brain Research, 1654, 165-170.

Russo, S. J.; Jenab, S.; Fabian, S. J.; Festa, E. D.; Kemen, L. M.; Quinones-Jenab, V. (2003). Sex differences in the conditioned rewarding effects of cocaine. Brain Research, 970, 214-220.

Schochet, T. L.; Kelley, A. E.; Landry, C. F. (2004). Differential behavioral effects of nicotine exposure in adolescent and adult rats. Psychopharmacology, 175, 265-273.

Schochet, T. L.; Kelley, A. E.; Landry, C. F. (2005). Differential expression of arc mRNA and other plasticity-related genes induced by nicotine in adolescent rat forebrain. Neuroscience, 135, 285-297.

Slawecki, C. J.; Gilder, A.; Roth, J.; Ehlers, C. L. (2003). Increased anxiety-like behavior in adult rats exposed to nicotine as adolescents. Pharmacology, Biochemistry, and Behavior, 75, 355-361.

Slotkin, T. A.; Card, J.; Seidler, F. J. (2014). Nicotine administration in adolescence reprograms the subsequent response to nicotine treatment and withdrawal in adulthood: sex-selective effects on cerebrocortical serotonergic function. Brain Research Bulletin, 102, 1-8.

Slotkin, T. A.; MacKillop, E. A.; Rudder, C. L.; Ryde, I. T.; Tate, C. A.; Seidler, F. J. (2007). Permanent, sex-selective effects of prenatal or adolescent nicotine exposure, separately or sequentially, in rat brain regions: indices of cholinergic and serotonergic synaptic function, cell signaling, and neural cell number and size at 6 months of age. Neuropsychopharmacology, 32, 1082-1097.

Slotkin, T. A.; Seidler, F. J. (2007). A unique role for striatal serotonergic systems in the withdrawal from adolescent nicotine administration. Neurotoxicology and Teratology, 29, 10-16.

Slotkin, T. A.; Seidler, F. J. (2009). Nicotine exposure in adolescence alters the response of serotonin systems to nicotine administered subsequently in adulthood. Developmental Neuroscience, 31, 58-70.

Trauth, J. A.; Seidler, F. J.; Ali, S. F.; Slotkin, T. A. (2001). Adolescent nicotine exposure produces immediate and long-term changes in CNS noradrenergic and dopaminergic function. Brain Research, 892, 269-280.

Trauth, J. A.; Seidler, F. J.; McCook, E. C.; Slotkin, T. A. (1999). Adolescent nicotine exposure causes persistent upregulation of nicotinic cholinergic receptors in rat brain regions. Brain Research, 851, 9-19.

Trauth, J. A.; Seidler, F. J.; Slotkin, T. A. (2000). Persistent and delayed behavioral changes after nicotine treatment in adolescent rats. Brain Research, 880, 167-172.

Vastola, B. J.; Douglas, L. A.; Varlinskaya, E. I.; Spear, L. P. (2002). Nicotine-induced conditioned place preference in adolescent and adult rats. Physiology, Behavior, 77.

Xu, Z.; Seidler, F. J.; Ali, S. F.; Slikker, W. J.; Slotkin, T. A. (2001). Fetal and adolescent nicotine administration: effects on CNS serotonergic systems. Brain Research, 914, 166-178.

Xu, Z.; Seidler, F. J.; Cousins, M. M.; Slikker, W. J.; Slotkin, T. A. (2002). Adolescent nicotine administration alters serotonin receptors and cell signaling mediated through adenylyl cyclase. Brain Research, 951, 280-292.

Zakharova, E.; Wade, D.; Izenwasser, S. (2009). Sensitivity to cocaine conditioned reward depends on sex and age. Pharmacology, Biochemistry, and Behavior, 92, 131-134.

Zipori, D.; Sadot-Sogrin, Y.; Goltseker, K.; Even-Chen, O.; Rahamim, N.; Shaham, O. et al. (2017). Re-exposure to nicotine-associated context from adolescence enhances alcohol intake in adulthood. Scientific Reports, 7, 2479.

4
传统卷烟和电子烟对大脑的影响

Ewelina Wawryk-Gawda, Marta Lis-Sochocka, Patrycja Chylińska-Wrzos, Beata Budzyńska, Barbara Jodłowska-Jędrych

Department of Histology and Embryology with Experimental Cytology Unit, Medical University, Lublin, Poland

缩略语

Bcl-2	B 细胞淋巴瘤 2	GLT-1	谷氨酸转运蛋白 -1
CREB/BDNF	环磷酸腺苷（cAMP）反应元件结合蛋白/脑源性神经营养因子	IL-1β	白介素 -1β
		nAChR	烟碱乙酰胆碱受体
fALFF	低频波动的分数振幅	NGF	神经生长因子
fMRI	功能性磁共振成像	RSFC	静息状态功能连接
FTND	Fagerström 烟碱依赖测试	TNF-α	肿瘤坏死因子 α
GABA	γ- 氨基丁酸		

4.1 引言

许多产品中都含有烟碱，最古老的含烟碱产品之一是传统卷烟（图 4.1）。如今，新的烟碱设备，如电子烟等新型烟碱装置越来越受欢迎（Oh, Kacker, 2014）。电子烟（图 4.2）上市的初衷是帮助吸烟者戒烟，从而治疗烟碱上瘾（Kaisar, Prasad, Liles, Cucullo, 2016）。然而，越来越多的数据表明，有些人，尤其是青少年，将电子烟作为获取烟碱的第一手段，从而开始吸烟成瘾。在年轻人中使用电子烟是"摩登"，被认为比传统吸烟健康（Cooper, Harell, Pérez, Delk, Perry, 2016; Kaisar et al. 2016; Lauterstein et al. 2016; Lee, Grana, Glantz, 2014; Makadia, Roper, Adrews, Tingen, 2017）。吸传统卷烟和使用电子烟的区别很大（表 4.1），但在这两种情况下，烟碱都会对身体产生不良影响（Geiss, Bianchi, Barahona, Barrero-Moreno, 2015）。电子烟不通过燃烧烟草来传递香味。相反，它们包含一种由电子元件热蒸发的液体调味剂（电子液体）。这种液体是水、甘油和/或丙二醇的混合物；有时，甲醛和其他混合物中含有精神活性物质。这种液体还含有烟碱和多种

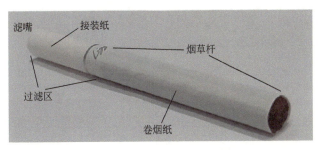

图 4.1 传统卷烟（图为带过滤嘴的传统卷烟）

香料（Bertholon et al. 2013）。虽然气溶胶是由烟油加热形成的，但它不含致癌燃烧产物，酚类和羰基化合物的数量是无法检测的。然而，电子烟的主动和被动"吸烟"都会对人体产生不良影响（Long, 2014; Tayyarah, Long, 2014）。与之前的观点相反，使用电子烟还会导致烟碱上瘾，甚至增加以后对传统卷烟上瘾的风险（Arane, Goldman, 2016）。

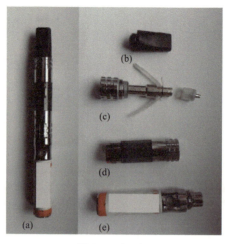

图4.2 电子烟

图中显示的是电子卷烟（a），它的吹口（b）与卷烟的滤嘴相似，它的雾化器（c）是一个加热元件，它使吹口中的液体蒸发，每吸一口烟就会产生雾。装有液体的墨盒（d）。该装置的主体：电池组件（e），其中包含可为雾化器提供动力的可充电电池。该装置的主体还装有一个电子空气流量传感器，用于在吸入时自动激活加热元件，并在每次吸入时亮起一个LED指示灯，发出激活该装置的信号。当用户按下按钮时，它通过吸入加热元件激活一个压力传感器，然后将液体雾化。电子液体在室内温度达到100～250℃，从而产生雾化蒸气（Polosa et al. 2011）。

表4.1 传统香烟与电子香烟的比较

特征	电子烟	传统香烟
呼气	气溶胶，蒸气	烟气
呼出气的主要成分	水，73%，3%～75%，7%；甘油，24%，2%～26%，7%（Long, 2014） 水，15%；甘油，73%（Tayyarah, Long, 2014）	水+甘油，83%±21%，卷烟样品的剩余呼出气溶胶质量归因于燃烧过程中产生的微粒，已知这些微粒占主流传统卷烟烟雾的70%以上（Long, 2014） 水，20%；甘油，2%，支持和燃烧产物，41%（Tayyarah, Long, 2014）
吸烟者环境中的烟碱	8～33μg/puff（Tayyarah, Long, 2014）	194～232μg（Tayyarah, Long, 2014）
吸烟者环境中的一氧化碳	无法检测到	20mg/支（Long, 2014） 34%（Tayyarah & Long, 2014）
吸烟者环境中的苯酚[①]	与呼出的呼吸量无显著差异	66μg/次（Tavvarah, Long, 2014） 22～32μg/次（Tayyarah, Long, 2014）
吸烟者环境中的羰基[②]		24μg/每次（Long, 2014） 211—251μg/每次（Tayyarah, Long, 2014）
吸烟者环境中的亚微米粒子	（1）比卷烟烟雾粒子还大 （2）仅在"吸烟"期间发生 （3）48%的沉积SMP非常小，以至于能够到达被动暴露受试者的肺泡区域（Bertholon et al. 2013; Protano et al. 2016）	（1）呼吸道中的沉积高于电子烟释放的沉积 （2）52%～53%的沉积SMP非常小，以至于能够到达被动暴露受试者的肺泡区域

① 酚类：对苯二酚、间苯二酚、邻苯二酚、苯酚、间/对甲酚和邻甲酚。
② 羰基：甲醛、乙醛、丙烯醛、丙醛、巴豆醛、MEK和丁醛。

4.2 烟碱使用者的大脑结构变化

传统卷烟对大脑的影响一直是许多研究的对象，但关于电子烟对中枢神经系统（CNS）的影响的文献相对较少。先前公布的数据显示，以电子烟形式使用烟碱的人与使用传统卷烟的人所观察到的变化相同的区域主要是额叶皮层、脑岛、丘脑和纹状体（图4.3）。这些变化可能与性别有关（Janes et al. 2017）。这些研究还表明，烟碱的使用会导致大脑结构和功能发生改变（Dumais et al. 2017）。通过磁共振成像（MRI）和功能性磁共振成像（fMRI）可以观察到由于对烟草（烟碱）上瘾而引起的结构和功能变化以及由于成瘾物质戒断而引起的变化。这些测试的结果表明，与不吸烟者相比，吸烟减少了双侧丘脑的体积。此外，根据Fagerström烟碱依赖测试（FTND）（Yu et al. 2018）的评估，年轻吸烟者的左丘脑体积与烟碱成瘾的严重程度相关。此外，Li等（2015）观察到年轻吸烟者的额叶皮层、左脑岛、左颞中回、右顶下小叶和右海马的皮质明显变薄。这些大脑结构的变化可能是认知控制和奖励驱动行为之间不平衡的原因，这些行为与烟碱成瘾和复发有关（Li et al. 2015）。

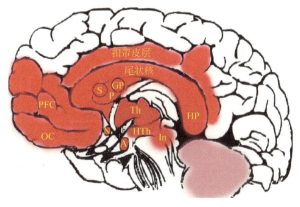

图4.3 传统吸烟和电子烟烟雾对大脑的影响区域

有关烟碱对大脑影响的数据显示，使用电子烟和吸烟会影响大脑的特定区域。它们是伏隔核（NAcc，图中以N表示）、杏仁核（A）、尾状核、扣带皮层、纹状体（S）、脑岛（In）、额叶皮层、前额叶皮层（PFC）、眶额皮层（OC）、丘脑（Th）、下丘脑（HTh）、海马（HP）、壳核（P）和苍白球（GP）。

4.3 传统吸烟者的大脑功能变化

静息状态功能性磁共振成像（fMRI）扫描被用于烟碱依赖的研究，提高了对烟碱依赖发展过程中神经可塑性变化的认识（Shen et al. 2016）。通过这些方法，研究人员发现与非吸烟者相比，吸烟者在眶额皮层、额上回、颞叶和脑岛之间的奖励回路中具有显著较低的静息状态功能连接性（RSFC）（Zhou et al. 2017）。Yuan等（2016）揭示了吸烟者的大脑结构和功能存在病理改变。在这项研究中，吸烟者的右尾状核体积增加，而在尾状体、背外侧前额叶皮层和眶额皮层之间的前纹状体回路RSFC减少。此外，Yuan等（2016）发现右尾状核体积与评估渴望状态的吸烟冲动（QSU）问题的结果之间存在显著的正相关关系。Wang等（2017）发现，吸烟者的丘脑与右侧背外侧前额叶皮层、前扣带皮层、脑岛和尾状核的静息状态功能连接性降低。他们还指出，丘脑在烟碱成瘾中也起作用。Shen等（2016）发现，与低依赖吸烟者相比，高依赖吸烟者在右侧杏仁核、左侧伏隔核和双侧海马体之间表现出更高的RSFC。Zhou等（2017）研究发现眶额皮层、颞叶、下顶叶皮层、枕叶和脑岛之间的RSFC与FTND呈正相关。功能性磁共振成像还可以评估大脑不同区域的低频波动的分数振幅（fALFF）。利用这项技术，Chu等（2014）观察到左侧枕中回、左侧边缘叶和左侧小脑后叶的fALFF增加，而右侧额中回、右侧颞上回、右侧核外回、左侧中央后回的fALFF减少，与不吸烟者相比，这些变化与累积烟碱摄入量和烟碱依赖程度有关。

4.4 电子烟使用者的大脑功能变化

目前，有关电子烟对大脑影响的数据有限；然而，Wall等（2017）的功能性磁共振成像研究显示，电子烟使用者的大脑皮层区域（运动皮层、脑岛、扣带回和杏仁核）和皮层下区域（壳核、丘脑、苍白球和小脑）网络中存在脑激活，而腹侧纹状体和眶额皮层中也存在相应的相对失活。Hobkirk等（2018）还报告称，除脑干外，电子烟使用者的右额极和额叶内侧皮层的两个簇的RSFC下降，具有注意力控制显著网络，左侧丘脑和脑岛的五个簇的RSFC下降，具有包含纹状体的奖励网络。此外，Hobkirk等（2018）指出，在戒断习惯后会出现戒断症状。

4.5 烟碱戒断症状

烟碱戒断症状是指停止摄入烟碱后出现的消极情绪。这些症状包括易怒、沮丧、焦虑、情绪低落、注意力难以集中、食欲增加、失眠和焦躁不安（McLaughlin, Dani, De Biasi, 2015）。fMRI测试显示，烟碱戒断综合征与前扣带皮层与楔前叶、脑岛、眶额回、额上回、后扣带皮层、颞上皮层和颞下叶之间的连接增加有关（Huang et al. 2014）。这些数据表明，吸烟会触发大脑中支持戒断诱发的渴望的结构性和功能性神经适应（Samochowiec, Rogoziński, Hajduk, Skrzypińska, Arentowicz, 2001）。戒断综合征的症状是烟碱输入引起某些神经递质受体活性变化的结果（图4.6）。烟碱通过激活N-胆碱能受体（nAChR，图4.4），刺激多巴胺能和谷胱甘肽能神经元的神经递质分泌（Ma, Liu, Neumann, Gao, 2017）。

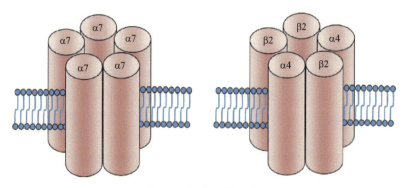

图4.4 烟碱胆碱能受体

N-胆碱能受体是由两种亚基单位（α和β）组成的五聚体结构。这些受体脱敏的倾向很大程度上取决于nAChR组件的亚基单位组成（同源或异源低聚）。

4.6 烟碱与奖励回路

烟碱通过增加中枢神经系统中多巴胺的释放（图4.5）和刺激奖励系统，以及增强运动耐力的活动和保持专注于寻求药物和自给药的食欲行为来激活中脑边缘系统（Berrendero, Robledo, Trigo, Martin-Garcia, Maldonado, 2010; Kostowski, 2001; Seo, Kim, Yu, Kang, 2016; Suchanecka, 2013）。此外，烟草烟雾的成分可以阻断单胺氧化酶A和B（Mao-A和Mao-B），并激活多巴胺能系统（Kostowski, 2001）。吸烟成瘾是一个复杂的过程（图4.6），主要与烟碱的上瘾作用有关，但传统卷烟的味道和香味也增强了人们的欲望和与吸烟有关的活动（仪式）（Kostowski, 2001）。

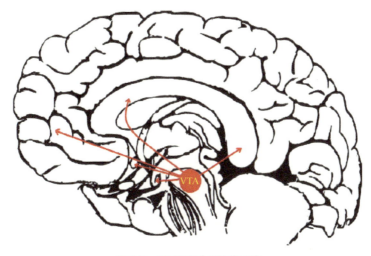

图 4.5　烟碱激活中脑边缘系统

烟碱激活腹侧被盖区（VTA）内的nAChR。多巴胺能投射器将信号从VTA传输到前额叶皮层、伏隔核、纹状体、海马体和杏仁核。多巴胺能投射靶区涉及强化（腹侧纹状体）、学习和陈述性记忆（海马体）、情感记忆（杏仁核）、习惯形成（背侧纹状体）、执行功能和工作记忆（前额叶皮层和眶额皮层）。慢性烟碱暴露通过改变阿片肽的合成和释放间接影响动机系统。成瘾过程产生细胞适应和大脑神经传递的改变，这些改变参与了烟碱戒断综合征。

受烟草成瘾影响的N-胆碱能受体是一种五聚体结构（图4.4），由α和β两种亚基组成。这些亚基有6个已知的α亚基和3个β亚基。烟碱对单个nAChR亚基的不同作用对神经系统产生了不同的影响。Baldassarri等（2018）发现，含36mg/mL（84%±3%）烟碱的电子烟蒸发后，平均β2-nAChR占用率高于8mg/mL（64%±17%），而吸烟后的平均β2-nAChR占用率为68%±18%。在Alasmari等（2017）的另一项研究中，吸入电子烟蒸气6个月会增加额叶皮层和纹状体中的α7-nAChR的表达，但不会增加海马体中的表达。此外，长期接触电子烟只会降低纹状体中谷氨酸转运蛋白1（GLT-1）的表达，但会导致额叶皮层、纹状体和海马体中胱氨酸/谷氨酸反向转运蛋白（xCT）的下调。在Hernandez和Terry Jr.（2005）的研究中，与对照组相比，雄性Wistar大鼠持续14天暴露于相对低剂量的烟碱（每12小时0.35mg/kg）中，其记忆性能有所改善。Hernandez和Terry Jr.（2005）认为，这种效果可能取决于烟碱诱导的特定乙酰胆碱受体亚型［受神经生长因子（NGF）调节的关键胆碱能蛋白］表达的变化。烟碱增加了不同学习和记忆相关大脑区域中nAChRs的表达，从而可能增强短期记忆功能的论点被用于建议基于烟碱型激动剂的记忆障碍治疗，如阿尔茨海默病（Xue et al. 2015）。

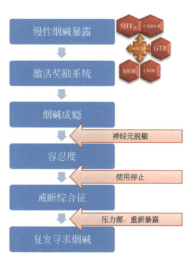

图 4.6 烟碱对中枢神经系统的影响

烟碱激活中脑边缘结构神经元上的 nAChR，从而增加奖励系统中多巴胺的分泌。另一种神经递质涉及奖励系统并在烟碱摄入后增加多巴胺的释放，它们是血清素（通过 5-HT_{2C} 受体亚型）、谷氨酸（谷氨酸能受体，GTR）、阿片肽（通过阿片受体，MOR）、大麻素（通过大麻素受体 1，CB1R）和 GABA。长期接触烟碱可诱发增强效应和卷烟渴望（烟碱成瘾）的发展。烟碱对奖励系统的长期激活导致神经元脱敏和感受器的上调，这是导致感受器发育的原因。停止使用烟碱会引起戒断综合征的行为和躯体症状。在戒断期间，暴露于应激源或烟碱环境中，会引发烟碱渴望，并复发寻求烟碱（Berrendero et al. 2010）。

4.7 烟碱对大脑发育的影响

另一方面，通过分析烟碱对大脑发育的影响得出的一些数据表明，该药物会导致神经退行性疾病，使用慢性烟碱对学习和认知功能有负面影响（Connor, Gould, 2017; Suter, Mastrobattista, Sachs, Aagaard, 2015）。此外，有数据表明，产前接触二手烟和烟碱可能会影响大脑发育（Peterson, Hecht, 2017; Protano, Manigrasso, Avino, Vitali, 2017; Smith et al. 2015）。然而，二手烟和电子烟对发育中的胎儿和幼儿的影响仅在少数研究中有描述（Protano, Manigrasso, Avino, Sernia, Vitali, 2016; Suter et al. 2015; Makadia et al. 2017）。然而，根据动物研究，烟碱导致前脑和中脑的血清素、多巴胺和去甲肾上腺素紊乱（Suter et al. 2015）。此外，根据 Lauterstein 等（2016）的研究，暴露于电子烟烟雾中的小鼠的后代在额叶皮层中出现了基因改变，这可能导致日后的认知和行为缺陷。事实上，Lavezzi 等（2017）指出，与 11% 对照组（不吸烟）相比吸烟母亲胎儿人脑某些区域的小脑胆碱能传递的改变可能是导致胎儿和婴儿猝死的原因，因为他们观察到 66% 的不明原因围产期猝死病例中，小脑皮质颗粒层中 α7-nAChR 表达阴性或低表达。此外，正如 Mohamed、Loy、Lim、Al Mamun 和 Jan Mohamed（2017）所见，产前烟碱浓度水平与沟通和精细运动技能呈负相关，而产后烟碱浓度水平与精细运动和解决问题技能呈负相关。

4.8 烟碱诱导的氧化应激和神经元凋亡

所描述的神经衰弱和大脑发育的改变可能是烟碱诱导的氧化应激和神经元凋亡的结果。在 Motaghinejad、Motevalian、Fatima、Faraji 和 Mozaffari（2017）的研究中，作者观察到烟碱治疗增加了脂质过氧化和 IL-1β、TNF-α 和促凋亡蛋白 Bax 的水平，同时降低了神经保护 CREB/BDNF

通路和海马区 Bcl-2 的水平。烟碱也降低了海马体中超氧化物歧化酶、谷胱甘肽过氧化物酶和谷胱甘肽还原酶的活性。添加到烟草或液体烟雾中的香料和其他物质可能会增加烟碱的毒性作用。薄荷醇是烟草和电子烟中常用的调味剂，可能导致烟碱敏感性（Fait et al. 2017; Thompson et al. 2017）。由于烟碱对大脑的毒性作用，意外摄入电子烟液体可能导致死亡。确实存在儿童和成人意外摄入电子烟液体的案例，表明摄入电子烟液体会导致严重的缺氧脑损伤、急性梗死和脑水肿，从而导致呼吸衰竭或死亡（Chen, Bright, Trivedi, Valento, 2015; Noble, Longstreet, Hendrickson, Gerona, 2017; Seo et al. 2016）。

4.9 结论

所提供的数据表明，传统卷烟和电子烟对使用者、附近的人以及未出生的人具有极大的危害。因此，最重要的是传播有关含有烟碱的不同产品的实际影响的知识，并提高公众的认识，即不仅是吸烟，而且电子烟或其他烟碱传递装置对使用者和旁观者都有害。因此，旨在促进健康和鼓励健康生活的活动应强调帮助停止烟碱消费。

术语解释	- 电子烟：电池驱动的提供烟碱的设备，看起来像卷烟，并释放蒸气（含烟碱的气溶胶）。这种蒸气是通过加热电子烟容器中的液体而产生的。这种液体含有不同浓度的烟碱、甘油、丙二醇、香料，有时还含有几种精神活性物质。 - 烟碱依赖：是一种成瘾综合征，因反复吸食烟碱而产生的行为和生理症状。 - 奖励系统：大脑中的神经系统是边缘系统的一部分，它与动机和行为控制有关。这个系统是通过满足"需要"（如饮酒、饮食和生殖）来激活的，也通过服用精神成瘾物质（如酒精、烟碱、安非他明和其他精神活性药物）来激活。 - 烟草燃烧产品：烟草制品（烟草、纤维素和其他物质）点燃时产生的烟雾含有不同直径的固体超细颗粒、自由基和致瘤气体（氮氧化物、一氧化碳等）。 - 传统（常规）卷烟：烟草和不同添加剂的组合物由薄纸包裹，然后将其点燃并由用户吸入烟气。除了烟碱之外，烟碱还含有多种燃烧产物。
奖励回路的关键事实	- 奖励回路是负责动机和行为控制的一组大脑结构。 - 奖励系统包括腹侧被盖区、纹状体、前额叶皮层、丘脑、苍白球、杏仁核和海马体等结构。 - 参与奖励系统的神经递质有多巴胺、乙酰胆碱、阿片类、大麻素、血清素、GABA 和谷氨酸。 - 每一次后续的需求满足都会带来"积极的强化"、刺激、愉悦和激励。 - 内在奖励（可口的食物和性）本质上是令人愉悦的，有助于提高生存和繁殖的可能性。 - 外在奖励（金钱）是一种具有吸引力和激励行为的条件性奖励。 - 精神活性药物和危险行为会激活奖励回路，导致成瘾。
要点总结	- 本章重点关注吸烟和电子烟烟液对使用者和二次接触者大脑的影响。 - 传统卷烟是一种长期合法的消费品。 - 电子烟是一种新型烟碱输送装置，部分取代了传统卷烟。

- 吸电子烟（使用电子烟）是通过加热含有烟碱、丙二醇、甘油、香料和其他物质的液体而吸入蒸气的行为。在吸电子烟过程中，不会发生燃烧。
- 传统卷烟吸烟和吸电子烟都会引起烟碱依赖戒断综合征。
- 通过这两种装置消耗烟碱会导致大脑中与奖励系统相关的特定区域的结构和功能变化。
- 当孕妇在产前或生命早期暴露于烟气或蒸气产品时，其烟碱的摄入会导致其后代的神经退化和大脑发育的改变。

参考文献

Alasmari, F.; Crotty, A. L. E.; Nelson, J. A.; Schiefer, I. T.; Breen, E,; Drummond, C. A. et al. (2017). Effects of chronic inhalation of electronic cigarettes containing nicotine on glial glutamate transporters and α-7 nicotinic acetylcholine receptor in female CD-1 mice. Progress in Neuro-Psychopharmacology & Biological Psychiatry, 77, 1-8.

Arane, K.; Goldman, R. D. (2016). Electronic cigarettes and adolescents. Canadian Family Physician M_edecin de famille canadien, 62(11), 897-898.

Baldassarri, S. R.; Hillmer, A. T.; Anderson, J. M.; Jatlow, P.; Nabulsi, N.; Labaree, D. et al. (2018). Use of electronic cigarettes leads to significant beta 2-nicotinic acetylcholine receptor occupancy: evidence from a PET imaging study. Nicotine & Tobacco Research, 20(4), 425-433. https://doi.org/10.1093/ntr/ntx091.

Berrendero, F.; Robledo, P.; Trigo, J. M.; Martín-García, E.; Maldonado, R. (2010). Neurobiological mechanisms involved in nicotine dependence and reward: participation of the endogenous opioid system. Neuroscience and Biobehavioral Reviews, 35(2), 220-231.

Bertholon, J. F.; Becquemin, M. H.; Roy, M.; Roy, F.; Ledur, D.; Annesi Maesano, I. et al. (2013). Comparison of the aerosol produced by electronic cigarettes with conventional cigarettes and the shisha. Revue des Maladies Respiratoires, 30(9), 752-757.

Chen, B. C.; Bright, S. B.; Trivedi, A. R. Valento, M. (2015). Death following intentional ingestion of e-liquid. Clinical Toxicology, 53(9), 914-916.

Chu, S.; Xiao, D.; Wang, S.; Peng, P.; Xie, T.; He, Y. et al. (2014). Spontaneous brain activity in chronic smokers revealed by fractional amplitude of low frequency fluctuation analysis: a resting state functional magnetic resonance imaging study. Chinese Medical Journal, 127(8), 1504-1509.

Connor, D. A.; Gould, T. J. (2017). Chronic fluoxetine ameliorates adolescent chronic nicotine exposure-induced long-term adult deficits in trace conditioning. Neuropharmacology, 2(125), 272-283.

Cooper, M.; Harrell, M. B.; P_erez, A.; Delk, J.; Perry, C. L. (2016). Flavorings and perceived harm and addictiveness of E-cigarettes among youth. Tobacco Regulatory Science, 2(3), 278-289.

Dumais, K. M.; Franklin, T. R.; Jagannathan, K.; Hager, N.; Gawrysiak, M.; Betts, J. et al. (2017). Multi-site exploration of sex differences in brain reactivity to smoking cues: consensus across sites and methodologies. Drug and Alcohol Dependence, 1(178), 469-476.

Fait, B. W.; Thompson, D. C.; Mose, T. N.; Jatlow, P.; Jordt, S. E.; Picciotto, M. R. et al. (2017). Menthol disrupts nicotine's psychostimulant properties in an age and sex-dependent manner in C57BL/6J mice. Behavioural Brain Research, 22(334), 72-77.

Geiss, O.; Bianchi, I.; Barahona, F.; Barrero-Moreno, J. (2015). Characterisation of mainstream and passive vapours emitted by selected electronic cigarettes. International Journal of Hygiene and Environmental Health, 218(1), 169-180.

Hernandez, C. M.; Terry, A. V.; Jr. (2005). Repeated nicotine exposure in rats: effects on memory function, cholinergic markers and nerve growth factor. Neuroscience, 130(4), 997-1012.

Hobkirk, A. L.; Nichols, T. T.; Foulds, J.; Yingst, J. M.; Veldheer, S. Hrabovsky, S. et al. (2018). Changes in resting state functional brain connectivity and withdrawal symptoms are associated with acute electronic cigarette use. Brain Research Bulletin, 138, 56-63.

Huang, W.; King, J. A.; Ursprung, W. W.; Zheng, S.; Zhang, N.; Kennedy, D. N. et al. (2014). The development and expression of physical nicotine dependence corresponds to structural and functional alterations in the anterior cingulate-precuneus pathway. Brain and Behawior, 4(3), 408-417.

Janes, A. C.; Gilman, J. M.; Radoman, M.; Pachas, G.; Fava, M.; Evins, A. E. (2017). Revisiting the role of the insula and smoking cue-reactivity in relapse: a replication and extension of neuroimaging findings. Drug and Alcohol Dependence, 12(179), 8-12.

Kaisar, M. A.; Prasad, S.; Liles, T.; Cucullo, L. (2016). A decade of e-cigarettes: limited research & unresolved safety concerns. Toxicology, 15(365), 67-75.

Kostowski, W. (2001). Współczesna farmakoterapia uzalez_ nienia od nikotyny. Alkoholizm i Narkomania, 14(l), 129-136.

Lauterstein, D. E.; Tijerina, P. B.; Corbett, K.; Akgol Oksuz, B.; Shen, S. S.; Gordon, T. et al. (2016). Frontal cortex transcriptome analysis of mice exposed to electronic cigarettes during early life stages. International Journal of Environmental Research and Public Health, 13(4), 417.

Lavezzi, A. M.; Ferrero, S.; Roncati, L.; Piscioli, F.; Matturri, L.; Pusiol, T. (2017). Nicotinic receptor abnormalities in the cerebellar cortex of sudden unexplained fetal and infant death victims-possible correlation with maternal smoking. American Society for Neurochemistry Neuro, 9(4), 1-10.

Lee, S.; Grana, R. A.; Glantz, S. A. (2014). Electronic cigarette use among Korean adolescents: a cross-sectional study of market penetration, dual use, and relationship to quit attempts and former smoking. The Journal of Adolescent Health, 54(6), 684-690.

Li, Y.; Yuan, K.; Cai, C.; Feng, D.; Yin, J.; Bi, Y. et al. (2015). Reduced frontal cortical thickness and increased caudate volume within fronto-striatal circuits in young adult smokers. Drug and Alcohol Dependence, 1(151), 211-219.

Long, G. A. (2014). Comparison of select analytes in exhaled aerosol from E-cigarettes with exhaled smoke from a conventional cigarette and exhaled

breaths. International Journal of Environmental Research and Public Health, 11, 11177-11191.
Ma, C.; Liu, Y.; Neumann, S.; Gao, X. (2017). Nicotine from cigarette smoking and diet and Parkinson disease: a review. Translational Neurodegeneration, 2(6), 18.
Makadia, L. D.; Roper, P. J.; Andrews, J. O.; Tingen, M. S. (2017). Tobacco use and smoke exposure in children: new trends, harm, and strategies to improve health outcomes. Current Allergy and Asthma Reports, 17(8), 55.
McLaughlin, I.; Dani, J. A.; De Biasi, M. (2015). Nicotine withdrawal. Current Topics in Behavioral Neurosciences, 24, 99-123.
Mohamed, N. N.; Loy, S. L.; Lim, P. Y.; Al Mamun, A.; Jan Mohamed, H. J. (2017). Early life secondhand smoke exposure assessed by hair nicotine biomarker may reduce children's neurodevelopment at 2 years of age. Science of the Total Environment, 10 (610-611), 147-153.
Motaghinejad, M.; Motevalian, M.; Fatima, S.; Faraji, F.; Mozaffari, S. (2017). The neuroprotective effect of curcumin against nicotine-induced neurotoxicity is mediated by CREB-BDNF signaling pathway. Neurochemical Research, 42(10), 2921-2932.
Noble, M. J.; Longstreet, B.; Hendrickson, R.G.; Gerona, R. (2017). Unintentional pediatric ingestion of electronic cigarette nicotine refill liquid necessitating intubation. Annals of Emergency Medicine, 69(1), 94-97.
Oh, A. Y.; Kacker, A. (2014). Do electronic cigarettes impart a lower potential disease burden than conventional tobacco cigarettes? Review on E-cigarette vapor versus tobacco smoke. Laryngoscope, 124(12), 2702-2706.
Peterson, L. A.; Hecht, S. S. (2017). Tobacco, e-cigarettes, and child health. Current Opinion in Pediatrics, 29(2), 225-230.
Polosa, R.; Caponnetto, P.; Morjaria, J. B.; Papale, G.; Campagna, D.; Russo, C. (2011). Effect of an electronic nicotine delivery device (e-Cigarette) on smoking reduction and cessation: a prospective 6-month pilot study. BMC Public Health, 11, 786.
Protano, C.; Manigrasso, M.; Avino, P.; Sernia, S.; Vitali, M. (2016). Second-hand smoke exposure generated by new electronic devices (IQOS® and e-cigs) and traditional cigarettes: submicron particle behaviour in human respiratory system. Annali di Igiene: Medicina Preventiva e di Comunita, 28(2), 109-112.
Protano, C.; Manigrasso, M.; Avino, P.; Vitali, M. (2017). Second-hand smoke generated by combustion and electronic smoking devices used in real scenarios: ultrafine particle pollution and age-related dose assessment. Environment International, 107, 190-195.
Samochowiec, J.; Rogozi_nski, D.; Hajduk, A.; Skrzypińska, A.; Arentowicz,G. (2001). Diagnostyka, mechanizm uzalez_ nienia i metody leczenia uzalez_ nienia od nikotyny. Alkoholizm i Narkomania, 14(3), 323-340.
Seo, A. D.; Kim, D. C.; Yu, H. J.; Kang, M. J. (2016). Accidental ingestion of E-cigarette liquid nicotine in a 15-month-old child: an infant mortality case of nicotine intoxication. Korean Journal of Pediatrics, 59(12), 490-493.
Shen, Z.; Huang, P.; Qian, W.; Wang, C.; Yu, H.; Yang, Y. et al. (2016). Severity of dependence modulates smokers' functional connectivity in the reward circuit: a preliminary study. Psychopharmacology, 233(11), 2129-2137.
Smith, D.; Aherrera, A.; Lopez, A.; Neptune, E.; Winickoff, J. P.; Klein, J. D. et al. (2015). Adult behavior in male mice exposed to E-cigarette nicotine vapors during late prenatal and early postnatal life. PLoS ONE, 10(9). e0137953.
Suchanecka, A. (2013). Rola dopaminy w procesach motywacyjnych i powstawaniu uzalez_ nień. Annales Academiae Medicae Stetinensis Roczniki Pomorksiej Akademii Medycznej w Szczecinie Neurokongwi Nistyka w patologii i zdrowiu, 158-161.
Suter, M. A.; Mastrobattista, J.; Sachs, M.; Aagaard, K. (2015). Is there evidence for potential harm of electronic cigarette use in pregnancy? Birth Defects Research Part A, 103(3), 186-195.
Tayyarah, R.; Long, G. A. (2014). Comparison of select analytes in aerosol from e-cigarettes with smoke from conventional cigarettes and with ambient air. Regulatory Toxicology and Pharmacology, 70 (3), 704-710.
Thompson, M. F.; Poirier, G. L.; Dávila-García, M. I.; Huang, W.; Tam, K.; Robidoux, M. et al. (2017). Menthol enhances nicotineinduced locomotor sensitization and in vivo functional connectivity in adolescence. Journal of Psychopharmacology, 1. 332-343.
Wall, M. B.; Mentink, A.; Lyons, G.; Kowalczyk, O. S.; Demetriou, L.; Newbould, R. D. (2017). Investigating the neural correlates of smoking: feasibility and results of combining electronic cigarettes with fMRI. Scientific Reports, 7(1), 11352.
Wang, C.; Bai, J.; Wang, C.; von Deneen, K. M.; Yuan, K.; Cheng, J. (2017). Altered thalamo-cortical resting state functional connectivity in smokers. Neuroscience Letters, 13(653), 120-125.
Xue, M.; Zhu, L.; Zhang, J.; Qiu, J.; Du, G.; Qiao, Z. et al. (2015). Low dose nicotine attenuates A β neurotoxicity through activation early growth response gene 1 pathway. PLoS ONE, 3, e0120267.
Yu, D.; Yuan, K.; Cheng, J.; Guan, Y.; Li, Y.; Bi, Y. et al. (2018). Reduced thalamus volume may reflect nicotine severity in young male smokers. Nicotine and Tobacco Research, 20(4), 434-439. https://doi.org/10.1093/ntr/ntx146.
Yuan, K.; Yu, D.; Bi, Y.; Li, Y.; Guan, Y.; Liu, J. et al. (2016). The implication of frontostriatal circuits in young smokers: a resting-state study. Human Brain Mapping, 37(6), 2013-2026.
Zhou, S.; Xiao, D.; Peng, P.; Wang, S. K.; Liu, Z.; Qin, H. Y. et al. (2017). Effect of smoking on resting-state functional connectivity in smokers: an fMRI study. Respirology, 22(6), 1118-1124.

5
减少烟草中的烟碱及其影响

Yael Abreu-Villaça[1], *Alex Christian Manhães*[1], *Anderson Ribeiro-Carvalho*[2]

1. Department of Physiological Sciences, Institute of Biology, State University of Rio de Janeiro, Rio de Janeiro, Brazil
2. Department of Sciences, Faculty of Teacher Training, State University of Rio de Janeiro, São Gonçalo, Brazil

缩略语

DAergic	多巴胺能	**nAChR**	烟碱乙酰胆碱受体
MAO	单胺氧化酶	**VTA**	腹侧被盖区
NAcc	伏隔核		

5.1 预防成瘾和减少烟草使用的战略

为了减少因需要处理与烟草消费相关的健康问题而对个人和社会造成的负担，自从首次发现吸烟构成健康危害的明确迹象以来，已经制订了若干旨在促进戒烟尝试和持续戒烟的策略（West, 2017）。这些策略可以分为两条主要行动线：第一条涉及预防成瘾，第二条旨在减少或完全停止烟草消费。例如，吸烟者可能会在意识到他们确实遭受了成瘾的有害影响后决定戒烟。在尝试这样做时，他们有多种选择，并取得了不同程度的成功（West, 2017）。他们可能会停止冷火鸡法这种充满严重戒断综合征后果的方法，或者他们可能会尝试通过逐渐减少消费、在戒烟前选择烟碱含量较低的品牌并诉诸于药物治疗和/或烟碱替代疗法来缓和戒烟。心理支持有时也用作戒烟尝试的辅助手段。鉴于与吸烟有关的疾病的社会经济影响，旨在预防或减少吸烟的公共政策也已实施（Hoffman, Tan, 2015）。其中包括限制在公共场所投放广告；确定合法购买的最低年龄；卷烟包装健康风险提示的义务；禁止在公共场所室内消费；最近，监管立法的实施要求将卷烟烟碱含量降低到不会导致成瘾的水平（World Health Organization, 2015）。例如，关于最后一项策略，美国的《家庭吸烟预防和烟草控制法》授权食品和药物管理局大幅降低香烟的烟碱含量，前提是这样做可以改善公众健康（United States Congress, 2009）。这一策略基于烟碱是香烟中主要的成瘾成分这一事实（United States Department of Health and Human Services, 1988），因此，前提是烟碱的减少将防止那些愿意尝试香烟的人形成成瘾吸烟并抑制吸烟者寻求烟碱的行为（Donny et al. 2012; Hatsukami, Benowitz, Donny, Henningfield, Zeller, 2013）。

如果强制降低卷烟中的烟碱含量被认为是解决与吸烟相关的健康问题的可行策略，那么极低烟碱卷烟的消费最终一定会导致以下结果中的一种，最好是两种：①从试验到继续使用的个体百分比降低，②减少吸烟量或成功戒烟的吸烟者百分比增加。简而言之，虽然通过严格限制卷烟中的烟碱含量确实可以减少消耗的烟碱总量，但在烟草烟雾中已确定的其他4000多种物质的含量，包括几种已知的致癌物质（Smith, Perfetti, Garg, Hansch, 2003），并没有受到太大影响（Denlinger-

Apte, Joel, Strasser, Donny, 2016）。尽管多年来吸烟可能导致严重健康后果的观念已经很普遍，甚至在吸烟者中也是如此，但有证据表明，人们对吸食烟碱含量极低的卷烟的有害影响存在错误认识。下面，在讨论了这些公众的看法之后，我们展示了人类和动物模型的研究结果，这些研究解决了降低卷烟中烟碱含量是否确实是管理吸烟及其健康后果的有利策略的问题。

5.2 公众对低烟碱卷烟健康风险的认知

减少卷烟中的烟碱含量的一个麻烦的方面是，它可能会产生不符合预期效果的结果，要么将当前吸烟者的卷烟消费量保持在与采用低烟碱卷烟之前观察到的水平相匹配的水平，要么实际上推动消费增长（Mercincavage et al. 2017）。更糟糕的是，非吸烟者，尤其是易受影响的青少年，以及那些已经成功戒烟的人开始吸烟，可能是因为一种错误的观点，即烟碱是与吸烟习惯相关的疾病的主要来源（Ambrose et al. 2014）。虽然许多吸烟者承认烟碱会导致上瘾，但他们可能没有意识到，吸烟导致的大多数疾病实际上是由烟草烟雾中存在的其他成分造成的。事实上，大约75%的美国成年人要么错误地认为烟碱会导致癌症，要么不确定这种因果关系是否存在（O'Brien, Nguyen, Persoskie, Hoffman, 2017）。在这种情况下，使用低烟碱卷烟可能被错误地认为危害较小，因此，吸烟者可能会选择低烟碱品牌而不是完全戒烟，认为使用低烟碱品牌对他/她的健康有益，同时可避免因戒烟而带来的不适。事实上，Denlinger-Apte等（2016）和O'Brien等（2017）表明，与普通的烟碱卷烟相比，受试者认为低烟碱卷烟对他们健康的整体危害较小，而且这种效应对特定的吸烟相关疾病也适用。

5.3 降低烟草产品中的烟碱含量是否有利？来自流行病学和人体实验研究的证据

与对低烟碱卷烟的不利看法可能最终推动消费增加的观点相反，这些卷烟产生了一系列理想的结果，包括增加戒烟的愿望、减少接触烟碱、减少吸烟和减少依赖（框5.1）。例如，Denlinger-Apte等（2016）证明，虽然他们的受试者认为极低烟碱卷烟的主观效果不如普通烟碱卷烟理想，但他们还预测，如果只有极低烟碱卷烟，他们将对戒烟有更大的兴趣。更重要的是，低烟碱卷烟的消费导致对这种成瘾药物的接触减少，这可能伴随着依赖性和渴望的减少（Donny et al. 2015; Higgins et al. 2017）。这些影响是在没有明显的补偿性消费迹象的情况下观察到的。在某些特殊情况下，在坚决尝试戒烟之前，使用低烟碱卷烟作为权宜之计可能特别有用。例如，想要减少接触烟草烟雾的有害后果但又不想应对烟碱戒断的影响，并发现吸烟行为在心理上非常有益的吸烟者就是这样一种情况（Benowitz, Donny, Hatsukami, 2017）。如果可以使用不燃烧的烟碱替代品（例如电子烟）以及使用极低烟碱卷烟，则他们的吸烟形态会发生改变，从而减少接触烟草烟雾（Hatsukami et al. 2017）。

在一些关于使用低烟碱卷烟的研究中观察到的有利结果似乎表明，广泛采用要求严格降低烟碱含量的法规是合理的。然而，也确定了几个不利方面（框5.2）。其中之一是补偿性消费（Strasser, Lerman, Sanborn, Pickworth, Feldman, 2007; Zacny, Stitzer, 1988）。当每天吸烟的卷烟总数增加（Mercincavage et al. 2017）和/或吸烟行为发生变化时，例如抽吸量、频率和次数增加时，就会出现这种补偿（Scherer, Lee, 2014）。例如，与高烟碱含量的卷烟相比，青少年在使用去烟碱香烟时会增加抽吸的次数，从而表现出部分补偿（Kassel et al. 2007）。成年人的补偿程度在不同研究中差异很大，尤其是在涉及品牌转换策略时（Scherer, Lee, 2014）。成年人吸烟形态变化最显著的方面是抽吸量，当品牌之间的烟碱产量差异较小时，发现该参数的补偿性增加更加明显。有迹象表明，在需要减少烟瘾的情况下，吸食低烟碱香烟可能会阻碍其继续使用。短期体重增加就是这样的一个例子。Rupprecht等（2017）证明，在持续使用极低烟碱卷烟的6周期间，男性和女性的体重可能增加1公斤以上。除了体重增加的美学影响外，肥胖也是一个健康问题，有其自身的一系列问题。另一个问题与认知能力的下降有关。还报道了与下层大脑功能改变相关的工作记忆缺陷（McClernon et al. 2016）。

框5.1

与低烟碱卷烟消费相关的有利方面

- 减少接触烟碱
- 降低从实验发展到依赖的可能性
- 减少依赖性
- 减少渴望
- 抑制烟碱寻求行为
- 减少吸烟
- 减少戒断症状
- 戒烟成功率较高

框5.2

与低烟碱卷烟消费相关的不利方面

- 认为低烟碱卷烟比一般卷烟危害小的错误看法
- 促进实验
- 补偿性吸烟
- 改变的吸烟形态（例如，体积、频率和抽吸次数的增加）
- 持续或增加接触有毒的非烟碱卷烟化合物
- 改变的情绪
- 认知能力下降

虽然我们对吸食低烟碱卷烟的潜在好处和坏处的认识一直在稳步增加，但仍有很多未知的地方，包括烟碱含量的逐渐变化与突然变化的影响，以及对脆弱人群特别是青少年的影响（Donny et al. 2014）。为了帮助弥补这一信息空白，已系统地使用动物模型来解决与低烟碱浓度烟草产品暴露相关的潜在问题（图5.1）。

5.4 降低烟草产品中的烟碱含量是否有利？大多数来自暴露动物模型的证据表明情况并非如此

除了烟碱外，吸烟者还会接触烟草烟雾中存在的几种其他物质，这些物质可能独立于烟碱作用或干扰烟碱作用。在这方面，烟草烟雾暴露的临床前模型是研究人类吸烟状况的相关方法。使用动物模型和体外研究产生的大多数数据表明，卷烟中烟碱含量的降低并不伴随着危害的明显减少（Deutsch, 2009）。例如，体外研究表明，与普通卷烟相比，烟碱含量低的卷烟产生的主流烟雾的化学成分的差异不会降低其致突变性和细胞毒性特性（Coffa, Coggins, Werley, Oldham, Fariss, 2016）。在大脑中，有证据表明，与普通卷烟相比，极低烟碱和不含烟碱的卷烟对血脑屏障内皮的损害更大，增加了脑血管和中枢神经系统疾病的风险（Naik et al. 2014）。鉴于迄今为止已确定的有害影响，使用低烟碱或去烟碱卷烟作为可能的减少危害的策略只有在这些卷烟的成瘾性低于普通卷烟的情况下才是合理的，因此可以显著减少消费。

烟瘾的发展不仅受卷烟烟碱含量的影响，还受非烟碱化合物的含量的影响，非烟碱化合物

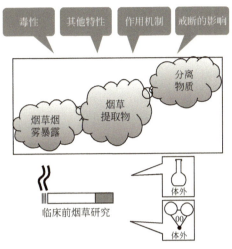

图 5.1 临床前烟草暴露模型

吸烟的影响最好通过暴露于烟草中发现的许多化合物来模拟,因此允许在人类中观察到的全方位的相互作用存在。含不同烟碱水平的卷烟和烟草提取物的研究已证明在这方面特别有用。然而,对烟碱以外的特定化合物的影响的研究也提供了有价值的信息。有证据表明,烟瘾不再仅仅被理解为对烟碱上瘾。

可能会促进或阻碍烟碱的作用。因此,仅接触烟碱并不能准确反映吸烟和接触烟草中存在的各种化合物的影响。例如,与只预先暴露于烟碱环境的老鼠相比,在青春期预先暴露于烟草烟雾环境的老鼠更容易受到后期(成年时)烟碱暴露的影响(de la Pena et al. 2014)。研究人员还调查了烟草中不同烟碱水平的影响。含有极低烟碱水平的卷烟产生的烟雾会对大脑功能产生显著的短期和长期影响,这与暴露于高烟碱水平烟草烟雾中的小鼠中所发现的结果不同(Abreu-Villaca et al. 2010, 2015, 2016)。即使烟碱含量大幅降低,也不能保护大脑。将青春期小鼠暴露于含有极低烟碱水平的卷烟烟雾中,会导致其猎奇行为减少,这一效应在暴露结束后仍会持续很长时间(Abreu-Villaca et al. 2015)。此外,暴露的中断会导致焦虑水平的增加,这是一个特别令人不安的事实,因为焦虑被认为是吸烟复发的相关因素(Abreu-Villaca et al. 2015)。作为乙酰胆碱的类似物,烟碱以胆碱能系统为主要靶点。有趣的是,尽管极低烟碱卷烟和传统卷烟之间的烟碱含量相差 10 倍,但暴露的胆碱能效应,如大脑皮层中的烟碱胆碱能受体 (nAChR) 上调,存在于暴露于这两种卷烟的小鼠中(Abreu-Villaca et al. 2016)。此外,暴露于极低烟碱卷烟烟雾中的小鼠在暴露期结束后很长时间内表现出大脑皮层中高亲和力胆碱转运蛋白的下调。这种转运蛋白是一种受神经冲动活动高度调节的胆碱能标记物,这表明当非常低水平的烟碱与其他烟草烟雾化合物结合时,仍然能够在戒断期间促进胆碱能突触损伤(Abreu-Villaca et al. 2016)。总的来说,这些数据表明,即使在烟碱暴露水平较低的情况下胆碱能系统仍然很脆弱,而烟碱的含量在吸烟时显著降低。

虽然动物模型是研究潜在的神经化学和行为影响以及烟草烟雾暴露的潜在机制的基础,但这些模型并未解决与含烟草产品的消费相关的奖励效应。在这方面,烟草提取物已被证明是特别有用的。可以训练啮齿动物自给药含有不同水平烟碱的烟草提取物,并且可以将它们的自给药模式与使用等效烟碱水平获得的模式进行比较。有趣的是,烟草提取物在自给药的获得和维持方面比单独的烟碱更有效,在应激诱导的恢复方面也更有效(Costello et al. 2014)。此外,单独的烟碱和烟草提取物对不同类型的 nAChR 具有相似的亲和力,但提取物在诱导 nAChR 上调的能力方面更有效(Ambrose et al. 2007)。此外,烟草提取物,而不是单独的烟碱,可以增加多巴胺转运蛋白的功能（Danielson, Putt, Truman, Kivell, 2014），引起比纹状体中的烟碱更强劲的细胞外多巴胺水平增加（Khalki, Navailles, Piron, De Deurwaerdere, 2013），并且在促进中缝神经元血清素活性抑制方面比烟碱更有效 (Touiki, Rat, Molimard, Chait, de Beaurepaire, 2007)。

临床前研究已经确定了许多可能导致烟草成瘾的神经活性非烟碱烟草成分（图5.2）。单胺氧化酶（MAO）抑制剂、乙醛和少量烟草生物碱在动物模型中模拟或增强烟碱的行为和神经药理学作用。MAO 催化包括多巴胺在内的单胺类物质的降解，而 MAO 抑制则主要在低剂量时增强烟碱的强化作用（Hogg, 2016）。烟草热解过程中产生的乙醛似乎也会增加烟碱的自给药（Belluzzi, Wang, Leslie, 2005）。此外，烟草还含有其他几种类似于烟碱的生物碱，例如降烟碱、可替宁和安那他滨，它们参与烟草的强化作用（Bardo, Green, Crooks, Dwoskin, 1999）。最后，还有一些能增强感官刺激的物质和最大限度减少吸入烟草烟雾引起的刺激的物质。例如，薄荷醇是一种常用的卷烟添加剂，可增加烟草产品的适口性（Fan et al. 2016），通过增加烟碱诱导的 nAChR 脱敏和上调，从而改变多巴胺神经元，从而改变烟碱在大脑中的作用兴奋性和运动敏感性（Henderson et al. 2017; Thompson et al. 2017）。

总之，这些数据表明，烟碱水平的降低既不能保护中枢神经系统免受烟草的毒性影响，也不能比烟碱含量正常的烟草更容易上瘾。考虑到越来越多的证据表明非烟碱化合物会影响烟草的成瘾特性，烟草成瘾不再被理解为烟碱成瘾。与烟碱具有协同作用或具有化学感觉效应的化合物可促进吸烟开始、阻止戒烟和促进复发，应加以管制。当考虑到烟草制造商已经开发出一系列物质来提高低烟碱卷烟的接受度和销量时，这一假设是至关重要的（Alpert, Agaku, Connolly, 2016; FDA, 1995）。

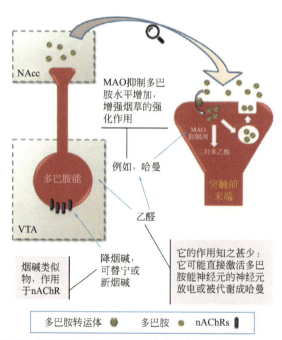

图 5.2 烟草烟雾中活性非烟碱化合物对中皮层边缘系统的影响

在这里，我们展示了中脑腹侧被盖区（VTA）多巴胺能（DAergic）投射到伏隔核（NAcc）的示意图。该通路在介导包括吸烟在内的滥用药物的奖励效应中发挥重要作用。烟草制品中的微量烟草生物碱（如降烟碱、可替宁和安那他滨）与位于多巴胺能神经元中的nAChR 直接相互作用。MAO 抑制剂（如哈曼）可增加多巴胺水平，增强烟草的强化作用。乙醛在烟草热解过程中产生，激活多巴胺能神经元的神经元放电或代谢成哈曼。

5.5 结论

降低烟草产品中的烟碱含量是基于这种策略可以防止成瘾的发展，抑制寻求烟碱的行为，并减少有害健康的影响这一前提的。我们发现，在人类和动物模型中都进行了流行病学和实验研究，证明使用低烟碱卷烟可以降低对这种药物的接触水平，有利于减少依赖性。然而，也有证据表明，这些卷烟可能不会抑制吸食烟碱的行为，并可能作为一种补偿策略而促使消费量上升，而且毒性效应非常明显。如果围绕这一问题的争议要得到最终解决，就需要继续进行研究。

术语解释	■ 脱敏：当受体降低其对激动剂分子的反应时发生的现象。 ■ 运动增敏：当随后接触药物时，引起比最初更大的运动过度活跃时发生的现象。 ■ 单胺氧化酶（MAO）抑制剂：抑制 MAO 酶家族活性的物质。这个家族的酶催化单胺类的氧化。 ■ 烟碱乙酰胆碱受体（nAChR）上调：烟碱等胆碱能激动剂促进的 nAChR 数量增加。 ■ 自给药：使用动物受试者对药物成瘾的各个方面进行建模的方法。一般来说，训练动物按下一个杠杆（通常通过静脉导管）输送一定剂量的药物。
烟草研究中烟碱减少的关键事实	■ 认识到烟碱是烟草烟雾中主要的成瘾成分，因此研制出了这种生物碱含量较低的卷烟。 ■ 这些卷烟包括由低烟碱含量的烟草混合物制成的卷烟，或烟碱（有意地）和其他成分（无意地）被部分或完全去除的卷烟。 ■ 这些卷烟已被研究团体用于确定烟草中的烟碱和非烟碱成分在健康中的作用。 ■ 没有完美的安慰剂卷烟，因为没有一种可供选择的卷烟在成分（不考虑烟碱）和感官特征上与普通卷烟完全相同。 ■ 使用低烟碱卷烟或烟草烟雾提取物的临床前研究，有助于目前对烟碱作用的认识。 ■ 动物模型允许研究烟草烟雾或烟草提取物中不同水平的烟碱的奖励和神经毒性作用，并进一步揭示烟草中存在的其他物质的作用。 ■ 来自评估烟草品牌毒性和添加剂潜力的临床和临床前研究的补充数据对政府机构烟草控制立法非常有用。
要点总结	■ 本章重点介绍降低烟草中烟碱含量的利弊。 ■ 烟碱是烟草产品中主要的成瘾成分。 ■ 烟碱含量的降低可能阻止成瘾机制的发生和/或可能抑制吸烟者寻求烟碱的行为。 ■ 因此，卷烟中烟碱含量低被认为是预防或减少吸烟的一种可能策略。 ■ 烟碱含量极低的卷烟可以减少烟碱的暴露，增加戒烟的欲望，减少依赖和渴望。 ■ 还有相反的证据表明，在管理吸烟习惯及其健康后果方面，降低烟碱含量可能不是一项有利的战略。 ■ 吸烟者可能会调整他们的吸烟吸入模式，以补偿低烟碱含量。 ■ 在"清淡烟"和低烟碱卷烟中，除烟碱外，烟草烟雾中有毒成分的含量没有减少。

- 烟草烟雾中除烟碱外的其他物质可能独立于或干扰烟碱对大脑的影响，并导致烟草毒性和/或成瘾。
- 卷烟中存在的一些物质可能会增强感官刺激和/或减少烟雾的过度刺激。
- 研究结果表明烟碱并不是导致烟草上瘾的唯一因素。

参考文献

Abreu-Villaca, Y.; Correa-Santos, M.; Dutra-Tavares, A. C.; PaesBranco, D.; Nunes-Freitas, A.; Manhaes, A. C. et al. (2016). A ten fold reduction of nicotine yield in tobacco smoke does not spare the central cholinergic system in adolescent mice. International Journal of Developmental Neuroscience, 52, 93-103.

Abreu-Villaca, Y.; Filgueiras, C. C.; Correa-Santos, M.; Cavina, C. C.; Naiff, V. F.; Krahe, T. E. et al. (2015). Tobacco smoke containing high or low levels of nicotine during adolescence: effects on noveltyseeking and anxiety-like behaviors in mice. Psychopharmacology, 232(10), 1693-1703.

Abreu-Villaca, Y.; Filgueiras, C. C.; Guthhierrez, M.; Medeiros, A. H.; Mattos, M. A.; Pereira Mdos, S. et al. (2010). Exposure to tobacco smoke containing either high or low levels of nicotine during adolescence: differential effects on choline uptake in the cerebral cortex and hippocampus. Nicotine, Tobacco Research, 12(7), 776-780.

Alpert, H. R.; Agaku, I. T.; Connolly, G. N. (2016). A study of pyrazines in cigarettes and how additives might be used to enhance tobacco addiction. Tobacco Control, 25(4), 444-450.

Ambrose, V.; Miller, J. H.; Dickson, S. J.; Hampton, S.; Truman, P.; Lea, R. A. et al. (2007). Tobacco particulate matter is more potent than nicotine at upregulating nicotinic receptors on SH-SY5Y cells. Nicotine, Tobacco Research, 9(8), 793-799.

Ambrose, B. K.; Rostron, B. L.; Johnson, S. E.; Portnoy, D. B.; Apelberg, B. J.; Kaufman, A. R. et al. (2014). Perceptions of the relative harm of cigarettes and e-cigarettes among U.S. youth. American Journal of Preventive Medicine, 47(2 Suppl. 1), S53-S60.

Bardo, M. T.; Green, T. A.; Crooks, P. A.; Dwoskin, L. P. (1999). Nornicotine is self-administered intravenously by rats. Psychopharmacology 38 5. REDUCTION OF NICOTINE IN TOBACCO AND IMPACT(Berl), 146(3), 290-296.

Belluzzi, J. D.; Wang, R.; Leslie, F. M. (2005). Acetaldehyde enhances acquisition of nicotine self-administration in adolescent rats. Neuropsychopharmacology, 30(4), 705-712.

Benowitz, N. L., Donny, E. C.; Hatsukami, D. K. (2017). Reduced nicotine content cigarettes, e-cigarettes and the cigarette end game. Addiction, 112(1), 6-7.

Coffa, B. G.; Coggins, C. R. E.; Werley, M. S.; Oldham, M. J.; Fariss, M. W. (2016). Chemical, physical, and in vitro characterization of research cigarettes containing denicotinized tobacco. Regulatory Toxicology and Pharmacology, 79, 64-73.

Costello, M. R.; Reynaga, D. D.; Mojica, C. Y.; Zaveri, N. T.; Belluzzi, J. D.; Leslie, F. M. (2014). Comparison of the reinforcing properties of nicotine and cigarette smoke extract in rats. Neuropsychopharmacology, 39(8), 1843-1851.

Danielson, K.; Putt, F.; Truman, P.; Kivell, B. M. (2014). The effects of nicotine and tobacco particulate matter on dopamine uptake in the rat brain. Synapse, 68(2), 45-60.

de la Pena, J. B.; Ahsan, H. M.; Botanas, C. J.; Sohn, A.; Yu, G. Y.; Cheong, J. H. (2014). Adolescent nicotine or cigarette smoke exposure changes subsequent response to nicotine conditioned place preference and self-administration. Behavioural Brain Research, 272, 156-164.

Denlinger-Apte, R. L.; Joel, D. L.; Strasser, A. A.; Donny, E. C. (2016). Low nicotine content descriptors reduce perceived health risks and positive cigarette ratings in participants using very low nicotine content cigarettes. Nicotine, Tobacco Research, 19(10), 1149-1154.

Deutsch, M. E. (2009). Less-toxic cigarette use may backfire. Science, 325 (5943), 944.

Donny, E. C.; Denlinger, R. L.; Tidey, J. W.; Koopmeiners, J. S.; Benowitz, N. L.; Vandrey, R. G. et al. (2015). Randomized trial of reduced-nicotine standards for cigarettes. The New England Journal of Medicine, 373(14), 1340-1349.

Donny, E. C.; Hatsukami, D. K.; Benowitz, N. L.; Sved, A. F.; Tidey, J. W.; Cassidy, R. N. (2014). Reduced nicotine product standards for combustible tobacco: building an empirical basis for effective regulation. Preventive Medicine, 68, 17-22.

Donny, E. C.; Taylor, T. G.; LeSage, M. G.; Levin, M.; Buffalari, D. M.; Joel, D. et al. (2012). Impact of tobacco regulation on animal research: new perspectives and opportunities. Nicotine, Tobacco Research, 14(11), 1319-1938.

Fan, L.; Balakrishna, S.; Jabba, S. V.; Bonner, P. E.; Taylor, S. R.; Picciotto, M. R. et al. (2016). Menthol decreases oral nicotine aversion in C57BL/6 mice through a TRPM8-dependent mechanism. Tobacco Control, 25(Suppl. 2), ii50-ii54.

FDA. (1995). Regulations restricting the sale and distribution of cigarettes and smokeless tobacco products to protect children and adolescents; proposed rule analysis regarding FDA's jurisdiction over nicotine-containing cigarettes and smokeless tobacco products; notice. Federal Register, 60, 41314-41792.

Hatsukami, D. K.; Benowitz, N. L.; Donny, E.; Henningfield, J.; Zeller, M. (2013). Nicotine reduction: strategic research plan. Nicotine, Tobacco Research, 15(6), 1003-1013.

Hatsukami, D. K.; Luo, X.; Dick, L.; Kangkum, M.; Allen, S. S.; Murphy, S. E. et al. (2017). Reduced nicotine content cigarettes and use of alternative nicotine products: exploratory trial. Addiction, 112(1), 156-167.

Henderson, B. J.; Wall, T. R.; Henley, B. M.; Kim, C. H.; McKinney, S.; Lester, H. A. (2017). Menthol enhances nicotine reward-related behavior by potentiating nicotine-induced changes in nAChR function, nAChR upregulation, and DA neuron excitability. Neuropsychopharmacology.

Higgins, S. T.; Heil, S. H.; Sigmon, S. C.; Tidey, J. W.; Gaalema, D. E.; Stitzer, M. L. et al. (2017). Response to varying the nicotine content of cigarettes in vulnerable populations: an initial experimental examination of acute effects. Psychopharmacology, 234(1), 89-98.

Hoffman, S. J.; Tan, C. (2015). Overview of systematic reviews on the health-related effects of government tobacco control policies. BMC Public Health, 15, 744.

Hogg, R. C. (2016). Contribution of monoamine oxidase inhibition to tobacco dependence: a review of the evidence. Nicotine, Tobacco Research, 18(5), 509-523.

Kassel, J. D.; Greenstein, J. E.; Evatt, D. P.; Wardle, M. C.; Yates, M. C.; Veilleux, J. C. et al. (2007). Smoking topography in response to denicotinized and high-yield nicotine cigarettes in adolescent smokers. The Journal of Adolescent Health, 40(1), 54-60.

Khalki, H.; Navailles, S.; Piron, C. L.; De Deurwaerdere, P. (2013). A tobacco extract containing alkaloids induces distinct effects compared to pure nicotine on dopamine release in the rat. Neuroscience Letters, 544, 85-88.

McClernon, F. J.; Froeliger, B.; Rose, J. E.; Kozink, R. V.; Addicott, M. A.; Sweitzer, M. M. et al. (2016). The effects of nicotine and nonnicotine smoking factors on working memory and associated brain function. Addiction Biology, 21(4), 954-961.

Mercincavage, M.; Saddleson, M. L.; Gup, E.; Halstead, A.; Mays, D.; Strasser, A. A. (2017). Reduced nicotine content cigarette advertising: how false beliefs and subjective ratings affect smoking behavior. Drug and Alcohol Dependence, 173, 99-106.

Naik, P.; Fofaria, N.; Prasad, S.; Sajja, R. K.; Weksler, B.; Couraud, P. O. et al. (2014). Oxidative and pro-inflammatory impact of regular and denicotinized cigarettes on blood brain barrier endothelial cells: is smoking reduced or nicotine-free products really safe? BMC Neuroscience, 23, 15-51.

O'Brien, E. K.; Nguyen, A. B.; Persoskie, A.; Hoffman, A. C. (2017). U. S. adults' addiction and harm beliefs about nicotine and low nicotine cigarettes. Preventive Medicine, 96, 94-100.

Rupprecht, L. E.; Koopmeiners, J. S.; Dermody, S. S.; Oliver, J. A.; al'Absi, M.; Benowitz, N. L. et al. (2017). Reducing nicotine exposure results in weight gain in smokers randomised to very low nicotine content cigarettes. Tobacco Control, 26(e1), e43-e48.

Scherer, G.; Lee, P. N. (2014). Smoking behaviour and compensation: a review of the literature with meta-analysis. Regulatory Toxicology and Pharmacology, 70(3), 615-628.

Smith, C. J.; Perfetti, T. A.; Garg, R.; Hansch, C. (2003). IARC carcinogens reported in cigarette mainstream smoke and their calculatedlog P values. Food and Chemical Toxicology, 41(6), 807-817.

Strasser, A. A.; Lerman, C.; Sanborn, P. M.; Pickworth, W. B.; Feldman, E. A. (2007). New lower nicotine cigarettes can produce compensatory smoking and increased carbon monoxide exposure. Drug and Alcohol Dependence, 86(2-3), 294-300.

Thompson, M. F.; Poirier, G. L.; Davila-Garcia, M. I.; Huang, W.; Tam, K.; Robidoux, M. et al. (2017). Menthol enhances nicotineinduced locomotor sensitization and in vivo functional connectivity in adolescence. Journal of Psychopharmacology.

Touiki, K.; Rat, P.; Molimard, R.; Chait, A.; de Beaurepaire, R. (2007). Effects of tobacco and cigarette smoke extracts on serotonergic raphe neurons in the rat. NeuroReport, 18(9), 925-929.

United States Congress. (2009). Family smoking prevention and tobacco control act. US Government Printing Office.

United States Department of Health and Human Services. (1988). The health consequences of smoking: nicotine addiction. a report of the surgeon general. US Department of Health and Human Services. DHHS Publication No. (CDC) 88-8406: Public Health Service, Centers for Disease Control, Center for Chronic Disease Prevention and Health Promotion, Office of Smoking and Health.

West, R. (2017). Tobacco smoking: Health impact, prevalence, correlates and interventions. Psychology and Health, 32(8), 1018-1036.

World Health Organization. (2015). Advisory note: Global nicotine reduction strategy: WHO study group on tobacco product regulation. Geneva: WHO Press.

Zacny, J. P.; Stitzer, M. L. (1988). Cigarette brand-switching: effects on smoke exposure and smoking behavior. The Journal of Pharmacology and Experimental Therapeutics, 246(2), 619-627.

6
产前烟碱暴露和神经前体细胞

Tursun Alkam[1,2], *Toshitaka Nabeshima*[1,3,4]

1. Japanese Drug Organization of Appropriate Use and Research, Nagoya, Japan
2. Department of Basic Medical Sciences, College of Osteopathic Medicine of the Pacific, Western University of Health Sciences, Pomona, CA, United States
3. Advanced Diagnostic System Research Laboratory, Graduate School of Health Sciences, Fujita Health University, Toyoake, Japan
4. Aino University, Ibaraki, Japan

缩略语

ACh	乙酰胆碱	NMDAR	N-甲基-D-天冬氨酸受体
CNS	中枢神经系统	NPC	神经前体细胞
DG	齿状回	NSC	神经干细胞
E	胚胎日	P	产后日
G	妊娠日	PNE	产前烟碱暴露
IPC	中间祖细胞	RGCs	放射状胶质细胞
mRNA	信使RNA	RT-PCR	逆转录-聚合酶链反应
nAChR	烟碱乙酰胆碱受体	SVZ	室下区

6.1 引言

怀孕期间吸烟的女性的后代会出现认知和情绪异常,包括注意力不集中、学习障碍、决策能力受损、冲动行为和躁动(Blood-Siegfried, Rende, 2010; Ernst, Moolchan, Robinson, 2001; Hamosh, Simon, Hamosh, 1979)。通过吸烟或在怀孕期间使用烟碱产品进行戒烟治疗而获得的烟碱,被认为是通过干扰nAChR的功能而干扰胎儿大脑的发育(Dempsey, Benowitz, 2001; Slotkin, 1998)。关于产前烟碱暴露(PNE)毒性的动物研究(图6.1)证实,烟碱在成年后代中诱发情绪和认知行为异常(Alkam, Kim, Mamiya, et al. 2013; Alkam, Kim, Hiramatsu, et al. 2013; Alkam et al. 2017; Berner et al. 2008; Britton, Vann, Robinson, 2007; Gold, Keller, Perry, 2009; Hall et al. 2016; Oliff, Gallardo, 1999)。这些行为异常与成人大脑中神经递质的产生和信号传导的缺陷有关(Alkam,

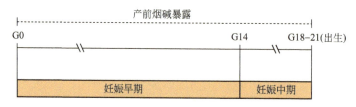

图 6.1 小鼠产前烟碱暴露期

啮齿动物的整个妊娠期为18~21天,包括人类妊娠早期和中期。改编自Dwyer等(2008)。

Kim, Mamiya, et al. 2013; Alkam et al. 2017; Huang, Liu, Griffith, Winzer-Serhan, 2007; Matta et al. 2007; Slotkin et al. 2005, 2007; Vaglenova et al. 2008; Vaglenova, Birru, Pandiella, Breese, 2004; Zhu et al. 2012; Zhu, Lee, Spencer, Biederman, Bhide, 2014），神经前体细胞增殖的中断和发育中大脑神经发生的损伤也与此有关（Abrous et al. 2002; Cohen et al. 2015; He, Wang, Wang, Shen, Yin, 2013; Scerri, Stewart, Breen, Balfour, 2006; Wei et al. 2012）。

6.2 大脑发育中的神经前体细胞

哺乳动物中枢神经系统（CNS）是胚胎发育过程中最早出现的系统之一。中枢神经系统来源于胚胎最外层的组织层，即外胚层。外胚层产生神经外胚层，形成神经板。神经板用一层神经上皮细胞形成神经管，即神经上皮。这些神经上皮细胞作为原代神经干细胞（NSC），在胚胎发育的早期产生分化的神经细胞类型，最初在早期产生神经元，但逐渐转变为产生不同类型的胶质细胞（Aaku-Saraste, Oback, Hellwig, Huttner, 1997; Kintner, 2002）。NSC被定义为具有无限自我更新能力的多能增殖细胞，具有两种有丝分裂途径，即对称分裂和不对称分裂。在对称分裂中，两个子细胞都成为多能神经干细胞。在不对称分裂中，一个子细胞变成多能神经干细胞，而另一个子细胞变成放射状神经胶质细胞，它可以自我更新并产生向神经元和神经胶质分化方向移动的中间祖细胞（IPC）（Gotz, Huttner, 2005; Potten, Loeffler, 1990; Seaberg, van der Kooy, 2003; Weiss et al. 1996）（图6.2）。

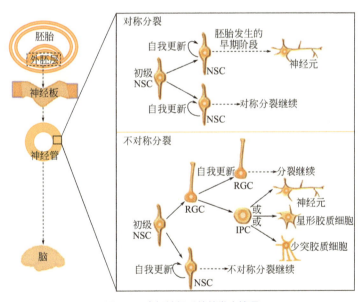

图 6.2 中枢神经系统的发育情况

神经管原代神经干细胞是一种具有无限自我更新能力的多能增殖细胞，具有对称分裂和不对称分裂两种有丝分裂途径。在对称分裂中，两个子细胞在早期产生神经元的同时成为多能神经干细胞。在不对称分裂中，一个子细胞成为多能神经干细胞，而另一个子细胞成为放射状神经胶质细胞，它能够自我更新并产生向神经元或神经胶质（星形胶质细胞或少突胶质细胞）分化方向移动的中间祖细胞。IPC，中间祖细胞；NSC，神经干细胞；RGC，放射状胶质细胞。

当皮层神经发生时，大约在小鼠胚胎第9天（E9）和第10天（E10）左右，神经干细胞开始获得与胶质细胞相关的特征（Kriegstein, Alvarez-Buylla, 2009）。放射状胶质细胞的不对称分裂导致自身的自我更新和神经元或胶质细胞（星形胶质细胞或少突胶质细胞）的诞生，这取决于细胞的分化（Fishell, Kriegstein, 2003）。这些细胞的增殖与分化以及细胞分裂的类型影响神经发生的比率（Gotz, Huttner, 2005）。在E15～E16的大鼠胚胎发生中，一个放射状胶质细胞在每个细胞周期中产生一个神经元和一个放射状胶质细胞（Noctor, Flint, Weissman, Dammerman, Kriegstein, 2001）。因此，NSCs通过自我更新和产生放射状胶质细胞（radial glial cells, RGCs），在发育中的大脑中产生大量分化细胞（包括神经元和胶质细胞）（Seaberg, van der Kooy, 2003; Weiss et al. 1996）。有趣的是，虽然在E14上从小鼠和大鼠的新皮层中分离出RGCs，当皮层神经发生处于高峰期时，主要在体外生成神经元，而当E18上皮层神经发生接近完成时，分离出的RGCs主要产生星形胶质细胞（Malatesta, Hartfuss, Gotz, 2000）。RGCs除了是神经元生成的来源外，还在脑组织发生过程中对其神经元后代的几代起着重要的指导作用，当大脑皮层中的神经元迁移完成时，RGCs会退化或变成星形胶质细胞，并且不再需要放射状胶质纤维作为神经元迁移的指南（Chanas-Sacre, Rogister, Moonen, Leprince, 2000; Mission, Takahashi, Caviness Jr., 1991; Noctor et al. 2001; Rakic, 1972）。

显然，在大脑的发育过程中，神经元不仅由NSCs直接产生，还来源于转运扩增的中间祖细胞RGCs（Kriegstein, Alvarez-Buylla, 2009）。因此，在胚胎和胎儿神经发生过程中，NSCs和RGCs都被认为是神经前体细胞（NPCs）（图6.2）。所有NPCs都可以通过巢蛋白（一种中间丝状蛋白）来识别，而表达巢蛋白的RGCs可以通过胶质纤维酸性蛋白（GFAP）与NSCs进行区分，GFAP也在星形胶质细胞中表达（Noctor et al. 2001）。

NPCs的协调增殖和分化是神经元发育过程中产生适当数量的神经元和胶质细胞以建立正常大脑功能的基础（Resende, Alves, Britto, Ulrich, 2008）。在胚胎和早期产后神经发生过程中，多能干细胞向RGCs的转变伴随着一系列细胞结构和功能的变化，包括放射状胶质细胞的"胶质"特征的出现，以及支持其新分配功能的新信号分子和蛋白质的出现（Kriegstein, Gotz, 2003; Urban, Guillemot, 2014）。作用于胚胎NPCs的多种信号的协调作用产生了大量不同的神经元和胶质细胞，这些细胞开始塑造大脑（Urban, Guillemot, 2014）。在这些信号分子和蛋白质的帮助下，新分化的神经元也会从出生地迁移到最终目的地，形成大脑的主要解剖区域，并在突触的帮助下，通过轴突、树突和棘与其他神经元建立终身功能通信路线。大脑的发育会在出生后持续到幼儿期才能完全完成。此后，除了脑室下区（SVZ）和海马齿状回（DG）内胚胎神经发生的延续之外，完整的大脑在成年期没有机会再生其神经元群。因此，在中枢神经系统的胚胎或产前发育期间，任何异常信号通路引起的神经发生的任何变化都会损害大脑的终生结构和功能。

6.3 NPCs中的烟碱乙酰胆碱受体

在胚胎期或出生后早期中枢神经系统的发育过程中，各种内在因素和细胞外信号通路驱动神经干细胞的增殖和分化（Urban, Guillemot, 2014）。在早期发育过程中，NPCs的增殖和分化需要在CNS形成的不同时间点通过模式化基因激活关键转录因子，这些基因受多种内在信号通路的控制（Kintner, 2002）。一旦胚胎神经发生启动，神经递质信号也会对神经发生的几个方面产生影响，包括增殖、迁移和中枢神经系统不同部位的分化（Berg, Belnoue, Song, Simon, 2013）。

乙酰胆碱（ACh）是参与胚胎和成人神经发生的一种神经递质，它通过烟碱乙酰胆碱受体（nAChR）发挥其功能（Itou et al. 2011）。NPCs中的nAChR的功能亚型在胚胎神经发生和早期脑发育的机制中起重要作用。

　　早在E10，在早期胚胎小鼠大脑皮层的神经前体细胞中就检测到了nAChR的α4和α7亚基的蛋白质，膜片钳电生理测量表明烟碱和乙酰胆碱能引起相当大的内向电流，这是烟碱受体诱发的细胞溶质Ca^{2+}信号的特征（Atluri et al. 2001），而早在E12就在大脑皮层中检测到了β2亚基的信使RNA（mRNA）(Zoli, Le Novere, Hill Jr., Changeux, 1995)。在未分化的巢蛋白阳性但GFAP阴性的NPCs中也检测到了nAChR的其他亚基，这些NPCs在胎儿后期从小鼠或大鼠新皮层中分离出来。从E15.5的新皮层中分离的胚胎小鼠NPCs的逆转录-聚合酶链反应（RT-PCR）分析揭示了nAChRs的α3、α4、α5、α7、α9、β2和β4亚基的mRNA表达，但不表达α2、α6和β3亚基。在同一研究中，检测到从E18胚胎大鼠新皮层制备的祖细胞中nAChR的α2、α3、α4、α5、α7、α9、β2和β4亚基的mRNA表达，而不是α6和β3亚基的mRNA表达（Takarada et al. 2012）。单个亚基的时间和区域表达及其各种组合可以形成神经元nAChRs的不同亚型。动态刺激nAChR的新兴功能亚型可调节NPCs的增殖、神经发生、神经元迁移、神经元成熟和可塑性，以及神经元存活和胶质生成（Abreu-Villaca, Filgueiras, Manhaes, 2011; Asrican, Paez-Gonzalez, Erb, Kuo, 2016）。

6.4　烟碱对产前神经发生的影响

　　nAChR的活性也受到其他外源性化学物质（如烟碱）的调节，并导致胎儿大脑发育的中断（Navarro et al. 1989）。有关烟碱影响的研究几乎一致报道了发育中的大脑神经发生的减少和成年生活中的认知缺陷（Abrous et al. 2002; Cohen et al. 2015; He et al. 2013; Scerri et al. 2006; Wei et al. 2012），这表明烟碱对胎儿大脑最直接的影响是破坏正在进行的神经发生。

　　在体内研究中，通过检测NPCs的增殖和新生细胞的神经元分化来研究神经发生（表6.1）。增殖细胞可以用注射的5-溴-2'-脱氧尿苷（BrdU）进行标记，BrdU是胸腺嘧啶的类似物。免疫组织化学中的抗BrdU抗体可以追踪到含有BrdU的新生细胞，而这些细胞的神经元分化可以通过将BrdU与单个神经元中的神经元标记物标记在一起来识别。从妊娠第3天（G3）到出生（产后第0天，P0），在子宫内通过渗透微型泵接触烟碱，然后通过母乳接触烟碱，直到P21，海马DG中P15的细胞增殖没有明显变化。在同一研究中，在P41检测中，烟碱组和对照组中（P15上）的BrdU标记的新生细胞均分化为海马DG中的神经元，表明神经发生没有改变（Mahar et al. 2012）。与对照后代相比，G7-P0期间通过渗透微型泵接触烟碱不会改变P14海马CA1、CA3或DG中的神经元数量（Wang, Gondre-Lewis, 2013）。G6-P21期间通过饮水暴露烟碱不会改变海马DG亚颗粒区增殖细胞指数，但会短暂抑制P21上大鼠后代NPCs的后期分化，而对P77的抑制作用则不明显（Ohishi et al. 2014）。但这些发现并不能反映烟碱对产前神经发生的直接影响，因为在这些研究中新生细胞并不是在出生前标记的，而是在烟碱的直接刺激作用微弱或不存在的围产期标记或检测的。在这些研究中，PNE缺乏对海马神经生成的影响，也可能是由于在不受烟碱直接影响的测试日，海马活跃的神经发生持续发挥作用。在出生后的早期，海马神经发生仍然很严重（Altman, Bayer, 1990），如果新生细胞在出生前某一特定时间窗内未被标记，这种强烈的神经发生可能会使评估PNE对胎儿神经发生的影响变得困难。此外，PNE后出生的孩子在出生后不久就会出现烟碱戒断现象，并可能改变nAChR的敏感度和功能（Slotkin, 1998）。如果在产后研究PNE对神经发生的影响，这些功能变化可能会使观察产前烟碱对NPCs的影响复杂化，使观察结果不那么有意义。因此，应在产前或出生前研究PNE对NPCs及其后续神经发生的影响，为成年后代的行为功能障碍提供支持性解释。当小鼠G14、G15和G16一系列时间窗期间的增殖细胞被标记为BrdU时，我们发现G14 P0期间的PNE通过抑制心室区和SVZ中的NPCs的增殖而损害神经发生（Aoyama et al. 2016）。这些损伤导致幼鼠P70 P84内侧前额叶皮层的谷氨酸能神经元减少。PNE的抗神经原作用被α7 nAChR拮抗剂甲基牛扁碱柠檬酸盐的预处理阻断，但不能被α4β2 nAChR拮抗剂二氢-β-刺桐定氢溴酸盐阻断（Aoyama et al. 2016）。这些结果表明，α7-nAChR介导的PNE诱导的产前神经前体细胞增殖的减少对于青少年和成年期观察到的后代行为功能障碍至关重要（Alkam, Kim, Mamiya et al. 2013; Alkam, Kim, Hiramatsu et al. 2013; Alkam et al. 2017; Aoyama et al. 2016）。

表6.1 产前烟碱暴露对神经发生的影响

时间曝光和路线	BrdU标记时间	检查时间	大脑区域	对神经发生的影响	参考文献
G3-P0，通过渗透微型泵，直到P21通过母乳	P15	P41	海马体	无变化	Mahar et al.（2012）
G7-P0，通过渗透微型泵	无标签	P14	海马体	神经元数量无变化	Wang, Gondre-Lewis（2013）
G6-P21，通过饮用水	无标签	P21和P77	海马体	暂时抑制P21的晚期神经元分化，但这种抑制在P77上消失	Ohishi et al.（2014）
G14-P0，通过饮用水	G14、G15、G16	P70-P84	内侧前额叶皮层	减少谷氨酸能神经元的数量	Aoyama et al.（2016）

在一项体外研究中，长期接触烟碱12天显著抑制了从E15.5或E18小鼠或大鼠新皮层中分离的未分化NPCs的增殖；NPCs随后分化为神经元（Takarada et al. 2012）。烟碱对增殖和神经元分化的这些影响被nAChR的α4β2亚型、二氢-β-刺桐定氢溴酸盐和4-(5-乙氧基-3-吡啶基)-N-甲基-(3E)-3-丁烯-1-胺的拮抗剂显著阻止，而不是被nAChR甲基牛扁碱柠檬酸盐的α7亚型拮抗剂阻止（Takarada et al. 2012）。虽然nAChR的亚型涉及NPCs的烟碱抑制增殖，但在体内和体外研究中有所不同，但这些发现证实了PNE的抗增殖作用。

6.5 涉及nAChR的相关功能

在神经元发育的关键产前和产后早期，nAChR不同亚型的区域和时间协调表达涉及与神经发生相关的机制。nAChR亚基的表达在大脑发育过程中受到强烈调节，当长期暴露于烟碱时，这些受体可以上调它们的表达（Abreu-Villaca et al. 2011）。α7亚型和α4β2亚型都是在与认知功能有关的大脑区域中发现的最丰富的nAChR类别（Corradi, Bouzat, 2016; Mazzaferro, Bermudez, Sine, 2017; Pandya, Yakel, 2011）。虽然nAChR的α4β2亚型在暴露于烟碱时强烈上调并显示出高亲和力的烟碱结合位点，但某些nAChR亚型甚至可能下调（Albuquerque, Pereira, Alkondon, Rogers, 2009）。已提出相对亚基关联和最终受体组装的差异来解释这些明显矛盾的结果（Albuquerque et al. 2009）。

来自不同亚基的nAChR组装的多样性导致了nAChR的功能差异，例如Ca^{2+}、Na^+和K^+离子渗透性和脱敏作用（Albuquerque et al. 2009）。已知由α7亚基组成的受体会迅速脱敏，并具有高于谷氨酸 N- 甲基 -D- 天冬氨酸受体（NMDAR）和大多数其他 nAChR 的高 Ca^{2+} 渗透率（Albuquerque et al. 2009）。在烟碱刺激 nAChR 后，细胞外 Ca^{2+} 进入细胞并诱导 Ca^{2+} 从细胞内储存中释放。钙信号在塑造 nAChR 介导的效应中至关重要（Abreu-Villaca et al. 2011）。众所周知，钙信号调节细胞周期的许多基本步骤，包括细胞周期各个阶段之间的转变、即刻早期基因的转录以及控制增殖、神经元分化和迁移的调节事件（Toth, Shum, Prakriya, 2016）。长期暴露于烟碱会显著抑制 NMDAR 亚基 1 缺陷的未分化 NPCs 的增殖，这表明 nAChR 的激活可能会通过独立于未分化 NPCs 中 NMDAR 信号的 Ca^{2+} 信号机制导致自我复制的负调节（Takarada et al. 2012）。有趣的是，从发育中的大鼠新皮层中分离的 NPCs 中 NMDAR 的激活会抑制增殖并导致随后的神经元谱系分化（Nakamichi, Takarada, Yoneda, 2009; Yoneyama et al. 2008）。

这些发现表明，钙信号可能介导了产前暴露的烟碱对 NPCs 的影响（图 6.3），而神经发生也可能受到发育中的大脑中其他信号输入的协调控制。

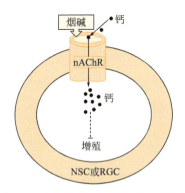

图 6.3　产前烟碱暴露对神经发生的影响

产前烟碱暴露通过增加 nAChR 钙内流抑制 NSC 和 RGC 的增殖。在胚胎和胎儿神经发生过程中，NSC 和 RGC 都是神经前体细胞。NSC，神经干细胞；RGC，放射状胶质细胞。

6.6　未来的发展方向

目前关于 PNE 对 NPCs 增殖和分化的抑制作用的文献表明，在啮齿动物大脑发育过程中，nAChR 的 α7 和 α4β2 亚型通过 Ca^{2+} 信号传导机制参与其中。然而，为个体 nAChR 亚型开发条件敲除和敲入模型动物将至关重要地有助于确定这些和其他 nAChR 亚型是如何参与调节 PNE 对发育中大脑神经发生的抑制作用的。

术语解释
- 细胞增殖：通过细胞分裂增加细胞数量的过程。
- 细胞分化：在中枢神经系统的发育过程中，中间祖细胞变成神经元、星形胶质细胞或少突胶质细胞的过程。
- 细胞自我更新：一个干细胞自身分裂成两个干细胞的过程，两个干细胞中至少有一个与原始干细胞具有相同的特性。
- 神经发生：胚胎和出生后早期大脑中由神经干细胞或神经前体细胞产生新神经元的过程。

产前接触烟草的关键事实

- 怀孕期间吸烟会破坏胎儿大脑的正常发育，并影响其一生中大脑的最佳功能。
- 产前被动吸烟也会破坏胎儿大脑的正常发育。
- 已在哺乳动物中鉴定出16个烟碱乙酰胆碱受体亚基。
- 哺乳动物的神经烟碱乙酰胆碱受体有11个亚基，可以调节大脑中的情绪、成瘾和认知相关的神经传递信号通路。
- 世界上80%以上的吸烟者生活在低收入和中等收入国家。除土耳其外，这些国家的孕妇烟草使用率较低。
- 基于人口的研究显示，美国和英国等高收入国家的孕妇吸烟率较高，而日本的孕妇吸烟率有所下降。
- 使用烟碱替代疗法在怀孕期间戒烟是有争议的，并不比安慰剂治疗更好。

要点总结

- 大脑发育期间暴露在烟草烟雾中与后来出现的认知问题有关。
- 在发育中的大脑中，神经前体细胞包括神经干细胞和放射状胶质细胞。
- 神经前体细胞表达烟碱乙酰胆碱受体。
- 产前暴露于烟碱（烟草的一种成分）通过抑制神经前体细胞的增殖而损害神经发生。
- 产前烟碱暴露对神经前体细胞增殖的抑制可能是通过烟碱乙酰胆碱受体的钙信号介导的。

参考文献

Aaku-Saraste, E.; Oback, B.; Hellwig, A.; Huttner, W. B. (1997). Neu-roepithelial cells downregulate their plasma membrane polarityprior to neural tube closure and neurogenesis. Mechanisms of Devel-opment, 69(1-2), 71-81.

Abreu-Villaca, Y.; Filgueiras, C. C.; Manhaes, A. C. (2011). Develop-mental aspects of the cholinergic system. Behavioural Brain Research, 221(2), 367-378.

Abrous, D. N.; Adriani, W.; Montaron, M. F.; Aurousseau, C.; Rougon, G.; Le Moal, M. et al. (2002). Nicotine self-administrationimpairs hippocampal plasticity. The Journal of Neuroscience, 22(9), 3656-3662.

Albuquerque, E. X.; Pereira, E. F.; Alkondon, M.; Rogers, S. W. (2009).Mammalian nicotinic acetylcholine receptors: from structure to func-tion. Physiological Reviews, 89(1), 73-120.

Alkam, T.; Kim, H. C.; Hiramatsu, M.; Mamiya, T.; Aoyama, Y.; Nitta, A. et al. (2013). Evaluation of emotional behaviors in young offspring of C57BL/6J mice after gestational and/or perinatal expo-sure to nicotine in six different time-windows. Behavioural Brain Research, 239, 80-89.

Alkam, T.; Kim, H. C.; Mamiya, T.; Yamada, K.; Hiramatsu, M.; Nabeshima, T. (2013). Evaluation of cognitive behaviors in young offspring of C57BL/6J mice after gestational nicotine exposureduring different time-windows.Psychopharmacology, 230(3), 451-463.

Alkam, T.; Mamiya, T.; Kimura, N.; Yoshida, A.; Kihara, D.; Tsunoda, Y.; et al. (2017). Prenatal nicotine exposure decreases the release of dopa-mine in the medial frontal cortex and induces atomoxetine responsive neurobehavioral deficits in mice. Psychopharmacology, 234(12), 1853-1869.

Altman, J.; Bayer, S. A. (1990). Migration and distribution of twopopulations of hippocampal granule cell precursors during the peri-natal and postnatal periods. The Journal of Comparative Neurology, 301(3), 365-381.

Aoyama, Y.; Toriumi, K.; Mouri, A.; Hattori, T.; Ueda, E.; Shimato, A.; et al. (2016). Prenatal nicotine exposure impairs the proliferation of neuronal progenitors, leading to fewer glutamatergic neuronsin the medial prefrontal cortex. Neuropsychopharmacology, 41(2), 578-589.

Asrican, B.; Paez-Gonzalez, P.; Erb, J.; Kuo, C. T. (2016). Cholinergiccircuit control of postnatal neurogenesis. Neurogenesis (Austin), 3(1).

Atluri, P.; Fleck, M. W.; Shen, Q.; Mah, S. J.; Stadfelt, D.; Barnes, W.; et al. (2001). Functional nicotinic acetylcholine receptor expression in stem and progenitor cells of the early embryonic mouse cerebralcortex. Developmental Biology, 240(1), 143-156.

Berg, D. A.; Belnoue, L.; Song, H.; Simon, A. (2013). Neurotransmitter-mediated control of neurogenesis in the adult vertebrate brain.Development, 140(12), 2548-2561.

Berner, J.; Ringstedt, T.; Brodin, E.; Hokfelt, T.; Lagercrantz, H.; Wickstrom, R. (2008). Prenatal exposure to nicotine affects substancep and preprotachykinin-A mRNA levels in newborn rat. PediatricResearch, 64(6), 621-624.

Blood-Siegfried, J.; Rende, E. K. (2010). The long-term effects of pre-natal nicotine exposure on neurologic development. Journal of Mid-wifery, Women's Health, 55(2), 143-152.

Britton, A. F.; Vann, R. E.; Robinson, S. E. (2007). Perinatal nicotineexposure eliminates peak in nicotinic acetylcholine receptor response in adolescent rats. The Journal of Pharmacology and Experi-mental Therapeutics, 320(2), 871-876.

Chanas-Sacre, G.; Rogister, B.; Moonen, G.; Leprince, P. (2000). Radialglia phenotype: origin, regulation, and transdifferentiation.Journal of Neuroscience Research, 61(4), 357-363.

Cohen, A.; Soleiman, M. T.; Talia, R.; Koob, G. F.; George, O.; Mandyam, C. D. (2015). Extended access nicotine self-administration with periodic deprivation increases immature neurons in the hippo-campus. Psychopharmacology, 232(2), 453-463.

Corradi, J.; Bouzat, C. (2016). Understanding the bases of function andmodulation of alpha7 nicotinic receptors: implications for drug dis-covery. Molecular Pharmacology, 90(3), 288-299.

Dempsey, D. A.; Benowitz, N. L. (2001). Risks and benefits of nicotineto aid smoking cessation in pregnancy. Drug Safety, 24(4), 277-322.

Dwyer, J. B.; Broide, R. S.; Leslie, F. M. (2008). Nicotine and brain development. Birth Defects Research. Part C, Embryo Today, 84(1), 30-44.

Ernst, M.; Moolchan, E. T.; Robinson, M. L. (2001). Behavioral and neural consequences of prenatal exposure to nicotine. Journal of the American Academy of Child and Adolescent Psychiatry, 40(6), 630-641.

Fishell, G.; Kriegstein, A. R. (2003). Neurons from radial glia: the con-sequences of asymmetric inheritance. Current Opinion in Neurobiol-ogy, 13(1), 34-41.

Gold, A. B.; Keller, A. B.; Perry, D. C. (2009). Prenatal exposure of rats to nicotine causes persistent alterations of nicotinic cholinergic recep-tors. Brain Research, 1250, 8 8-100.

Gotz, M.; Huttner, W. B. (2005). The cell biology of neurogenesis.Nature Reviews: Molecular Cell Biology, 6(10), 777-788.

Hall, B. J.; Cauley, M.; Burke, D. A.; Kiany, A.; Slotkin, T. A.; Levin, E. D. (2016). Cognitive and behavioral impairments evoked by low-level exposure to tobacco smoke components: comparison with nic-otine alone. Toxicological Sciences, 151(2), 236-244.

Hamosh, M.; Simon, M. R.; Hamosh, P. (1979). Effect of nicotine on thedevelopment of fetal and suckling rats.Biology of the Neonate, 35(5-6), 290-297.

He, N.; Wang, Z.; Wang, Y.; Shen, H.; Yin, M. (2013). ZY-1, a novelnicotinic analog, promotes proliferation and migration of adult hip-pocampal neural stem/progenitor cells. Cellular and Molecular Neu-robiology, 33(8), 1149-1157.

Huang, L. Z.; Liu, X.; Griffith, W. H.; Winzer-Serhan, U. H. (2007).Chronic neonatal nicotine increases anxiety but does not impair cog-nition in adult rats. Behavioral Neuroscience, 121(6), 1342-1352.

Itou, Y.; Nochi, R.; Kuribayashi, H.; Saito, Y.; Hisatsune, T. (2011).Cholinergic activation of hippocampal neural stem cells in aged den-tate gyrus. Hippocampus, 21(4), 446-459.

Kintner, C. (2002). Neurogenesis in embryos and in adult neural stemcells. The Journal of Neuroscience, 22(3), 639-643.

Kriegstein, A.; Alvarez-Buylla, A. (2009). The glial nature of embry-onic and adult neural stem cells. Annual Review of Neuroscience, 32, 149-184.

Kriegstein, A. R.; Gotz, M. (2003). Radial glia diversity: a matter of cellfate. Glia, 43(1), 37-43.

Mahar, I.; Bagot, R. C.; Davoli, M. A.; Miksys, S.; Tyndale, R. F.; Walker, C. D. et al. (2012). Developmental hippocampal neuroplas-ticity in a model of nicotine replacement therapy during pregnancyand breastfeeding. PLoS ONE, 7(5), e37219.

Malatesta, P.; Hartfuss, E.; Gotz, M. (2000). Isolation of radial glialcells by fluorescent-activated cell sorting reveals a neuronal lineage.Development, 127(24), 5253-5263.

Matta, S. G.; Balfour, D. J.; Benowitz, N. L.; Boyd, R. T.; Buccafusco, J. J.; Caggiula, A. R. et al. (2007). Guidelines on nicotine dose selection forin vivo research. Psychopharmacology, 190(3), 269-319.

Mazzaferro, S.; Bermudez, I.; Sine, S. M. (2017). Alpha4beta2 nicotinicacetylcholine receptors: relationships between subunit stoichiometry and function at the single channel level.The Journal of Biological Chem-istry, 292(7), 2729-2740.

Mission, J. P.; Takahashi, T.; Caviness, V. S.; Jr. (1991). Ontogenyof radial and other astroglial cells in murine cerebral cortex. Glia, 4(2), 138-148.

Nakamichi, N.; Takarada, T.; Yoneda, Y. (2009). Neurogenesis medi-ated by gamma-aminobutyric acid and glutamate signaling. Journalof Pharmacological Sciences, 110(2), 133-149.

Navarro, H. A.; Seidler, F. J.; Eylers, J. P.; Baker, F. E.; Dobbins, S. S.; Lappi, S. E. et al. (1989). Effects of prenatal nicotine exposure on development of central and peripheral cholinergic neurotransmitter systems. Evidence for cholinergic trophic influences in developingbrain. The Journal of Pharmacology and Experimental Therapeutics, 251(3), 894-900.

Noctor, S. C.; Flint, A. C.; Weissman, T. A.; Dammerman, R. S.; Kriegstein, A. R. (2001). Neurons derived from radial glial cells estab-lish radial units in neocortex. Nature, 409(6821), 714-720.

Ohishi, T.; Wang, L.; Akane, H.; Shiraki, A.; Itahashi, M.; Mitsumori, K.; et al. (2014). Transient suppression of late-stage neuronal progenitorcell differentiation in the hippocampal dentate gyrus of rat offspringafter maternal exposure to nicotine. Archives of Toxicology, 88(2), 443-454.

Oliff, H. S.; Gallardo, K. A. (1999). The effect of nicotine on developingbrain catecholamine systems. Frontiers in Bioscience, 4, D883-D897.

Pandya, A.; Yakel, J. L. (2011). Allosteric modulators of the alpha4-beta2 subtype of neuronal nicotinic acetylcholine receptors. Biochem-ical Pharmacology, 82(8), 952-958.

Potten, C. S.; Loeffler, M. (1990). Stem cells: attributes, cycles, spirals, pitfalls and uncertainties. Lessons for and from the crypt.Development, 110(4), 1001-1020.

Rakic, P. (1972). Mode of cell migration to the superficial layers of fetalmonkey neocortex. The Journal of Comparative Neurology, 145(1), 61-83.

Resende, R. R.; Alves, A. S.; Britto, L. R.; Ulrich, H. (2008). Role of ace-tylcholine receptors in proliferation and differentiation of P19embryonal carcinoma cells. Experimental Cell Research, 314(7), 1429-1443.

Scerri, C.; Stewart, C. A.; Breen, K. C.; Balfour, D. J. (2006). The effectsof chronic nicotine on spatial learning and bromodeoxyuridineincorporation into the dentate gyrus of the rat. Psychopharmacology, 184(3-4), 540-546.

Seaberg, R. M.; van der Kooy, D. (2003). Stem and progenitor cells: thepremature desertion of rigorous definitions. Trends in Neurosciences, 26(3), 125-131.

Slotkin, T. A. (1998). Fetal nicotine or cocaine exposure: which one isworse? The Journal of Pharmacology and Experimental Therapeutics, 285(3), 931-945.

Slotkin, T. A.; MacKillop, E. A.; Rudder, C. L.; Ryde, I. T.; Tate, C. A.; Seidler, F. J. (2007). Permanent, sex-selective effects of prenatal oradolescent nicotine exposure, separately or sequentially, in rat brainregions: indices of cholinergic and serotonergic synaptic function, cell signaling, and neural cell number and size at 6 months of age.Neuropsychopharmacology, 32(5), 1082-1097.

Slotkin, T. A.; Seidler, F. J.; Qiao, D.; Aldridge, J. E.; Tate, C. A.; Cousins, M. M. et al. (2005). Effects of prenatal nicotine exposureon primate brain development and attempted amelioration withsupplemental choline or vitamin C: neurotransmitter receptors, cell signaling and cell development biomarkers in fetal brain regions of rhesus monkeys. Neuropsychopharmacology, 30(1), 129-144.

Takarada, T.; Nakamichi, N.; Kitajima, S.; Fukumori, R.; Nakazato, R.; Le, N. Q. et al. (2012). Promoted neuronal differentiation after acti-vation of alpha4/beta2 nicotinic acetylcholine receptors in undiffer-entiated neural progenitors. PLoS ONE, 7(10), e46177.

Toth, A. B.; Shum, A. K.; Prakriya, M. (2016). Regulation of neurogen-esis by calcium signaling. Cell Calcium, 59(2-3), 124-134.

Urban, N.; Guillemot, F. (2014). Neurogenesis in the embryonic andadult brain: same regulators, different roles. Frontiers in Cellular Neu-roscience, 8, 396.

Vaglenova, J.; Birru, S.; Pandiella, N. M.; Breese, C. R. (2004). Anassessment of the long-term developmental and behavioral teratoge-nicity of prenatal nicotine exposure. Behavioural Brain Research, 150(1-2), 159-170.

Vaglenova, J.; Parameshwaran, K.; Suppiramaniam, V.; Breese, C. R.; Pandiella, N.; Birru, S. (2008). Long-lasting teratogenic effects of nicotine on cognition: gender specificity and role of AMPA receptor function. Neurobiology of Learning and Memory, 90(3), 527-536.

Wang, H.; Gondre-Lewis, M. C. (2013). Prenatal nicotine and maternaldeprivation stress de-regulate the development of CA1, CA3, anddentate gyrus neurons in hippocampus of infant rats. PLoS ONE, 8(6), e65517.

Wei, Z.; Belal, C.; Tu, W.; Chigurupati, S.; Ameli, N. J.; Lu, Y.; et al. (2012). Chronic nicotine administration impairs activation of cyclic AMP-response element binding protein and survival of new-born cells in the dentate gyrus. Stem Cells and Development, 21(3), 411-422.

Weiss, S.; Reynolds, B. A.; Vescovi, A. L.; Morshead, C.; Craig, C. G.; van der Kooy, D. (1996). Is there a neural stem cell in the mammalianforebrain? Trends in Neurosciences, 19(9), 387-393.

Yoneyama, M.; Nakamichi, N.; Fukui, M.; Kitayama, T.; Georgiev, D.D.; Makanga, J. O. et al. (2008). Promotion of neuronal differ-entiation through activation of N-methyl-D-aspartate receptorstransiently expressed by undifferentiated neural progenitor cells in fetal rat neocortex. Journal of Neuroscience Research, 86(11), 2392-2402.

Zhu, J.; Lee, K. P.; Spencer, T. J.; Biederman, J.; Bhide, P. G. (2014).Transgenerational transmission of hyperactivity in a mouse modelof ADHD. The Journal of Neuroscience, 34(8), 2768-2773.

Zhu, J.; Zhang, X.; Xu, Y.; Spencer, T. J.; Biederman, J.; Bhide, P. G. (2012). Prenatal nicotine exposure mouse model showing hyperactivity, reduced cingulate cortex volume, reduced dopamine turnover, andresponsiveness to oral methylphenidate treatment. The Journal ofNeuroscience, 32(27), 9410-9418.

Zoli, M.; Le Novere, N.; Hill, J. A.; Jr.; Changeux, J. P. (1995).Developmental regulation of nicotinic ACh receptor subunitmRNAs in the rat central and peripheral nervous systems. The Journal of Neuroscience, 15(3 Pt 1), 1912-1939.

7
烟碱依赖性神经元中突触定位的烟碱乙酰胆碱受体亚基

Kristi A. Kohlmeier

Department of Drug Design and Pharmacology, Faculty of Health and Medical Sciences,
University of Copenhagen, Copenhagen, Denmark

7.1 引言

烟碱不会在哺乳动物体内自然产生。然而，对烟碱强烈激活内源性信号递质乙酰胆碱（ACh）受体之一的能力的认识导致将该ACh受体命名为烟碱乙酰胆碱受体（nAChR）。烟碱被认为是哺乳动物nAChR的原型激动剂，事实上，与烟碱天然激动剂ACh相比，烟碱在某些方面能更有效地激活该受体（Whiteaker, Sharples, Wonnacott, 1998）。nAChR遍布人体各处，虽然被内源性乙酰胆碱酯酶激活，但它们也可以通过传统的可燃香烟和电子烟的蒸气以及戒断辅助剂（例如透皮烟碱贴片和含烟碱的口香糖）激活。烟碱的精神药理作用是由于大脑中nAChR的激活，因此，检查nAChR如何在中枢神经系统内的突触中发挥作用与考虑含烟碱产品引起的神经生物学效应有关，除了在认知增强和唤醒增加的潜在积极作用的基础上，也诱发产生心理依赖的消极作用。

7.2 nAChR的结构和结合

位于突触位置的nAChR是五聚体、配体门控的膜结合蛋白结构，在N-端结构域包含一个胞外二硫键，可产生其他"cysloop"配体门控受体的半胱氨酸环特征，例如与nAChR相关的可渗透氯的GABAA受体和甘氨酸受体。nAChR可以形成同型或异型五聚体结构，五个亚基形成一个中央离子可渗透孔（Albuquerque, Pereira, Alkondon, Rogers, 2009）。迄今为止，已鉴定了nAChR的16个同源哺乳动物亚基，它们被指定为α或β：α2～α10和β2～β10（图7.1）。五个亚基与由两个或三个α亚基和两个或三个β亚基组成的异聚受体共组装，形成对激动剂具有高亲和力的受体复合物。低亲和力受体通常是同源的，最常见的是五个α7亚基。存在α8和α9亚基的同源nAChR；然而，这些亚基也可以参与异聚体。有趣的是，虽然长期以来α7亚基被认为仅作为人脑内同源结构的一部分存在，但最近的数据表明，α7亚基也可以与功能性nAChR簇中的其他亚基一起表达（Moretti et al. 2014）。与β亚基的共表达显然是含有α2～α6的nAChR功能的必要条件，与α9亚基的结合是含有α10亚基的nAChR活性的先决条件（Elgoyhen et al. 2001）。

正构配体（包括乙酰胆碱和外源应用的烟碱）的结合位点位于亚基之间的界面，根据亚基的化学计量数，还确定了多个变构结合位点（图7.2）。在与激动剂结合后，nAChR会发生一种

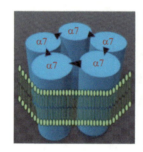

图7.1 神经元烟碱受体

神经元烟碱受体是由决定受体亲和力的亚基组成的同型和异型五聚体受体家族。

改变,使钠离子和钾离子传导,这种改变可以通过与试剂在变构位点结合而改变(Albuquerque et al. 2009)。钙的渗透性可以通过包含在亚基的五聚体结构中而被赋予,这允许通过沿着孔隙的带电残基和位于孔隙外部区域的极性残基来通过阳离子,例如存在于含有α9的nAChR异构体中(Dani, 1986)。一般而言,nAChR被认为会迅速脱敏,长期接触烟碱可能导致nAChR显著脱敏,使其关闭并处于无反应状态(Dani, Radcliffe, Pidoplichko, 2000)。

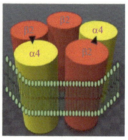

图7.2 神经元烟碱受体(nAChR)的结构

乙酰胆碱的结合位点位于亚基界面(黑色箭头),亚基的组成决定了离子的渗透性。

然而,这个不应期发病率和恢复率的速度高度依赖于亚基组成(McGehee, Role, 1995)。此外,多个时间常数似乎与脱敏的寿命有关。对烟碱的依赖的特点是血液中的药物水平恒定,而习惯性使用者造成的持续暴露很可能将nAChR的脱敏动力学转变为长寿命状态(Dani, Heinemann, 1996)。因此,除了赋予离子渗透性外,亚基群还定义了激动剂和调节剂结合的药代动力学特性,并且烟碱暴露的动态时间模式赋予了动力学特征的进一步复杂性。

尽管表达系统暗示了过多的亚基组合,但在天然系统中,只有少数亚基群已被明确确定,高亲和力α4β2和低亲和力同源α7被认为是最丰富的,毫无疑问,也是最好的表征。α4β2与α7的区别在于其对低水平激动剂的脱敏速度更快,其动力学相对较慢,两者的药理学敏感性不同。在含有α和β的nAChR中,亚基相对于彼此的定位会导致对ACh的敏感性不同,其中(α4)2(β2)3(或Ⅰ型)星座对ACh表现出高亲和力,而(α4)3(β2)2(或Ⅱ型)关系导致对天然存在的激动剂的亲和力较低(Miwa, Freedman, Lester, 2011; Moroni, Bermudez, 2006)。其他调节因素包括钙、蛋白激酶以及细胞内和细胞外多肽也可以改变nAChR的动力学功能(Miwa et al. 2011; Parri, Dineley, 2010)。

一个非常有趣的特征是,长期暴露于激动剂会导致突触定位的、膜结合的α4β2受体的数量上调,这是其他半胱氨酸环受体没有表现出来的现象(Fenster, Whitworth, Sheffield, Quick, Lester,

1999）。研究发现，对含烟碱产品的长期暴露提高了人脑中高亲和力标记的烟碱结合位点；然而，这一发现背后的机制尚不清楚（Marks, Burch, Collins, 1983）。后来的研究表明在孤立系统中脱敏和上调之间存在关系（Fenster et al.1999）。这项研究的含义是，长期暴露在烟碱激动剂的环境中，比如经常使用烟碱产品的经历，很可能会导致大脑突触的nAChR增加，这些突触可能在成瘾、耐受和戒断的过程中发挥作用（Fenster et al. 1999）。

7.3 位置

7.3.1 突触前

在人类大脑中，nAChRs在突触前位点表现出很强的存在性（图7.3），在突触前位点，它们可以通过突触前膜释放乙酰胆碱或在突触外位点释放乙酰胆碱而被内源性激活，在突触外位点，乙酰胆碱的较慢的作用量传递或溢出可能发挥作用（Bennett, Arroyo, Berns, Hestrin, 2012）。然而，这种效应在由乙酰胆碱控制的过程中的生物学意义可能不像物理介导的快速突触信号那样相关（Sarter, Parikh, Howe, 2009）。无论乙酰胆碱的作用如何，外源使用烟碱都可能激活突触前神经元，无论是突触前膜内还是突触外，都可能导致细胞兴奋性的改变。如果突触前nAChR能渗透钙离子，那么该离子末端的增加可能会导致特征神经递质的释放（Alkondon, Pereira, Eisenberg, Albuquerque, 1999）。即使在nAChR孔没有钙通透性的情况下，也可以产生递质的增加，因为预计nAChR的激活将导致末端去极化，这将间接导致电压门控钙通道的激活，从而导致神经递质的释放。这些突触前nAChR所在的神经元的表型决定了它们的激活是否会导致兴奋性调节剂或递质（如谷氨酸）或抑制性递质（如GABA）释放到突触后细胞上。通过这种方式，尽管激动剂与突触前nAChR结合后的细胞作用几乎完全是兴奋的，但事实上，如果位于抑制细胞上，它们的激活可能会通过对突触后细胞的下游抑制作用导致网络的净抑制。

7.3.2 突触后

虽然最常被认为位于突触前，但许多研究已经确定了位于突触后膜上的nAChR（图7.3）。除了它们在树突和轴突上的存在之外，钙可渗透的α7同源受体还定位在胞体上，在那里它们介导钙依赖性事件，包括细胞内信使的激活，这可能导致基因表达的刺激，从而在突触可塑性中发挥

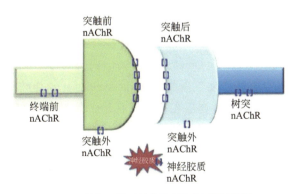

图7.3 神经元烟碱受体位于几个不同的位置

nAChR可以在神经元突触前、突触后和突触外的位置发现。

作用（Lagostena, Trocme-Thibierge, Morain, Cherubini, 2008）。与其他一些nAChR亚基群相比，含同源α7的受体表现出快速的脱敏速度和较低的乙酰胆碱的亲和力。然而，认识到这种nAChR亚基群与膜运输事件的耦合导致了这种受体的出现，尽管该受体迅速脱敏，但可能在比以前认为的更长的时间线上参与细胞事件（Liu, Tearle, Nai, Berg, 2005），并且阐明该受体与其他细胞内运输蛋白之间的关联可以暗示突触后细胞的其他功能。在突触后也发现了nAChR的α4β2亚基群。然而，高亲和力和低亲和力的配置似乎在细胞上表现出不同的解剖定位。低亲和力受体（Ⅰ型）主要存在于轴突上，高亲和力受体（Ⅱ型）存在于树突和胞体上（Alkondon et al. 1999）。

7.4 中脑边缘通路中的nAChR

尽管nAChR在整个大脑的突触前和突触后被发现，但它们在中脑边缘通路中的位置被认为在烟碱的依赖性诱导特性中起着重要作用。中脑边缘回路由含有多巴胺（DA）的投影组成，从腹侧被盖区（VTA）到伏隔核（NAcc）。nAc向前额叶皮层（PFC）发送兴奋性投射。VTA-nAc-PFC通路中的活动已被证明与涉及动机选择和情绪的决策有关。虽然涉及整个大脑的多个回路（Koob, Volkow, 2016），但由于年龄、遗传或外部行为引起的中脑边缘通路功能的功能障碍或改变与多种基于心理和认知的障碍有关，包括药物-寻求行为（Volkow, Koob, McLellan, 2016）。

尽管滥用药物的作用机制多种多样，但大多数依赖诱导药物的一个共同特征是能够刺激NAcc壳内DA的大阶段性上升，NAcc接收从VTA投射的含DA的传入（Grace, 1991; Schultz, 2007a, 2007b; Zhang et al. 2009）。DA VTA细胞的基础放电导致强直DA释放；然而，由这种阶段性放电介导的DA的大幅上升会激励刺激，并且DA的阶段性上升被认为参与了药物依赖性基础过程的启动（Grace, 1991）。烟碱已被证明可以通过各种由nAChR作用引起的突触前和突触后介导机制刺激中脑边缘通路中DA的增加。吸烟会导致大脑中烟碱水平升高至100nmol/L（Henningfield, Stapleton, Benowitz, Grayson, London, 1993），该浓度足以激活并导致nAChR的显著脱敏（Mansvelder, Keath, McGehee, 2002; Mansvelder, McGehee, 2002）。

VTA内nAChR亚基mRNA的定量分析表明，在多种VTA细胞类型中存在高水平的α4、α6、α7、β2和β3转录物，包括该细胞核中存在的DA和GABA细胞（Champtiaux et al. 2002; Klink, de Kerchove d'Exaerde, Zoli, Changeux, 2001; Wooltorton, Pidoplichko, Broide, Dani, 2003）。因此，预计烟碱会以动力学上不同的nAChR亚型激发VTA细胞（Dani et al. 2000; Fisher, Pidoplichko, Dani, 1998; Klink et al. 2001; Pidoplichko, DeBiasi, Williams, Dani, 1997; Wooltorton et al. 2003）。在VTA中，高亲和力α4β2 nAChRs存在于含有DA和GABA的神经元的突触后。VTA内的GABA能神经元已显示向DA VTA细胞发送投射（Omelchenko, Sesack, 2009）。作用于DA和GABA能VTA神经元上的nAChR的烟碱会直接激发这些细胞（Mansvelder et al. 2002; Mansvelder, McGehee, 2000）。含有α7的nAChR存在于源自皮层和皮层下区域的突触前谷氨酸能末端(Omelchenko, Sesack, 2007)，烟碱对它的激发会导致兴奋性传导增强，直接传递到突触后VTA细胞 (Dani et al. 2000; Mansvelder et al. 2002; Mansvelder, McGehee, 2000）。突触后α4β2 nAChR的激活将导致阳离子流动，与作用于突触后NMDA和AMPA受体的谷氨酸能增强相结合，将诱导细胞去极化，足以引发动作电位，这被认为是NAcc壳内DA阶段性上升的基础（Zhang et al. 2009）。有趣的是，同时减少强直DA释放将确保增强从DA传入到伏隔核外壳的信噪比（Zhang et al. 2009）。

GABA能nAChR的激发不仅来自烟碱暴露，还来自内源性ACh传入（Mansvelder, McGehee, 2000）。然而，α4β2 nAChR对GABA能VTA细胞的脱敏被认为会导致针对DA VTA细胞的抑制驱动减少（Dani, 2015; Mansvelder, McGehee, 2002）。已经提供了质疑这种被广泛接受的模型的证据，这表明行为相关的DA细胞功能也可能需要GABA能nAChR的协调活动（Tolu et al. 2013）。尽管α4β2可迅速脱敏，但由于长期突触增强（LTP）的发展，DA VTA细胞的兴奋持续存在，这表明烟碱暴露可在DA VTA细胞的突触内诱发（Mansvelder, McGehee, 2000）。除了需要含有功能性α7的受体外，烟碱诱导DA VTA细胞LTP的机制部分取决于突触后去极化和随后突触后NMDA受体镁阻滞的去除。

　　除了含有α4β2和α7的nAChR外，α6亚基已被证明在持久性DA VTA细胞兴奋性的细胞机制中发挥作用；然而，该亚基对烟碱反应的必要性受到了质疑。这些亚基已被证明是在投射到NAcc壳的DA神经元上突触后表达的，它们的激活是持久的，并且由低浓度的烟碱产生（Zhao-Shea et al. 2011），数据表明α6亚基包含在α4β2复合物中（Grady, Wageman, Patzlaff, Marks, 2012; Zhao-Shea et al. 2011）。迄今为止，这种复合物对烟碱的敏感性是所有已鉴定的天然nAChR中最高的（Grady et al. 2007; Salminen et al. 2007），被认为在面对脱敏和摄入药物后烟碱浓度降低的情况下，对DA VTA神经元的持续兴奋性起着重要作用（Gotti et al. 2010; Zhao-Shea et al. 2011）。然而，复合物中的α4或α6亚基是否对烟碱诱导的DA VTA细胞放电增强至关重要仍然是一个有争议的问题（Exley et al. 2011）。α6亚基还显示参与增强AMPA受体功能和改变DA VTA细胞上的AMPA/NMDA比率，表明其在LTP诱导中起作用（Berry, Engle, McIntosh, Drenan, 2015; Engle, McIntosh, Drenan, 2015; Engle, Shih, McIntosh, Drenan, 2013）。综上所述，这些研究表明，α6亚基可能在中脑边缘通路内nAChR介导的细胞激活中发挥作用；然而，对该作用背后的确切机制的阐明仍然存在。

7.5　内源性ACh和nAChR

　　尽管DA VTA神经元上的nAChR对外源性烟碱的应用反应良好，但它们会被ACh自然激活（Mameli-Engvall et al. 2006），并且这种内源性ACh在自然动机行为中起着重要作用（Forster, Blaha, 2000; Forster, Falcon, Miller, Heruc, Blaha, 2002; Jerlhag, Janson, Waters, Engel, 2012; Lammel et al. 2012; Schmidt, Famous, Pierce, 2009; Shinohara, Kihara, Ide, Minami, Kaneda, 2014; Steidl, Veverka, 2015）。一种模型假设乙酰胆碱的内源性作用在某些方面被烟碱篡夺，因为烟碱的持续存在导致乙酰胆碱作用的nAChR脱敏，从而减少正常胆碱能信号的影响（Dani, Kosten, Benowitz, 2014）。然而，药物刺激的乙酰胆碱升高也可能在激励药物刺激方面发挥作用，导致继续使用。来自VTA中间神经元的局部ACh输入源，如果受到刺激，会导致DA VTA细胞的兴奋，足以在伏隔核（NAcc）中释放DA，并且烟碱很可能会激活这些细胞上的nAChR（Cachope et al. 2012）。VTA的胆碱能输入还来自两个脑桥核的含ACh的投射：背外侧被盖（LDT）和脚桥被盖（Omelchenko, Sesack, 2005, 2006）（图7.4）。来自LDT的大部分VTA胆碱能输入形成解剖学定义的兴奋性突触，这些突触优先存在于投射到NAcc的DA VTA细胞上（Omelchenko, Sesack, 2005, 2006）。有趣的是，已经发现这种投射的完整性对于阶段性爆发背后的DA神经元的放电模式至关重要，而这种放电模式被认为是NAcc中与行为相关的、大量DA外流所必需的（Chen,

Lodge, 2013; Grace, 1991; Grace, Floresco, Goto, Lodge, 2007; Lodge, Grace, 2006; Maskos, 2008）。谷氨酸投射也从LDT发送到VTA（Omelchenko, Sesack, 2007），这种兴奋性神经递质可能参与将DA VTA细胞的强直放电转换为爆发放电（Lammel et al. 2012）。综合来看，最近的研究坚定地将LDT作为DA VTA细胞和行为功能的重要调节器（Chen, Lodge, 2013; Forster et al. 2002; Forster, Blaha, 2000; Lammel et al. 2012; Steidl, Veverka, 2015; Xiao et al. 2016）。

烟碱可通过作用于VTA中的nAChR直接导致DA VTA细胞的激活，但DA活性的增强也可能来自向VTA发送兴奋性投射的细胞上的nAChR的激活。nAChR存在于LDT中，它们可以被足以诱导细胞放电的烟碱功能激活（Christensen, Ishibashi, Nielsen, Leonard, Kohlmeier, 2014）。LDT的胆碱能细胞和推定的谷氨酸能细胞可以被烟碱充分激活，以刺激这些细胞输出到它们的目标结构，包括VTA内的结构（Christensen et al. 2014）。含有α7和β2亚基的突触后nAChR与LDT细胞的烟碱激活有关（Kohlmeier, 2013）。因此，烟碱在促进NAcc中DA释放方面的作用可能包括激活胆碱能和谷氨酸能脑桥神经元组中的nAChR，这将有助于将DA VTA细胞的放电从基础水平转移到行为相关的、神经编码奖励的阶段性模式特征（Kohlmeier, 2013）。

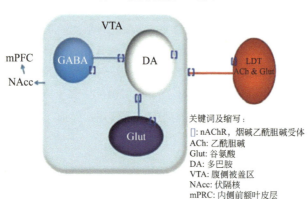

图7.4 中边缘神经元回路

来自背外侧被盖（LDT）的乙酰胆碱激活位于腹侧被盖区（VTA）GABA能、谷氨酸能和多巴胺神经元上的nAChR。

7.6 结论

烟碱的心理生物学作用是由于它对神经中枢的作用。这些受体遍布整个大脑；然而，它们是由烟碱在中伏隔神经回路中激活的，这对动机失效行为至关重要，这被认为是该药物成瘾特性的基础。位于神经元区域的nAChR的激活也可能与此有关，nAChR投射到腹侧被盖区，并控制该区域细胞的行为相关放电活动。nAChR由多个亚基组成；然而，α4β2、α7和α6亚基似乎在烟碱奖励特性背后的细胞行为中发挥了至关重要的作用。包含这些亚基的nAChR位于中伏隔回路内的多个神经元表型上，它们可以通过这些细胞上的突触前或突触后位置发挥作用。nAChR是基于烟碱戒断计划最突出和最有前途的目标之一。然而，尽管已经获得了很多关于烟碱如何作用于这些中伏隔通路受体的信息，但如果我们想在戒烟策略中有效地以这些受体为药物靶点，我们还需要在突触水平了解更多关于烟碱成瘾的基础。

致谢

作者感谢 A. Sabina Kristensen 在制作数据时提供的帮助。

术语解释

- nAChR: 内源性神经递质乙酰胆碱（ACh）是两种受体的激动剂，一种是离子型受体即烟碱乙酰胆碱受体（nAChR），另一种是代谢型受体即毒蕈碱受体。
- VTA: 腹侧被盖区（VTA）是一个主要由多巴胺（DA）和含有 GABA 的细胞组成的中脑核。从腹侧被盖区释放 DA 是触发刺激的突出信号。
- 伏隔核（NAcc）：由多刺的 GABA 细胞组成，是含 DA VTA 细胞的主要靶点，DA 大幅升高激活参与信号显著性。
- LDT：背外侧被盖是一个由乙酰胆碱、GABA 能和谷氨酸能神经元组成的脑桥核，这些神经元向腹侧被盖区发送投射物。尽管几十年来人们已经认识到 LDT 在唤醒中的作用，但最近 LDT 被添加到大脑奖励通路的回路模型中。
- 后突触：在一个三方突触中，受体在树突或体细胞间隔上的定位表明该受体位于突触后或突触的接收端。
- 前突触：在一个三方突触中，受体在细胞轴突末端的位置指定该受体为前突触，它经常参与从末端释放神经活性化学物质。

nAChR 的关键事实

- 乙酰胆碱（ACh）可内源性刺激 nAChR。
- 外源性使用烟碱可刺激 nAChRs。
- nAChR 由 α 和/或 β 类型的 5 个亚基组成。
- nAChR 的两个主要亚基群与药物成瘾有关，即 α4β2 亚基群和一个由 5 个 α7 亚基组成的同质亚基群。
- nAChR 受体在突触前和突触后末端定位的差异以及亚基的组成导致了 GABA 能、谷氨酸能和多巴胺神经元在成瘾相关回路中的不同激活。

药物成瘾回路的关键事实

- 从 VTA 向 NAcc 释放 DA 是刺激（如滥用药物）信号突出的关键成分。
- 烟碱激活 nAChR 会改变其对内源性乙酰胆碱的反应。
- ACh 由来自 LDT 的传入物内源性提供给 VTA，通过这种连接，LDT 改变了 DA VTA 细胞的兴奋性。
- nAChR 存在于 LDT 中，外源性烟碱除了激活 VTA 中的受体外，还激活了这些受体。因此，大脑暴露于烟碱会改变 VTA 内的 LDT 传入对内源性乙酰胆碱的释放。

要点总结

- 烟碱的心理生物学行为是由于 nAChR 的激活。
- nAChR 的亚基组成赋予激动剂激活反应动力学。
- 大脑中最常见的亚基群是异质 α4β2 组合和同质 α7 组合。
- nAChR 可以位于突触前、突触后和突触外。
- 烟碱的成瘾特性是通过激活中伏隔神经回路中的突触前和突触后 nAChR 而获得的。
- 烟碱通过激活位于突触前 GABA 能和谷氨酸能末端的 nAChR 以及位于突触后含有多巴胺的 VTA 细胞的 nAChR，诱导多巴胺大幅上升。
- 来自 LDT 的胆碱能传入物也受到烟碱的影响，导致 VTA 内 nAChR 的内源性激活剂的释放发生变化。

参考文献

Albuquerque, E. X.; Pereira, E. F.; Alkondon, M.; Rogers, S. W. (2009). Mammalian nicotinic acetylcholine receptors: from structure to func-tion. Physiological Reviews, 89, 7 3-120.

Alkondon, M.; Pereira, E. F.; Eisenberg, H. M.; Albuquerque, E.X. (1999). Choline and selective antagonists identify two subtypesof nicotinic acetylcholine receptors that modulate GABA releasefrom CA1 interneurons in rat hippocampal slices. The Journal of Neuroscience, 19, 2693-2705.

Bennett, C.; Arroyo, S.; Berns, D.; Hestrin, S. (2012). Mechanismsgenerating dual-component nicotinic EPSCs in cortical interneurons.The Journal of Neuroscience, 32, 17287-17296.

Berry, J. N.; Engle, S. E.; McIntosh, J. M.; Drenan, R. M. (2015). alpha6-Containing nicotinic acetylcholine receptors in midbrain dopamineneurons are poised to govern dopamine-mediated behaviors and synaptic plasticity. Neuroscience, 304, 161-175.

Cachope, R.; Mateo, Y.; Mathur, B. N.; Irving, J.; Wang, H. L.; Morales, M. et al. (2012). Selective activation of cholinergic interneu-rons enhances accumbal phasic dopamine release: setting the tonefor reward processing. Cell Reports, 2, 33-41.

Champtiaux, N.; Han, Z. Y.; Bessis, A.; Rossi, F. M.; Zoli, M.; Marubio, L. et al. (2002). Distribution and pharmacology of alpha 6-containing nicotinic acetylcholine receptors analyzed with mutant mice. The Journal of Neuroscience, 22, 1208-1217.

Chen, L.; Lodge, D. J. (2013). The lateral mesopontine tegmentumregulates both tonic and phasic activity of VTA dopamine neurons.Journal of Neurophysiology, 110, 2287-2294.

Christensen, M. H.; Ishibashi, M.; Nielsen, M. L.; Leonard, C. S.; Kohlmeier, K. A. (2014). Age-related changes in nicotine response of cholinergic and non-cholinergic laterodorsal tegmental neurons:implications for the heightened adolescent susceptibility to nicotineaddiction. Neuropharmacology, 85, 263-283.

Dani, J. A. (1986). Ion-channel entrances influence permeation. Net charge, size, shape, and binding considerations.Biophysical Journal, 49, 607-618.

Dani, J. A. (2015). Neuronal nicotinic acetylcholine receptor structureand function and response to nicotine. International Review ofNeurobiology, 124, 3-19.

Dani, J. A.; Heinemann, S. (1996). Molecular and cellular aspects ofnicotine abuse. Neuron, 16, 905-908.

Dani, J. A.; Kosten, T. R.; Benowitz, N. L. (2014). The pharmacology ofnicotine and tobacco. In: Ries R.K.; Fiellin D.A.; Miller S.C.; Saitz R. (Eds.), The ASAM principles of addiction medicine (pp. 201-216). Philadelphia, PA: Lippincott Williams, Wilkins, Wolters Kluwer. (Chapter 12).

Dani, J. A.; Radcliffe, K. A.; Pidoplichko, V. I. (2000). Variations indesensitization of nicotinic acetylcholine receptors from hippocam-pus and midbrain dopamine areas. European Journal of Pharmacology, 393, 31-38.

Elgoyhen, A. B.; Vetter, D. E.; Katz, E.; Rothlin, C. V.; Heinemann, S. F.; Boulter, J. (2001). alpha10: a determinant of nicotinic cholinergicreceptor function in mammalian vestibular and cochlear mechano-sensory hair cells. Proceedings of the National Academy of Sciences ofthe United States of America, 98, 3501-3506.

Engle, S. E.; McIntosh, J. M.; Drenan, R. M. (2015). Nicotine and eth-anol cooperate to enhance ventral tegmental area AMPA receptorfunction via alpha6-containing nicotinic receptors. Neuropharmacol-ogy, 91, 13-22.

Engle, S. E.; Shih, P. Y.; McIntosh, J. M.; Drenan, R. M. (2013). alpha4al-pha6beta2*nicotinic acetylcholine receptor activation on ventral teg-mental area dopamine neurons is sufficient to stimulate adepolarizing conductance and enhance surface AMPA receptorfunction. Molecular Pharmacology, 84, 393-406.

Exley, R.; Maubourguet, N.; David, V.; Eddine, R.; Evrard, A.; Pons, S. et al. (2011). Distinct contributions of nicotinic acetylcholine receptorsubunit alpha4 and subunit alpha6 to the reinforcing effects of nicotine. Proceedings of the National Academy of Sciences of the United States of America, 108, 7577-7582.

Fenster, C. P.; Whitworth, T. L.; Sheffield, E. B.; Quick, M. W.; Lester, R. A. (1999). Upregulation of surface alpha4beta2 nicotinic receptors is initiated by receptor desensitization after chronic expo-sure to nicotine. The Journal of Neuroscience, 19, 4804-4814.

Fisher, J. L.; Pidoplichko, V. I.; Dani, J. A. (1998). Nicotine modifiesthe activity of ventral tegmental area dopaminergic neurons andhippocampal GABAergic neurons. Journal of Physiology, Paris, 92, 209-213.

Forster, G. L.; Blaha, C. D. (2000). Laterodorsal tegmental stimulationelicits dopamine efflux in the rat nucleus accumbens by activation ofacetylcholine and glutamate receptors in the ventral tegmental area. The European Journal of Neuroscience, 12, 3596-3604.

Forster, G. L.; Falcon, A. J.; Miller, A. D.; Heruc, G. A.; Blaha, C.D. (2002). Effects of laterodorsal tegmentum excitotoxic lesions on behavioral and dopamine responses evoked by morphine andd-amphetamine. Neuroscience, 114, 817-823.

Gotti, C.; Guiducci, S.; Tedesco, V.; Corbioli, S.; Zanetti, L.; Moretti, M. et al. (2010). Nicotinic acetylcholine receptors in the mesolimbic pathway: primary role of ventral tegmental area alpha6beta2*receptors in mediating systemic nicotine effects on dopamine release, locomotion, and reinforcement. The Journal of Neuroscience, 30, 5311-5325.

Grace, A. A. (1991). Phasic versus tonic dopamine release and the mod-ulation of dopamine system responsivity: a hypothesis for the etiol-ogy of schizophrenia. Neuroscience, 41, 1-24.

Grace, A. A.; Floresco, S. B.; Goto, Y.; Lodge, D. J. (2007). Regulation of firing of dopaminergic neurons and control of goal-directed behav-iors. Trends in Neurosciences, 30, 220-227.

Grady, S. R.; Salminen, O.; Laverty, D. C.; Whiteaker, P.; McIntosh, J. M.; Collins, A. C. et al. (2007). The subtypes of nicotinic acetylcholine receptors on dopaminergic terminals of mouse striatum. Biochemical Pharmacology, 74, 1235-1246.

Grady, S. R.; Wageman, C. R.; Patzlaff, N. E.; Marks, M. J. (2012). Lowconcentrations of nicotine differentially desensitize nicotinic acetyl-choline receptors that include alpha5 or alpha6 subunits and thatmediate synaptosomal neurotransmitter release. Neuropharmacology, 62, 1935-1943.

Henningfield, J. E.; Stapleton, J. M.; Benowitz, N. L.; Grayson, R. F.; London, E. D. (1993). Higher levels of nicotine in arterial than in venous blood after cigarette smoking. Drug and Alcohol Dependence, 33, 2 3-29.

Jerlhag, E.; Janson, A. C.; Waters, S.; Engel, J. A. (2012). Concomitantrelease of ventral tegmental acetylcholine and accumbal dopamineby ghrelin in rats. PLoS One, 7, e49557.

Klink, R.; de Kerchove d'Exaerde, A.; Zoli, M.; Changeux, J. P. (2001). Molecular and physiological diversity of nicotinic acetylcholinereceptors in the midbrain dopaminergic nuclei. The Journal of Neuro-science, 21, 1452-1463.

Kohlmeier, K. A. (2013). Off the beaten path: drug addiction and thepontine laterodorsal tegmentum. ISRN Neuroscience, 2013, 604847.

Koob, G. F.; Volkow, N. D. (2016). Neurobiology of addiction: a neu-rocircuitry analysis. Lancet Psychiatry, 3, 760-773.

Lagostena, L.; Trocme-Thibierge, C.; Morain, P.; Cherubini, E. (2008). The partial alpha7 nicotine acetylcholine receptor agonist S 24795enhances long-term potentiation at CA3-CA1 synapses in the adult mouse hippocampus. Neuropharmacology, 54, 676-685.

Lammel, S.; Lim, B. K.; Ran, C.; Huang, K. W.; Betley, M. J.; Tye, K. M. et al. (2012). Input-specific control of reward and aversion in the ven-tral tegmental area. Nature, 491, 212-217.

Liu, Z.; Tearle, A. W.; Nai, Q.; Berg, D. K. (2005). Rapid activity-drivenSNARE-dependent trafficking of nicotinic receptors on somatic spines. The Journal of Neuroscience, 25, 1159-1168.

Lodge, D. J.; Grace, A. A. (2006). The laterodorsal tegmentum isessential for burst firing of ventral tegmental area dopamineneurons. Proceedings of the National Academy of Sciences of the United States of America, 103, 5167-5172.

Mameli-Engvall, M.; Evrard, A.; Pons, S.; Maskos, U.; Svensson, T. H.; Changeux, J. P. et al. (2006). Hierarchical control of dopamine neuron-firing patterns by nicotinic receptors. Neuron, 50, 911-921.

Mansvelder, H. D.; Keath, J. R.; McGehee, D. S. (2002). Synaptic mech-anisms underlie nicotine-induced excitability of brain reward areas.Neuron, 33, 905-919.

Mansvelder, H. D.; McGehee, D. S. (2000). Long-term potentiation ofexcitatory inputs to brain reward areas by nicotine. Neuron, 27, 349-357.

Mansvelder, H. D.; McGehee, D. S. (2002). Cellular and synapticmechanisms of nicotine addiction. Journal of Neurobiology, 53, 606-617.

Marks, M. J.; Burch, J. B.; Collins, A. C. (1983). Effects of chronic nic-otine infusion on tolerance development and nicotinic receptors.The Journal of Pharmacology and Experimental Therapeutics, 226, 817-825.

Maskos, U. (2008). The cholinergic mesopontine tegmentum is a rela-tively neglected nicotinic master modulator of the dopaminergic sys-tem: relevance to drugs of abuse and pathology. British Journal of Pharmacology, 153 (Suppl. 1), S438-S445.

McGehee, D. S.; Role, L. W. (1995). Physiological diversity of nicotinicacetylcholine receptors expressed by vertebrate neurons. AnnualReview of Physiology, 57, 521-546.

Miwa, J. M.; Freedman, R.; Lester, H. A. (2011). Neural systems gov-erned by nicotinic acetylcholine receptors: emerging hypotheses.Neuron, 70, 2 0-33.

Moretti, M.; Zoli, M.; George, A. A.; Lukas, R. J.; Pistillo, F.; Maskos, U.et al. (2014). The novel alpha7beta2-nicotinic acetylcholine receptorsubtype is expressed in mouse and human basal forebrain: biochem-ical and pharmacological characterization. Molecular Pharmacology, 86, 306-317.

Moroni, M.; Bermudez, I. (2006). Stoichiometry and pharmacology of two human alpha4beta2 nicotinic receptor types. Journal of Molecular Neuroscience, 30, 9 5-96.

Omelchenko, N.; Sesack, S. R. (2005). Laterodorsal tegmental projec-tions to identified cell populations in the rat ventral tegmental area. The Journal of Comparative Neurology, 483, 217-235.

Omelchenko, N.; Sesack, S. R. (2006). Cholinergic axons in the rat ven-tral tegmental area synapse preferentially onto mesoaccumbens dopamine neurons. The Journal of Comparative Neurology, 494, 863-875.

Omelchenko, N.; Sesack, S. R. (2007). Glutamate synaptic inputs to ventral tegmental area neurons in the rat derive primarily from sub-cortical sources. Neuroscience, 146, 1259-1274.

Omelchenko, N.; Sesack, S. R. (2009). Ultrastructural analysis of localcollaterals of rat ventral tegmental area neurons: GABA phenotype and synapses onto dopamine and GABA cells. Synapse, 63, 895-906.

Parri, R. H.; Dineley, T. K. (2010). Nicotinic acetylcholine receptorinteraction with beta-amyloid: molecular, cellular, and physiological consequences. Current Alzheimer Research, 7, 2 7-39.

Pidoplichko, V. I.; DeBiasi, M.; Williams, J. T.; Dani, J. A. (1997). Nic-otine activates and desensitizes midbrain dopamine neurons.Nature, 390, 401-404.

Salminen, O.; Drapeau, J. A.; McIntosh, J. M.; Collins, A. C.; Marks, M. J.; Grady, S. R. (2007). Pharmacology of alpha-conotoxin MII-sensitive subtypes of nicotinic acetylcholine receptors isolatedby breeding of null mutant mice. Molecular Pharmacology, 71, 1563-1571.

Sarter, M.; Parikh, V.; Howe, W. M. (2009). Phasic acetylcholinerelease and the volume transmission hypothesis: time to move on.Nature Reviews Neuroscience, 10, 383-390.

Schmidt, H. D.; Famous, K. R.; Pierce, R. C. (2009). The limbic circuitryunderlying cocaine seeking encompasses the PPTg/LDT. The Euro-pean Journal of Neuroscience, 30, 1358-1369.

Schultz, W. (2007a). Behavioral dopamine signals. Trends in Neurosci-ences, 30, 203-210.

Schultz, W. (2007b). Multiple dopamine functions at different timecourses. Annual Review of Neuroscience, 30, 259-288.

Shinohara, F.; Kihara, Y.; Ide, S.; Minami, M.; Kaneda, K. (2014). Crit-ical role of cholinergic transmission from the laterodorsal tegmentalnucleus to the ventral tegmental area in cocaine-induced place pref-erence. Neuropharmacology, 79, 573-579.

Steidl, S.; Veverka, K. (2015). Optogenetic excitation of LDTg axons in theVTA reinforces operant responding in rats.Brain Research, 1614, 86-93.

Tolu, S.; Eddine, R.; Marti, F.; David, V.; Graupner, M.; Pons, S. et al. (2013). Co-activation of VTA DA and GABA neurons mediatesnicotine reinforcement. Molecular Psychiatry, 18, 382-393.

Volkow, N. D.; Koob, G. F.; McLellan, A. T. (2016). Neurobiologicadvances from the brain disease model of addiction. The New England Journal of

Medicine, 374, 363-371.

Whiteaker, P.; Sharples, C. G.; Wonnacott, S. (1998). Agonist-induced up-regulation of alpha4beta2 nicotinic acetylcholine receptors inM10 cells: pharmacological and spatial definition. Molecular Pharma-cology, 53, 950-962.

Wooltorton, J. R.; Pidoplichko, V. I.; Broide, R. S.; Dani, J. A. (2003). Differential desensitization and distribution of nicotinic acetylcho-line receptor subtypes in midbrain dopamine areas. The Journal of Neuroscience, 23, 3176-3185.

Xiao, C.; Cho, J. R.; Zhou, C.; Treweek, J. B.; Chan, K.; McKinney, S. L. et al. (2016). Cholinergic mesopontine signals govern locomotion and reward through dissociable midbrain pathways. Neuron, 90, 333-347.

Zhang, T.; Zhang, L.; Liang, Y.; Siapas, A. G.; Zhou, F. M.; Dani, J.A. (2009). Dopamine signaling differences in the nucleus accumbensand dorsal striatum exploited by nicotine. The Journal of Neuroscience, 29, 4035-4043.

Zhao-Shea, R.; Liu, L.; Soll, L. G.; Improgo, M. R.; Meyers, E. E.; McIntosh, J. M. et al. (2011). Nicotine-mediated activation of dopa-minergic neurons in distinct regions of the ventral tegmental area.Neuropsychopharmacology, 36, 1021-1032.

8
在不同模型中，可替宁作为一种可能的烟碱效应的变构调节剂

Oné R. Pagán

Department of Biology, West Chester University, West Chester, PA, United States

缩略语

CYP2A6	细胞色素P450 2A6	**nAChR**	烟碱乙酰胆碱受体
LGIC	配体门控离子通道	**PMR**	微观可逆性原理

8.1 引言

烟碱最活跃的异构体［3-（1-甲基-2-吡咯烷基）吡啶的S-异构体］被广泛认为是人类已知的最容易上瘾的化合物之一，至少一直被列为这方面的"五大"物质之一（Stolerman, Jarvis, 1995）。烟碱使用和滥用的历史、科学重要性、管理模式等在本书的其他地方进行了回顾。该化合物的主要天然来源是烟草植物，即烟草以及相关的烟草种类（Firn, 2011）。然而，有一种令人惊讶的相关植物（主要但不限于茄科的其他成员）含有可检测到的烟碱水平，尽管与烟草相比，其烟碱的含量要低得多。这些其他植物种类包括可食用植物，如西红柿、茄子和花椰菜（Domino, Hornbach, Demana, 1993）。与许多植物次生代谢物相似，烟碱在自然界中的作用似乎是作为杀虫剂（Soloway, 1976）。有目的地向作物喷洒烟碱和选择烟碱产量较高的烟草植物是公认的农业实践（Jackson, Johnson, Stephenson, 2002; Schmeltz, 1971），其目的是抗击农业害虫。这一想法的直接调查支持的一个例子包括一份研究报告，在该报告中，淡化烟草的烟碱产生途径被沉默，使它们的烟碱产生减少了95%以上。与野生型植物相比，这些改良植物对昆虫捕食的抵抗力明显降低（Steppuhn, Gase, Krock, Halitschke, Baldwin, 2004）。

8.2 烟碱乙酰胆碱受体

烟碱定义了一类统称为烟碱乙酰胆碱受体（nAChR）的大分子，它们属于配体门控离子通道（LGIC）的一般家族。有趣的是，除了nAChR，烟碱似乎在几个模型中与蛋白泛素复合物相互作用（Caldeira, Salazar, Curcio, Canzoniero, Duarte, 2014; Chapman, 2009; Kane, Konu, Ma, Li, 2004; Massaly, Francès, Moulédous, 2014; Rezvani, Teng, Shim, De Biasi, 2007）。对这些替代烟碱靶点的研究可能会导致新的药物疗法的发展。尽管如此，到目前为止，对烟碱最了解的分子靶标仍然是nAChRs。

到目前为止，最了解的LGIC是肌肉型nAChR。该受体在离子通道中占有独特的历史地位。它是第一个被纯化的，第一个确定其一级结构的，第一个在人工脂质双分子层中进行功能

重组的，也是第一个获得单通道记录的（Hucho, Tsetlin, Machold, 1996; Karlin, Akabas, 1995）。nAChRs也是描述变构受体的原型模型之一（Bertrand, Changeaux, 1995）。毫无疑问的是，该受体将是第一个在原子水平上被理解的LGIC（Chen, 2010; Giastas, Zouridakis, Tzartos, 2018; Gu, Zhong, Wei, 2011; Tsetlin, Hucho, 2009）。nAChRs有两种广泛定义的类型：肌肉型受体（主要负责导致横纹肌收缩的生理事件）和异质性神经元型（主要存在于神经组织中，涉及多种神经系统功能）（Dani, 2015; Hogg, Bertrand, 2004; Hurst, Rollema, Bertrand, 2013）。

在过去40年左右的时间里，神经元nAChR作为治疗各种神经精神疾病的可能靶点得到了深入研究（Freedman, 2014; Pogocki, Ruman, Danilczuk, Celuch, Wałajtys-Rode, 2007; Rollema, Bertrand, Hurst, 2015; Terry, Callahan, Hall, Webster, 2011; Terry, Callahan, Hernandez, 2015）。尽管对迄今为止已知的每种神经元nAChR亚型的特定结构、生化和生理特征的理解取得了很大进展，但开发有用的药物疗法的前景充其量只是适度的，除了戒烟疗法［一种相当有见地的疗法，Bertrand, Terry（2018）最近发表了对该领域总体状况的评论］。

所有nAChR都是形成离子通道的五聚体蛋白质。肌肉型nAChR是一种异聚复合物，由α、β、γ和δ亚基形成，显示出化学计量的α2βγδ。在肌肉型nAChR的情况下，在发育时，γ亚基被ε亚基取代。按照惯例，肌肉型α和β亚基被认为是同类中的第一个（即α1和β1）。相比之下，神经元nAChR存在于由两个α亚基（α2～α10）和三个β亚基（β2～β4）组成的异聚体组合中；或者，同源nAChR由五个相同的α亚基组成。例如，最好理解的同型烟碱受体是由五个α7亚基组成的受体。几种类型的nAChR上的各种突变与各种神经肌肉和神经元通道疾病有关（Wu, Lukas, 2011; Zoli, Pistillo, Gotti, 2015）。

nAChR在本书的其他地方进行了更详细的讨论。但是，我想在此指出的主要点是，由于11种神经元亚基α2～α10/β2～β4的多种可能组合，神经元nAChR在脊椎动物神经系统中表现出丰富的亚型。每种不同的组合优先在特定的神经元结构和组织中表达，使每种受体类型具有微妙的生理特性和调节域。这一点对于讨论烟碱及其主要代谢产物可替宁的相互作用特别重要。

8.3 可替宁

在人类中，烟碱被代谢成大约25种代谢物（Benowitz, Hukkanen, Jacob, 2009）。这种代谢大多是由一种叫做细胞色素P450 2A6（CYP2A6）的肝酶完成的，该酶催化约80%被吸收的烟碱转化为可替宁（Grizzell, Echeverría, 2015）。因此，可替宁被广泛认为是人类的主要烟碱代谢物。反过来，可替宁被CYP2A6进一步代谢成一系列化合物，尽管其代谢率低于烟碱。在结构上，可替宁和烟碱非常相似，它们之间的唯一区别是羰基（图8.1）。尽管烟碱和可替宁在结构上非常相似，但这两种化合物对神经系统的影响存在显著差异（Grizzell, Echeverría, 2015）。这一事实很可能反映了它们各自与神经元nAChR的相互作用，并且对本章中的思想特别重要。

从药代动力学上看，可替宁的半衰期比烟碱更长（De Schepper, Van Hecken, Daenens, Van Rossum, 1987），这证明了这样一种观点，即烟碱产生的大多数长期（而不是直接）胆碱能效应实际上归因于可替宁（Grizzell, Echeverría, 2015）。此外，可替宁似乎显示出烟碱的许多有益作用，但缺乏大多数的负面作用，包括其成瘾性（Hatsukami, Grillo, Pentel, Oncken, Bliss, 1997; Moran, 2012; Grizzell, Echeverría, 2015）。研究可替宁的最初动力是烟草消费的指标（Benowitz et al. 2009; Moran, 2012）。最近，可替宁引起了追求新型药物治疗的研究人员的兴趣。可替宁正在被研究作为一种抗炎药（Echeverría, Grizzell, Barreto, 2016）和帕金森病（Barreto, Yarkov, Avila-Rodriguez, Aliev, Echeverría, 2015）、阿尔茨海默病（Echeverría, Zeitlin et al. 2012）、创伤后应激障碍（Barreto, Iarkov, Moran, 2014; Barreto et al. 2015; Mendoza et al. 2018）的一种可能治疗方法。有趣的是，可替宁也已显示出具有抗抑郁作用（Grizzell et al. 2014）。

尽管可替宁通常会表现出与烟碱类似的生理作用（即烟碱激动剂；Grizzell, Echeverría, 2015; Moran, 2012），但在某些情况下，根据模型系统和所研究烟碱受体的具体类型，可替宁和烟碱表现出相反的生理作用（Grizzell, Echeverría, 2015），并且相互拮抗，尤其是在放射性配体结合研究中（Vainio, Tuominen, 2001; Vainio, Törnquist, Tuominen, 2000; Vainio, Viluksela, Tuominen, et al. 1998a, b）。

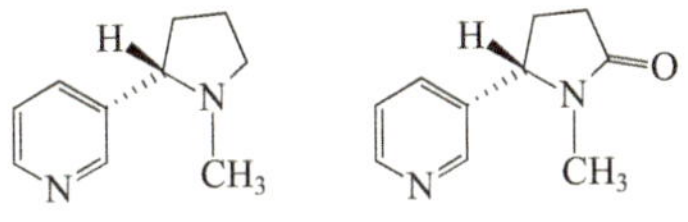

图 8.1 这项工作中审查过的化合物

8.4 烟碱/可替宁和涡虫

直到最近，可替宁仅在脊椎动物模型中进行了体内研究，或在体外使用了来源于脊椎动物的细胞系进行了研究。然而，由于烟碱代谢，在某些无脊椎动物中也检测到了可替宁。这些无脊椎动物包括一种蝇类（*Calliphora vomitoria*, Magni et al. 2016）、烟青虫（*Heliothis virescens*, Orth, Head, Mierkowski, 2007）和蜜蜂（du Rand, Pirk, Nicolson, Apostolides, 2017）。在撰写本文时，尚未在任何无脊椎动物模型中对可替宁的生理和行为影响进行系统研究。本实验室的数据表明，可替宁在特定的无脊椎动物系统（涡虫）中起烟碱拮抗剂的作用。涡虫是再生和发育生物学中公认的模式生物。自20世纪70年代以来，已经在药理学和神经生物学方面对它们进行了越来越多的研究，尤其是滥用药物的行为影响及其作用机理（Pagán, 2017）。我们最近报道了可替宁以浓度依赖的方式阻止了涡虫 *Girardia tigrina* 中三种不同的烟碱诱导的行为的诱导（Bach et al. 2016）。研究的行为包括运动减少、癫痫样运动和戒断样行为。此外，我们正在进一步探索可替宁对涡虫行为的拮抗作用。初步结果表明，可替宁在该生物体中是烟碱的非竞争性抑制剂（Pagán 等，未发表的数据）。据我们所知，我们的结果代表了对无脊椎动物模型中烟碱/可替宁相互作用的首次研究，为从生态毒理学到农业的一系列有趣的可能性打开了大门。目前尚不清楚涡虫是否将烟碱代谢成可替宁。一些研究已经证实了涡虫中胆碱能系统的存在。乙酰胆碱和烟碱会诱发涡虫的行为效应（Buttarelli, Pellicano, Pontieri, 2008; Buttarelli, Pontieri, Margotta, Palladini, 2000; Pagán et al. 2009, 2013; Pagán, Montgomery, Deats, Bach, Baker, 2015; Rawls et al. 2011）。使用原位杂交（Cebrià et al. 2002）、微阵列技术（Nakazawa et al. 2003）和表达序列标签（Mineta et al. 2003）发现了在涡虫中候选 nAChR 实例的间接证据。此外，使用涡虫 *Schmidtea mediterranea* 数据库（http://smedgd.neuro.utah.edu/; Robb, Gotting, Ross, Sánchez Alvarado, 2015），我们发现了几种烟碱样受体候选序列。这些推定的涡虫烟碱结合位点尚未直接鉴定。因此，迄今为止，尚不清楚在涡虫中烟碱的特定分子靶标。尽管如此，还是可以合理地预期这些扁虫在其nAChR上将表现出相似程度的多样性。我们在涡虫中对烟碱和可替宁的研究（Bach et al. 2016）表明，可替宁本身不会引起任何明显的行为影响，但可替宁可拮抗此类生物中烟碱诱导的行为。基于此，假设调节位点至少存在于一种推定的涡虫nAChR亚型中，当其与可替宁结合时会抑制烟碱的行为作用。

总之，在包括涡虫在内的各种模型中，烟碱和可替宁之间体内和体外药理学相互作用的异质性表明，与烟碱类似，可替宁与神经元nAChR的多种亚型相互作用。可替宁的某些作用似乎是模仿烟碱的（即胆碱能激动剂），因此最简单的解释是，在这些情况下，可替宁与烟碱的结合位点相同或至少重叠。另一方面，可替宁表现为烟碱拮抗剂的情况表明存在更复杂的相互作用。一种可能的解释是变构调节模型。

8.5 微观可逆性原理

微观可逆性原理（PMR）是由Gilbert N. Lewis于1925年以热力学为基础提出的。最初，Lewis称其为"整体平衡法则"。他将其表述为"对应于每个过程都有一个逆向过程，在平衡状态下，每个过程的平均速率等于其逆向过程的平均速率"（Lewis, 1925）。在Lewis的论文发表的同一年，Richard C. Tolman试图反驳Lewis的想法，但奇怪的是，在此过程中，他最终将其更名为"微观可逆性原理"（Tolman, 1925）。尽管Tolman面临挑战，但仍获得了PMR的实验证据，具有讽刺意味的是，Tolman对该概念的命名永远与模型联系在一起。PMR已被证明不仅适用于平衡条件，而且还适用于远离平衡的系统，找到了使用瞬态动力学技术建模酶促反应以及最终配体-受体系统的方法（Astumian, 2012; Blackmond, 2009a; Hess, 2003）。在这种情况下，PMR本质上表明，配体与其受体靶标结合所需的自由能与化合物是否与受体的活性形式或非活性形式结合无关。换句话说，无论采取何种结合或酶促途径，合成产品或激活受体系统的能量消耗都是恒定的（Kenakin, 1997）。Katz和Thesleff（1957）提出了该原理的最早应用之一，以描述电动机端板模型中对乙酰胆碱的脱敏。对该原理的进一步研究提出了nAChR激活和失活的机制（图8.2；Hess, 2003）。最终，这是假设nAChR中存在调节域的基础。据预测，化合物结合受体非活性构象的调节位点比结合受体活性状态的替代位点具有更高的亲和力，将使平衡转向受体的非活性构象。相反，优先与活性受体调节位点结合的化合物不会抑制该受体。此外，这样的配体将取代受体上的抑制剂。这是预测该受体先前未知的激活剂和抑制剂以及扩展到其他相关受体系统的理论基础。使用瞬态动力学技术提供的支持这些预测的证据，以研究可卡因和谷氨酸能药物(+)地佐西平对nAChR的抑制机制（Hess et al. 2000），最终确定了减轻这种抑制的化合物（Hess et al. 2003; Sivaprakasam, Pagán, Hess, 2010）。有趣的是，发现促性腺甲酯（一种主要的可卡因代谢物）和类似物3-乙酰促性腺甲酯是可卡因肌肉型nAChR的缓解剂（Ambre, Ruo, Smith, Backes, Smith, 1982, 图8.3），可缓解可卡因对肌肉型nAChR（Chen, Banerjee, Hess, 2004）和神经元型nAChR（Krivoshein, Hess, 2004）的抑制作用。此外，nAChR的紧密结构类似物γ型氨基丁酸受体A型和抑制性受体也证明了类似的机制（GABA-A, Ramakrishnan, Hess, 2004, 2005, 2010）。

至少在某些nAChR亚型中，代谢物（芽子碱甲酯）充当其母体化合物（可卡因）的抑制剂的观点与可替宁可以充当烟碱拮抗剂的观点是一致的。这一观点的间接证据是可替宁在各种系统中的生理效应的异质性（Grizzell, Echeverría, 2015）以及我们自己使用涡虫的研究。PMR的进化意义在生化和药理学文献中很少被明确提及除了一些明显的例外，特别是考虑到许多酶的聚合物性质（Blackmond, 2009b; Burbaum, Raines, Albery, Knowles, 1989; Ricard, 1978）。从这个角度出发，进化论的解释暗示了催化效率和调节能力的最大化（Ricard, 1978）。将这些原理应用于调节受体功能的新调节机制的发现是一个令人兴奋的研究领域，它有可能获得针对各种病理状况的新药物疗法。对nAChR和相关蛋白的进一步研究以及使用已建立的模型生物（如涡虫）的新应用，可以为理解可替宁如何充当调节配体提供重要的帮助，这可能有助于阐明神经递质变构调节的一般机制。

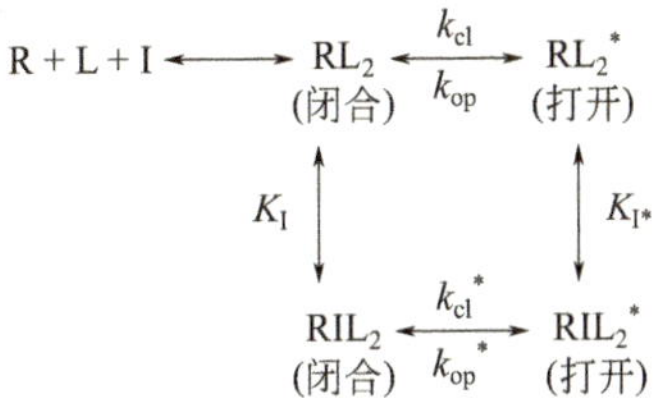

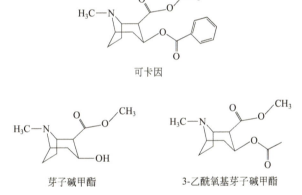

图8.2 拟议的烟碱乙酰胆碱受体抑制机制

I为变构配体（抑制剂或活化剂）；K_I和K_{I^*}分别为观察到的闭合通道和打开通道形式的变构配体的解离常数；k_{op}和k_{cl}分别为通道开启和关闭的速率常数；k_{op}^*和k_{cl}^*分别为当变构配体与开放通道结合时，通道打开和关闭的速率常数；L为配体；R为受体；RL、RIL_2和RL_2为闭合通道构象；RL_2^*和RIL_2^*为打开通道构象。参考Hess等（2000）。

可卡因

芽子碱甲酯　　　　　3-乙酰氧基芽子碱甲酯

图8.3 可卡因的变构抑制剂实例

致谢

我谨将本章献给我的博士生导师，康奈尔大学的George P. Hess教授，从他那里我了解了微观可逆性原理。他是我的一位良师益友。我非常感谢西切斯特大学生物系、赞助研究办公室、科学与数学学院以及国立卫生研究院（NIH; R03DA026518）的财政支持。我声明没有利益冲突。

术语解释
- 可替宁：人体主要烟碱代谢物。
- 烟碱乙酰胆碱受体：是目前最著名的配体门控离子通道。由被烟碱激活的能力来定义。
- 涡虫：是一种无脊椎动物，属于扁形动物门。这些生物是生物化学和行为药理学中一个新兴的模型。
- 微观可逆性原理：描述了酶或变构受体不同激活途径的生物能量等效性。

关键事实
- 可替宁正在被研究作为一种药物制剂，用于治疗帕金森病、阿尔茨海默病、创伤后应激障碍和抑郁症等。
- 可替宁可以作为烟碱的激动剂或拮抗剂，这取决于具体的模型。
- 烟碱乙酰胆碱受体是迄今为止最著名的蛋白质受体。
- 涡虫是神经药理学中越来越流行的模型。

要点总结
- 可替宁和烟碱结合在同一个蛋白质目标上：烟碱乙酰胆碱受体（nAChR）。
- 烟碱/烟碱特异性相互作用机制尚不完全清楚。
- 当可替宁作为nAChR的激动剂时，最可能的解释是烟碱和可替宁结合在这个受体上的相同位置。
- 当可替宁作为nAChR的拮抗剂时，最可能的解释是烟碱和可替宁的结合位点显示出变构作用。
- 微观可逆性原理可以提供一个合适的机制模型来阐明可替宁/烟碱的相互作用。
- 涡虫是研究可替宁/烟碱相互作用的合适体内模型。

参考文献

Ambre, J. J.; Ruo, T. I.; Smith, G. L.; Backes, D.; Smith, C. M. (1982). Ecgonine methyl ester, a major metabolite of cocaine. Journal of Analytical Toxicology, 6 (1), 26-29.

Astumian, R. D. (2012). Microscopic reversibility as the organizing principle of molecular machines. Nature Nanotechnology, 7 (11), 684-688.

Bach, D. J.; Tenaglia, M.; Baker, D. L.; Deats, S.; Montgomery, E.; Pagán, O. R. (2016). Cotinine antagonizes the behavioral effects of nicotine exposure in the planarian Girardia tigrina. Neuroscience Letters, 632, 204-208.

Barreto, G. E.; Iarkov, A.; Moran, V. E. (2014). Beneficial effects of nicotine, cotinine and its metabolites as potential agents for Parkinson's disease. Frontiers in Aging Neuroscience, 6, 340.

Barreto, G. E.; Yarkov, A.; Avila-Rodriguez, M.; Aliev, G.; Echeverría, V. (2015). Nicotine-derived compounds as therapeutic tools against post-traumatic stress disorder. Current Pharmaceutical Design, 21 (25), 3589-3595.

Benowitz, N. L.; Hukkanen, J.; Jacob, P. (2009). Nicotine chemistry, metabolism, kinetics and biomarkers. Handbook of Experimental Pharmacology, 192, 29-60.

Bertrand, D.; Changeaux, J. P. (1995). Nicotinic receptor: an allosteric protein specialized for intercellular communication. Seminars in the Neurosciences, 7, 75-90.

Bertrand, D.; Terry, A. V.; Jr. (2018). The wonderland of neuronal nicotinic acetylcholine receptors. Biochemical Pharmacology, 151, 214-225.

Blackmond, D. G. (2009a). Challenging the concept of "recycling" as a mechanism for the evolution of homochirality in chemical reactions. Chirality, 21 (3), 359-362.

Blackmond, D. G. (2009b). "If pigs could fly" chemistry: a tutorial on the principle of microscopic reversibility. Angewandte Chemie (International Ed. in English), 48 (15), 2648-2654.

Burbaum, J. J.; Raines, R. T.; Albery, W. J.; Knowles, J. R. (1989). Evolutionary optimization of the catalytic effectiveness of an enzyme. Biochemistry, 28 (24), 9293-9305.

Buttarelli, F. R.; Pellicano, C.; Pontieri, F. E. (2008). Neuropharmacology and behavior in planarians: translations to mammals. Comparative Biochemistry and Physiology, Part C: Toxicology, Pharmacology, 147 (4), 399-408.

Buttarelli, F. R.; Pontieri, F. E.; Margotta, V.; Palladini, G. (2000). Acetylcholine/dopamine interaction in planaria. Comparative Biochemistry and Physiology, Part C: Toxicology, Pharmacology, 125 (2), 225-231.

Caldeira, M. V.; Salazar, I. L.; Curcio, M.; Canzoniero, L. M.; Duarte, C. B. (2014). Role of the ubiquitin-proteasome system in brain ischemia: friend or foe? Progress in Neurobiology, 112, 50-69.

Cebrià, F.; Kudome, T.; Nakazawa, M.; Mineta, K.; Ikeo, K.; Gojobori, T. et al. (2002). The expression of neural-specific genes reveals the structural and molecular complexity of the planarian central nervous system. Mechanisms of Development, 116 (1-2), 199-204.

Chapman, M. A. (2009). Does smoking reduce the risk of Parkinson's disease through stimulation of the ubiquitin-proteasome system? Medical Hypotheses, 73 (6), 887-891.

Chen, L. (2010). In pursuit of the high-resolution structure of nicotinic acetylcholine receptors. The Journal of Physiology, 588 (Pt 4), 557-564.

Chen, Y.; Banerjee, A.; Hess, G. P. (2004). Mechanism-based discovery of small molecules that prevent noncompetitive inhibition by cocaine and MK-801 mediated by two different sites on the nicotinic acetylcholine receptor. Biochemistry, 43 (31), 10149-10156.

Dani, J. A. (2015). Neuronal nicotinic acetylcholine receptor structure and function and response to nicotine. International Review of Neurobiology, 124, 3-19.

De Schepper, P. J.; Van Hecken, A.; Daenens, P.; Van Rossum, J.M. (1987). Kinetics of cotinine after oral and intravenous administration to man. European Journal of Clinical Pharmacology, 31 (5), 583-588.

Domino, E. F.; Hornbach, E.; Demana, T. (1993). The nicotine contentof common vegetables. The New England Journal of Medicine, 329 (6), 437.

du Rand, E. E.; Pirk, C. W. W.; Nicolson, S. W.; Apostolides, Z. (2017).The metabolic fate of nectar nicotine in worker honey bees. Journal of Insect Physiology, 98, 14-22.

Echeverría, V.; Grizzell, J. A.; Barreto, G. E. (2016). Neuroinflammation:a therapeutic target of cotinine for the treatment of psychiatricdisorders? Current Pharmaceutical Design, 22 (10), 1324-1333.

Echeverría, V.; Zeitlin, R. (2012). Cotinine: a potential new therapeuticagent against Alzheimer's disease. CNS Neuroscience, Therapeutics, 18 (7), 517-523.

Firn, R. (2011). Nature's chemicals: The natural products that shaped ourworld. New York: Oxford University Press.Freedman, R. (2014). α7-nicotinic acetylcholine receptor agonists for cognitiveenhancement in schizophrenia. Annual Review of Medicine, 65, 245-261.

Giastas, P.; Zouridakis, M.; Tzartos, S. J. (2018). Understandingstructure-function relationships of the human neuronal acetylcholine receptor: insights from the first crystal structures of neuronalsubunits. British Journal of Pharmacology, 175 (11), 1880-1891.

Grizzell, J. A.; Echeverría, V. (2015). New insights into the mechanismsof action of cotinine and its distinctive effects from nicotine.Neurochemical Research, 40 (10), 2032-2046.

Grizzell, J. A.; Mullins, M.; Iarkov, A.; Rohani, A.; Charry, L. C.; Echeverría, V. (2014). Cotinine reduces depressive-like behaviorand hippocampal vascular endothelial growth factor downregulationafter forced swim stress in mice. Behavioral Neuroscience, 128 (6), 713-721.

Gu, R. X.; Zhong, Y. Q.; Wei, D. Q. (2011). Structural basis of agonistselectivity for different nAChR subtypes: insights from crystal structures, mutation experiments and molecular simulations. CurrentPharmaceutical Design, 17 (17), 1652-1662.

Hatsukami, D. K.; Grillo, M.; Pentel, P. R.; Oncken, C.; Bliss, R. (1997).Safety of cotinine in humans: physiologic, subjective, and cognitive effects. Pharmacology, Biochemistry, and Behavior, 57 (4), 643-650.

Hess, G. P. (2003). Rapid chemical reaction techniques developed for usein investigations of membrane-bound proteins (neurotransmitter receptors). Biophysical Chemistry, 100 (1-3), 493-506.

Hess, G. P.; Gameiro, A. M.; Schoenfeld, R. C.; Chen, Y.; Ulrich, H.; Nye, J. A. et al. (2003). Reversing the action of noncompetitive inhibitors (MK-801 and cocaine) on a protein (nicotinic acetylcholinreceptor)-mediated reaction. Biochemistry, 42 (20), 6106-6114.

Hess, G. P.; Ulrich, H.; Breitinger, H. G.; Niu, L.; Gameiro, A. M.Grewer, C. et al. (2000). Mechanism-based discovery of ligands that counteract inhibition of the nicotinic acetylcholine receptor bycocaine and MK-801. Proceedings of the National Academy of Sciences of the United States of America, 97 (25), 13895-13900.

Hogg, R. C.; Bertrand, D. (2004). Nicotinic acetylcholine receptors asdrug targets. Current Drug Targets. CNS and Neurological Disorders, 3 (2), 123-130.

Hucho, F.; Tsetlin, V. I.; Machold, J. (1996). The emerging threedimensionalstructure of a receptor. The nicotinic acetylcholine receptor. European Journal of Biochemistry, 239 (3), 539-557.

Hurst, R.; Rollema, H.; Bertrand, D. (2013). Nicotinic acetylcholinereceptors: from basic science to therapeutics. Pharmacology, Therapeutics, 137 (1), 22-54.

Jackson, D. M.; Johnson, A. W.; Stephenson, M. G. (2002). Survival anddevelopment of Heliothis virescens (Lepidoptera: Noctuidae) larvaeon isogenic tobacco lines with different levels of alkaloids. Journalof Economic Entomology, 95 (6), 1294-1302.

Kane, J. K.; Konu, O.; Ma, J. Z.; Li, M. D. (2004). Nicotine coregulatesmultiple pathways involved in protein modification/degradation inrat brain. Brain Research Molecular Brain Research. 132 (2), 181-191.

Karlin, A.; Akabas, M. H. (1995). Toward a structural basis for thefunction of nicotinic acetylcholine receptors and their cousins.Neuron, 15 (6), 1231-1244.

Katz, B.; Thesleff, S. (1957).Astudy of the desensitization produced byacetylcholine at the motor end-plate. The Journal of Physiology, 138 (1), 63-80.

Kenakin, T. (1997). Molecular pharmacology:Ashort course (1st ed.). Wiley-Blackwell.

Krivoshein, A. V.; Hess, G. P. (2004). Mechanism-based approach to the successful prevention of cocaine inhibition of the neuronal (alpha 3 beta 4) nicotinic acetylcholine receptor. Biochemistry, 43 (2), 481-489.

Lewis, G. N. (1925). A new principle of equilibrium. Proceedings of theNational Academy of Sciences of the United States of America, 11 (3), 179-183.

Magni, P. A.; Pazzi, M.; Vincenti, M.; Alladio, E.; Brandimarte, M.; Dadour, I. R. (2016). Development and validation of a GC-MSmethod for nicotine detection in Calliphora vomitoria (L.) (Diptera:Calliphoridae). Forensic Science International, 261, 53-60.

Massaly, N.; Francès, B.; Mouledous, L. (2014). Roles of the ubiquitinproteasome system in the effects of drugs of abuse. Frontiers in MolecularNeuroscience, 7, 99.

Mendoza, C.; Barreto, G. E.; Iarkov, A.; Tarasov, V. V.; Aliev, G.; Echeverría, V. (2018). Cotinine: a therapy for memory extinction inpost-traumatic stress disorder. Molecular Neurobiology. https://doi.org/10.1007/s12035-018-0869-3.

Mineta, K.; Nakazawa, M.; Cebria, F.; Ikeo, K.; Agata, K.; Gojobori, T. (2003). Origin and evolutionary process of the CNS elucidatedby comparative genomics analysis of planarian ESTs. Proceedingsof the National Academy of Sciences of the United States ofAmerica, 100 (13), 7666-7671.

Moran, V. E. (2012). Cotinine: beyond that expected, more than a biomarkerof tobacco consumption. Frontiers in Pharmacology, 3, 173.

Nakazawa, M.; Cebrià, F.; Mineta, K.; Ikeo, K.; Agata, K.; Gojobori, T. (2003). Search for the evolutionary origin of a brain: planarianbrain characterized by microarray. Molecular Biology and Evolution, 20 (5), 784-791.

Orth, R. G.; Head, G.; Mierkowski, M. (2007). Determining larval hostplant use by a polyphagous lepidopteran through analysis of adultmoths for plant secondary metabolites. Journal of Chemical Ecology, 33 (6), 1131-1148.

Pagán, O. R. (2017). Planaria: an animal model that integrates development, regeneration and pharmacology. The International Journal of Developmental Biology, 61 (8-9), 519-529.

Pagán, O. R.; Deats, S.; Baker, D.; Montgomery, E.; Wilk, G.; Tenaglia, M. et al. (2013). Planarians require an intact brain to behaviorallyreact to cocaine, but not to react to nicotine. Neuroscience, 246, 265-270.

Pagán, O. R.; Montgomery, E.; Deats, S.; Bach, D.; Baker, D. (2015). Evidence of nicotine-induced, curare-insensitive, behavior in planarians. Neurochemical Research, 40 (10), 2087-2090.

Pagán, O. R.; Rowlands, A. L.; Fattore, A. L.; Coudron, T.; Urban, K. R.; Bidja, A. H. et al. (2009). A cembranoid from tobacco prevents theexpression of nicotine-induced withdrawal behavior in planarian worms. European Journal of Pharmacology, 615 (1-3), 118-124.

Pogocki, D.; Ruman, T.; Danilczuk, M.; Celuch, M.; Wałajtys-Rode, E. (2007). Application of nicotine enantiomers, derivativesand analogues in therapy of neurodegenerative disorders. EuropeanJournal of Pharmacology, 563 (1-3), 18-39.

Ramakrishnan, L.; Hess, G. P. (2004). On the mechanism of a mutated and abnormally functioning gamma-aminobutyric acid (A) receptorlinked to epilepsy. Biochemistry, 43 (23), 7534-7540.

Ramakrishnan, L.; Hess, G. P. (2005). Picrotoxin inhibition mechanismof a gamma-aminobutyric acid A receptor investigated by a laserpulsephotolysis technique. Biochemistry, 44 (23), 8523-8532.

Ramakrishnan, L.; Hess, G. P. (2010). Mechanism of potentiation of dysfunctional epilepsy-linked mutated GABA (A) receptor by a neurosteroid (3alpha, 21-dihydroxy-5alpha-pregnan-20-one): Transientkinetic investigations. Biochemistry, 49 (36), 7892-7901.

Rawls, S. M.; Patil, T.; Tallarida, C. S.; Baron, S.; Kim, M.; Song, K.; et al. (2011). Nicotine behavioral pharmacology: clues from planarians. Drug and Alcohol Dependence, 118(2-3), 274-279.

Rezvani, K.; Teng, Y.; Shim, D.; De Biasi, M. (2007). Nicotine regulates multiple synaptic proteins by inhibiting proteasomal activity. The Journal of Neuroscience, 27(39), 10508-10519.

Ricard, J. (1978). Generalized microscopic reversibility, kinetic co-operativity of enzymes and evolution. The Biochemical Journal, 175(3), 779-791.

Robb, S. M.; Gotting, K.; Ross, E.; Sánchez Alvarado, A. (2015). SmedGD 2.0: the Schmidtea mediterranea genome database. Genesis, 53(8), 535-546.

Rollema, H.; Bertrand, D.; Hurst, R. S. (2015). Nicotinic agonists and antagonists. In I. Stolerman, & L. Price (Eds.), Encyclopedia of psychopharmacology. Berlin, Heidelberg: Springer.

Schmeltz, I. (1971). Nicotine and other tobacco alkaloids. In M. Jacobson, & D. G. Crosby (Eds.), Naturally occurring insecticides (pp. 99-136). New York, NY: Marcel Dekker.

Sivaprakasam, K.; Pagán, O. R.; Hess, G. P. (2010). Minimal RNA aptamer sequences that can inhibit or alleviate noncompetitive inhibition of the muscle-type nicotinic acetylcholine receptor. The Journal of Membrane Biology, 233(1-3), 1-12.

Soloway, S. B. (1976). Naturally occurring insecticides. Environmental Health Perspectives, 14, 109-117.

Steppuhn, A.; Gase, K.; Krock, B.; Halitschke, R.; Baldwin, I. T. (2004). Nicotine's defensive function in nature. PLoS Biology, 2(8), E217.

Stolerman, I. P.; Jarvis, M. J. (1995). The scientific case that nicotine is addictive. Psychopharmacology, 117(1), 2-10 (discussion 14-20).

Terry, A. V.; Callahan, P. M.; Hall, B.; Webster, S. J. (2011). Alzheimer's disease and age-related memory decline (preclinical). Pharmacology, Biochemistry, and Behavior, 99(2), 190-210.

Terry, A. V.; Callahan, P. M.; Hernandez, C. M. (2015). Nicotinic ligands as multifunctional agents for the treatment of neuropsychiatric disorders. Biochemical Pharmacology, 97(4), 388-398.

Tolman, R. C. (1925). The principle of microscopic reversibility. Proceedings of the National Academy of Sciences of the United States of America, 11(7), 436-439.

Tsetlin, V.; Hucho, F. (2009). Nicotinic acetylcholine receptors at atomic resolution. Current Opinion in Pharmacology, 9(3), 306-310.

Vainio, P. J.; Törnquist, K.; Tuominen, R. K. (2000). Cotinine and nicotine inhibit each other's calcium responses in bovine chromaffin cells. Toxicology and Applied Pharmacology, 163(2), 183-187.

Vainio, P. J.; Tuominen, R. K. (2001). Cotinine binding to nicotinic acetylcholine receptors in bovine chromaffin cell and rat brain membranes. Nicotine Tobacco Research, 3(2), 177-182.

Vainio, P. J.; Viluksela, M.; Tuominen, R. K. (1998a). Inhibition of nicotinic responses by cotinine in bovine adrenal chromaffin cells. Pharmacology & Toxicology, 83(5), 188-193.

Vainio, P. J.; Viluksela, M.; Tuominen, R. K. (1998b). Nicotine-like effects of cotinine on protein kinase C activity and noradrenaline release in bovine adrenal chromaffin cells. Journal of Autonomic Pharmacology, 18(4), 245-250.

Wu, J.; Lukas, R. J. (2011). Naturally-expressed nicotinic acetylcholine receptor subtypes. Biochemical Pharmacology, 82(8), 800-807.

Zoli, M.; Pistillo, F.; Gotti, C. (2015). Diversity of native nicotinic receptor subtypes in mammalian brain. Neuropharmacology, 96(Pt B), 302-311.

9
烟碱、神经可塑性和烟碱的治疗潜力

Russell W. Brown, W. Drew Gill

Department of Biomedical Sciences, East Tennessee State University, James H. Quillen College of Medicine, Johnson City, TN, United States

缩略语

AD	阿尔茨海默病	**GDNF**	胶质细胞源性神经营养因子
BDNF	脑源性神经营养因子	**nAChR**	烟碱乙酰胆碱受体
CREB	环磷酸腺苷反应元件结合蛋白	**NGF**	神经生长因子
FGF	成纤维细胞生长因子	**PD**	帕金森病

9.1 引言

本综述的重点是探索烟碱对神经可塑性的影响。本文旨在分析烟碱对神经可塑性的两个最终后果：①与烟碱成瘾相关的神经营养因子的增加所起的作用；②神经可塑性蛋白的变化对烟碱和抗神经炎性作用所产生的神经保护作用的可能作用。另一个分析领域将是烟碱对行为的影响，以支持烟碱对神经可塑性的影响。大部分综述将集中在临床前文献上，尽管强调了这项工作的翻译影响。

烟碱（1-甲基-2-[3-吡啶基]吡咯烷）是一种生物碱，是烟草中的主要成分，会产生生理和心理效应，导致烟碱被吸收到血液中，最终导致烟草使用成瘾。1988年，美国卫生局局长提议将烟碱与酒精、鸦片类药物、安非他明和可卡因一起列入成瘾或依赖毒品类别（USPHS,1988）。值得注意的是，烟草使用在被诊断为不同精神障碍的个体中也特别普遍，在精神病患者中，尤其是被诊断为精神分裂症的个体中，烟草滥用的发生率尤其高（Prochaska, Das, Young-Wolff, 2017）。

9.2 烟碱作为神经保护剂

烟碱是一种在对大脑造成伤害的情况下具有潜在优势的药物。烟碱是烟碱乙酰胆碱受体（nAChR）的激动剂，这些受体存在于大脑中大多数小分子神经递质的末端。烟碱已被证明能增加所有这些神经递质的活性（McGehee, Role, 1996）。烟碱可以增强神经元活性的事实可能在其增加神经营养因子蛋白方面发挥了作用，其中许多蛋白是活性依赖的（Mitre, Mariga, Chao, 2017）。烟碱与神经营养因子蛋白的相互作用使研究人员推测，烟碱的这些增加可能是烟碱在脑损伤模型中增强认知能力、减少认知缺陷的基础，也可能是吸烟人群中帕金森病（PD）发病率较低的机制（Mudo, Belluardo, Fuxe, 2007）。换句话说，烟碱与吸烟导致的肺癌有关，单独服用时可能具有治疗潜力，而且在过去的30年里，有足够的证据表明情况可能就是如此。虽然烟碱本身不太可能是一种治疗药物，但在过去的几十年里，有一些非常有趣的发现可能会改变我们对待烟碱及其神经保护潜力的方式。

9.3 烟碱和神经营养因子

有很多研究分析了神经营养因子在神经保护、脑损伤和中风后的功能恢复以及阿尔茨海默病（AD）、PD等神经退行性疾病中的作用。神经营养因子是支持发育和成熟神经元生长、存活、分化和维持的生物分子家族（Koskela et al. 2017）。此外，由于它们的活动依赖释放，神经营养因子非常适合通过在突触前终端的直接作用来增强突触活动，从而改变神经元连接的强度（Tyler, Perrett, Pozzo-Miller, 2002）。神经营养因子与酪氨酸激酶（Trk）受体亚型结合，产生从末端到细胞体的逆行信号，导致细胞整体功能的改变（Friedman, Greene, 1999）。虽然神经营养因子的增加通常被视为一种特定药物在神经保护方面的积极作用，但它也可能是其成瘾特性的潜在机制（Pickens et al. 2011）。一些成瘾的精神刺激剂，包括安非他明、可卡因和甲基苯丙胺，已经被证明可以增加介导成瘾的大脑区域的神经营养因子（Angelucci et al. 2009）。

9.4 烟碱、nAChR及其与神经营养因子的关系

烟碱是烟碱受体的乙酰胆碱能激动剂，并且很容易穿过血脑屏障。在大脑中，同聚α7和异聚α4/β2是数量最多的nAChR（Dineley, Anshul, Yakel, 2015）。已经分离和鉴定了多种nAChR，这些受体具有α（α2～α7、α9和α10）和β（β2～β4）亚基，尽管并非所有受体都包含这两个亚基。构成受体的这些亚基围绕一个中央亲水孔组装，该孔介导钾离子（K^+）、钠离子（Na^+）和钙离子（Ca^{2+}）等阳离子的流动，这些都在神经元传递中起着至关重要的作用。此外，这些亚基以不同的组合组装以产生具有不同电生理特性和大脑定位的各种nAChR亚型（Brown et al. 2017）。然而，在我们实验室的一项研究中，我们在24h时分析了GDNF，并且有证据表明烟碱对GDNF的影响可能是时间锁定的，因为另一项研究报告称，烟碱在给药1h后GDNF会增加（Takarada et al. 2012）。此外，烟碱和/或烟碱激动剂也显示出会增加许多这些神经营养因子的受体表达，包括结合NGF的Trk A和结合BDNF的Trk B。

9.5 烟碱、BDNF和成瘾

关于成瘾，大多数研究的兴趣在于研究BDNF在烟碱的有益方面的作用（Perna, Brown, 2013）。对BDNF的关注可能部分是因为它不仅在大脑区域中普遍存在，而且在其他精神疾病中也起重要作用，其中吸烟是一种常见的共病，包括精神分裂症和重度抑郁症（Jamal, Van der Does, Penninx, 2015）。烟碱和脑区BDNF之间似乎有很强的关系，BDNF介导药物奖励无疑对成瘾行为有影响（Naha, Gandhi, Gautam, Prakash, 2017）。几项研究表明，在正常大鼠给药后72h内，烟碱可增加不同脑区BDNF的表达（Kenny, File, Rattray, 2000）。然而，这些研究大多集中在海马体和前额叶皮层，在我们实验室工作之外，很少有研究分析大脑区域中介导药物成瘾的BDNF。Maggio等（1997）首次证明烟碱增强了背侧纹状体中的BDNF，但这项研究更多的是针

对烟碱在PD与成瘾中潜在的神经保护作用。我们在一系列研究中表明，新生儿喹吡洛（多巴胺D_2受体激动剂）治疗大鼠，在其一生中多巴胺D_2受体敏感性增加，从而在脑组织被破坏时增强伏隔核和海马中的BDNF对烟碱的反应。在最后一次烟碱治疗后24小时进行测定（Brown et al. 2012）。因此，烟碱可以增加脑内多个区域的BDNF。

烟碱和大多数其他神经营养因子在成瘾中的作用的信息很少。然而，已经有几项研究分析了MAPK/ERK通路上神经营养因子的几种下游调节剂，包括环AMP反应元件结合蛋白（CREB）。CREB是一种细胞转录因子，它与称为cAMP反应元件（CRE）的某些DNA序列结合，可增加或减少下游基因的转录。CREB调节多种基因，包括BDNF和酪氨酸羟化酶（去甲肾上腺素和多巴胺生物合成的前体），这可能与烟碱的神经可塑性后果有关。Brunzell、Mineur、Neve和Picciotto（2009）证明烟碱增加了小鼠伏隔核中CREB的活性，表现出烟碱条件性位置偏好（CPP）。重要的是，通过病毒载体实验诱导的伏隔CREB表达下降足以阻断烟碱CPP的表达。另一项研究重复了这种效应，并使用nAChR通用拮抗剂美加明阻断了CPP和CREB的表达（Pascual, Pastor, Bernabeu, 2009）。此外，烟碱已被证明会在行为致敏后增加前额叶皮层中的CREB-ser133（Gomez, Midde, Mactutus, Booze, Zhu, 2012）。从本质上讲，烟碱在已知对成瘾很重要的大脑区域（例如伏隔核和前额叶皮层中的多巴胺末端区域）产生的CREB增加可能是BDNF增加甚至多巴胺水平变化的潜在机制。无论如何，其他神经营养因子可能在烟碱对成瘾的影响中发挥作用，需要更彻底地探索这种研究途径，以更好地了解这些影响。

9.6　动物模型的功能改善：帕金森病

由于烟碱对神经营养因子和突触生成的影响，烟碱对神经保护的作用一直是研究的重点。当然，烟碱改善功能的大部分工作都是在帕金森病中进行的。在过去的20年里，有相当多的流行病学证据一直表明，帕金森病在吸烟者中的患病率低于从不吸烟的人。Maryka Quik博士和他的同事已经证明烟碱和/或nAChR激动剂可以保护黑质纹状体免受损害，这一发现可能有助于解释吸烟导致帕金森病发病率明显下降（Quik, 2004）。基于这些观察，已经有几项研究分析了烟碱是否可能是预防帕金森病风险或可能减缓疾病进展的有前途的药物。这种方法的理论基础是nAChR和纹状体中的多巴胺能系统之间的密切关系。众所周知，nAChRs定位于伏隔核和纹状体的多巴胺能神经元终末。烟碱在这些nAChR中扮演激动剂的角色，增加多巴胺的释放，这最终不仅是对药物成瘾的基础，而且还增加了这些区域的整体神经元活动。在帕金森病的动物模型中，烟碱已被证明能保护1-甲基-4-苯基-1,2,3,6-四氢吡啶（MPTP）引起的纹状体损伤并改善运动功能（Janson, Fuxe, Goldstein, 1992）。此外，研究表明，烟碱可以减少左旋多巴诱导的异常不自主运动，这是左旋多巴治疗帕金森病的一个令人衰弱的并发症（Quik, Bordia, Zhang, Perez, 2015）。这些联合观察表明，nAChR刺激可能代表了一种有效的治疗帕金森病的策略，并减轻了与该疾病相关的行为缺陷。

烟碱作为帕金森病治疗靶点的进一步支持是，这种效应也是剂量依赖性的。Tanner等（2002）发现，在双胞胎中，帕金森病的风险与吸烟量呈负相关。然而，一些作者认为，环境因素"吸烟"与帕金森病之间的联系可能部分是由于帕金森病易感个体的特定个性特征引起的一种附带现象（Evans et al. 2006）。另一方面，支持烟碱可能对帕金森病具有神经保护作用的进一步证据是，烟碱可以上调已被证明可以防止或减缓神经退化的抗凋亡蛋白（Dasgupta et al. 2006），并增加可以防止神经毒性的细胞色素P450酶（Miksys, Tyndale, 2006）。似乎有足够的证据支持烟碱可能对帕金森病有神经保护作用，尽管这些发现存在局限性，特别是涉及α7nAChR激动剂。

9.7 动物模型的功能改善：阿尔茨海默病

自然，介于烟碱在乙酰胆碱能nAChR上的激动剂作用，有相当多的研究重点分析了烟碱是否可以对AD产生类似的神经保护，其中胆碱能激动剂（乙酰胆碱酯酶抑制剂）是一种常见的治疗选择。AD的特点是几个神经病理特征，包括淀粉样蛋白β肽（Aβ）的积累、tau蛋白的细胞内沉积、神经元丢失和显著的突触丢失（Spires-Jones, Attems, Thal, 2017）。使用[^{3}H]-烟碱和[^{3}H]-ACh进行的结合研究表明，AD患者大脑皮层中烟碱和ACh结合位点显著减少，表明nAChR和毒蕈碱乙酰胆碱受体（mAChR）群体均减少（Lombardo, Maskos,2015）。考虑到大量关于ACh在认知中的作用的文献，AD中乙酰胆碱能神经元的退化导致了老年性疾病的"胆碱能假说"的形成（Bartus,Dean,Beer, Lippa,1982;Davies, Maloney,1976），根据该假说，胆碱能神经支配的减少是观察到的AD患者认知功能下降的原因。

一系列研究表明，α7nAChR与淀粉样蛋白β肽共定位（Wang et al. 2000），而α4nAChR亚基则没有显示出这一点。nAChR和Aβ相互作用启动了与神经保护、突触可塑性和认知相关的分子通路（Dineley et al. 2015）。例如，Akt磷酸化介导了抗凋亡通路的下游激活，该通路也可被烟碱治疗激活（Maldifassi et al. 2014）。在离体海马切片制备中，在Aβ$_{1-42}$单体和低聚物的浓度孵育后，观察到海马长期增强（LTP）的增加。LTP是一种与长期记忆储存有关的细胞现象（Kumar, 2011）。研究发现，LTP和细胞内通路的激活是由α7nAChRs的激活介导的（Puzzo et al. 2008）。从功能上讲，体内Aβ注入小鼠背侧海马能够提高对海马依赖的任务的表现，如莫里斯水迷宫和情境恐惧条件反射。有趣的是，Aβ-nAChR的相互作用也被证明可以抑制生存途径，一项研究表明Aβ可以抑制α7nAChR激活的神经保护作用（Liu et al. 2007）。显然，作为AD的一个可能的治疗靶点，这是一个非常复杂的相互作用，值得进一步研究。

9.8 烟碱对脑损伤造成的认知损害的神经保护

烟碱已被证明可以增加大脑区域的神经营养因子，这些神经营养因子介导了由创伤性脑损伤（TBI）或其他神经退行性疾病（特别是海马结构）造成的认知损害。基于这些效应，一直以来的研究重点是分析没有成瘾特性的nAChR激动剂，目的是神经保护（Jurado-Coronel et al. 2016）。重要的是要确定，如果烟碱已经被证明可以增加可能与神经保护有关的神经营养因子，那么就必须确定烟碱也可以减轻与脑损伤相关的行为缺陷。在正常的对照组动物中，烟碱已被证明可以提高没有接受过任何脑损伤和/或创伤的啮齿动物的认知能力。杜克大学的Ed Levin博士和他的同事已经通过多项研究证明，烟碱对胆碱能和谷氨酸能突触的作用似乎介导了它对认知的增强作用（Levin, Bradley, Addy, Sigurani, 2002）。因此，长期以来，单独使用烟碱可以提高认知能力，这导致这种药物有可能减轻创伤性脑损伤的认知损害。

虽然这些增强作用的机制尚未完全阐明，但似乎α7 nAChR是重要的。激活α7 nAChR可以改善老年大鼠的认知能力（Arendash, Sanberg, Sengstock, 1995），而阻断这些受体则会损害认知能力（Levin et al. 2002）。与这些动物研究相一致的是，来自临床研究的最新数据表明，α7 nAChR 部分激动剂 ABT-126 对被诊断为认知障碍的精神分裂症患者的记忆和注意力产生了积极影响（Haig, Bain, Robieson, Baker, Othman, 2016）。临床前，在莫里斯水迷宫上测试的大鼠中，慢性间歇给予烟碱可以减轻穹窿损伤或创伤性脑损伤引起的认知障碍，这是一种主要由海马形态功能介导的空间记忆任务（Brown, Gonzalez, Wishaw, Kolb, 2001; Verbois, Hopkins, Scheff, Pauly, 2003）。Verbois、Scheff 和 Pauly（2003）也报道了烟碱减弱了动物海马中创伤产生的 α7 nAChR 的减少。虽然最近关于 nAChR 在创伤性脑损伤中的作用的研究还不多，但这是一个具有治疗潜力的领域，特别是考虑到烟碱的抗炎特性。

9.9 烟碱和神经炎症

神经炎症在许多疾病中都很常见，不仅包括 AD 和 PD，还包括精神疾病，如精神分裂症、重度抑郁症和双相情感障碍。只有 α7 nAChR 在单核细胞和巨噬细胞中均有表达，这一事实促进了对 α7 nAChR 在小胶质细胞/巨噬细胞活化级联反应中的作用的研究（Wang et al. 2003）。有强有力的证据表明，烟碱和 nAChR 激动剂对 α7 nAChR 的激活降低了小胶质细胞的异常激活，这在神经炎症中非常普遍。由此得出结论，烟碱对小胶质细胞激活的抑制作用一定介导了烟碱的部分神经保护作用（Morioka et al. 2015）。

我们已经了解到，α7 nAChR 的激活在介导抗炎和激活抗凋亡通路方面有很重要的作用。此外，乙酰胆碱能活性的增加会导致几种促炎细胞因子的释放减弱，包括 TNF、IL-1β 和 IL-6（Marrero, Bencherif, 2009）。大脑中由 α7 nAChR 介导的胆碱能抗炎通路的存在，为以神经炎症为特征的神经疾病提供了新的治疗途径。此外，在诊断为 AD 和精神分裂症的患者的海马体结构中发现的 α7 nAChR 存在缺陷（Olincy, Freedman, 2012），导致人们侧重于将 α7 nAChR 作为治疗靶点。然而，这一靶点的缺点是 α7 nAChR 会被其激动剂迅速脱敏，因此对结合没有反应，从而不响应结合。α7 nAChR 的这一特性限制了直接增加乙酰胆碱水平的药物的疗效，如上述的乙酰胆碱酯酶抑制剂和受体激动剂（Williams, Wang, Papke, 2011）。

另一方面，众所周知，不仅 α7 nAChR 被竞争性拮抗剂以及完全和部分激动剂等配体引起的构象变化激活，而且 α7 nAChR 还受到与变构位点结合的变构调节剂的正或负调节（Echeverria, Yarkov, Aliev, 2016）。通过在变构结合位点结合，变构调节剂会改变受体的构象，从而增强受体在功能状态下的表现，在没有正构激动剂的情况下允许更高的自发打开率。此外，α7 nAChR 变构结合位点的调节剂将通过抑制 α7 nAChR 的脱敏状态，提高激动剂在整个激活通道中诱导阳离子（如 Na^+、Ca^{2+}）电流的功效。正变构调节剂（PAM）可以将受体的构象从不可激活状态转换为可激活状态，并且可能有能力规避 α7 nAChR 快速脱敏状态的问题。

9.10 结论

烟碱和 nAChR 激动剂本质上构成了一把通往成瘾和神经保护的双刃剑。然而，烟碱和 nAChR 激动剂可以增加神经营养因子，从而导致突触发生和神经保护。α7 nAChR 作为一个特定的靶点，由于其抗炎特性以及在避免烟碱成瘾特性的同时增强认知能力的潜力，人们似乎对其给予了大量关注。正如Echeverria和他的同事们所提出的那样，由于α7 nAChR独特的脱敏特性，药物研发可能被推向PAMs，这可能导致nAChR成为治疗靶点。

要点总结

- 烟碱和烟碱乙酰胆碱受体（nAChR）激动剂可以增加大脑的神经营养因子。
- 突触发生和突触维持的变化是烟碱成瘾和神经保护特性的基础。
- 烟碱的神经保护特性的最有力证据出现在帕金森病研究领域。
- α7 nAChR的激动剂似乎具有最强的治疗潜力。
- 当分析烟碱神经保护的潜力时，应牢记烟碱的抗炎特性。

参考文献

Angelucci, F.; Ricci, V.; Spalletta, G.; Caltagirone, C.; Mathé, A. A.; Bria, P. (2009). Effects of psychostimulants on neurotrophins implications for psychostimulant-induced neurotoxicity. International Reviews in Neurobiology, 88, 1-24.

Arendash, G. W.; Sanberg, P. R.; Sengstock, G. J. (1995). Nicotine enhances the learning and memory of aged rats. Pharmacology Biochemistry, Behavior, 52, 517-523.

Bartus, R. T.; Dean, R. L.; Beer, B.; Lippa, A. S. (1982). The cholinergic hypothesis of geriatric memory dysfunction. Science, 217, 408-414.

Brown, R. W.; Gonzalez, C. L.; Whishaw, I. Q.; Kolb, B. (2001). Nicotine improvement of Morris water task performance after fimbriafornix lesion is blocked by mecamylamine. Behavioural Brain Research, 119, 185-192.

Brown, R. W.; Kirby, S. L.; Denton, A. R.; Dose, J. M.; Cummins, E. D.; Gill, W. D. et al. (2017). An analysis of the rewarding and aversive associative properties of nicotine in the neonatal quinpirole model: effects on glial cell line-derived neurotrophic factor (GDNF). Schizophrenia Research, 17, 30161-30165.

Brown, R. W.; Maple, A. M.; Perna, M. K.; Sheppard, A. B.; Cope, Z. A.; Kostrzewa, R. M. (2012). Schizophrenia and substance abuse comorbidity: nicotine addiction and the neonatal quinpirole model. Developmental Neuroscience, 34, 140-151.

Brunzell, D. H.; Mineur, Y. S.; Neve, R. L.; Picciotto, M. R. (2009). Nucleus accumbens CREB activity is necessary for nicotine conditioned place preference. Neuropsychopharmacology, 34, 1993-2001.

Dasgupta, P.; Kinkade, R.; Joshi, B.; Decook, C.; Haura, E.; Chellappan, S. (2006). Nicotine inhibits apoptosis induced by chemotherapeutic drugs by up-regulating XIAP and survivin. Proceeding of the National Academy of Science of the United States of America, 103, 6332-6337.

Davies, P.; Maloney, A. J. (1976). Selective loss of central cholinergic neurons in Alzheimer's disease. Lancet, 2, 1403.

Dineley, K. T.; Anshul, A. P.; Yakel, J. L. (2015). Nicotinic ACh receptors as therapeutic targets in CNS disorders. Trends in Pharmacological Sciences, 36(2), 96-108.

Echeverria, V.; Yarkov, A.; Aliev, G. (2016). Positive modulators of the α7 nicotinic receptor against neuroinflammation and cognitive impairment in Alzheimer's disease. Progress in Neurobiology, 144, 142-157.

Evans, A. H.; Lawrence, A. D.; Potts, J.; MacGregor, L.; Katzenschlager, R.; Shaw, K. et al. (2006). Relationship between impulsive sensation seeking traits, smoking, alcohol and caffeine intake, and Parkinson's disease. Journal of Neurology, Neurosurgery and Psychiatry, 77, 317-321.

Friedman, W. J.; Greene, L. A. (1999). Neurotrophin signaling via Trks and p75. Experimental Cell Research, 253, 131-142.

Gomez, A. M.; Midde, N. M.; Mactutus, C. F.; Booze, R. M.; Zhu, J. (2012). Environmental enrichment alters nicotine-mediated locomotor sensitization and phosphorylation of DARPP-32 and CREB in rat prefrontal cortex. PLoS One, 7, e44149.

Haig, G. M.; Bain, E. E.; Robieson, W. Z.; Baker, J. D.; Othman, A. A. (2016). A randomized trial to assess the efficacy and safety of ABT-126, a selectiveα7 nicotinic acetylcholine receptor agonist, in the treatment of cognitive impairment in schizophrenia. American Journal of Psychiatry, 173, 827-835.

Jamal, M.; Van der Does, W.; Penninx, B. W. (2015). Effect of variation in BDNF Val(66)Met polymorphism, smoking, and nicotine dependence on symptom severity of depressive and anxiety disorders. Drug Alcohol Dependence, 1(148), 150-157.

Janson, A. M.; Fuxe, K.; Goldstein, M. (1992). Differential effects of acute and chronic nicotine treatment on MPTP-(1-methyl-4-phenyl-1, 2, 3, 6-tetrahydropyridine) induced degeneration of nigrostriatal dopamine neurons in the black mouse. Clinical Investigations, 70, 232-238.

Jurado-Coronel, J. C.; Avila-Rodriguez, M.; Capani, F.; Gonzalez, J.; Moran, V. E.; Barreto, G. E. (2016). Targeting the nicotinic acetylcholine receptors (nAChRs) in astrocytes as a potential therapeutic target in Parkinson's disease. Current Pharmaceutical Design, 22, 1305-1311.

Kenny, P. J.; File, S. E.; Rattray, M. (2000). Acute nicotine decreases, and chronic nicotine increases the expression of brain-derived neurotrophic factor mRNA in rat hippocampus. Brain Research Molecular Brain Research, 85, 234-238.

Koskela, M.; Bäck, S.; Võikar, V.; Richie, C. T.; Domanskyi, A.; Harvey, B. K. et al. (2017). Update of neurotrophic factors in neurobiology of addiction and future directions. Neurobiology, 97(Pt B), 189-200.

Kumar, A. (2011). Long-term potentiation at CA3-CA1 hippocampal synapses with special emphasis on aging, disease, and stress. Frontiers in Aging Neuroscience, 3, 7-11.

Levin, E. D.; Bradley, A.; Addy, N.; Sigurani, N. (2002). Hippocampal alpha 7 and alpha 4 beta 2 nicotinic receptors and working memory. Neuroscience, 109, 757-765.

Liu, Q.; Zhang, J.; Zhu, H.; Qin, C.; Chen, Q.; Zhao, B. (2007). Dissecting the signaling pathway of nicotine-mediated neuroprotection in a mouse Alzheimer disease model. FASEB Journal, 21, 61-73.

Lombardo, S.; Maskos, U. (2015). Role of the nicotinic acetylcholine receptor in Alzheimer's disease pathology and treatment. Neuropharmacology, 96(Pt B), 255-262.

Maggio, R.; Riva, M.; Vaglini, F.; Fornai, F.; Racagni, G.; Corsini, G. U(1997). Striatal increase of neurotrophic factors as a mechanism of nicotine protection in experimental parkinsonism. Journal of Neural Transmission, 104, 1113-1123.

Maldifassi, M. C.; Atienza, G.; Arnalich, F.; López-Collazo, E.; Cedillo, J. L.; Martín-Sánchez, C. et al. (2014). A new IRAK-M-mediated mechanism implicated in the anti-inflammatory effect of nicotine viaα7 nicotinic receptors in human macrophages. PLoS One, 9(9), e108397.

Marrero, M. B.; Bencherif, M. (2009). Convergence of alpha 7 nicotinic acetylcholine receptor-activated pathways for anti-apoptosis and anti-inflammation: central role for JAK2 activation of STAT3 and NF-kappaB. Brain Research, 1256, 1-7.

McGehee, D. S.; Role, L. W. (1996). Neurobiology: memories of nicotine. Nature, 383, 670-671.

Miksys, S.; Tyndale, R. F. (2006). Nicotine induces brain CYP enzymes: relevance to Parkinson's disease. Journal of Neural Transmission, 70, 177-180.

Mitre, M.; Mariga, A.; Chao, M. V. (2017). Neurotrophin signalling: novel insights into mechanisms and pathophysiology. Clinical Science, 131, 13-23.

Morioka, N.; Harano, S.; Tokuhara, M.; Idenoshita, Y.; Zhang, F. F.; Hisaoka-Nakashima, K. et al. (2015). Stimulation of α7 nicotinic acetylcholine receptor regulates glutamate transporter GLAST via basic fibroblast growth factor production in cultured cortical microglia. Brain Research, 1625, 111-120.

Mudo, G.; Belluardo, N.; Fuxe, K. (2007). Nicotinic receptor agonists as neuroprotective/neurotrophic drugs. Progress in molecular mechanisms. Journal of Neural Transmission, 114, 135-147.

Naha, N.; Gandhi, D. N.; Gautam, A. K.; Prakash, J. R. (2017). Nicotine and cigarette smoke modulate Nrf2-BDNF-dopaminergic signal and neurobehavioral disorders in adult rat cerebral cortex. Human Experimental Toxicology 37, 540-566.

Olincy, A.; Freedman, R. (2012). Nicotinic mechanisms in the treatment of psychotic disorders: a focus on theα7 nicotinic receptor. Handbook of Experimental Pharmacology, 213, 211-232.

Pascual, M. M.; Pastor, V.; Bernabeu, R. O. (2009). Nicotineconditioned place preference induced CREB phosphorylation and Fos expression in the adult rat brain. Psychopharmacology, 207, 57-71.

Perna, M. K.; Brown, R. W. (2013). Adolescent nicotine sensitization and effects of nicotine on accumbal dopamine release in a rodent model of increased dopamine D2 receptor sensitivity. Behavioural Brain Research, 242, 102-109.

Pickens, C. L.; Airavaara, M.; Theberge, F.; Fanous, S.; Hope, B. T.; Shaham, Y. (2011). Neurobiology of the incubation of drug craving. Trends in Neuroscience, 34, 411-420.

Prochaska, J. J.; Das, S.; Young-Wolff, K. C. (2017). Smoking, mental Illness, and public Health. Annual Review of Public Health, 38, 165-185.

Puzzo, D.; Privitera, L.; Leznik, E.; Fà, M.; Staniszewski, A.; Palmeri, A. et al. (2008). Picomolar amyloid-βpositively modulates synaptic plasticity and memory in hippocampus. Journal of Neuroscience, 28, 14537-14545.

Quik, M. (2004). Smoking, nicotine and Parkinson's disease. Trends in Neuroscience, 27, 561-568.

Quik, M.; Bordia, T.; Zhang, D.; Perez, X. A. (2015). Nicotine and nicotinic receptor drugs: potential for Parkinson's disease and druginduced movement disorders. International Review of Neurobiology, 124, 247-271.

Spires-Jones, T. L.; Attems, J.; Thal, D. R. (2017). Interactions of pathological proteins in neurodegenerative diseases. Acta Neuropathology, 134, 187-205.

Takarada, T.; Nakamichi, N.; Kawagoe, H.; Ogura, M.; Fukumori, R.; Nakazato, R. et al. (2012). Possible neuroprotective property of nicotinic acetylcholine receptors in association with predominant upregulation of glial cell line-derived neurotrophic factor in astrocytes. Journal of Neuroscience Research, 90, 2074-2085.

Tanner, C. M.; Goldman, S. M.; Aston, D. A.; Ottman, R.; Ellenberg, J.; Mayeux, R. et al. (2002). Smoking and Parkinson's disease in twins. Neurology, 58, 581-588.

Tyler, W. J.; Perrett, S. P.; Pozzo-Miller, L. D. (2002). The role of neurotrophins in neurotransmitter release. Neuroscientist, 8, 524-531.

United States Department of Health and Human Services. (1988). The Health Consequences of Smoking: A Report of the Surgeon General (pp. 1-643). United States Department of Health and Human Services.

Verbois, S. L.; Hopkins, D. M.; Scheff, S. W.; Pauly, J. R. (2003). Chronic intermittent nicotine administration attenuates traumatic brain injury-induced cognitive dysfunction. Neuroscience, 119, 1199-1208.

Verbois, S. L.; Scheff, S. W.; Pauly, J. R. (2003). Chronic nicotine treatment attenuates alpha 7 nicotinic receptor deficits following traumatic brain injury. Neuropharmacology, 44, 224-233.

Wang, H. -Y.; Lee, D. H. S.; D'Andrea, M. R.; Peterson, P. A.; Shank, R. P.; Reitz, A. B. (2000). β-Amyloid1-42 binds toα7 nicotinic acetylcholine receptor with high affinity implications for Alzheimer's disease pathology. Journal of Biological Chemistry, 275, 5626-5632.

Wang, H.; Yu, M.; Ochani, M.; Amella, C. A.; Tanovic, M.; Susarla, S. et al. (2003). Nicotinic acetylcholine receptor alpha7 subunit is an essential regulator of inflammation. Nature, 421, 384-388.

Williams, D. K.; Wang, J.; Papke, R. L. (2011). Positive allosteric modulators as an approach to nicotinic acetylcholine receptor-targeted therapeutics: advantages and limitations. Biochemical Pharmacology, 82, 915-930.

10
缰状突触和烟碱

Jessica L. Ables[1], *Beatriz Antolin-Fontes*[2], *Ines Ibañez-Tallon*[3]

1. Department of Psychiatry, The Icahn School of Medicine at Mount Sinai, New York, NY, United States
2. Faculty of Medicine, Imperial College London, Hammersmith Hospital Campus, London, United Kingdom
3. Laboratory of Molecular Biology, The Rockefeller University, New York, NY, United States

缩略语

3V	第三脑室	LDTg	被盖背外侧核
4V	第四脑室	LHb	外侧缰核
ACh	乙酰胆碱	LV	侧脑室
AP	动作电位	MHb	内侧缰核
BAC	细菌人工染色体	MHbD	内侧缰核背侧
ChAT	胆碱乙酰转移酶	MHbS	内侧缰核上
cKO	条件性敲除	MHbV	内侧缰核腹侧
CPA	条件性位置厌恶	MHbVc	内侧缰核腹中区
DR	中缝背核	MHbVl	内侧缰核腹外侧
DTg	背侧被盖核	MHbVm	内侧缰核腹内侧
EC	内嗅皮层	MnR	中缝
EPSP	兴奋性突触后电位	MS	内侧隔
FR	反折束	nAChR	烟碱乙酰胆碱受体
GWAS	全基因组关联研究	NDB	对角带核
Hb-IPN	缰核脚间	NI	不确定核
HC	海马	OPRM	μ-阿片受体
HCN	超极化激活环核苷酸门控	PAG	中脑导水管周围灰质
Hyp	下丘脑	sEPSC	自发兴奋性突触后电流
IL-18	白介素18	SFi	隔伞核
IPA	脚间核尖	SNP	单核苷酸多态性
IPC	脚间核中央	SP	物质P
IPDL	脚间核背外侧	SV	突触小泡
IPDM	脚间核背中线	Thal	丘脑
IPI	脚间核中间	TRAP	翻译核糖体亲和纯化
IPL	脚间外侧核	TS	三角隔
IPN	喙间核	VACHT	囊泡乙酰胆碱转运体
IPR	脚间核	VGLUT	囊泡谷氨酸转运体
KCC2 K^+/Cl^-	共转运蛋白2	VTA	腹侧被盖区
LC	位点蓝斑		

10.1 引言

人类全基因组关联研究（GWAS）已经证实，遗传因素参与了药物成瘾的发展。2008年，有两项研究报道，编码α3β4α5烟碱受体的基因簇CHRNA3-B4-A5的变异与肺癌疾病易感性有关（Hung et al. 2008），并与烟碱依赖型肺癌和外周疾病相关（Thorgeirsson et al. 2008）。这是一个值得注意的发现，因为虽然α4β2和α7 nAChR是存在于大脑和外周的主要烟碱受体亚型，但GWAS并没有将这些基因与烟碱滥用联系起来。相反，他们指出，α3β4α5 nAChR亚型在MHb-IPN中高度富集，对于烟碱依赖的获得和戒烟困难是至关重要的。许多研究小组在不同的人群中复制了这些GWAS（Bierut, 2010; Bierut et al. 2008; Liu et al. 2010），最近对啮齿类动物的研究揭示了其分子机制（Fowler, Lu, Johnson, Marks, Kenny, 2011; Frahm et al. 2011）。这些研究重新唤起了人们对这一古老大脑结构的兴趣，并导致了人们对理解这一回路及其对成瘾的意义的重大努力（Antolin-Fontes, Ables, Gorlich, Ibanez-Tallon, 2015）。在本章中，我们将讨论目前对MHb的理解及其在烟碱依赖中的作用。

10.2 缰核：一个高度保守的回路

缰核是上丘脑中的一对结构，在脊椎动物中高度保守，将新皮层和边缘前脑中参与执行功能的最近进化的结构与中脑和后脑中处理睡眠、疼痛和奖励的古老区域连接起来（Antolin-Fontes et al. 2015; Boulos, Darcq, Kieffer, 2017）。虽然所有脊椎动物都有缰核，但哺乳动物和低等脊椎动物在靶结构和组织方面是有区别的。鱼类、爬行动物和鸟类的缰骨的左右两侧是不对称的，而哺乳动物的缰骨基本上是对称的。在鱼类和两栖动物中，缰核被组织成背核和腹核，这两个核都通过反折束（FR）投射到IPN，它们都与哺乳动物的MHb同源，而鱼类中是否存在哺乳动物外侧缰核（LHb）的同源物则尚不清楚。在两栖动物中，腹侧缰核似乎相当于高等脊椎动物的LHb（Aizawa, Amo, Okamoto, 2011）。爬行动物、鸟类和哺乳动物既有围绕IPN投射到更多嘴部结构的LHb，包括腹侧被盖区（VTA）、被盖嘴内侧（RMTg）以及中缝正中核和中缝背核，也有MHb投射到IPN，后者进而投射到中缝、被盖背外侧核（LDTg）和终核。LHb和MHb都通过正中前脑束接受来自隔膜、前额叶皮层和下丘脑的输入，尽管每个核的输入不同（有关连接的详细综述，请参见 Boulos et al. 2017）。因此，缰核处于战略位置，以调节多巴胺能、5-羟色胺能和肾上腺素能张力，以响应来自更高结构的输入，并将皮层决策与奖励和外部刺激相结合（图10.1）。

事实上，一些动物研究已经证明了缰核在精神疾病和药物成瘾中的作用。在动物模型中的研究表明，在长期服用烟碱和可卡因后，受体发生退化，并且退化分别发生在MHb或LHb神经元，这表明缰核可能是大脑的一个"薄弱环节"，特别容易受到药物滥用的影响（Ciani, Severi, Bartesaghi, Contestabile, 2005）。在更多的功能水平上，LHb和MHb都被发现在戒断的表达中发挥作用，这与它们在厌恶刺激中的激活是一致的。戒掉可卡因或烟碱会分别增加LHb或MHb的活性（Ciani et al. 2005）。依赖于MHb的IPN的激活对于烟碱戒断的行为表达是必要的，相反，抑制IPN的活性会减弱烟碱戒断（Zhao-Shea, Liu, Pang, Gardner, Tapper, 2013）。在接下来的章节中，我们将更详细地讨论MHb-IPN通路在烟碱成瘾中的作用，这在很大程度上是由于它高表达多种nAChR。

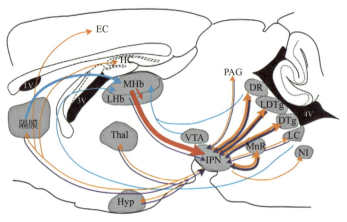

图 10.1 MHb-IPN 连接

小鼠大脑矢状面示意图，显示 MHb 传入（蓝色）、MHb 传出（红色）、IPN 传入（紫色）和 IPN 传出（橙色）。箭头的粗细反映了连接的强度。图片来自 Antolin-Fontes 等（2015），神经药理学，经出版商许可。

10.3 MHb-IPN 中的烟碱乙酰胆碱受体多样性

MHb-IPN 回路在哺乳动物的大脑中表达最高密度的 nAChR（Le Novere, Zoli, Changeux, 1996; Marks et al. 1992; Yeh et al. 2001）。除 α9 和 α10 外，所有已知的神经元 nAChR 亚基均存在于 MHb-IPN 中。α3 和 β4 nAChR 亚基在整个腹侧 MHb 和 IPN 中高度富集（Gorlich et al. 2013; Quick, Ceballos, Kasten, McIntosh, Lester, 1999; Salas, Pieri, Fung, Dani, De Biasi, 2003; Sheffield, Quick, Lester, 2000; Shih et al. 2014），而 α4、α6、β2、和 β3 亚基选择性地存在于腹侧 MHb 的某些亚基中（Shih et al. 2014）。具体地说，α4 亚基定位于 vMHb 的外侧（Fonck et al. 2009; Nashmi et al. 2007; Shih et al. 2014），α6 亚基主要位于 vMHb 的下部，β2 和 β3 亚基位于 vMHb 的中心和下部（Shih et al. 2014）。辅助 α5 亚基不仅在 MHb 和 IPN 中与 α3β4* 结合组装，而且还可以掺入 α4β2* 复合物中，并在 IPN 中强表达（图 10.2）。

与人类 GWAS 一致，动物模型的累积证据表明，在 MHb-IPN 中表达的 α3、β4 和 α5 nAChR 是烟碱摄取和烟碱戒断的关键调节因子（Fowler et al. 2011; Frahm et al. 2011; Salas, Sturm, Boulter, De Biasi, 2009）。利用在内源性位点过表达 β4 nAChR 亚基的转基因小鼠，发现了 β4 在烟碱厌恶中的关键作用。这些被称为 Tabac 小鼠的小鼠对烟碱的敏感度增强，消耗减少（Frahm et al. 2011）。β4 的表达具有速率限制性，并与 α5 竞争形成五聚体 α3β4α5 nAChR（Frahm et al. 2011; Slimak et al. 2014）。因此，过表达 β4 导致 α3β4* 受体数量增加，并在体外和体内增强 α3β4* 电流（Frahm et al. 2011）。β4 增加烟碱诱发电流的能力取决于位于受体细胞内前庭的独特的单一残基 S435（Frahm et al. 2011）（图 10.3）。序列比对发现了细胞内前庭的其他 SNP 映射，其中之一是与人类烟碱依赖高风险相关的最常见的多态性，即 CHRNA5 中的 rs16969968（Bierut et al. 2008）。对 α5 亚基的这一单核苷酸多态性功能 [导致天冬氨酸被天冬氨酸取代为天冬酰胺（D398N）] 的分析表明，烟碱诱发的电流显著减少。在行为上，这种非同义变体有深远的影响：在过表达 β4 的 Tabac 小鼠中观察到的烟碱厌恶情绪在病毒介导的 MHb 中 α5 D398N 变体的表达后被逆转（Frahm et al. 2011）（图 10.3）。

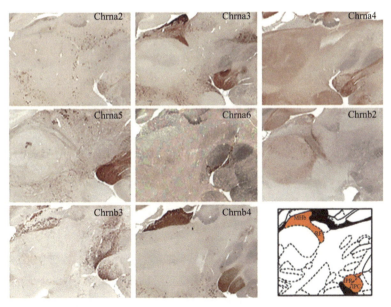

图 10.2　nAChR 亚基在 MHb-IPN 中表达

在 BAC 转基因小鼠（Gensat.org）中，大麻素和 IPN 在相应的基因调控区域下的矢状面切片图中显示了 MHb 和 IPN 区域。在获得 GENSAT 许可的情况下使用。Chrn 表示致病基因定位分析整体图。

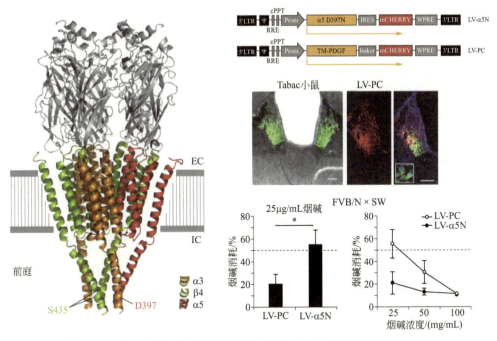

图 10.3　Tabac 小鼠对烟碱的厌恶情绪被 MHb 中 α5 D397N 变体的表达逆转

（左）$α3_2β4_2α5_1$ nAChR 模型显示了 α3（橙色）、α5（红色）和 β4（绿色）亚基的跨膜和胞内结构域，以及 β4 中的特定残基 S435 和 α5 中的 D397，这是与重度吸烟有关的最常见的变异。（右）用于注射 Tabac 小鼠 MHb 的慢病毒（LV）结构。Tabac 小鼠的 eGFP 荧光与注射小鼠的 LV 对照（LV-PC）或表达 α5 D397N 基因变异的 LV（LV-α5N）的 mCherry 荧光共定位。与注射 LV-PC 的 Tabac 小鼠相比，注射 LV-α5N 的 Tabac 小鼠不再表现出烟碱厌恶。经出版商许可，由 Frahm 等（2011），Neuron 修改而成。

在缺乏 α5 亚基的动物中观察到的表型支持 α5 nAChR 亚基在烟碱厌恶中的作用。这些小鼠继续以通常在野生型动物中引起厌恶的剂量进行烟碱自给药，当 α5 nAChR 亚基在 MHb 或 IPN 中重新表达时，烟碱自给药又回到了野生型水平。此外，病毒介导的MHb-IPN回路中α5 nAChR亚基的敲除并没有改变低剂量烟碱的奖励增强特性，但显著降低了高剂量烟碱在大鼠体内的厌恶效应（Fowler et al. 2011）。

α3β4*或α3β4α5 nAChR对烟碱的亲和力低于α4β2受体，在吸烟者中发现的烟碱水平的脱敏程度可能低于α4β2 nAChR，因为它们保持了对吸烟者烟碱水平波动的敏感性（Rose et al. 2007）。这与α3、β4和α5亚基在烟碱厌恶中的作用一起，产生了一个模型，在该模型中，烟碱奖励和烟碱厌恶是由不同的回路介导的（Fowler, Kenny, 2014）：低剂量的烟碱会激活中伏隔核通路中高亲和力的α4α6β2β3* nAChR亚型（Grady et al. 2007），而高剂量的烟碱激活亲和力较低的α3β4*或α5* nAChR，从而导致厌恶（Fowler, Kenny, 2014）。

除烟碱厌恶外，位于MHb-IPN回路中的β4和α5 nAChR均与烟碱戒断的生理症状有关。β4或α5亚基缺失的小鼠在长期服用烟碱和减弱戒断诱导的痛觉过敏后有较少的躯体戒断迹象（Jackson, Martin, Changeux, Damaj, 2008; Salas et al. 2009; Salas, Pieri, De Biasi, 2004）。烟碱戒断的表现在α2、β2和β6亚基缺失的小鼠中也发生了改变（Jackson et al. 2008; Lotfipour et al. 2013），这些亚基也存在于MHb-IPN轴中（Shih et al. 2014）。

10.4 缰核神经元的电生理学

缰核神经元的解剖学和电生理特性是非常独特的。在MHb中，有两个不同的种群：腹侧MHb的胆碱能种群投射到吻侧（IPR）、中间（IPI）和中央（IPC）亚核，背侧MHb的肽能（P物质阳性）种群投射到IPN（IPL）的外侧部分（图10.4）。这两种类型的投射都释放谷氨酸，但胆碱能群体也共释放乙酰胆碱，最近一项里程碑式的研究证明了这一点，该研究使用通道视紫红质-2转基因小鼠研究蓝光刺激下的突触传递。短暂刺激MHb传出引起谷氨酸能而不是胆碱能反应，而强直刺激需要产生由nAChR介导的缓慢内向电流，从而确立缰核神经元使用两种传递模式：谷氨酸的有线传递和ACh的体积传递（Ren et al. 2011）。

与这种共释放一致，通过共聚焦显微镜（图10.4）、免疫沉淀分析（Frahm et al. 2015; Ren et al. 2011）和电子显微镜（Frahm et al. 2015），在IPN的相同MHb末端发现了ACh（VACHT）和谷氨酸（VGLUT1/2）的囊泡转运蛋白。值得注意的是，在同一缰核末端，这两种转运蛋白也一起出现在相同的突触小泡中（Frahm et al. 2015）（图10.5）。

两种神经递质的共同释放在神经系统中并不少见（有关综述请参见El Mestikawy, Wallen-Mackenzie, Fortin, Descarries, Trudeau, 2011; Hnasko, Edwards, 2012），并允许对单个突触的兴奋性-抑制性平衡进行精确的局部控制（Shabel, Proulx, Piriz, Malinow, 2014）。ChAT-cKO小鼠MHb神经元ACh的局部消除降低了IPN神经元的谷氨酸能微型兴奋性突触后电位（mEPSCs）的幅度，因为在缺乏ACh的情况下，VACHT不再能促进谷氨酸通过VGLUT1/2进入囊泡，从而降低了谷氨酸的囊泡含量。在其他突触中也观察到了囊泡协同作用，例如纹状体突触小泡、胆碱能基底前脑神经元和脊髓运动神经元（El Mestikawy et al. 2011; Hnasko, Edwards, 2012）。因此，ACh和谷氨酸的共传递可能被认为是规则而不是例外，这提出了一个关于协同递质释放和神经递质协同在胆碱能突触中的作用的基本问题，并表明这些递质的囊泡协同作用一定增加了适应优势。除了缰核神经元在胞体中含有高浓度的突触后nAChR外（Frahm et al. 2011; Gorlich et al. 2013），大脑中存在的大多数nAChR都是突触前的，以促进谷氨酸的释放（Girod, Role, 2001; McGehee, Heath, Gelber, Devay, Role, 1995）。这种突触前易化也发生在Hb-IPN中，因为MHb神经元也沿着它们到IPN的轴突投射表达特别高水平的nAChR（表10.1和表10.2）。

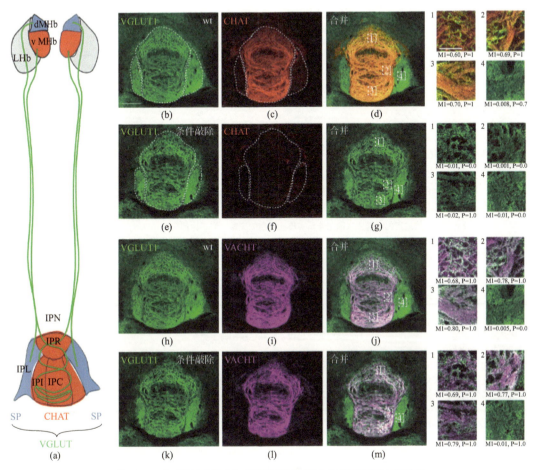

图10.4 胆碱能轴突终末和谷氨酸能轴突终末在IPN亚核中的分布

（a）MHb神经元向IPN亚核的分离投射示意图。MHb背侧（蓝色）的肽能（物质P，SP）神经元投射到外侧IPN（IPL，蓝色）。腹侧MHb（vMHb，红色）的胆碱能（ChAT阳性）神经元投射到IPN的脚间核（IPR）、脚间核中间（IPI）和中央亚核（IPC）（红色）。这两种类型的投射共同释放谷氨酸（VGLUT，绿色）。（b）～（m）IPN不同亚核谷氨酸能和胆碱能标记物的双重免疫染色和Manders'共存系数分析。该图取自Frahm等（2015），eLife，经出版商许可。

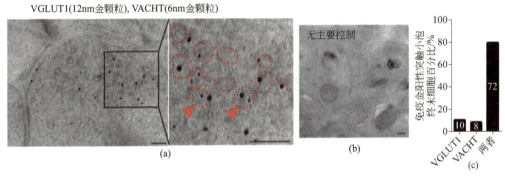

图10.5

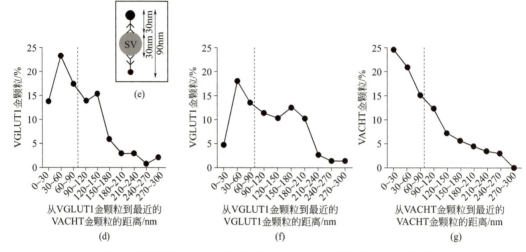

图10.5　VACHT 和 VGLUT1 共定位于中央 IPN 轴突终末的相同突触小泡中

（a）和（b）免疫金电镜观察谷氨酸（VGLUT，12nm 金颗粒）和乙酰胆碱（VACHT，6nm 金颗粒）的囊泡转运蛋白在同一缰核突触小泡（SV，红色部分）的共定位。箭头表示包含两种转运蛋白的突触小泡。比例尺，100nm。（c）仅 VGLUT1 和/或 VACHT 囊泡转运蛋白 SV 阳性的轴突终末百分比。（d）、（f）和（g）免疫金颗粒之间距离分布的频率直方图。（e）根据 SV 和结合抗体的大小，两个免疫金颗粒之间潜在标记同一突触小泡的最大距离为 90nm。该图取自 Frahm 等（2015），eLife，经出版商许可。

表10.1　缰核-IPN 回路的关键事实

- 缰核-IPN 回路在所有脊椎动物中都是保守的
- 缰核的主要功能是连接前脑和后脑，调节大脑中的多巴胺、5-羟色胺和肾上腺素
- 缰核的主要输出轨迹称为反屈束
- 缰核可分为外侧核和内侧核。外侧缰核投射到 VTA、中缝和其他中脑核，而内侧缰核的主要目标是脚间核
- 来自外侧缰核的纤维被分离到反屈束的外侧，而来自内侧缰核的纤维形成核心
- 内侧缰核由肽能、胆碱能和谷氨酸能神经元组成，外侧缰核由谷氨酸能和 GABA 能神经元组成

注：本表列出了缰核-IPN 回路的关键事实，包括其一般功能和解剖结构。

表10.2　MHb-IPN 中 nAChR 的关键事实

- MHb 和 IPN 一起表达哺乳动物大脑中 nAChR 的最高密度
- nAChR 高度富集于 MHb-IPN 束的三个部分：MHb 神经元胞体、IPN 内 MHb 神经元突触前终末和突触后 IPN 神经元。
- 在 MHb 和 IPN 中主要表达的 nAChR 亚基是 α3、β4 和 α5
- α5 和 α4 nAChR 亚基介导对烟碱摄取和戒断的厌恶反应
- 突触前 nAChRs 促进 MHb 终末释放谷氨酸

注：本表列出了 MHb-IPN 束的 nAChRs 的关键事实，包括在 MHb 和 IPN 神经元中表达的主要亚基及其定位和在烟碱厌恶中的作用。

术语解释

- 成瘾：人类吸毒的一种行为模式，其特征是缺乏对摄取或强制使用的控制，不断增加使用，产生耐受性，并不顾不良后果使用。成瘾通常与食用有问题的物质后的内疚有关，而不是一种获得感。成瘾是反复使用某种物质的结果，被认为是大脑回路中神经适应性变化的结果。
- 共同传递：当神经元在刺激时释放两种不同的神经递质时的传递。在大多数情况下，共同传递需要两个不同的囊泡神经递质转运蛋白在同一末端共存。如果两个转运蛋白都在同一个突触小泡中，它们就可以协同将这两种神经递质填满囊泡，这一过程被称为囊泡协同作用。

术语解释

- **GWAS**：全基因组关联研究寻找在人类群体中发现的遗传变异（单核苷酸多态性）与特定性状或疾病之间的关联。

- **缰核-脚间环路**：脊椎动物上丘脑中保守的脑结构，其特点是缰核内高密度的神经元通过反屈束将轴突投射发送到脚间核。缰绳源于拉丁语中的"缰绳"，意为"鞭子"或"缰绳"，因为反屈束有明显的长突起。脚间核是指位于大脑脚之间的核。

- **突触前易化**：通过位于突触前的受体促进神经递质的释放。大脑中的nAChRs大多是突触前的，它们通过ACh的体积传递激活，促进了突触前的钙内流，进而促进了神经递质的释放。

- **戒断**：突然停止使用一种长期使用的物质时身体和/或心理症状的经历。戒断不是成瘾的同义词，在没有成瘾的情况下可能会发生。戒断是长期使用时发生的神经适应性变化的结果，在没有这种物质的情况下，这种变化是不适应的。

要点总结

- 缰核-脚间环路在表达对高剂量烟碱的厌恶和对烟碱戒断的负面体验中起作用。
- 缰核-脚间环路表达广泛的烟碱乙酰胆碱受体亚基，包括与烟碱成瘾有关的亚基。
- 慢性烟碱暴露、戒断烟碱和再次暴露烟碱会改变缰核的基线放电速率。
- 乙酰胆碱和谷氨酸由缰核胆碱能神经元共同释放。
- 在胆碱能MHb末端可以观察到谷氨酸和乙酰胆碱之间的囊泡协同作用。
- MHB终末释放ACh是nAChR介导的突触前易化所必需的。

参考文献

Aizawa, H.; Amo, R.; Okamoto, H. (2011). Phylogeny and ontogeny of he habenular structure. Frontiers in Neuroscience, 5, 138.

Antolin-Fontes, B.; Ables, J. L.; Gorlich, A.; Ibanez-Tallon, I. (2015). he habenulo-interpeduncular pathway in nicotine aversion and ithdrawal. Neuropharmacology, 96(Pt B), 213-222.

Bierut, L. J. (2010). Convergence of genetic findings for nicotine depen dence and smoking related diseases with chromosome 15q24-25. Trends in Pharmacological Sciences, 31(1), 46-51.

Bierut, L. J.; Stitzel, J. A.; Wang, J. C.; Hinrichs, A. L.; Grucza, R. A.; uei, X. et al. (2008). Variants in nicotinic receptors and risk for nic otine dependence. The American Journal of Psychiatry, 165(9), 1163-1171.

Boulos, L. J.; Darcq, E.; Kieffer, B. L. (2017). Translating the Habenula from rodents to humans. Biological Psychiatry, 81(4), 296-305.

Ciani, E.; Severi, S.; Bartesaghi, R.; Contestabile, A. (2005). Neuro chemical correlates of nicotine neurotoxicity on rat habenulo interpeduncular cholinergic neurons. Neurotoxicology, 26(3), 67-474.

El Mestikawy, S.; Wallen-Mackenzie, A.; Fortin, G. M.; Descarries, L.; Trudeau, L. E. (2011). From glutamate co-release to vesicular synergy: vesicular glutamate transporters. Nature Reviews Neuroscience, 2(4), 204-216.

Fonck, C.; Nashmi, R.; Salas, R.; Zhou, C.; Huang, Q.; De Biasi, M. et al. (2009). Demonstration of functional alpha4-containing icotinic receptors in the medial habenula. Neuropharmacology, 56(1), 247-253.

Fowler, C. D.; Kenny, P. J. (2014). Nicotine aversion: neurobiological echanisms and relevance to tobacco dependence vulnerability. europharmacology, 76(Pt B), 533-544.

Fowler, C. D.; Lu, Q.; Johnson, P. M.; Marks, M. J.; Kenny, P. J. (2011). Habenular alpha5 nicotinic receptor subunit signalling controls nic otine intake. Nature, 471(7340), 597-601.

Frahm, S.; Antolin-Fontes, B.; Gorlich, A.; Zander, J. F.; Ahnert Hilger, G.; Ibanez-Tallon, I. (2015). An essential role of cetylcholine-glutamate synergy at habenular synapses in nicotine dependence. eLife, 4, e11396.

Frahm, S.; Slimak, M. A.; Ferrarese, L.; Santos-Torres, J.; Antolin Fontes, B.; Auer, S. et al. (2011). Aversion to nicotine is regulatedby the balanced activity of beta4 and alpha5 nicotinic receptor sub units in the medial habenula. Neuron, 70(3), 522-535.

Girod, R.; Role, L. W. (2001). Long-lasting enhancement of glutama tergic synaptic transmission by acetylcholine contrasts withresponse adaptation after exposure to low-level nicotine. The Journal of Neuroscience, 21(14), 5182-5190.

Gorlich, A.; Antolin-Fontes, B.; Ables, J. L.; Frahm, S.; Slimak, M. A.; Dougherty, J. D. et al. (2013). Reexposure to nicotine during with drawal increases the pacemaking activity of cholinergic habenular neurons. Proceedings of the National Academy of Sciences of the United States of America, 110(42), 17077-17082.

Grady, S. R.; Salminen, O.; Laverty, D. C.; Whiteaker, P.; McIntosh, J. M.; Collins, A. C. et al. (2007). The subtypes of nicotinic acetylcholine receptors on dopaminergic terminals of mouse striatum. Biochemical Pharmacology, 74(8), 1235-1246.

Hnasko, T. S.; Edwards, R. H. (2012). Neurotransmitter corelease: mechanism and physiological role. Annual Review of Physiology, 74, 225-243.

Hung, R. J.; McKay, J. D.; Gaborieau, V.; Boffetta, P.; Hashibe, M.; Zaridze, D. et al. (2008). A susceptibility locus for lung cancer maps to nicotinic acetylcholine receptor subunit genes on 15q25. Nature, 452(7187), 633-637.

Jackson, K. J.; Martin, B. R.; Changeux, J. P.; Damaj, M. I. (2008). Differential role of nicotinic acetylcholine receptor subunits in physical and affective nicotine withdrawal signs. The Journal of Pharmacology and Experimental Therapeutics, 325(1), 302-312.

Le Novere, N.; Zoli, M.; Changeux, J. P. (1996). Neuronal nicotinic receptor alpha 6 subunit mRNA is selectively concentrated in cate cholaminergic nuclei of the rat brain. The European Journal of Neuro science, 8(11), 2428-2439.

Liu, J. Z.; Tozzi, F.; Waterworth, D. M.; Pillai, S. G.; Muglia, P.; Middleton, L. et al. (2010). Meta-analysis and imputation refines the association of 15q25 with smoking quantity. Nature Genetics, 42(5), 436-440.

Lotfipour, S.; Byun, J. S.; Leach, P.; Fowler, C. D.; Murphy, N. P.; Kenny, P. J. et al. (2013). Targeted deletion of the mouse alpha2 nic otinic acetylcholine receptor subunit gene (Chrna2) potentiates nicotine-modulated behaviors. The Journal of Neuroscience, 33(18), 7728-7741.

Marks, M. J.; Pauly, J. R.; Gross, S. D.; Deneris, E. S.; Hermans Borgmeyer, I.; Heinemann, S. F. et al. (1992). Nicotine binding and nicotinic receptor subunit RNA after chronic nicotine treatment. The Journal of Neuroscience, 12(7), 2765-2784.

McGehee, D. S.; Heath, M. J.; Gelber, S.; Devay, P.; Role, L. W. (1995). Nicotine enhancement of fast excitatory synaptic transmission in CNS by presynaptic receptors. Science, 269(5231), 1692-1696.

Nashmi, R.; Xiao, C.; Deshpande, P.; McKinney, S.; Grady, S. R.; Whiteaker, P. et al. (2007). Chronic nicotine cell specifically upregu lates functional alpha 4* nicotinic receptors: basis for both tolerance in midbrain and enhanced long-term potentiation in perforant path. The Journal of Neuroscience, 27(31), 8202-8218.

Quick, M. W.; Ceballos, R. M.; Kasten, M.; McIntosh, J. M.; Lester, R. A. (1999). Alpha3beta4 subunit-containing nicotinic receptors dom inate function in rat medial habenula neurons. Neuropharmacology, 38(6), 769-783.

Ren, J.; Qin, C.; Hu, F.; Tan, J.; Qiu, L.; Zhao, S. et al. (2011). Habenula"cholinergic" neurons co-release glutamate and acetylcholine and activate postsynaptic neurons via distinct transmission modes. Neuron, 69(3), 445-452.

Rose, J. E.; Behm, F. M.; Salley, A. N.; Bates, J. E.; Coleman, R. E.; Hawk, T. C. et al. (2007). Regional brain activity correlates of nico tine dependence. Neuropsychopharmacology, 32(12), 2441-2452.

Salas, R.; Pieri, F.; De Biasi, M. (2004). Decreased signs of nicotine withdrawal in mice null for the beta4 nicotinic acetylcholine receptor subunit. The Journal of Neuroscience, 24(45), 10035-10039.

Salas, R.; Pieri, F.; Fung, B.; Dani, J. A.; De Biasi, M. (2003). Altered anxiety-related responses in mutant mice lacking the beta4 subunit of the nicotinic receptor. The Journal of Neuroscience, 23(15), 6255-6263.

Salas, R.; Sturm, R.; Boulter, J.; De Biasi, M. (2009). Nicotinic receptors in the habenulo-interpeduncular system are necessary for nicotine withdrawal in mice. The Journal of Neuroscience, 29(10), 3014-3018.

Shabel, S. J.; Proulx, C. D.; Piriz, J.; Malinow, R. (2014). Mood regula tion. GABA/glutamate co-release controls habenula output and is modified by antidepressant treatment. Science, 345(6203), 1494-1498.

Sheffield, E. B.; Quick, M. W.; Lester, R. A. (2000). Nicotinic acetylcho line receptor subunit mRNA expression and channel function in medial habenula neurons. Neuropharmacology, 39(13), 2591-2603.

Shih, P. Y.; Engle, S. E.; Oh, G.; Deshpande, P.; Puskar, N. L.; Lester, H. A. et al. (2014). Differential expression and function of nicotinic ace tylcholine receptors in subdivisions of medial habenula. The Journal of Neuroscience, 34(29), 9789-9802.

Slimak, M. A.; Ables, J. L.; Frahm, S.; Antolin-Fontes, B.; Santos Torres, J.; Moretti, M. et al. (2014). Habenular expression of rare mis sense variants of the beta4 nicotinic receptor subunit alters nicotine consumption. Frontiers in Human Neuroscience, 8, 12.

Thorgeirsson, T. E.; Geller, F.; Sulem, P.; Rafnar, T.; Wiste, A.; Magnusson, K. P. et al. (2008). A variant associated with nicotine dependence, lung cancer and peripheral arterial disease. Nature, 452(7187), 638-642.

Yeh, J. J.; Yasuda, R. P.; Davila-Garcia, M. I.; Xiao, Y.; Ebert, S.; Gupta, T.; et al. (2001). Neuronal nicotinic acetylcholine receptor alpha3 subu nit protein in rat brain and sympathetic ganglion measured using a subunit-specific antibody: regional and ontogenic expression. Journal of Neurochemistry, 77(1), 336-346.

Zhao-Shea, R.; Liu, L.; Pang, X.; Gardner, P. D.; Tapper, A. R. (2013). Activation of GABAergic neurons in the interpeduncular nucleus triggers physical nicotine withdrawal symptoms. Current Biology, 23(23), 2327-2335.

11
烟碱对大脑神经元的神经保护：烟碱成瘾的另一面

Dzejla Bajrektarevic[1], *Silvia Corsini*[2], *Andrea Nistri*[1], *Maria Tortora*[3]

1. Department of Neuroscience, SISSA, Trieste, Italy
2. Neuroscience Paris Seine—Institute of Biology Paris Seine, CNRS, UMR 8246—Inserm U1130, Universite Pierre et Marie Curie (UPMC), Sorbonne Universites, Paris, France
3. MRC London Institute of Medical Science, Imperial College of London, London, United Kingdom

缩略语

ACh	乙酰胆碱	Hsp70	热休克蛋白70
AD	阿尔茨海默病	MAPK	丝裂原活化蛋白激酶
AIF	凋亡诱导因子	MPTP	线粒体通透性转换孔
Akt	蛋白激酶B	nAChR	烟碱乙酰胆碱受体
ALS	肌萎缩侧索硬化症	NFT	神经原纤维缠结
BDNF	脑源性神经营养因子	NGF	神经生长因子
CaKM II	Ca^{2+}/钙调蛋白依赖性蛋白激酶II	PI3K	磷脂酰肌醇3-激酶
CREB	环磷酸腺苷反应元件结合蛋白	PLC	磷脂酶C
cyt-c	细胞色素c	ROS	活性氧物种
ERK1/2	细胞外调节蛋白激酶1/2	SP	老年斑
FGF-2	成纤维细胞生长因子2	TBOAD	L-苏氨酸-β-苄氧天冬氨酸
HMs	舌下运动神经元	Trk A	酪氨酸激酶A

11.1 引言

烟碱乙酰胆碱受体（nAChR；主要是α4β2和α7亚型；第2章和第4章）是与神经退行性疾病相关的药物研究和开发的重要靶点，其中高亲和力烟碱结合位点的丢失是重要的（Newhouse, Potter, Singh, 2004; Picciotto, Zoli, 2008）。目前，乙酰胆碱酯酶抑制剂是唯一可用于治疗认知衰退的胆碱能药物（Pepeu, Giovannini, 2009），因为它们有望提高乙酰胆碱（ACh）的浓度及其对nAChR的作用（Anand, Gill, Mahdi, 2014; Geldenhuys, Darvesh, 2015）。正如第1章所述，烟草和烟碱研究领域已经强调了它们与主要神经疾病的联系。因此，这些数据为一种自上而下的方法提供了动力，以了解烟碱是否可以通过特定分子或细胞机制改变病程，更好地探索临床前模型。

11.2 神经退行性疾病的流行病学研究：烟碱与吸烟

在16世纪，Jean Nicot将烟碱得名的烟草植物带到了法国，并提出了它的医学用途。尽管烟碱作为一种有效的胆碱能激动剂激活和脱敏nAChR的作用已得到证实（Giniatullin, Nistri, Yakel, 2005），但持续服用烟碱预计会引起更复杂的效应，包括大幅上调nAChR的表达（Parker et al.

2004）。吸烟是一种非常有效的管理烟碱的方式，早期流行病学研究表明，吸烟与帕金森病的发病率呈负相关，其到达大脑的速度是静脉注射途径的两倍（Tyas，1996）。烟碱对阿尔茨海默病（AD）的影响仍是一个尚未完全解决的复杂课题。如表11.1所示，检验AD风险因素的荟萃分析报告了吸烟和AD之间的负相关关系。尽管早期的研究表明吸烟者的烟碱结合位点密度可能更高，从而保护他们免受AD的侵袭，但许多研究都有方法学上的局限性，如病例异质性、样本量小以及未被评估为无AD的对照（Tyas，1996）。随后的前瞻性研究没有显示吸烟者AD发病率降低，甚至没有增加AD风险（表11.1）。尽管如此，这些前瞻性研究的有效性也受到随访时间长短、间接诊断、戒烟和发病之间的可变间隔以及吸烟量的限制。尽管存在这些悬而未决的问题，烟碱（和相关激动剂）在临床神经保护方面的工作已经开展，目的是增强AD和一般神经退行性变中nAChR的活性。

表11.1　神经元nAChRs在阿尔茨海默病（AD）中的建议作用

临床结果	研究方案
吸烟者较低的AD发病率	病例-对照研究的荟萃分析[1]，流行病学证据的综述[2]
吸烟者较高的AD发病率	系统回顾[3]和荟萃分析，基于前瞻性人群的队列研究[4]，观察性研究[5]
烟碱给药的临床研究	急性皮下烟碱[6][7]，静脉注射烟碱[8]，烟碱贴片[9]-[11]
烟碱激动剂应用的临床研究	α4β2受体激动剂[12]，α7受体激动剂[13]
吸烟对AD神经病理的影响	尸检发现[14]

[1] Graves et al. Int J Epidemiol, 1991, 2, S48-S57.
[2] Lee, Neuroepidemiology, 1994, 4, 131-144.
[3] Peters et al. BMC Geriatr.; 2008, 23, 8-36.
[4] Reitz et al. Neurology, 2007, 10, 998-1005.
[5] Almeida et al. Am J Geriatr Psychiatry, 2008, 16, 92-98.
[6] Jones et al. Psychopharmacology, 1992, 108, 485-494.
[7] Sahakian et al. Br J Psychiatry, 1989, 154, 797-800.
[8] Newhouse et al. Psychopharmacology, 1988, 95, 171-217.
[9] Newhouse et al. Neurology, 2012, 10 (78), 91-101.
[10] White and Levin, Psychopharmacology, 1999, 143, 158-165.
[11] Wilson et al. Pharmacol Biochem Behav, 1995, 51, 509-514.
[12] Dunbar et al. Psychopharmacology, 2007, 191, 919-929.
[13] Haydar et al. Bioorg Med Chem, 2009, 17, 5247-5258.
[14] Urlich et al. Acta Neuropathol, 1997, 94, 450-454.

11.3　神经退行性疾病的临床研究：烟草与烟碱的影响

虽然有一些报告表明烟碱本身可以激活人的nAChR（表11.1），但烟碱对AD的影响的病理学研究并没有提供明确的结论。因此，慢性吸烟直接影响神经元功能，对神经元的长期存活有负面影响，因为几个大脑区域的灰质密度降低（表11.1），而另一项尸检研究表明，吸烟仅能减少女性的老年斑（SP）和神经原纤维缠结（NFT）的数量（表11.1）。相反，Swan和Lessov-Schlaggar（2007）提出吸烟与执行功能和言语记忆领域的认知加速下降和痴呆症风险增加有关，尽管观察到烟碱可以提高警觉性、记忆力和注意力。由于烟草中存在有毒化合物，了解烟碱对阿尔茨海默病或其他神经退行性疾病的作用应该基于烟碱本身的数据。

皮下或经皮给药烟碱和烟碱激动剂（表11.1）治疗AD的前瞻性研究似乎支持潜在的认知益处。其他小规模试验表明，皮下烟碱（表11.1）可改善视觉注意力、信息处理、知觉和活力。与这一观点一致的是，据报道，慢性经皮烟碱（表11.1）能显著改善注意力，且副作用最小。烟碱经皮吸收（表11.1）可以安全地用于6个月以上有轻度认知障碍的非吸烟受试者，并改善注意力、记忆力和精神处理能力。

还进行了nAChR激动剂的大型试验（表11.1）。例如，异普利克林（AZD3480；原TC-1734）对α4β2受体具有高亲和力和选择性，而SEN12333/WAY317538对α7受体具有高亲和力（表11.1）。由于AZD3480和SEN12333/WAY317538明显改善了人类的认知能力，它们可能是治疗AD和其他认知障碍的候选药物（表11.1）。

尽管目前有关于烟碱和nAChR激动剂在AD中作用的数据，但当实质性的神经元损伤早在临床表现之前就开始出现时，就很难治疗像AD这样的慢性疾病。由于SP和NFTs的主要原因尚不清楚，损伤限制而不是阻止疾病进展通常是目标，而且是有时间限制的。原则上，处理疾病的早期阶段可能更有用，因为此时改变疾病的方法更现实。

对于另一种神经退行性疾病，即肌萎缩侧索硬化症（ALS；卢伽雷氏症），其伴有进行性运动神经元变性和肌肉无力，可以提供不同的情况（Rothstein, Martin, Kuncl, 1992）。大规模研究表明吸烟与肌萎缩侧索硬化症之间存在正相关（Alonso, Logroscino, Hernán, 2010; de Jong et al. 2012），可能是由于已知烟草引起的伴随的呼吸和心血管缺陷。然而，由于在大量患者中，ALS最早的病理生理学可能是由于兴奋性递质谷氨酸的运输受损（Rothstein et al. 1992），所以有可能检查烟碱对从先兆到神经退化的初级细胞过程的影响。为此，在假设nAChR的调节对延缓病理恶化具有重要意义的前提下，了解烟碱对简单的神经退行性变模型的体内外细胞效应，对临床应用具有一定的价值。

11.4 烟碱对体外模型的细胞效应

nAChRs在突触（第2章）和突触前扣上表达，在那里它们调节其他神经递质的分泌（Alkondon, Albuquerque, 2004），并调节尖峰放电（Mulle, Vidal, Benoit, Changeux, 1991）。因此，烟碱的作用在不同的脑区是不同的，因为它依赖于局部nAChR的表达。烟碱的纳摩尔浓度与吸烟后血浆中的浓度相似，它通过作用于突触前nAChR增加突触前Ca^{2+}内流，从而增强GABA能、谷氨酸能和胆碱能传递，例如大鼠海马（Gray, Rajan, Radcliff, Yakehiro, Dani, 1996）、小鼠杏仁核（Barazangi, Role, 2001）和小鸡缰核（McGehee, Heath, Gelber, 2001）。在鸡脑切片中，烟碱以剂量依赖的方式调节GABA能突触传递，低浓度（50～100nmol/L）可增强电诱发的GABA能电流，而高剂量（0.5～1.0μmol/L）则不影响或减弱诱发的GABA传递（Zhu, Chiappinelli, 1999）。

体外研究支持烟碱给药的神经保护作用的概念，烟碱对nAChRs的影响是时间和剂量依赖的（表11.2）。关于烟碱对谷氨酸兴奋性毒性的神经保护作用，Dajas-Bailador, Lima和Wonnacott（2000）报道，激活α7受体可以保护海马神经元对抗NMDA诱导的细胞死亡。根据这一发现，烟碱强烈地保护脑干舌下运动神经元（HMs），防止它们在接触谷氨酸转运阻滞剂DL-苏氨酸-β-苄氧天冬氨酸后丢失（TBOA；表11.2）。通过使用TBOA模拟ALS的早期病理生理阶段（Urushitani et al. 1998），细胞外谷氨酸的逐渐积聚伴随着随后的网络破裂和延迟性死亡的触发（Sharifullina, Nistri, 2006）。烟碱（1～10μmol/L）抑制TBOA诱发的HMs的爆裂活动，减少兴奋性神经传递，并加强突触抑制（表11.2）。烟碱的神经保护可能是由于增加了Ca^{2+}通过nAChR

的内流（图11.1），特别是α7亚型，它们对这种阳离子相当敏感（Shen, Yakel, 2009）。α7 nAChR 基因敲除小鼠的神经保护失败证实了α7受体在介导神经保护中起主导作用（表11.2）。根据这一观察，选择性α7激动剂PNU282987通过恢复线粒体膜电位、降低超氧阴离子水平和减少器官型海马培养中活性氧（ROS）的产生来保护毒性（表11.2）。

表11.2 烟碱对体外制剂的影响

动物模型或细胞类型	制备	烟碱的神经保护作用
大鼠	皮层神经元原代培养	提高细胞生存能力[①-③]
大鼠	舌下神经核片	通过激活nAChR降低活性氧和线粒体能量障碍[④,⑤]
大鼠	舌下神经核片	连接蛋白36活性降低，Hsp70表达增加[⑥]
小鼠	从小鼠肝脏中分离出线粒体	通过激活PI3K/Akt调控MPTP相关信号通路[⑦]
大鼠和α7 nAChR敲除小鼠	海马切片	在体外缺血模型中，LDH释放的减少作为神经元损伤的参数。α7 nAChR敲除小鼠细胞释放LDH的对比失败[⑧]
大鼠	大脑线粒体	非胆碱能受体介导的ROS减少[⑨]
小鼠	腹侧中脑培养	减少UPR信号通路下游效应子（CHOP）及其激活子（eIF2α）。两种应激因子XBP1和ATF6的核迁移功能受损[⑩]
小鼠	海马器官培养	在存在神经炎症刺激（LPS, 1ng/mL）和线粒体功能障碍（使用线粒体复合物Ⅲ阻断剂抗霉素A）的情况下，烟碱通过激活PI3K/Akt信号通路降低毒性[⑪]
细胞系	PC12细胞	预防神经生长因子剥夺引起的细胞死亡[⑫]
大鼠	原代神经元培养	通过 与烟碱（0.5μmol/L, 7d）、谷氨酸（20μmol/L）、A$β_{1-40}$（1nmol/L）和 A$β_{1-42}$（100pmol/L）共孵育24h来降低毒性。烟碱的保护作用是通过激活PI3K，导致Akt磷酸化，并增加生存前蛋白Bcl-2[⑬]
大鼠	中脑原代培养	烟碱（0.1～100μmol/L）和鱼藤酮（100nmol/L）共给药24h，通过激活PI3K-Akt通路，对比鱼藤酮的毒性[⑭]
细胞系	人SH-SY5Y神经母细胞瘤细胞	烟碱（0.01～100μmol/L）预处理12h后，A$β_{25-35}$暴露可降低caspase-3的激活，并以时间依赖的方式增加Bcl-2、Bcl-xL和Mcl-1的表达[⑮]
小鼠	原代皮层小胶质细胞培养，原代海马和皮层神经元培养	烟碱维持小胶质细胞处于不活跃状态。烟碱在脂多糖处理的小胶质细胞中保留神经元[⑯]
小鼠	原代星形胶质细胞培养	减少星形胶质细胞的激活，抑制磷酸化Erk和p38在线粒体或炎症应激源存在时的增加[⑰]

① Akaike et al. Brain Res, 1994, 644, 181-187.
② Semba et al. Brain Res, 1996, 735, 335-338.
③ Kaneko et al. Brain Res, 1997, 765, 135-140.
④ Corsini et al. J Physiol, 2016, 594, 6777-6798.
⑤ Tortora et al. Neurosci Lett, 2017, 639, 43-48.
⑥ Corsini et al. Cell Death Dis, 2017, 8, e2881.
⑦ Gergalova et al. Int J Biochem Cell Biol, 2014, 49, 26-31.
⑧ Egea et al. Neuroscience, 2007, 145, 866-872.
⑨ Cormier et al. Brain Res, 2001, 900, 72-79.
⑩ Srinivasan et al. J Neurosci, 2016, 36, 65-79.
⑪ Navarro et al. Biochem Pharmacol, 2015, 97, 473-481.
⑫ Yamashita et al. Neurosci Lett, 1996, 213, 145-147.
⑬ Kihara et al. J Biol Chem, 2001, 276, 13541-13546.
⑭ Takeuchi et al. J Neurosci Res, 2009, 87, 576-585.
⑮ Xue et al. Int J Mol Med, 2014, 33, 925-933.
⑯ Noda and Kobayashi, J Physiol Sci, 2017, 67, 235-245.
⑰ Liu et al. J Neuroinflam, 2017, 141, 473-474.

11.5 烟碱对小鼠、大鼠、猴模型的神经保护作用

体内实验也证实了烟碱激活神经保护的分子和细胞机制。如表11.3所示，烟碱（皮下或静脉注射）的有益作用已在体内的一系列动物模型中被报道。

药理学策略（表11.3；Bitner et al. 2010; Li, Arias, Jonnala, Mruthinti, Buccafusco, 2005）和对基因敲除小鼠的实验（表11.3）已经证实，α7和α4β2受体介导神经保护，其相对贡献取决于动物模型、年龄和大脑区域。例如，包含α7的受体的神经保护作用已经在海马和内嗅皮层中观察到，但在大鼠AD模型的大脑皮层或下丘脑中没有观察到（Li et al. 2005）。选择性α7 nAChR激动剂还可以根据在各种记忆测试方案中检测到的改进的性能来增强AD模型的认知性能（Bitner et al. 2010）。

使用药理学工具（α4β2或α7 nAChR激动剂）和分子工具（$\beta_2^{-/-}$或$\alpha_7^{-/-}$基因敲除小鼠），已经观察到α4β2 nAChR参与了新生小鼠兴奋性中毒性脑损伤的神经保护作用，而在成年动物中具有神经保护作用的α7受体在这个早期则没有（表11.3）。α7 nAChR在新生儿和成人模型中的不同作用可能是由于这种高Ca^{2+}渗透性受体类型在出生后期间在皮层内瞬时过度表达（表11.3）。

11.6 烟碱影响细胞内信号传递

烟碱激活受体后的下游效应器仍不完全清楚，可能涉及存活和凋亡信号级联反应（Buckingham, Jones, Brown, Sattelle, 2009），如图11.1所示。在脑干运动神经元中，烟碱导致连接蛋白36缝隙

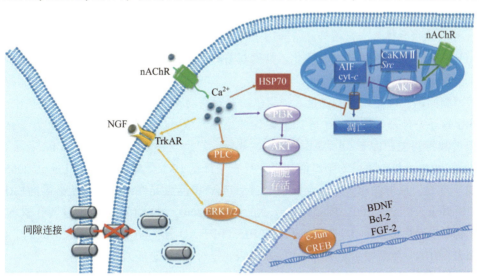

图11.1 说明烟碱对体外和体内模型的神经保护作用的理想化图

烟碱诱导位于细胞膜和线粒体膜上的烟碱乙酰胆碱受体（nAChR）开放。由此产生的Ca^{2+}内流激活了一系列促进细胞存活和阻止细胞凋亡的复杂途径。线粒体nAChR激活磷脂酰肌醇3-激酶/蛋白激酶B（PI3K/Akt）通路，阻止凋亡诱导因子（AIF）和细胞色素c（cyt-c）释放，抑制Ca^{2+}/钙调蛋白依赖性蛋白激酶Ⅱ（CaKMⅡ）和酪氨酸蛋白激酶Src相关通路。致死性AIF的释放/转位也受到热休克蛋白70（Hsp70）水平升高的限制。细胞外调节蛋白激酶1/2（ERK1/2）途径可通过磷脂酶C（PLC）直接激活，或通过细胞外神经生长因子（NGF）结合的酪氨酸激酶A（TrkA）受体表达增加而间接激活。在细胞核中，ERK1/2激活c-Jun和cAMP反应元件结合蛋白（CREB）等转录因子，上调与细胞生存相关的基因，如脑源性神经营养因子（BDNF）、B细胞淋巴瘤2（Bcl-2）和成纤维细胞生长因子2（FGF-2）。此外，烟碱阻止缝隙连接通信，并有利于连接蛋白36从膜到胞浆的重新分布，从而在集体兴奋过程中将神经元解耦。S. Corsini未发表。

连接蛋白从膜到胞浆的重新分布，从而解耦HMs，防止死亡刺激从受伤的运动神经元扩散到未受伤的运动神经元（表11.2）。此外，在兴奋性应激过程中，烟碱可促进保护因子热休克蛋白70（Hsp70）的表达，以阻止导致细胞死亡的凋亡诱导因子（AIF）通过DNA损伤的核迁移。在β-淀粉样蛋白诱导的神经毒性存在的情况下，烟碱通过激活α7 nAChR触发磷脂酰肌醇3-激酶（PI3K）通路，减少AIF的释放/转位（Yu, Mechawar, Krantic, Quirion, 2011）。PI3K蛋白激酶B（Akt）和丝裂原活化蛋白激酶（MAPK）通路通过抑制凋亡信号的关键步骤，在促进细胞存活中发挥重要作用（Datta, Brunet, Greenberger, 1999; Erhardt, Schremser, Cooper, 1999）。烟碱（通过α7受体）通过调节PI3K活性显著降低了谷氨酸和β-淀粉样蛋白在原代神经元培养中引起的毒性（表11.2）。重要的是，烟碱还诱导细胞外调节蛋白激酶1/2（ERK1/2）、p38和c-Jun MAPK等抗凋亡蛋白显著增强（表11.2）。在一个由线粒体复合物Ⅰ抑制剂鱼藤酮引起的氧化应激模型中，α7和α4β2 nAChR信号通过激活PI3K-Akt通路对比了未折叠蛋白的聚集和凋亡通路的激活。

烟碱激活的神经保护性MAPK/ERK通路（Hetman, Gozdz, 2004）通过磷脂酶C（PLC）激活在体外和体内模型中发挥假定作用（表11.2和表11.3；Bitner et al. 2010; Brunzell, Russell, Picciotto, 2003; Jonnala, Terry Jr., Buccafusco, 2002; Li et al. 2005; Toborek et al. 2007）。长期服用烟碱可以通过Ca^{2+}的内流和释放或脑源性神经营养因子（BDNF；Brunzell et al. 2003）等神经营养因子的调节来调节ERK信号。已经在培养的脊髓神经元中观察到由于ERK通路的激活而产生的神经保护作用，这些神经元被认为是脊髓损伤（Toborek et al. 2007）和AD（表11.2；Bitner et al. 2010）的模型，并且它似乎依赖于抗凋亡蛋白Bcl-2的上调（表11.2和表11.3；Heusch, Maneckjee, 1998）。此外，烟碱增加酪氨酸激酶A（TrkA）受体的表达（Jonnala et al. 2002; Li et al. 2005），该受体是酪氨酸激酶家族的成员，通过激活几个信号级联影响神经元的可塑性、分化和存活。具体地说，TrkA是一种膜结合受体，一旦被神经营养因子样神经生长因子（NGF）激活，就会使自身和某些与MAPK/ERK通路相关的蛋白磷酸化。烟碱与TrkA相关的神经保护作用主要在AD模型中报道（Jonnala et al. 2002; Li et al. 2005）。

基底前脑胆碱能神经元的丢失是人类阿尔茨海默病的一个标志；在大鼠的基底核中，它与α7 nAChRs的丢失有关，并且显然与TrkA阳性神经元的减少相一致（Li et al. 2005）。因此，胆碱能缺陷的起源可能归因于Aβ肽$Aβ_{1-42}$的毒性效应，它是一种高亲和力α7 nAChR阻滞剂（Li, Buccafusco, 2004），并在随后的胆碱能神经元死亡中降低TrkA受体的表达（Li et al. 2005）。为了抵消这一现象，值得注意的是，烟碱引起激活环AMP反应元件结合蛋白所必需的ERK磷酸化（CREB; Brunzell et al. 2003; Pandey, Roy, Xu, Mittal, 2001; 图11.1），后者通过调节BDNF的转录在认知功能中发挥重要作用（Bitner et al. 2010）。由于AD病理与CREB磷酸化形式的下调有关（Bitner et al. 2010），用烟碱激动剂增强CREB的表达是对比AD进展的潜在策略。

烟碱还作用于线粒体外膜表达的α7 nAChR，后者通过不依赖离子的机制激活线粒体内的PI3K/Akt途径，并抑制酪氨酸蛋白激酶Src和Ca^{2+}/钙调蛋白依赖性蛋白激酶Ⅱ（CaKMⅡ；表11.2；图11.1）。这些效应防止了凋亡前事件的发生，如线粒体通透性转换孔（MPTP）的形成和随之而来的细胞色素c（cyt-c）的释放（表11.2）。与这些观察结果一致，βA肽（$Aβ_{25-35}$）通过人SH-SY5Y神经母细胞瘤细胞凋亡、caspase-3激活和cyt-c释放的毒性作用可被烟碱阻断（表11.2）。

除了促进细胞存活，nAChR激活还可抑制活性氧的形成和线粒体能量功能障碍，这是谷氨酸介导的兴奋毒性的两个关键下游效应因子（表11.2）。固有的nAChR活性不足以对比这两个过程

（表11.2）。在大鼠脑线粒体上，烟碱的抗氧化特性不是由受体介导的；事实上，烟碱可以通过抑制NADPH与呼吸链的复合物Ⅰ直接相互作用，从而通过nAChR不依赖的过程诱导超氧阴离子生成减少（表11.2）。Linert等（1999）实际上提出了烟碱对帕金森病和阿尔茨海默病的有益/保护作用至少部分是由于抗氧化机制。表11.2列出了一些可能参与烟碱介导的神经保护的其他机制。

其他几个与烟碱神经保护相关的基因还参与表达调控、早期生长反应、转录因子和同源框活性（Belluardo et al. 2005）。这些在烟碱受体控制下的基因可能在受体激活与包括烟碱的神经保护-神经营养作用在内的长期神经元反应的耦合中发挥重要作用（Belluardo et al. 2005）。其中，重要的是要考虑神经营养成纤维细胞生长因子2（FGF-2）的作用，它在几种体外和体内损伤模型中都与神经保护和神经元存活有关（表11.3）。

表11.3 烟碱对体内动物模型的影响

实验条件	动物模型	烟碱的神经保护作用
帕金森病	C57BL/6J 小鼠	激活nAChR可保护多巴胺能神经元抗变性[1]
阿尔茨海默病	C57BL/6J 小鼠	烟碱通过上调抗凋亡蛋白（Bcl-2）抑制A β_{25-35} 诱导的神经毒性[2]
脑内出血	C57BL/6J 小鼠	α7 nAChR的激活增加了存活神经元的数量，减少了激活的小胶质细胞/巨噬细胞[3]
兴奋性中毒	小鼠nAChR亚基的基因敲除	烟碱通过激活α4β2 nAChR降低新生小鼠皮层损伤[4]
炎症	B6（H-2^b），nAChRα7$^{-/-}$，FoxP3^{GFP} 和 CX$_3$CR1$^{+/GFP}$小鼠	α7 nAChR对烟碱对脑炎症的影响仅起部分作用。非α7 nAChR参与了烟碱的抗炎特性[5]
衰老	SD大鼠	烟碱上调胶质细胞和神经元细胞的FGF-2 mRNA[6]
学习和记忆障碍	SD大鼠	在记忆测试中，烟碱可以防止表现受损[7]

[1] Takeuchi et al. J Neurosci Res, 2009, 87, 576-585.
[2] Xue et al. Int J Mol Med, 2014, 33, 925-933.
[3] Hijioka et al. Neuroscience, 2012, 222, 10-19.
[4] Laudenbach et al. FASEB J, 2002, 16, 423-425.
[5] Hao et al. Exp Neurol, 2011, 227, 110-119.
[6] Belluardo et al. Neurobiol Aging, 2004, 25, 1333-1342.
[7] Hiramatsu et al. J Neural Transm, 2002, 109, 361-375.

近年来，研究了nAChR在胶质细胞，特别是小胶质细胞和星形胶质细胞中的作用。小胶质细胞由中枢神经系统的免疫细胞组成，在缺血、创伤和中风等病理条件下，随着形态的变化，小胶质细胞迅速激活（Kettenmann, Hanish, Noda, Verkhratsky, 2011）。烟碱可防止由炎症过程和神经元损伤刺激的小胶质细胞的形态变化（表11.2）。此外，由于胶质细胞是复杂大脑网络的活跃成分，了解烟碱对小胶质细胞的保护是否会对神经元产生影响将是一件有趣的事情。此外，抑制星形胶质细胞已被提出为治疗神经退行性疾病的一种新策略（表11.2），因为烟碱预处理通过α7 nAChR抑制化学应激源激活星形胶质细胞。这些问题显然需要进一步调查。

术语解释

- 细胞凋亡：是发生在多细胞生物体中的程序性细胞死亡过程。
- 兴奋性中毒：细胞外高谷氨酸引起兴奋性受体过度活性的病理过程。它可以破坏或杀死神经细胞。
- 体外研究：在实验室条件下，对生物环境之外的有机体、细胞或分子进行的研究。

	- 体内研究：在整个活的有机体上进行的研究。
- 氧化应激：由于细胞内活性氧的产生和清除不匹配，细胞能量代谢失衡。
- 突触前专用区：位于轴突末端，含有要释放到突触间隙中的神经递质的特殊区域。
烟碱神经保护的关键事实	- nAChR是药物研究和开发的重要靶点。
- 通过吸烟给药的烟碱到达大脑的速度是通过静脉给药的两倍。
- 流行病学研究报告吸烟与帕金森病或阿尔茨海默病的发病率呈负相关。
- 烟碱可能会提高警觉性、记忆力、注意力和心理处理能力。
- 烟碱神经元效应与对血管和呼吸系统的损伤相平衡。
要点总结	- 尽管吸烟固有着严重的健康风险，但烟碱可以保护脑神经元免受细胞死亡的影响。
- 神经元死亡可能是由过量的细胞外谷氨酸引起的兴奋性毒性，也可能是由有毒的肽（如β-淀粉样蛋白片段）引起的。
- 烟碱的这种作用是通过激活由细胞膜和线粒体膜表达的神经元烟碱受体介导的。
- 烟碱受体的激活触发了多条细胞内途径，以防止DNA损伤。
- 某些合成的烟碱受体激动剂可以模仿烟碱的神经保护作用。
- 烟碱受体的神经保护作用勾勒出一种未来的药理学策略，可以在早期阶段阻止神经退化。

参考文献

Alkondon, M.; Albuquerque, E. X. (2004). The nicotinic acetylcholine receptor subtypes and their function in the hippocampus and cerebral cortex. Progress in Brain Research, 145, 109-120.

Alonso, A.; Logroscino, G.; Hernán, M. A. (2010). Smoking and the risk of amyotrophic lateral sclerosis: a systematic review and metaanalysis. Journal of Neurology Neurosurgery, and Psychiatry, 81, 1249-1252.

Anand, R.; Gill, K. D.; Mahdi, A. A. (2014). Therapeutics of Alzheimer's disease: past, present and future. Neuropharmacology, 76, 27-50.

Barazangi, N.; Role, L. (2001). Nicotine-induced enhancement of glutamatergic and GABAergic synaptic transmission in the mouse amygdala. Journal of Neurophysiology, 86, 463-474.

Belluardo, N.; Olsson, P. A.; Mudò, G.; Sommer, W. H.; Amato, G.; Fuxe, K. (2005). Transcription factor gene expression profiling after acute intermittent nicotine treatment in the rat cerebral cortex. Neuroscience, 133, 787-796.

Bitner, R. S.; Bunnelle, W. H.; Decker, M. W.; Drescher, K. U.; Kohlhaas, K. L.; Markosyan, S. et al. (2010). In vivo pharmacological characterization of a novel selective α7 neuronal nicotinic acetylcholine receptor agonist ABT-107: preclinical considerations in Alzheimer's disease. The Journal of Pharmacology and Experimental Therapeutics, 334, 875-886.

Brunzell, D. H.; Russell, D. S.; Picciotto, M. R. (2003). In vivo nicotine treatment regulates mesocorticolimbic CREB and ERK signaling in C57Bl/6J mice. Journal of Neurochemistry, 84, 1431-1441.

Buckingham, S.; Jones, A.; Brown, L. A.; Sattelle, B. D. (2009). Nicotinic acetylcholine receptor signalling: roles in Alzheimer's disease and amyloid neuroprotection. Pharmacological Reviews, 61, 39-61.

Dajas-Bailador, F. A.; Lima, P. A.; Wonnacott, S. (2000). The α7 nicotinicacetylcholine receptor subtypemediatesnicotineprotection against NMDA excitotoxicity in primary hippocampal cultures through a Ca^{2+} dependent mechanism. Neuropharmacology, 39, 2799-2807.

Datta, S. R.; Brunet, A.; Greenberger, M. E. (1999). Cellular survival: a play in three Akts. Genes and Development, 13, 2905-2927.

de Jong, S. W.; Huisman, M. H.; Sutedja, N. A.; van der Kooi, A. J.; de Visser, M.; Schelhaas, H. J. et al. (2012). Smoking, alcohol consumption, and the risk of amyotrophic lateral sclerosis: a population-based study. American Journal of Epidemiology, 176, 233-239.

Erhardt, P.; Schremser, E. J.; Cooper, G. M. (1999). B-Raf inhibits programmed cell death downstream of cytochrome c release from mitochondria by activating the MEK/Erk pathway. Molecular and Cellular Biology, 19, 5308-5315.

Geldenhuys, W. J.; Darvesh, A. S. (2015). Pharmacotherapy of Alzheimer's disease: current and future trends. Expert Review of Neurotherapeutics, 15, 3-5.

Giniatullin, R.; Nistri, A.; Yakel, J. L. (2005). Desensitization of nicotinic ACh receptors: shaping cholinergic signaling. Trends in Neurosciences, 28,

371-378.

Gray, R.; Rajan, A.; Radcliff, K.; Yakehiro, M.; Dani, J. (1996). Hippocampal synaptic transmission enhanced by low concentrations of nicotine. Nature, 383, 713-716.

Hetman, M.; Gozdz, A. (2004). Role of extracellular signal regulated kinases 1 and 2 in neuronal survival. European Journal of Biochemistry, 271, 2050-2055.

Heusch, W. L.; Maneckjee, R. (1998). Signalling pathways involved in nicotine regulation of apoptosis of human lung cancer cells. Carcinogenesis, 19, 551-556.

Jonnala, R. R.; Terry, A. V.; Jr.; Buccafusco, J. J. (2002). Nicotine increases the expression of high affinity nerve growth factor receptors in both in vitro and in vivo. Life Sciences, 70, 1543-1554.

Kettenmann, H.; Hanish, U. K.; Noda, M.; Verkhratsky, A. (2011). Physiology of microglia. American Physiological Society, 91, 461-553.

Li, X. D.; Arias, E.; Jonnala, R. R.; Mruthinti, S.; Buccafusco, J. J. (2005). Effect of amyloid peptides on the increase in TrkA receptor expression induced by nicotine in vitro and in vivo. Journal of Molecular Neuroscience, 27, 325-336.

Li, X. D.; Buccafusco, J. J. (2004). Role of α7 nicotinic acetylcholine receptors in the pressor response to intracerebroventricular injection of choline: blockade by amyloid peptide Aβ1-42. Journal of Pharmacology and Experimental Therapeutics, 309, 1206-1212.

Linert, W.; Bridge, M. H.; Huber, M.; Bjugstad, K. B.; Grossman, S.; Arendash, G. W. (1999). In vitro and in vivo studies investigating possible antioxidant actions of nicotine: relevance to Parkinson's and Alzheimer's diseases. Biochimica et Biophysica Acta, 1454, 143-152.

Mai, H.; May, W. S.; Gao, F.; Jin, Z.; Deng, X. (2003). A functional role for nicotine in Bcl2 phosphorylation and suppression of apoptosis. The Journal of Biological Chemistry, 278, 1886-1891.

McGehee, D. S.; Heath, M. J.; Gelber, S.; Devay, P.; Role, L. W. (1995). Nicotine enhancement of fast excitatory synaptic transmission in CNS by presynaptic receptors. Science, 269, 1692-1696.

Mulle, C.; Vidal, C.; Benoit, P.; Changeux, J. P. (1991). Existence of different subtypes of nicotinic acetylcholine receptors in the rat habenulo-interpeduncular system. The Journal of Neuroscience, 11, 2588-2597.

Newhouse, P. A.; Potter, A.; Singh, A. (2004). Effects of nicotinic stimulation on cognitive performance. Current Opinion in Pharmacology, 1, 36-46.

Pandey, U. C.; Roy, A.; Xu, T.; Mittal, N. (2001). Effects of protracted nicotine exposure and withdrawal on the expression and phosphorylation of the CREB gene transcription factor in rat brain. Journal of Neurochemistry, 77, 943-952.

Parker, S. L.; Fu, Y.; McAllen, K.; Luo, J.; McIntosh, J. M.; Lindstrom, J. M. (2004). Sharp BM Up-regulation of brain nicotinic acetylcholine receptors in the rat during long-term self administration of nicotine: disproportionate increase of the α6 subunit. Molecular Pharmacology, 65, 611-622.

Pepeu, G.; Giovannini, M. G. (2009). Cholinesterase inhibitors and beyond. Current Alzheimer Research, 2, 86-96.

Picciotto, M. R.; Zoli, M. (2008). Neuroprotection via nAChRs: the role of nAChRs in neurodegenerative disorders such as Alzheimer's and Parkinson's disease. Frontiers in Bioscience, 13, 492-504.

Rothstein, J. D.; Martin, L. J.; Kuncl, R. W. (1992). Decreased glutamate transport by the brain and spinal cord in amyotrophic lateral sclerosis. The New England Journal of Medicine, 326, 1464-1468.

Sharifullina, E.; Nistri, A. (2006). Glutamate uptake block triggers deadly rhythmic bursting of neonatal rat hypoglossal motoneurons. The Journal of Physiology, 572, 407-423.

Shen, J. X.; Yakel, J. L. (2009). Nicotinic acetylcholine receptormediated calcium signaling in the nervous system. Acta Pharmacological Sinica, 30, 673-680.

Swan, G. E.; Lessov-Schlaggar, C. N. (2007). The effects of tobacco smoke and nicotine on cognition and the brain. Neuropsychology review, 17, 259-273.

Toborek, M.; Son, K. W.; Pudelko, A.; King-Pospisil, K.; Wylegala, E.; Malecki, A. (2007). ERK 1/2 signaling pathway is involved in nicotine-mediated neuroprotection in spinal cord neurons. Journal of Cellular Biochemistry, 100, 279-292.

Tyas, S. L. (1996). Are tobacco and alcohol use related to Alzheimer's disease? A critical assessment of the evidence and its implications. Addiction Biology, 1, 237-254.

Urushitani, M.; Shimohama, S.; Kihara, T.; Sawada, H.; Akaike, A.; Ibi, M. et al. (1998). Mechanism of selective motor neuronal death after exposure of spinal cord to glutamate: involvement of glutamate-induced nitric oxide in motor neuron toxicity and nonmotor neuron protection. Annals of Neurology, 44, 796-807.

Yu, W.; Mechawar, N.; Krantic, S.; Quirion, R. (2011). α7 Nicotinic receptor activation reduces β-amyloid-induced apoptosis by inhibiting caspase-independent death through phosphatidylinositol 3-kinase signaling. Journal of Neurochemistry, 119, 848-858.

Zhu, P. J.; Chiappinelli, V. A. (1999). Nicotine modulates evoked GABAergic transmission in the brain. Journal of Neurophysiology, 82, 3041-3045.

12
将烟碱、薄荷醇和大脑变化联系起来

Brandon J. Henderson

Department of Biomedical Sciences, Marshall University, Joan C. Edwards School of Medicine, Huntington, WV, United States

缩略语

GABA	γ-氨基丁酸	**SNr**	黑质网状部
nAChR	烟碱乙酰胆碱受体	**VTA**	腹侧被盖区
SNc	黑质致密部		

12.1 引言

薄荷醇是世界上最受欢迎的烟草香料。在美国和欧洲国家，吸薄荷醇卷烟的人占吸烟人口的30%（Caraballo, Asman, 2011）。在其他地方，吸薄荷醇卷烟的比率各不相同，最高的是菲律宾（60%）（WHO, 2016）。非裔美国人表现出令人难以置信的高吸薄荷醇卷烟的比率：75%的成年人和90%的青年吸烟者（D'Silva, Boyle, Lien, Rode, Okuyemi, 2012）。美国一般吸烟的年轻人也更喜欢薄荷醇卷烟，而不是无香卷烟（Villanti et al. 2016）。薄荷醇不仅在高剂量（3～20mg/支）的卷烟中发现，而且在98%的非薄荷醇卷烟的低剂量（2～70μg/支）中也存在（Ai et al. 2015）。

薄荷醇是从薄荷油中提取的一种芳香的单萜类化合物。它通过对瞬时受体电位melastatin-8（TrpM8）的激动剂活性产生局部降温感觉（Journigan, Zaveri, 2013）。对薄荷醇作用的研究目前正在扩大，因为公众对薄荷醇在降低戒烟率、心血管效应和吸烟相关癌症事件中的作用的担忧日益增加（下面将进一步讨论）。在这里，我们讨论薄荷醇、烟碱以及它们的联合作用对大脑的影响。

12.2 薄荷醇卷烟简史

第一支薄荷醇卷烟很可能是由Axton-Fisher于1926年销售的"Spud"（Proctor, 2012）。不久之后（1933），烟草公司的Brown和Williamson推出了他们的库尔牌薄荷醇卷烟。自20世纪50年代以来，薄荷醇卷烟是否不成比例地向非裔美国人销售一直存在一些争论。讨论这一点会偏离本章的重点，但可以在其他地方找到彻底的评论（Lochlann Jain, 2003）。最值得注意的公共卫生问题涉及薄荷醇在烟碱成瘾中的作用。当我们检查所有年龄段的吸烟者时，与非薄荷醇卷烟的吸烟者相比，薄荷醇卷烟的吸烟者的戒烟率明显降低（Delnevo, Gundersen, Hrywna, Echeverria, Steinberg, 2011; D'Silva et al. 2012）。当然，这会增加与吸烟相关的负面结果的风险：肺癌、食道癌、口腔癌和喉癌，且心脏病和高血压的发病率更高。这一担忧已经变得如此严重，以至于美国食品和药物管理局（FDA）和世界卫生组织（WHO）进行了独立调查，并得出薄荷醇确实会增加吸烟的开始，并导致更强烈的成瘾的结论（FDA, 2012; WHO, 2016）。

薄荷醇卷烟的年轻吸烟者过渡到终身吸烟的可能性是非薄荷醇卷烟的年轻吸烟者的两倍（D'Silva et al. 2012）。随着电子烟越来越受欢迎，加味产品（包括薄荷醇）的吸烟率也在增加，特别是在年轻吸烟者中（CDC, 2016; Villanti et al. 2016）。这困扰着许多公共卫生专家，因为他们担心这可能会助长新一代烟碱成瘾者。

12.3　薄荷醇和烟碱：早期临床发现

薄荷醇如何降低吸烟者的戒烟率？一些研究表明，薄荷醇可以减少气道刺激，使吸烟者吸入更多烟碱。临床报告显示，使用薄荷醇卷烟可以显著增加吸食时间、吸烟量和吸食次数（Ahijevych, Parsley, 1999）。还有证据表明，薄荷醇降低烟碱的新陈代谢，使血浆中烟碱浓度升高（Alsharari et al. 2015; Benowitz, Herrera, Jacob, 2004）。尽管如此，还是有相反的论点，因为其他报告表明，随着薄荷醇的使用，血浆烟碱水平没有显著增加（Ashley, Dixon, Sisodiya, Prasad, 2012）。

关于吸食薄荷醇和非薄荷醇卷烟最引人注目的发现是对烟碱乙酰胆碱受体（nAChR）上调的影响。含有β2的（β2*）nAChRs的上调是慢性烟碱暴露的一个很好的特征。这发生在人类吸烟者（Jasinska, Zorick, Brody, Stein, 2013）、啮齿动物（Henderson et al. 2017）和细胞系（Srinivasan et al. 2011）中。这被认为是烟碱成瘾的生物标志物，因为这一事件在改变多巴胺奖励途径方面发挥着重要作用（Faure, Tolu, Valverde, Naude, 2014; Nashmi et al. 2007）。在吸食薄荷醇或非薄荷醇卷烟的人类中，Brody 等（2013）发现，与不吸薄荷醇卷烟的人相比，吸薄荷醇卷烟的人在几个大脑区域表现出更多的β2*. nAChR 上调。这些大脑区域包括前额叶皮层、胼胝体、下丘脑、小脑和脑干。这些区域中有许多在多巴胺奖励途径中发挥着重要作用（图 12.1），这一发现是理解为什么薄荷醇卷烟吸烟者戒烟率较低的关键一步。

12.4　薄荷醇对Cys-loop受体的作用

薄荷醇在几类离子通道上的分子作用已经被研究过（有关完整的综述，请参阅 Oz, El Nebrisi, Yang, Howarth, Al Kury, 2017），包括 Cys-loop 受体家族。许多这些研究使用相当高的剂量（>50μmol/L）的薄荷醇（表 12.1），而少数使用被认为与吸烟有关的较低剂量（<1μmol/L）的薄荷醇（讨论如下）。Cys-loop 配体门控离子通道家族包括 nAChR、γ-氨基丁酸（GABA）、甘氨酸、5-羟色胺3（5-HT$_3$）和锌激活的离子通道受体。这些受体中的每一个都由一个五聚体蛋白组件组成，并具有一个特征良好的环，该环由两个半胱氨酸（Cys）残基之间的高度保守的氨基酸组成，这些残基形成一个二硫键（Sine, Engel, 2006）。薄荷醇被发现是α4β2 nAChR 的负变构调节剂，是α7和α3β4 nAChR 的非竞争性拮抗剂，IC$_{50}$值分别为 111μmol/L、35μmol/L 和 70μmol/L（Ashoor et al. 2013b; Hans et al. 2012; Ton et al. 2015）（表 12.1）。此外，薄荷醇已被证明是 5-HT$_3$ 受体的非竞争性拮抗剂（IC$_{50}$, 163μmol/L）、GABA$_A$ 受体的正变构调节剂（EC$_{50}$, 60～160μmol/L）和甘氨酸受体的正变构调节剂（EC$_{50}$, 50μmol/L）（Ashoor et al. 2013a; Hall et al. 2004; Lau, Karim, Goodchild, Vaughan, Drew, 2014）。尽管许多研究仅考察了（−）-薄荷醇，但一项研究却发

现了（+）-薄荷醇和（-）-薄荷醇的药理作用存在显著差异（Hall et al. 2004）。在此，（+）-薄荷醇和（-）-薄荷醇均作为$GABA_A$电流的增强剂，但是（+）-薄荷醇比（-）-薄荷醇更有效。因此，薄荷醇在Cys-loop受体上可能存在更多的立体特异性相互作用尚待发现。这些研究中使用的浓度可能会超过体内发现的浓度，因为与吸烟相关的薄荷醇浓度可能<8μmol/L（Benowitz et al. 2004）。这些使用高浓度（μmol/L）薄荷醇的发现可能无法解释薄荷醇吸烟者中β2* nAChR上调增强的观察结果（Brody et al. 2013），但是从这些观察结果中可以得出一些启示。GABA神经元在烟碱奖励途径中起着重要作用；因此，薄荷醇增强GABA信号的能力可能会在大脑中产生导致烟碱成瘾的显著变化（下面将进一步讨论）。

鉴于薄荷醇在药理上操纵Cys-loop受体的能力，人们对确定其结合位点非常感兴趣。在将薄荷醇与苯二氮䓬类药物和麻醉剂异丙酚的作用进行比较的研究中，发现薄荷醇和异丙酚可能在$GABA_A$受体上共享相同的结合位点（Watt et al. 2008）。鉴于薄荷醇和异丙酚之间保守的化学特性，薄荷醇以类似于异丙酚的方式与$GABA_A$受体结合并不令人难以置信。已经使用计算方法来确定nAChR上的变构结合位点（Ashoor et al. 2013b）。由于肌肉型nAChR与α7 nAChR有相似之处，故以肌肉型nAChR为模型，它是当时唯一具有可解的全长晶体结构的nAChR。在此，薄荷醇的结合被发现在跨膜区，类似于Watt等（2008）的发现。尽管如此，该领域仍远未确定nAChRs上的薄荷醇结合位点。

表12.1 薄荷醇对Cys-loop受体的急性作用

受体	作用	IC_{50}或者EC_{50}	立体选择？
$GABA_A$	正变构调节剂[1],[2]	约60μmol/L，（+）-薄荷醇 约160μmol/L，（-）-薄荷醇	是
甘氨酸	正变构调节剂[1]	75μmol/L	否
5-HT_3	非竞争性拮抗剂[3]	163μmol/L	否
α3β4 nAChR	非竞争性拮抗剂[4]	69～100μmol/L	未知
α7 nAChR	非竞争性拮抗剂[5]	33μmol/L	否
α4β2 nAChR	负变构调节剂[6]	111μmol/L	未知

[1] Hall et al. (2004).
[2] Corvalan, Zygadlo, Garcia (2009).
[3] Ashoor et al. (2013a).
[4] Ton et al. (2015).
[5] Ashoor et al. (2013b).
[6] Hans, Wilhelm, Swandulla (2012).

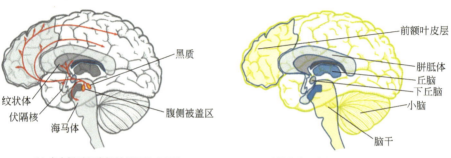

(a) 来自黑质和腹侧被盖区的多巴胺神经元投射示意图（红色）

(b) 吸烟者大脑中显示β2* nAChR上调的大脑区域示意图（见Jasinska et al. 2013）

图12.1 人类吸烟者在大脑成瘾行为的几个区域表现出β2* nAChR的上调

12.5 薄荷醇通过改变中脑多巴胺神经元增强烟碱奖励

为了了解薄荷醇如何与烟碱作用来增强nAChR上调（如Brody等所观察到的那样），并可能降低戒烟率，完成了几项研究，以考查薄荷醇改变烟碱在大脑中的行为的能力。在啮齿动物模型中，我们知道nAChR亚基对于烟碱奖励和强化很重要：单独缺失α4、α6或β2 nAChR亚基可阻止小鼠烟碱的自给药，而这些缺失的亚基在VTA（而不是SNc或SNr）中的选择性重新表达可恢复自给药行为（Pons et al. 2008）（有关VTA多巴胺神经元的神经元输入示意图，请参见图12.2）。吸烟相关浓度的烟碱选择性激活α6β2*或α4β2* nAChR，可刺激VTA DA神经元的去极化并提高放电频率（Engle, Shih, McIntosh, Drenan, 2013; Liu, Zho-Shea, McIntosh, Gardner, Tapper, 2012）。综上所述，这些结果清楚地表明，VTA α4β2*、α6β2*和α4α6β2* nAChR是烟碱的主要靶标，并介导其奖励和增强特性。

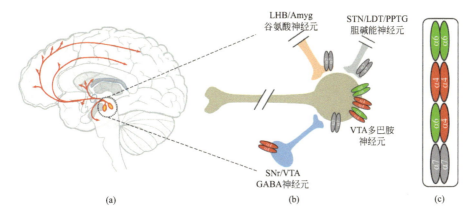

图12.2 （a）多巴胺奖励途径示意图；（b）中脑和 nAChR 亚型中参与烟碱奖励的神经元示意图；
（c）分图（b）中 nAChR 亚型的关键字

其他缩略语：Amyg, 杏仁核；LDT, 背外侧被盖；LHB, 外侧系带；PPTG, 桥足被盖核；STN, 丘脑下核

12.5.1 薄荷醇增强烟碱引起的nAChR上调

烟碱对大脑的作用已得到很好的表征。烟碱上调nAChR，改变多巴胺和GABA神经元的放电频率和兴奋性，并增强伏隔核中多巴胺的释放（有关完整的综述，请参见Faure et al. 2014）。最近，关于薄荷醇对这些特征明确的烟碱诱发的大脑变化的影响的研究已经完成（Henderson et al. 2017）。使用小鼠进行的实验表明，薄荷醇和烟碱在VTA和SNr中上调α4β2*和α4α6β2* nAChR（不是α6β2* nAChR）明显比单独使用烟碱要高得多（Henderson et al. 2017）（见图12.3）。另一项使用小鼠的研究还报道，薄荷醇可增强烟碱对前额叶皮层中β2* nAChR亚基的上调（Alsharari et al. 2015）。这些研究为使用人脑成像的检测提供了nAChR亚型特异性、区域特异性和细胞特异性相关性（Brody et al. 2013）。

薄荷醇可增强烟碱的奖励和强化条件位置偏好分析已用于检查薄荷醇如何改变与烟碱奖励相关的行为（Henderson et al. 2017）。条件位置偏好是一种基于Pavlovian训练的实验方法，用于研究与药物奖励相关的行为。这种方法经常被用于研究烟碱奖励相关行为（Henderson et al. 2017;Tapper et al. 2004）。在该测定中，将薄荷醇以被认为与吸烟相关的剂量添加到烟碱中，并显著增加了烟碱奖励相关行为（Henderson et al. 2017）。

大鼠自给药实验还用于考查薄荷醇对烟碱奖励和强化的作用。像条件位置偏好一样，这些实验用于考查药物奖励，但与条件位置偏好不同，药物传递取决于啮齿动物触发机制的可能性。

在大鼠静脉内烟碱自给药实验中，据报道薄荷醇还可以提高烟碱摄入量（Biswas et al. 2016; Wang, Wang, Chen, 2014）。假定薄荷醇本身无益，因为这些研究还表明使用条件位置偏好测定法，许多剂量的薄荷醇无法在小鼠中产生奖励（Henderson et al. 2017）。总之，这些实验清楚地证明了薄荷醇增强了烟碱的奖励和强化作用。更重要的是，这表明在吸食薄荷醇卷烟的人群中戒烟率降低可能是由于薄荷醇使烟碱更具奖励作用（更容易上瘾）。当然，还有其他特征可能是戒烟率降低的基础，因为最近发现薄荷醇还可以提高烟碱戒断率（Alsharari et al. 2015）。

尽管有报道称薄荷醇增强了烟碱引起的多个大脑区域的β2* nAChR上调（Alsharari et al. 2015; Henderson et al. 2017），但这些研究并没有改变薄荷醇或烟碱的浓度的奖励相关行为。当使用足以改变奖励相关行为的烟碱和薄荷醇剂量重复进行上调测定时（Henderson et al. 2017），VTA中烟碱诱导的α4α6β2* nAChR上调仅增强了（见图12.3）。鉴于α4α6β2* nAChRs对烟碱最敏感，并在中脑的多巴胺神经元上选择性表达，这表明这些nAChRs的选择性上调会显著改变多巴胺神经元的兴奋性和信号传导（下文将进一步讨论）。这标志着α4α6β2* nAChRs是薄荷醇增强烟碱奖励和强化能力的主要贡献者。

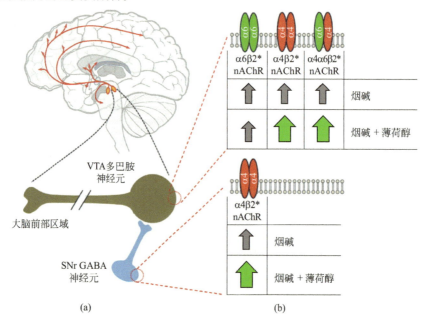

图12.3 VTA多巴胺神经元上的α4β2*、α6β2*和α4α6β2* nAChR被烟碱和烟碱加薄荷醇上调
（a）从中脑向大脑前部区域（伏隔核，前额叶皮层和纹状体）突出的VTA多巴胺神经元的示意图。
（b）由烟碱或烟碱加薄荷醇上调的细胞表面nAChR示意图。箭头的大小指示上调的程度。

12.5.2 薄荷醇增强烟碱引起的多巴胺神经元兴奋性变化

中脑多巴胺神经元表现出两种不同类型的自发活动：一种以缓慢、有规律的尖峰（强音）为特征，另一种以活动爆发（阶段）为特征。烟碱通过其以细胞特异性方式上调nAChR的能力（Nashmi et al. 2007），改变了多巴胺神经元的强直性和阶段性活性（全文请参见Faure et al. 2014）。对于观察到的烟碱诱导的多巴胺神经元放电变化，GABA神经元至关重要。来自VTA和SNr的GABA神经元为投射到大脑前部区域的VTA多巴胺神经元提供抑制性输入。在长期暴露于烟碱之后，α4* nAChR在VTA和SNr GABA能神经元上调（Nashmi et al. 2007）。GABA神经元上调的α4* nAChR提供增强的抑制信号，并减少强直多巴胺神经元的放电。但是，急性烟碱暴露会暂时增强GABA能的活性，随后由于α4* nAChR脱敏作用上调而导致活性长期降低。这触发了多巴胺神经元爆发放电（Mansvelder, Keath, McGehee, 2002）（总结在图12.4中）。这可能是由于烟碱诱导的α4α6β2* nAChR多巴胺神经元放电的增强取决于同时含有α4和α6亚基的nAChR（Engle et al. 2013; Liu et al. 2012）。

还发现薄荷醇与烟碱结合可以改变多巴胺神经元的放电（图12.4）。薄荷醇和烟碱会使烟碱刺激的多巴胺神经元放电频率增加，其频率明显高于单独的烟碱。再次，这可能是由于增强了α4α6β2* nAChR的上调 [见图12.3（a）]。尽管薄荷醇增强了烟碱对多巴胺神经元的作用，但发现薄荷醇逆转了烟碱对GABA神经元放电的作用。如前所述，长期暴露于烟碱会使GABA神经元在急性暴露于烟碱时表现出持续的活动抑制（图12.4）。在薄荷醇加烟碱的情况下，GABA神经元放电频率瞬时增加，但缓慢返回类似于基线放电频率的状态。因此，没有观察到活动持续降低的迹象。已显示薄荷醇（单独）可降低α4β2* nAChR脱敏作用（Henderson et al. 2016）。这可能解释了长期暴露于薄荷醇和烟碱中的GABA神经元在烟碱应用过程中可能无法脱敏，因为它们仅具有α4（非α6）β2* nAChR。总而言之，当我们考虑烟碱对多巴胺神经元放电的特征性影响时，薄荷醇会增强多巴胺神经元放电的这些变化，最终导致兴奋性增强。

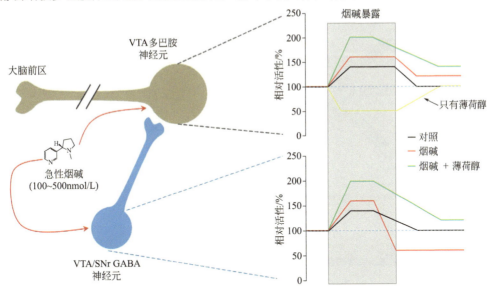

图12.4　烟碱具有很好的特征，可以瞬时增强多巴胺和GABA神经元的放电（用透明的灰色阴影表示）

还已知在长期暴露于烟碱后（>7d），GABA神经元迅速脱敏并表现出降低的放电频率（长达1h）。这导致对多巴胺神经元的抑制。这有助于增加多巴胺神经元的兴奋性。薄荷醇和烟碱的慢性治疗可防止GABA神经元脱敏，但多巴胺神经元的兴奋性增强。

参见Henderson等（2017）。

12.6　薄荷醇本身会改变中脑多巴胺神经元上的nAChR

我们对薄荷醇作用的大部分了解来自对薄荷醇与烟碱结合使用的研究。从这些研究来看，尚不清楚薄荷醇是否会自己产生作用，并且是烟碱的添加剂还是薄荷醇本身会引起明显的大脑变化。为此，已经完成了一些调查以解决这个问题。

12.6.1 单独的薄荷醇上调nAChR

为更好地了解薄荷醇如何在吸烟者中产生增强的nAChR上调，研究了薄荷醇在不存在烟碱的情况下对上调的作用（Henderson et al. 2016）。在此，发现薄荷醇上调了瞬时转染到神经2a细胞中的α4β2和α6β2β3 nAChR。更重要的是，这是通过薄荷醇的浓度（0.5μmol/L）实现的，该浓度远低于变构拮抗作用或Cys-loop受体增强所必需的浓度（见表12.1）。在小鼠中，使用浓度<2.5μmol/L的薄荷醇观察到nAChR的上调（Henderson et al. 2016）。薄荷醇还表现出与烟碱诱导的上调不同的中脑α4* nAChR的细胞特异性上调。烟碱强烈上调SNr和VTA GABA神经元上的α4* nAChR（Nashmi et al. 2007），但薄荷醇上调SNc和VTA DA神经元上的α4* nAChR，而不上调SNr α4* nAChR（Henderson et al. 2016）。

当将薄荷醇和烟碱与单独的薄荷醇进行比较时，nAChR的上调也有所不同：烟碱和薄荷醇上调高敏感性nAChR，而单独的薄荷醇仅上调低敏感性nAChR（图12.5）。这仅在体外制剂中观察到，因为使用小鼠进行的研究无法提供有关nAChR化学计量的信息。

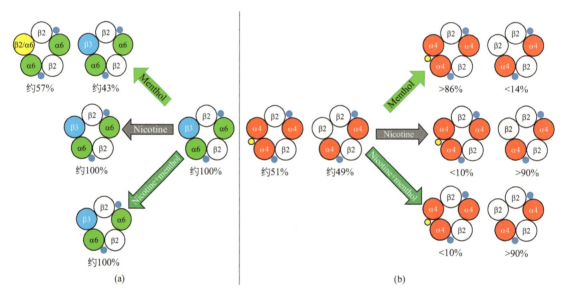

图12.5 薄荷醇、烟碱和薄荷醇加烟碱改变（a）α6* 和（b）α4* nAChR 的化学计量

该图显示了从瞬时转染了 α6、β2和β3 nAChR 亚基或α4和β2 nAChR 亚基的培养神经2a细胞中获得的发现（Henderson et al. 2017, 2016）。单独的薄荷醇可稳定低灵敏性 nAChRs［α6β2（非β3）和α4$_{(2)}$β2$_{(3)}$］。烟碱和烟碱加薄荷醇可稳定高敏感性 nAChRs［α6β2β3 和α4$_{(2)}$β2$_{(3)}$］。蓝点表示烟碱和乙酰胆碱的激动剂结合位点。黄点表示最近已针对ACh表征的非典型结合位点。

12.6.2 单独的薄荷醇可消除烟碱奖励相关行为

有趣的是，在使用小鼠的条件位置偏好试验中，在烟碱之前暴露于薄荷醇可防止烟碱奖励相关行为（Henderson et al. 2016）。在该测定中，在条件位置偏好训练之前，仅用薄荷醇对小鼠治疗10d。因此，预防烟碱奖励相关行为的原因可能是薄荷醇上调低亲和力nAChR的能力。结果是，由于存在低亲和力而不是高亲和力的nAChR，烟碱无法有效激活中脑多巴胺和GABA神经元。

12.7 结论

薄荷醇、烟碱及其组合会引起大脑的若干变化。尽管已证明薄荷醇可作用于几种 Cys-loop 受体，但长期作用仅在 nAChR 上得以表征。烟碱和薄荷醇单独或一起上调大脑 nAChR。高烟碱敏感性 nAChR 的上调引起多巴胺奖励信号的显著变化（总结见表12.2）。最值得注意的是，这些神经元表现出对烟碱的兴奋性增加。这可能是与单独的烟碱相比，薄荷醇与烟碱结合会产生更大的积极奖励的原因。总之，这些变化突出了一个事实，即薄荷醇卷烟吸烟者戒烟率的下降至少可以部分归因于薄荷醇诱导的烟碱奖励的提高。

表12.2 烟碱、烟碱＋薄荷醇、薄荷醇引起的大脑变化的比较

	烟碱	烟碱＋薄荷醇	薄荷醇
上调			
α4* nAChR 上调	腹侧被盖区[1]，黑质致密部[1]，黑质网状部[1],[4]，纹状体[2]	腹侧被盖区[1]，黑质致密部[1]，黑质网状部[1],[4]，纹状体[2]	腹侧被盖区[3]，黑质致密部[3]，纹状体[3]
α6* nAChR 上调	腹侧被盖区[1]，黑质致密部[1]	前额叶皮层[2]腹侧被盖区[2]	前额叶皮层[3]
α4α6* nAChR 上调	腹侧被盖区[1]，黑质致密部[1]	腹侧被盖区[1]，黑质致密部[1]	腹侧被盖区[3]，黑质致密部[3]尚未检查
神经元基线放电			
多巴胺神经元	发射减少[1],[4]	发射减少[1]	发射减少[3]
γ-氨基丁酸神经元	发射增加[1]	发射增加[1]	尚未检查
神经元兴奋性			
多巴胺神经元	兴奋性增加[1],[4]	兴奋性增加[1]	兴奋性减少[3]
γ-氨基丁酸神经元	兴奋性减少[1]	兴奋性增加[1]	尚未检查

[1] Henderson et al. (2017).
[2] Alsharari et al. (2015).
[3] Henderson et al. (2016).
[4] Nashmi et al. (2007).

术语解释

- 条件位置偏好：一种与工具/动物反应无关的药物奖励相关行为的测定。
- 药物奖励和强化：使用动物模型对成瘾的研究非常复杂。因此，对测定法进行了优化以测量成瘾的各个组成部分：奖励、强化、恢复、戒断等。
- 电生理学：细胞和神经元电学性质的研究。
- 烟碱乙酰胆碱受体（nAChR）：对烟碱敏感的胆碱能受体。这些受体存在于周围和中枢神经系统中。乙酰胆碱（ACh）是 nAChR 和毒蕈碱 ACh 受体的内源性神经递质。
- 伏隔核：腹侧纹状体的区域，其中中脑边缘多巴胺神经元的末端终止于 GABA 能中型多刺神经元。
- 前额叶皮层：大脑皮层的区域，覆盖前脑区域，并与认知行为的许多方面有关。
- 自给药：自我管理药物增强相关行为的测定，取决于动物的行为（选择）。
- 黑质肉质网：中脑区主要由抑制性 GABA 能神经元组成。

- 上调：是一个复杂的过程，但是该术语最广泛地用于表示特定蛋白质数量的增加。这可能发生在许多蛋白质上，但这是烟碱的标志性特征：烟碱增加了nAChR的数量（上调）。
- 腹侧被盖区：靠近腹侧中脑中线的脑区，是中脑边缘和黑质纹状体途径的多巴胺投射的起源。该区域对于奖励回路至关重要。

薄荷醇的关键事实
- 薄荷醇是美国非电子烟中唯一允许使用的合法调味剂。
- 甚至98%的非薄荷醇卷烟中都含有薄荷醇。
- 薄荷标记的卷烟中薄荷醇的含量≥3mg/支。
- 在非薄荷醇卷烟中，薄荷醇以痕量（＜0.1mg）存在。
- 薄荷醇除用作烟草调味剂外，还用作薄荷和薄荷调味产品（口香糖、糖果等）的调味剂、局部麻醉剂、减充血剂、止痒剂。

要点总结
- 烟碱和薄荷醇均上调中脑多巴胺和GABA神经元的nAChRs。
- 当烟碱与薄荷醇混合使用时，所发生的上调明显大于单独使用的任何一种。
- 个别地，烟碱会增加阶段性多巴胺神经元的放电，而薄荷醇会降低这种放电模式。
- 薄荷醇和烟碱的结合可增强阶段性多巴胺神经元的放电，使其水平高于单独的烟碱。
- 最终，这些变化增加了多巴胺神经元的兴奋性，并增强了烟碱的奖励。

参考文献

Ahijevych, K.; Parsley, L. A. (1999). Smoke constituent exposure and stage of change in black and white women cigarette smokers. Addictive Behaviors, 24, 115-120.

Ai, J.; Taylor, K. M.; Lisko, J. G.; Tran, H.; Watson, C. H.; Holman, M. R. (2015). Menthol content in US marketed cigarettes. Nicotine, Tobacco Research. https://doi.org/10.1093/ntr/ntv162.

Alsharari, S. D.; King, J. R.; Nordman, J. C.; Muldoon, P. P.; Jackson, A.; Zhu, A. Z. X. et al. (2015). Effects of menthol on nicotine pharmacokinetic, pharmacology and dependence in mice. PLoS One, 10, e0137070.

Ashley, M.; Dixon, M.; Sisodiya, A.; Prasad, K. (2012). Lack of effect of menthol level and type on smokers' estimated mouth level exposures to tar and nicotine and perceived sensory characteristics of cigarette smoke. Regulatory toxicology and pharmacology: RTP, 63, 381-390.

Ashoor, A.; Nordman, J. C.; Veltri, D.; Yang, K. H.; Shuba, Y.; Al Kury, L. et al. (2013a). Menthol inhibits 5-HT3 receptor-mediated currents. The Journal of Pharmacology and Experimental Therapeutics, 347, 398-409.

Ashoor, A.; Nordman, J. C.; Veltri, D.; Yang, K. -H. S.; Al Kury, L.; Shuba, Y. et al. (2013b). Menthol binding and inhibition of α7-nicotinic acetylcholine receptors. PLoS One, 8, e67674.

Benowitz, N. L.; Herrera, B.; Jacob, P.; 3rd (2004). Mentholated cigarette smoking inhibits nicotine metabolism. The Journal of Pharmacology and Experimental Therapeutics, 310, 1208-1215.

Biswas, L.; Harrison, E.; Gong, Y.; Avusula, R.; Lee, J.; Zhang, M. et al. (2016). Enhancing effect of menthol on nicotine selfadministration in rats. Psychopharmacology, 233, 3417-3427.

Brody, A.; Mukhin, A.; La Charite, J.; Ta, K.; Farahi, J.; Sugar, C. et al. (2013). Up-regulation of nicotinic acetylcholine receptors in menthol cigarette smokers. The International Journal of Neuropsychopharmacology, 16, 957-966.

Caraballo, R. S.; Asman, K. (2011). Epidemiology of menthol cigarette use in the United States. Tobacco Induced Diseases, 9(Suppl 1), S1.

CDC. (2016). Tobacco use among middle and high school students—United States, 2011-2015. Morbidity and Mortality Weekly Report, 65, 361-367.

Corvalan, N. A.; Zygadlo, J. A.; Garcia, D. A. (2009). Stereo-selective activity of menthol on GABA(A) receptor. Chirality, 21, 525-530.

Delnevo, C. D.; Gundersen, D. A.; Hrywna, M.; Echeverria, S. E.; Steinberg, M. B. (2011). Smoking-cessation prevalence among U. S. smokers of menthol versus non-menthol cigarettes. American Journal of Preventive Medicine, 41, 357-365.

D'Silva, J.; Boyle, R. G.; Lien, R.; Rode, P.; Okuyemi, K. S. (2012). Cessation outcomes among treatment-seeking menthol and nonmenthol smokers. American Journal of Preventive Medicine, 43, S242-S248.

Engle, S. E.; Shih, P. Y.; McIntosh, J. M.; Drenan, R. M. (2013). alpha4 alpha6 beta2* nicotinic acetylcholine receptor activation on ventral tegmental area dopamine neurons is sufficient to stimulate a depolarizing conductance and enhance surface AMPA receptor function. Molecular

Pharmacology, 84, 393-406.

Faure, P.; Tolu, S.; Valverde, S.; Naude, J. (2014). Role of nicotinic acetylcholine receptors in regulating dopamine neuron activity. Neuroscience, 282, 86-100.

FDA. (2012). Priliminary scientific evaluation of the possible public health effects of menthol versus nonmenthol cigarettes. (2012). https://www.fda.gov/downloads/ucm361598.pdf.

Hall, A. C.; Turcotte, C. M.; Betts, B. A.; Yeung, W. Y.; Agyeman, A. S.; Burk, L. A. (2004). Modulation of human GABAA and glycine receptor currents by menthol and related monoterpenoids. European Journal of Pharmacology, 506, 9-16.

Hans, M.; Wilhelm, M.; Swandulla, D. (2012). Menthol suppresses nicotinic acetylcholine receptor functioning in sensory neurons via allosteric modulation. Chemical Senses, 37, 463-469.

Henderson, B. J.; Wall, T.; Henley, B. M.; Kim, C. H.; Nichols, W. A.; Moaddel, R. et al. (2016). Menthol alone upregulates midbrain nAChRs, alters nAChR sybtype stoichiometry, alters dopamine neuron firing frequency, and prevents nicotine reward. The Journal of Neuroscience, 36, 2957-2974.

Henderson, B. J.; Wall, T. R.; Henley, B. M.; Kim, C. H.; McKinney, S.; Lester, H. A. (2017). Menthol enhances nicotine reward-related behavior by potentiating nicotine-induced changes in nAChR function, nAChR upregulation, and DA neuron excitability. Neuropsychopharmacology. https://doi.org/10.1038/npp.2017.72.

Jasinska, A. J.; Zorick, T.; Brody, A. L.; Stein, E. A. (2013). Dual role of nicotine in addiction and cognition: a review of neuroimaging studies in humans. Neuropharmacology, 84, 111-122.

Journigan, V. B.; Zaveri, N. T. (2013). TRPM8 ion channel ligands for new therapeutic applications and as probes to study menthol pharmacology. Life Sciences, 92, 425-437.

Lau, B. K.; Karim, S.; Goodchild, A. K.; Vaughan, C. W.; Drew, G. M. (2014). Menthol enhances phasic and tonic GABAA receptor mediated currents in midbrain periaqueductal grey neurons. British Journal of Pharmacology, 171, 2803-2813.

Liu, L.; Zhao-Shea, R.; McIntosh, J. M.; Gardner, P. D.; Tapper, A. R. (2012). Nicotine persistently activates ventral tegmental area dopaminergic neurons via nicotinic acetylcholine receptors containing alpha4 and alpha6 subunits. Molecular Pharmacology, 81, 541-548.

Lochlann Jain, S. S. (2003). "Come up to the Kool taste": African American upward mobility and the semiotics of smoking menthols. Public Culture, 15, 295-322.

Mansvelder, H. D.; Keath, J. R.; McGehee, D. S. (2002). Synaptic mechnisms underlie nicotine-induced excitability of brain reward areas. Neuron, 33, 905-919.

Nashmi, R.; Xiao, C.; Deshpande, P.; McKinney, S.; Grady, S. R. Whiteaker, P. et al. (2007). Chronic nicotine cell specifically upregulates functional α4* nicotinic receptors: basis for both tolerance in midbrain and enhanced long-term potentiation in perforant path. The Journal of Neuroscience, 27, 8202-8218.

Oz, M.; El Nebrisi, E. G.; Yang, K. S.; Howarth, F. C.; Al Kury, L. T. (2017). Cellular and molecular targets of menthol actions. Frontiers in Pharmacology, 8, 472.

Pons, S.; Fattore, L.; Cossu, G.; Tolu, S.; Porcu, E.; McIntosh, J. M. et al. (2008). Crucial role of α4 and α6 nicotinic acetylcholine receptor subunits from ventral tegmental area in systemic nicotine self-administration. The Journal of Neuroscience, 28, 12318-12327.

Proctor, R. N. (2012). Golden holocaust: Origins of the cigarette catastrophe and the case for abolition. University of California Press. Sine, S. M.; Engel, A. G. (2006). Recent advances in Cys-loop receptor structure and function. Nature, 440, 448-455.

Srinivasan, R.; Pantoja, R.; Moss, F. J.; Mackey, E. D. W.; Son, C.; Miwa, J. et al. (2011). Nicotine upregulates α4β2 nicotinic receptors and ER exit sites via stoichiometry-dependent chaperoning. The Journal of General Physiology, 137, 59-79.

Tapper, A. R.; McKinney, S. L.; Nashmi, R.; Schwarz, J.; Deshpande, P.; Labarca, C. et al. (2004). Nicotine activation of α4* receptors: sufficient for reward, tolerance and sensitization. Science, 306, 1029-1032.

Ton, H. T.; Smart, A. E.; Aguilar, B. L.; Olson, T. T.; Kellar, K. J.; Ahern, G. P. (2015). Menthol enhances the desensitization of human alpha3 beta4 nicotinic acetylcholine receptors. Molecular Pharmacology, 88, 256-264.

Villanti, A. C.; Mowery, P. D.; Delnevo, C. D.; Niaura, R. S.; Abrams, D. B.; Giovino, G. A. (2016). Changes in the prevalence and correlates of menthol cigarette use in the USA, 2004-2014. Tobacco Control, 25, ii14-ii20.

Wang, T.; Wang, B.; Chen, H. (2014). Menthol facilitates the intravenous self-administration of nicotine in rats. Frontiers in Behavioral Neuroscience, 8, 437.

Watt, E. E.; Betts, B. A.; Kotey, F. O.; Humbert, D. J.; Griffith, T. N.; Kelly, E. W. et al. (2008). Menthol shares general anesthetic activity and sites of action on the GABA(A) receptor with the intravenous agent, propofol. European Journal of Pharmacology, 590, 120-126.

WHO (2016) Banning menthol in tobacco products. http://apps.who.int/iris/bitstream/10665/205928/1/9789241510332_eng.pdf.

13
吸烟与烟碱：对多发性硬化症的影响

Insa Backhaus, Alice Mannocci, Giuseppe La Torre, Aldo Liccardi

Department of Public Health and Infectious Diseases, Sapienza University of Rome, Piazzale Aldo Moro, Rome, Italy

缩略语

Anti-EBNA	爱泼斯坦-巴尔病毒核抗原的血清抗体滴度	EU	欧盟
		HLA	人白细胞抗原
CI	置信区间	MS	多发性硬化症
CNS	中枢神经系统	OR	比值比
EBV	爱泼斯坦-巴尔病毒		

13.1 引言

吸烟是全球可预防疾病的主要原因。仅在欧盟，每年就有70万人因吸烟而过早死亡。众所周知，吸烟是呼吸系统疾病、心血管疾病和自身免疫性疾病的主要原因，但越来越多的数据表明，烟碱（一种具有成瘾性的卷烟成分）可能会降低帕金森病等疾病的发病率和严重程度（Quik et al. 2007）和多发性硬化症（MS）。

MS是一种复杂的中枢神经系统（CNS）的进行性疾病，是一种炎症性脱髓鞘疾病，是年轻人中最常见的神经系统疾病和非创伤性残疾的原因之一。全世界范围内受MS影响的人数在110万～250万之间。MS的发病通常在成年初期，即20～50岁之间，这是生产力的最高峰。因此，MS是一个紧迫的公共卫生问题。MS的表现从无害疾病到迅速发展的致残疾病，需要严格的生活方式调整。MS的病程可以是复发缓解型或进展型（Hauser, Goodin, 2012）。

当免疫系统错误地攻击人体自身的健康组织时，就会发生诸如MS的自身免疫性疾病（Longo et al. 2012）。对于MS，在CNS内，免疫系统会攻击髓磷脂，髓磷脂是一种围绕并隔离神经纤维的脂肪物质，称为轴突。在此过程中，大脑和脊髓的这些绝缘覆盖层被损坏（图13.1）。此过程也称为脱髓鞘。髓鞘变薄，最终破裂；因此，轴突不能再正常工作了。往返于大脑和脊髓的神经冲动被打断，导致一系列症状，如刺痛感、虚弱、平衡受损和视力模糊（Hauser, Goodin, 2012）（表13.1）。尽管自1868年发现MS以来已经有200多年的历史了，但MS的病因尚不完全清楚（Gohil, 2015）。研究人员认为，遗传易感性和某些环境因素在疾病发展中起主要作用。例如，环境因素包括感染爱泼斯坦-巴尔病毒、纬度和吸烟。特别地，吸烟已被不利地提出，并且正在成为诸如MS的慢性炎症疾病的强烈危险因素。对26项研究的系统回顾和荟萃分析显示，与不吸烟者相比，经常吸烟者的患病风险增加了55%（Zhang et al. 2016）。对34个研究的另一项荟萃分析显示了相似的结果。该荟萃分析称，与不吸烟者相比，经常吸烟者的OR估计值为1.46（1.33和1.59），当前吸烟者的OR估计值为1.57（1.34和1.80），而前吸烟者的OR估计值为1.36

（1.27和1.46）（Poorolajal, Bahrami, Karami, Hooshmand, 2016）。许多研究支持以下论点：吸烟不仅是一种增加MS风险的重要风险因素，而且也对MS的发展和进程有影响（Hernán et al. 2005）。

本章对吸烟、烟碱和MS之间关系的发现进行了全面回顾。本章讨论的具体问题如下：①吸烟与多发性硬化症易感性之间是否存在关联？②烟碱与多发性硬化症易感性之间是否存在关联？③将吸烟与MS联系起来的可能机制是什么？

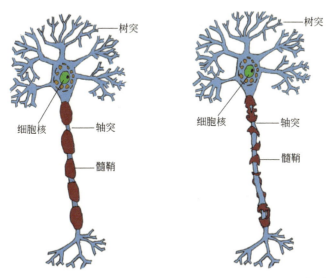

图13.1 没有MS的健康神经元（左）和患有MS的受损神经元（右）

左侧显示正常神经元，右侧显示MS中发现的脱髓鞘神经元。轴突负责从神经元细胞体传递到中枢神经系统和周围神经系统的电脉冲。称为髓磷脂的脂肪保护层围绕着轴突，并有助于电脉冲沿着轴突的传递。MS导致髓磷脂脱髓鞘、丢失或分解，因此会中断或扭曲沿轴突到达CNS的信息。

表13.1 多发性硬化症的主要事实

- 多发性硬化症是一种影响中枢神经系统的自身免疫性疾病
- 多发性硬化症的典型发病年龄在20～40岁之间
- 北部的MS患病率高于南部
- 病程可以是复发缓解型或进展型
- 有四种类型：复发缓解型多发性硬化症、继发进展型多发性硬化症、原发进展型多发性硬化症、进展复发型多发性硬化症
- 研究人员认为，遗传易感性和环境在疾病发展中起关键作用
- 症状包括麻木或刺痛感、虚弱、平衡受损、视力模糊、膀胱或肠道问题以及认知和情绪变化

注：该表列出了多发性硬化症的关键事实，包括流行病学、MS的病程和类型以及患者可能遇到的危险因素和症状。

13.2 吸烟和MS风险

建立多发性硬化症和吸烟之间可能联系的历史可以追溯到20世纪60年代，当时的观察性研究首次发表。（Antonovsky et al. 1965; Simpson, Newell, Schapira, 1966）。Antonovsky等（1965）和Simpson等（1966）是最早独立发表有关吸烟和MS风险研究的研究团队之一。但是，这些研究的结果有争议，并没有得出任何有意义的结论。Antonovsky等（1965）和他的研究小组询问了来自以色列的241名MS患者是否在发病前吸烟。结果表明，在MS病例中，发病年龄之前吸烟的比例明显高于对照组（44%和36%，$p=0.02$）（Antonovsky et al. 1965）。相反，Simpson及其

同事得出的结论是，在英格兰的病例和对照组中，患者和对照组中吸烟者的比例没有总体差异（Simpson et al. 1966）。

在过去的几十年中，MS与吸烟之间可能存在的关系这一话题引起了许多研究团队的关注，并且在过去的十年中，已发表文章的数量激增。表13.2概述了观察性研究（病例对照研究、队列研究和横断面研究）。在20世纪90年代，英国发表了两项纵向研究。这两项研究均观察到经常吸烟的女性患MS的风险更高，尽管这些发现并不显著（Thorogood, Hannaford, 1998; Villard-Mackintosh, Vessey, 1993）。然而，必须指出的是，这两项研究均主要关注口服避孕药与MS风险之间的关系，而吸烟仅被视为次要因素。Hernán、Oleky和Ascherio（2001）在美国护士健康研究（121700名女性）和美国护士健康研究Ⅱ（116671名女性）中队列研究了MS发病率与吸烟之间的关系。结果表明，在对年龄、纬度和血统进行调整之后，当前吸烟者的相对发病率为1.6（95% CI: 1.2～2.1）。例如，来自加拿大的一项回顾性病例对照研究发现，吸烟与MS风险之间存在直接且显著的关联（Ghadirian et al. 2001）。研究人员研究了200个人以及202个年龄和性别匹配的对照者的吸烟习惯。结果表明，与从未吸烟者相比，曾经吸烟者的OR为1.6（95% CI: 1.0～2.4）。每天吸20～40支卷烟的重度吸烟者，其风险增加了近两倍，OR为1.9（95% CI: 1.2～3.2）（Ghadirian et al. 2001），这证明了吸烟数量和患MS风险之间的剂量反应相关性。Ghadirian等（2001）基于对MS诊断前一年中报告的吸烟情况进行了分析，并根据年龄、性别和教育程度进行了调整。贝尔格莱德的一项病例对照研究证实了这些发现。Pekmezovic等（2006）表明，与对照组相比，MS患者中的吸烟者更为普遍（Pekmezovic et al. 2006）。此外，研究人员观察到MS风险与吸烟持续时间（年）（$p = 0.027$）和每日吸烟量（$p = 0.021$）之间的剂量反应关系。尽管如此，MS是一种复杂的疾病，吸烟可能与其他MS危险因素相互作用，并且这种可能的相互作用甚至可能增加MS风险。Simon和他的同事（Simon et al. 2010）恰好研究了这种相互作用。

研究人员研究了吸烟如何与爱泼斯坦-巴尔病毒核抗原（anti-EBNA）和HLA-DR15的血清抗体滴度相互作用（Simon et al., 2010）。他们对来自三项MS病例对照研究的约440例病例和860例对照进行了单独分析和汇总分析。结果表明，与"从未吸烟者"相比，"永远吸烟者"与更高的anti-EBNA滴度相关的MS风险更高。但是，这仅在抗EBNA滴度高的人群中观察到。事实上，在研究吸烟和抗EBNA抗体滴度的联合作用时，曾经吸烟者具有最高的EBNA滴度，其MS风险增加了7倍（RR: 7.4; 95% CI: 3.6～15.0）（Simon et al. 2010）。确定任何环境因素的成因的关键点是敏感性与剂量之间的相互作用（van der Mei, Simpson, Stankovich, Taylor, 2011）。尽管许多研究报告称，随着吸烟量的增加，MS易感性增加（Carlens et al. 2010; Throgood, Hannaford, 1998），但其他研究显示没有影响（Antonovsky et al. 1965; Jafari et al. 2009）。

然而，在结合病例对照研究时发现，"曾经吸烟者"与"从未吸烟者"的OR值为1.40（95% CI: 1.29～1.52），而"当前吸烟者"与"不吸烟者"的OR值为1.42（95% CI: 1.26～1.60）（Backhaus, Mannocci, Lemmens, La Torre, 2016）。图13.2显示了Backhaus等（2016）最近进行的荟萃分析的森林图。在其他荟萃分析中也证明了类似的结果（Handel et al. 2011; Hawkes, 2007; Poorolajal et al. 2016; Zhang et al. 2016）。例如，Poorolajal等（2016）研究显示，长期吸烟者MS的估计OR为1.46（95% CI: 1.33～1.59），当前吸烟者为1.57（95% CI: 1.34～1.80）。Zhang等（2016）将他们的分析分为保守分析和非保守分析，提出吸烟是MS的一个危险因素。保守模

型仅包括描述在疾病发病前吸烟行为的研究，而非保守模型包括所有研究，无论吸烟行为是在发病前还是同时发生。两项分析均表明，吸烟是MS的一个危险因素，对于保守分析，OR值为1.55（95% CI：1.48～1.62），对于非保守分析，OR值则为1.57（95% CI：1.50～1.64）。此外，当使用多发性硬化McDonald标准对研究进行汇总分析以确定MS病例时，可以观察到可比的结果（OR：1.41；95% CI：1.14～1.75）（图13.3）。

表13.2 评估吸烟和多发性硬化症风险的观察性研究的特点

参考文献	国家	研究方向	诊断标准	案例数量	对照组数量	RR/OR	置信区间	男女比例（女性/男性）
Antonovsky et al. (1965)	以色列	病例-对照	未声明	241	964	1.4	1.05～1.86	1.2
Alonso, Cook, Maghzi, Divani (2011)	爱尔兰	病例-对照	McDonald诊断标准	394	394	1.7	0.9～3.07	3.7
Al-Afasy et al. (2013)	科威特	病例-对照	神经科医生诊断	101	202	1.7	0.9～3.4	1.2
Briggs et al. (2014)	美国/瑞典	病例-对照	神经科医生诊断	1506	1070	1.97	1.29～3.00	NA
Carlens et al. (2010)	瑞典	一批	病例诊断	277777（总人数）		1.9	1.4～2.6	全男性
Engdahl et al. (2014)	瑞典	病例-对照	McDonald诊断标准	466	487	1.57	1.16～2.12	2.5
Ghadirian, Dadgostar, Azani, Maisonneuve (2001)	加拿大	病例-对照	未声明	200	202	1.6	1～2.4	2.2
Healy et al. (2009)	美国	横断面研究	McDonald诊断标准	1465		2.41	1.09～5.34	NA
Hedström, Bäärnhielm, Olsson, Alfredsson (2009)	瑞典	病例-对照	McDonald诊断标准	902	1855	1.5	1.3～1.8	2.6
Hedström et al. (2011)	瑞典	病例-对照	McDonald诊断标准	843	1209	1.6	1.3～2.0	NA
Hedström, Hillert, Olsson, Alfredsson (2013)	瑞典	病例-对照	McDonald诊断标准	7883	9264	1.5	1.4～1.6	2.6
Hernán et al. (2001)	美国	一批	Poser准则	238371（总人数）		1.6	1.2～2.1	全女性
Hernán et al. (2005)	美国	病例-对照	Poser准则	201	1913	1.3	1～1.7	2.4
Jafari, Hoppenbrouwers, Hop, Breteler, Hintzen (2009)	荷兰	病例-对照	McDonald诊断标准	136	204	1.09	0.68～1.73	1.7

续表

参考文献	国家	研究方向	诊断标准	案例数量	对照组数量	RR/OR	置信区间	男女比例（女性/男性）
Mansouri et al. (2014)	爱尔兰	病例-对照	Poser和McDonald诊断标准	1403	883	1.93	1.31～2.73	3.11
Maghzi et al. (2011)	爱尔兰	病例-对照	McDonald诊断标准	516	1090	2.67	1.70～4.21	3.7
Kotzamani et al. (2012)	希腊	病例-对照	临床核磁共振成像	657	593	1.9（f：1.8, 2.0）		1.6
Pekmezovic et al. (2006)	塞尔维亚	病例-对照	Poser准则	210	210	2.4	1.3～4.2	NA
O'Gorman, Bukhari, Todd, Freeman, Broadley (2014)	澳大利亚	病例-对照	McDonald诊断标准	560	480	1.9	1.5～2.5	4.5
Rodríguez Regal et al. (2009)	西班牙	病例-对照	McDonald诊断标准	138	138	2.18	1.3～3.6	2.2
Roudbari, Ansar, Yousefzad (2013)	爱尔兰	病例-对照	Poser和McDonald诊断标准	514		危险比率2.25	95%CI：（1.3～3.88）	1.4
Ramagopalan et al. (2013)	加拿大	病例-对照	未声明	3157	756	1.32	1.10～1.60	3.3
Salzer et al. (2013)	瑞典	病例-对照	ICD	192	384	1.5	0.98～2.3	NA
da Silva et al. (2009)	巴西	病例-对照	Poser准则	81	81	7.6	2.1～28.2	N/A
Simon et al. (2010)	美国	病例-对照	Poser准则和成像	442	865	1.5	1～2.4	2.1
Sundström, Nyström, Hallmans (2008)	瑞典	病例-对照	Poser准则	109	218	1.4	0.78～2.6	1.3
Simpson et al. (1966)	澳大利亚	病例-对照	未声明	584	无数据	1.1	0.9～1.3	1.5
Thorogood, Hannaford (1998)	美国	一批	GP诊断	无数据		1.2	0.8～1.8	女性
Villard-Mackintosh, Vessey (1993)	美国	一批	专家诊断	无数据		1.5	0.94～2.53	女性
Zorzon et al. (2003)	美国		未声明	140	131	1.9OR(最近的吸烟者)	1.1～3.2	1.8

注：它显示了1965年至2014年间进行的观察研究的特征。大多数研究在欧洲进行(如瑞典)。

表13.3 评估瑞典鼻烟、烟碱和多发性硬化症风险的研究特点

参考文献	国家	研究方向	诊断标准	案例数量	对照组数量	RR/OR	较低的95%和较高的CI
Carlens et al. (2010)	瑞典	一批	未声明	2777777		1	0.8～1.4
Hedström et al. (2009)	瑞典	病例-对照	McDonald诊断标准	902	1855	0.3	0.1～0.8
Hedström et al. (2013)	瑞典	病例-对照	McDonald诊断标准	7883	9437	0.83	0.75～0.92

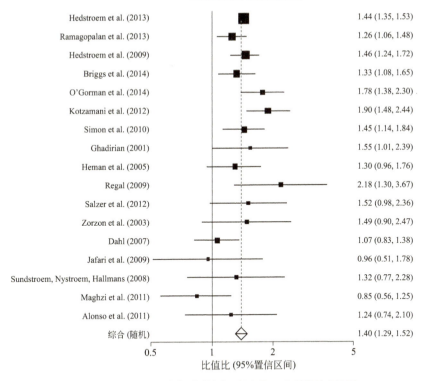

图 13.2 "曾经吸烟者"对"从未吸烟者" MS 风险的森林图

森林图显示曾经吸烟者和从未吸烟者的汇总分析。每条水平线显示每个研究的估计值的 95% CI。空心菱形代表总体概要估计。该图摘自 Backhaus 等（2016）。

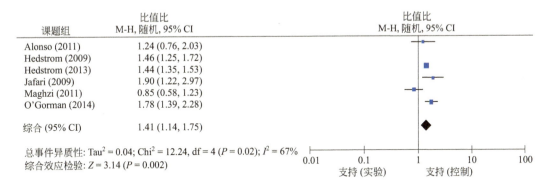

图 13.3 使用多发性硬化 McDonald 诊断标准研究的"永远"与"从未"吸烟者的 MS 风险森林图

它显示了使用 McDonald 标准对曾经吸烟和从不吸烟的人进行比较的汇总分析。每条水平线显示每个研究的估计值的 95% CI。空心菱形代表总体概要估计。

13.3 吸烟、MS的进展和症状恶化

吸烟与疾病进展之间的关联仍不确定。有些研究表明风险增加，而另一些则没有。Hernán 等（2005）进行了一项嵌套的病例对照研究，包括 MS 201 名患者和 1913 个对照。吸烟患者发生复发缓解性临床症状的可能性是发生继发性症状的 3 倍。Courville、Maschmeyer 和 Delay

（1964）证明吸烟后症状立即恶化。一项包括来自美国的1465例患者在内的横断面调查报告称，在基线时，就扩大的残疾状态量表评分和多发性硬化症严重程度评分而言，与不吸烟者相比，目前的吸烟者的病情明显差（Healy et al. 2009）。与不吸烟者相比，目前的吸烟者更可能患有原发进展型多发性硬化症。与以前进行的研究相比，该研究的样本量更大，并且具有更大的统计能力。

13.4 吸烟和多发性硬化症之间的联系机制

吸烟通常会对免疫系统产生各种有害影响，从而引起相对免疫缺陷和较高的感染率。然而，吸烟如何影响多发性硬化症的风险还没有完全被了解。已经提出了几种机制，包括吸烟对血脑屏障的免疫调节和直接作用、卷烟烟雾的神经毒性作用以及对呼吸道的影响（Pugliatti et al. 2008）。

卷烟烟雾中含有6000多种潜在有毒成分，如烟碱、一氧化碳和氰化氢（Arnson, Shoenfeld, Amital, 2010）。其中一些成分可能对中枢神经系统有直接的毒性作用（Costenbader, Karlson, 2006）。引起关注的一种主要且可能是最具影响力的成分是氰化氢。在20世纪60年代末，Levine（1967）发现烟草烟雾的某些成分，如氰化氢及其主要代谢产物硫氰酸盐可能对包括CNS在内的中枢神经系统有毒性作用。有趣的是，胼胝体不仅在大多数MS病例中经常异常，而且最容易受到氰化物的损害（Evangelou et al. 2000; Ozturk et al. 2010）。吸入卷烟烟雾是氰化氢的主要来源。这可以解释吸烟是增加MS风险的主要因素的想法。另一个可能的解释是，吸烟与呼吸系统疾病的易感性增加有关，而这又是与MS风险升高相关的另一个危险因素（Egesten et al. 2008; Jafari, Hintzen, 2011）。这与瑞典的研究相一致，即吸烟而不是烟碱是造成这种现象的原因。通过气道介导的烟草烟雾成分可能引起肺部刺激（Hedström et al. 2009）。

使用动物模型进行的实验研究表明，卷烟的成分会影响免疫系统的各个部分，包括先天免疫、B细胞和T细胞以及自然杀伤细胞（Fusby et al. 2010; Handel et al. 2011）。最后，吸烟与其他自身免疫性疾病（如格雷夫斯病和克罗恩病）有关，这些疾病可以与MS进行类比（Costenbader, Karlson, 2006）。

13.5 烟碱和多发性硬化症

大量证据表明，吸烟会增加患MS的风险，甚至可能加速疾病的发展。这是否也适用于无烟烟草和烟碱以及烟草中的成瘾成分仍然未知。与卷烟烟雾不同，烟碱尚未被认为具有致癌性，甚至可能对炎症性疾病具有治疗和保护作用（Piao et al. 2009）。与吸烟相比，缺乏关于烟碱及其对MS影响的文献。表13.3概述了针对瑞典鼻烟、烟碱和MS风险的研究。瑞典的两项研究探讨了烟碱可能对MS的病因具有保护作用（Hedström et al. 2009; Hedström et al. 2013）。在一项病例对照研究中，研究小组研究了约7880名MS患者和9440名对照的鼻烟习惯。结果表明，与从未使用过鼻烟的人相比，使用鼻烟的人患MS的风险降低（17%）（Hedström et al. 2013）。此外，研究小组证明了鼻烟使用累积剂量的增加与患病风险之间存在反比关系（Hedström et al. 2013），这表明鼻烟使用次数越多，患MS的风险越低。像吸烟一样，这种关联背后的机制尚未完全被理解。除了烟碱，可咀嚼的烟草还包含许多不同的物质，这些物质可能导致所观察到的效果（Hedström et al. 2013）。一个可能的解释是烟碱对髓磷脂抗原的影响。伊朗的一个研究小组研究了烟碱在实验性自身免疫性脑脊髓炎模型中的作用。他们使用动物模型证明，接受烟碱治疗的小鼠在组织病理学评估中具有较少的炎症反应，同时具有髓鞘保护作用（Naddafi, Reza Haidari, Azizi, Sedaghat, Mirshafiey, 2013）。

13.6 结论

与卷烟烟雾不同，烟碱尚未被认为具有致癌性，甚至可能具有作为神经保护和抗炎剂的治疗潜力。必须意识到MS是一种非常复杂的疾病，危险因素最有可能受到与其他环境和遗传因素相互作用的影响。此外，观察研究有一些必须承认的局限性。回顾性研究和基于问卷的研究容易产生回忆偏倚（Hassan, 2005）。回忆偏倚的问题对于有关多发性硬化症的研究尤为重要，因为回忆信息完全取决于记忆，而记忆可能在MS病例中受到限制。还需要其他研究来解释吸烟和烟碱如何影响免疫系统及其在MS发展和进展中的作用。然而，根据研究结果，戒烟将使人和患者受益。内科医生、卫生保健专业人员和政策制定者应仔细考虑这种关联，尤其是因为吸烟仍然是主要的可改变危险因素。

术语解释

- 自身免疫性疾病：身体组织受到自身免疫系统的攻击。这可能导致被攻击的身体组织受损。
- B细胞：也称为B淋巴细胞。负责产生抗体。
- 动因：因果之间的关系，也称为因果关系。
- 胼胝体：连接左右半球，并负责它们的通信。
- McDonald标准：多发性硬化症的诊断标准。这些标准于2001年引入，并于2005年进行了修订，重点是在不同时间和不同区域的病变的临床、放射学和实验室证据。
- 多发性硬化症：一种影响中枢神经系统的自身免疫性炎症性脱髓鞘疾病。
- 比值比：一种对暴露和结果之间关联的测量。表示疾病与暴露之间关联强度的指标，指暴露者的疾病危险性为非暴露者的多少倍。
- 流行率：在给定时间段内具有或具有特定特征的人口比例。
- 鼻烟/湿鼻烟：通常通过鼻腔吸入或吸入的无烟烟草。它也被称为蘸烟。它是一种精细研磨和润湿的烟草产品。
- T细胞：也称为T淋巴细胞，对于细胞介导的免疫很重要。

要点总结

- 本章重点讨论吸烟、烟碱和多发性硬化症之间的关系。
- 观察性研究的数据表明，吸烟是多发性硬化症发展的重要因素。
- 另一方面，烟碱可能具有保护作用。
- 瑞典的一个研究小组证明，与不使用鼻烟的人相比，使用鼻烟的人患多发性硬化症的风险降低17%。
- 需要进行更多的研究以充分了解这种关联背后的机制。

参考文献

Al-Afasy, H. H.; Al-Obaidan, M. A.; Al-Ansari, Y. A.; Al-Yatama, S. A.; Al-Rukaibi, M. S.; Makki, N. I. et al. (2013). Risk factors for multiple sclerosis in Kuwait: a population-based case-control study. Neuroepidemiology, 40(1), 30-35. (2013).

Alonso, A.; Cook, S. D.; Maghzi, A. -H.; Divani, A. A. (2011). A casecontrol study of risk factors for multiple sclerosis in Iran. Multiple Sclerosis (Houndmills, Basingstoke, England), 17(5), 550-555. (2011).

Antonovsky, A.; Leibowitz, U.; Smith, H. A.; Medalie, J. M.; Balogh, M.; Kats, R. et al. (1965). Epidemiologic study of multiple sclerosis in Israel. I. An overall review of methods and findings. Archives of Neurology, 13, 183-193.

Arnson, Y.; Shoenfeld, Y.; Amital, H. (2010). Effects of tobacco smoke on immunity, inflammation and autoimmunity. Journal of Autoimmunity, 34(3), J258-J265.

Backhaus, I.; Mannocci, A.; Lemmens, P. H. H. M.; La Torre, G. (2016). Smoking as a risk factor for developing multiple sclerosis: a metaanalysis of observational studies. La Clinica Terapeutica, 167(3), 82-92.

Briggs, F. B. S.; Acuna, B.; Shen, L.; Ramsay, P.; Quach, H.; Bernstein, A. et al. (2014). Smoking and risk of multiple sclerosis: evidence of modification by NAT1 variants. Epidemiology (Cambridge, Mass), 25(4), 605-614.

Carlens, C.; Hergens, M. -P.; Grunewald, J.; Ekbom, A.; Eklund, A.; Höglund, C. O. et al. (2010). Smoking, use of moist snuff, and risk of chronic inflammatory diseases. American Journal of RespiratoryandCriticalCareMedicine, 181(11), 1217-1222.

Costenbader, K. H.; Karlson, E. W. (2006). Cigarette smoking and autoimmune disease: what can we learn from epidemiology Lupus, 15(11), 737-745.

Courville, C. B.; Maschmeyer, J. E.; Delay, C. P. (1964). Effect of smoking on the acute exacerbations of multiple sclerosis. Bulletin of the Los Angeles Neurological Society, 29, 1-6.

da Silva, K. R. P.; Alvarenga, R. M. P.; Fernandez, Y.; Fernandez, O.; Alvarenga, H.; Thuler, L. C. S. (2009). Potential risk factors for multiple sclerosis in Rio de Janeiro: a case-control study. Arquivos de Neuro-Psiquiatria, 67(2A), 229-234.

Egesten, A.; Brandt, L.; Olsson, T.; Granath, F.; Inghammar, M.; Löfdahl, C. -G. et al. (2008). Increased prevalence of multiple sclerosis among COPD patients and their first-degree relatives: a population-based study. Lung, 186(3), 173-178.

Engdahl, E.; Gustafsson, R.; Ramanujam, R.; Sundqvist, E.; Olsson, T.; Hillert, J. et al. (2014). HLA-A(*)02, gender and tobacco smoking, but not multiple sclerosis, affects the IgG antibody response against human herpesvirus 6. Human Immunology, 75(6), 524-530.

Evangelou, N.; Konz, D.; Esiri, M. M.; Smith, S.; Palace, J.; Matthews, P. M. (2000). Regional axonal loss in the corpus callosum correlates with cerebral white matter lesion volume and distribution in multiple sclerosis. Brain: A Journal of Neurology, 123(Pt 9), 1845-1849.

Fusby, J. S.; Kassmeier, M. D.; Palmer, V. L.; Perry, G. A.; Anderson, D. K.; Hackfort, B. T. et al. (2010). Cigarette smoke-induced effects on bone marrow B-cell subsets and CD4+:CD8+ T-cell ratios are reversed by smoking cessation: influence of bone mass on immune cell response to and recovery from smoke exposure. Inhalation Toxicology, 22(9), 785-796.

Ghadirian, P.; Dadgostar, B.; Azani, R.; Maisonneuve, P. (2001). A case-control study of the association between socio-demographic, lifestyle and medical history factors and multiple sclerosis. Canadian Journal of Public Health, 92(4), 281-285.

Gohil, K. (2015). Multiple sclerosis: progress, but no cure. Pharmacy and Therapeutics, 40(9), 604-605.

Handel, A. E.; Williamson, A. J.; Disanto, G.; Dobson, R.; Giovannoni, G.; Ramagopalan, S. V. (2011). Smoking and multiple sclerosis: an updated meta-analysis. PLoS One, 6(1), e16149.

Hassan, E. (2005). Recall Bias can be a threat to retrospective and prospective research designs. The Internet Journal of Epidemiology, 3(2)Retrieved from (2005). http://ispub.com/IJE/3/2/13060.

Hauser, S. L.; Goodin, D. S. (2012). Chapter 380. Multiple sclerosis and other demyelinating diseases. In D. L. Longo, A. S. Fauci, D. L. Kasper, S. L. Hauser, J. L. Jameson, J. Loscalzo (Eds.), Harrison's Principles of Internal Medicine (18th ed.). New York, NY: TheMcGraw-Hill Companies.

Hawkes, C. H. (2007). Smoking is a risk factor for multiple sclerosis:a metanalysis. Multiple Sclerosis (Houndmills, Basingstoke, England), 13(5), 610-615.

Healy, B. C.; Ali, E.; Guttmann, C. R. G.; Chitnis, T.; Glanz, B. I.; Buckle, G. et al. (2009). Smoking and disease progression in multiple sclerosis. Archives of Neurology, 66(7), 858-864.

Hedström, A. K.; Bäärnhielm, M.; Olsson, T.; Alfredsson, L. (2009). Tobacco smoking, but not Swedish snuff use, increases the risk of multiple sclerosis. Neurology, 73(9), 696-701.

Hedström, A. K.; Hillert, J.; Olsson, T.; Alfredsson, L. (2013). Nicotine might have a protective effect in the etiology of multiple sclerosis. Multiple Sclerosis (Houndmills, Basingstoke, England), 19(8), 1009-1013.

Hedström, A. K.; Sundqvist, E.; Bäärnhielm, M.; Nordin, N.; Hillert, J.; Kockum, I. et al. (2011). Smoking and two human leukocyte antigen genes interact to increase the risk for multiple sclerosis. Brain: A Journal of Neurology, 134(Pt 3), 653-664.

Hernán, M. A.; Jick, S. S.; Logroscino, G.; Olek, M. J.; Ascherio, A.; Jick, H. (2005). Cigarette smoking and the progression of multiple sclerosis. Brain: A Journal of Neurology, 128(Pt 6), 1461-1465.

Hernán, M. A.; Oleky, M. J.; Ascherio, A. (2001). Cigarette smoking and incidence of multiple sclerosis. American Journal of Epidemiology, 154(1), 69-74.

Jafari, N.; Hintzen, R. Q. (2011). The association between cigarette smoking and multiple sclerosis. Journal of the Neurological Sciences, 311(1-2), 78-85.

Jafari, N.; Hoppenbrouwers, I. A.; Hop, W. C. J.; Breteler, M. M. B.; Hintzen, R. Q. (2009). Cigarette smoking and risk of MS in multiplex families. Multiple Sclerosis (Houndmills, Basingstoke, England), 15(11), 1363-1367.

Kotzamani, D.; Panou, T.; Mastorodemos, V.; Tzagournissakis, M.; Nikolakaki, H.; Spanaki, C. et al. (2012). Rising incidence of multiple sclerosis in females associated with urbanization. Neurology, 78(22), 1728-1735.

Levine, S. (1967). Experimental cyanide encephalopathy: Gradients of susceptibility in the corpus callosum. Journal of Neuropathology and Experimental Neurology, 26(2), 214-222.

Longo, H.; Longo, D. L.; Harrison, T. R. (2012). In D. L. Longo (Ed.), Harrison's principles of internal medicine. (18th ed.). New York: McGraw-Hill.

Maghzi, A. H.; Etemadifar, M.; Heshmat-Ghahdarijani, K.; Moradi, V.; Nonahal, S.; Ghorbani, A. et al. (2011). Cigarette smoking and the risk of multiple sclerosis: a sibling case-control study in Isfahan, Iran. Neuroepidemiology, 37(3-4), 238-242.

Mansouri, B.; Asadollahi, S.; Heidari, K.; Fakhri, M.; Assarzadegan, F.; Nazari, M. et al. (2014). Risk factors for increased multiple sclerosis susceptibility in the Iranian population. Journal of Clinical Neuroscience: Official Journal of the Neurosurgical Society of Australasia, 21(12), 2207-2211.

Naddafi, F.; Reza Haidari, M.; Azizi, G.; Sedaghat, R.; Mirshafiey, A. (2013). Novel therapeutic approach by nicotine in experimental model of multiple sclerosis. Innovations in Clinical Neuroscience, 10(4), 20-25.

O'Gorman, C.; Bukhari, W.; Todd, A.; Freeman, S.; Broadley, S. A. (2014). Smoking increases the risk of multiple sclerosis in Queensland, Australia. Journal of Clinical Neuroscience: Official Journal of the Neurosurgical Society of Australasia, 21(10), 1730-1733.

Ozturk, A.; Smith, S. A.; Gordon-Lipkin, E. M.; Harrison, D. M.; Shiee, N.; Pham, D. L. et al. (2010). MRI of the Corpus callosum in multiple sclerosis: association with disability. Multiple Sclerosis (Houndmills, Basingstoke, England), 16(2), 166. (2010).

Pekmezovic, T.; Drulovic, J.; Milenkovic, M.; Jarebinski, M.; Stojsavljevic, N.; Mesaros, S. et al. (2006). Lifestyle factors and multiple sclerosis: a case-control study in Belgrade. Neuroepidemiology, 27(4), 212-216.

Piao, W. -H.; Campagnolo, D.; Dayao, C.; Lukas, R. J.; Wu, J.; Shi, F. -D. (2009). Nicotine and inflammatory neurological disorders. Acta Pharmacologica Sinica, 30(6), 715-722.

Poorolajal, J.; Bahrami, M.; Karami, M.; Hooshmand, E. (2016). Effect of smoking on multiple sclerosis: a meta-analysis. Journal of Public Health, 2010, fdw030.

Pugliatti, M.; Harbo, H. F.; Holmøy, T.; Kampman, M. T.; Myhr, K. -M.; Riise, T. et al. (2008). Environmental risk factors in multiple sclerosis. Acta Neurologica Scandinavica. Supplementum, 188, 34-40.

Quik, M.; Bordia, T.; O'Leary, K. (2007). Nicotinic receptors as CNS targets for Parkinson's disease. Biochemical Pharmacology, 74(8), 1224-1234.

Ramagopalan, S. V.; Lee, J. D.; Yee, I. M.; Guimond, C.; Traboulsee, A. L.; Ebers, G. C. et al. (2013). Association of smoking with risk of multiple sclerosis: A population-based study. Journal of Neurology, 260 (7), 1778-1781.

Rodríguez Regal, A.; del Campo Amigo, M.; Paz-Esquete, J.; Martínez Feijoo, A.; Cebrián, E.; Suárez Gil, P. et al. (2009). A case-control study of the influence of the smoking behaviour in multiple sclerosis. Neurologia (Barcelona, Spain), 24(3), 177-180.

Roudbari, S. A.; Ansar, M. M.; Yousefzad, A. (2013). Smoking as a risk factor for development of secondary progressive multiple sclerosis: a study in IRAN, Guilan. Journal of the Neurological Sciences, 330(1-2), 52-55.

Russo, C.; Morabito, F.; Luise, F.; Piromalli, A.; Battaglia, L.; Vinci, A. et al. (2008). Hyperhomocysteinemia is associated with cognitive impairment in multiple sclerosis. Journal of Neurology, 255(1), 64-69.

Salzer, J.; Hallmans, G.; Nyström, M.; Stenlund, H.; Wadell, G.; Sundström, P. (2013). Smoking as a risk factor for multiple sclerosis. Multiple Sclerosis (Houndmills, Basingstoke, England), 19(8), 1022-1027.

Simon, K. C.; van der Mei, I. A. F.; Munger, K. L.; Ponsonby, A.; Dickinson, J.; Dwyer, T. et al. (2010). Combined effects of smoking, anti-EBNA antibodies, and HLA-DRB1*1501 on multiple sclerosis risk. Neurology, 74(17), 1365-1371.

Simpson, C. A.; Newell, D. J.; Schapira, K. (1966). Smoking and multiple sclerosis. Neurology, 16(10), 1041-1043.

Sundström, P.; Nyström, L.; Hallmans, G. (2008). Smoke exposure increases the risk for multiple sclerosis. European Journal of Neurology, 15(6), 579-583.

Thorogood, M.; Hannaford, P. C. (1998). The influence of oral contraceptives on the risk of multiple sclerosis. British Journal of Obstetrics and Gynaecology, 105(12), 1296-1299.

van der Mei, I. A. F.; Simpson, S.; Stankovich, J.; Taylor, B. V. (2011). Individual and joint action of environmental factors and risk of MS. Neurologic Clinics, 29(2), 233-255.

Villard-Mackintosh, L.; Vessey, M. P. (1993). Oral contraceptives and reproductive factors in multiple sclerosis incidence. Contraception, 47(2), 161-168.

Zhang, P.; Wang, R.; Li, Z.; Wang, Y.; Gao, C.; Lv, X. et al. (2016). The risk of smoking on multiple sclerosis: a meta-analysis based on 20, 626 cases from case-control and cohort studies. PeerJ, 4, e1797.

Zorzon, M.; Zivadinov, R.; Nasuelli, D.; Dolfini, P.; Bosco, A.; Bratina, A. et al. (2003). Risk factors of multiple sclerosis: a case-control study. Neurological Sciences: Official Journal of the Italian Neurological Society and of the Italian Society of Clinical Neurophysiology, 24(4), 242-247.

14
多巴胺能系统的烟草和正电子发射断层扫描（PET）：人类研究综述

Chidera C. Chukwueke[1], Bernard Le Foll[1,2]

1. Department of Pharmacology and Toxicology, University of Toronto, Toronto, ON, Canada
2. Translational Addiction Research Laboratory, Centre for Addiction and Mental Health, Toronto, ON, Canada

缩略语			
BP_{ND}	结合潜力（不可替代）	MDD	重度抑郁症
$D_1/D_2/D_3$	多巴胺受体亚型 1/2/3	Nic	烟碱化卷烟
DA	多巴胺	PET	正电子发射断层扫描
Denic	去烟碱化卷烟		

14.1 吸烟和多巴胺能系统

在美国吸烟是可预防的死亡的主要原因（Surgeon General, 2014），因此迫切需要更好地了解维持吸烟的机制以改善治疗。烟碱是烟草中的精神活性成分，据报道可通过调节多巴胺（DA）的神经传递来发挥其奖励和强化作用（Di Chiara, 2000）。正电子发射断层扫描（PET）的出现目前使得评估人体对烟碱使用的反应中的DA活性成为可能。

14.1.1 正电子发射断层扫描

这项技术的早期迭代可以追溯到20世纪50年代，PET成像已经发展成为能够生成用于评估神经化学脑活动的高分辨率图像（Portnow et al. 2013）。PET扫描仪通过检测使用正电子发射放射性示踪剂产生的光子或伽马射线来重建空间密度的图像。通过使用与感兴趣受体结合的放射性示踪剂，PET成像可以评估区域受体密度和神经递质波动。这是通过测量放射性示踪剂结合潜力（BP）来完成的，该电位被定义为 B_{max}（受体密度）与 K_D（放射性示踪剂平衡解离常数）之比（Mintun et al. 1984）。放射性示踪剂的结合亲和力是 K_D 的倒数，因此 BP_{ND} 可以看作受体密度和放射性示踪剂亲和力的乘积。

在PET研究中，BP_{ND} 是指平衡状态下组织中特异性结合的放射性示踪剂与不可替代的放射性示踪剂之比。BP_{ND} 在参考组织方法中经常使用，它比较了富含受体与不含受体的区域的放射性示踪剂的浓度。在调查吸烟者大脑活动的PET研究中，BP_{ND} 提供了一种间接测量神经传递和受体可用性的方法。通过研究放射性示踪剂 BP_{ND} 在急性刺激（如吸烟）前后的差异，可以推断出DA神经递质浓度的变化是刺激引起的放射性示踪剂与内源性神经递质之间竞争加剧的结果。因此，与基线 BP_{ND} 值相比，在急性刺激后观察到的 BP_{ND} 降低被认为反映了DA浓度的增加（而 BP_{ND} 的升高也反映了神经递质的减少）。另一方面，可以通过比较吸烟者和非吸烟者之间的基线

BP_{ND}来观察受体的利用率。这种设计可以推断出在稳定的基线条件下区域受体的可用性，因此组间的差异可能反映了对慢性烟草使用的神经适应性变化。在本章中，我们将回顾使用PET评估吸烟或烟碱对人类DA活性的影响的研究。

14.1.2 多巴胺

DA与药物成瘾有关（Volkow et al. 2012），因此有必要评估其在烟草依赖中的作用。像大多数滥用药物一样，吸烟会增加细胞外DA的浓度，尤其是在纹状体中（Brody, Mandelkern et al. 2009）。药物引起的DA浓度通常也与药物的奖励作用有关（Volkow et al. 2012）。本文着重综述了烟碱PET研究，通过使用具有不同区域BP_{ND}和受体亲和力的放射性示踪剂推断出DA合成、神经传递和DA受体（如亚型D_1、D_2和D_3）的可用性。使用放射性示踪剂$[^{11}C]$-雷氯必利和$[^{18}F]$-氟利德（fallypride）测定D_2活性，使用放射性示踪剂$[^{11}C]$-SCH 23390测定D_1活性。此外，本章还介绍了使用$[^{11}C]$-(+)-PHNO测量的纹状体D_3活性，使用$[^{11}C]$-FLB-457测量的皮质D_2活性以及使用$[^{18}F]$-氟多巴测量的DA合成。

尽管这里回顾的研究使用了各种放射性示踪剂，但仍存在一些方法上的共性。首先，一些研究通过研究急性烟碱给药前后放射性示踪剂BP_{ND}之间的差异来评估DA的释放。如上所述，通过推断放射性示踪剂BP_{ND}中刺激诱导的变化按比例反映了刺激诱导的DA浓度变化，间接测量了DA释放。其次，一些研究比较了慢性吸烟者和非吸烟者之间的基线BP_{ND}，以评估长期使用烟碱后DA受体的水平。但是，值得注意的是，使用这种设计，仍然难以确定观察到的BP_{ND}差异是否反映了先前存在的神经形态或它们是否是烟碱使用的后果。

14.2 对人类吸烟者进行的PET研究

14.2.1 $[^{11}C]$-雷氯必利

（1）DA释放

$[^{11}C]$-雷氯必利是一种D_2/D_3受体拮抗剂，对纹状体D_2的偏好程度高于D_3（Lammertsma, Hume, 1996），已成为PET研究烟碱相关D_2活性的主要放射性示踪剂。使用该示踪剂的研究（表14.1）表明，在室外休息期间，与不吸烟者相比，吸烟者的腹侧纹状体中释放DA（Brody et al., 2004）。一项双盲、随机的安慰剂对照研究证实，吸烟者（而非非吸烟者）摄入烟碱口香糖后，其腹侧纹状体释放DA（Takahashi et al. 2008）。最近的报道显示吸烟引起DA在背侧纹状体中释放（Weinstein et al. 2016）。这些研究提供了支持烟碱诱导的DA释放的多模式证据。在使用$[^{11}C]$-雷氯必利（Cosgrove et al. 2014）和不同放射性示踪剂的研究中也报道了性别差异（Brown et al. 2012; Okita, Petersen et al. 2016）。使用$[^{11}C]$-雷氯必利后，男性吸烟者在腹侧纹状体中释放DA，而女性吸烟者在常规吸烟后在背侧纹状体中显示出较快的吸烟反应（Cosgrove et al. 2014）。该报道增加了对烟碱的不同性别特定区域和时间DA反应。相比之下，一些研究报告称，在扫描仪中定期吸烟或鼻内烟碱给药后均未释放DA（Barrett et al. 2004; Montgomery et al. 2007）。尽管使用相同的放射性示踪剂，但这些结果可能归因于方法不同。支持烟碱诱导的DA释放的研究表明，在腹侧纹状体（Brody et al. 2004; Takahashi et al. 2008）和背侧纹状体（Weinstein et al. 2016），男性更多地体现在腹侧纹状体，而女性则在背侧纹状体表现出时间进程敏感的DA反应（Cosgrove et al. 2014）。

表14.1 [^{11}C]-雷氯必利研究

参考文献	学科	研究目的	干预手段	结论
Wiers et al. (2017)	8名当前吸烟者(每天7.4支)、10名戒烟者和18名不吸烟者	评估吸烟状态对基线D_2受体可用性和DA释放的影响	回顾分析安慰剂或哌醋甲酯注射后进行一次PET扫描的受试者的数据	吸烟者的受体水平显著较低,而戒烟者和不吸烟者没有区别。注射哌醋甲酯后吸烟者与非吸烟者DA释放无显著差异
Weinstein et al. (2016)	10名吸烟者,平均每天吸烟21支	使用[^{11}C]-雷氯必利评估预处理卷烟使用与吸烟诱导的DA释放之间的关联	安非他酮治疗第七周的一次PET扫描,受试者在扫描中途休息期间在另一个房间吸烟	吸烟诱导尾状核和壳核中的DA释放
Cosgrove et al. (2014); Albrecht et al. (2013)	16名吸烟者(8名男性,8名女性)共81名受试者。34名不寻求治疗的酗酒者,21名饮酒吸烟者,26名饮酒不吸烟者	使用[^{11}C]-雷氯必利评估了吸烟对男性和女性的不同影响 使用[^{11}C]-雷氯必利PET数据进行了一项回顾性研究,以评估酒精和烟草在纹状体多巴胺浓度的慢性共病使用中的不同作用	一次PET扫描,受试者在扫描中抽一支或两支烟 N/A	在男性中发现显著的右侧腹侧纹状体激活,而在女性中没有。女性在背侧壳核对吸烟的反应更快 发现吸烟但与非吸烟组相比,主要在背侧纹状体和背侧壳核的结合较低。腹侧纹状体没有发现差异
Domino et al. (2012)	20名男性吸烟者,每天吸烟15~40支	使用[^{11}C]-雷氯必利抽吸烟碱化卷烟和去烟碱化卷烟后,检查OPRM1 A118G多态性对DA释放的调节作用	两次PET扫描。先抽两支去烟碱化卷烟,再抽两支烟碱化卷烟	与具有纯合AA等位基因的个体相比,具有G等位基因的个体在右侧尾状核和腹侧苍白球中表现出更多的烟碱诱导DA释放
Brody, Mandelkern et al. (2009)	62名依赖吸烟者,每天吸烟24.2支	在烟碱化卷烟中使用[^{11}C]-雷氟必利与在去烟碱化卷烟中比较吸烟诱导的DA释放	一次PET扫描,在此期间他们吸食了烟碱化或去烟碱化的卷烟	两种卷烟都减轻了烟瘾;然而,只有含烟碱的卷烟会增加腹侧纹状体的DA释放并改善情绪
Brody, Olmstead et al. (2009)	56名吸烟者,每天吸烟24.7支,有和没有MDD	使用[^{11}C]-雷氯必利来检查有和没有抑郁发作的吸烟者之间吸烟引起的DA释放	一次PET扫描,在此期间受试者抽了一支普通卷烟	与MDD相比,MDD+受试者表现出吸烟诱导的DA释放增加。更多的吸烟诱导的DA释放与更多的扫描前抑郁和焦虑水平相关
Busto et al. (2009)	17名MDD+/−吸烟者,平均每天吸16.65支卷烟,相比之下,21名MDD+/−不吸烟者	使用[^{11}C]-雷氯必利比较了急性安非他明激发对健康对照组和有或没有烟草依赖的抑郁受试者的影响	两次PET扫描,一次基线扫描,然后是口服安非他明后的一次扫描	吸烟者,但不是MDD+受试者,在基线时表现出较低的结合。MDD+吸烟者表现出最大的安非他明诱导的结合减少
Takahashi et al. (2008)	6名吸烟者,每天吸烟超过15支,和6名不吸烟者	一项双盲、随机、安慰剂对照研究,调查使用烟碱口香糖的吸烟者和非吸烟者之间[^{11}C]-雷氯必利结合的差异	两次PET扫描。两次扫描都完成了,而受试者在整个扫描过程中咀嚼烟碱或安慰剂口香糖	与安慰剂相比,烟碱口香糖在吸烟者纹状体区域的结合显著降低,而非吸烟者则不然。纹状体结合与烟碱依赖程度相关
Scott et al. (2007)	6名吸烟者,平均每天吸烟16.7支,和6名年龄和性别匹配的非吸烟者	使用[^{11}C]-雷氯必利和[^{11}C]-卡芬太尼检查吸食烟碱化和去烟碱化卷烟对D_2和μ-阿片受体的影响	一次PET扫描。在扫描期间,受试者以平衡的方式依次注射两种放射性示踪剂。吸烟者在扫描的前半部分抽吸脱烟碱卷烟,在扫描后半部分抽吸含烟碱卷烟	与不吸烟者相比,吸烟者在D_2结合方面没有显著差异。与烟碱化香烟相比,烟碱化香烟在左腹基底神经节中的D_2/D_3结合率较低

续表

参考文献	学科	研究目的	干预手段	结论
Montgomery et al. (2007)	10名吸烟者，平均每天吸烟10.9支	使用[^{11}C]-雷氯必利确定了通过鼻腔喷雾给予烟碱对DA释放的影响	一次PET扫描，中期烟碱鼻腔喷雾给药	烟碱给药前后的结合没有显著差异。发现烟碱引起的情绪变化与背侧纹状体结合之间存在多种关联
Brody et al. (2006)	45名吸烟者，每天吸烟23.9支	使用[^{11}C]-雷氯必利评估DA活性检查涉及吸烟诱导的DA释放的遗传变异性	在吸烟或不吸烟的情况下进行一次PET扫描	发现特定基因多态性与更大的吸烟诱导的DA释放之间的关联
Barrett et al. (2004)	10名男性吸烟者，平均每天吸烟18支	使用[^{11}C]-雷氯必利评估DA活性对急性吸烟的反应，以及与烟碱渴望和吸烟的快感效应的关联	吸烟条件下的两次PET扫描，受试者在扫描仪中反复吸烟，在非吸烟条件下不吸烟	吸烟和不吸烟条件之间的DA结合没有显著差异；然而，吸烟的快感效应与背侧纹状体中的DA结合显著相关
Brody et al. (2004)	20名吸烟者，每天至少抽15支烟	使用[^{11}C]-雷氯必利评估通过普通卷烟给予烟碱对DA释放的影响	一次PET扫描，其中一半受试者处于吸烟状态，而另一半处于对照状态	吸烟条件导致腹侧纹状体结合显著减少，这与自我报告的渴望减少有关

注：此表概述了使用放射性示踪剂[^{11}C]-雷氯必利的烟碱PET研究的主题、目的和结论。DA，多巴胺；MDD+/−，重度抑郁症阳性或阴性；PET，正电子发射断层扫描。

然而，烟碱给药不一致地诱导明显的DA释放（Barrett et al. 2004; Montgomery et al. 2007）。文献中的这种不一致可能表明，烟碱引起的DA释放对烟碱的给药途径（如吸烟与喷鼻）、吸烟方法（如在户外与在扫描仪中）或其他因素（如戒断和烟草中的多种化学物质）敏感。应当指出的是，大多数此类研究中的样本量较小且缺乏对某些因素的系统控制，因此目前很难对这些因素的影响得出结论。

（2）烟碱化卷烟与去烟碱化卷烟

为了阐明烟碱对DA释放的特定贡献，研究采用了烟碱化（nic；含有一定量的烟碱）与去烟碱化（denic；含有大量减少的烟碱，即几乎没有烟碱）的卷烟范例。这种范例是有益的，因为如果测试了适当的控制条件，则抽根卷烟可以让我们检查吸烟线索（即吸烟行为减去烟碱的释放）对DA活动的影响。采用这种范例的研究产生了相对一致的结果。一项研究表明，与去烟碱化卷烟相比，吸烟者（$N=6$）抽吸烟碱化卷烟后，其腹侧纹状体中显示出DA释放（Scott et al. 2007）。这些发现在另一项更大样本的研究中得到了证实（$N=62$; Brody, Mandelkern et al. 2009）。有趣的是，另一项评估烟碱化卷烟与去烟碱化卷烟对DA释放的反应的研究证实，尽管在整个纹状体中（即腹侧和背侧），同时也显示出去烟碱化卷烟诱导的右背纹状体DA释放（Domino et al. 2013）。总的来说，这些研究为吸烟引起的DA释放提供了进一步的证据。烟碱本身可能促进吸烟引起的腹侧纹状体DA的释放，而背侧纹状体DA的释放可能与吸烟提示有关。药物成瘾的文献支持腹侧纹状体DA的释放与药物奖励强化效应有关，而背侧纹状体DA的释放与习惯学习和接触药物相关线索有关这一观点（Volkow et al. 2009; Volkow et al. 2012）。

（3）主观上相互关联

据报道，渴望、情绪调节和烟碱依赖严重程度的主观测量与烟碱诱导的多巴胺活性有关。据报道，吸烟引起的情绪变化和愉悦效应与背侧纹状体中DA的释放相关（Barrett et al. 2004;

Montgomery et al. 2007）。另一方面，研究表明腹侧纹状体DA的释放与主观渴望分数的降低和情绪改善有关（Brody et al. 2004; Brody, Mandelkern et al. 2009; Takahashi et al. 2008）。此外，据报道，烟碱依赖严重程度的主观测量与腹侧纹状体DA释放（Scott et al. 2007; Takahashi et al. 2008）和基线背侧纹状体DA受体可用性（Montgomery et al. 2007）相关，这使得区域差异不那么明显。虽然需要更多的研究来区分烟碱依赖的区域贡献，但这些结果确实支持这一观点，即这两个区在成瘾的行为成分中都发挥着重要作用（Volkow et al. 2012）。

（4）烟碱和抑郁症

烟草依赖可能发生在共病的重度抑郁症（MDD）的背景下。在使用[^{11}C]-雷氯必利的研究中，与那些没有抑郁发作的吸烟者相比，有抑郁发作的吸烟者表现出更多的吸烟诱导的DA释放（Brody, Olmstead et al. 2009）。另一方面，与患有或不患有MDD的非吸烟者相比，患有MDD的吸烟者表现出钝化的苯丙胺激发的DA反应（Busto et al. 2009）。研究设计中的明显差异可能是导致结果不一致的原因。然而，有可能的是，在患有精神健康问题的吸烟者中，使用依赖物质（如吸烟者的烟碱）会刺激过度活跃的DA反应，而不太熟悉的物质（如吸烟者的苯丙胺）会产生较弱的反应，这一点以前已经报道过（Parsey et al. 2001）。总而言之，很明显，MDD和烟碱依赖的并存比任何一种疾病单独存在更会导致DA系统的失调。

（5）遗传变异

使用[^{11}C]-雷氯必利检测吸烟者的遗传变异性的研究表明，它与各种遗传多态性有关（Brody et al. 2006; Domino et al. 2012）。根据这些研究，μ-阿片受体的G等位基因和与低静息DA张力相关的基因（多巴胺转运体的9个重复等位基因、儿茶酚-O-甲基转移酶的Val/Val基因型和D4受体的7个重复等位基因）的携带者在吸烟诱导的DA释放方面表现出更大的幅度。这些研究以男性为主，因此有必要进行进一步的研究。虽然还远没有定论，但遗传变异可能能够解释吸烟诱导的多巴胺释放的个体差异的很大一部分原因。

（6）受体可用性

使用[^{11}C]-雷氯必利评估烟草依赖中受体可用性变化的研究产生了好坏参半的结果。虽然早期的研究表明吸烟者和不吸烟者的基线受体可用性没有差异（Scott et al. 2007; Takahashi et al. 2008），但最近的研究对这些发现提出了挑战。研究表明，与不吸烟者相比，同时存在酒精使用和抑郁问题的吸烟者表现出更低的D_2受体可用性（Albrecht, Kareken, Yoder, 2013; Busto et al. 2009）。这一发现最近得到了Wiers等（2017）的支持。使用回顾性研究设计发现，与不吸烟者相比，当前吸烟者的D_2受体可用性较低。在这项研究中，戒烟者和不吸烟者在D_2受体可用性方面没有区别，这表明戒烟期可能会使受体水平正常化。虽然这些报告不一致，但成瘾诱导的DA受体下调是有很充分的记录的（Volkow et al. 2009），并在使用不同放射性示踪剂的烟碱PET研究中看到（Dagher et al. 2001; Fehr et al. 2008; Yasuno et al. 2007），因此支持烟草依赖确实会降低DA受体的可用性以及在戒烟后恢复的可能性。有趣的是，最近的一项研究表明，每天吸烟与背侧纹状体DA释放呈负相关，表明神经适应性耐受吸烟（Weinstein et al. 2016）；然而，这些发现是初步的。

14.2.2 [^{18}F]-氟利德

烟碱PET研究利用[^{18}F]-氟利德（表14.2），一种高亲和力D_2放射性配体（Riccardi et al. 2008, 2005），来评估纹状体和纹状体外区域D_2/D_3受体的可用性。[^{18}F]-氟利德研究显示吸烟者的背侧

纹状体 D_2 受体可用性较低，但不吸烟者没有（Fehr et al. 2008）。然而，性别差异使这一发现复杂化，因为研究报告称，男性吸烟者的背侧纹状体 D_2 可用性较低（Brown et al. 2012），而女性吸烟者的中脑 D_2 可用性较高，与背侧纹状体 D_2 可用性呈正相关（Okita, Petersen et al. 2016）。这表明烟碱依赖的DA系统活性低下，男性比女性经历更多的DA受体下调。$[^{18}F]$-氟利德研究证实DA系统与渴望、吸烟和依赖严重程度之间存在关联。研究表明渴望与腹侧纹状体受体的可用性呈正相关，而与前扣带回和颞叶下部皮层呈负相关（Fehr et al. 2008）。此外，一项研究表明，腹侧纹状体中较低的 D_2 可用性与较高的卷烟使用和依赖严重程度相关（Okita, Mandelkern, London, 2016），而另一项研究显示依赖分数与背侧纹状体 D_2 可用性呈负相关（Okita, Petersen et al. 2016）。这表明渴望可能是通过纹状体和纹状体外区域进行调节的，根据 $[^{11}C]$-雷氯必利的研究，依赖程度可能与两个纹状体区域的DA受体可用性有关。

表14.2 $[^{18}F]$-氟利德研究

作者	研究对象	研究目的	干预手段	结论
Okita, Mandelkern et al. (2016)	20名非独立吸烟者	与日常吸烟和烟碱依赖相关的 $[^{18}F]$-氟利德结合	一次PET扫描	腹侧纹状体中较低的结合与较高的卷烟使用量相关。较高的依赖性与整个纹状体（腹侧和背侧纹状体）的较低结合相关。这表明随着卷烟使用的升级和依赖性的发展，DA受体下调
Okita, Petersen et al. (2016)	18名吸烟者，每天吸烟 5～20 支，和19名不吸烟者	使用 $[^{18}F]$-氟利德评估中脑DA受体可用性的性别差异	一次PET扫描	女性吸烟者表现出比男性吸烟者更高的中脑结合。中脑结合与纹状体结合呈正相关，与依赖性呈负相关
Brown et al. (2012)	19名轻度吸烟者，每天吸烟 4～14 支，和18名不吸烟者	使用 $[^{18}F]$-氟利德调查轻度吸烟者与非吸烟者的性别差异	一次PET扫描	与女性和非吸烟者相比，男性吸烟者尾状核和壳核中 D_2/D_3 受体的可用性显著降低。女性在受体可用性方面与非吸烟者没有区别
Fehr et al. (2008)	17名吸烟者，平均每天吸烟19.5支，和21名不吸烟者	使用 $[^{18}F]$-氟利德比较吸烟者和非吸烟者在纹状体和纹状体外区域的 D_2/D_3 受体可用性	两次PET扫描，第一次是定期吸烟后，第二次是24小时禁欲后	在定期吸烟和戒烟后，吸烟者在壳核中显示出较低的 D_2/D_3 受体可用性，但在纹状体外区域则不然。这项研究发现了几个大脑区域的结合与行为测量之间的相关性

14.2.3 $[^{11}C]$-FLB-457

一项单一研究使用 $[^{11}C]$-FLB-457（表14.3）研究了吸烟诱导的皮层DA释放。$[^{11}C]$-FLB-457是一种高亲和力的 D_2/D_3 受体配体，在DA受体密度较低的皮层区域对DA变化显示出更高的敏感性（Narendran et al. 2009）。研究大脑皮层多巴胺传递的唯一研究表明，吸烟主要在扣带皮层释放多巴胺（Winget al. 2015）。在本研究中，渴望与皮层DA释放无关，因此，皮层DA传递在烟碱渴望中的作用尚不清楚。然而，这确实使吸烟会导致纹状体DA释放，也会导致皮质DA释放的文献增多。

表14.3 $[^{11}C]$-FLB-457研究

作者	研究对象	研究目的	干预手段	结论
Wing et al. (2015)	10名吸烟者，平均每天吸烟16支	使用 $[^{11}C]$-FLB-457调查吸烟在纹状体外和皮质脑区引起的DA释放	两次PET扫描。禁欲16小时后的第一次扫描，吸烟至饱食后的第二次扫描	发现主要是扣带回的结合显著减少。更大的抽吸量与更大的结合减少相关

14.2.4 [^{11}C]-(+)-PHNO

[^{11}C]-(+)-PHNO是一种D_2/D_3激动剂,据报道比[^{11}C]-雷氯必利对DA的急性波动更敏感(Shotbolt et al. 2012),并且是纹状体外区域(如黑质)的D_3首选激动剂(Tziortzi et al. 2011)。为了确定D_3在烟碱依赖中的具体作用,有关[^{11}C]-(+)-PHNO(表14.4)的研究表明,经常吸烟会增加边缘(即腹侧)纹状体和富含D_3的腹侧苍白球中DA的释(图14.1)(Le Foll et al. 2014)。吸烟的动机、渴望和戒断症状与边缘纹状体中DA的释放有关(Le Foll et al. 2014)。然而,在一项先导研究中,仅呈现与吸烟相关的线索,并没有引起可检测到的DA反应(Chiuccariello et al. 2013)。在这一点上,这些研究支持纹状体的参与,并表明富含D_3的区域(腹侧苍白球)参与了对吸烟的反应,而不涉及与吸烟相关的环境线索。

表14.4 [^{11}C]-(+)-PHNO研究

参考文献	研究对象	研究目的	干预手段	结论
Le Foll et al. (2014)	10名吸烟者,每天吸烟13.2支	使用[^{11}C]-(+)-PHNO研究吸烟诱导的纹状体、腹侧苍白球和黑质中的DA释放	在吸烟和戒烟条件下进行两次PET扫描	与戒烟条件相比,吸烟条件导致边缘纹状体和腹侧苍白球的结合显著减少。PHNO结合与吸烟行为之间也存在相关性
Chiuccariello et al. (2013)	18名吸烟者,每天吸烟18.2支	通过使用[^{11}C]-(+)-PHNO呈现吸烟提示与中性提示来研究DA释放	带有吸烟提示与中性提示(视觉和触觉成分)的PET扫描	在吸烟和中性提示呈现之间,任何大脑区域的DA水平没有显著差异

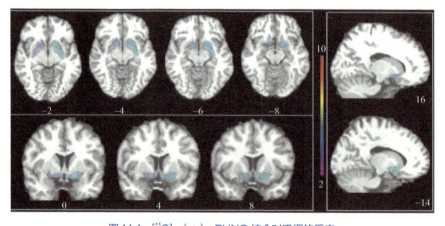

图14.1 [^{11}C]-(+)-PHNO结合对吸烟的反应

T-统计叠加平均T1 MRI显示吸烟后[^{11}C]-(+)-PHNO BP_{ND}明显降低。[^{11}C]-(+)-PHNO BP_{ND}簇在纹状体腹侧部分和对应于腹侧苍白球的区域下降最大。出于可视化目的,图像的阈值为$P<0.05$未校正。改编自Le Foll等(2014)。

14.2.5 [^{11}C]-SCH23390

使用D_1受体拮抗剂[^{11}C]-SCH23390测量D_1受体可用性的研究(表14.5)显示吸烟者腹侧纹状体D_1受体可用性明显低于非吸烟者(Dagher et al. 2001)。Yasuno等(2007)重复了这些发现,显示吸烟者腹侧纹状体D_1受体的可用性较低,戒烟6个月后增加。Yasuno等(2007)发现腹侧纹状体D_1受体与线索诱导的渴望得分也呈负相关,表明较低的D_1受体密度与更大的渴望之间存在关联。这些研究表明，虽然长期吸烟会导致D_1受体的下调，这与更大的渴望有关，但这种下调可能在戒烟后逆转，就像D_2受体一样（Wiers et al., 2017）。

表14.5 [^{11}C]-SCH23390 研究

参考文献	研究对象	研究目的	干预手段	结论
Yasuno et al. (2007)	18名吸烟者，每天至少抽15支烟，和12名不吸烟者	使用[^{11}C]-SCH23390研究调查吸烟者与非吸烟者在常规吸烟期间和戒烟数月后D_1受体的结合水平	受试者在基线时接受了一次PET扫描，达到禁欲的受试者接受了随后的PET扫描	吸烟者的D_1受体结合显著低于非吸烟者。禁欲3个月和6个月后，双侧伏隔核中的D_1受体结合增加。最后，伏隔核在吸烟诱导的大脑激活、渴望评分和D_1受体结合之间存在显著的负相关
Dagher et al. (2001)	11名吸烟者平均，每天吸烟19.4支，和18名不吸烟者	使用[^{11}C]-SCH23390研究调查吸烟者与非吸烟者的D_1受体密度	两次PET扫描，一次在隔夜禁欲后，另一次在正常吸烟率期间	吸烟者在整个纹状体中的D1受体结合显著低于非吸烟者；然而，隔夜禁欲和经常吸烟之间的D_1受体结合没有差异

14.2.6 [^{18}F]-氟多巴

使用[^{18}F]-氟多巴调查吸烟者DA合成能力的研究结果喜忧参半（表14.6）。一项研究报告称，男性吸烟者背侧纹状体的DA活性明显高于不吸烟者（Salokangas et al. 2000），而Bloomfield等（2014）发现与吸烟状况相关的整个纹状体没有差异。这些不一致的结果可能是由于样本总体不一致。Salokangas等（2000）只研究了男性重度吸烟者，而Bloomfield等（2014）研究了男性和女性中度吸烟者。因此，重度吸烟者的多巴胺合成可能会改变，而中度吸烟者则不会。

表14.6 [^{18}F]-氟多巴

参考文献	研究对象	研究目的	干预手段	结论
Bloomfield et al. (2014)	15名吸烟者（平均每天8.1支卷烟）与之相匹配的15名非吸烟者	使用[^{18}F]氟多巴比较吸烟者和非吸烟者的DA合成	一次PET扫描；吸烟者在扫描前戒烟3小时	在任何纹状体区域发现DA合成与吸烟者状态、每日吸烟或性别之间没有关联
Salokangas et al. (2000)	9名吸烟者，每天吸19.8支烟，和10名不吸烟者	使用[^{18}F]-氟多巴调查吸烟者和非吸烟者的基底神经节中的多巴胺合成是否不同	一次PET扫描	吸烟者在壳核和尾状核中显示出增加的DA合成，特别是在右尾状核和左壳核中

14.3 结论

利用多种放射性示踪剂，PET研究已经阐明了烟碱与多巴胺的关系。首先，烟碱似乎能诱导纹状体（腹侧和背侧）、皮层（主要是扣带回）和富含D_3的区域（腹侧苍白球）释放DA。虽然烟碱本身可能是DA释放的主要贡献者，但与吸烟有关的线索也可能发挥重要作用。然而，烟碱诱导的DA释放并没有一致的报道，而且可能对烟碱的给药途径、吸烟方法和其他因素敏感。此外，烟碱诱导的多巴胺释放可能在性别、不同的遗传多态性和共病疾病之间有所不同。

其次，长期使用烟草会导致D_1和D_2受体表达下调，尽管这对于戒烟者来说可能是可逆的。

与DA释放一样，DA受体的下调也可能在不同性别之间有不同的经历。随着烟碱依赖的发展，DA合成也可能受到影响，尽管这可能会对重度使用者造成更严重的影响。

最后，DA活性与几种吸烟行为存在区域相关性。渴望似乎与腹侧纹状体DA活性和受体（D_1和D_2）的可用性有关，但也可能与皮层区域有关。吸烟引起的情绪变化和愉悦效应可能与背侧纹状体有关，而依赖的严重程度可能与两个纹状体区域的活动有关。这些行为和烟草依赖作为一个整体与药物治疗（如伐伦克林和安非他酮）有效对抗。有趣的是，安非他酮（Brody et al. 2010）和伐伦克林（Di Ciano et al. 2016）似乎对DA传递的影响不同。

由于烟草依赖仍然是一个相当大的临床问题，需要更多的研究来了解复杂的烟草与DA的关系。总体而言，在这一领域进行的PET研究非常有限，我们对DA合成和受体如何随时间进化知之甚少。显然有必要进行更多、更大规模的研究。重要的是要描述吸烟对不同脑区DA传递的影响，并探索个别因素对所测量信号的可变性的作用。更好地了解受试者对临床使用的药物的反应也将更好地理解这些药物在人类吸烟者身上的作用机制。

术语解释	
	■ 急性挑战：物质的管理，以便在定义的参数上引起可测量的变化。
	■ 结合潜力：放射性标记配体结合能力的量度。这种测量通常是受体可用性和配体亲和力的组合。
	■ 去烟碱化卷烟：一种烟碱含量显著降低的卷烟，通常用于研究目的。
	■ 背侧纹状体：是皮层下基底神经节的一部分。这个区域通常由尾状核和壳核组成。
	■ 诱导性多巴胺释放：一种物质或行为引起的多巴胺浓度变化的量度。例如，吸烟诱导多巴胺释放是指吸烟后会使多巴胺释放。
	■ 边缘纹状体：类似于腹侧纹状体，有时可互换使用。这个大脑区域指的是纹状体中接受边缘结构（如杏仁核和海马）的神经元投射的部分。
	■ 烟碱化卷烟：一种含有固定浓度烟碱的卷烟。这种卷烟类似于商业购买的卷烟，但也可能是专门为研究目的而生产的。
	■ 受体可用性：配体可能结合的特定大脑区域内受体的密度或数量。
	■ 与吸烟有关的提示：这是指与吸烟有关的刺激。例如，卷烟或打火机的图片或者卷烟烟雾的气味。
	■ 腹侧纹状体：是皮层下基底神经节的一部分。这个区域通常包括伏隔核。

PET中放射性示踪剂的关键事实	
	■ PET中使用的放射性示踪剂是与目标受体结合的发射正电子的化学配体。
	■ 许多放射性示踪剂对几种受体的亲和力不同。
	■ 通过与内源性神经递质竞争受体结合，可以间接测量神经递质的浓度。
	■ 放射性示踪剂允许在静止状态下通过估算BP_{ND}来测量受体密度。

要点总结	
	■ 本章使用正电子发射断层扫描（PET）回顾了人类多巴胺（DA）在烟碱依赖性中的活性。
	■ PET使用不同的放射性示踪剂评估体内不同大脑区域的DA神经传递以及体内不同受体亚型的可用性。

要点总结

- 研究表明，烟草施用会增加纹状体、富含D_3的纹状体区域和皮层区域的DA水平。
- 关于烟草提高DA水平的能力的报道不一致。
- 性别和遗传变异可能会影响这些影响。
- 长期使用烟草会下调DA受体，戒断一段时间后可能会逆转。
- 与DA变化相关的几种与烟草相关的表型：戒断、渴望、情绪变化和依赖性严重程度。
- 未来的研究应集中于阐明个体变异的机制基础，因为它涉及对慢性烟草使用引起的急性神经传递和神经适应性变化，以改善治疗效果。

参考文献

Albrecht, D. S.; Kareken, D. A.; Yoder, K. K. (2013). Effects of smoking on D2/D3 striatal receptor availability in alcoholics and social drinkers. Brain Imaging and Behavior, 7(3), 326-334. https://doi.org/10.1007/s11682-013-9233-4.

Barrett, S. P.; Boileau, I.; Okker, J.; Pihl, R. O.; Dagher, A. (2004). The hedonic response to cigarette smoking is proportional to dopamine release in the human striatum as measured by positron emission tomography and [11C]raclopride. Synapse, 54(2), 65-71. https://doi.org/10.1002/syn.20066.

Bloomfield, M. A.; Pepper, F.; Egerton, A.; Demjaha, A.; Tomasi, G.; Mouchlianitis, E. et al. (2014). Dopamine function in cigarette smokers: an [18F]-DOPA PET study. Neuropsychopharmacology, 39(10), 2397-2404.

Brody, A. L.; London, E. D.; Olmstead, R. E.; Allen-Martinez, Z.; Shulenberger, S.; Costello, M. R. et al. (2010). Smoking-induced change in intrasynaptic dopamine concentration: effect of treatment for tobacco dependence. Psychiatry Research: Neuroimaging, 183(3), 218-224.

Brody, A. L.; Mandelkern, M. A.; Olmstead, R. E.; Allen-Martinez, Z.; Scheibal, D.; Abrams, A. L. et al. (2009). Ventral striatal dopamine release in response to smoking a regular vs a denicotinized cigarette. Neuropsychopharmacology, 34(2), 282-289.

Brody, A. L.; Mandelkern, M. A.; Olmstead, R. E.; Scheibal, D.; Hahn, E.; Shiraga, S. et al. (2006). Gene variants of brain dopamine pathways and smoking-induced dopamine release in the ventral caudate/nucleus accumbens. Archives of General Psychiatry, 63(7), 808.

Brody, A. L.; Olmstead, R. E.; Abrams, A. L.; Costello, M. R.; Khan, A.; Kozman, D. et al. (2009). Effect of a history of major depressive disorder on smoking-induced dopamine release. Biological Psychiatry, 66(9), 898-901.

Brody, A. L.; Olmstead, R. E.; London, E. D.; Farahi, J.; Meyer, J. H.; Grossman, P. et al. (2004). Smoking-induced ventral striatum dopamine release. American Journal of Psychiatry, 161(7), 1211-1218.

Brown, A. K.; Mandelkern, M. A.; Farahi, J.; Robertson, C.; Ghahremani, D. G.; Sumerel, B. et al. (2012). Sex differences in striatal dopamine D2/D3 receptor availability in smokers and non-smokers. The International Journal of Neuropsychopharmacology, 15(07), 989-994.

Busto, U. E.; Redden, L.; Mayberg, H.; Kapur, S.; Houle, S.; Zawertailo, L. A. (2009). Dopaminergic activity in depressed smokers: a positron emission tomography study. Synapse, 63(8), 681-689.

Chiuccariello, L.; Boileau, I.; Guranda, M.; Rusjan, P. M.; Wilson, A. A.; Zawertailo, L. et al. (2013). Presentation of smoking-associated cues does not elicit dopamine release after one-hour smoking abstinence: a [^{11}C]-(+)-PHNO PET study. PLoS ONE, 8(3), e60382.

Cosgrove, K. P.; Wang, S.; Kim, S.-J.; McGovern, E.; Nabulsi, N.; Gao, H. et al. (2014). Sex differences in the brain's dopamine signature of cigarette smoking. Journal of Neuroscience, 34(50), 16851-16855.

Dagher, A.; Bleicher, C.; Aston, J. A.; Gunn, R. N.; Clarke, P.; Cumming, P. (2001). Reduced dopamine D1 receptor binding in the ventral striatum of cigarette smokers. Synapse, 42(1), 48-53.

Di Chiara, G. (2000). Role of dopamine in the behavioural actions of nicotine related to addiction. European Journal of Pharmacology, 393(1), 295-314. https://doi.org/10.1016/S0014-2999(00)00122-9.

Di Ciano, P.; Guranda, M.; Lagzdins, D.; Tyndale, R. F.; Gamaleddin, I.; Selby, P. et al. (2016). Varenicline-induced elevation of dopamine in smokers: a preliminary [^{11}C]-(+)-PHNO PET study. Neuropsychopharmacology. Retrieved from: (2016). http://www.nature.com/npp/journal/vaop/ncurrent/full/npp2015305a.html.

Domino, E. F.; Evans, C. L.; Ni, L.; Guthrie, S. K.; Koeppe, R. A.; Zubieta, J.-K. (2012). Tobacco smoking produces greater striatal dopamine release in G-allele carriers with mu opioid receptor A118G polymorphism. Progress in Neuro-Psychopharmacology and Biological Psychiatry, 38(2), 236-240.

Domino, E. F.; Ni, L.; Domino, J. S.; Yang, W.; Evans, C.; Guthrie, S. et al. (2013). Denicotinized versus average nicotine tobacco cigarette smoking differentially releases striatal dopamine. Nicotine, Tobacco Research, 15(1), 11-21.

Fehr, C.; Yakushev, I.; Hohmann, N.; Buchholz, H.-G.; Landvogt, C.; Deckers, H. et al. (2008). Association of low striatal dopamine D 2receptor availability with nicotine dependence similar to that seenwith other drugs of abuse. American Journal of Psychiatry, 165(4), 507-514.

Lammertsma, A. A.; Hume, S. P. (1996). Simplified reference tissue model for PET receptor studies. NeuroImage, 4(3), 153-158.

Le Foll, B.; Guranda, M.; Wilson, A. A.; Houle, S.; Rusjan, P. M.; Wing, V. C. et al. (2014). Elevation of dopamine induced by cigarette smoking: novel insights from a [^{11}C]-(+)-PHNO PET study in humans. Neuropsychopharmacology, 39(2), 415-424.

Mintun, M. A.; Raichle, M. E.; Kilbourn, M. R.; Wooten, G. F.; Welch, M. J. (1984). A quantitative model for the in vivo assessment of drug binding sites with positron emission tomography. Annals of Neurology, 15(3), 217-227.

Montgomery, A. J.; Lingford-Hughes, A. R.; Egerton, A.; Nutt, D. J.; Grasby, P. M. (2007). The effect of nicotine on striatal dopamine release in man: a [^{11}C]raclopride PET study. Synapse, 61(8), 637-645.

Narendran, R.; Frankle, W. G.; Mason, N. S.; Rabiner, E. A.; Gunn, R. N.; Searle, G. E. et al. (2009). Positron emission tomography imaging of amphetamine-induced dopamine release in the human cortex: acomparative evaluation of the high affinity dopamine D2/3 radiotracers [^{11}C]FLB 457 and [^{11}C]fallypride. Synapse, 63(6), 447-461.

Okita, K.; Mandelkern, M. A.; London, E. D. (2016). Cigarette use and striatal dopamine D2/3 receptors: possible role in the link between smoking and nicotine dependence. International Journal of Neuropsychopharmacology, 19(11). pyw074.

Okita, K.; Petersen, N.; Robertson, C. L.; Dean, A. C.; Mandelkern, M. A.; London, E. D. (2016). Sex differences in midbrain dopamine D2-type receptor availability and association with nicotine dependence. Neuropsychopharmacology, 41(12), 2913-2919.

Parsey, R. V.; Oquendo, M. A.; Zea-Ponce, Y.; Rodenhiser, J.; Kegeles, L. S.; Pratap, M. et al. (2001). Dopamine D(2) receptor availability and amphetamine-induced dopamine release in unipolar depression. Biological Psychiatry, 50(5), 313-322.

Portnow, L. H.; Vaillancourt, D. E.; Okun, M. S. (2013). The history of cerebral PET scanning from physiology to cutting-edge technology. Neurology, 80(10), 952-956.

Riccardi, P.; Baldwin, R.; Salomon, R.; Anderson, S.; Ansari, M. S.; Li, R. et al. (2008). Estimation of baseline dopamine D2 receptor occupancy in striatum and extrastriatal regions in humans with positron emission tomography with [^{18}F] fallypride. Biological Psychiatry, 63(2), 241-244.

Riccardi, P.; Li, R.; Ansari, M. S.; Zald, D.; Park, S.; Dawant, B. et al. (2005). Amphetamine-induced displacement of [^{18}F] fallypride in striatum and extrastriatal regions in humans. Neuropsychopharmacology, 31(5), 1016-1026.

Salokangas, R. K.; Vilkman, H.; Ilonen, T.; Taiminen, T.; Bergman, J.; Haaparanta, M. et al. (2000). High levels of dopamine activity in the basal ganglia of cigarette smokers. American Journal of Psychiatry, 157(4), 632-634.

Scott, D. J.; Domino, E. F.; Heitzeg, M. M.; Koeppe, R. A.; Ni, L.; Guthrie, S. et al. (2007). Smoking modulation of μ-opioid and dopamine D2 receptor-mediated neurotransmission in humans. Neuropsychopharmacology, 32(2), 450-457.

Shotbolt, P.; Tziortzi, A. C.; Searle, G. E.; Colasanti, A.; van der Aart, J.; Abanades, S. et al. (2012). Within-subject comparison of [^{11}C]-(+)-PHNO and [^{11}C]raclopride sensitivity to acute amphetamine challenge in healthy humans. Journal of Cerebral Blood Flow, Metabolism, 32(1), 127-136.

Surgeon General (2014). The health consequences of smoking—50 years of progress: a report of the surgeon general. US Department of Health and Human Services.

Takahashi, H.; Fujimura, Y.; Hayashi, M.; Takano, H.; Kato, M.; Okubo, Y. et al. (2008). Enhanced dopamine release by nicotine in cigarette smokers: a double-blind, randomized, placebo-controlled pilot study. The International Journal of Neuropsychopharmacology, 11(03). https://doi.org/10.1017/S1461145707008103.

Tziortzi, A. C.; Searle, G. E.; Tzimopoulou, S.; Salinas, C.; Beaver, J. D.; Jenkinson, M. et al. (2011). Imaging dopamine receptors in humans with [^{11}C]-(+)-PHNO: dissection of D3 signal and anatomy. NeuroImage, 54(1), 264-277.

Volkow, N. D.; Fowler, J. S.; Wang, G. J.; Baler, R.; Telang, F. (2009). Imaging dopamine's role in drug abuse and addiction. Neuropharmacology, 56, 3-8.

Volkow, N. D.; Wang, G. -J.; Fowler, J. S.; Tomasi, D. (2012). Addiction circuitry in the human brain. Annual Review of Pharmacology and Toxicology, 52(1), 321-336.

Weinstein, A. M.; Freedman, N.; Greif, J.; Yemini, Z.; Mishani, E.; London, E. et al. (2016). Negative association of pretreatmentcigarette use with smoking-induced striatal dopamine release in smokers receiving bupropion treatment: pre-treatment cigarette use and dopamine release. The American Journal on Addictions, 25(6), 486-492.

Wiers, C. E.; Cabrera, E. A.; Tomasi, D.; Wong, C. T.; Demiral, Ş. B.; Kim, S. W. et al. (2017). Striatal dopamine D2/D3 receptor availability varies across smoking status. Neuropsychopharmacology, https://doi.org/10.1038/npp.2017.131.

Wing, V. C.; Payer, D. E.; Houle, S.; George, T. P.; Boileau, I. (2015). Measuring cigarette smoking-induced cortical dopamine release: a [^{11}C] FLB-457 PET study. Neuropsychopharmacology, 40(7), 1417-1427.

Yasuno, F.; Ota, M.; Ando, K.; Ando, T.; Maeda, J.; Ichimiya, T. et al. (2007). Role of ventral striatal dopamine D1 receptor in cigarette craving. Biological Psychiatry, 61(11), 1252-1259.

15
静止状态功能连接成像和烟碱依赖

Victor M. Vergara, Vince D. Calhoun

The Mind Research Network, Albuquerque, NM, United States

缩略语

ACC	前扣带皮层	ECN	执行控制网络
BART	气球模拟风险任务	fMRI	功能磁共振成像
BOLD	血氧水平依赖	rsFC	静止状态功能连接
dlPFC	背外侧前额叶皮层	SN	显著性网络
DMN	默认模式网络		

15.1 引言

烟碱对神经系统的影响不仅局限于需要完成任务的大脑活动，还会延伸到毫无挑战的静止状态。即使在这种静止状态下，大脑仍处于不断活动的状态，表现出对身体健康很重要的行为。在低频率时可以观察到静止状态的波动，表现出通过大脑的重要协同激活模式。大脑不同区域之间的协同激活被认为是功能连接（van den Heuvel, Hulshoff Pol, 2010）。不同的全脑连接模式已经被发现可以自发地通过时间进行迭代。这些全脑模式和点对点连接的中断与患有不同类型成瘾症的患者的神经功能障碍有关（Sutherland, McHugh, Pariyadath, Stein, 2012）。特别是烟碱会影响通常与烟碱成瘾相关的区域的功能连接，如脑岛和前扣带皮层。下面的汇编展示了通过研究静止状态下大脑的功能连接而获得的最相关的结果和结论。

15.2 评估静止状态下的功能连接

静止状态功能连接（rsFC）的评估基于对大脑活动的动态变化的测量。功能磁共振成像（fMRI）是用于功能连接估计的几种方法中应用最广泛的一种，其具有相对较高的时间分辨率和最小的侵袭作用。在本节中，我们将用 fMRI 来描述 rsFC。

15.2.1 fMRI 数据中的感兴趣区域和静止状态网络

由于血液的磁化特性，神经元的活动可以通过 fMRI 数据进行评估。根据氧合血和缺氧血的顺磁差异，选择静脉血中的脱氧血红蛋白作为 BOLD 造影剂（Ogawa et al. 1990）。瞬时 BOLD 测量提供了关于氧代谢随时间变化的突触活动的信息（Ekstrom, 2010; Heeger, Ress, 2002）。结构上独立的大脑区域显示同步神经元活动，可以使用 BOLD 信号进行评估（Biswal et al. 1995）。测量到的不同神经元群体之间的一致性活动表明了它们的功能连接，这已经被证明与白质束相关

(Honey et al. 2009）。关注特定脑区的BOLD信号是评估rsFC的一项重要技术，该方法在一个特定的位置进行标记，并估计与其他大脑区域的共激活（Biswal et al. 1995）。这种方法在有先验信息的情况下使用。标记与假设检验相关。另一个重要的选择促进了识别功能和空间上不同的BOLD信号。脑源识别通常是用盲源分离方法（单词"blind"表示先验信息的缺乏）来实现的，其中我们可以提及字典学习（Lee et al. 2016）和独立成分分析（Calhoun, Adali, 2012）。由于没有先验信息或假设，这些方法被用于探索性和数据驱动的研究。

15.2.2 使用fMRI的静态rsFC

相关性是最早用于估计rsFC的方法之一（van den Heuvel, Hulshoff Pol, 2010）。最简单的方法是假设rsFC在fMRI扫描期间保持不变。在实践中，fMRI扫描时间最短为5min（Allen et al. 2011），但扫描时间越长越好，10min扫描时间被认为在捕获信号功率方面足够高（Murphy et al. 2007）。扫描时间将决定相关估计中的数据量，从而对评估的意义有重要的影响。图15.1显示了一个典型的rsFC相关矩阵和涉及的大脑领域。这些大脑区域最近才被用于烟碱和酒精的研究（Vergara, Liu, et al. 2017）。盲源分离技术，如独立成分分析，往往更能抵御干扰，允许预处理的单次通过（Vergara, Mayer et al. 2017），而其他技术可能需要更精细的清洁预处理（Power et al. 2014）。

15.2.3 使用fMRI的动态rsFC

通过文献收集的证据表明，在静止状态实验中功能连接不会保持不变。相反，大脑的连通性出现了明显的时间变化，这可以在典型的扫描长度内观察到（Chang, Glover, 2010）。捕获这种动态需要在相对较短的时间内使用协同激活评估。时间间隔越短，时间分辨率越好；然而，较短的时间跨度会减少可用于相关性的数据样本的数量，从而降低连接的评估。建议使用40~100s的时间间隔来评估功能连接（Leonardi, Van De Ville, 2015; Zalesky, Breakspear, 2015）。

动态rsFC研究已经确定了一组有限的连接模式，随着全脑动态的演变，这些连接模式会随时间不断迭代（Allen et al. 2014; Sakoğlu et al. 2010）。这些模式被称为动态状态，并且是高度可复制的（Abrol, Chaze, Damaraju, Calhoun, 2016）。有证据支持状态与心理和情绪精神状态之间的联系（Cribben, Haraldsdottir, Atlas, Wager, Lindquist, 2012）。图15.1给出了一项涉及烟碱、酒精和大麻的研究中发现的一组动态状态（Vergara, Weiland, Hutchison, Calhoun, 2018）。连接分析可以在每个状态上隔离rsFC后应用，其方式与应用于静态rsFC的方式类似。在这种情况下，分析的数量与确定的状态一样多。最常见的度量是每个状态的频率和持续时间。更频繁发生的状态对整体rsFC有更强的影响。这些动态状态的特征无法通过静态rsFC获得，但会对rsFC人口统计学和神经病学测量的分析产生影响。

15.3 静止状态功能连接

在大脑的一些重要区域，包括背外侧前额叶皮层（dlPFC）、脑岛、前扣带皮层（ACC）、感觉运动区、执行控制网络（ECN）和默认模式网络（DMN），已经观察到与烟碱使用相关的异常功能连接。这些区域属于涉及外感受、内感受、渴望和一般静止状态动力学的网络。本节总结了大脑中与烟碱有关的静止状态的发现。

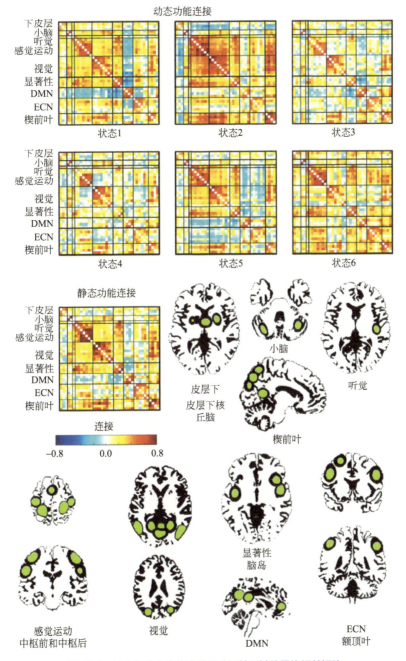

图 15.1 静态和动态功能连接和脑相关区域的平均相关矩阵

图中显示了静态（Vergara, Liu et al. 2017）和动态（Vergara et al. 2018）功能连接的平均相关矩阵。包括代表每个功能组的区域的位置：皮层下、小脑、听觉、感觉运动、视觉、显著性、默认模式网络（DMN）、执行控制网络（ECN）和楔前叶。这一数据是根据先前发表的 534 名受试者的数据重新计算的（Vergara et al. 2018）

15.3.1 脑岛

脑岛在烟碱成瘾中占有重要地位，因为它在感知身体的生理状态方面的作用，这是一种被称为内感受的特征（Craig, 2009）。脑岛可以解决身体的感觉，包括疼痛、温度、痒、触摸、饥饿、口渴、需求空气、肌肉感觉（Craig, 2003）。这种内感受的结合会影响感觉和决策，从而导致烟碱成瘾（Naqvi, Bechara, 2009），在某种程度上，这一区域的创伤使有意识的冲动停止，从而导致戒烟（Naqvi, Rudrauf, Damasio, Bechara, 2007）。这些观察结果表明脑岛是维持吸烟冲动的关键区域，这种冲动源于大脑和身体之间的内感受关系。

除了它在内感受系统中的作用外，脑岛和植根于躯体感觉皮层的"外感受"系统之间的关系可能与吸烟行为的维持有关。例如，复发的吸烟者在脑岛和双侧前、后中枢脑回表现出较弱的rsFC（Addicott, Sweitzer, Froeliger, Rose, McClernon, 2015）。这种影响与吸烟者较差的抑制控制有关，这与去/不去研究的观察结果一致（Perry, Carroll, 2008）。脑岛和躯体感觉皮层与ACC、前额叶皮层、基底神经节和丘脑共同参与反应抑制网络（Congdon et al. 2010; Janes et al. 2010）。在Congdon的研究中发现的网络（Congdon et al. 2010）与其他静止状态研究中的网络紧密匹配，进一步证明rsFC和与烟碱有关的要求任务效应涉及类似的大脑结构。

烟碱对脑岛的影响表现为纵向的戒断成分。除了烟碱对多巴胺的调节作用（Marshall, Redfern, Wonnacott, 2002），与健康对照组相比，经常吸烟的人在扫描前吸了一根烟，在注射烟碱后观察到岛叶-dlPFC和岛叶-颞叶皮层之间的负功能连接（以负相关衡量）。（Stoeckel, Chai, Zhang, Whitfield-Gabrieli, Evins, 2016）。该研究还发现，与健康对照组相比，吸烟者在上述大脑区域的灰质密度有所下降。通过dlPFC和岛叶之间的功能连接预测24小时后成功戒断（Zelle, Gates, Fiez, Sayette, Wilson, 2017）。这些功能连接效应是大脑中烟碱存在的反应，当试图保持戒断时，这也会调节未来的自我控制。

脑岛具有内感受和外感受处理的双重功能，这可以被烟碱改变（Addicott et al. 2015）。脑岛rsFC的变化扩展到已知的大脑网络，如ECN（Stoeckel et al. 2016）和DMN（Wilcox et al. 2017），这是静止状态下最具影响力的网络（Buckner, Andrews-Hanna, Schacter, 2008）。脑岛是竞争网络状态的中心，它提供了在对立网络之间切换的显著处理功能（Sutherland et al. 2013）。脑岛与其他重要大脑区域的相互作用使得它成为成瘾的一个有高度兴趣的区域（Naqvi, Bechara, 2009）。

15.3.2 前扣带皮层

ACC是rsFC与烟碱相关的另一个大脑区域。脑岛-ACC静止状态连接的增加与在收集静止数据后执行任务时测量到的吸烟线索反应性增强有关（Janes, Farmer et al. 2015）。烟碱的影响在ACC和脑岛之间产生了重要的变化，因为它们的功能关系可能有助于激发吸烟的冲动。脑岛和ACC是显著性网络的核心部分，在自我参照脑功能中与DMN相互作用（Spreng, Stevens et al. 2010）。DMN在需要外部注意的任务中不那么活跃，而在静止状态下更活跃（Buckner et al. 2008）。然而，在暴露于外部吸烟环境期间，DMN表现出异常高的活性，是因为其被ACC中的谷氨酸调节，导致更高的反应性。不正常的ACC使静止状态区域与任务相关区域共同激活，从而增加吸烟提示反应并促进吸烟行为。

吸烟者的ACC除了与自我感知区域的失调有关外，还被发现与认知控制区域有异常的联系。几项研究表明，烟碱依赖者的行为风险更大（Galvan et al. 2013）。使用气球模拟风险任务（BART）的风险行为测量（Lejuez et al. 2002）已经能够区分吸烟者和非吸烟者（Lejuez et al. 2003）。BART实验数据表明，ACC是危险行为的重要组成部分（Rao, Korczykowski, Pluta, Hoang, Detre, 2008）。虽然大脑和危险行为之间的关系必须通过任务设计来测量，但在任务中观察到的效果会在静息状态中反映出来。在以ACC和丘脑为主要节点的网络中，烟碱依赖、危险行为（使用BART测量）和rsFC之间的三方关系已被确定（Wei et al. 2016）。同样的研究确定，在任务中大脑的激活与任务本身或烟碱依赖无关。

ACC与烟碱的关系似乎可以通过它与大脑其他区域形成网络的关系来解释。烟碱成瘾也与ACC-纹状体连接强度有关（Hong et al. 2009），表明ACC的作用达到奖励调节区域。在这个功能失调的网络中重要的节点是ACC、脑岛、丘脑和腹侧纹状体。一些研究表明，参与显著情绪处理的杏仁核可以加入到这个网络中（Bi et al. 2017）。

15.3.3 默认模式网络

一组很好识别的大脑区域在被动休息期间是活跃的，这表明存在默认的大脑活动（Buckner, Vincent, 2007）。相关区域形成了一个大脑区域网络，包括扣带皮层、顶叶和前额叶皮层以及其他区域（Buckner et al. 2008）。DMN是静止状态实验的主要研究重点。DMN功能已经被发现受到烟碱摄入的影响。大脑中烟碱的存在降低了静止状态下DMN的活性（Tanabe et al. 2011; Weiland et al. 2015）。DMN活性降低有助于增强对任务有要求的功能，如视觉空间注意（Hahn et al. 2007; Thiel, Zilles, Fink, 2005）和工作记忆（Bentley, Husain, Dolan, 2004）。DMN功能的这些改变并不是免费的。在吸烟提示暴露期间，烟碱产生一种减少DMN抑制的抵消作用（Janes et al. 2016; Wilcox et al. 2017）。烟碱的双重作用是显而易见的，它虽然增强了一些认知能力，但也促进了成瘾（Jasinska, Zorick, Brody, Stein, 2014）。此外，随着吸烟者年龄的增长，认知能力的下降也与烟碱摄入的负面影响有关（Kalmijn, 2002）。

15.3.4 执行控制和显著性网络

在静止状态下的成瘾研究中，另外两个高度相关的网络是ECN和显著性网络（SN）。SN的中心部分是脑岛，这是一个与烟碱成瘾高度相关的区域（Naqvi et al. 2007）。与DMN类似，静止状态实验发现顶叶皮层和dlPFC区域这两个主要的ECN区域的功能连接降低。与ECN、认知和烟碱相关的有害影响并没有持续观察到，但是它们可能与戒断相互作用。例如，烟碱戒断会导致注意力难以集中和烦躁不安（Hughes, 2007），与烟碱给药后注意力和记忆的增强形成对比（Bentley et al. 2004; Hahn et al. 2007; Thiel et al. 2005）。除了认知改变，功能失调的ECN还会导致成瘾行为，因为它有更强的线索反应（Goldstein, Volkow, 2002）以及抑制控制过程中更高的激活（Luijten et al. 2013; Zhang et al. 2011）。

15.3.5 DMN-SN-ECN——烟碱成瘾网络模型

三种静止状态网络（DMN、SN、ECN）保持交互作用的功能平衡。大脑中烟碱的影响改变了这种平衡，从而促进了成瘾行为。烟碱成瘾网络模型（Sutherland et al. 2012）描述了这些静止状态网络之间的交互更改。该模型描述的烟碱给药效应如图15.2所示。在给药期间，烟碱使大脑的处理过程远离DMN。由于DMN的影响减弱，ECN中的rsFC及其与SN的相互作用得到了增强。更多的注意力被导向外在刺激，导致基于任务的活动的性能改进。该模型与在未接触烟碱中观察到的认知增强效应一致（Heishman, et al. 2010）以及烟碱抑制非吸烟者DMN活动的证据（Tanabe et al. 2011）。图 15.3 示出了烟碱戒断的网络交互作用。在戒断期间，模型（Sutherland et al., 2012）预测，（1）脑岛和 DMN 之间的 rsFC 增加与戒断症状和任务表现受损相关，（2）ECN 和脑岛之间的 rsFC 减少，（3）DMN 内的 rsFC 增加，（4）ECN 内的 rsFC 减少，（5）导致 DMN 和 ECN 之间功能失调，降低了它们的负耦合（Cole et al. 2010）。

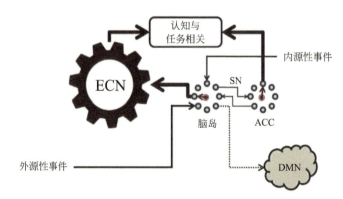

图 15.2　烟碱给药后的静止状态相互作用

烟碱会抑制默认模式网络（DMN）（Tanabe et al. 2011），从而促进执行控制网络（ECN）与注意力和记忆的增强相一致（Bentley et al. 2004; Hahn et al. 2007）。

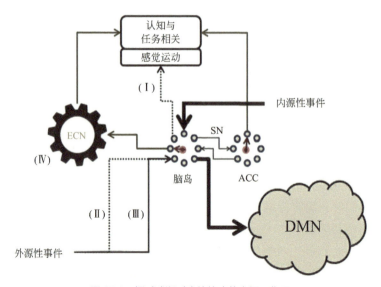

图 15.3　烟碱戒断对应的静止状态相互作用

内源性事件和外源性事件的处理方式不同。在烟碱戒断期间，前默认模式网络（DMN）抑制（由于烟碱给药）减弱（Janes et al. 2016; Wilcox et al. 2017）以及其他效应：（Ⅰ）脑岛-感觉运动连接性弱（Addicott et al. 2015），（Ⅱ）包括枕区在内的感觉输入连接性降低（Addicott et al. 2015）；Vergara, Liu, et al. 2017）等，（Ⅲ）增强视觉空间注意区域的功能（Hahn et al. 2007; Vergara, Liu et al. 2017），（Ⅳ）降低执行控制网络（ECN）的静止状态功能（Weiland et al. 2015）。

15.4　静止状态功能连接的处理意义

与传统卷烟差别很大的烟碱给药产品的出现，给临床医生带来了新的挑战（Schick et al. 2017）。20 世纪开发的烟碱依赖测试的重点是卷烟使用的准确性，这已被重复多次，最近有证据表明，一种新的修改可能是可取的（Chabrol, Niezborala, Chastan, Montastruc, Mullet, 2003）。另外，大脑主要网络（DMN、ECN、SN）和大脑中的烟碱之间的相互作用为基于神经成像的成瘾生物标记提供了重要特征，从而导致识别烟碱成瘾的可能性（Pariyadath, Stein, Ross, 2014）。生物标记发展包括预测和跟踪治疗结果的可能性。壳核、ACC、尾状核和dlPFC中较高的rsFC（Wilcox et al. 2017）被发现是烟碱治疗结果的预测因子，可以识别出复发风险较高的个体。在类似的情况下，rsFC提供了证据，证明至少存在三个烟碱使用者亚群（Ding et al. 2018）。这些结果表明，rsFC是一个重要的工具来调查大脑烟碱状态，进一步评估成瘾行为。

术语解释

- BOLD：基于氧合血与脱氧血顺磁差异的血氧水平依赖性造影剂。
- 默认模式网络：与需要大量活动的任务相比，静止状态下需要更活跃的大脑区域网络。其主要组成部分是内侧前额叶皮层、角回和后扣带皮层。
- 动态静止状态功能连接：在相对较短（小于100s）的时间内测量同步激活。
- 执行控制网络：一种对行为控制和目标导向任务所必需的执行和认知功能的大脑区域网络。其关键组成部分是背外侧前额叶和顶叶皮层。
- 静止状态功能连接：基于同步神经元激活的脑区间的静止状态关系。在fMRI中，神经元激活是通过血氧浓度依赖性信号来测量的。
- 静止状态：大脑不受挑战的休息时刻，大脑没有内测量同步激活忙于艰巨的任务。
- 静态静止状态功能连接：在相对较长时间（5min）内对同步激活的测量。

静止状态大脑网络的关键事实

- 默认模式网络和任务正网络的活动以一种反相关的方式波动。
- 积极任务网络是在工作期间所需要的外部要求的任务。
- 积极任务网络包括执行控制、体感和视觉网络。
- 反相关对大脑的健康运行很重要。

要点总结

- 静止状态的大脑激活是通过血氧浓度依赖性的对比来测量的。
- 静止状态功能连接与休息时大脑区域的同步激活有关。
- 烟碱成瘾的三个重要的静止状态网络分别是默认模式网络、执行控制网络和显著性网络。
- 在静止状态研究中发现的大脑网络的功能平衡受烟碱的影响。
- 烟碱的使用可以增强执行控制网络的功能。
- 烟碱戒断增强了默认模式网络的功能。
- 静止状态网络间失调的相互作用促进烟碱寻求行为。

参考文献

Abrol, A.; Chaze, C.; Damaraju, E.; Calhoun, V. D. (2016). The chronnectome: evaluating replicability of dynamic connectivity patterns in 7500 resting fMRI datasets (pp. 5571-5574)Conference Proceedings: Annual International Conference of the IEEE Engineering in Medicine and Biology Society, 2016. https://doi.org/10.1109/EMBC.2016.7591989.

Addicott, M. A.; Sweitzer, M. M.; Froeliger, B.; Rose, J. E.; McClernon, F. J. (2015). Increased functional connectivity in an insula-based network is associated with improved smoking cessation outcomes. Neuropsychopharmacology, 40(11), 2648-2656.

Allen, E. A.; Damaraju, E.; Plis, S. M.; Erhardt, E. B.; Eichele, T.; Calhoun, V. D. (2014). Tracking whole-brain connectivity dynamics in the resting state. Cerebral Cortex, 24(3), 663-676.

Allen, E. A.; Erhardt, E. B.; Damaraju, E.; Gruner, W.; Segall, J. M.; Silva, R. F. et al. (2011). A baseline for the multivariate comparison of resting-state networks. Frontiers in Systems Neuroscience, 5, 2.

Bentley, P.; Husain, M.; Dolan, R. J. (2004). Effects of cholinergic enhancement on visual stimulation, spatial attention, and spatial working memory. Neuron, 41(6), 969-982.

Bi, Y.; Yuan, K.; Guan, Y.; Cheng, J.; Zhang, Y.; Li, Y. et al. (2017). Altered resting state functional connectivity of anterior insula in young smokers. Brain Imaging and Behavior, 11(1), 155-165.

Biswal, B.; Zerrin Yetkin, F.; Haughton, V. M.; Hyde, J. S. (1995). Functional connectivity in the motor cortex of resting human brain using echo-planar MRI. Magnetic Resonance in Medicine, 34(4), 537-541.

Buckner, R. L.; Andrews-Hanna, J. R.; Schacter, D. L. (2008). The brain's default network: anatomy, function, and relevance to disease. Annals of the New York Academy of Sciences, 1124(1), 1-38.

Buckner, R. L.; Vincent, J. L. (2007). Unrest at rest: default activity and spontaneous network correlations. NeuroImage, 37(4), 1091-1096.

Calhoun, V. D.; Adali, T. (2012). Multisubject independent component analysis of fMRI: a decade of intrinsic networks, default mode, and neurodiagnostic discovery. IEEE Reviews in Biomedical Engineering, 5, 60-73.

Chabrol, H.; Niezborala, M.; Chastan, E.; Montastruc, J. -L.; Mullet, E. (2003). A study of the psychometric properties of the Fagestrom Test for Nicotine Dependence. Addictive Behaviors, 28(8), 1441-1445.

Chang, C.; Glover, G. H. (2010). Time-frequency dynamics of restingstate brain connectivity m easured with fMRI. NeuroImage, 50(1), 81-98.

Cole, D. M.; Beckmann, C. F.; Long, C. J.; Matthews, P. M.; Durcan, M. J.; Beaver, J. D. (2010). Nicotine replacement in abstinent smokers improves cognitive withdrawal symptoms with modulation of resting brain network dynamics. Neuroimage, 52(2), 590-599.

Congdon, E.; Mumford, J. A.; Cohen, J. R.; Galvan, A.; Aron, A. R.; Xue, G. et al. (2010). Engagement of large-scale networks is related to individual differences in inhibitory control. NeuroImage, 53(2), 653-663.

Craig, A. (2003). Interoception: the sense of the physiological condition of the body. Current Opinion in Neurobiology, 13(4), 500-505.

Craig, A. D. (2009). How do you feel-now? The anterior insula and human awareness. Nature Reviews Neuroscience, 10(1), 59-70.

Cribben, I.; Haraldsdottir, R.; Atlas, L. Y.; Wager, T. D.; Lindquist, M. A. (2012). Dynamic connectivity regression: determining staterelated changes in brain connectivity. NeuroImage, 61(4), 907-920.

Ding, X.; Salmeron, B. J.; Wang, J.; Yang, Y.; Stein, E. A.; Ross, T. J. (2018). Evidence of subgroups in smokers as revealed in clinical measures and evaluated by neuroimaging data: a preliminary study. Addiction Biology. https://doi. org/10. 1111/adb. 12620.

Ekstrom, A. (2010). How and when the fMRI BOLD signal relates to underlying neural activity: the danger in dissociation. Brain Research Reviews, 62(2), 233-244.

Fedota, J. R.; Stein, E. A. (2015). Resting-state functional connectivity and nicotine addiction: prospects for biomarker development. Annals of the New York Academy of Sciences, 1349(1), 64-82.

Galvan, A.; Schonberg, T.; Mumford, J.; Kohno, M.; Poldrack, R. A.; London, E. D. (2013). Greater risk sensitivity of dorsolateral prefrontal cortex in young smokers than in nonsmokers. Psychopharmacology, 229(2), 345-355.

Goldstein, R. Z.; Volkow, N. D. (2002). Drug addiction and its underlying neurobiological basis: neuroimaging evidence for the involvement of the frontal cortex. The American Journal of Psychiatry, 159(10), 1642-1652.

Hahn, B.; Ross, T. J.; Yang, Y.; Kim, I.; Huestis, M. A.; Stein, E. A. (2007). Nicotine enhances visuospatial attention by deactivating areas of the resting brain default network. The Journal of Neuroscience, 27(13), 3477-3489.

Heeger, D. J.; Ress, D. (2002). What does fMRI tell us about neuronal activity? Nature Reviews Neuroscience, 3(2), 142-151.

Heishman, S. J.; Kleykamp, B. A.; Singleton, E. G. (2010). Metaanalysis of the acute effects of nicotine and smoking on human performance. Psychopharmacology, 210(4), 453-469.

Honey, C.; Sporns, O.; Cammoun, L.; Gigandet, X.; Thiran, J. -P.; Meuli, R. et al. (2009). Predicting human resting-state functional connectivity from structural connectivity. Proceedings of the National Academy of Sciences, 106(6), 2035-2040.

Hong, L. E.; Gu, H.; Yang, Y.; Ross, T. J.; Salmeron, B. J.; Buchholz, B. et al. (2009). Association of nicotine addiction and nicotine's actions with separate cingulate cortex functional circuits. Archives of General Psychiatry, 66(4), 431-441.

Hughes, J. R. (2007). Effects of abstinence from tobacco: valid symptoms and time course. Nicotine, Tobacco Research, 9(3), 315-327.

Janes, A. C.; Betts, J.; Jensen, J. E.; Lukas, S. E. (2016). Dorsal anterior cingulate glutamate is associated with engagement of the default mode network during exposure to smoking cues. Drug and Alcohol Dependence, 167, 75-81.

Janes, A. C.; Farmer, S.; Peechatka, A. L.; deB Frederick, B.; Lukas, S. E. (2015). Insula-dorsal anterior cingulate cortex coupling is associated with enhanced brain reactivity to smoking cues. Neuropsychopharmacology, 40(7), 1561-1568.

Janes, A. C.; Pizzagalli, D. A.; Richardt, S.; deB Frederick, B.; Chuzi, S.; Pachas, G. et al. (2010). Brain reactivity to smoking cues prior to smoking cessation predicts ability to maintain tobacco abstinence. Biological Psychiatry, 67(8), 722-729.

Jasinska, A. J.; Zorick, T.; Brody, A. L.; Stein, E. A. (2014). Dual role of nicotine in addiction and cognition: a review of neuroimaging studies in humans. Neuropharmacology, 84, 111-122.

Kalmijn, S. (2002). Cigarette smoking and alcohol consumption in relation to cognitive performance in middle age. American Journal of Epidemiology, 156(10), 936-944.

Lee, Y. B.; Lee, J.; Tak, S.; Lee, K.; Na, D. L.; Seo, S. W. et al. (2016). Sparse SPM: group sparse-dictionary learning in SPM framework for resting-state functional connectivity MRI analysis. NeuroImage, 125, 1032-1045.

Lejuez, C. W.; Aklin, W. M.; Jones, H. A.; Richards, J. B.; Strong, D. R.; Kahler, C. W. et al. (2003). The balloon analogue risk task (BART) differentiates smokers and nonsmokers. Experimental and Clinical Psychopharmacology, 11(1), 26-33.

Lejuez, C. W.; Read, J. P.; Kahler, C. W.; Richards, J. B.; Ramsey, S. E.; Stuart, G. L. et al. (2002). Evaluation of a behavioral measure of risk taking: the Balloon Analogue Risk Task (BART). Journal of Experimental Psychology: Applied, 8(2), 75-84.

Leonardi, N.; Van De Ville, D. (2015). On spurious and real fluctuations of dynamic functional connectivity during rest. NeuroImage, 104, 430-436.

Luijten, M.; O'Connor, D. A.; Rossiter, S.; Franken, I. H.; Hester, R. (2013). Effects of reward and punishment on brain activations associated with inhibitory control in cigarette smokers. Addiction, 108(11), 1969-1978.

Marshall, D. L.; Redfern, P. H.; Wonnacott, S. (2002). Presynaptic nicotinic modulation of dopamine release in the three ascending pathways studied by in vivo microdialysis: comparison of naive and chronic nicotine-treated rats. Journal of Neurochemistry, 68(4), 1511-1519.

Murphy, K.; Bodurka, J.; Bandettini, P. A. (2007). How long to scan? The relationship between fMRI temporal signal to noise ratio and necessary scan duration. NeuroImage, 34(2), 565-574.

Naqvi, N. H.; Bechara, A. (2009). The hidden island of addiction: the insula. Trends in Neurosciences, 32(1), 56-67.

Naqvi, N. H.; Rudrauf, D.; Damasio, H.; Bechara, A. (2007). Damage to the insula disrupts addiction to cigarette smoking. Science, 315(5811), 531-534.

Ogawa, S.; Lee, T. M.; Kay, A. R.; Tank, D. W. (1990). Brain magnetic resonance imaging with contrast dependent on blood oxygenation. Proceedings of the National Academy of Sciences of the United States of America, 87(24), 9868-9872.

Pariyadath, V.; Stein, E. A.; Ross, T. J. (2014). Machine learning classification of resting state functional connectivity predicts smoking status. Frontiers in Human Neuroscience, 8, 425.

Perry, J. L.; & Carroll, M. E. (2008). The role of impulsive behavior in drug abuse. Psychopharmacology, 200(1), 1-26.

Power, J. D.; Mitra, A.; Laumann, T. O.; Snyder, A. Z.; Schlaggar, B. L.; Petersen, S. E. (2014). Methods to detect, characterize, and remove motion artifact in resting state fMRI. NeuroImage, 84, 320-341.

Rao, H.; Korczykowski, M.; Pluta, J.; Hoang, A.; Detre, J. A. (2008). Neural correlates of voluntary and involuntary risk taking in the human brain: an fMRI study of the Balloon Analog Risk Task (BART). NeuroImage, 42(2), 902-910.

Sakoğlu, ü.; Pearlson, G. D.; Kiehl, K. A.; Wang, Y. M.; Michael, A. M.; Calhoun, V. D. (2010). A method for evaluating dynamic functional network connectivity and task-modulation: application to schizophrenia. Magnetic Resonance Materials in Physics, Biology and Medicine, 23(5-6), 351-366.

Schick, S. F.; Blount, B. C.; Jacob, P. R.; Saliba, N. A.; Bernert, J. T.; El Hellani, A. et al. (2017). Biomarkers of exposure to new and emerging tobacco delivery products. American Journal of Physiology Lung Cellular and Molecular Physiology, 313(3), L425-L452.

Spreng, R. N.; Mar, R. A.; Kim, A. S. (2009). The common neural basis of autobiographical memory, prospection, navigation, theory of mind, and the default mode: a quantitative meta-analysis. Journal of Cognitive Neuroscience, 21(3), 489-510.

Spreng, R. N.; Stevens, W. D.; Chamberlain, J. P.; Gilmore, A. W.; Schacter, D. L. (2010). Default network activity, coupled with the frontoparietal control network, supports goal-directed cognition. NeuroImage, 53(1), 303-317.

Stoeckel, L. E.; Chai, X. J.; Zhang, J.; Whitfield-Gabrieli, S.; Evins, A. E. (2016). Lower gray matter density and functional connectivity in the anterior insula in smokers compared with never smokers. Addiction Biology, 21(4), 972-981.

Sutherland, M. T.; Carroll, A. J.; Salmeron, B. J.; Ross, T. J.; Hong, L. E.; Stein, E. A. (2013). Down-regulation of amygdala and insula functional circuits by varenicline and nicotine in abstinent cigarette smokers. Biological Psychiatry, 74(7), 538-546.

Sutherland, M. T.; McHugh, M. J.; Pariyadath, V.; Stein, E. A. (2012). Resting state functional connectivity in addiction: lessons learned and a road ahead. NeuroImage, 62(4), 2281-2295.

Tanabe, J.; Nyberg, E.; Martin, L. F.; Martin, J.; Cordes, D.; Kronberg, E. et al. (2011). Nicotine effects on default mode network during resting state. Psychopharmacology, 216(2), 287-295.

Thiel, C. M.; Zilles, K.; Fink, G. R. (2005). Nicotine modulates reorienting of visuospatial attention and neural activity in human parietal cortex. Neuropsychopharmacology, 30(4), 810-820.

van den Heuvel, M. P.; Hulshoff Pol, H. E. (2010). Exploring the brain network: a review on resting-state fMRI functional connectivity. European Neuropsychopharmacology, 20(8), 519-534.

Vergara, V. M.; Liu, J.; Claus, E. D.; Hutchison, K.; Calhoun, V. (2017). Alterations of resting state functional network connectivity in the brain of nicotine and alcohol users. NeuroImage, 151, 45-54.

Vergara, V. M.; Mayer, A. R.; Damaraju, E.; Hutchison, K.; Calhoun, V. D. (2017). The effect of preprocessing pipelines in subject classification and detection of abnormal resting state functional network connectivity using group ICA. Neuroimage, 145(Pt B), 365-376.

Vergara, V. M.; Weiland, B. J.; Hutchison, K. E.; Calhoun, V. D. (2018). The impact of combinations of alcohol, nicotine, and cannabis on dynamic brain connectivity. Neuropsychopharmacology, 43(4), 877-890.

Wei, Z.; Yang, N.; Liu, Y.; Yang, L.; Wang, Y.; Han, L. et al. (2016). Resting-state functional connectivity between the dorsal anterior cingulate cortex and thalamus is associated with risky decision-making in nicotine addicts. Scientific Reports, 6, 21778.

Weiland, B. J.; Sabbineni, A.; Calhoun, V. D.; Welsh, R. C.; Hutchison, K. E. (2015). Reduced executive and default network functional connectivity in cigarette smokers. Human Brain Mapping, 36(3), 872-882.

Wilcox, C. E.; Calhoun, V. D.; Rachakonda, S.; Claus, E. D.; Littlewood, R. A.; Mickey, J. et al. (2017). Functional network connectivity predicts treatment outcome during treatment of nicotine use disorder. Psychiatry Research, 265, 45-53.

Zalesky, A.; Breakspear, M. (2015). Towards a statistical test for functional connectivity dynamics. NeuroImage, 114, 466-470.

Zelle, S. L.; Gates, K. M.; Fiez, J. A.; Sayette, M. A.; Wilson, S. J. (2017). The first day is always the hardest: functional connectivity during cue exposure and the ability to resist smoking in the initial hours of a quit attempt. NeuroImage, 151, 24-32.

Zhang, X.; Salmeron, B. J.; Ross, T. J.; Gu, H.; Geng, X.; Yang, Y. et al. (2011). Anatomical differences and network characteristics underlying smoking cue reactivity. NeuroImage, 54(1), 131-141.

16
急性烟碱效应的功能磁共振成像

Christiane M. Thiel

Biological Psychology Lab, Department of Psychology, Department for Medicine and Health Sciences, Carl von Ossietzky University Oldenburg, Oldenburg, Germany

缩略语

BOLD	血氧水平依赖性	PET	正电子发射断层扫描
fMRI	功能磁共振成像		

16.1 引言

神经成像技术，如功能磁共振成像（fMRI）或正电子发射断层扫描（PET），允许研究烟碱对人类的影响背后的神经生物学机制。fMRI于1991年引入，通过所谓的血氧水平依赖性（BOLD）对比来测量大脑活动，该对比利用了含氧和脱氧血液的不同磁性（Belliveau et al. 1991）。尽管这是一种依赖于神经血管耦合的神经元活动的间接测量方法，但它与神经元的局部场电位密切相关（Logothetis, 2008）。用这种方法研究药物在人类大脑中的作用的研究被归入"药理学fMRI"或"药学fMRI"。然而，也有不同的药理学fMRI方法需要区分。大多数药理学fMRI研究了给药结合认知、感觉或运动任务的作用。参与者或患者在接受常规fMRI研究之前，会被给予药物或安慰剂。这种方法能够研究大脑的哪些区域或者网络会对任务做出反应，以及它们是如何被药物调节的。例如，人们可以分析在注意力任务中烟碱的作用下，哪些大脑区域的活动增加或减少。需要注意的是，通过这种方法识别出的大脑区域不一定与那些受体密度高的区域对应。显示药物引起的调节的区域与任务相关的活动在很大程度上取决于所使用的范式。例如，如果受试者执行运动任务，烟碱可能会影响运动皮层内的BOLD的活跃程度，但如果执行工作记忆任务，则是在前额叶皮质层。

最近，越来越多的fMRI研究已经研究了烟碱对所谓的静止状态网络的影响。在这种方法中，参与者或患者在fMRI检查前接受药物治疗。与基于任务的功能磁共振成像不同的是，静止状态研究测量的是当受试者在休息时的大脑活动，也就是说，睁着眼睛或闭着眼睛，在功能磁共振成像中什么都没有。在这样的休息期间，BOLD信号显示低频（<0.1Hz）自发性波动在大脑分布区域中表现出强烈的时间相干性（Buckner, Vincent, 2007; Greicius, 2008; Lu, Stein, 2014）。几个静止状态网络已经被分离出来，它们与任务诱导的激活和失活以及结构连接相一致（Beckmann et al. 2005）。三种网络经常被报道与烟碱的作用有关，是默认模式网络，其中包括内侧前额叶皮层、后扣带皮层和海马旁回，通常在任务执行过程中失效；前额叶背外侧和后顶叶外侧有节点的执行控制网络；突出网络由背侧前扣带回和额岛叶皮层组成。

另一种不太常见的方法尝试衡量药物诱导的BOLD活动的变化，考虑药代动力学参数而不是基于任务的参数（Bloom et al. 1999）。因为烟碱表现出快速起效和抵消效应，这种药代动力学方法是可行的。利用这种方法，Stein等（1998）的研究表明烟碱可诱导大脑边缘区域的BOLD活动的剂量依赖性增加。药代动力学方法和进一步的进展可能对药物开发具有特殊的意义（Black, Koller, Miller, 2013）。

在本章中，我们将总结在非吸烟者或吸烟者中使用安慰剂控制的急性烟碱应用的任务型和静止状态功能磁共振成像研究的主要发现。主要关注奖励相关过程和烟碱依赖的功能磁共振成像研究的结果，这在其他地方进行了回顾，不会详细说明（Fedota, Stein, 2015; Sutherland, Stein, 2018）。在fMRI研究中，烟碱或烟碱化合物被用于治疗精神疾病中的功能失调的神经回路，如精神分裂症，也没有得到解决（Smucny, Tregellas, 2017）。

16.2 基于任务的fMRI研究

急性烟碱给药对非吸烟者或最低限度剥夺吸烟者的精细运动能力、警觉性、注意力定向、短期情景记忆和工作记忆有有益的行为影响（Heishman, Kleykamp, Singleton, 2010）。因此，大多数基于任务的fMRI研究的目的是识别急性烟碱效应与注意力和记忆力相关的神经关联。下面我们将重点讨论这些问题；Newhouse、Potter、Dumas和Thiel（2011）对神经烟碱对认知功能的影响进行了更广泛的综述。

关于烟碱影响的首批fMRI研究之一是由Lawrence、Ross和Stein（2002）进行的，其专注于持续的注意力。非剥夺吸烟者在进入核磁共振检查前2h前接受了21mg烟碱或安慰剂贴片。在MRI中，他们执行了一个快速的视觉信息处理和控制任务，同时测量了大脑活动。主要的发现是，在持续注意力任务中，烟碱增加了几个注意力相关区域的神经活动，包括顶叶和枕叶皮层、丘脑和尾状核。然而，在行为上，烟碱只有在第二次实验中才会改善任务表现。在随后的一项研究中，同一组研究了在服用21mg烟碱或安慰剂贴片的情况下，轻度剥夺吸烟者在一项提示目标检测任务中的视觉空间注意定向（Hahn et al. 2007）。当受试者将注意力转向一个可能即将到来的目标时，数据分析集中在提示期的BOLD活动。结果显示，包括前扣带皮层和后扣带皮层、左角回、左前中额回和双边楔叶等多个大脑区域失活。这些大脑区域是所谓的默认模式网络的一部分，在任务执行过程中表现出失活，通常与任务积极网络的活动增加有关（Fox et al. 2005）。这一解释得到了一项发现的支持，即失活的增加与烟碱作用下的工作表现改善有关。在烟碱的作用下，默认模式网络中增加的失活部分以类似的方法重现，但略有不同的范式，利用了基于特征的选择性视觉注意、分散注意和简单的目标检测（Hahn et al. 2009）。第二个发现是，独立于任务条件，烟碱会减少额叶、颞叶、丘脑和视觉区域的神经活动。这个结果与上述报道中发现的与注意力相关的大脑区域的BOLD活动增加的结果形成对比（Lawrence et al. 2002）。由于使用了同样的受试者人群和烟碱给药模式，作者认为神经烟碱效应的方向性可能取决于任务要求。与注意力相关的大脑区域的神经活动的增加可能主要发生在需要最大处理能力的快速刺激呈现的任务中。

到目前为止，研究调查了烟碱对吸烟者的影响。对吸烟者的研究的一个局限性是烟碱作用下神经活动的变化可能反映了戒断效应的逆转，尽管上述研究试图通过将戒断时间减少到2～3h来减少这种影响。第二个局限性是有证据表明吸烟者的大脑结构和功能发生了变化，如前额叶灰质受损，这可能扰乱对烟碱的反应（Fritz et al. 2014; Zhang et al. 2011）。对非吸烟者的烟碱影响的测试避免了这些混淆。

我们实验室研究了烟碱对非吸烟者的神经影响。一些研究集中在视觉空间注意的定向和重定向。受试者在进入MRI前咀嚼2mg烟碱或安慰剂口香糖30min，他们进行了具有有效和无效提示目标的目标检测任务（Thiel, Fink, 2008; Thiel, Zilles, Fink, 2005; Vossel, Thiel, Fink, 2008）。数据分析侧重于比较在烟碱和安慰剂的有效提示试验中的无效神经活动。所有这些研究的主要发现是，烟碱会降低与注意力相关的大脑区域的神经活动，包括右顶叶皮层（右角回和右楔前叶）、颞中回和额中回。在行为上，烟碱通过减少反应时间来改善注意力的重新定向，尽管烟碱的行为影响很小，特别是在线索有效性低的情况下。在非吸烟者中，在使用0.5mg烟碱鼻喷剂（Rusted, Ruest, Gray, 2011）后的前瞻性记忆试验中，也发现下顶叶皮层的BOLD活动减少。因此，在非吸烟者和Hahn等（2009）观察到的与注意力相关的大脑区域中，烟碱引起的神经活动减少的影响似乎与吸烟状况和药物使用模式无关。

Smucny等（2015）对不吸烟者使用7mg烟碱或安慰剂贴片研究了烟碱对听觉注意的影响。这个任务是一个持续的注意力任务听觉刺激的呈现。另外还有两个因素被操纵：任务难度和注意力分散。独立于任务条件，烟碱增加了BOLD运动和躯体感觉皮层的活动（见Wylie et al. 2013；因为在敲击手指时，这些区域没有烟碱的影响）。根据任务条件的不同，在前扣带皮层、海马体和下顶叶皮层中都发现了烟碱引起的BOLD活动的增加和减少。在前扣带皮层和顶叶皮层，在没有分心的最简单条件下，BOLD反应的增幅最大。Hahn等（2009）认为，如果刺激被快速呈现并需要最大的处理能力，那么烟碱作用下与注意力相关的大脑区域的BOLD信号会增加。

Warbrick等（2011）研究了通过鼻喷雾剂给予1mg烟碱后，BOLD信号的增减与行为益处的关系。他们研究了一组最低限度剥夺吸烟者和不吸烟者的混合视觉古怪任务。虽然烟碱会导致大脑不同区域的神经活动的整体增加，但存在很大的个体差异，一些受试者的BOLD活动有所增加，而另一些受试者则减少。额叶、顶叶和枕脑区域BOLD活动的减少与反应时间和反应时间可变性的降低有关，这可能表明神经活动的减少是有益的行为表现。然而，存在一个悬而未决的问题：为什么神经活动的减少会有利于表现？Thiel和Fink（2008）测试了一个关于选择性注意的益处的建议。该假说认为，与注意力相关的活动减少可能反映了在无效提示试验中注意力重新定位需求的减少，因为烟碱可能减少了对线索提供的自上而下信息的依赖（Yu, Dayan, 2005）。然而，神经数据不能提供任何证据证明烟碱对自上而下信息的依赖性降低。

与注意力相关的大脑区域在很大程度上与在工作记忆过程中被招募的大脑区域重叠（Mayer et al. 2007）。因此，我们可以期待类似的烟碱引起的工作记忆任务的变化。然而，烟碱对工作记忆的影响的研究很少。Kumari等（2003）使用视觉n-back任务对不吸烟者进行了皮下注射12μg/kg烟碱或相应安慰剂的测试。烟碱改善了任务表现，增加了前扣带皮层、额叶上皮层和上顶叶皮层的BOLD活动，这与吸烟者在烟碱的作用下执行持续的注意力任务的结果相似（Lawrence et al. 2002）。一项新的研究测试了吸烟者在烟碱作用下的工作记忆，没有任何证据表明烟碱引起的变化大脑活动（Sutherland, et al. 2011）。因此，工作记忆和注意力共享的共同神经网络是否同样受到烟碱的调节，这一问题仍然悬而未决。

尽管已经发表了一些关于烟碱的药理学功能磁共振成像研究，并且上面已经描述了一些一致的模式，但仍有许多不一致之处。为了汇总不同烟碱神经成像研究的结果，Sutherland等（2015）对所有给予急性烟碱激动剂的安慰剂对照研究进行了基于坐标的激活病灶荟萃分析。尽管这样的分析将会漏掉特定于某些认知任务的烟碱调节，并显示出对那些与研究最多的认知功能相关的大脑区域的偏见，不过，它是查明跨任务共同机制的一种宝贵方法。对吸烟者和非吸烟者进行元分析和各种各样的任务的结果都显示出一种烟碱诱导的BOLD活动增加和减少的普遍模式（图16.1）。下降主要出现在默认模式网络和与注意力相关的右后顶叶皮层中，其他与注意力相关的大脑区域［包括皮层和皮层下（丘脑）区域］大多在烟碱作用下BOLD活动增加。

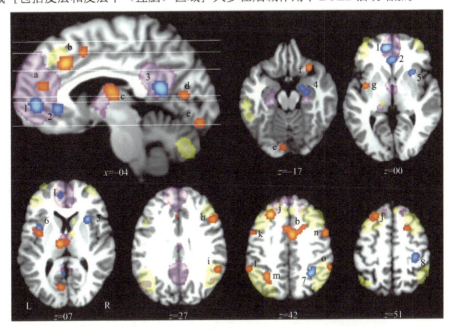

图16.1 给予烟碱乙酰胆碱受体激动剂后活性和失活性的概述

描述了38项研究的估计激活图（ALE元分析），涉及796名参与者（汇集了吸烟者和非吸烟者，包括少数精神分裂症患者的研究）。红色区域表示在药物作用下神经活动增加的区域；蓝色区域表示活动减少。紫色区域描绘了默认模式网络；黄色区域描绘了执行控制网络。活动减少的区域：1+2，前扣带皮层；3，后扣带皮层；4，海马旁回；5+6，脑岛；7，顶叶上叶；8，中央后回/脑岛。活动增加的区域：a，内侧额回；b，前扣带；c，丘脑；d，楔片；e，舌回；f，额下回；g，脑岛；h+j，额中回；i，缘上回；k+n，中央前回；l+o，下顶叶；m，上顶叶。经爱思唯尔授权，Sutherland, M.T., Ray, K.L., Riedel, M.C., Yanes, J.A., Stein, E.A., Laird, A.R. (2015)转载。烟碱乙酰胆碱受体激动剂的神经生物学影响：药理学神经成像研究的激活似然估计荟萃分析。生物精神病学，78（10），711-720。生物精神病学协会版权所有。

16.3 静止状态fMRI研究

在任务执行过程中，BOLD信号的变化受任务触发的神经活动和低频范围内的内源性BOLD信号波动的潜在状态的影响（Buckner, Vincent, 2007）。静止状态网络在理解精神和神经疾病的大规模改变方面受到了越来越多的关注。内源性BOLD信号波动也是在了解药物在系统层面的作用时应考虑的一个重要方面。

Tanabe等（2011）对烟碱影响进行了静止状态、fMRI研究。非吸烟者在进入MRI 90min前接受7mg烟碱或安慰剂贴片。在MRI中，实验对象被要求闭眼休息。fMRI数据分析采用独立成分分析方法来识别静止状态网络。烟碱减少了默认模式网络区域的活动，包括楔前叶、后扣带皮层和额叶内侧皮层。烟碱给药后在纹状体外静止状态网络中观察到了活动的增加。研究人员在服用安慰剂和4mg烟碱口香糖的被剥夺吸烟者（8h）中分析了默认静止状态网络和执行静止状态网络之间的耦合（Cole et al. 2010）。结果显示，网络耦合与戒烟的认知症状之间存在相关性。Hong

等（2009）进行了以扣带皮层为中心的基于兴趣的功能连接分析。温和剥夺烟民根据吸烟习惯接受21mg或35mg烟碱贴剂，然后进行静止状态MRI扫描。烟碱增加了不同扣带皮层与顶叶皮层和额叶皮层的功能连接（图16.2）。但请注意后，两项研究在较长时间的任务型fMRI后进行静止状态扫描，这可能会影响静止状态活动（Breckel et al. 2013）。

烟碱静止状态连接的两个进一步研究选择了基于图论的分析方法（Giessing et al. 2013; Wylie et al. 2012）。与上述的静止状态分析相反，此方法描述了由节点和边缘组成的功能连接的大脑网络的拓扑结构（Bullmore, Sporns, 2009）。大脑区域通常构成节点，而边缘与它们之间的功能交互有关。关于药物效应，拓扑方法允许量化药物是否改变网络拓扑结构，促进或阻碍信息处理（Giessing, Thiel, 2012）。使用这种方法和4mg烟碱口香糖，对轻度剥夺吸烟者进行睁眼静止状态扫描，Giessing等（2013）表明，烟碱倾向于提高整个大脑网络的效率，即整个网络的信息交换程度，显著降低平均聚类，即大脑后部区域的邻居之间的信息交换程度。因此，功能远程连接的数量增加。研究结果表明，大脑网络在烟碱的作用下会发生变化，转向更一体化的网络配置。Wylie等（2012）研究了非吸烟者在静止状态下闭眼服用7mg烟碱（经皮）的情况。这项研究也显示出烟碱作用下全球大脑网络效率的增加趋势，以及与聚类有关的局部效率的提高。需要注意的是，烟碱的作用可能会因在睁眼或闭眼下研究静止状态的活动而有所不同（Ran zi et al. 2016），这可能是这种差异的一种解释。

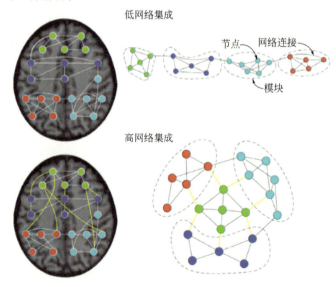

图16.2　烟碱作用后脑功能图整合增强

该图描述了拓扑结构不同的分别具有较低和较高的网络集成的两个图。左边的部分描绘了大脑物理空间内的图形。在烟碱条件下，网络集成增加的特征是串行处理减少和并行信息传输能力提高，即提高了全球脑网络的效率。模块通过更短的路径长度连接，且较少聚集。此外，在烟碱作用下，功能性远距离连接（黄色）的数量也有所增加。节点：大脑中唯一的同质部分，如解剖学上定义的大脑区域；边缘：两个节点之间的功能连接；模块：小的子网。转载自Giessing和Thiel（2012）。

16.4　前景

即使神经成像方法的可用性使我们在过去的几十年里使用这些技术在人脑的水平上来绘制烟碱对人体的影响，我们还远远没有画出一幅令人信服的图片来说明烟碱在休息或工作时调节神经回路的方向的性能。除了不同的药物应用模式外，比较不同研究的主要问题是广泛使用的不同范例和/或数据分析技术。此外，许多早期的药理学fMRI研究使用小受试者数量和宽松的统计阈值，这可能容易出现假阳性和偏倚的叙述审查或基于已发表的激活焦点的元分析。在神经成像领域，数据共享已经成为跨范式和主题的发现的一个重要的方面，药理学fMRI方法可能受益于这些发展（Poldrack, Gorgolewski, 2014）。由于与基于任务的研究相比，静止状态的可变性较小，第一种方法是公开分享原始静止状态烟碱数据，以便进行更大规模的分析。最近的方法为标准化数据采集和分析提供了指导，这是这项工作所需要的（Khalili-Mahani et al. 2017）。汇集不同的研究对象也可以调查烟碱影响的个体间的巨大差异（Newhouse et al. 2004）。

术语解释

- **注意力相关的大脑区域**：当受试者在基于任务的fMRI中执行一项注意力任务时，这些区域通常是活跃的。它们包括顶叶和额叶皮层区域以及皮层下区域，如丘脑。如果在视觉模式中测试注意力，更高的视觉区域也很活跃。
- **BOLD效应**：是与神经活动有关的fMRI研究中获得的信号。它取决于氧和脱氧血红蛋白的相对水平，磁共振成像可以检测到这两种血红蛋白，从而绘制出人类大脑中的神经活动。
- **默认模式网络**：这个网络由一系列大脑区域组成，大部分集中在大脑的中部，当一个人不参与任务，而是在休息或做白日梦时，这些区域就会非常活跃。
- **图论**：是一个允许的数学框架，为对象之间的成对关系建模。它已经被引入神经成像领域来模拟大脑的功能和结构连接。
- **药理学fMRI研究**：药理学fMRI本身不是一种技术；它是所有fMRI研究的总称（如基于任务和静止状态），这些研究包括给药以研究其对神经活动和回路的影响。
- **静止状态fMRI研究**：在这些研究中，受试者被要求睁眼或闭眼，同时测量他们的大脑活动。数据分析了低频自发波动，在空间分离的大脑区域中表现出很强的时间相干性。
- **基于任务的fMRI研究**：在这些研究中，受试者在执行运动、感觉或认知任务时，同时测量他们的大脑活动。数据分析比较了任务执行时的大脑活动和各自的控制条件或任务中不同刺激之间的大脑活动。

fMRI的关键事实

- 追踪人类大脑中无创神经活动的主要技术。
- 自20世纪90年代以来，使用该技术识别认知功能的神经关联的研究数量大幅增加。
- fMRI信号是一种对神经系统活动的间接测量方法，测量出现在细胞活跃的大脑区域的氧合和脱氧血红蛋白的变化的。
- 为了发现信号，各种数据分析步骤都是必要的，包括信号的重建、预处理和统计分析方法。
- 近年来，不同分析和建模方法的数量大量增加。
- 对fMRI数据的分析从分析局部神经活动的变化转变为广泛分布的大脑网络中功能连接的变化。

要点总结

- 本章重点研究烟碱对人脑的急性影响，在认知任务或急性状态下，以测量功能连接的变化。
- 在非吸烟者的几项视觉空间选择性注意任务中，以及在一项针对吸烟者的研究中，发现烟碱导致的大脑顶叶和额叶区域的失活。
- 在持续的视觉注意力和工作记忆任务中，烟碱诱导的激活增加在大脑的顶叶和额叶区域被发现。

- 一项对吸烟者和非吸烟者的烟碱神经成像研究的荟萃分析显示，烟碱下的默认模式网络和后顶叶皮层的神经活动减少，而与注意力相关的大脑区域的神经活动增加。
- 静止状态fMRI研究提供了在烟碱条件下非吸烟者的默认模式网络活动减少的证据。
- 基于图表的静止状态数据分析方法表明，吸烟者和非吸烟者在烟碱作用下的全球网络效率有所提高。

参考文献

Beckmann, C. F.; DeLuca, M.; Devlin, J. T.; Smith, S. M. (2005). Investigations into resting-state connectivity using independent component analysis. Philosophical Transactions of the Royal Society London B Biological Sciences, 360(1457), 1001-1013.

Belliveau, J. W.; Kennedy, D. N.; Jr.; McKinstry, R. C.; Buchbinder, B. R.; Weisskoff, R. M.; Cohen, M. S. et al. (1991). Functional mapping of the human visual cortex by magnetic resonance imaging. Science, 254 (5032), 716-719.

Black, K. J.; Koller, J. M.; Miller, B. D. (2013). Rapid quantitative pharmacodynamic imaging by a novel method: theory, simulation testing and proof of principle. PeerJ, 1. e117.

Bloom, A. S.; Hoffmann, R. G.; Fuller, S. A.; Pankiewicz, J.; Harsch, H. H.; Stein, E. A. (1999). Determination of drug-induced changes in functional MRI signal using a pharmacokinetic model. Human Brain Mapping, 8(4), 235-244.

Breckel, T. P.; Thiel, C. M.; Bullmore, E. T.; Zalesky, A.; Patel, A. X.; Giessing, C. (2013). Long-term effects of attentional performance on functional brain network topology. PLoS ONE, 8(9), e74125.

Buckner, R. L.; Vincent, J. L. (2007). Unrest at rest: default activity and spontaneous network correlations. NeuroImage, 37(4), 1091-1096. discussion 1097-1099.

Bullmore, E.; Sporns, O. (2009). Complex brain networks: graph theoretical analysis of structural and functional systems. Nature Reviews. Neuroscience, 10(3), 186-198.

Cole, D. M.; Beckmann, C. F.; Long, C. J.; Matthews, P. M.; Durcan, M. J.; Beaver, J. D. (2010). Nicotine replacement in abstinent smokers improves cognitive withdrawal symptoms with modulation of resting brain network dynamics. NeuroImage, 52(2), 590-599.

Fedota, J. R.; Stein, E. A. (2015). Resting-state functional connectivity and nicotine addiction: prospects for biomarker development. Annals of the New York Academy of Sciences, 1349, 64-82.

Fox, M. D.; Snyder, A. Z.; Vincent, J. L.; Corbetta, M.; Van Essen, D. C.; Raichle, M. E. (2005). The human brain is intrinsically organized into dynamic, anticorrelated functional networks. Proceedings of the National Academy of Sciences of the United States of America, 102(27), 9673-9678.

Fritz, H. C.; Wittfeld, K.; Schmidt, C. O.; Domin, M.; Grabe, H. J.; Hegenscheid, K. et al. (2014). Current smoking and reduced gray matter volume-a voxel-based morphometry study. Neuropsychopharmacology, 39(11), 2594-2600.

Giessing, C.; Thiel, C. M. (2012). Pro-cognitive drug effects modulate functional brain network organization. Frontiers in Behavioral Neuroscience, 6, 53.

Giessing, C.; Thiel, C. M.; Alexander-Bloch, A. F.; Patel, A. X.; Bullmore, E. T. (2013). Human brain functional network changes associated with enhanced and impaired attentional task performance. The Journal of Neuroscience, 33(14), 5903-5914.

Greicius, M. (2008). Resting-state functional connectivity in neuropsychiatric disorders. Current Opinion in Neurology, 21(4), 424-430.

Hahn, B.; Ross, T. J.; Wolkenberg, F. A.; Shakleya, D. M.; Huestis, M. A.; Stein, E. A. (2009). Performance effects of nicotine during selective attention, divided attention, and simple stimulus detection: an fMRI study. Cerebral Cortex, 19(9), 1990-2000.

Hahn, B.; Ross, T. J.; Yang, Y.; Kim, I.; Huestis, M. A.; Stein, E. A. (2007). Nicotine enhances visuospatial attention by deactivating areas of the resting brain default network. The Journal of Neuroscience, 27(13), 3477-3489.

Heishman, S. J.; Kleykamp, B. A.; Singleton, E. G. (2010). Metaanalysis of the acute effects of nicotine and smoking on human performance. Psychopharmacology, 210(4), 453-469.

Hong, L. E.; Gu, H.; Yang, Y.; Ross, T. J.; Salmeron, B. J.; Buchholz, B. et al. (2009). Association of nicotine addiction and nicotine's actions with separate cingulate cortex functional circuits. Archives of General Psychiatry, 66(4), 431-441.

Khalili-Mahani, N.; Rombouts, S. A.; van Osch, M. J.; Duff, E. P.; Carbonell, F.; Nickerson, L. D. et al. (2017). Biomarkers, designs, and interpretations of resting-state fMRI in translational pharmacological research: a review of state-of-the-art, challenges, and opportunities for studying brain chemistry. Human Brain Mapping, 38(4), 2276-2325.

Kumari, V.; Gray, J. A.; ffytche, D. H.; Mitterschiffthaler, M. T.; Das, M.; Zachariah, E. et al. (2003). Cognitive effects of nicotine in humans: an fMRI study. NeuroImage, 19(3), 1002-1013.

Lawrence, N. S.; Ross, T. J.; Stein, E. A. (2002). Cognitive mechanisms of nicotine on visual attention. Neuron, 36(3), 539-548.

Logothetis, N. K. (2008). What we can do and what we cannot do with fMRI. Nature, 453(7197), 869-878.

Lu, H.; Stein, E. A. (2014). Resting state functional connectivity: its physiological basis and application in neuropharmacology. Neuropharmacology, 84, 79-89.

Mayer, J. S.; Bittner, R. A.; Nikolic, D.; Bledowski, C.; Goebel, R.; Linden, D. E. (2007). Common neural substrates for visual working memory and attention. NeuroImage, 36(2), 441-453.

Newhouse, P. A.; Potter, A. S.; Dumas, J. A.; Thiel, C. M. (2011). Functional brain imaging of nicotinic effects on higher cognitive processes. Biochemical Pharmacology, 82(8), 943-951.

Newhouse, P. A.; Potter, A.; Singh, A. (2004). Effects of nicotinic stimulation on cognitive performance. Current Opinion in Pharmacology, 4(1), 36-46.

Poldrack, R. A.; Gorgolewski, K. J. (2014). Making big data open: data sharing in neuroimaging. Nature Neuroscience, 17(11), 1510-1517.

Ranzi, P.; Thiel, C. M.; Herrmann, C. S. (2016). EEG source reconstruction in male nonsmokers after nicotine administration during the resting state. Neuropsychobiology, 73(4), 191-200.

Rusted, J.; Ruest, T.; Gray, M. A. (2011). Acute effects of nicotine administration during prospective memory, an event related fMRI study. Neuropsychologia, 49(9), 2362-2368.

Smucny, J.; Olincy, A.; Eichman, L. S.; Tregellas, J. R. (2015). Neuronal effects of nicotine during auditory selective attention. Psychopharmacology, 232(11), 2017-2028.

Smucny, J.; Tregellas, J. R. (2017). Targeting neuronal dysfunction in schizophrenia with nicotine: evidence from neurophysiology to neuroimaging. Journal of Psychopharmacology, 31(7), 801-811.

Stein, E. A.; Pankiewicz, J.; Harsch, H. H.; Cho, J. K.; Fuller, S. A.; Hoffmann, R. G. et al. (1998). Nicotine-induced limbic cortical activation in the human brain: a functional MRI study. The American Journal of Psychiatry, 155(8), 1009-1015.

Sutherland, M. T.; Ray, K. L.; Riedel, M. C.; Yanes, J. A.; Stein, E. A.; Laird, A. R. (2015). Neurobiological impact of nicotinic acetylcholine receptor agonists: an activation likelihood estimation meta-analysis of pharmacologic neuroimaging studies. Biological Psychiatry, 78(10), 711-720.

Sutherland, M. T.; Ross, T. J.; Shakleya, D. M.; Huestis, M. A.; Stein, E. A. (2011). Chronic smoking, but not acute nicotine administration, modulates neural correlates of working memory. Psychopharmacology, 213(1), 29-42.

Sutherland, M. T.; Stein, E. A. (2018). Functional neurocircuits and neuroimaging biomarkers of tobacco use disorder. Trends in Molecular Medicine, 24(2), 129-143.

Tanabe, J.; Nyberg, E.; Martin, L. F.; Martin, J.; Cordes, D.; Kronberg, E. et al. (2011). Nicotine effects on default mode network during resting state. Psychopharmacology.

Thiel, C. M.; Fink, G. R. (2008). Effects of the cholinergic agonist nicotine on reorienting of visual spatial attention and top-down attentional control. Neuroscience, 152(2), 381-390.

Thiel, C. M.; Zilles, K.; Fink, G. R. (2005). Nicotine modulates reorienting of visuospatial attention and neural activity in human parietal cortex. Neuropsychopharmacology, 30(4), 810-820.

Vossel, S.; Thiel, C. M.; Fink, G. R. (2008). Behavioral and neural effects of nicotine on visuospatial attentional reorienting in non-smoking subjects. Neuropsychopharmacology, 33(4), 731-738.

Warbrick, T.; Mobascher, A.; Brinkmeyer, J.; Musso, F.; Stoecker, T.; Shah, N. J. et al. (2011). Direction and magnitude of nicotine effects on the fMRI BOLD response are related to nicotine effects on behavioral performance. Psychopharmacology (Berl), 215(2), 333-344.

Wylie, K. P.; Rojas, D. C.; Tanabe, J.; Martin, L. F.; Tregellas, J. R. (2012). Nicotine increases brain functional network efficiency. NeuroImage, 63(1), 73-80.

Wylie, K. P.; Tanabe, J.; Martin, L. F.; Wongngamnit, N.; Tregellas, J. R. (2013). Nicotine increases cerebellar activity during finger tapping. PLoS ONE, 8(12), e84581.

Yu, A. J.; Dayan, P. (2005). Uncertainty, neuromodulation, and attention. Neuron, 46(4), 681-692.

Zhang, X.; Salmeron, B. J.; Ross, T. J.; Geng, X.; Yang, Y.; Stein, E. A. (2011). Factors underlying prefrontal and insula structural alterations in smokers. NeuroImage, 54(1), 42-48.

17
精神分裂症中的烟碱依赖：烟碱乙酰胆碱受体的贡献

Robert D. Cole, Vinay Parikh

Department of Psychology and Neuroscience Program, Temple University, Philadelphia, PA, United States

缩略语

DA 多巴胺   **PFC** 前额叶皮层
nAChR 烟碱乙酰胆碱受体

17.1 引言

烟碱是烟草中发现的精神活性成分，尽管它对健康造成了毁灭性的影响，但它仍是世界上滥用最广泛的药物之一。"健康"人口烟碱消费率在20%～35%，但据报道，患有精神分裂症（一种使人衰弱的慢性精神疾病）的人口的发生率是健康人口的3～4倍。患有精神分裂症的吸烟者不仅吸烟更多，而且可以从每支卷烟中提取更多的烟碱。此外，与没有精神分裂症的吸烟者相比，精神分裂症患者在戒断期间经历了更强的强化作用和更严重的戒断症状。因此，精神分裂症患者更容易发展为烟碱依赖，且他们的戒烟仍然非常具有挑战性。

烟碱依赖也被发现与精神分裂症患者的症状的严重程度和不良的结果有关。此外，大量吸烟的这些人非常容易患上各种疾病，如心血管疾病和肺部疾病，从而导致过早死亡。因此，对精神分裂症患者同时使用烟碱的神经生物学机制的基础理解，对于制订治疗策略以改善精神分裂患者的戒烟、治疗结果和寿命至关重要。本章的重点是在神经基础上，即改变神经元烟碱乙酰胆碱受体（nAChR）的功能可能导致精神分裂症的烟碱依赖。被诊断患有精神分裂症的人表现出积极（幻觉、妄想和思维障碍）、消极（情绪表达减少、动机丧失和社会心理障碍）和认知（思维混乱、注意力和工作记忆缺陷以及执行力功能障碍）的症状。支持这些症状和nAChR功能障碍之间联系的经验证据将被回顾。最后，本章将深入探究将nAChR靶向治疗作为探讨精神分裂症的临床症状及改善其戒烟效果的新方法。

17.2 nAChR药理学

烟碱主要通过与遍布整个中枢神经系统的nAChR结合而发挥其行为和神经调节作用。nAChR是一个配体门控的离子性受体家族，通过改变阳离子通道电流来介导快速突触传递。这些受体属于内源性神经递质ACh激活的两类胆碱能受体之一。乙酰胆碱刺激的其他类型的胆碱能受体是毒蕈碱受体，即G蛋白偶联受体。

神经元nAChR是五聚体结构，由五种跨膜单位组合而成，包括九种α亚基（α2～α10）和三种β亚基（β2～β4），其排列为异构体组装或同构体组装（Gotti et al. 2009）。在哺乳动物的大脑中，同质α7和异质α4β2是最占优势和分布最广泛的nAChRs。对烟碱具有更高亲和力的α4β2 nAChR已被证明在持续使用烟碱的情况下会脱敏和上调（Marks, Grady, Collins, 1993）。另一方面，α7 nAChR具有更快的受体动力学和增强的Ca^{2+}渗透性，但对烟碱的亲和力较低（Castro, Albuquerque, 1995）。由于较高的Ca^{2+}渗透性，α7 nAChR被认为可以促进下游信号通路，如作为细胞外信号调节酶和cAMP反应元件结合蛋白（Bitner et al. 2007）。nAChRs定位于突触前和突触后两个部位。突触前nAChR既存在于自身受体，也存在于异质受体，已知它可以直接或与其他共存的受体在末端相互作用调节多种神经递质的释放，包括多巴胺（DA）和谷氨酸（Parikh, Ji, Decker, Sarter, 2010; Wonnacott, 1997）。涉及α4β2和α7 nAChR的基因和药物操作的动物研究表明，这些受体参与了特定的行为过程，如烟碱的强化和奖励效应（Dani, De Biasi, 2001）、情绪与焦虑（Picciotto et al. 2015）和认知（Guillem et al. 2011; Young et al. 2007）。现在开始的持续研究发现了包含三元亚基复合体的其他nAChR的作用，如α3β4α5和α4β2α5，以及它们对特定神经生理和行为过程的贡献。

17.3 精神分裂症中nAChR的表达

伴随着与精神分裂症相关的无数神经递质功能障碍，神经元nAChR表达的改变已经通过各种死后成像和基因图谱研究被揭示。精神分裂症患者的脑解剖评估显示，与健康对照组相比，病人在多个大脑区域的α7 nAChR的表达降低（Court et al. 1999; Freedman et al. 1995; Guan et al. 1999）。然而，在精神分裂症吸烟者和健康吸烟者之间未观察到α7 nAChR mRNA和蛋白质水平的差异，这提示烟碱的使用可能改善了这些受体在精神分裂症中的异常翻译后修饰或转运（Mexal et al. 2010）。

受体放射自显影研究表明，精神分裂症吸烟者大脑中高亲和力的α4β2 nAChR没有上调，这在正常吸烟者中很常见（Breese et al. 2000; Durany et al. 2000）。另外，使用正电子发射断层扫描的人类神经成像研究也显示，与正常吸烟者相比，精神分裂症吸烟者的β2* nAChR可用性降低（Brasic et al. 2012; D'Souza et al. 2012），但与不吸烟的精神分裂症患者相比，其上调水平更高（Esterlis et al. 2014）。这些发现表明，在精神分裂症患者中，α4β2 nAChR的脱敏或转换是不正常的。

遗传研究中积累的证据表明，精神分裂症和nAChR亚基基因之间存在联系，这可能解释了nAChR表达和功能的改变。在精神分裂症患者中，位于15号染色体（15q13—14）上的α7（*CHRNA7*）亚基的基因多态性已被报道（Freedman et al. 2001）。此外，在精神分裂症患者的背外侧前额叶皮层（PFC）中发现了嵌合基因α7 nAChR（*CHRFAM7A*）的过表达，该基因被认为是α7 nAChR功能的显性负调控因子（Kunii et al. 2015）。α4和β2亚基与精神分裂症之间的遗传相互作用也有报道，精神分裂症与α4β2 nAChR之间可能存在联系（De Luca et al. 2006; Voineskos et al. 2007）。此外，有新的证据表明，在15号染色体上编码α3、α5和β4亚基的*CHRNA5/A3/B4*基因簇中的变异可能与吸烟行为有关（Lassi et al. 2016）。总之，这些研究表明，精神分裂症患者的nAChR失调，这些受试者吸烟的高发生率可能代表着其试图恢复nAChR功能。表17.1提供了评估吸烟和非吸烟精神分裂症患者nAChR密度的临床研究总结。

表17.1 精神分裂症患者吸烟和不吸烟人群中nAChR密度的研究

nAChRs	技术	比较	脑区	影响	参考文献
α7 nAChR	放射自显影术	SZ与正常	海马体、丘脑和前额叶皮层	减少了α7 nAChR密度	Freedman et al.（1995） Court et al.（1999） Guan et al.（1999）
	荧光原位杂交法	SZ与正常	背外侧前额叶皮层	嵌合基因α7 nAChR（CHRFAM7A）的过表达	Kunii et al.（2015）
	蛋白免疫印迹法	SZ与正常	背外侧前额叶皮层	减少了α7 nAChR蛋白的表达	Mexal et al.（2010）
α4β2 nAChR	放射自显影术	SZ吸烟者与正常吸烟者	皮层、纹状体和海马体	降低了α4β2 nAChR密度	Breese et al.（2000） Durany et al.（2000）
	正电子发射断层扫描	SZ吸烟者与正常吸烟者	额叶皮层、顶叶皮层和丘脑	降低了β2 nAChR的可用性	Brasic et al.（2012） D'Souza et al.（2012）
	正电子发射断层扫描	SZ吸烟者与SZ不吸烟者	额叶皮层，顶叶皮层和纹状体	β2 nAChR上调	Esterlis et al.（2014）

注：1. SZ表示精神分裂症。
2. 改编自Parikh et al.（2016）。

17.4 nAChRs和精神分裂症的阳性症状

据报道，少量的烟碱摄入可降低精神分裂症患者的阳性症状（精神病）评分（Aguilar et al. 2005）。此外，*CHRFAM7A*和*CHRNA7*的较高比率被认为与精神分裂症临床诊断之前烟碱依赖的发展和精神病症状本身有关（Kunii et al. 2015）。过量的*CHRFAM7A*表达通过减少阳离子通道功能破坏突触前和突触后隔室的α7 nAChR信号，因此可能导致阳性症状。虽然高亲和性nAChR α4β2*与精神分裂症的发展没有直接关系，β2* nAChR mRNA转录在经历精神病症状的双相情感障碍患者中发生改变（Severance, Yolken, 2007）。另一方面，有研究发现精神分裂症患者的阳性症状没有变化（Patkar et al. 2002），或这些症状的强度随吸烟而增加（Ziedonis et al. 1994）。这样，因此，关于nAChR在调节精神分裂症阳性症状方面的确切作用的证据尚不明确，还需在这个方面进行更多的研究。

17.5 精神分裂症的烟碱和认知：nAChRs的神经调节

认知缺陷被认为是精神分裂症的一个中心特征。与正常受试者相比，精神分裂症患者的感觉门控减少，这种效应被发现与*CHRNA7*基因的多态性有关（Freedman et al. 2001）。感觉门控的缺陷会导致更高的认知过程的中断，如注意力和工作记忆。在α7 nAChR基因纯合子缺失的小鼠中进行的动物研究报道了在认识任务中的障碍，包括五选择连续反应时间的任务和与延时不匹配的样本任务（Fernandes et al. 2006; Young et al. 2007）。此外，急性全身给药SSR180711（一种α7 nAChR部分激动剂），改善了新生大鼠海马体腹侧损伤模型的注意移位，再现了精神分裂症的许多发展方面（Brooks et al. 2012）。精神分裂症吸烟者表现出P50感觉门控功能明显改善（Adler, Hoffer, Wiser, Freedman, 1993）。此外，吸烟的精神分裂症患者在持续、选择性注意和工作记忆任务上的表现优于非吸烟者（Segarra et al. 2011）。总的来说，这些研究结果表明，α7 nAChR信号的干扰可能解释了精神分裂症患者的认知缺陷，精神分裂症患者较高烟碱的使用可能代表了通过保持低亲和力的nAChR激活来使认知缺陷正常化的一种尝试。虽然缺乏直接的临床证据支持α4β2 nAChR参与精神分裂症的认知症状，但推测吸烟诱导的这些高亲和力nAChR的激活可以改善精神分裂症受试者的注意力。在此背景下，利用β2 nAChR亚基基因缺失的小鼠进行的动物研究报道了在注意力处理和冲突解决方面的不足（Granon, Faure, Changeux, 2003; Guillem et al. 2011）。

DA缺失和PFC中通过D_1受体传递的信号传导中断都与精神分裂症患者的认知缺陷有关（Goldman-Rakic, Castner, Svensson, Siever, Williams, 2004）。含有α7和β2亚基的nAChRs均存在于前额叶多巴胺能末端，并调节DA的释放（Livingstone et al. 2009）。此外，nAChRs在中脑DA神经元的细胞体上也有表达，并可能通过调节这些神经元的放电速率来影响DA的释放。因此，吸烟或摄入烟碱可能通过激活α7 nAChR和α4β2* nAChR，并使PFC中DA的传输正常化，从而部分缓解精神分裂症的认知症状。

有令人信服的证据表明nAChR也调节突触谷氨酸信号的传导。投射到PFC的V层锥体神经元的丘脑皮层谷氨酸能传入神经具有功能性的含β2*亚基的nAChRs。此外，在缺乏β2 nAChR的小鼠局部应用烟碱后，PFC中的谷氨酸释放和自发兴奋性突触后电流被消除（Lambe et al. 2003; Parikh et al. 2010）。这些研究表明，α4β2 nAChRs调节丘脑皮层谷氨酸能传递，这对注意处理至关重要。Andre和他的同事们（Andre, Leach, Gould, 2011）发现，NMDA受体拮抗剂MK-801诱导的恐惧条件反射缺陷被烟碱改善，这种作用是由海马体中含有β2*亚基的nAChR介导的。这份报告提供了明确的证据，表明烟碱对海马依赖记忆的有益认知作用涉及通过α4β2 nAChRs促进突触后NMDA介导的谷氨酸信号传导。α7 nAChR的激活也被证明对前额叶网络中的突触后NMDA受体的兴奋至关重要（Yang et al. 2013）。此外，NMDA谷氨酸受体介导的信号通路的畸变也被认为是导致精神分裂症认知症状的潜在机制之一（Moghaddam, Javitt, 2012）。因此，与nAChR激活相关的前额叶谷氨酸信号通路的增强可能会纠正精神分裂症患者的注意缺陷。

DA和谷氨酸神经递质系统相互作用，促进PFC的突触可塑性。特别是D_1受体的激活通过细胞内Ca^{2+}和蛋白激酶A促进NMDA反应，这两种受体之间的协同作用对正常的皮质锥体细胞兴奋性和PFC功能至关重要（Tseng, O'Donnell, 2004）。如上所述，nAChR的药理拮抗作用扰乱了依赖于PFC的认知功能。因此，烟碱或特异性的α4β2/α7 nAChR激动剂刺激前额叶nAChR，可使DA-谷氨酸释放正常化，恢复D1/NMDA受体信号转导和协同作用，从而改善精神分裂症患者的部分认知障碍（Parikh, Kutlu, Gould, 2016）。图17.1显示了一个假设模型，该模型说明了nAChR介导的PFC中DA-谷氨酸串扰促进如何微调精神分裂症患者的认知功能。

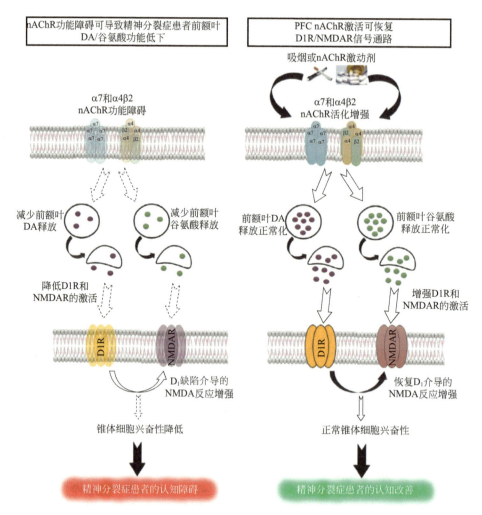

图 17.1 前额叶 nAChR 在精神分裂症认知缺陷中的作用

（左）精神分裂症患者的 nAChR 功能障碍导致 DNA 和 PFC 中谷氨酸释放的缺乏，导致 D1 和 NMDA 受体信号传导减少。D_1 和 NMDA 受体之间的协同作用减弱会破坏 PFC 兴奋性和认知功能。（右）吸烟（烟碱）或激活 α4β2 和/或 α7 nAChR 增加 PFC 中 DA/谷氨酸的释放，并恢复两者之间的协同作用。DA 和谷氨酸信号使 PFC 功能正常化并改善精神分裂症患者的认知。

17.6 nAChRs 对精神分裂症的阴性症状的贡献

精神分裂症的阴性症状包括缺乏追求目标的动力、快感缺乏、社会交往戒断和对情感刺激的情绪反应减少，这些都预示着精神分裂症患者的吸烟行为（Patkar et al. 2002）。奖励处理缺陷被认为是导致精神分裂症阴性症状的表现之一。此外，已知 α4β2 nAChR 可调节奖励动机行为，并在精神分裂症患者中发现 *CHRNA4* 基因多态性与重度吸烟之间存在显著关联（Voineskos et al. 2007）。最近的核成像研究中使用了一种名为 β2 nAChR 的激动剂示踪剂 [^{123}I]5-IA-85380，与正常吸烟者相比，精神分裂症吸烟者的 α4β2 nAChR 可用性较低，而且受体可用性和阴性症状之间呈负相关（D'Souza et al. 2007; Esterlis et al. 2014）。因此，精神分裂症患者体内的高烟碱强化作用可能与 α4β2 nAChR 功能障碍引起的阴性症状有关。α7 nAChR 突变小鼠获得自然奖励的动机不受影响（Young et al. 2007）。此外，给药时使用 α7 激动剂或 α7 nAChR 亚基缺失均不影烟碱的奖励和强化（Grottick et al. 2000; Pons et al. 2008）。然而，在具有精神分裂症特征的转基因小鼠模型中使用 TC-5619（α7 nAChR 全激动剂）改善了这些动物的社会行为（Hauser et al. 2009）。基于现有的证据，α7 nAChR 的中断似乎不会改变精神分裂症患者的奖励敏感性，它们与阴性症状的联系可能与奖励处理缺陷无关。

17.7 nAChR 调节作为精神分裂症的可能治疗方法

虽然烟碱可以缓解精神分裂症患者的症状，但高成瘾特性和长期治疗后的耐受性的发展限制了其作为候选药物的使用。大量证据表明，α7 nAChR 可作为精神分裂症的治疗靶点，一些 α7 nAChR 配体已经在临床研究中。涉及用部分 α7 nAChR 激动剂 GTS-21 治疗精神分裂症的 II 期临床试验显示，精神分裂症患者 P50 感觉门控功能、注意力、工作记忆和阴性症状得到改善（Olincy, Freedman, 2012）。在精神分裂症患者中，使用选择性 α7 nAChR 部分激动剂如 Encenicline 和托烷司琼进行的临床研究，报告了对各认知指标的积极作用（Noroozian et al. 2013; Preskorn et al. 2014）。此外，α7 nAChR 全激动剂 TC-5619 也被发现对精神分裂症吸烟者的工作记忆表现有有益的影响（Lieberman et al. 2013）。

研究 α7 nAChR 的正变构调节剂（PAMs）是控制精神分裂症认知症状的新途径。PAMs 的作用是独特的，因为它们优先结合到受体的变构位点，使内源性配体位点开放。PAMs 也能增强内源性配体的作用，而不直接激活受体信号通路。使用这种方法的一个关键优势是，α7 nAChR 调节不仅可以放大 α7 nAChR 激活产生的行为/认知效应，而且还可以防止对这些受体脱敏可能发生的这些效应的耐受性。在这方面，加兰他敏，一种胆碱酯酶抑制剂，也是一种 α7 nAChR PAM，已在精神分裂症患者中显示出神经认知功能的改善（Buchanan et al. 2008）。

伐伦克林是一种 α4β2 nAChR 部分激动剂，作为抗精神病的辅助治疗药物，在威斯康星卡分类测试和数字符号替代测试中显著改善了精神分裂症吸烟者的认知表现（Shim et al. 2012）另一项临床研究报道，伐伦克林维持治疗增加了精神分裂症患者的戒烟率（Evins et al. 2014）。此外，情感扁平化基线症状较低的精神分裂症患者更有可能实现戒烟，并在伐伦克林治疗期间表现出更大的奖励敏感性增加（Dutra, Stoeckel, Carlini, Pizzagalli, Evins, 2012）。根据现有的证据，似乎 α7 和 α4β2 nAChR 配体都有希望成为精神分裂症阴性和认知症状的潜在的治疗靶点。此外，α4β2 nAChRs 为靶点可能也有利于减少精神分裂症患者的吸烟复发。表 17.2 描述了 nAChR 调节剂在精神分裂症患者中的临床试验结果。最近的全基因组关联研究表明，编码 α5 nAChR 亚基的人类 *CHRNA5* 基因的多态性会增加吸烟和精神分裂症的风险。此外，具有 α5 nAChR 基因单核苷酸多态性的小鼠表现出 PFC 依赖的行为缺陷，而慢性烟碱则逆转了这些动物的低额状态（Koukouli et al. 2017）。准确定位 α5 nAChR 能否提高已知与 PFC 功能障碍相关的精神分裂症认知症状和改善精神分裂症患者的烟碱依赖仍有待观察。

表17.2　nAChR 配体对精神分裂症患者认知、阴性症状及吸烟的影响的临床研究

nAChR 配体	特异性	临床阶段	神经行为的影响
GTS-21	α7 nAChR 部分激动剂	II 期临床试验	改善 P50 感觉门控功能、注意力、工作记忆和阴性症状
Encenicline	α7 nAChR 部分激动剂	II 期临床试验	对错配负性、P300 电位、视觉注意、非语言工作记忆和决策有积极作用
托烷司琼	α7 nAChR 部分激动剂	II 期临床试验	改善听觉感觉门控和注意力

续表

nAChR配体	特异性	临床阶段	神经行为的影响
TC-5619	α7 nAChR 全激动剂	探索性试验	增强工作记忆性能
加兰他敏	α7 nAChR PAM	Ⅲ期临床试验	提高注意力和记忆力
伐伦克林	α7 nAChR 部分激动剂	Ⅲ期临床试验	提高认知灵活性、视觉空间工作记忆表现，增加戒烟率，增加奖励敏感性，减少阴性症状

注：改编自 Parikh et al.（2016）。

17.8 结论

精神分裂症患者吸烟的比例远远高于正常人群。有相当多的证据支持烟碱消费的急剧增加可能源于大脑中 nAChRs 的失调，这可能是通过改变 DA 和谷氨酸等神经递质系统及其下游靶点而导致精神分裂症病理的各种症状。因此，nAChRs 亚型特异性激动剂的发展为减轻精神分裂症症状提供了一种可行的治疗选择。此外，nAChR 调节剂也可以有效地改善戒烟，以规避患有精神分裂症的吸烟者与吸烟有关的健康危害。

术语解释

- 激动剂：一种与受体结合并激活受体以产生生物反应的化学物质。
- 认知：获得知识的心理过程，包括知觉、注意力、记忆力和判断力。
- 多巴胺：一种儿茶酚胺神经递质，参与奖励动机行为和认知。成瘾性药物会增加大脑中的多巴胺释放。
- 基因多态性：在 DNA 序列的等位基因中发生的变异。
- 谷氨酸：大脑中主要的兴奋性神经递质。谷氨酸参与突触可塑性以及学习和记忆。
- 异聚体受体：由不同类型的蛋白质亚基组成的受体。
- 同源受体：由相似的蛋白质亚基组成的受体。
- 烟碱：一种存在于烟草植物叶片中的生物碱。烟碱具有精神活性，极易上瘾。
- 烟碱乙酰胆碱受体：对神经递质乙酰胆碱或烟碱有反应的受体蛋白。这些蛋白质与离子通道相连，在激活状态下，离子通道允许细胞内的阳离子通过，产生去极化。
- 五聚物蛋白质：由五个蛋白质亚单位组成的蛋白质结构。

精神分裂症的关键事实

- 精神分裂症是一种致残的异质精神障碍，其干扰正常社交、清晰思考和区分现实各方面的能力。
- 精神分裂症的症状可分为三类：积极型、消极型和认知型。
- 遗传因素和环境因素的相互作用导致了患精神分裂症的风险。
- 包括神经递质多巴胺和谷氨酸在内的大脑化学物质的不平衡与精神分裂症的症状有关。
- 精神分裂症没有治愈方法，但症状可以通过抗精神病药物和心理治疗来控制。

要点总结
- 那些被诊断为精神分裂症的人摄入烟碱的比例是健康人的3～4倍。
- 烟碱与烟碱乙酰胆碱受体（nAChR）相互作用产生不同的行为效果。
- nAChRs在精神分裂症患者的大脑中表达失调。
- nAChRs影响谷氨酸和多巴胺的作用，以改变精神分裂症的认知症状。
- 发展特定的nAChR激动剂可以控制精神分裂症的症状和改善戒烟。

参考文献

Adler, L. E.; Hoffer, L. D.; Wiser, A.; Freedman, R. (1993). Normalization of auditory physiology by cigarette smoking in schizophrenic patients. The American Journal of Psychiatry, 150(12), 1856-1861.

Aguilar, M. C.; Gurpegui, M.; Diaz, F. J.; de Leon, J. (2005). Nicotine dependence and symptoms in schizophrenia: naturalistic study of complex interactions. The British Journal of Psychiatry, 186, 215-221.

Andre, J. M.; Leach, P. T.; Gould, T. J. (2011). Nicotine ameliorates NMDA receptor antagonist-induced deficits in contextual fear conditioning through high-affinity nicotinic acetylcholine receptors in the hippocampus. Neuropharmacology, 60(4), 617-625.

Bitner, R. S.; Bunnelle, W. H.; Anderson, D. J.; Briggs, C. A.; Buccafusco, J.; Curzon, P. et al. (2007). Broad-spectrum efficacy across cognitive domains by α7 nicotinic acetylcholine receptoragonism correlates with activation of ERK1/2 and CREB phosphorylation pathways. Journal of Neuroscience, 27(39), 10578-10587.

Brasic, J. R.; Cascella, N.; Kumar, A.; Zhou, Y.; Hilton, J.; Raymont, V. et al. (2012). Positron emission tomography experience with 2-[^{18}F]fluoro-3-(2(S)-azetidinylmethoxy)pyridine (2-[^{18}F]FA) in the living human brain of smokers with paranoid schizophrenia. Synapse, 66(4), 352-368.

Breese, C. R.; Lee, M. J.; Adams, C. E.; Sullivan, B.; Logel, J.; Gillen, K. M.; et al. (2000). Abnormal regulation of high affinity nicotinic receptors in subjects with schizophrenia. Neuropsychopharmacology, 23(4), 351-364.

Brooks, J. M.; Pershing, M. L.; Thomsen, M. S.; Mikkelsen, J. D.; Sarter, M.; Bruno, J. P. (2012). Transient inactivation of the neonatal ventral hippocampus impairs attentional set-shifting behavior: reversal with an alpha7 nicotinic agonist. Neuropsychopharmacology, 37(11), 2476-2486.

Buchanan, R. W.; Conley, R. R.; Dickinson, D.; Ball, M. P.; Feldman, S.; Gold, J. M. et al. (2008). Galantamine for the treatment of cognitive impairments in people with schizophrenia. The American Journal of Psychiatry, 165(1), 82-89.

Castro, N. G.; Albuquerque, E. X. (1995). Alpha-bungarotoxinsensitive hippocampal nicotinic receptor channel has a high calcium permeability. Biophysical Journal, 68(2), 516-524.

Court, J.; Spurden, D.; Lloyd, S.; McKeith, I.; Ballard, C.; Cairns, N. et al. (1999). Neuronal nicotinic receptors in dementia with Lewy bodies and schizophrenia: alpha-bungarotoxin and nicotine binding in the thalamus. Journal of Neurochemistry, 73(4), 1590-1597.

Dani, J. A.; De Biasi, M. (2001). Cellular mechanisms of nicotine addiction. Pharmacology, Biochemistry, and Behavior, 70(4), 439-446.

De Luca, V.; Voineskos, S.; Wong, G.; Kennedy, J. L. (2006). Genetic interaction between alpha4 and beta2 subunits of high affinity nicotinic receptor: analysis in schizophrenia. Experimental Brain Research, 174(2), 292-296.

D'Souza, D. C.; Esterlis, I.; Carbuto, M.; Krasenics, M.; Seibyl, J.; Bois, F. et al. (2012). Lower ss2*-nicotinic acetylcholine receptor availability in smokers with schizophrenia. The American Journal of Psychiatry, 169(3), 326-334.

Durany, N.; Zochling, R.; Boissl, K. W.; Paulus, W.; Ransmayr, G.; Tatschner, T. et al. (2000). Human post-mortem striatal alpha4beta2 nicotinic acetylcholine receptor density in schizophrenia and Parkinson's syndrome. Neuroscience Letters, 287(2), 109-112.

Dutra, S. J.; Stoeckel, L. E.; Carlini, S. V.; Pizzagalli, D. A.; Evins, A. E. (2012). Varenicline as a smoking cessation aid in schizophrenia: effects on smoking behavior and reward sensitivity. Psychopharmacology, 219(1), 25-34.

Esterlis, I.; Ranganathan, M.; Bois, F.; Pittman, B.; Picciotto, M. R.; Shearer, L. et al. (2014). In vivo evidence for beta2 nicotinic acetylcholine receptor subunit upregulation in smokers as compared with nonsmokers with schizophrenia. Biological Psychiatry, 76(6), 495-502.

Evins, A. E.; Cather, C.; Pratt, S. A.; Pachas, G. N.; Hoeppner, S. S.; Goff, D. C. et al. (2014). Maintenance treatment with varenicline for smoking cessation in patients with schizophrenia and bipolar disorder: a randomized clinical trial. JAMA, 311(2), 145-154.

Fernandes, C.; Hoyle, E.; Dempster, E.; Schalkwyk, L. C.; Collier, D. A. (2006). Performance deficit of alpha7 nicotinic receptor knockout mice in a delayed matching-to-place task suggests a mild impairment of working/episodic-like memory. Genes, Brain, and Behavior, 5(6), 433-440.

Freedman, R.; Hall, M.; Adler, L. E.; Leonard, S. (1995). Evidence in postmortem brain tissue for decreased numbers of hippocampal nicotinic receptors in schizophrenia. Biological Psychiatry, 38(1), 22-33.

Freedman, R.; Leonard, S.; Gault, J. M.; Hopkins, J.; Cloninger, C. R.; Kaufmann, C. A. et al. (2001). Linkage disequilibrium for schizophrenia at the chromosome 15q13-14 locus of the alpha7-nicotinic acetylcholine receptor subunit gene (CHRNA7). American Journal of Medical Genetics, 105(1), 20-22.

Goldman-Rakic, P. S.; Castner, S. A.; Svensson, T. H.; Siever, L. J.; Williams, G. V. (2004). Targeting the dopamine D1 receptor in schizophrenia: Insights for cognitive dysfunction. Psychopharmacology, 174(1), 3-16.

Gotti, C.; Clementi, F.; Fornari, A.; Gaimarri, A.; Guiducci, S.; Manfredi, I. et al. (2009). Structural and functional diversity of native brain neuronal nicotinic receptors. Biochemical Pharmacology, 78(7), 703-711.

Granon, S.; Faure, P.; Changeux, J.-P. (2003). Executive and social behaviors under nicotinic receptor regulation. Proceedings of the National Academy of Sciences, 100(16), 9596-9601.

Grottick, A. J.; Trube, G.; Corrigall, W. A.; Huwyler, J.; Malherbe, P.; Wyler, R. et al. (2000). Evidence that nicotinic alpha(7) receptors are not involved in the hyperlocomotor and rewarding effects of nicotine. The Journal of Pharmacology and Experimental Therapeutics, 294(3), 1112-1119.

Guan, Z. Z.; Zhang, X.; Blennow, K.; Nordberg, A. (1999). Decreased protein level of nicotinic receptor alpha7 subunit in the frontal cortex from schizophrenic brain. NeuroReport, 10(8), 1779-1782.

Guillem, K.; Bloem, B.; Poorthuis, R. B.; Loos, M.; Smit, A. B.; Maskos, U. et al. (2011). Nicotinic acetylcholine receptor beta2 subunits in the medial prefrontal cortex control attention. Science, 333(6044), 888-891.

Hauser, T. A.; Kucinski, A.; Jordan, K. G.; Gatto, G. J.; Wersinger, S. R.; Hesse, R. A. et al. (2009). TC-5619: an alpha7 neuronal nicotinic receptor-selective agonist that demonstrates efficacy in animal models of the positive and negative symptoms and cognitive dysfunction of schizophrenia. Biochemical Pharmacology, 78(7), 803-812.

Koukouli, F.; Rooy, M.; Tziotis, D.; Sailor, K. A.; O'Neill, H. C.; Levenga, J. et al. (2017). Nicotine reverses hypofrontality in animal models of addiction and schizophrenia. Nature Medicine, 23(3), 347-354.

Kunii, Y.; Zhang, W.; Xu, Q.; Hyde, T. M.; McFadden, W.; Shin, J. H. et al. (2015). CHRNA7 and CHRFAM7A mRNAs: Co-localized and their expression levels altered in the postmortem dorsolateral prefrontal cortex in major psychiatric disorders. The American Journal of Psychiatry, 172(11), 1122-1130.

Lambe, E. K.; Picciotto, M. R.; Aghajanian, G. K. (2003). Nicotine induces glutamate release from thalamocortical terminals in prefrontal cortex. Neuropsychopharmacology, 28(2), 216-225.

Lassi, G.; Taylor, A. E.; Timpson, N. J.; Kenny, P. J.; Mather, R. J.; Eisen, T. et al. (2016). The CHRNA5-A3-B4 gene cluster and smoking: From discovery to therapeutics. Trends in Neurosciences, 39(12), 851-861.

Lieberman, J. A.; Dunbar, G.; Segreti, A. C.; Girgis, R. R.; Seoane, F.; Beaver, J. S. et al. (2013). A randomized exploratory trial of an alpha-7 nicotinic receptor agonist (TC-5619) for cognitive enhancement in schizophrenia. Neuropsychopharmacology, 38(6), 968-975.

Livingstone, P. D.; Srinivasan, J.; Kew, J. N.; Dawson, L. A.; Gotti, C.; Moretti, M. et al. (2009). Alpha7 and non-alpha7 nicotinic acetylcholine receptors modulate dopamine release in vitro and in vivo in the rat prefrontal cortex. The European Journal of Neuroscience, 29(3), 539-550.

Marks, M. J.; Grady, S. R.; Collins, A. C. (1993). Downregulation of nicotinic receptor function after chronic nicotine infusion. The Journal of Pharmacology and Experimental Therapeutics, 266(3), 1268-1276.

Mexal, S.; Berger, R.; Logel, J.; Ross, R. G.; Freedman, R.; Leonard, S. (2010). Differential regulation of alpha7 nicotinic receptor gene (CHRNA7) expression in schizophrenic smokers. Journal of Molecular Neuroscience, 40(1-2), 185-195.

Moghaddam, B.; Javitt, D. (2012). From revolution to evolution: the glutamate hypothesis of schizophrenia and its implication for treatment. Neuropsychopharmacology, 37(1), 4-15.

Noroozian, M.; Ghasemi, S.; Hosseini, S. M.; Modabbernia, A.; KhodaieArdakani, M. R.; Mirshafiee, O. et al. (2013). A placebo-controlled study of tropisetron added to risperidone for the treatment of negative symptoms in chronic and stable schizophrenia. Psychopharmacology, 228(4), 595-602.

Olincy, A.; Freedman, R. (2012). Nicotinic mechanisms in the treatment of psychotic disorders: a focus on the alpha7 nicotinic receptor. Handbook of Experimental Pharmacology, (213), 211-232.

Parikh, V.; Ji, J.; Decker, M. W.; Sarter, M. (2010). Prefrontal beta2 subunit-containing and alpha7 nicotinic acetylcholine receptors differentially control glutamatergic and cholinergic signaling. The Journal of Neuroscience, 30(9), 3518-3530.

Parikh, V.; Kutlu, M. G.; Gould, T. J. (2016). nAChR dysfunction as a common substrate for schizophrenia and comorbid nicotine addiction: current trends and perspectives. Schizophrenia Research, 171(1-3), 1-15.

Patkar, A. A.; Gopalakrishnan, R.; Lundy, A.; Leone, F. T.; Certa, K. M.; Weinstein, S. P. (2002). Relationship between tobacco smoking and positive and negative symptoms in schizophrenia. The Journal of Nervous and Mental Disease, 190(9), 604-610.

Picciotto, M. R.; Lewis, A. S.; van Schalkwyk, G. I.; Mineur, Y. S. (2015). Mood and anxiety regulation by nicotinic acetylcholine receptors: a potential pathway to modulate aggression and related behavioral states. Neuropharmacology, 96(Pt B), 235-243.

Pons, S.; Fattore, L.; Cossu, G.; Tolu, S.; Porcu, E.; McIntosh, J. M. et al. (2008). Crucial role of alpha4 and alpha6 nicotinic acetylcholine receptor subunits from ventral tegmental area in systemic nicotine self-administration. The Journal of Neuroscience, 28(47), 12318-12327.

Preskorn, S. H.; Gawryl, M.; Dgetluck, N.; Palfreyman, M.; Bauer, L. O.; Hilt, D. C. (2014). Normalizing effects of EVP-6124, an alpha-7 nicotinic partial agonist, on event-related potentials and cognition: a proof of concept, randomized trial in patients with schizophrenia. Journal of Psychiatric Practice, 20(1), 12-24.

Segarra, R.; Zabala, A.; Eguiluz, J. I.; Ojeda, N.; Elizagarate, E.; Sanchez, P. et al. (2011). Cognitive performance and smoking in first-episode psychosis: the self-medication hypothesis. European Archives of Psychiatry and Clinical Neuroscience, 261(4), 241-250.

Severance, E. G.; Yolken, R. H. (2007). Lack of RIC-3 congruence with beta2 subunit-containing nicotinic acetylcholine receptors in bipolar disorder. Neuroscience, 148(2), 454-460.

Shim, J. C.; Jung, D. U.; Jung, S. S.; Seo, Y. S.; Cho, D. M.; Lee, J. H. et al. (2012). Adjunctive varenicline treatment with antipsychotic medications for cognitive impairments in people with schizophrenia: a randomized double-blind placebo-controlled trial. Neuropsychopharmacology, 37(3), 660-668.

Tseng, K. Y.; O'Donnell, P. (2004). Dopamine-glutamate interactions controlling prefrontal cortical pyramidal cell excitability involve multiple signaling mechanisms. The Journal of Neuroscience, 24(22), 5131-5139.

Voineskos, S.; De Luca, V.; Mensah, A.; Vincent, J. B.; Potapova, N.; Kennedy, J. L. (2007). Association of alpha4beta2 nicotinic receptor and heavy smoking in schizophrenia. Journal of Psychiatry Neuroscience, 32(6), 412-416.

Wonnacott, S. (1997). Presynaptic nicotinic ACh receptors. Trends in Neurosciences, 20(2), 92-98.

Yang, Y.; Paspalas, C. D.; Jin, L. E.; Picciotto, M. R.; Arnsten, A. F.; Wang, M. (2013). Nicotinic alpha7 receptors enhance NMDA cognitive circuits in dorsolateral prefrontal cortex. Proceedings of the National Academy of Sciences of the United States of America, 110(29), 12078-12083.

Young, J. W.; Crawford, N.; Kelly, J. S.; Kerr, L. E.; Marston, H. M.; Spratt, C. et al. (2007). Impaired attention is central to the cognitive deficits observed in alpha 7 deficient mice. European Neuropsychopharmacology, 17(2), 145-155.

Ziedonis, D. M.; Kosten, T. R.; Glazer, W. M.; Frances, R. J. (1994). Nicotine dependence and schizophrenia. Hospital & Community Psychiatry, 45(3), 204-206.

18
注意偏向和吸烟

David J. Drobes[1], *Jason A. Oliver*[2], *John B. Correa*[1], *David E. Evans*[1]

1. Tobacco Research and Intervention Program, Department of Health Outcomes and Behavior, Moffitt Cancer Center, Tampa, FL, United States
2. Center for Addiction Science and Technology, Department of Psychiatry and Behavioral Sciences, Duke University School of Medicine, Durham, NC, United States

缩略语

AB	注意偏向	**EEG**	脑电图
ABR	注意偏向再训练	**RT**	反应时间

18.1 引言

长期以来，人们发现与食欲或所需物质或物体有关的刺激和思想会过多地吸引人的注意力。爱吃甜食的人倾向于看巧克力蛋糕，强迫性赌徒在地板上发现扑克筹码，或者严重依赖的吸烟者在街上发现有人在抽烟。这些观察结果是注意偏向（AB）的例子，这种现象似乎在成瘾行为的现象学和治疗中具有关键的重要性。在某种程度上，与物质有关的刺激会吸引或引起人们的注意，这可能会引发或扩展与成瘾有关的观念和行为的动机。在过去的几十年中，关于AB主题的理论和实证研究都大量地来自认知心理学领域，并且近年来已扩展到吸烟和其他成瘾行为的研究。

基于学习的成瘾理论断言，与药物有关的环境刺激通过经典条件的过程，成为促进药物动机状态的条件刺激。基于这些理论，传统的提示反应性研究范式向用户提供了显著的药物配对提示，典型的响应模式包括主观渴望、生理唤起和/或寻求药物或摄入行为。成瘾者对药物线索反应的增强越来越多地从成瘾的认知（如信息处理）或神经理论的角度进行解释，在这种情况下，线索显著性与信息处理和早期阶段的注意力捕获和/或维持增加有关（如Franken, 2003; Robinson, Berridge, 1993; Tiffany, 1990）。对药物相关线索的注意偏向的过程被认为是药物寻求和摄入的发展和表达的基础。本章将回顾已用于研究与吸烟相关的AB的范式，并将讨论这项工作的临床意义。此外，我们将讨论该领域当前的研究挑战以及研究和应用的未来方向。

18.2 范式和措施

修改后的Stroop任务。在经典的Stroop任务（Stroop, 1935）中，颜色词以一致（如蓝色字体的"蓝色"）和不一致（如蓝色字体的"红色"）表示。与不一致词相比，参与者可以更快速地识别一致词的字体颜色，这反映了单词语义内容自动处理的认知干扰，尽管这对于执行任务不是必需的。此任务已被修改，以研究显著词的处理偏向，包括与药物使用和滥用有关的偏向。在吸烟领域，这是通过吸烟和中性词（如工具和家用物品）的呈现来实现的，目的是识别字体颜色而忽略词的内容。值得注意的是，Stroop 任务的改编从原始 Stroop 中提取不同的过程，从而在阅读和看到颜色之间引发了更直接的冲突。研究结果通常证实，吸烟者比非吸烟者需要更长的时间来识别与中性词相关的吸烟相关词的颜色（如 Johnsen et al. 1997），但是与原始的 Stroop 任务的干扰效应相比，这些影响相对微妙。此外，其他成瘾的 Stroop 效应似乎至少部分取决于设计因素。在一项使用酒精相关 Stroop 任务的研究中，只有在指示参与者压制酒精相关思想时才存在干扰效应，这表明 Stroop 效应可能更多是由于避免处理语义内容而引起的，而不是注意力捕获中的偏向（Klein,2007）。另一项研究发现，在使用药物的诊所中，患者和医护人员之间的模棱两可的干扰作用表明，这种影响本身可能是由熟悉度而不是成瘾引起的（Ryan,2002）。迄今为止，这两个问题都尚未在吸烟研究中得到明确的审查。

一项关于吸烟 Stroop 研究的荟萃分析（Cox et al. 2006）表明，当使用卡片格式（所有单词同时出现在一张卡片上）时，相对于单次试验格式（即与吸烟有关的和控制词以随机或伪随机的顺序出现），或者当单词以块的形式出现时（即一个类别中的所有单词连续出现，其次是一个单独的块控制类别的词）作为比较，随机穿插的顺序。情绪 Stroop 任务也存在类似的发现（Kindt et al.1996）。如果响应是针对整个吸烟单词块，而不是针对每个单词的最初定向响应，则这可能会质疑吸烟 Stroop 范式作为注意偏向的纯粹度量（即早期定向刺激）的有效性。因此，尽管在普通吸烟者中存在对吸烟言语做出反应的干扰效应似乎是可靠的，并且尚无科学论据，但这些发现的基本含义仍不确定。

视觉/点探针。评估对成瘾刺激的注意偏向的另一个常见任务是视觉（或点）探针任务。在这项任务中，与吸烟有关的刺激和中性刺激并排呈现。在设定的时间段后，图像消失，其中一个图像会被参与者必须响应的"探针"代替，例如，通过指示箭头指向的方向或仅指示探针的位置。通过对比参与者对替代吸烟刺激和中性刺激的探针的反应速度，可以推断出个体在刺激抵消时将注意力转移的位置。也就是说，定向于吸烟刺激导致对替换吸烟图像的探针的响应时间减少，而对替代中性刺激的探针的响应时间延长。此外，通过改变刺激表现的持续时间，研究人员试图解析注意力的各个组成部分（即初始捕获与维持）。许多研究已经使用该任务来检验吸烟提示的注意偏向是否随吸烟状况而变化（如 Ehrman et al. 2002）。有趣的是，一些研究表明，较轻或较少依赖的吸烟者的注意偏向更大（Hogarth et al. 2003; Mogg et al. 2005）。但是，与成瘾的 Stroop 一样，也提出了围绕解释的问题。例如，关于评估注意力定向所需的刺激表现的确切持续时间存在争论。一些研究人员认为，只有不到200ms的持续时间才能反映定向响应（Field, Cox, 2008），而另一些研究人员则认为，持续时间长达500ms才能捕获定向响应（Robbins, Ehrman, 2004）。

眼动追踪。眼动追踪是一种已在神经科学、心理学、广告学和市场研究中广泛使用的方法（Duchowski, 2007），并且已经证明了它在识别与各种类型的心理病理学（如情绪障碍和焦虑症）相关的注意偏向的功效（Armstrong, Olatunji, 2012）。眼动追踪任务主要基于计算机，涉及测量在计算机屏幕上向个体展示视觉刺激时其直接注视的位置。与修改的 Stroop 或视觉/点探针任务相比，眼动跟踪任务可能会产生更直接的注意力分配度量，从而产生更有效的AB估计值，它们均依赖于响应的产生，而这可能需要认知工作，而不仅仅是简单的注意力分配。许多当代的眼动追踪系统都是基于视频的，并利用高分辨率相机、红外或近红外光源、头戴式摄像机以及先进的图像处理硬件和软件。典型的眼动追踪系统可以产生几种视觉注意力的客观衡量指标（如定向和维持），如总注视时间（注视刺激所花费的时间）、注视等待时间（注视指向刺激之前经过的时间）以及初始注视的区域（注视最初指向的刺激类型）。眼动追踪研究显示，与吸烟有关的AB与当前吸烟（Kwak et al. 2007）、自我报告的渴望（Kang et al. 2012）和烟碱剥夺（Field, Mogg, Bradley, 2004）之间存在关联。

神经指数。对药物提示的注意偏向的神经标记可能比行为标记（如RT）更敏感，因为行为可能反映了多个认知过程的总和。一项fMRI研究的荟萃分析（Engelmann et al. 2012）检查了更长的吸烟线索反应，证实了许多受影响的大脑区域（如楔前叶、前扣带和后扣带皮层、前额叶和顶叶皮层、背侧纹状体和脑岛）。虽然这些发现有助于我们理解吸烟线索的反应，但更广泛地说，fMRI的时间分辨率不足以捕获对吸烟相关刺激的初始定向或注意偏差。相比之下，基于EEG的事件相关电位（ERP）具有更高的时间分辨率，更适合于在刺激暴露后的最初几百毫秒内标记神经事件（Van Veen, Carter, 2002），因此可以捕获对吸烟/药物线索的早期定向反应（如Oliver et al. 2016）。特别的是，情感线索（如Schupp et al. 2000）和吸烟相关线索（如Littel, Franken, 2011; Oliver et al. 2016; Versace et al. 2010）使LPP增加。然而，关于吸烟线索的研究结果参差不齐，一些研究发现吸烟者和非吸烟者的LPP与吸烟和控制线索的LPP相等（Bloom et al. 2013; Warren, McDonough, 1999）。然而，最近的发现表明，吸烟线索的LPP幅度与吸烟行为呈正相关（Littel, Franken, 2011; Versace et al. 2011）。

其他ERP组件似乎也受到吸烟者吸烟线索的影响。例如，与不吸烟者相比，吸烟者对吸烟提示的"N300"反应减少了（Warren, McDonough, 1999），甚至在戒烟期间减少了更多（McDonough, Warren, 2001）。枕骨P1（峰值140ms）对吸烟线索的反应与吸烟水平呈正相关，甚至观察到吸烟线索的更早处理（Versace et al. 2011）。这些早期的ERP组件（P1和N300）可能反映了无意识/前意识活动（Dehaene, 2014），而LPP可能反映了对刺激的有意识关注。

其他范式。已经开发或修改了许多其他范式来评估AB在吸烟行为中的作用。这些范式包括：①双重任务（如Sayette, Hufford, 1994）：吸烟者会看到视觉上的吸烟或中性提示，但被要求对以不同方式呈现的刺激做出反应。②注意眨眼（Chanon, Sours, Boettiger, 2010）：参与者对目标刺激的反应叠加在吸烟和中性线索的快速序列。③N-black工作记忆（Evans et al. 2011）：提出了一系列吸烟和中性的单词，并且参与者必须回答该单词是否与先前提出的一项、两项或三项试验相匹配。④视觉搜索（Oliver, Drobes, 2012）：吸烟和中性线索被嵌入分散注意力的刺激网格中。对这些范式和其他范式的详细描述超出了本文的范围，但这显然是一个活跃的研究领域，这些范式继续为关注的各个组成部分如何控制吸烟行为提供证据。

18.3 临床相关性

大量文献研究了AB、吸烟相关行为与戒烟之间的关系。利用修改后的Stroop任务进行的研究发现，与吸烟有关的线索中的AB可能与当前吸烟（Munafò et al. 2003）、自我报告的渴望（Mogg, Bradley, 2002）、吸烟的期望值（Werers et al. 2009）和吸烟的预期机会有关（Wertz, Sayette, 2001）。视觉/点探针研究证实了其中的某些关系并确定了其他关系（如Ehrman et al. 2002; Vollstädt-Klein et al. 2011; Waters et al. 2003）。最后，眼动追踪研究已将与吸烟有关的线索中的AB与临床相关结果联系起来，包括渴望、吸烟行为和烟碱剥夺效应（Field et al. 2004; Kang et al. 2012; Kwak et al. 2007）。荟萃分析支持 AB 和渴望/冲动的测量是相关的，尽管这种关系的强度似乎不高（Field, Munafò, Franken, 2009）。

鉴于在所有范式中，与吸烟有关的线索中的 AB 似乎与临床相关的吸烟行为有关，因此可以合理地假设，与吸烟有关的线索中的 AB 可能是成功戒烟的潜在障碍。事实上，一项研究发现，与吸烟有关的单词的 AB（在修改的 Stroop 任务中）预计在戒烟后 1 周复发，尽管在戒烟后 1 个月或 3 个月没有复发（Powell et al. 2010）。另一项经过改进的 Stroop 研究发现，将 RT 延长至第一个与吸烟相关的单词可以预测复发时间，但是在随后的试验中 RT 并未显示出这种效果（Waters et al. 2003）。尽管重复这些发现将是有价值的，但研究人员已开始制订干预策略，以减少吸烟相关线索中的吸烟者的 AB，并认为这将减少吸烟行为并改善戒烟效果。注意偏向再训练（ABR）已显示出在改善与其他类型的精神病理学有关的症状方面的功效（Hakamata et al. 2010），已成为戒烟研究领域中一种有趣的新方法。评估 ABR 的研究利用了传统的 AB 方法（主要是视觉/点探针任务），并试图重新训练吸烟者的自动注意过程。对吸烟者进行训练，以使其在出现时避免吸烟相关的刺激，或者将吸烟相关的刺激与负面的描述语联系起来。

早期的 ABR 研究发现，至少在有时间限制的实验室环境中，吸烟者确实可以接受训练以减少与吸烟相关的刺激中的 AB（Attwood et al. 2008; Field et al. 2009; Lopes, Pires, Bizarro, 2014）。然而，最近的研究对于成功地重新吸引吸烟者的注意力产生了不同的发现（如 Begh et al. 2015; Elfeddali et al. 2016），并且这些培训程序并不易于概括戒烟结果（如 Begh et al. 2015; Kerst, Waters, 2014）。ABR 对卷烟渴望的影响也存在不一致之处，一些研究发现 ABR 可以有效减少烟瘾（如 Attwood et al. 2008; Kerst, Waters, 2014），而其他人则没有发现这种影响（如 Begh et al. 2015; Field, Duka, et al. 2009; Field, Munafò, et al. 2009; McHugh et al. 2010）。尽管如此，仍需要继续进行有关 AB 潜在临床应用的研究。正如 Franken 和 van de Wetering（2015）所建议的那样，应该在更大、更系统的研究工作中评估 AB（和其他神经认知措施）的临床效用，这些研究将这些指标作为诊断、治疗选择、治疗结果以及治疗效果的调节剂。AB 措施在任何这些临床领域都可能被证明是有用的，并且要使 AB 程序从实验室有效地转向临床，应更加着重于完善实验程序并应用合理的方法来测量自然环境中的这种结构。

18.4 当前的挑战

在 AB 的研究中显然存在多种心理上和解释上的挑战。例如，对 7 项与药物相关的 AB 的独立研究的结果进行重新分析后发现，视觉/点探针任务表现出的内部一致性远低于可接受的水平（Ataya et al. 2012）。在这些研究中无法评估重测的可靠性，但在使用视觉/点探针任务进行威胁处理的研究中，重测的可靠性一直很低（Schmukle, 2005）。对 AB 文献中通常采用的其他认知措施和操作也提出了类似的关注（例如，戒烟过夜；Rhodes, Hawk, 2016）。

另一个设计问题是 AB 文献中缺少"积极的"或"主动的"控制条件。尽管有几个显著的例外（Drobes, Elibero, Evans, 2006; Oliver et al. 2016; Versace et al. 2011），但典型的 AB 研究对比了对吸烟线索的注意和对情绪惰性的"控制"刺激的注意。当包括其他情绪（显著）类别时，研究结果表明，对 AB 任务的传统解释是与物质有关的提示获得了引起这些提示"吸引"注意力的激励性动机特性，并不一定是驱动效果的因素（Field, Cox, 2008）。事实上，明显的线索（即那些被认为具有食欲或厌恶情绪的线索）通常会产生相似水平的AB。例如，在一项研究中，吸烟者对吸烟和令人愉悦的图像均表现出AB，这表明AB的发现可能是由于吸烟者自身的潜在诱因或"食欲过高"引起的，而这本身并不是吸烟的功能（Oliver et al. 2016）。

18.5 总结与展望

已经开发出多种范式来评估对吸烟线索的初步定向和维持。除了证明吸烟者中存在AB之外，研究还显示AB与临床相关的吸烟相关变量之间存在关系，如渴望、烟碱依赖和戒烟/复发。在这些文献中，一个新的重点领域是研究旨在在戒烟的背景下将AB降低为吸烟线索的培训程序。迄今为止，ABR研究产生了混合的证据，需要更多的工作来确定其作为戒烟治疗的组成部分的潜在作用。许多方法学问题，包括低可靠性和注意偏向与吸烟行为之间关联的重复性不足，表明有必要进行较大规模的精心设计的研究，以便更好地阐明AB的性质以及如何最佳地测量AB的过程并制订有效的治疗策略，从而解决其在吸烟成瘾中的作用。除了用于个人理解和干预吸烟行为的AB范式之外，这些方法现在正在烟草政策和法规环境中应用。例如，眼动追踪范例已显示出图形警告标签和卷烟包装的其他特征是如何吸引吸烟者的注意力的（如Strasser et al. 2012）。类似的AB方法被用于评估各种与卷烟相关的消息传递格式，包括印刷广告（如Lochbuehler et al. 2016）和销售点展示（如Dutra et al. 2018）。

术语解释	■ 注意偏向再训练：指减少对相关提示的注意偏向的方法。 ■ 注意偏向：注意偏向是指对某些个体或群体的刺激与注意力或相关性增强。注意偏向的关键子组件包括信息处理的初始定向和维持阶段。 ■ 眼动追踪：眼动追踪包括测量当个体在计算机屏幕上受到视觉刺激时直接注视的位置，从而提供对注意力分配的直接评估。 ■ 修改后的Stroop任务：此任务涉及命名单词的颜色，当单词具有引起注意的显著性或相关性时，该颜色将延迟。 ■ 视觉/点探针：此任务涉及检测替换视野中两个刺激之一的目标的存在。当目标检测取代具有更大相关性的刺激并因此受到更多关注时，目标检测的速度会更快。
注意偏向评估的关键事实	■ AB是成瘾的一种重要现象，最初是在专注于药物配对线索的自动处理理论中得到强调的，如Tiffany（1990）对药物冲动和药物使用的认知理论。 ■ AB评估捕获显著线索的隐式（或无意识）处理，这被认为反映了药物配对线索的激励显著性。这可以提供成瘾的关键指标。 ■ AB评估要求对与药物相关的重要线索进行有控制的陈述，并同时衡量对这些线索的关注程度。 ■ 自20世纪90年代以来，文献中就出现了对吸烟者进行AB评估的范式，最早的研究使用了经典Stroop任务的修改版本。 ■ 许多后续范式已用于评估吸烟者的AB，包括视觉/点探针任务、眼动追踪任务以及对显著线索的神经处理的测量。

要点总结

- 本章重点关注与吸烟有关的线索的注意偏向（AB），该注意偏向采用了认知心理学和神经科学的模型和范式。
- 对于持续吸烟的人和试图戒烟的人来说，注意偏向可能是吸烟动机的基础。
- 评估与吸烟相关的AB的常用方法包括修改后的Stroop任务、视觉/点探针任务、眼动追踪和直接神经指标。
- AB任务处理关注的不同子组件，每个子组件都受到方法论和解释性问题的影响。
- 我们建议解决方法上的局限性将改善AB发现的概念清晰性。
- 最近对个人进行再培训以减少注意力偏向的尝试尚未确定这些方法与戒烟结果的改善相关。
- AB模式越来越多地用于解决烟草政策和法规问题。

参考文献

Armstrong, T.; Olatunji, B. O. (2012). Eye tracking of attention in the affective disorders: a meta-analytic review and synthesis. Clinical Psychology Review, 32, 704-723.

Ataya, A. F.; Adams, S.; Mullings, E.; Cooper, R. M.; Attwood, A. S.; Munafò, M. R. (2012). Internal reliability of measures of substancerelated cognitive bias. Drug and Alcohol Dependence, 121, 148-151.

Attwood, A. S.; O'Sullivan, H.; Leonards, U.; Mackintosh, B.; Munafò, M. R. (2008). Attentional bias training and cue reactivity in cigarette smokers. Addiction, 103, 1875-1882.

Begh, R.; Munafò, M. R.; Shiffman, S.; Ferguson, S. G.; Nichols, L.; Mohammed, M. A. et al. (2015). Lack of attentional retraining effects in cigarette smokers attempting cessation: a proof of concept doubleblind randomised controlled trial. Drug and Alcohol Dependence, 149, 158-165.

Bloom, E. L.; Potts, G. F.; Evans, D. E.; Drobes, D. J. (2013). Cue reactivity in smokers: an event-related potential study. International Journal of Psychophysiology, 90(2), 258-264.

Chanon, V. W.; Sours, C. R.; Boettiger, C. A. (2010). Attentional bias toward cigarette cues in active smokers. Psychopharmacology, 212, 309-320.

Cox, W. M.; Fadardi, J. S.; Pothos, E. M. (2006). The addiction-stroop test: theoretical considerations and procedural recommendations. Psychological Bulletin, 132, 443-476.

Dehaene, S. (2014). Consciousness and the brain: Deciphering how the brain codes our thoughts. New York: Penguin.

Drobes, D. J.; Elibero, A.; Evans, D. E. (2006). Attentional bias for smoking and affective stimuli: a Stroop task study. Psychology of Addictive Behaviors, 20, 490-495.

Duchowski, A. T. (2007). Eye tracking methodology: Theory and practice (2nd ed.). London: Springer.

Dutra, L. M.; Nonnemaker, J.; Guillory, J.; Bradfield, B.; Taylor, N.; Kim, A. (2018). Smokers' attention to point-of-sale antismoking ads: an eye-tracking study. Tobacco Regulatory Science, 4, 631-643.

Ehrman, R. N.; Robbins, S. J.; Bromwell, M. A.; Lankford, M. E.; Monterosso, J. R.; O'Brien, C. P. (2002). Comparing attentional bias to smoking cues in current smokers, former smokers, and nonsmokers using a dot-probe task. Drug and Alcohol Dependence, 67, 185-191.

Elfeddali, I.; de Vries, H.; Bolman, C.; Pronk, T.; Wiers, R. W. (2016). A randomized controlled trial of web-based attentional bias modification to help smokers quit. Health Psychology, 35, 870-880.

Engelmann, J. M.; Versace, F.; Robinson, J. D.; Minnix, J. A.; Lam, C. Y.; Cui, Y. et al. (2012). Neural substrates of smoking cue reactivity: a meta-analysis of fMRI studies. NeuroImage, 60, 252-262.

Evans, D. E.; Craig, C.; Oliver, J. A.; Drobes, D. J. (2011). The smoking N-back: a measure of biased cue processing at varying levels of cognitive load. Nicotine, Tobacco Research, 13, 88-93.

Field, M.; Cox, W. M. (2008). Attentional bias in addictive behaviors: a review of its development, causes, and consequences. Drug and Alcohol Dependence, 97, 1-20.

Field, M.; Duka, T.; Tyler, E.; Schoenmakers, T. (2009). Attentional bias modification in tobacco smokers. Nicotine, Tobacco Research, 11, 812-822.

Field, M.; Mogg, K.; Bradley, B. P. (2004). Eye movements to smokingrelated cues: effects of nicotine deprivation. Psychopharmacology, 173, 116-123.

Field, M.; Munafò, M. R.; Franken, I. H. (2009). A meta-analytic investigation of the relationship between attentional bias and subjective craving in substance abuse. Psychological Bulletin, 135, 589-607.

Franken, I. H. (2003). Drug craving and addiction: Integrating psychological and neuropsychopharmacological approaches. Progress in Neuro-Psychopharmacology, Biological Psychiatry, 27, 563-579.

Franken, I. H.; van de Wetering, B. J. (2015). Bridging the gap between the neurocognitive lab and the addiction clinic. Addictive Behaviors, 44, 108-114.

Hakamata, Y.; Lissek, S.; Bar-Haim, Y.; Britton, J. C.; Fox, N. A.; Leibenluft, E. et al. (2010). Attention bias modification treatment: a meta-analysis toward the establishment of novel treatment for anxiety. Biological Psychiatry, 68, 982-990.

Hogarth, L. C.; Mogg, K.; Bradley, B. P.; Duka, T.; Dickinson, A. (2003). Attentional orienting towards smoking-related stimuli. Behavioural Pharmacology, 14, 153-160.

Johnsen, B. H.; Thayer, J. F.; Laberg, J. C.; Asbjornsen, A. E. (1997). Attentional bias in active smokers, abstinent smokers, and nonsmokers. Addictive Behaviors, 22, 813-817.

Kang, O. S.; Chang, D. S.; Jahng, G. H.; Kim, S. Y.; Kim, H.; Kim, J. W. et al. (2012). Individual differences in smoking-related cue reactivityin smokers: an eye-tracking and fMRI study. Progress in NeuroPsychopharmacology and Biological Psychiatry, 38, 285-293.

Kerst, W. F.; Waters, A. J. (2014). Attentional retraining administered in the field reduces smokers' attentional bias and craving. Health Psychology, 33, 1232-1240.

Kindt, M.; Bierman, D.; Brosschot, J. F. (1996). Stroop versus Stroop: comparison of a card format and a single-trial format of the standard color-word Stroop task and the emotional Stroop task. Personality and Individual Differences, 21, 653-661.

Klein, A. A. (2007). Suppression-induced hyperaccessibility of thoughts in abstinent alcoholics: a preliminary investigation. Behaviour Research and Therapy, 45, 169-177.

Kwak, S. M.; Na, D. L.; Kim, G.; Kim, G. S.; Lee, J. H. (2007). Use of eye movement to measure smokers' attentional bias to smoking-related cues. Cyberpsychology, Behavior, 10, 299-304.

Littel, M.; Franken, I. H. (2011). Implicit and explicit selective attention to smoking cues in smokers indexed by brain potentials. Journal of Psychopharmacology, 25, 503-513.

Lochbuehler, K.; Tang, K. Z.; Souprountchouk, V.; Campetti, D.; Cappella, J. N.; Kozlowski, L. T. et al. (2016). Using eye-tracking to examine how embedding risk corrective statements improves cigarette risk beliefs: implications for tobacco regulatory policy. Drug and Alcohol Dependence, 164, 97-105.

Lopes, F. M.; Pires, A. V.; Bizarro, L. (2014). Attentional bias modification in smokers trying to quit: a longitudinal study about the effects of number of sessions. Journal of Substance Abuse Treatment, 47, 50-57.

McDonough, B. E.; Warren, C. A. (2001). Effects of 12-h tobacco deprivation on event-related potentials elicited by visual smoking cues. Psychopharmacology, 154, 282-291.

McHugh, R. K.; Murray, H. W.; Hearon, B. A.; Calkins, A. W.; Otto, M. W. (2010). Attentional bias and craving in smokers: the impact of a single attentional training session. Nicotine, Tobacco Research, 12, 1261-1264.

Mogg, K.; Bradley, B. P. (2002). Selective processing of smokingrelated cues in smokers: manipulation of deprivation level and comparison of three measures of processing bias. Journal of Psychopharmacology, 16, 385-392.

Mogg, K.; Field, M.; Bradley, B. P. (2005). Attentional and approach biases for smoking cues in smokers: an investigation of competing theoretical views of addiction. Psychopharmacology, 180, 333-341.

Munafò, M.; Mogg, K.; Roberts, S.; Bradley, B. P.; Murphy, M. (2003). Selective processing of smoking-related cues in current smokers, ex-smokers and never-smokers on the modified Stroop task. Journal of Psychopharmacology, 17, 310-316.

Oliver, J. A.; Drobes, D. J. (2012). Visual search and attentional bias for smoking cues: the role of familiarity. Experimental and Clinical Psychopharmacology, 20, 489-496.

Oliver, J. A.; Jentink, K. G.; Drobes, D. J.; Evans, D. E. (2016). Smokers exhibit biased neural processing of smoking and affective images. Health Psychology, 35, 866-869.

Powell, J.; Dawkins, L.; West, R.; Powell, J.; Pickering, A. (2010). Relapse to smoking during unaided cessation: clinical, cognitive and motivational predictors. Psychopharmacology, 212, 537-549.

Rhodes, J. D.; Hawk, L. W. (2016). Smoke and mirrors: the overnight abstinence paradigm as an index of disrupted cognitive function. Psychopharmacology, 233, 1395-1404.

Robbins, S. J.; Ehrman, R. N. (2004). The role of attentional bias in substance abuse. Behavioral and Cognitive Neuroscience Reviews, 3, 243-260.

Robinson, T. E.; Berridge, K. C. (1993). The neural basis of drug craving: an incentive-sensitization theory of addiction. Brain Research, 18, 247-291.

Ryan, F. (2002). Attentional bias and alcohol dependence: a controlled study using the modified Stroop paradigm. Addictive Behaviors, 27, 471-482.

Sayette, M. A.; Hufford, M. R. (1994). Effects of cue exposure and deprivation on cognitive resources in smokers. Journal of Abnormal Psychology, 103, 812-818.

Schmukle, S. C. (2005). Unreliability of the dot probe task. European Journal of Personality, 19, 595-605.

Schupp, H. T.; Cuthbert, B. N.; Bradley, M. M.; Cacioppo, J. T.; Ito, T.; Lang, P. J. (2000). Affective picture processing: the late positive potential is modulated by motivational relevance. Psychophysiology, 37, 257-261.

Strasser, A. A.; Tang, K. Z.; Romer, D.; Jepson, C.; Cappella, J. N. (2012). Graphic warning labels in cigarette advertisements: recall and viewing patterns. American Journal of Preventive Medicine, 43, 41-47.

Stroop, J. R. (1935). Studies of interference in serial verbal reactions. Journal of Experimental Psychology, 18, 643. Tiffany, S. T. (1990). A cognitive model of drug urges and drug-usebehavior: role of automatic and nonautomatic processes. Psychological Review, 97, 147-168.

Van Veen, V.; Carter, C. S. (2002). The anterior cingulate as a conflict monitor: fMRI and ERP studies. Physiology and Behavior, 77, 477-482.

Versace, F.; Minnix, J. A.; Robinson, J. D.; Lam, C. Y.; Brown, V. L.; Cinciripini, P. M. (2011). Brain reactivity to emotional, neutral and cigarette-related stimuli in smokers. Addiction Biology, 16, 296-307.

Versace, F.; Robinson, J. D.; Lam, C. Y.; Minnix, J. A.; Brown, V. L.; Carter, B. L. et al. (2010). Cigarette cues capture smokers' attention: Evidence from event-related potentials. Psychophysiology, 47, 435-441.

Vollstädt-Klein, S.; Loeber, S.; Winter, S.; Lemenager, T.; von der Goltz, C.; Dinter, C. et al. (2011). Attention shift towards smoking cues relates to severity of dependence, smoking behavior and breath carbon monoxide. European Addiction Research, 17, 217-224.

Warren, C. A.; McDonough, B. E. (1999). Event-related brain potentials as indicators of smoking cue-reactivity. Clinical Neurophysiology, 110, 1570-

1584.

Waters, A. J.; Carter, B. L.; Robinson, J. D.; Wetter, D. W.; Lam, C. Y.; Kerst, W. et al. (2009). Attentional bias is associated with incentive-related physiological and subjective measures. Experimental and Clinical Psychopharmacology, 17, 247-257.

Waters, A. J.; Shiffman, S.; Bradley, B. P.; Mogg, K. (2003). Attentional shifts to smoking cues in smokers. Addiction, 98, 1409-1417.

Waters, A. J.; Shiffman, S.; Sayette, M. A.; Paty, J. A.; Gwaltney, C. J.; Balabanis, M. H. (2003). Attentional bias predicts outcome in smoking cessation. Health Psychology, 22, 378-387.

Wertz, J. M.; Sayette, M. A. (2001). Effects of smoking opportunity on attentional bias in smokers. Psychology of Addictive Behaviors, 15, 268-271.

19
烟碱对人体抑制控制的影响

Ulrich Ettinger[1], Veena Kumari[2]

1. Department of Psychology, University of Bonn, Bonn, Germany
2. Centre for Cognitive Neuroscience, Division of Psychology, College of Health and Life Sciences, Brunel University London, Uxbridge, United Kingdom

缩略语

ADHD	注意缺陷多动障碍	**RT**	反应时间
ANT	注意网络测试	**SSRT**	停止信号响应时间

19.1 引言

抑制不必要的行为、思想或情感的能力是服务于目标导向行为的重要功能。日常生活中经常需要抑制冲动和不适当的（再）动作，而这种能力与有利的个人和社会功能有关。因此，提高抑制不想要的行为的能力一直是一些研究的重点。一些研究人员通过训练来改善抑制控制，另一种广泛采用的方法是应用增强认知的物质，如烟碱乙酰胆碱受体激动剂烟碱。

研究抑制控制的药理学影响是很重要的。第一，此类研究具有识别认知领域的潜力，可以在健康的人类中增强认知领域，以改善在职业、教育和其他社会环境中的功能。第二，在一些精神和神经病学的患者群体中观察到抑制性损伤，开发一些治疗方法来缓解这些缺陷是一个尚未得到满足的临床需求。第三，对于烟碱来说，重要的是要了解导致吸烟和维持吸烟的因素。这些可能包括对认知方面的有益影响。最后，药物对抑制控制作用的实验研究可能会为认知和脑功能模型提供参考。

本章重点介绍烟碱对抑制控制的影响。抑制控制包括抑制运动反应和注意控制分散信息的干扰。本章讨论烟碱对研究最广泛的抑制范式的影响，即抑制作用、反扫视任务、停止信号任务、go/no-go任务、Stroop任务和侧翼任务。考虑到该文献在方法学上的巨大异质性，讨论了在烟民匮乏的人群中受控烟碱应用（如贴剂、片剂、注射剂或口香糖）和吸烟的发现。出于篇幅考虑，仅考虑对人类的研究。

19.2 烟碱对响应抑制和干扰控制的影响

19.2.1 反扫视任务

在反扫视任务（图19.1）中，指示参与者进行快速眼球扫视，远离突然出现的周围目标，同时避免扫视。抑制控制此任务的主要措施是方向错误率，即参与者首先看向外围目标的试验百分比。此外，经常会报道正确响应的等待时间（RT）。通常将前扫视任务作为感觉运动控制条件。

大量研究提供了烟碱对反扫视任务表现的有益作用的证据。据报道，这些研究效果在任务特征（如阻滞或混合的反扫视/前扫视任务）、烟碱施用方法（如戒断后吸烟、口香糖、鼻喷雾剂、注射剂和贴剂）、临床特征（如精神分裂症患者、分裂型个体和对照）以及吸烟状况（如吸烟者和非吸烟者）方面存在显著差异。

在大多数但不是所有的研究中，已经观察到烟碱方向误差的减少（Dawkins et al. 2009; Dawkins et al. 2007; Dépatie et al. 2002; Larrison, Briand, Sereno, 2004; Larrison-Faucher, Matorin, Sereno, 2004; Petrovsky et al. 2012, 2013; Pettiford et al. 2007; Powell, Dawkins, Davis, 2002; Rycroft, Hutton, Rusted, 2006; Schmechtig et al. 2013; Ettinger et al.2009, 2017; Rycroft et al 2007; Thaker et al. 1991; Wachter, Gilbert, 2013）。烟碱还可能减少反扫视潜伏期（Bowling, Donnelly, 2010; Ettinger et al. 2009; Larrison et al. 2004; Larrison-Faucher et al. 2004; Petrovsky et al. 2013; Rycroft et al. 2006, 2007; Wachter, Gilbert, 2013），尽管并非所有研究都观察到了这种效应（Dépatie et al. 2002; Ettinger et al. 2017; Petrovsky et al. 2012; Schmechtig et al. 2013; Thaker et al. 1991）。应当指出，并非所有研究都报道了潜伏期。

尽管这些影响通常独立于临床（精神分裂症组、分裂人格组和对照组）和吸烟（吸烟者组和非吸烟者组）状态，但对于反扫视能力可能会有基线依赖性的影响（Ettinger et al. 2017）。例如，一项对精神分裂症患者的研究表明，表现不佳的患者的改善更大（Larrison-Faucher et al. 2004）。此外，Petrovsky等（2012）报道，烟碱减少了表现不佳的健康参与者的反扫视误差，但并未降低表现良好的健康参与者的反扫视误差，而不会影响反扫视潜伏期或前扫视性能。Wachter和Gilbert（2013）也观察到基线依赖性，他们报道了表现较差和中等（但不高）的吸烟者在烟碱贴剂处理后反扫视的潜伏期降低，但前扫视的潜伏期未降低，对错误率没有任何影响。

总而言之，在大多数研究中，烟碱对方向错误或反扫视潜伏期都有有益的影响。鉴于大多数研究报告显示，对前程控制任务的表现没有显著影响（Dawkins et al. 2007; Dépatie et al. 2002; Ettinger et al. 2009; Larrison et al. 2004; Larrison-Faucher et al. 2004; Petrovsky et al. 2012; Pettiford et al. 2007; Schmechtig et al. 2013; Thaker et al. 1991; Wachter, Gilbert, 2013; Ettinger et al. 2017; Petrovsky et al. 2013），这些发现可能反映了对自上而下控制眼跳运动的有益效果。

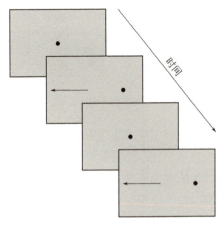

图 19.1 反扫视任务的流程图

在反扫视任务中，必须在与周围刺激相反的方向上进行快速的眼球运动（此处用灰色箭头表示）。如本例所示，反扫视试验可以被屏蔽显示，也可以与扫视试验交错显示（针对目标的扫视）。

19.2.2 停止信号任务

停止信号任务（图19.2）是一种停止或取消运动响应的措施。该任务已被广泛用于建模的认知和神经机制反应精神病学和神经病患者的反应抑制以及抑制控制缺陷。关键的因变量是SSRT，它是停止过程速度的间接度量，但是在一些研究中也报道了RTs和正确反应的百分比。

在患有注意缺陷多动障碍（ADHD）的非吸烟青少年（Potter, Newhouse, 2004）和成人（Potter, Newhouse, 2008）中观察到了烟碱对SSRT的有益作用。在非吸烟的年轻人中，他们的冲动性很高（Potter et al. 2012）；在健康的不吸烟者中也更弱势（Logemann et al. 2014b）。然而，其他研究未能观察到对健康的非吸烟者的影响（在吸烟者和非吸烟者的样本中进行比较）（Ettinger et al. 2017; Wignall, De Wit, 2011; Bekker et al.2005; Logemann et al. 2014a）。

烟碱对SSRT有益作用的更一致的证据来自对戒烟状态下吸烟者的研究。在大多数研究中，与戒烟相比，正常吸烟后的表现更好（Ashare, Hawk, 2012; Charles-Walsh et al. 2014; Tsaur et al. 2015）。一项研究表明，吸烟者吸烟后SSRT升高，这表明烟碱具有去抑制作用（Austin et al.2014）。

总体而言，烟碱可改善具有抑制功能障碍的个体（即ADHD和抽烟的吸烟者）的停止信号任务表现。然而，对健康吸烟者和非吸烟者实验控制的烟碱应用似乎不能可靠地提高这项任务的表现。

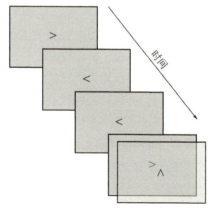

图19.2　停止信号任务的流程图

在停止信号任务中，当出现突然停止信号时，必须停止选择反应任务中的响应。在此，参与者必须通过指示目标箭头的方向（左或右）做出响应，但在目标之后不久显示停止信号（此处为向上的箭头）时，参与者必须停止此响应。停止信号也可以是听觉刺激。

19.2.3 go/no-go任务

go/no-go任务（图19.3）被广泛用于评估抑制主导运动反应的能力。抑制任务控制的最常见方法是错误率，即no-go试验的反应百分比，尽管研究也经常报道go试验的反应时间。

尽管有证据表明吸烟对吸烟者的继续不吸烟有有益影响（Kozink et al. 2010），但大多数研究似乎并未发现烟碱有显著影响，包括使用无烟吸烟者的设计（Ettinger et al. 2017; Evans et al. 2009; Giessing et al. 2013; Harrison, Coppola, McKee, 2009; Smucny et al. 2015）。一项对ADHD吸烟者和吸烟控制的吸烟者的研究发现，与饱食状态相比，戒断患者的错误更多，戒断状态下的患者比对照组犯更多的错误（McClernon et al. 2008）。

在缺乏烟碱的吸烟者中，对烟碱进行短时间、低变量的即时 RTs 试验也有证据（Giessing et al. 2013; Harrison et al. 2009; Houlihan et al. 1996; Ettinger et al. 2017; Kozink et al. 2010; Smucny et al. 2015）。

总而言之，大多数研究未能提供烟碱对 go/no-go 任务中反应抑制的有益作用的证据，而关于去 RTs 的作用方面的证据还很混杂。

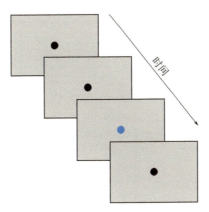

图 19.3　go/no-go 任务的流程图

在 go/no-go 任务中，参与者必须对频繁执行的刺激做出响应（此处为黑色圆圈），但在显示为不执行刺激时（此处为蓝色圆圈）保留响应。在任务的变体中，包括了奇数球刺激 oddbal 范式。这些在一个刺激维度上也与围棋刺激 go 刺激不同 [如颜色；因此在该示例中，奇数球刺激 oddbal 范式可以是绿色圆圈（未示出）]，但是必须像围棋刺激 go 刺激一样被响应。

19.2.4　Stroop 任务

在 Stroop 任务（图 19.4）中，需禁止以颜色词命名，而是对单词的打印颜色进行命名。Stroop 任务及其变体已广泛应用于认知神经科学、精神药理学和精神病理学研究。关键性能指标是 Stroop 效应，即不一致条件和一致条件之间的 RTs 或错误率的差异。

大量研究考查了烟碱对 Stroop 效应的影响。研究采用了实验控制的应用程序和自然方法，这些方法涉及吸烟者在不同剥夺时间后吸烟。总体而言，大多数研究未能观察到吸烟或烟碱的受控应用对 Stroop 效应的影响（Cook et al. 2003; Della et al. 1999; Ettinger et al. 2017; Evins et al. 2005; Foulds et al. 1996; George et al. 2002; Ilan, Polich, 2001; Kos, Hasenfratz, Bättig, 1997; Levin et al. 1996; Mancuso et al. 1999; Parrott, Craig, 1992; Poltavski, Petros, 2006; Rusted et al. 2000; Suter et al.1983; Tsaur et al. 2015; Wesnes, Revell, 1984; Xu et al. 2007; Xu, Domino, 2000; Zack et al. 2001）。

然而，其他研究也报道了任务性能的总体提高（Atzori et al. 2008; Azizian et al. 2010; Mancuso et al. 1999; Pomerleau et al. 1994; Potter, Newhouse, 2008; Rusted et al. 2000; Zack et al. 2001）。然而，其他研究也观察到了健康个体（Domier et al. 2007; Hasenfratz, Bättig, 1992; Landers et al. 1992; Provost, Woodward, 1991; Wesnes, Warburton, 1978; Wignall, De Wit, 2011）和患有 ADHD（Potter, Newhouse, 2004）和精神分裂症的患者（Barr et al. 2008）的 Stroop 效应有选择性的改善。也有证据表明烟碱对 Stroop 表现的影响可能取决于 *CHRNA5* 基因型（Jensen et al. 2015）和吸烟者的状况，在吸烟者中观察到有益的影响，但在非吸烟者中则没有（Grundey et al. 2015）。因此，总的来说，烟碱对 Stroop 任务中抑制控制的影响似乎并不可靠。其原因尚不清楚，因为在吸烟者和非吸烟者的样本以及使用方法（如吸烟者中的卷烟与受控贴剂的使用）中都获得了正面和负面影响。

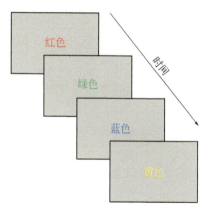

图 19.4　Stroop 任务的流程图

在 Stroop 任务中，要求参与者命名刺激词的印刷颜色。流程图显示了不一致和一致刺激的随机序列。刺激也可能被屏蔽显示，即在一致和不一致刺激的单独列表中。Stroop 任务通常还包括一个色条条件，以测量简单的颜色命名时间，并经常在刺激发生之前使用中心固定的十字（此处未显示）。

19.2.5　侧翼任务

侧翼任务（图 19.5）是注意干扰的常用度量。在侧翼任务中，需要对中央刺激做出反应，而外围侧翼则被忽略。与一致或中立条件相比，当外围侧翼与中央刺激不一致时，侧翼效应描述了性能的下降。侧翼任务的一种变体是注意网络测试（ANT），除了冲突由于侧翼不协调而产生的效果会激发警觉和定向注意力。

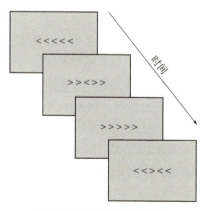

图 19.5　侧翼任务的流程图

在该侧翼任务的变体中，要求参与者用按钮指示按下中心箭头的方向（向右或向左），而忽略侧翼干扰器。此流程图显示了一致和不一致试验的随机序列。试验还可能包括中性的侧翼，并经常在刺激开始之前使用中央的十字（此处未显示）。

而一项研究发现，精神分裂症吸烟者和吸烟对照者使用 21mg 烟碱贴片后，对 ANT 的干扰控制更为有效（AhnAllen et al. 2008），其他研究未能观察到烟碱对鼻烟使用者（Lindren et al. 1996）和非吸烟者（Ettinger et al. 2017; Kleykamp et al. 2005; Wignall, De Wit, 2011）或吸烟者和非吸烟者样本（Myers et al. 2013）的侧翼干扰控制的影响。但是，Lindgren 及其同事的研究报告称，口服鼻烟后，RT 总体降低，正确反应率得到改善，这表明烟碱具有总体性能增强作用（Lindren et al. 1996）。

侧翼任务也已用于调查戒烟吸烟者的烟碱效应。一项研究发现，与自由吸烟相比，过夜戒烟后吸烟者的 RTs（通常与同伴侧翼一致性无关）较高（Schlienz, Hawk, Rosch, 2013）。在另一项研究中，与正常吸烟相比，吸烟者在戒烟期间的戒烟速度准确性降低（Schlienz, Hawk, 2017）。因此，总的来说，烟碱给药对侧翼任务的干扰控制的影响可能很小，多数研究未能报道干扰特异性作用或任何作用。

19.3　结论

总体而言，尽管有证据表明烟碱对抑制控制有有益作用，但文献却参差不齐。在反扫视任务中观察到了最一致的效果，其中大多数研究报道了错误率和/或潜伏期的改善。大多数研究还报道了对SSRT的有益影响，尤其是在受损人群中。有力的证据表明，对go/no-go任务、Stroop任务和侧翼任务对是否执行始终具有积极影响。

这些发现可能与较早的结论相吻合，即烟碱改善了注意力的更多基本功能，如警觉和定向，比注意力的选择性功能更强（Heishman et al. 2010; Provost, Woodward, 1991）。然而，应该指出的是，烟碱对基础的、自下而上的注意力处理的改善可能会导致自上而下的控制受损（Ettinger et al. 2017; Rycroft et al. 2006），这种情况很少见。这表明烟碱可能对信息处理的组成部分产生积极影响，不仅有益于基本注意功能，而且可以在自上而下的控制过程中发挥作用。

go/no-go任务、Stroop任务和侧翼任务的影响不一致的原因尚不清楚，但可能与任务因素、参与者因素、药物剂量因素以及它们之间的相互作用有关。

诸如抑制负荷、注意力负荷或一般任务复杂性之类的任务因素可能会导致跨任务的烟碱效应变化。有趣的是，反扫视和停止信号任务的效果似乎比其他任务更为一致。此问题尚未得到系统的调查。需要有选择地改变相关任务特征和抑制要求的设计。

在一些研究中发现，参与者因素在反扫视、停止信号和Stroop任务中发挥作用。这些因素包括基线表现（反扫视）、临床状况和/或冲动程度（停止信号和go/no-go）、基因型（Stroop）和吸烟状况（Stroop）。这些因素可能在解释烟碱反应的个体差异和整体结果的研究差异（考虑到研究之间参与者招募和选择的差异）方面起重要作用。

最后，在某些研究中（Larrison-Faucher et al. 2004; Poltavski, Petros, Holm, 2012）已观察到烟碱对抑制作用的剂量依赖性，但在其他研究中却未观察到（Bekker et al. 2005; Foulds et al. 1996; Kleykamp et al. 2005; Meyers et al. 2015; Parrott, Craig, 1992）。一个相关的问题是，某些烟碱给药方法比其他方法（如注射与吸烟）具有更好的滴定度，可以达到最佳剂量以满足个体参与者的需求。然而，一般而言，剂量依赖性问题值得进一步关注。此外，剂量依赖性可能与参与者和任务因素相互作用。

术语解释

- 反扫视：与突然发生的周围刺激方向相反的扫视。
- 佣金错误：对不应被回应的刺激的回应。
- 侧翼效应：在侧翼任务中，不一致条件和一致条件之间的RT差异。
- 反应时间（RT）：从刺激出现到参与者的行为反应的时间，通常以ms为单位。
- 扫视：眼睛快速的共轭运动。
- 停止信号响应时间（SSRT）：停止信号任务中停止过程的等待时间。无法直接观察到SSRT，但可以对其进行估算。

- Stroop效应：色彩词的含义对其打印颜色的响应的干扰。与打印颜色和单词不对应（如以绿色打印单词黄色）相比，当打印颜色对应于该单词（如以蓝色打印单词蓝色）时，命名打印颜色单词的颜色更快且更不易出错。

抑制控制的关键事实

- 抑制一词表示一种异质构建体，包含神经科学和心理学领域的许多不同现象。
- 在认知心理学中，抑制控制是一种关键的执行功能，是指抑制行为、思想和情感的能力。
- 在日常生活中，必须抑制不必要的反应、冲动或情绪。
- 在许多神经和精神疾病中都发现了抑制控制的不足。
- 抑制控制通常显示出良好的时间稳定性和显著的遗传力。
- 抑制控制的神经网络包括前额叶皮层及其后皮层和皮层下的投射目标。

要点总结

- 本章回顾了烟碱对人体抑制控制的影响的文献。
- 包含的抑制控制范式是反扫视、停止信号、go/no-go、Stroop和侧翼任务。
- 包括对抽烟者中受控应用（如贴剂、片剂、注射剂、锭剂、喷雾剂或口香糖）和被剥夺的吸烟者的研究。
- 大部分反扫视任务研究都显示出有益的效果。
- 在抑制性障碍人群中观察到了对停止信号任务的有益影响。
- 对go/no-go、Stroop和侧翼任务的影响不太一致。
- 总的来说，文献表明烟碱对抑制控制的影响可能是微妙的，任务、参与者和剂量因素可能起一定作用。

参考文献

AhnAllen, C. G.; Nestor, P. G.; Shenton, M. E.; McCarley, R. W.; Niznikiewicz, M. A. (2008). Early nicotine withdrawal and transdermal nicotine effects on neurocognitive performance in schizophrenia. Schizophrenia Research, 100(1), 261-269.

Ashare, R. L.; Hawk, L. W. (2012). Effects of smoking abstinence on impulsive behavior among smokers high and low in ADHD-like symptoms. Psychopharmacology, 219(2), 537-547.

Atzori, G.; Lemmonds, C. A.; Kotler, M. L.; Durcan, M. J.; Boyle, J. (2008). Efficacy of a nicotine (4mg)-containing lozenge on the cognitive impairment of nicotine withdrawal. Journal of Clinical Psychopharmacology, 28(6), 667-674.

Austin, A. J.; Duka, T.; Rusted, J.; Jackson, A. (2014). Effect of varenicline on aspects of inhibitory control in smokers. Psychopharmacology, 231(18), 3771-3785.

Azizian, A.; Nestor, L. J.; Payer, D.; Monterosso, J. R.; Brody, A. L.; London, E. D. (2010). Smoking reduces conflict-related anterior cingulate activity in abstinent cigarette smokers performing a Stroop task. Neuropsychopharmacology, 35(3), 775-782.

Barr, R. S.; Culhane, M. A.; Jubelt, L. E.; Mufti, R. S.; Dyer, M. A.; Weiss, A. P. et al. (2008). The effects of transdermal nicotine on cognition in nonsmokers with schizophrenia and nonpsychiatric controls. Neuropsychopharmacology, 33(3), 480-490.

Bekker, E. M.; Böcker, K. B. E.; Van Hunsel, F.; van den Berg, M. C.; Kenemans, J. L. (2005). Acute effects of nicotine on attention and response inhibition. Pharmacology, Biochemistry, and Behavior, 82(3), 539-548.

Bowling, A. C.; Donnelly, J. F. (2010). Effect of nicotine on saccadic eye movement latencies in non-smokers. Human Psychopharmacology, 25 (5), 410-418.

Charles-Walsh, K.; Furlong, L.; Munro, D. G.; Hester, R. (2014). Inhibitory control dysfunction in nicotine dependence and the influence of short-term abstinence. Drug and Alcohol Dependence, 143, 81-86.

Cook, M. R.; Gerkovich, M. M.; Graham, C.; Hoffman, S. J.; Peterson, R. C. (2003). Effects of the nicotine patch on performance during the first week of smoking cessation. Nicotine, Tobacco Research, 5(2), 169-180.

Dawkins, L.; Powell, J. H.; Pickering, A.; Powell, J.; West, R. (2009). Patterns of change in withdrawal symptoms, desire to smoke, reward motivation and response inhibition across 3 months of smoking abstinence. Addiction, 104(7), 850-858.

Dawkins, L.; Powell, J. H.; West, R.; Powell, J.; Pickering, A. (2007). A double-blind placebo-controlled experimental study of nicotine: II--effects on response inhibition and executive functioning. Psychopharmacology, 190(4), 457-467.

Della Casa, V.; Höfer, I.; Weiner, I.; Feldon, J. (1999). Effects of smoking status and schizotypy on latent inhibition. Journal of Psychopharmacology, 13(1), 45-57.

Dépatie, L.; O'Driscoll, G. A.; Holahan, A. -L. V.; Atkinson, V.; Thavundayil, J. X.; Kin, N. N. Y. et al. (2002). Nicotine and behavioral markers of risk for schizophrenia: a double-blind, placebo-controlled, cross-over study. Neuropsychopharmacology, 27(6), 1056-1070.

Domier, C. P.; Monterosso, J. R.; Brody, A. L.; Simon, S. L.; Mendrek, A.; Olmstead, R. et al. (2007). Effects of cigarette smoking and abstinence on stroop task performance. Psychopharmacology, 195(1), 1-9.

Ettinger, U.; Faiola, E.; Kasparbauer, A. -M.; Petrovsky, N.; Chan, R. C. K.; Liepelt, R. et al. (2017). Effects of nicotine on response inhibition and interference control. Psychopharmacology, 234(7), 1093-1111.

Ettinger, U.; Williams, S. C. R. R.; Patel, D.; Michel, T. M.; Nwaigwe, A.; Caceres, A. et al. (2009). Effects of acute nicotine on brain function in healthy smokers and non-smokers: estimation of inter-individual response heterogeneity. NeuroImage, 45(2), 549-561.

Evans, D. E.; Park, J. Y.; Maxfield, N.; Drobes, D. J. (2009). Neurocognitive variation in smoking behavior and withdrawal: genetic and affective moderators. Genes, Brain and Behavior, 8(1), 86-96.

Evins, A. E.; Deckersbach, T.; Cather, C.; Freudenreich, O.; Culhane, M. A.; Henderson, D. C. et al. (2005). Independent effects of tobacco abstinence and bupropion on cognitive function in schizophrenia. Journal of Clinical Psychiatry, 66(9), 1184-1190.

Foulds, J.; Stapleton, J.; Swettenham, J.; Bell, N.; McSorley, K.; Russell, M. A. (1996). Cognitive performance effects of subcutaneous nicotine in smokers and never-smokers. Psychopharmacology, 127(1), 31-38.

George, T.; Vessicchio, J. C.; Termine, A.; Sahady, D. M.; Head, C. A.; Pepper, W. T. et al. (2002). Effects of smoking abstinence on visuospatial working memory function in schizophrenia. Neuropsychopharmacology, 26(1), 75-85.

Giessing, C.; Thiel, C. M.; Alexander-Bloch, A. F.; Patel, A. X.; Bullmore, E. T. (2013). Human brain functional network changesassociated with enhanced and impaired attentional task performance. Journal of Neuroscience, 33(14), 5903-5914.

Grundey, J.; Amu, R.; Ambrus, G. G.; Batsikadze, G.; Paulus, W.; Nitsche, M. A. (2015). Double dissociation of working memoryand attentional processes in smokers and non-smokers with and without nicotine. Psychopharmacology, 232(14), 2491-2501.

Harrison, E. L. R.; Coppola, S.; McKee, S. A. (2009). Nicotine deprivation and trait impulsivity affect smokers' performance on cognitive tasks of inhibition and attention. Experimental and Clinical Psychopharmacology, 17(2), 91-98.

Hasenfratz, M.; Bättig, K. (1992). Action profiles of smoking and caffeine: Stroop effect, EEG, and peripheral physiology. Pharmacology, Biochemistry, and Behavior, 42(1), 155-161.

Heishman, S. J.; Kleykamp, B. A.; Singleton, E. G. (2010). Meta-analysis of the acute effects of nicotine and smoking on human performance. Psychopharmacology, 210(4), 453-469.

Houlihan, M. E.; Pritchard, W. S.; Krieble, K. K.; Robinson, J. H.; Duke, D. W. (1996). Effects of cigarette smoking on EEG spectralband power, dimensional complexity, and nonlinearity during reaction-time task performance. Psychophysiology, 33(6), 740-746.

Ilan, A. B.; Polich, J. (2001). Tobacco smoking and event-related brain potentials in a Stroop task. International Journal of Psychophysiology, 40 (2), 109-118.

Jensen, K. P.; DeVito, E. E.; Herman, A. I.; Valentine, G. W.; Gelernter, J.; Sofuoglu, M. (2015). A CHRNA5 smoking risk variant decreases the aversive effects of nicotine in humans. Neuropsychopharmacology, 40(12), 2813-2821.

Kleykamp, B. A.; Jennings, J. M.; Blank, M. D.; Eissenberg, T. (2005). The effects of nicotine on attention and working memory in neversmokers. Psychology of Addictive Behaviors, 19(4), 433-438.

Kos, J.; Hasenfratz, M.; Bättig, K. (1997). Effects of a 2-day abstinence from smoking on dietary, cognitive, subjective, and physiologic parameters among younger and older female smokers. Physiology, Behavior, 61(5), 671-678.

Kozink, R. V.; Kollins, S. H.; McClernon, F. J. (2010). Smoking withdrawal modulates right inferior frontal cortex but not presupplementary motor area activation during inhibitory control. Neuropsychopharmacology, 35(13), 2600-2606.

Landers, D. M.; Crews, D. J.; Boutcher, S. H.; Skinner, J. S.; Gustafsen, S. (1992). The effects of smokeless tobacco on performance and psychophysiological response. Medicine and Science in Sports and Exercise, 24(8), 895-903.

Larrison, A. L.; Briand, K. A.; Sereno, A. B. (2004). Nicotine improves antisaccade task performance without affecting prosaccades. Human Psychopharmacology, 19(6), 409-419.

Larrison-Faucher, A. L.; Matorin, A. A.; Sereno, A. B. (2004). Nicotine reduces antisaccade errors in task impaired schizophrenic subjects. Progress in Neuro-Psychopharmacology, Biological Psychiatry, 28(3), 505-516.

Levin, E. D.; Conners, C. K.; Sparrow, E.; Hinton, S. C.; Erhardt, D.; Meck, W. H. et al. (1996). Nicotine effects on adults with attentiondeficit/ hyperactivity disorder. Psychopharmacology, 123(1), 55-63.

Lindgren, M.; Stenberg, G.; Rosen, I. (1996). Effects of nicotine in visual attention tasks. Human Psychopharmacology: Clinical and Experimental, 11(1), 47-51.

Logemann, H. N. A.; Böcker, K. B. E.; Deschamps, P. K. H.; Kemner, C.; Kenemans, J. L. (2014a). Differences between nicotine-abstinent smokers and non-smokers in terms of visuospatial attention and inhibition before and after single-blind nicotine administration. Neuroscience, 277, 375-382.

Logemann, H. N. A.; Böcker, K. B. E.; Deschamps, P. K. H.; Kemner, C.; Kenemans, J. L. (2014b). The effect of enhancing cholinergic neurotransmission by nicotine on EEG indices of inhibition in the human brain. Pharmacology Biochemistry and Behavior, 122, 89-96.

Mancuso, G.; Warburton, D. M.; Melen, M.; Sherwood, N.; Tirelli, E. (1999). Selective effects of nicotine on attentional processes. Psychopharmacology, 146(2), 199-204.

McClernon, F. J.; Kollins, S. H.; Lutz, A. M.; Fitzgerald, D. P.; Murray, D. W.; Redman, C. et al. (2008). Effects of smoking abstinence on adult smokers with and without attention deficit hyperactivity disorder: results of a preliminary study. Psychopharmacology, 197(1), 95-105.

Meyers, K. K.; Crane, N. A.; O'Day, R.; Zubieta, J. K.; Giordani, B.; Pomerleau, C. S. et al. (2015). Smoking history, and not depression, is related to deficits in detection of happy and sad faces. Addictive Behaviors, 41, 210-217.

Myers, C. S.; Taylor, R. C.; Salmeron, B. J.; Waters, A. J.; Heishman, S. J. (2013). Nicotine enhances alerting, but not executive, attention in smokers and nonsmokers. Nicotine, Tobacco Research, 15(1), 277-281.

Parrott, A. C.; Craig, D. (1992). Cigarette smoking and nicotine gum (0, 2 and 4mg): effects upon four visual attention tasks. Neuropsychobiology, 25(1), 34-43.

Petrovsky, N.; Ettinger, U.; Quednow, B. B.; Landsberg, M. W.; Drees, J.; Lennertz, L. et al. (2013). Nicotine enhances antisaccade performance in schizophrenia patients and healthy controls. International Journal of Neuropsychopharmacology, 16(7), 1473-1481.

Petrovsky, N.; Ettinger, U.; Quednow, B. B.; Walter, H.; Schnell, K.; Kessler, H. et al. (2012). Nicotine differentially modulates antisaccade performance in healthy male non-smoking volunteers stratified for low and high accuracy. Psychopharmacology, 221(1), 27-38.

Pettiford, J.; Kozink, R. V.; Lutz, A. M.; Kollins, S. H.; Rose, J. E.; McClernon, F. J. (2007). Increases in impulsivity following smoking abstinence are related to baseline nicotine intake and boredom susceptibility. Addictive Behaviors, 32(10), 2351-2357.

Poltavski, D. V.; Petros, T. (2006). Effects of transdermal nicotine on attention in adult non-smokers with and without attentional deficits. Physiology, Behavior, 87(3), 614-624.

Poltavski, D. V.; Petros, T. V.; Holm, J. E. (2012). Lower but not higher doses of transdermal nicotine facilitate cognitive performance in smokers on gender non-preferred tasks. Pharmacology Biochemistry and Behavior, 102(3), 423-433.

Pomerleau, C. S.; Teuscher, F.; Goeters, S.; Pomerleau, O. F. (1994). Effects of nicotine abstinence and menstrual phase on task performance. Addictive Behaviors, 19(4), 357-362.

Potter, A. S.; Bucci, D. J.; Newhouse, P. A. (2012). Manipulation of nicotinic acetylcholine receptors differentially affects behavioral inhibition in human subjects with and without disordered baseline impulsivity. Psychopharmacology, 220(2), 331-340.

Potter, A. S.; Newhouse, P. A. (2004). Effects of acute nicotine administration on behavioral inhibition in adolescents with attentiondeficit/hyperactivity disorder. Psychopharmacology, 176(2), 182-194.

Potter, A. S.; Newhouse, P. A. (2008). Acute nicotine improves cognitive deficits in young adults with attention-deficit/hyperactivity disorder. Pharmacology Biochemistry and Behavior, 88(4), 407-417.

Powell, J.; Dawkins, L.; Davis, R. E. (2002). Smoking, reward responsiveness, and response inhibition: tests of an incentive motivational model. Biological Psychiatry, 51(2), 151-163.

Provost, S. C.; Woodward, R. (1991). Effects of nicotine gum on repeated administration of the stroop test. Psychopharmacology, 104 (4), 536-540.

Rusted, J. M.; Caulfield, D.; King, L.; Goode, A. (2000). Moving out of the laboratory: does nicotine improve everyday attention? Behavioural Pharmacology, 11(7-8), 621-629.

Rycroft, N.; Hutton, S. B.; Clowry, O.; Groomsbridge, C.; Sierakowski, A.; Rusted, J. M. (2007). Non-cholinergic modulation of antisaccade performance: a modafinil-nicotine comparison. Psychopharmacology, 195(2), 245-253.

Rycroft, N.; Hutton, S. B.; Rusted, J. M. (2006). The antisaccade task as an index of sustained goal activation in working memory: modulation by nicotine. Psychopharmacology, 188(4), 521-529.

Schlienz, N. J.; Hawk, L. W. (2017). Probing the behavioral and neurophysiological effects of acute smoking abstinence on drug and nondrug reinforcement during a cognitive task. Nicotine, Tobacco Research, 19(6), 729-737.

Schlienz, N. J.; Hawk, L. W.; Rosch, K. S. (2013). The effects of acute abstinence from smoking and performance-based rewards on performance monitoring. Psychopharmacology, 229(4), 701-711.

Schmechtig, A.; Lees, J.; Grayson, L.; Craig, K. J.; Dadhiwala, R.; Dawson, G. R. et al. (2013). Effects of risperidone, amisulpride and nicotine on eye movement control and their modulation by schizotypy. Psychopharmacology, 227(2), 331-345.

Smucny, J.; Olincy, A.; Eichman, L. S.; Tregellas, J. R. (2015). Neuronal effects of nicotine during auditory selective attention. Psychopharmacology, 232(11), 2017-2028.

Suter, T. W.; Buzzi, R.; Woodson, P. P.; Bättig, K. (1983). Psychophysiological correlates of conflict solving and cigarette smoking. Activitas Nervosa Superior, 25(4), 261-272.

Thaker, G. K.; Ellsberry, R.; Moran, M.; Lahti, A.; Tamminga, C. (1991). Tobacco smoking increases square-wave jerks during pursuit eye movements. Biological Psychiatry, 29(1), 82-88.

Tsaur, S.; Strasser, A. A.; Souprountchouk, V.; Evans, G. C.; Ashare, R. L. (2015). Time dependency of craving and response inhibition during nicotine abstinence. Addiction Research and Theory, 23(3), 205-212.

Wachter, N. J.; Gilbert, D. G. (2013). Nicotine differentially modulates antisaccade eye-gaze away from emotional stimuli in nonsmokers stratified by pre-task baseline performance. Psychopharmacology, 225(3), 561-568.

Wesnes, K.; Revell, A. (1984). The separate and combined effects of scopolamine and nicotine on human information processing. Psychopharmacology, 84(1), 5-11.

Wesnes, K.; Warburton, D. M. (1978). The effect of cigarette smoking and nicotine tablets upon human attention. In R. E. Thornton (Ed.), Smoking behaviour: Physiological and psychological influences (pp. 131-147). Edinburgh: Churchill Livingstone.

Wignall, N. D.; DeWit, H. (2011). Effects of nicotine on attention and inhibitory control in healthy nonsmokers. Experimental and Clinical Psychopharmacology, 19(3), 183-191.

Xu, X.; Domino, E. F. (2000). Effects of tobacco smoking on topographic EEG and Stroop test in smoking deprived smokers. Progress in Neuro-Psychopharmacology, Biological Psychiatry, 24(4), 535-546.

Xu, J.; Mendrek, A.; Cohen, M. S.; Monterosso, J.; Simon, S.; Jarvik, M. et al. (2007). Effect of cigarette smoking on prefrontal cortical function in nondeprived smokers performing the Stroop task. Neuropsychopharmacology, 32(6), 1421-1428.

Zack, M.; Belsito, L.; Scher, R.; Eissenberg, T.; Corrigall, W. A. (2001). Effects of abstinence and smoking on information processing in adolescent smokers. Psychopharmacology, 153(2), 249-257.

20
烟碱、促肾上腺皮质激素释放因子和焦虑样行为

Adriaan W. Bruijnzeel

Department of Psychiatry, University of Florida, Gainesville, FL, United States

缩略语

CeA	中央杏仁核	**ICSS**	颅内自我刺激
CRF	促肾上腺皮质激素释放因子	**IPN**	脚间核
CRF1	促肾上腺皮质激素释放因子1型受体	**PVN**	下丘脑室旁核
CRF2	促肾上腺皮质激素释放因子2型受体	**VTA**	腹侧被盖区

20.1 引言

烟草成瘾的特征是失去对吸烟的控制和强烈的渴望，并且在戒烟后会出现负面的情感性戒断症状。全世界大约有10亿烟民，并且绝大多数人希望戒烟（WHO, 2011）。西方社会的吸烟率正在下降（WHO, 2015）。吸烟的人越来越少，戒烟的人越来越多（Kulik, Glantz, 2016）。在20世纪90年代末，近25%的美国成年人吸烟，而在2014年，这一比例还不到16%（Clarke, Norris, Schiller, 2017）。在受过高等教育、富裕的人群中，吸烟率的下降尤为明显。然而，在经济弱势群体和精神疾病患者中，吸烟率仍然很高（Bruijnzeel, 2017; de Leon et al.2002; Hughes et al. 1986）。Hughes及其同事是最早调查精神病患者吸烟率的人之一（Hughes et al. 1986）。他们报道称，几乎90%的精神分裂症患者和50%的抑郁症患者吸烟。患有焦虑症也会增加吸烟的风险。一项针对青少年的大型研究表明，在以后的生活中，有社交恐惧症的非吸烟者和非独立吸烟者依赖烟碱的风险增加（Sonntag et al. 2000）。

临床研究表明，吸烟、抑郁和焦虑症之间存在关联（Bruijnzeel, 2012）。对来自新西兰的儿童进行的一项研究表明，青少年和年轻人的抑郁与烟碱依赖性之间存在很强的联系（Fergusson, Goodwin, Horwood, 2003）。这与美国另一项调查吸烟、抑郁和焦虑症之间的关系的大型研究一致（Johnson et al. 2000）。在这项研究中，青少年在16岁（1985—1986）和22岁时接受了采访。16岁时抑郁会增加在同一发育阶段对烟碱依赖的风险。在此期间，青少年时期的焦虑症与吸烟之间没有关联。但是，在青春期大量吸烟（每天吸烟超过20支）会增加成年后患恐惧症、广泛性焦虑症和恐慌症的风险。这表明青春期吸烟会诱发大脑变化，从而增加以后生活中患焦虑症的可能性。尝试戒烟时，患有焦虑症也会增加复发的风险。焦虑敏感性高的吸烟者比焦虑敏感性低的吸烟者更容易戒烟（Zvolensky et al. 2017）。

总的来说，戒烟会导致焦虑的增加，从而导致吸烟的复发（Bruijnzeel, 2012）。吸烟者比不吸烟者更容易患焦虑症，患有焦虑症的烟民戒烟动机更弱（Johnson et al. 2000; Zvolensky et al. 2007）。在本章的概述中，将讨论CRF在烟碱戒断引起的焦虑样行为中的作用。

20.2 促肾上腺皮质激素释放因子（CRF）

促肾上腺皮质激素释放因子在调节下丘脑-垂体-肾上腺（HPA）轴、对应激的自主反应和行为中发挥作用。CRF在下丘脑产生并转运至中位隆起。在门脉循环中释放后，它刺激垂体前叶释放前体阿黑皮素（POMC）的神经肽类激素（如ACTH）。ACTH刺激糖皮质激素从肾上腺皮质释放。CRF也在下丘脑外脑部位表达。在中央杏仁核（CeA）、纹状体尾部（BNST）、蓝斑核、臂旁核、背迷走神经复合体和前额叶皮层均检测到CRF阳性细胞（Swanson et al. 1983）。有研究表明，应激源可诱导下丘脑和CeA释放CRF（Cook, 2004; Hand et al. 2002; Merali et al. 1998; Merlo Pich et al. 1993）。

尿皮质素1是被发现的CRF受体家族的第二个成员（Vaughan et al. 1995）。尿皮质素1在大脑中的分布与CRF有很大的不同。尿皮质素1在动眼神经副核和外侧上橄榄体中表达。从动眼神经副核到外侧上橄榄体的尿皮质素1投射可能介导焦虑样行为（Radulovic et al. 1999）。在外周也检测到了高水平的尿皮质素1。尿皮质素1在胃肠道、肾上腺和睾丸中表达（Oki et al. 1998）。最近发现的CRF家族成员是尿皮质素2和尿皮质素3（Hauger et al. 2003; Hsu, Hsueh, 2001; Lewis et al. 2001; Reyes et al. 2001）。已在蓝斑核、下丘脑室旁核（PVN）和弓状核中检测到尿皮质素2。在胃肠道、肾上腺、心脏、血细胞和睾丸中也检测到高水平的尿皮质素2（Hsu, Hsueh, 2001）。已在下丘脑、脑干、侧间隔、BNST、胃肠道、肾上腺和皮肤中检测到尿皮质素3（Hsu, Hsueh, 2001; Lewis et al. 2001）。

20.3 促肾上腺皮质激素释放因子受体

在垂体前叶、杏仁核、大脑皮层和海马体中已检测到CRF结合位点（De Souza et al. 1985; De Souza, Perrin, Rivier, Vale, Kuhar, 1984）。在发现CRF结合位点十年后，克隆了两个CRF受体（Chen, Lewis, Perrin, Vale, 1993; Lovenberg, Liaw et al. 1995; Perrin, Donaldson, Chen, Lewis, Vale, 1993）。CRF1受体在垂体前叶表达并调节HPA轴活性。CRF1受体也在皮层区域、海马和基底外侧杏仁核中表达（Potter et al. 1994）。CRF2受体主要表达于皮层下脑区域，包括侧间核、PVN和下丘脑腹内侧核（Lovenberg, Chalmers, Liu, De Souza, 1995）。CRF和尿皮质素1以高亲和力结合CRF1受体，并且尿皮质素1也以高亲和力结合CRF2受体（Vaughan et al. 1995）。尿皮质素2和尿皮质素3对CRF1受体的亲和力低，对CRF2受体的亲和力高（Lewis et al. 2001）。

20.4 研究烟碱戒断引起的焦虑样行为的动物模型

已开发出广泛的动物模型来研究烟碱戒断引起的焦虑样行为。在大多数研究中，对通过渗透性微型泵或注射非连续性烟碱给药的大鼠或小鼠的焦虑样行为进行了研究（Epping-Jordan et al. 1998; Malin, 2001）。在小鼠的研究中，烟碱经常被添加到饮用水中以诱导依赖（Grabus et al. 2005）。有大量证据表明，可以通过非连续性烟碱给药来建立烟碱依赖性。在停止使用泵或注射剂烟碱给药后，在大鼠和小鼠中观察到自发的和沉淀的躯体体征（Epping-Jordan et al. 1998; Malin, 2001）。在停止口服烟碱后，小鼠体内也有体征（Grabus et al. 2005）。颅内自我刺激

(ICSS)范例已被广泛用于研究与烟碱戒断相关的快感不足。在此过程中,将电极植入前脑内侧束中,大鼠可以在手术室中自我刺激其奖励系统。停止给予烟碱会导致快感不足,这反映在大脑奖励阈值的升高上。停止给予烟碱后,大鼠对奖励性电刺激的敏感性降低,因此需要更高的电流来维持ICSS行为。停止非连续性烟碱给药会导致大鼠和小鼠的大脑奖励阈值升高(即快感不足)(Epping-Jordan et al. 1998; Johnson, Hollander, Kenny, 2008)。停止给予烟碱也已显示出增加大鼠和小鼠的焦虑样行为。Damaj及其同事表明,停止给予烟碱[24mg/(kg·d)和48mg/(kg·d),共14d,微型泵]会导致烟碱、促肾上腺皮质激素释放因子和焦虑样行为,同时增加了小鼠在高架迷宫测试中的焦虑样行为(Damaj, Kao, Martin, 2003)。较低的烟碱剂量[6mg/(kg·d)]不会引起依赖性,也不会增加焦虑样行为。在这项研究中,研究了停止烟碱给药24h后的焦虑样行为。与此类似,在停止慢性烟碱给药(注射7d或14d)后72h,大鼠在社交互动测试中显示出更多的焦虑样行为(Irvine, Cheeta, File, 1999)。大多数研究调查了停止非连续性烟碱自给药后大鼠和小鼠的焦虑样行为。然而,一些研究也研究了烟碱自给药后的焦虑样行为。Irvine及其同事在停止烟碱自给药4周后的0h、24h和72h的社交互动测试中研究了焦虑样行为(Irvine et al. 2001)。在最后一次自给药后,大鼠表现出增加的焦虑样行为,但在24h或48h后不再表现出这种症状。这表明慢性烟碱自给药会增加焦虑样行为,但停止烟碱自给药不会增加焦虑样行为。最近的研究表明,在停止烟碱自给药后,大鼠是否表现出焦虑样行为取决于烟碱自给药的范式。Cohen及其同事研究了短期和长期烟碱自给药停止后大鼠的焦虑样行为(Cohen et al. 2015)。短期访问的大鼠每天1h自给药烟碱,长期访问的大鼠每天21h自给药烟碱。在这项研究中,大鼠被允许自给药烟碱14周,并且在最后一次自给药后72h调查焦虑样行为。停止长期烟碱自给药后,大鼠表现出焦虑样行为,但停止短期烟碱自给药则没有。长期接触的大鼠在烟碱自给药停止后表现出躯体戒断迹象,而短期接触的大鼠则没有。这表明烟碱自给药在长期范式下会导致依赖,而在短期范式下则不会。这表明,只有发展出烟碱依赖的老鼠,在烟碱自给药停止后,才会表现出焦虑样行为。

20.5 促肾上腺皮质激素释放因子、烟碱戒断和焦虑症

一些关于CRF的初步研究表明,它会增加焦虑样行为(Dunn, File, 1987; Swerdlow, Geyer, Vale, Koob, 1986)。CRF主要通过激活CRF1受体来介导焦虑样行为。已在大脑和血脑屏障外部(如胃肠道和垂体前叶)发现了CRF1受体(Van Pett et al. 2000; Yuan et al. 2012)。最近的一项研究表明,CRF诱导的焦虑样行为的增加是由大脑中的CRF1受体介导的,而不是由血脑屏障外部的CRF1受体介导的(Tanaka et al. 2017)。停止烟碱给药后,CRF还有助于产生焦虑样行为。Cohen及其同事发现,长时间服用烟碱(21h)的大鼠在最后一次自给药后72h显示出焦虑样行为(Cohen et al. 2015)。全身性和CeA内CRF1受体拮抗剂MPZP的给药可以阻止这种焦虑样行为的增加。

缰核-脚间核回路在调节情绪状态和药物成瘾中起着至关重要的作用(Hikosaka 2010)。内侧缰核接受来自隔膜和斜角带核的输入,并通过后屈束连接到脚间核(IPN)。缰核和IPN在烟碱依赖性的发展中发挥作用。nAChR在烟碱依赖小鼠的缰核和IPN中的阻滞导致躯体戒断症状(Salas, Sturm, Boulter, De, 2009)。此外,在缰核中表达超灵敏α6/α4β2 nAChR的小鼠比对照小鼠更焦虑(Pang et al. 2016)。Zhao-Shea及其同事探讨了CRF在烟碱戒断期间焦虑样行为中的缰核-

脚间核回路中的作用（Zhao-Shea et al. 2015）。他们报道称，IPN中的CRF释放介导了焦虑样行为。IPN中CRF的输注增加了焦虑样行为，而IPN中CRF1受体的阻滞减少了烟碱戒断所引起的焦虑样行为。用短发夹RNA降低腹侧被盖区（VTA）中的CRF水平，可减少烟碱戒断所致IPN的激活和焦虑样行为。这表明烟碱摄入停止后焦虑样行为的增加是由从VTA到IPN的CRF投射的激活介导的。VTA中的CRF受体也与可卡因在大鼠中的致焦虑作用有关（Ettenberg et al. 2015）。总体而言，这些发现表明CRF在VTA和IPN中的传输有助于具有药物摄入史的动物的焦虑样行为。

20.6 CRF2受体在烟碱戒断中的作用

Bagosi和他的同事研究了CRF2受体在烟碱戒断中的作用。给小鼠注射烟碱7d，在最后一次注射24h后，研究烟碱戒断对焦虑和抑郁样行为的影响（Bagosi et al. 2016）。摄入烟碱的小鼠在升高的迷宫测试中表现出增加的焦虑样行为，在强迫游泳测试中表现出抑郁样行为。尿皮质素2或尿皮质素3的中枢给药阻止了烟碱戒断引起的焦虑和抑郁样行为增加。CRF2受体激动剂的使用也减少了烟碱戒断小鼠皮质酮水平的升高。刺激CRF2受体可以减少酒精戒断期间的焦虑样行为，这与研究结果一致（Valdez, Sabino, Koob, 2004）。应当指出，并非所有研究都发现对CRF2受体的刺激会减少与停药有关的焦虑样行为。一项研究报道称，用antisauvagine-30（拮抗剂）阻断CRF2受体可减少苯丙胺戒断期间的焦虑样行为（Reinbold et al. 2014）。同样，CRF2受体敲除小鼠在阿片类药物戒断期间不表现出快感缺乏样状态（Ingallinesi et al. 2012）。因此，关于CRF2受体在药物戒断中的作用的研究结果相互矛盾。然而，所讨论的研究表明，刺激CRF2受体可能减少与烟碱和酒精戒断有关的焦虑和抑郁样行为。

20.7 与烟碱戒断有关的CRF和快感缺乏

我们实验室探究了CRF在烟碱戒断引起的快感缺乏中的作用。在我们的第一个实验中，我们研究了阻断CRF1和CRF2受体是否会降低与烟碱戒断相关的脑阈值的升高。(Bruijnzeel et al. 2007)。中枢（icv）给予非选择性CRF1/CRF2受体拮抗剂 D-Phe CRF$_{(12-41)}$减少了美加明引起的大脑奖励阈值升高。在后续实验中，研究了CRF1和CRF2受体在与沉淀的烟碱戒断相关的快感缺乏症中的作用（Bruijnzeel, Prado, Isaac, 2009）。CRF1受体被R278995/CRA0450阻断，CRF2受体被astressin 2B阻断。受体阻断CRF1，而不是CRF2，阻止了与烟碱戒断相关的大脑奖励阈值的升高。这些发现表明，CRF1受体在与戒烟有关的快感缺乏症中发挥作用。然后，研究人员研究了大脑的调节介导了烟碱戒断有关的快感缺乏的大脑区域（Marcinkiewcz et al. 2009）。非选择性CRF受体拮抗剂 D-Phe CRF$_{(12-41)}$进入CeA和NAcc壳层可防止烟碱依赖性大鼠的脑奖励阈值升高。相反，在BNST中阻断CRF1/CRF2受体是无效的。为了研究CeA中的CRF1受体是否在烟碱戒断中发挥作用，我们使用选择性CRF1受体拮抗剂 R278995/CRA0450进行了一项研究（Bruijnzeel et al. 2012）。我们发现，CeA中CRF1受体的阻滞减少了与烟碱戒断相关的快感不足。总体而言，这些研究表明，CeA和Nacc壳层中的CRF信号在与烟碱戒断相关的消极情绪状态中发挥作用。

20.8 结论

临床研究表明，吸烟与焦虑之间存在正相关关系，而高水平的焦虑会导致复发。回顾的动物研究表明，停止非持续性烟碱给药和停止长期烟碱自给药会导致焦虑样行为的增加。长时间暴露于烟碱会使大脑CRF系统失调，对CRF1受体的阻滞或对CRF2受体的刺激会减少与烟碱戒断相关的焦虑样行为。因此，阻断CRF1受体或刺激CRF2受体的药物可以减少戒烟过程中的焦虑，从而降低复发的风险。

术语解释
- 成瘾性脑部疾病：其特征是失去对药物使用的控制，并在停止使用药物后出现戒断症状。
- 快感缺乏：情绪低落，使人们无法享受愉悦。它是抑郁症的核心症状之一。
- 促肾上腺皮质激素释放因子（CRF）：在大脑中产生的神经肽，在应激反应、焦虑和抑郁中起重要作用。
- 颅内自我刺激（ICSS）：一种用于确定啮齿动物大脑奖励系统状态的方法。
- 大鼠药物自给药：其中使用大鼠静脉内置导管制备大鼠以研究滥用药物的积极增强作用。

吸烟的关键事实
- 全世界大约有10亿人吸烟。
- 当人们停止吸烟时，他们会感到焦虑和沮丧，并有强烈的吸烟冲动。
- 大多数人需要经过几次尝试才能戒烟。
- 在20世纪30年代，科学家开始意识到吸烟对健康有不利影响。
- 戒烟有几种治疗方法，但是复发率仍然很高。
- 富裕的健康人群中的吸烟率正在下降，但是精神疾病患者更难以戒烟。

要点总结
- 本章重点介绍CRF在与烟碱戒断相关的焦虑和抑郁样行为中的作用。
- 在精神疾病患者中吸烟更为普遍。
- 停止烟碱给药会导致焦虑和抑郁样行为的增加。
- CRF释放的增加有助于烟碱戒断期间的焦虑和抑郁样行为。
- CRF通过与CRF1和CRF2受体结合来介导其在大脑中的作用。
- 阻断CRF1受体可减少与烟碱戒断相关的焦虑和抑郁样行为。
- 刺激CRF2受体可减少与烟碱戒断相关的焦虑和抑郁样行为。

致谢

A.B.在撰写本章时，获得了美国国立卫生研究院国家药物滥用研究所的支持，证书编号为R01DA042530。

参考文献

Bagosi, Z.;Palotai, M.;Simon, B.; Bokor, P.;Buzás, A.;Balangó, B. et al. (2016). Selective CRF2 receptor agonists ameliorate the anxiety- and depression-like state developed during chronic nicotinetreatment and consequent acute withdrawal in mice. Brain Research, 1652, 2 1-29.

Bruijnzeel, A. W. (2012). Tobacco addiction and the dysregulation of brain stress systems. Neuroscience and Biobehavioral Reviews, 36, 1418-1441.

Bruijnzeel, A. W. (2017). Reducing the prevalence of smoking: policy measures and focusing on specific populations. Nicotine, Tobacco Research 19, 1003-1004.

Bruijnzeel, A. W.; Ford, J.; Rogers, J. A.; Scheick, S.; Ji, Y.; Bishnoi, M. et al. (2012). Blockade of CRF1 receptors in the central nucleus of the amygdala attenuates the dysphoria associated with nicotine withdrawal in rats. Pharmacology, Biochemistry, and Behavior, 101(1), 62-68.

Bruijnzeel, A. W.; Prado, M.; Isaac, S. (2009). Corticotropin-releasing factor-1 receptor activation mediates nicotine withdrawal-induced deficit in brain reward function and stress-induced relapse. Biological Psychiatry, 66, 110-117.

Bruijnzeel, A. W.; Zislis, G.; Wilson, C.; Gold, M. S. (2007). Antago-nism of CRF receptors prevents the deficit in brain reward function associated with precipitated nicotine withdrawal in rats. Neuropsy-chopharmacology, 32(4), 955-963.

Chen, R.; Lewis, K. A.; Perrin, M. H.; Vale, W. W. (1993). Expression cloning of a human corticotropin-releasing-factor receptor. Proceedings of the National Academy of Sciences of the United States of America, 90(19), 8967-8971.

Clarke, T. C.; Norris, T.; Schiller, J. S. (2017). Early release of selected estimates based on data from the 2016 National Health Interview Survey. National Center for Health Statistics. Retrieved from: https://www. cdc. gov/nchs/data/nhis/earlyrelease/earlyrelease201705. pdf.

Cohen, A.; Treweek, J.; Edwards, S.; Leao, R. M.; Schulteis, G.; Koob, G. F. et al. (2015). Extended access to nicotine leads to a CRF1 receptor dependent increase in anxiety-like behavior and hyperalgesia in rats. Addiction Biology, 20(1), 56-68.

Cook, C. J. (2004). Stress induces CRF release in the paraventricular nucleus, and both CRF and GABA release in the amygdala. Physiol-ogy, Behavior, 82(4), 751-762.

Damaj, M. I.; Kao, W.; Martin, B. R. (2003). Characterization of spontaneous and precipitated nicotine withdrawal in the mouse. The Journal of Pharmacology and Experimental Therapeutics, 307(2), 526-534.

de Leon, J.; Diaz, F. J.; Rogers, T.; Browne, D.; Dinsmore, L. (2002). Initiation of daily smoking and nicotine dependence in schizophrenia and mood disorders. Schizophrenia Research, 56(1), 47-54.

De Souza, E. B.; Insel, T. R.; Perrin, M. H.; Rivier, J.; Vale, W. W.; Kuhar, M. J. (1985). Corticotropin-releasing factor receptors are widely distributed within the rat central nervous system: an autoradiographic study. The Journal of Neuroscience, 5(12), 3189-3203.

De Souza, E. B.; Perrin, M. H.; Rivier, J.; Vale, W. W.; Kuhar, M. J. (1984). Corticotropin-releasing factor receptors in rat pituitary gland: autoradiographic localization. Brain Research, 296(1), 202-207.

Dunn, A. J.; File, S. E. (1987). Corticotropin-releasing factor has an anxiogenic action in the social interaction test. Hormones and Behavior, 21(2), 193-202.

Epping-Jordan, M. P.; Watkins, S. S.; Koob, G. F.; Markou, A. (1998). Dramatic decreases in brain reward function during nicotine withdrawal. Nature, 393(6680), 76-79.

Ettenberg, A.; Cotten, S. W.; Brito, M. A.; Klein, A. K.; Ohana, T. A.; Margolin, B. et al. (2015). CRF antagonism within the ventral tegmental area but not the extended amygdala attenuates the anxio-genic effects of cocaine in rats. Pharmacology, Biochemistry, and Behavior, 138, 148-155.

Fergusson, D. M.; Goodwin, R. D.; Horwood, L. J. (2003). Major depression and cigarette smoking: results of a 21-year longitudinal study. Psychological Medicine, 33(8), 1357-1367.

Grabus, S. D.; Martin, B. R.; Batman, A. M.; Tyndale, R. F.; Sellers, E.; Damaj, M. I. (2005). Nicotine physical dependence and tolerance in the mouse following chronic oral administration. Psychopharmacol-ogy, 178(2-3), 183-192.

Hand, G. A.; Hewitt, C. B.; Fulk, L. J.; Stock, H. S.; Carson, J. A.; Davis, J M. et al. (2002). Differential release of corticotropin-releasing hormone (CRH) in the amygdala during different types of stressors. Brain Research, 949(1-2), 122-130.

Hauger, R. L.; Grigoriadis, D. E.; Dallman, M. F.; Plotsky, P. M.; Vale, W. W.; Dautzenberg, F. M. (2003). International Union of Pharmacol- ogy. XXXVI. Current status of the nomenclature for receptors forcorticotropin-releasing factor and their ligands. Pharmacological Reviews, 55(1), 21-26.

Hikosaka, O. (2010). The habenula: from stress evasion to value-based decision-making. Nature Reviews Neuroscience, 11(7), 503-513.

Hsu, S. Y.; Hsueh, A. J. (2001). Human stresscopin and stress copin related peptide are selective ligands for the type 2 corticotropin-releasing hormone receptor. Nature Medicine, 7(5), 605-611.

Hughes, J. R.; Hatsukami, D. K.; Mitchell, J. E.; Dahlgren, L. A. (1986). Prevalence of smoking among psychiatric outpatients. The American Journal of Psychiatry, 143(8), 993-997.

Ingallinesi, M.; Rouibi, K.; Le Moine, C.; Papaleo, F.; Contarino, A. (2012). CRF2 receptor-deficiency eliminates opiate withdrawal distress without impairing stress coping. Molecular Psy-chiatry, 17(12), 1283.

Irvine, E.; Bagnalasta, M.; Marcon, C.; Motta, C.; Tessari, M.; File, S. et al. (2001). Nicotine self-administration and withdrawal: modula-tion of anxiety in the social interaction test in rats. Psychopharmacol-ogy, 153(3), 315-320.

Irvine, E. E.; Cheeta, S.; File, S. E. (1999). Time-course of changes in the social interaction test of anxiety following acute and chronic admin-istration of nicotine. Behavioural Pharmacology, 10(6-7), 691-697.

Johnson, J. G.; Cohen, P.; Pine, D. S.; Klein, D. F.; Kasen, S.; Brook, J. S. (2000). Association between cigarette smoking and anxiety disor- ders during adolescence and early adulthood. JAMA, 284(18), 2348-2351.

Johnson, P. M.; Hollander, J. A.; Kenny, P. J. (2008). Decreased brain reward function during nicotine withdrawal in C57BL6 mice: evidence from intracranial self-stimulation (ICSS) studies. Pharmacol-ogy, Biochemistry, and Behavior, 90(3), 409-415.

Kulik, M. C.; Glantz, S. A. (2016). The smoking population in the USA and EU is softening not hardening. Tobacco Control, 25(4), 470-475.

Lewis, K.; Li, C.; Perrin, M. H.; Blount, A.; Kunitake, K.; Donaldson, C. et al. (2001). Identification of urocortin III, an additional member of the corticotropin-releasing factor (CRF) family with high affinity for the CRF2 receptor. Proceedings of the National Academy of Sciences of the United States of America, 98(13), 7570-7575.

Lovenberg, T. W.; Chalmers, D. T.; Liu, C; De Souza, E. B. (1995). CRF2 alpha and CRF2 beta receptor mRNAs are differentially distributed between the rat central nervous system and peripheral tis-sues. Endocrinology, 136(9), 4139-4142.

Lovenberg, T. W.; Liaw, C. W.; Grigoriadis, D. E.; Clevenger, W.; Chalmers, D. T.; De Souza, E. B. et al. (1995). Cloning and characterization of a functionally distinct corticotropin-releasing factor receptor subtype from rat brain. Proceedings of the National Academy of Sciences of the United States of America, 92(3), 836-840.

Malin, D. H. (2001). Nicotine dependence: studies with a laboratory model. Pharmacology, Biochemistry, and Behavior, 70(4), 551-559.

Marcinkiewcz, C. A.; Prado, M. M.; Isaac, S. K.; Marshall, A.; Rylkova, D.; Bruijnzeel, A. W. (2009). Corticotropin-releasing factor within the central nucleus of the amygdala and the nucleus accumbens shell mediates the negative affective state of nicotine withdrawal in rats. Neuropsychopharmacology, 34(7), 1743-1752.

Merali, Z.; McIntosh, J.; Kent, P.; Michaud, D.; Anisman, H. (1998). Aversive and appetitive events evoke the release of corticotropin-releasing hormone and bombesin-like peptides at the central nucleus of the amygdala. The Journal of Neuroscience, 18(12), 4758-4766.

Merlo Pich, E.; Koob, G. F.; Heilig, M.; Menzaghi, F.; Vale, W.; Weiss, F. (1993). Corticotropin-releasing factor release from the mediobasal hypothalamus of the rat as measured by microdialysis. Neuroscience, 55(3), 695-707.

Oki, Y.; Iwabuchi, M.; Masuzawa, M.; Watanabe, F.; Ozawa, M.; Iino, K. et al. (1998). Distribution and concentration of urocortin, and effect of adrenalectomy on its content in rat hypothalamus. Life Sciences, 62(9), 807-812.

Pang, X.; Liu, L.; Ngolab, J.; Zhao-Shea, R.; McIntosh, J. M.; Gardner, P. D. et al. (2016). Habenula cholinergic neurons regulate anxiety during nicotine withdrawal via nicotinic acetylcholine receptors. Neuropharmacology, 107, 294-304.

Perrin, M. H.; Donaldson, C. J.; Chen, R.; Lewis, K. A.; Vale, W. W. (1993). Cloning and functional expression of a rat brain corticotropin releasing factor (CRF) receptor. Endocrinology, 133(6), 3058-3061.

Potter, E.; Sutton, S.; Donaldson, C.; Chen, R.; Perrin, M.; Lewis, K. et al. (1994). Distribution of corticotropin-releasing factor receptor mRNA expression in the rat brain and pituitary. Proceedings of the National Academy of Sciences of the United States of America, 91(19), 8777-8781.

Radulovic, J.; Ruhmann, A.; Liepold, T.; Spiess, J. (1999). Modulation of learning and anxiety by corticotropin-releasing factor (CRF) and stress: differential roles of CRF receptors 1 and 2. The Journal of Neu- roscience, 19(12), 5016-5025.

Reinbold, E. D.; Scholl, J. L.; Oliver, K. M.; Watt, M. J.; Forster, G. L. (2014). Central CRF 2 receptor antagonism reduces anxiety states during amphetamine withdrawal. Neuroscience Research, 89, 37-43.

Reyes, T. M.; Lewis, K.; Perrin, M. H.; Kunitake, K. S.; Vaughan, J.; Arias, C. A. et al. (2001). Urocortin II: a member of the corticotropin-releasing factor (CRF) neuropeptide family that is selectively bound by type 2 CRF receptors. Proceedings of the National Academy of Sciences of the United States of America, 98(5), 2843-2848.

Salas, R.; Sturm, R.; Boulter, J.; De, B. M. (2009). Nicotinic receptors in the habenulo-interpeduncular system are necessary for nicotine withdrawal in mice. The Journal of Neuroscience, 29(10), 3014-3018.

Sonntag, H.; Wittchen, H.; Höfler, M.; Kessler, R.; Stein, M. (2000). Are social fears and DSM-IV social anxiety disorder associated with smoking and nicotine dependence in adolescents and young adults ?European Psychiatry, 15(1), 67-74.

Swanson, L. W.; Sawchenko, P. E.; Rivier, J.; Vale, W. W. (1983). Organization of ovine corticotropin-releasing factor immunoreactive cells and fibers in the rat brain: an immunohistochemical study. Neuroendocrinology, 36, 165-186.

Swerdlow, N. R.; Geyer, M. A.; Vale, W. W.; Koob, G. F. (1986). Corticotropin-releasing factor potentiates acoustic startle in rats: blockade by chlordiazepoxide. Psychopharmacology, 88(2), 147-152.

Tanaka, M.; Tomimatsu, Y.; Sakimura, K.; Ootani, Y.; Sako, Y.; Kojima, T. et al. (2017). Characterization of Crf1 receptor antagonists with differential peripheral vs central actions in Crf challenge in rats. Peptides, 95, 40-50.

Valdez, G. R.; Sabino, V.; Koob, G. F. (2004). Increased anxiety-like behavior and ethanol self-administration in dependent rats: reversal via corticotropin-releasing factor-2 receptor activation. Alcoholism, Clinical and Experimental Research, 28(6), 865-872.

Van Pett, K.; Viau, V.; Bittencourt, J. C.; Chan, R. K.; Li, H. Y.; Arias, C. et al. (2000). Distribution of mRNAs encoding CRF receptors in brain and pituitary of rat and mouse. The Journal of Comparative Neurology, 428(2), 191-212.

Vaughan, J.; Donaldson, C.; Bittencourt, J.; Perrin, M. H.; Lewis, K.; Sutton, S. et al. (1995). Urocortin, a mammalian neuropeptide related to fish urotensin I and to corticotropin-releasing factor. Nature, 378(6554), 287-292.

WHO (2011). Systematic review of the link between tobacco and poverty. Retrieved from:http://www. who. int/tobacco/publications/syst_rev_ tobacco_ poverty/en/index. html.

WHO (2015). WHO report on the global tobacco epidemic, 2015: raising taxeson tobacco. Retrieved from:http://www. who. int/tobacco/global_report 2015/en/.

Yuan, P. -Q.; Wu, S. V.; Elliott, J.; Anton, P. A.; Chatzaki, E.; Million, M. et al. (2012). Expression of corticotropin releasing factor receptortype 1 (CRF 1) in the human gastrointestinal tract and upregulationin the colonic mucosa in patients with ulcerative colitis. Peptides, 38 (1), 62-69.

Zhao-Shea, R.; DeGroot, S. R.; Liu, L.; Vallaster, M.; Pang, X.; Su, Q. et al. (2015). Increased CRF signalling in a ventral tegmental area-interpeduncular nucleus-medial habenula circuit induces anxiety during nicotine withdrawal. Nature Communications, 6, 6770.

Zvolensky, M. J.; Rodríguez-Cano, R.; Paulus, D. J.; Kotov, R.; Bromet, E.; Gonzalez, A. et al. (2017). Respiratory problems and anxiety sensitivity in smoking lapse among treatment seeking smokers. Addictive Behaviors, 75, 25-29.

Zvolensky, M. J.; Vujanovic, A. A.; Miller, M. O.; Bernstein, A.; Yartz, A. R.; Gregor, K. L. et al. (2007). Incremental validity of anxiety sensitivity in terms of motivation to quit, reasons for quitting, and barriers to quitting among community-recruited daily smokers. Nicotine, Tobacco Research, 9(9), 965-975.

21

6-羟基-L-烟碱和记忆障碍

Lucian Hritcu, Marius Mihasan

Department of Biology, Alexandru Ioan Cuza University of Iasi, Iasi, Romania

缩略语

2,3,6-THP	2,3,6-三羟基吡啶	CHL	氯磺胺
2,6-DHP	2,6-二羟基吡啶	DHPH	2,6-二羟基吡啶-3-羟化酶
2,6-DHPON	2,6-二羟基伪氧烟碱	DHPONH	2,6-二羟基伪氧烟碱水解酶
6HDNO	6-羟基-D-烟碱氧化酶	KDH	酮脱氢酶
6HLN	6-羟基-L-烟碱	MGABA	γ-N-甲基氨基丁酸酯
6HLNO	6-羟基-L-烟碱氧化酶	nAChBP	烟碱样受体结合域同源物
6-HMM	6-羟甲基肌司明	nAChR	烟碱乙酰胆碱受体
6-HPON	6-羟基伪氧烟碱	NB	烟碱蓝
AD	阿尔茨海默病	NDH	烟碱脱氢酶

21.1 引言

阿尔茨海默病（AD）是一种进行性神经退行性疾病，认知能力逐渐下降。它被认为是痴呆症的最常见病理原因（Sase, Yamamoto, Kawashima, Tan, Sawa, 2017）。据报道，2016年，80岁或85岁以上的老年人约有200万人患有老年痴呆症，占所有患有AD的人群的37%（Hebert, Weuve, Scherr, Evans, 2013）。到2050年，可能有多达700万的85岁及以上AD患者，占所有65岁及以上AD患者的51%（Hebert et al. 2013）。据报道，烟碱样受体是神经系统中的治疗靶点（Taly et al. 2009）。此外，烟碱乙酰胆碱受体（nAChR）亚型α7和α4β2在AD的参与也有一定的临床意义（Parri, Hernandez, Dineley, 2011）。AD的特征是基底前脑、大脑皮层和海马中的烟碱型和毒蕈碱型乙酰胆碱受体表达均显著降低（Kása, Rakonczay, Gulya, 1997）。因此，在大脑皮层中有明显的α4β2 nAChR亚型丧失（Aubert et al. 1992），而在海马中，α7 nAChR的缺失与记忆功能的逐步改变有关（Nordberg, 2001）。

一些流行病学研究显示，数据表明烟草消费与AD的发展呈反比关系（Echeverria Moran, 2013）。烟草的推定有益作用主要归因于烟碱，据报道烟碱可改善认知能力并减少AD小鼠模型中的斑块（Nordberg et al. 2002）。大量研究表明，急性烟碱给药可显著改善AD患者在认知任务中的表现（Taly et al. 2009）。nAChRs在注意力、学习和记忆中起着重要作用，因此烟碱对记忆的积极作用主要归因于这些受体的激活（Sabbagh, Lukas, Sparks, Reid, 2002）。此外，在验尸中发现，与患有该病的非吸烟者相比，吸烟的AD患者的大脑中神经毒性剂的β-淀粉样蛋白的验尸水平显著降低（Boopathi, Kolandaivel, 2014）。烟碱作为认知增强剂和AD治疗策略的高效力（Murray, Abeles, 2002）不仅可以通过其结合和调节nAChR的能力来解释，还可以通过低浓度下的抗氧化作用来解释（Newman et al. 2002），以及通过其与β-淀粉样肽相互作用的能力来解释。但是，烟碱尚未在临床研究中证明是治疗AD的有效方法（López-Arrieta, Sanz, 2001）。其半衰期短（约2h），因此已证明对其他各种器官（如肺脏）的负面影响（Hecht, Hochalter, Villalta, Murphy, 2000），这与卷烟的联系以及与吸烟相关的负面宣传相关（Buccafusco, 2004），而烟碱并未强加自己作为AD的可行治疗剂。

许多研究主要集中在哺乳动物细胞中发现的烟碱和烟碱代谢物的作用上，因为它们对烟碱暴露引起的神经药理作用具有潜在的贡献（Pogocki et al. 2007; Riveles, Huang, Quik, 2008）。在哺乳动物细胞中，烟碱在肝脏中广泛代谢为六种主要代谢物（烟碱葡糖苷酸、烟碱-N-氧化物、去甲烟碱、异乙氧基离子、可替宁和2-羟基烟碱）。第一次代谢过程中的主要途径产生可替宁（70%～80%的烟碱在人体代谢为可替宁），这可能与吸烟作为nAChR的配体的多种神经生物学效应有关（Dome, Lazary, Kalapos, Rihmer, 2010）。此外，还有其他一些迹象表明可替宁是一种药理活性物质。它在细胞培养模型中具有神经保护和/或细胞保护作用、注意力增强作用、类抗精神病药作用（在脉冲前抑制中）、纹状体组织样品中的多巴胺释放作用等（O'Leary, Parameswaran, McIntosh, Quik, 2008）。

所有这些结果表明，烟碱和烟碱代谢物对脑功能的影响不可忽略。因此，获得更多有关各种来源的烟碱代谢物的生物学效应的信息变得越来越重要，以便可能处理某些神经退行性疾病中的神经系统异常。

21.2 对治疗的影响

对于对烟碱/烟草产品成瘾的受试者有许多可用的治疗方法，如烟碱替代疗法（贴剂和烟碱胶）、烟碱喷雾剂和吸入剂、药物。此外，还提到了不同的心理和行为疗法，如催眠疗法、认知行为疗法和神经语言编程，以帮助人们对抗烟草成瘾。

21.3 细菌中烟碱的衍生物

烟碱受体结合域同系物（nAChRs）的晶体结构测定（Celie et al. 2004）以及α7 nAChRs的结构测定（Mowrey et al. 2013）激发了多个学术和制药实验室对设计新烟碱药物可能性的兴趣。从这个角度来看，烟碱衍生物是理想的候选者，提供了多种可能性。困难首先在于鉴定具有烟碱有益作用但没有其副作用的分子（Pogocki et al. 2007），其次在于提供用于生产和分离所鉴定化合物的简单可靠的方法。在这种情况下，降解烟碱的细菌具有使用这种生物碱作为唯一碳源的能力，可提供具有生物技术潜力的广泛烟碱衍生物。大量报道表明，细菌包括假单胞菌（Liu et al. 2014; Tang et al. 2011）、芽孢杆菌和假单胞菌（Ma et al. 2015; Yu, Tang, Zhu, Li, Xu, 2015）、根癌农杆菌S33（Wang, Liu, Xu, 2009）、无色菌（Hylin, 1958）和烟酸无色杆菌（Hylin, 1958）可以通过以下三种相关途径降解烟碱：吡啶途径（Brandsch, 2006）、吡咯烷途径（Tang et al. 2013）和VPP途径（吡啶和吡咯烷途径的变异）（Wang, Huang, Xie, Xu, 2012）。Brandsch（2006）以及Gurusamy和Natarajan（2013）分别在两篇综述中广泛介绍了在每条途径中涉及的中间体和酶。

21.4 烟草节杆菌中的烟碱代谢

到目前为止，研究最广泛的是烟曲霉pAO1的烟碱代谢。该细菌利用吡啶途径降解烟碱。简而言之，烟碱降解始于吡啶环被烟碱脱氢酶（NDH）羟基化为6-羟基-L-烟碱（6HLN）（Andreesen, Fetzner, 2002）。接下来，吡咯烷环被6-羟基-L-烟碱氧化酶（6HLNO）氧化（Schenk, Decker, 1999），并形成了6-羟甲基肌司明（6-HMM）。该化合物与水自发反应，转化为6-羟基伪氧烟碱［6-HPON；N-甲基氨基丙基-(6-羟基吡啶基-3)-酮］。6HLNO具有高立体选择性，仅作用于6-羟基-L-烟碱。烟草植物可以产生少量的D-烟碱，因此烟曲霉pAO1可以产生6-羟基-D-烟碱氧化酶（6HDNO），它可以将6-羟基-L-烟碱转化为6-HMM，然后连续生成6-HPON（Decker, Bleeg, 1965）。在6-HPON的C2处进行的第二次羟基化反应生成2,6-二羟基伪氧烟碱（2,6-DHPON）。此步骤由多聚酮脱氢酶（KDH）编码。烟碱分解代谢的关键步骤是2,6-二羟基伪氧烟碱水解酶（DHPONH）（Sachelaru, Schiltz, Igloi, Brandsch, 2005）将2,6-DHPON裂解为两种主要代谢物：2,6-二羟基吡啶（2,6-DHP）和γ-N-甲基氨基丁酸酯（MGABA）。2,6-DHP被一种称为2,6-二羟基吡啶-3-羟化酶（DHPH）的FAD依赖性单加氧酶进一步羟基化，生成2,3,6-三羟基吡啶（2,3,6-THP）。在氧气存在的情况下，2,3,6-THP表现出明显的自发二聚作用。二聚化发生在细胞内部，反应产物为4,4′,5,5′-四羟基-3,3′-二氮杂-2,2′-二苯醌，其排出后聚集形成烟碱特征性蓝色的培养基（NB）。即使德国弗莱堡大学的Roderich Brandsch教授的小组已详细描述了烟曲霉的代谢途径，但到目前为止，已鉴定的代谢产物尚未在生物技术上得到应用。

21.5 6HLN能够与nAChR相互作用

我们很感兴趣地发现在烟曲霉分解代谢途径中发现的任何烟碱中间体对nAChRs都具有亲和力，并且我们在计算机模拟实验中评估了它们的结合潜力（Mihasan, Capatina, Neagu, Stefan, Hritcu, 2013）。为此，可从PubChem（Kim et al. 2016）下载烟曲霉烟碱降解途径中发现的所有中间体的3D结构，并将其转换为适合使用FROG v.1.01进行对接的格式在线药物构象生成（Leite et al. 2007）。定向对接所需的所有步骤（分子表面生成、球体生成和能量网格生成）均使用ADT 1.5.4实现（Morris et al. 2009）。以乙酰胆碱结合蛋白（AChBP, PDB ID: 1UW6）为受体，采用Auto-dock 4进行硅对接（Celie et al. 2004）。受体保持刚性，并且所有配体都是柔性的。允许配体分子内的所有键旋转。对接的目标区域是一个中心位于AChBP亚基a的Tyr143上的约150Å（1Å = 10^{-10}m）的立方体。

首先，将L-烟碱停靠在结合位点。将计算机确定的AChBP结合位点中L-烟碱的方向与Celie等（2004）在实验中观察到的方向进行了比较。计算得出的L-烟碱位与实验确定的位姿［对于配体的12个重叠原子，均方根偏差（RMSD）为0.2Å］之间有很好的拟合，表明了所用对接方法的可靠性。

结果表明，6HLN的理论结合位与实验中观察到的12个配体原子的RMSD为0.19 Å非常相似。这种化合物不仅可以装入结合袋，而且AutoDockTools计算的6HLN相互作用能的增加是由于6HLN的羟基和Tyr185残基之间增加了一个氢键。利用Rastija和Medić-Šarić(2009)提出的量子化学定量构效关系（QSAR）方程评价了6HLN的抗氧化活性。结果表明，6HLN对烟碱的抗氧化活性（IC_{50}为43.06）较IC_{50}为54.54有所提高。

21.6 使用基于烟草节杆菌的生物技术生产的6HLN

由于这项初步计算研究产生的有希望的数据,人们可能很容易看到6HLN的高生物技术潜力。目前,这种化合物可以通过重氮化反应在6-氨基烟碱上进行化学合成,可以从不同的供应商处(Santa Cruz Biotechnology或Carbosynth)以相当昂贵的价格购买。尽管如此,烟草节杆菌还提供了一种利用烟草废料和副产品生产这种化合物的替代方法。

烟草节杆菌生长培养基的HPLC分析显示,在烟碱存在下,细菌生长过程中有少量的6HLN积累(Boiangiu, Guzun, Mihasan, 2014)。先前发表的两篇文章指出,不仅在烟草节杆菌的烟碱生长培养基中可以发现6HLN(Hochstein, Rittenberg, 1959),而且可能存在涉及便利运输系统的出口机制(Ganas, Igloi, Brandsch, 2009)。6HLN的积累只是暂时的,培养基中的烟碱一旦耗尽,6HLN含量就会下降(图21.1)。显然,这涉及代谢失衡。

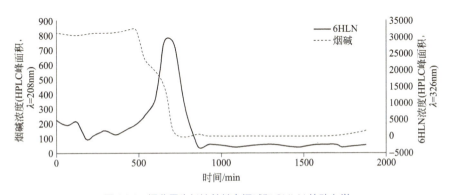

图21.1 烟曲霉生长培养基中烟碱和6HLN的动力学

可以观察到6HLN的暂时积累(实线)。培养基中的烟碱一旦耗尽(虚线),6HLN含量就会下降。

NDH是一种三聚体酶,它含有钼吡喃蝶呤二核苷酸辅因子FAD和两个铁硫簇(Andreesen, Fetzner, 2002),负责将L-烟碱转化为6HNLO,对其底物具有大致相同的亲和力(K_m为0.037mmol/L),但亲和力和反应速率[比活为29.2μmol/(min·mg)]与下游酶6-羟基-L-烟碱氧化酶(6HLNO)相比更高(Hochstein, Dalton, 1967)。二聚体酶6HLNO的每个亚基包含一个FAD(Schenk, Decker, 1999),K_m为0.02mmol/L,比NDH活性低得多,为4.73μmol/(min·mg)(Decker, Dai, Möhler, Brühmüller, 1972; Kachalova et al. 2010)。基本上,只要烟碱仍在介质中,NDH就会以相当快的速度将其转换为6HLN,6HLNO无法跟上转换,并且6HLN会在介质中积累。烟碱耗尽后,6HLNO可以迅速恢复,6HLN被消耗(图21.2)。

观察到的代谢失衡可用于产生6HLN。为了增加产量,创建了基因工程烟曲霉菌株。将ndh基因克隆到定制的pART2表达载体中(Andrei, Mihasan, 2013; Sandu, Chiribau, Sachelaru, Brandsch, 2005),该基因允许NDH以烟碱依赖性方式过度表达(图21.3)。目前,我们的实验室使用低密度烟曲霉pART2ndh细胞培养物在烧瓶中于28℃恒定搅拌下培养,以产生6HLN。通过过表达NDH并使用0.05mmol/L $ZnSO_4$化学抑制6HLNO,我们通常能够在每100mL培养基中产生50~60mg 6HLN。

生产的6HLN具有增强记忆的作用。

接下来,在雄性Wistar大鼠体内对6HLN进行了测试,并证明其对记忆过程和大脑氧化状态具有令人惊讶的积极影响。Hritcu 等（2013）证明，对 6HLN 的体内慢性治疗（0.3mg/kg，连续 7 天）显著增加了 Y 型迷宫任务的自发交替和八臂迷宫任务的工作记忆，在八臂迷宫任务中的参考记忆探索结果表明，在不影响长期记忆的情况下 6HLN 可以对短期记忆产生影响。此外，Y 迷宫测试中的手臂进入次数证明了 6HLN 可显著改善运动能力（表 21.1）。此外，6HLN 可增加大鼠颞叶匀浆中的抗氧化酶活性（SOD 和 GPX）并减少脂质过氧化（MDA）的产生，表明其具有抗氧化作用（表 21.2）。我们得出的结论是 6HLN 对空间记忆的积极影响可能是由抗氧化作用引起的。

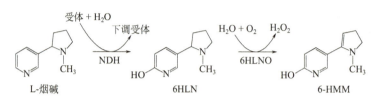

图 21.2 烟曲霉烟碱分解代谢途径中 6HLN 的上下游反应

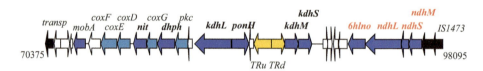

图 21.3 *ndh* 和 *6hlno* 基因（红色）在烟曲霉 pAO1 巨质粒的 *nic* 基因簇中的位置

暗蓝色，经实验证明与烟碱代谢有关的基因；淡蓝色，推测参与烟碱代谢的基因；白色，无实验或推定功能的基因；黑色，转座子和插入元件；黄色，假定的转录因子

表 21.1 6HLN 在记忆实验模型中的作用

烟碱衍生物	药物施用	动物种类	行为学测试	影响	参考文献
6-羟基-L-烟碱	初次给药大鼠腹腔注射 0.3mg/kg	大鼠	Y 迷宫	改善短期记忆和运动活动	Hritcu et al. (2013)
	初次给药大鼠腹腔注射 0.3mg/kg	大鼠	横臂迷宫	增强工作记忆，不影响参考记忆	Hritcu et al. (2013)
	东莨菪碱（0.7mg/kg）处理的大鼠腹腔注射 0.3mg/kg	大鼠	Y 迷宫	持续短期记忆和运动活动	Hritcu, Stefan, Brandsch, Mihasan (2015)
	东莨菪碱（0.7 mg/kg）处理的大鼠腹腔注射 0.3mg/kg	大鼠	横臂迷宫	增强工作记忆和参考记忆	Hritcu et al. (2015)
	氯异丙肾上腺素（10 mg/kg）处理的大鼠腹腔注射 0.3 mg/kg	大鼠	Y 迷宫	增强自发交替	Hritcu et al. (2017)
	氯异丙肾上腺素（10 mg/kg）处理的大鼠腹腔注射 0.3mg/kg	大鼠	横臂迷宫	改进工作记忆和参考记忆	Hritcu et al. (2017)

Hritcu 等（2015）证明 6HLN 改善了东莨菪碱引起的空间记忆障碍（表 21.1）。与对照组相比，东莨菪碱处理的大鼠海马匀浆中超氧化物歧化酶、谷胱甘肽过氧化物酶和过氧化氢酶活性降低，还原型谷胱甘肽总含量降低。与对照组相比，东莨菪碱处理的大鼠海马匀浆中丙二醛（脂质过氧化）的产生显著增加，这是抗氧化酶活性受损的结果。因此，我们的研究结果表明，通过减轻大鼠海马中的氧化应激，给予 6HLN 可以减轻东莨菪碱所致的空间记忆障碍。

最近，Hritcu 等（2017）报道称，6HLN 给药可以减轻氯磺胺（CHL）大鼠模型海马中的认知缺陷（表21.1），并恢复其抗氧化能力（表21.2）。综上所述，与烟碱相比，6HLN给药可以显著改善Y型迷宫和八臂迷宫中的空间记忆能力，这项任务减少了CHL处理的大鼠海马中脂质过氧化作用，并增强了其抗氧化状态。观察到的这种作用可能提示烟碱和6HLN都可能具有神经保护作用。但是，在CHL治疗的大鼠中，与烟碱相比，6HLN的作用明显增强。在这项研究的观察中，我们可以认为6HLN可能在诸如AD之类的记忆障碍的治疗和/或管理中起有益作用，并表明烟碱乙酰胆碱系统在脑功能障碍中具有重要意义。此外，还报道了（Hritcu et al.2017）烟碱和6HLN均在氯磺胺大鼠模型中充当抗焦虑药和抗抑郁药。所观察到的作用可能是由烟碱乙酰胆碱受体介导的。

总之，我们的数据为烟碱和烟碱代谢产物在记忆过程和脑氧化状态中的作用提供了额外的支持。此外，应考虑6HLN的有益药理特性和相对于烟碱改善的安全性。最后，我们在图21.4中总结了6HLN作为记忆增强剂和抗氧化剂的作用机理。

表21.2 6HLN对氧化应激的影响

烟碱衍生物	药物施用	动物种类	生化标记	影响	参考文献
6-羟基-L-烟碱	初次给药大鼠腹腔注射0.3mg/kg	大鼠	SOD、GPX、MDA	SOD活性增加，GPX和MDA水平降低	Hritcu et al. (2013)
	东莨菪碱（0.7mg/kg）处理的大鼠腹腔注射0.3mg/kg	大鼠	SOD、GPX、CAT、GSH、MDA	提高SOD、GPX、CAT和GSH水平，降低MDA水平	Hritcu et al. (2013)
	氯异丙肾上腺素（10mg/kg）处理的大鼠腹腔注射0.3mg/kg	大鼠	SOD、GPX、CAT、GSH、MDA	提高SOD、GPX、CAT和GSH水平，降低MDA水平	Hritcu et al. (2017)

注：SOD，超氧化物歧化酶；GPX，谷胱甘肽过氧化物酶；CAT，过氧化氢酶；GSH，谷胱甘肽；MDA，丙二醛。

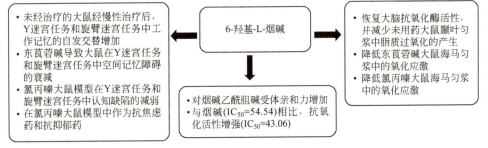

图21.4 6HLN可能具有增强记忆力和抗氧化活性的作用机理

术语解释

- 烟草节杆菌（Arthrobacter nicotinovorans）：从土壤中分离出来的革兰氏阳性放线菌，具有降解烟碱的能力。以前曾被描述为 *A. oxydans*。
- 脑氧化应激：氧化剂和抗氧化剂之间的不平衡，其特征在于大脑抵抗自由基产生的能力下降。
- 计算机方法：一种基于计算机程序和算法的方法。
- pAO1巨质粒：从烟草节杆菌中分离出的大型细菌质粒，其中包含负责细菌降解烟碱的基因。
- 八臂迷宫测试：一种用于评估啮齿动物的工作记忆和参考记忆的行为测试。
- Y型迷宫测试：一种用于评估啮齿动物的空间短期记忆的行为测试。

记忆障碍的关键事实	■ 阿尔茨海默病（AD）是一种进行性神经退行性疾病，主要特征是学习和记忆丧失。
	■ 已证实在AD期间胆碱能神经元丧失和乙酰胆碱水平显著下降，从而导致记忆障碍。
	■ AD中可能会由于抗氧化酶活性降低而导致脑氧化应激增加。
	■ 寻找新的治疗选择引起了人们的极大兴趣。

要点总结	■ 本章重点介绍烟碱代谢物6-羟基-L-烟碱（6HLN）。
	■ 6HLN是由烟曲霉pAO1菌株中的烟碱降解产生的。
	■ 使用计算机模拟和体内行为学方法以及使用认知障碍动物模型评估靶标-配体相互作用以及对6HLN的记忆过程和脑氧化应激的影响。
	■ 6HLN是烟碱乙酰胆碱受体的有效激动剂，具有增强记忆力和抗氧化的作用。
	■ 但是，我们认为6HLN可能是改善AD记忆障碍的有价值的治疗剂。

致谢

这项工作得到了PED-PN-III-P2-2.1-PED-2016-0177的支持。

参考文献

Andreesen, J. R.; Fetzner, S. (2002). The molybdenum-containing hydroxylases of nicotinate, isonicotinate, and nicotine. Metal Ions in Biological Systems, 39, 405-430.

Andrei, A.; Mihasan, M. (2013). Molecular gene cloning of nicotine-dehidrogenase from the pAO1 megaplasmid of Arthrobacter nicotinovorans. Analele Stiintifice ale Universitatii "Alexandru Ioan Cuza" dinIasi Sec. Ⅱ a. Genetica si Biologie Moleculara, 14, 15-19.

Aubert, I.; Araujo, D. M.; Cecyre, D.; Robitaille, Y.; Gauthier, S.; Quirion, R. (1992). Comparative alterations of nicotinic and muscarinic binding sites in Alzheimer's and Parkinson's diseases. Journal of Neurochemistry, 58(2), 529-541.

Boiangiu, R.; Guzun, D.; Mihasan, M. (2014). Time dependent accumulation of nicotine derivatives in the culture medium of Arthrobacter nicotinovoranspAO1. Analele Stiintifice ale Universitatii"Alexandru Ioan Cuza"din Iasi Sec. Ⅱ a. Genetica si Biologie Moleculara, 15, 19-25.

Boopathi, S.; Kolandaivel, P. (2014). Targeted studies on the interaction of nicotine and morin molecules with amyloid β-protein. Journal of Molecular Modeling, 20(3), 1-15. https://doi. org/10. 1007/s00894-014-2109-8.

Brandsch, R. (2006). Microbiology and biochemistry of nicotine degradation. Applied Microbiology and Biotechnology, 69, 493-498.

Buccafusco, J. (2004). Neuronal nicotinic receptor subtypes: defining therapeutic targets. Molecular Interventions, 4, 285-295.

Celie, P. H. N.; van Rossum-Fikkert, S. E.; van Dijk, W. J.; Brejc, K.; Smit, A. B.; Sixma, T. K. (2004). Nicotine and carbamylcholine binding to nicotinic acetylcholine receptors as studied in AChBP crystal structures. Neuron, 41(6), 907-914.

Decker, K.; Bleeg, H. (1965). Induction and purification of stereospecific nicotine oxidizing enzymes from Arthrobacter oxidans. Biochimicaet Biophysica Acta (BBA): Enzymology and Biological Oxidation, 105, 313-324.

Decker, K.; Dai, V.; Möhler, H.; Brühmüller, M. (1972). D- and L-6-hydroxynicotine oxidase, enantiozymes of Arthrobacter oxidans. Zeitschrift fur Naturforschung. Teil B. Anorganische Chemie, organische Chemie, Biochemie, Biophysik, Biologie, 27, 1072-1073.

Dome, P.; Lazary, J.; Kalapos, M. P.; Rihmer, Z. (2010). Smoking, nicotine and neuropsychiatric disorders. Neuroscience, Biobehavioral Reviews, 34(3), 295-342.

Echeverria Moran, V. (2013). Brain effects of nicotine and derived compounds. Frontiers in Pharmacology, 4, 60.

Ganas, P.; Igloi, G. L.; Brandsch, R. (2009). The megaplasmid pAO1 of Arthrobacter nicotinovoransand nicotine catabolism. In E. Schwartz (Ed.), Microbial Megaplasmids(pp. 271-282). Berlin, Heidelberg: Springer Berlin Heidelberg.

Gurusamy, R.; Natarajan, S. (2013). Current status on biochemistry and molecular biology of microbial degradation of nicotine. The Scientific World Journal, 2013, 125385.

Hebert, L. E.; Weuve, J.; Scherr, P. A.; Evans, D. A. (2013). Alzheimer disease in the United States (2010-2050) estimated using the 2010 census. Neurology, 80(19), 1778-1783.

Hecht, S. S.; Hochalter, J. B.; Villalta, P. W.; Murphy, S. E. (2000). 20-Hydroxylation of nicotine by cytochrome P450 2A6 and human liver microsomes: Formation of a lung carcinogen precursor. Proceedings of the National Academy of Sciences of the United States of America, 97(23), 12493-12497.

Hochstein, L. I.; Dalton, B. P. (1967). The purification and properties of nicotine oxidase. Biochimica et Biophysica Acta (BBA): Enzymology, 139(1), 56-68.

Hochstein, L. I.; Rittenberg, S. C. (1959). The bacterial oxidation of nicotine: I. Nicotine oxidation by cell-free preparations. Journal of Biological Chemistry, 234(1), 151-155.

Hritcu, L.; Ionita, R.; Motei, D. E.; Babii, C.; Stefan, M.; Mihasan, M. (2017). Nicotine versus 6-hydroxy-L-nicotine against chlorisond amine induced memory impairment and oxidative stress in the rat hippocampus. Biomedicine, Pharmacotherapy, 86, 102-108. (2017).

Hritcu, L.; Stefan, M.; Brandsch, R.; Mihasan, M. (2013). 6-hydroxy-l-nicotine from Arthrobacter nicotinovoranssustain spatial memory formation by decreasing brain oxidative stress in rats. Journal of Physiology and Biochemistry, 69(1), 25-34.

Hritcu, L.; Stefan, M.; Brandsch, R.; Mihasan, M. (2015). Enhanced behavioral response by decreasing brain oxidative stress to 6-hydroxy-L-nicotine in Alzheimer's disease rat model. Neuroscience Letters, 591, 41-47.

Hylin, J. W. (1958). Microbial degradation of nicotine I. Achromobacter nicotinophagumn. sp. : morphology and physiology. Journal of Bacteriology, 76(1), 36-40.

Kachalova, G. S.; Bourenkov, G. P.; Mengesdorf, T.; Schenk, S.; Maun, H. R.; Burghammer, M. et al. (2010). Crystal structure analysis of free and substrate-bound 6-hydroxy-L-nicotine oxidase from Arthrobacter nicotinovorans. Journal of Molecular Biology, 396(3), 785-799.

Kása, P.; Rakonczay, Z.; Gulya, K. (1997). The cholinergic system in Alzheimer's disease. Progress in Neurobiology, 52(6), 511-535.

Kim, S.; Thiessen, P. A.; Bolton, E. E.; Chen, J.; Fu, G.; Gindulyte, A. et al. (2016). PubChem substance and compound databases. Nucleic Acids Research, 44 (Database issue), D1202-D1213.

Leite, T. B.; Gomes, D.; Miteva, M. A.; Chomilier, J.; Villoutreix, B. O.; Tufféry, P. (2007). Frog: a FRee online drug 3D conformation generator. Nucleic Acids Research, 35 (Web Server issue), W568-W572.

Liu, Y.; Wang, L.; Huang, K.; Wang, W.; Nie, X.; Jiang, Y. et al. (2014). Physiological and biochemical characterization of a novel nicotine degrading bacteriumPseudomonas geniculataN1. PLoS One, 9(1), e84399.

López-Arrieta, J.; Sanz, F. J. S. (2001). Nicotine for Alzheimer's disease. Cochrane Database of Systematic Reviews. 2, https:/ /doi. org/10. 1002/14651858. CD001749.

Ma, Y.; Wei, Y.; Qiu, J.; Wen, R.; Hong, J.; Liu, W. (2014). Isolation, transposon mutagenesis, and characterization of the novel nicotine degrading strain Shinellasp. HZN7. Applied Microbiology and Biotechnol-ogy, 98(6), 2625-2636.

Ma, Y.; Wen, R.; Qiu, J.; Hong, J.; Liu, M.; Zhang, D. (2015). Biodegradation of nicotine by a novel strain Pusillimonas . Research in Microbiology, 166(2), 67-71.

Mihasan, M.; Capatina, L.; Neagu, E.; Stefan, M.; Hritcu, L. (2013). In silicoidentification of 6-hydroxy-L-nicotine as a novel neuroprotective drug. Romanian Biotechnological Letters, 18, 8333-8340.

Morris, G. M.; Huey, R.; Lindstrom, W.; Sanner, M. F.; Belew, R. K.; Goodsell, D. S. et al. (2009). AutoDock4 and AutoDockTools4: automated docking with selective receptor flexibility. Journal of Computational Chemistry, 30(16), 2785-2791.

Mowrey, D. D.; Liu, Q.; Bondarenko, V.; Chen, Q.; Seyoum, E.; Xu, Y. et al. (2013). Insights into distinct modulation ofα7 and α7β2 nicotinic acetylcholine receptors by the volatile anesthetic isoflurane Journal of Biological Chemistry, 288(50), 35793-35800.

Murray, K. N.; Abeles, N. (2002). Nicotine's effect on neural and cognitive functioning in an aging population. Aging, Mental Health, 6(2), 129-138.

Newman, M. B.; Arendash, G. W.; Shytle, R. D.; Bickford, P. C.; Tighe, T.; Sanberg, P. R. (2002). Nicotine's oxidative and antioxidant properties in CNS. Life Sciences, 71(24), 2807-2820.

Nordberg, A. (2001). Nicotinic receptor abnormalities of Alzheimer's disease: Therapeutic implications. Biological Psychiatry, 49, 200-210.

Nordberg, A.; Hellström-Lindahl, E.; Lee, M.; Johnson, M.; Mousavi, M.; Hall, R. et al. (2002). Chronic nicotine treatment reduces β-amyloidosis in the brain of a mouse model of Alzheimer's disease (APPsw). Journal of Neurochemistry, 81(3), 655-658.

O'Leary, K.; Parameswaran, N.; McIntosh, J. M.; Quik, M. (2008). Cotinine selectively activates a subpopulation of alpha3/alpha6beta2 nicotinic receptors in monkey striatum. Journal of Pharmacology and Experimental Therapeutics, 325, 646-654.

Parri, H. R.; Hernandez, C. M.; Dineley, K. T. (2011). Research update: alpha7 nicotinic acetylcholine receptor mechanisms in Alzheimer's disease. Biochemical Pharmacology, 82(8), 931-942. (2011).

Pogocki, D.; Ruman, T.; Danilczuk, M.; Danilczuk, M.; Celuch, M.; Wałajtys-Rode, E. (2007). Application of nicotine enantiomers, derivatives and analogues in therapy of neurodegenerative disorders. European Journal of Pharmacology, 563, 18-39.

Rastija, V.; Medić-Šarić, M. (2009). QSAR study of antioxidant activity of wine polyphenols. European Journal of Medicinal Chemistry, 44(1), 400-408.

Riveles, K.; Huang, L. Z.; Quik, M. (2008). Cigarette smoke, nicotine and cotinine protect against 6-hydroxydopamine-induced toxicity in SH-SY5Y cells. Neurotoxicology, 29, 421-427. Sabbagh, M.; Lukas, R.; Sparks, D.; Reid, R. (2002). The nicotinic acetylcholine receptor, smoking, and Alzheimer's disease. Journal of Alzheimer's disease: JAD, 4, 317-325.

Sachelaru, P.; Schiltz, E.; Igloi, G. L.; Brandsch, R. (2005). Anα/β-fold C—C bond hydrolase is involved in a central step of nicotine catabolism by Arthrobacter nicotinovorans. Journal of Bacteriology, 187(24), 8516-8519.

Sandu, C.; Chiribau, C. -B.; Sachelaru, P.; Brandsch, R. (2005). Plasmids for nicotine-dependent and -independent gene expression in Arthrobacter nicotinovorans and other arthrobacter species. Applied and Environmental Microbiology, 71(12), 8920-8924.

Sase, S.; Yamamoto, H.; Kawashima, E.; Tan, X.; Sawa, Y. (2017). Discrimination between patients with Alzheimer disease and healthy subjects using layer analysis of cerebral blood flow and xenon solubility coefficient in xenon-enhanced computed tomography . Journal of Computer Assisted Tomography, 41(3), 477-483.

Schenk, S.; Decker, K. (1999). Horizontal gene transfer involved in the convergent evolution of the plasmid-encoded enantioselective 6-hydroxynicotine oxidases. Jounal of Molecular Evolution, 48, 178-186.

Taly, A.; Corringer, P. -J.; Guedin, D.; Lestage, P.; Changeux, J. -P. (2009). Nicotinic receptors: allosteric transitions and therapeutic targets in the nervous system. Nature Reviews Drug Discovery, 8, 733.

Tang, H.; Wang, L.; Wang, W.; Yu, H.; Zhang, K.; Yao, Y. et al. (2013). Systematic unraveling of the unsolved pathway of nicotine degradation in Pseudomonas. PLoS Genetics, 9(10), e1003923.

Tang, H.; Yao, Y.; Zhang, D.; Meng, X.; Wang, L.; Yu, H. et al. (2011). A novel NADH-dependent and FAD-containing hydroxylase is crucial for nicotine degradation byPseudomonas putida. The Journal of Biological Chemistry, 286(45), 39179-39187.

Wang, S.; Huang, H.; Xie, K.; Xu, P. (2012). Identification of nicotine biotransformation intermediates by Agrobacterium tumefaciens strain S33 suggests a novel nicotine degradation pathway. Applied Microbiology and Biotechnology, 95(6), 1567-1578.

Wang, S. N.; Liu, Z.; Xu, P. (2009). Biodegradation of nicotine by a newly isolated Agrobacteriumsp. strain S33. Journal of Applied Microbiology, 107(3), 838-847.

Yu, H.; Tang, H.; Zhu, X.; Li, Y.; Xu, P. (2015). Molecular mechanism of nicotine degradation by a newly isolated strain, Ochrobactrumsp. strain SJY1. Applied and Environmental Microbiology, 81(1), 272-281.

22
可替宁与记忆：为忘而忆

Valentina Echeverria[1,2], *Ross Zeitlin*[1]

1. Research, Development Service, Bay Pines VA Healthcare System, Bay Pines, FL, United States
2. Fac. Cs de la Salud, Universidad San Sebastián, Lientur 1457, Concepción, Chile

缩略语

AD	阿尔茨海默病	**nAChR**	烟碱乙酰胆碱受体
ASDs	自闭症谱系障碍	**NFAT**	活化T细胞核因子
Aβ	淀粉样β肽	**NFκB**	核因子κB
BDNF	脑源性神经营养因子	**NT-3**	神经营养素3
CNS	中枢神经系统	**PD**	帕金森病
FXS	脆性X染色体综合征	**PTSD**	创伤后应激障碍
GFAP	胶质原纤维酸性蛋白	**SCHZ**	精神分裂症
GSK3	糖原合酶激酶3	**STAT**	信号转导子和转录因子激活剂
IL	白介素	**Tg**	转基因
KO	敲除	**VEGFR**	血管内皮生长因子受体
mGluR5	代谢型谷氨酸受体5		

22.1 引言

大量研究强调了PTSD、精神分裂症（SCHZ）和重度抑郁症患者中烟草消费的高发生率。曾经有人认为，从这些疾病相关的不良症状中得到缓解的希望会导致患有这些疾病的人吸烟（Echeverria, Grizzell, Barreto, 2016; Moran, 2012）。可替宁是烟碱的主要代谢产物，在正常和病理条件下对大脑功能具有有益作用（Grizzell, Echeverria, 2015; Moran, 2012; Zevin et al. 2000）。安全性研究证实了可替宁的安全性及其与烟碱在哺乳动物成瘾、毒性和血管功能方面的不同作用（Benowitz et al. 1983; Benowitz, Sharp, 1989; Hatsukami et al. 1998; Hatsukami et al. 1998; Hatsukami et al. 1997; Keenan et al. 1994; Kuo et al. 1989）。在不同病理状况和衰老的动物模型中广泛记录了可替宁在促进高级认知功能方面的积极作用（Buccafusco, Terry Jr., 2003; Echeverria, Grizzell, Barreto, 2016; Echeverria, Zeitlin, 2012; Grizzell, Echeverria, 2015）（图22.1）。二十多年前的一项研究表明，可替宁提高了猕猴延迟匹配样本任务的性能准确性（Buccafusco, Terry Jr., 2003）。然而，可能是由于可获得更有效的nAChR激动剂，因此不鼓励其发展为治疗药物。考虑到吸烟与帕金森病（PD）和阿尔茨海默病（AD）以及其他影响记忆力的精神疾病（如PTSD和严重抑郁症）的发生率较低相关，可替宁对记忆力的影响已得到越来越多的研究（表22.1）。

表22.1 临床前研究显示可替宁对记忆力有有益作用

动物模型/条件	年份	信号相关因素	参考文献
猴子/老龄	2005	—	Terry AV Jr. et al.
猴子/SCHZ	2009	—	Buccafusco JJ et al.
Tg6799老鼠/AD	2011	Akt，GSK3	Echeverria V et al.
雄性Wistar老鼠/SCHZ	2012	—	Terry AV Jr. et al.
老鼠/PTSD	2014	ERK	Zeitlin R et al.
老鼠/抑郁	2014	GSK3, 突触素	Grizzell JA et al.
老鼠/抑郁	2014	VEGF, Erb	Grizzell JA et al.
雄性年轻老鼠/PTSD	2014	α7, α4β2 nAChRs, ERK	de Aguiar RB
DBA/2老鼠/感觉门控	2014	α7, α4β2 nAChRs	Wildeboer-Andrud KM et al.
Tg6799老鼠/AD	2014	PSD95	Patel et al.
雄性Sprague-Dawley老鼠/多奈哌齐治疗	2015	α7, α4β2 nAChRs	Terry AV Jr. et al
Wistar雌性/化疗	2016	—	Iarkov A et al.
FXM(−/−)老鼠/自闭症	2017	Akt, GSK3	Pardo M et al.
Tg6799老鼠/AD	2017	Tau, CREB	Grizzell JA et al.
C57BL/6老鼠/抑郁	2017	GFAP	Perez-Urrutia et al.

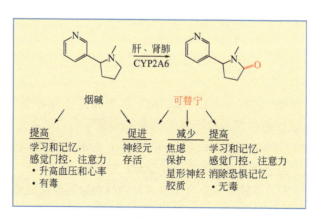

图22.1 可替宁对烟碱具有特性

可替宁是烟碱的主要衍生物，可被细胞色素P450代谢。这种转化提供了可替宁新的有益作用。

22.2 可替宁可改善AD小鼠的记忆力

我们的记忆定义了我们，它的可塑性影响着我们生活的方方面面。正如Gabriel García Márquez所说，"生活不是一个人生活过什么，而是一个人记住什么以及如何记住它以重新叙述它"（García Márquez, 2003）。

可替宁抗AD病理学的第一个证据来自毒性研究，试图证明它会加剧淀粉样β肽（Aβ）的神经毒性作用。出乎意料的是，这些研究表明可替宁可通过抑制Aβ的聚集来降低Aβ的毒性（Burgess, et al. 2008; Echeverria et al. 2011）。后来其他小组也报道了类似的结果（Gao, La, Chapman, Bertrand, Terry, 2012）（图22.2）。在这些研究之后，使用转基因（Tg）6799 AD小鼠进行了研究，结果表明可替宁在疾病的各个阶段均可有效减少Aβ聚集和tau过度磷酸化。这些效应伴随着工作记忆的改善，包括在圆形平台、八臂迷宫、干扰和新颖的物体识别测试等数项测试中进行（Echeverria et al. 2011; Echeverria, Zeitlin, 2012; Grizzell et al. 2017）。可替宁不仅有助于改善记忆，而且减少了Tg6799小鼠的抑郁样行为（Patel et al. 2014）。

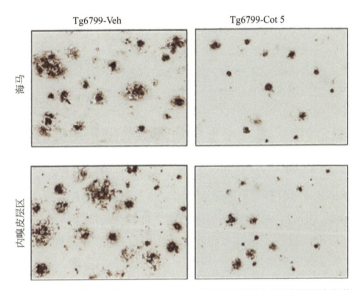

图 22.2　可替宁可抑制 Tg6799 AD 小鼠海马和皮层中的淀粉样蛋白负荷

该图描述了用媒介物（Veh）或可替宁5mg/kg（Cot 5）处理的转基因（Tg）6799小鼠大脑中Aβ斑块的免疫组织化学分析。各组之间的差异是显著的，可替宁治疗的Tg小鼠明显降低。摘自Patel等（2014）。

22.3　可替宁预防创伤后应激障碍小鼠模型中的记忆力丧失

创伤后应激障碍是由于遭受痛苦或目睹暴力状况（如车祸、战争、自然灾害、强奸或谋杀）而遭受无法逃避的恐怖而引起的（Young, 2017）。PTSD的实际治疗药物具有副作用，其积极作用仅限于部分患者（Thomas, Stein, 2017）。此外，它们通常具有短期疗效，其中很大一部分患者复发。最近的临床研究报道了哌唑嗪在减轻PTSD患者的噩梦方面的令人鼓舞的结果（Breen, Blankley, Fine, 2017; Singh et al. 2016）。目前已经研究了寻找副作用少、能永久消除恐惧的新疗法。

PTSD患者中烟草消费的高发生率（Kelly, Jensen, Sofuoglu, 2015）及其对记忆的影响促使了可替宁对PTSD的研究。可替宁在强迫游泳、约束应激和恐惧条件引起的PTSD动物模型中显示出抗抑郁、抗焦虑和增强记忆的作用。此外，可替宁增强了条件性啮齿动物的情景恐惧消除（de Aguiar et al. 2013; Echeverria et al. 2017; Grizzell et al. 2014; Patel et al. 2014; Perez-Urrutia et al. 2017; Zeitlin et al. 2012）（图22.3）。

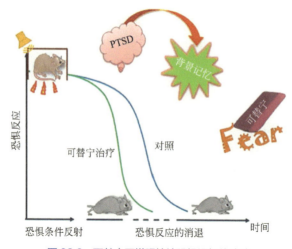

图 22.3 可替宁可增强情境恐惧记忆的消除

促进小鼠恐惧消除的示意图。请注意，烟碱无助于消除情景恐惧。

22.4 可替宁恢复慢性应激对星形胶质细胞数量和功能的影响

最近的研究表明，啮齿动物的星形胶质细胞受到恐惧条件反射和约束应激的严重影响（Perez-Urrutia et al. 2017; Saur et al. 2016）。星形胶质细胞被认为是中枢神经系统（CNS）的多功能照顾者（Moraga-Amaro et al. 2014）。星形胶质细胞将中枢神经系统的灰质细分为包含血管、神经元和突触的区域。它们对于大脑的正常发育必不可少；调节神经元信号；并在维持离子、神经递质、水和能量稳态方面发挥中心作用，并可以发挥神经祖细胞的功能。在大鼠中，恐惧条件降低了 GFAP + 星形胶质细胞的密度并改变了星形胶质细胞的形态，减少了它们的初级突起总数，并减少了海马区CA1区树突的复杂性（Saur et al. 2016）。应激会降低星形胶质细胞标记物GFAP的表达（Czeh et al. 2006; Gomez-Galan et al. 2013; Perez-Urrutia et al. 2017）。此外，在受到束缚应激的动物的血脑屏障中也发现了GFAP表达的变化（Santha et al. 2015）。最近的研究表明，可替宁可增加受限小鼠海马的突触密度（Grizzell, Echeverria, 2015; Grizzell, Iarkov et al. 2014）。令人惊讶的是，鼻内可替宁的后处理诱导了受限制的小鼠海马和额叶皮层星形胶质细胞的恢复（Perez-Urrutia et al. 2017）。这是一个相关的发现，因为啮齿动物的固定应激和恐惧条件都会在与记忆有关的大脑区域引起认知障碍和星形胶质细胞的缺乏。因此，由于星形胶质细胞在支持神经元可塑性、能量平衡和大脑损伤后恢复方面起着重要作用，记忆力减退、抑郁症和星形胶质细胞缺乏症似乎是相关的。这些功能是通过释放能量化合物和神经营养因子来实现的。基于这一证据，可以认为星形胶质细胞功能的恢复是可替宁在大脑中起作用的一种细胞机制。

22.5 可替宁在抑郁症和PTSD啮齿动物模型中激活的信号通路

22.5.1 可替宁通过调节nAChR具有抗炎作用

神经炎症涉及一系列影响神经元、内皮细胞和神经胶质细胞的事件，这些事件发生在PTSD、AD和抑郁症中（Echeverria, Grizzell, Barreto, 2016; Echeverria, Yarkov, Aliev, 2016; Mendoza et al.

2016; Wager-Smith, Markou, 2011)。如上所述，神经胶质细胞具有有益的作用。然而，它们的慢性激活通过诱导神经炎症和细胞死亡来损害大脑功能（Cabezas et al. 2017）。

可替宁激活的下游效应子的生化研究和使用表达人α7nAChR的非洲爪蟾卵母细胞的初步电生理研究（由Zeitlin博士于2009年9月28日传达）被允许假设可替宁是α7 nAChR的PAM（Echeverria, Zeitlin, 2012）（图22.4）。后来，可替宁的药效学得到了证实，结果表明，可替宁对PAM具有预期的作用，可增强乙酰胆碱酯酶抑制剂（如多奈哌齐）在大鼠中的作用（Terry Jr., Callahan, Bertrand, 2015）。α7 nAChR具有抗炎作用并能抑制免疫细胞释放炎性因子（Han et al. 2014），因此激活该受体的可替宁在大脑中可能具有相似的作用。另一方面，已经表明可替宁促进大鼠恐惧消退需要激活α7和α4β2 nAChRs（de Aguiar et al. 2013）。这种依赖性可以基于以下事实：胆碱能系统会影响前额叶皮层和海马的突触可塑性，增强PFC对杏仁核的抑制作用以及海马对抑制性记忆的巩固作用（Liberzon, Sripada, 2008）。对小鼠的另一项研究还发现，可替宁可通过调节nAChR来影响感觉门控能力（Wildeboer-Andrud et al. 2014）。

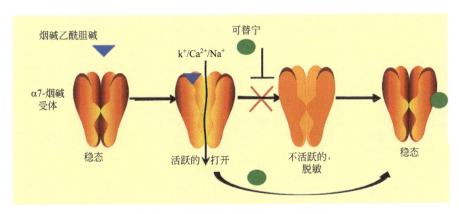

图 22.4 可替宁正变构调节 α7 nAChR

可替宁对α7烟碱受体进行正变构调节的示意图，可替宁增加膜上可被乙酰胆碱（ACh）激活的受体数量。

22.5.2 可替宁刺激Akt和ERK信号通路

可替宁对认知的有益作用似乎还取决于VEGF表达的增强（Echeverria et al. 2017）和对下游效应蛋白激酶B（Akt）的刺激（Echeverria, Grizzell, Barreto, 2016）。该激酶调节大脑中的蛋白质合成、神经发生、神经元存活和神经元可塑性，并且由于许多精神病和神经病而在大脑中被下调。Akt由nAChR、酪氨酸受体激酶B、脑源性神经营养因子（BDNF）、神经营养素（NT）-3生长因子受体（Wang et al. 2017）和血管内皮生长因子受体（VEGFR）激活，可促进大脑可塑性、神经元存活、神经发生和血管生成（Fournier et al. 2012; Wu et al. 2008）。可替宁会增加VEGF的表达，因此可能会刺激大脑中的VEGFRs（Conklin, Zhao, Zhong, Chen, 2002; Echeverria et al. 2017; Grizzell et al. 2014）。根据这一发现，可替宁刺激了AktGSK3途径并促进了神经元的存活和突触素在小鼠大脑中的表达（Grizzell, Iarkov et al. 2014）。此外，可替宁对Akt的激活伴随着Tg6799小鼠大脑中突触后密度蛋白95（PSD95）水平的增加。同样，可替宁通过在丝氨酸9位点的磷酸化抑制GSK3β。Akt抑制GSK3可以解释细胞凋亡和tau磷酸化的降低。GSK3也是细胞因子表达和T细胞增殖、分化和存活的关键调节剂，通过控制核因子κB（NFκβ）、活化T细胞核因子（NFAT）以及信号转导子和转录激活因子（STAT）的表达来调节（图22.5）。神经炎症与包括AD在内的几种精神疾病的进展有关。因此，可替宁和锂等GSK3抑制剂可减少神经炎症，减少tau病理和神经元细胞死亡（Gates, Dunnett, 2001）。可替宁抑制GSK3活化、tau磷酸化和Aβ聚集的附加作用值得其用于抗AD疗法的临床研究。

海马中另一种蛋白激酶ERK1/2的激活在促进情境恐惧消退和神经可塑性中起关键作用（Fischer et al. 2007; Guedea et al. 2011; Herry et al. 2006; Matsuda et al. 2010）。与该作用一致的是，可替宁通过磷酸化增加ERK活化，同时促进啮齿动物的恐惧消退（de Aguiar et al. 2013; Zeitlin et al. 2012）（图22.5）。

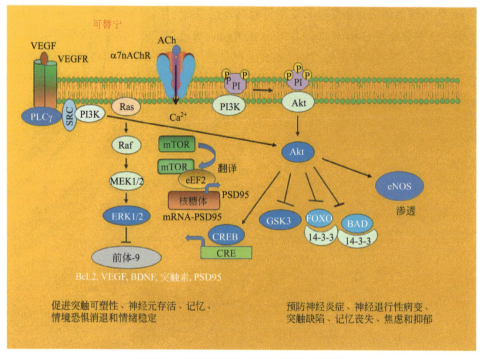

图22.5　可替宁刺激健康大脑功能的信号通路

可替宁通过激活nAChR和VEGF信号传导可刺激存活因子（如Akt）的表达，并抑制凋亡因子（如GSK3β），从而促进tau过度磷酸化和神经元细胞死亡以及突触蛋白的表达。

22.6　可替宁可恢复雌性大鼠化疗后的工作记忆能力

化疗对认知能力有深远影响，包括注意力缺陷、工作记忆减弱和思维减慢，这是一种被称为"化疗脑"的综合征（Simo et al. 2013）。使用化学疗法诱发的认知障碍的大鼠模型，已显示可替宁增强了化学疗法治疗的大鼠的参考记忆并降低了抑郁样行为（Iarkov, Appunn, Echeverria, 2016）。这项研究表明，可替宁可以帮助癌症患者从"化疗脑"中康复。

22.7　可替宁可恢复自闭症谱系障碍和精神分裂症动物模型的记忆

自闭症谱系障碍（ASDs）影响全球数百万人（Prevalence of autism mspectrum disorders——Autism and Developmental Disabilities Monitoring Network, 14 sites, United States, 2008, 2012）。

ASDs涉及错误的突触发育和功能（Spooren et al. 2012）。脆性X染色体综合征（FXS）是导致智力障碍的主要原因，也是自闭症最普遍的原因（Garber et al. 2008），FXS是脆性X智力发育迟缓蛋白（FMRP）表达缺失所致。患有FXS的儿童表现出认知和行为缺陷，包括社交退缩、注意力缺陷、多动和刻板行为（Chudley et al. 1983）。FMR1基因敲除（KO）小鼠（FXS小鼠）是ASD最具特征的动物模型之一（Moy et al. 2006）。这些小鼠表现出类似自闭症的核心症状，包括学习范式中的错误增加。FXS小鼠表现出突触可塑性和脊柱密度的降低，以及大脑中代谢型谷氨酸受体5（mGluR5）的过度激活。mGluR5刺激GSK3β信号。FXS小鼠中FMRP介导的GSK3β失调被认为是ASD病理中的关键事件，因为GSK3β的过度激活会导致神经炎症，并对神经发生、认知能力（King et al. 2013）和大脑发育（Martel et al. 2013）产生负面影响。因此，GSK3β信号传导可能是AD、FXS和相关ASD的疾病缓解干预措施的新型治疗靶点（Hooper, Killick, Lovestone, 2008）。先前的研究表明，烟碱刺激胆碱能系统对自闭症症状（如重复行为和社交退缩）具有积极作用。有趣的是，我们先前发现可替宁可抑制小鼠大脑中的GSK3β。使用$Fmr1^{-/-}$敲除小鼠和对照组的同窝仔小鼠，已显示可替宁在$Fmr1^{-/-}$小鼠的海马中增加了Akt对GSK3β的丝氨酸磷酸化的抑制（Portis et al. 2012）。可替宁治疗改善了$Fmr1^{-/-}$的空间处理、新颖物体识别和时间顺序方面的认知能力。此外，他们使用遗传工具证明了可替宁的有益作用取决于Akt对GSK3的抑制。该证据表明可替宁可以成为ASD的有前途的疗法。多项研究表明，可替宁可预防精神分裂症大鼠和猴子模型中的工作记忆丧失（Buccafusco, Terry Jr. 2009; Terry Jr. et al. 2012）。这些研究与烟碱受体的正构调节剂可能构成SCHZ记忆障碍的有效疗法的想法相符。

关键事实
- 精神病患者的烟草消费较高，并且新证据表明，烟草消费可能是一种自我药物治疗形式，旨在获得烟碱主要衍生物可替宁的益处。
- 目前的证据表明，可替宁可能是一种针对以胆碱能缺乏和/或神经炎症为特征的记忆障碍的有效疗法。
- 在正常和病理条件下，可替宁在哺乳动物中具有抗炎、帮助记忆、抗抑郁和抗焦虑作用。
- 大量临床研究表明，可替宁在人体中的安全性和非成瘾性的作用和在哺乳动物中的治疗作用的剂量相当。
- 需要临床研究以确认可替宁对改善人类记忆的有效性。

要点总结
- 可替宁通过一种涉及额叶皮层和海马中ERK激活和Akt / GSK3途径激活的机制来预防认知障碍。
- 可替宁通过刺激PTSD和AD小鼠海马和额叶皮层中突触素和PSD95，从而刺激突触发生。
- 可替宁可刺激应激小鼠的VEGF因子表达。
- 可替宁通过一种涉及激活nAChR信号及其下游效应子ERK1/2的机制来增强情景恐惧记忆的消除。
- 可替宁可恢复受慢性应激影响的星形胶质细胞的数量和形态。

术语解释
- 阿尔茨海默病：进行性神经退行性疾病和老年痴呆症的主要病因，其特征是突触丧失、神经元细胞死亡、星形胶质细胞增多、tau病理和聚集性Aβ老年斑形成。

- 星形胶质细胞增多：星形胶质细胞形态改变和数量增加可能会导致神经炎症以及氧气和一氧化氮的氧化性物质的释放。
- 灭绝：重复暴露于与创伤事件有关的线索后恐惧反应的减轻。
- 恐惧条件：对环境线索和有害的、令人恐惧的刺激进行配对，以使其进一步暴露于线索之下，从而引发条件恐惧反应。
- 药效学：对包括受体和其他蛋白质结合在内的引起其抑制或激活的药物作用机理的研究。
- 药代动力学：药物在体内的吸收、分布、代谢和排泄。
- 创伤后应激障碍（PTSD）：这是一种轻度神经退行性疾病，是痴呆症的主要病因，是由于暴露于创伤事件而引起的，而创伤事件会对自己或他人的生命造成不可避免的危险。
- 精神分裂症：一种以认知缺陷为特征的精神病性疾病，包括脉冲前抑制、工作记忆受损以及妄想和谵妄等症状。
- 突触神经元结构：代表神经元之间的神经化学联系，涉及突触前位点和突触后位点，突触前位点包含突触小泡，突触后位点周围有离子通道、受体和信号传导因子。
- 突触形成：神经元中出现新的突触。

参考文献

Benowitz, N. L.; Kuyt, F.; Jacob, P.; 3rd, Jones, R. T.; Osman, A. L. (1983). Cotinine disposition and effects. Clinical Pharmacolog and Therapeutics, 34(5), 604-611.

Benowitz, N. L.; Sharp, D. S. (1989). Inverse relation between serum cotinine concentration and blood pressure in cigarette smokers. Circulation, 80(5), 1309-1312.

Breen, A.; Blankley, K.; Fine, J. (2017). The efficacy of prazosin for the treatment of posttraumatic stress disorder nightmares in U. S. military veterans. Journal of the American Association of Nurse Practitioners, 29(2), 65-69.

Buccafusco, J. J.; Terry, A. V.; Jr. (2003). The potential role of cotinine in the cognitive and neuroprotective actions of nicotine. Life Sciences, 72 (26), 2931-2942.

Buccafusco, J. J.; Terry, A. V.; Jr. (2009). A reversible model of the cognitive impairment associated with schizophrenia in monkeys: potential therapeutic effects of two nicotinic acetylcholine receptor agonists. Biochemical Pharmacology, 78(7), 852-862.

Burgess, S.; Zeitlin, R. S.; Gamble-George, J.; Echeverria Moran, V. (2008). P2-319: Cotinine is neuroprotective against beta-amyloid toxicity. Alzheimer's and Dementia, 4(4).

Cabezas, R.; Vega-Vela, N. E.; Gonzalez-Sanmiguel, J. et al. (2017). PDGF-BB preserves mitochondrial morphology, attenuates ROS production, and upregulates neuroglobin in an astrocytic model under rotenone insult. Molecular Neurobiology. https://doi.org/10.1007/s12035-017-0567-6.

Chudley, A. E.; Knoll, J.; Gerrard, J. W.; Shepel, L.; McGahey, E., Anderson, J. (1983). Fragile (X) X-linked mental retardation I: relationship between age and intelligence and the frequency of expression of fragil (X)(q28). American Journal of Medical Genetics, 14(4), 699-712.

Conklin, B. S.; Zhao, W.; Zhong, D. S.; Chen, C. (2002). Nicotine and cotinine up-regulate vascular endothelial growth factor expression in endothelial cells. The American Journal of Pathology, 160(2), 413-418.

Czeh, B.; Simon, M.; Schmelting, B.; Hiemke, C.; Fuchs, E. (2006). Astroglial plasticity in the hippocampus is affected by chronic psychosocial stress and concomitant fluoxetine treatment. Neuropsychopharmacology, 31(8), 1616-1626.

de Aguiar, R. B.; Parfitt, G. M.; Jaboinski, J.; Barros, D. M. (2013). Neuroactive effects of cotinine on the hippocampus: behavioral and biochemical parameters. Neuropharmacology, 71, 292-298.

Echeverria, V.; Barreto, G. E.; Avila-Rodriguez, M.; Tarasov, V. V.; Aliev, G. (2017). Is VEGF a key target of cotinine and other potential therapies against Alzheimer disease? Current Alzheimer Research. https://doi.org/10.2174/1567205014666170329113007.

Echeverria, V.; Grizzell, J. A.; Barreto, G. E. (2016). Neuroinflammation: a therapeutic target of cotinine for the treatment of psychiatric disorders? Current Pharmaceutical Design, 22(10), 1324-1333.

Echeverria, V.; Yarkov, A.; Aliev, G. (2016). Positive modulators of the alpha7 nicotinic receptor against neuroinflammation and cognitive impairment in Alzheimer's disease. Progress in Neurobiology, 144, 142-157.

Echeverria, V.; Zeitlin, R. (2012). Cotinine: a potential new therapeutic agent against Alzheimer's disease. CNS Neuroscience, Therapeutics, 18(7), 517-523.

Echeverria, V.; Zeitlin, R.; Burgess, S.; Patel, S.; Barman, A.; Thakur, G. et al. (2011). Cotinine reduces amyloid-beta aggregation and improves memory in Alzheimer's disease mice. Journal of Alzheimer's Disease, 24(4), 817-835.

Fischer, A.; Radulovic, M.; Schrick, C.; Sananbenesi, F.; Godovac Zimmermann, J.; Radulovic, J. (2007). Hippocampal Mek/Erk signaling mediates extinction of contextual freezing behavior. Neurobiology of Learning and Memory, 87(1), 149-158.

Fournier, N. M.; Lee, B.; Banasr, M.; Elsayed, M.; Duman, R. S. (2012). Vascular endothelial growth factor regulates adult hippocampal cell proliferation through MEK/ERK- and PI3K/Akt-dependent signaling. Neuropharmacology, 63(4), 642-652.

J. Gao, B. La, J. M. Chapman, D. Bertrand, A. V. Terry; (2012). Neuroprotective effects of the nicotine metabolite, cotinine, and several structural analogs of cotinine paper presented at the Society for Neuroscience, New Orleans, LA.

Garber, K. B.; Visootsak, J.; Warren, S. T. (2008). Fragile X syndrome. European Journal of Human Genetics, 16(6), 666-672.

Márquez G. G.; Living to Tell the Tale(2003) (Edith Grossman, translator), New York, 2004, Vintage International, pp 1-493. ISBN 1-4000-3454.

Gates, M. A.; Dunnett, S. B. (2001). The influence of astrocytes on the development, regeneration and reconstruction of the nigrostriatal dopamine system. Restorative Neurology and Neuroscience, 19(1-2), 67-83.

Gomez-Galan, M.; De Bundel, D.; Van Eeckhaut, A.; Smolders, I.; Lindskog, M. (2013). Dysfunctional astrocytic regulation of glutamate transmission in a rat model of depression. Molecular Psychiatry, 18(5), 582-594.

Grizzell, J. A.; Echeverria, V. (2015). New insights into the mechanisms of action of cotinine and its distinctive effects from nicotine. Neurochemical Research, 40(10), 2032-2046.

Grizzell, J. A.; Iarkov, A.; Holmes, R.; Mori, T.; Echeverria, V. (2014). Cotinine reduces depressive-like behavior, working memory deficits, and synaptic loss associated with chronic stress in mice. Behavioural Brain Research, 268, 55-65.

Grizzell, J. A.; Mullins, M.; Iarkov, A.; Rohani, A.; Charry, L. C.; Echeverria, V. (2014). Cotinine reduces depressive-like behavior and hippocampal vascular endothelial growth factor downregulation after forced swim stress in mice. Behavioral Neuroscience, 128 (6), 713-721.

Grizzell, J. A.; Patel, S.; Barreto, G. E.; Echeverria, V. (2017). Cotinine improves visual recognition memory and decreases cortical Tau phosphorylation in the Tg6799 mice. Progress in Neuro Psychopharmacology, Biological Psychiatry, 78, 75-81.

Guedea, A. L.; Schrick, C.; Guzman, Y. F.; Leaderbrand, K.; Jovasevic, V.; Corcoran, K. A. et al. (2011). ERK-associated changes of AP-1 proteins during fear extinction. Molecular and Cellular Neurosciences, 47(2), 137-144.

Han, Z.; Li, L.; Wang, L.; Degos, V.; Maze, M.; Su, H. (2014). Alpha-7 nicotinic acetylcholine receptor agonist treatment reduces neuroinflammation, oxidative stress, and brain injury in mice with ischemic stroke and bone fracture. Journal of Neurochemistry, 131(4), 498-508.

Hatsukami, D.; Lexau, B.; Nelson, D.; Pentel, P. R.; Sofuoglu, M.; Goldman, A. (1998). Effects of cotinine on cigarette self-administration. Psychopharmacology, 138(2), 184-189.

Hatsukami, D.; Pentel, P. R.; Jensen, J.; Nelson, D.; Allen, S. S.; Goldman, A. et al. (1998). Cotinine: effects with and without nicotine. Psychopharmacology, 135(2), 141-150.

Hatsukami, D. K.; Grillo, M.; Pentel, P. R.; Oncken, C.; Bliss, R. (1997)Safety of cotinine in humans: physiologic, subjective, and cognitive effects. Pharmacology, Biochemistry, and Behavior, 57(4), 643-650.

Herry, C.; Trifilieff, P.; Micheau, J.; Luthi, A.; Mons, N. (2006). Extinction of auditory fear conditioning requires MAPK/ERK activation in the basolateral amygdala. The European Journal of Neuroscience, 24(1), 261-269.

Hooper, C.; Killick, R.; Lovestone, S. (2008). The GSK3 hypothesis of Alzheimer's disease. Journal of Neurochemistry, 104(6), 1433-1439.

Iarkov, A.; Appunn, D.; Echeverria, V. (2016). Post-treatment with cotinine improved memory and decreased depressive-like behavior after chemotherapy in rats. Cancer Chemotherapy and Pharmacology, 78(5), 1033-1039.

Keenan, R. M.; Hatsukami, D. K.; Pentel, P. R.; Thompson, T. N.; Grillo, M. A. (1994). Pharmacodynamic effects of cotinine in abstinent cigarette smokers. Clinical Pharmacology and Therapeutics, 55(5), 581-590.

Kelly, M. M.; Jensen, K. P.; Sofuoglu, M. (2015). Co-occurring tobacco use and posttraumatic stress disorder: Smoking cessation treatment implications. The American Journal on Addictions, 24(8), 695-704.

King, M. K.; Pardo, M.; Cheng, Y.; Downey, K.; Jope, R. S.; Beurel, E. (2013). Glycogen synthase kinase-3 inhibitors: rescuers of cognitive impairments. Pharmacology, Therapeutics. https:/ /doi. org/10. 1016/j. pharmthera. 2013. 07. 010.

Kuo, B. S.; Dryjski, M.; Bjornsson, T. D. (1989). Influence of nicotine and cotinine on the expression of plasminogen activator activity in bovine aortic endothelial cells. Thrombosis and Haemostasis, 61(1), 70-76.

Liberzon, I.; Sripada, C. S. (2008). The functional neuroanatomy of PTSD: a critical review. Progress in Brain Research, 167, 151-169.

Martel, C.; Allouche, M.; Esposti, D. D.; Fanelli, E.; Boursier, C.; Henry, C. et al. (2013). Glycogen synthase kinase 3-mediated voltage-dependent anion channel phosphorylation controls outer mitochondrial membrane permeability during lipid accumulation. Hepatology, 57(1), 93-102.

Matsuda, S.; Matsuzawa, D.; Nakazawa, K.; Sutoh, C.; Ohtsuka, H.; Ishii, D. et al. (2010). d-serine enhances extinction of auditory cued fear conditioning via ERK1/2 phosphorylation in mice. Progress in Neuro-Psychopharmacology, Biological Psychiatry, 34(6), 895-902.

Mendoza, C.; Barreto, G. E.; Avila-Rodriguez, M.; Echeverria, V. (2016). Role of neuroinflammation and sex hormones in war-related PTSD. Molecular and Cellular Endocrinology, 434, 266-277.

Moraga-Amaro, R.; Jerez-Baraona, J. M.; Simon, F.; Stehberg, J. (2014). Role of astrocytes in memory and psychiatric disorders. Journal of Physiology, Paris, 108(4-6), 240-251.

Moran, V. E. (2012). Cotinine: beyond that expected, more than a biomarker of tobacco consumption. Frontiers in Pharmacology, 3, 173.

Moy, S. S.; Nadler, J. J.; Magnuson, T. R.; Crawley, J. N. (2006). Mouse models of autism spectrum disorders: the challenge for behavioral genetics. American Journal of Medical Genetics Part C, Seminars in Medical Genetics, 142C(1), 40-51.

Patel, S.; Grizzell, J. A.; Holmes, R.; Zeitlin, R.; Solomon, R.; Sutton, T. L. et al. (2014). Cotinine halts the advance of Alzheimer's disease-like pathology and associated depressive-like behavior in Tg6799 mice. Frontiers in Aging Neuroscience, 6, 162.

Perez-Urrutia, N.; Mendoza, C.; Alvarez-Ricartes, N.; Oliveros- Matus, P.; Echeverria, F.; Grizzell, J. A. et al. (2017). Intranasal cotinine improves memory, and reduces depressive-like behavior, and GFAP+ cells loss induced by restraint stress in mice. Experimental Neurology, 295, 211-221.

Portis, S.; Giunta, B.; Obregon, D.; Tan, J. (2012). The role of glycogen synthase kinase-3 signaling in neurodevelopment and fragile X syndrome.

International Journal of Physiology, Pathophysiology, and Pharmacology, 4(3), 140-148.

Prevalence of autism spectrum disorders—Autism and Developmental Disabilities Monitoring Network, 14 sites, United States, 2008 (2012). MMWR Surveillance Summaries, 61(3), 1-19.

Santha, P.; Veszelka, S.; Hoyk, Z.; Meszaros, M.; Walter, F. R.; Toth, A. E. et al. (2015). Restraint stress-induced morphological changes at the blood-brain barrier in adult rats. Frontiers in Molecular Neuroscience, 8, 88.

Saur, L.; Baptista, P. P.; Bagatini, P. B.; Neves, L. T.; de Oliveira, R. M.; Vaz, S. P. et al. (2016). Experimental post-traumatic stress disorder decreases astrocyte density and changes astrocytic polarity in the CA1 Hippocampus of male rats. Neurochemical Research, 41(4), 892-904.

Simo, M.; Rifa-Ros, X.; Rodriguez-Fornells, A.; Bruna, J. (2013). Chemobrain: a systematic review of structural and functional neuroimaging studies. Neuroscience and Biobehavioral Reviews. https://doi.org/10.1016/j.neubiorev.2013.04.015.

Singh, B.; Hughes, A. J.; Mehta, G.; Erwin, P. J.; Parsaik, A. K. (2016). Efficacy of prazosin in posttraumatic stress disorder: a systematic review and meta-analysis. Prime Care Companion to CNS Disorders. 18(4). https://doi.org/10.4088/PCC.16r01943.

Spooren, W.; Lindemann, L.; Ghosh, A.; Santarelli, L. (2012). Synapse dysfunction in autism: a molecular medicine approach to drug discovery in neurodevelopmental disorders. Trends in Pharmacological Sciences.

Terry, A. V.; Jr.; Buccafusco, J. J.; Schade, R. F.; Vandenhuerk, L.; Callahan, P. M.; Beck, W. D. et al. (2012). The nicotine metabolite, cotinine, attenuates glutamate (NMDA) antagonist-related effects on the performance of the five choice serial reaction time task (5C-SRTT) in rats. Biochemical Pharmacology, 83(7), 941-951.

Terry, A. V.; Jr.; Callahan, P. M.; Bertrand, D. (2015). R-(+) and S-(-) isomers of cotinine augment cholinergic responses in vitro and in vivo. The Journal of Pharmacology and Experimental Therapeutics, 352(2), 405-418.

Thomas, E.; Stein, D. J. (2017). Novel pharmacological treatment strategies for posttraumatic stress disorder. Expert Review of Clinical Pharmacology, 10(2), 167-177.

Wager-Smith, K.; Markou, A. (2011). Depression: a repair response to stress-induced neuronal microdamage that can grade into a chronic neuroinflammatory condition? Neuroscience and Biobehavioral Reviews, 35(3), 742-764.

Wang, Z. G.; Li, H.; Huang, Y.; Li, R.; Wang, X. F.; Yu, L. X. et al. (2017). Nerve growth factor-induced Akt/mTOR activation protects the ischemic heart via restoring autophagic flux and attenuating ubiquitinated protein accumulation. Oncotarget, 8(3), 5400-5413.

Wildeboer-Andrud, K. M.; Zheng, L.; Choo, K. S.; Stevens, K. E. (2014). Cotinine impacts sensory processing in DBA/2 mice through changes in the conditioning amplitude. Pharmacology, Biochemistry, and Behavior, 117, 144-150.

Wu, H.; Lu, D.; Jiang, H.; Xiong, Y.; Qu, C.; Li, B. et al. (2008). Simvastatin-mediated upregulation of VEGF and BDNF, activation of the PI3K/Akt pathway, and increase of neurogenesis are associated with therapeutic improvement after traumatic brain injury. Journal of Neurotrauma, 25(2), 130-139.

Young, G. (2017). PTSD in court II: Risk factors, endophenotypes, and biological underpinnings in PTSD. International Journal of Law and Psychiatry, 51, 1-21.

Zeitlin, R.; Patel, S.; Solomon, R.; Tran, J.; Weeber, E. J.; Echeverria, V. (2012). Cotinine enhances the extinction of contextual fear memory and reduces anxiety after fear conditioning. Behavioural Brain Research, 228(2), 284-293.

Zevin, S.; Jacob, P.; Geppetti, P.; Benowitz, N. L. (2000). Clinical pharmacology of oral cotinine. Drug and Alcohol Dependence, 60(1), 13-18.

23
烟碱在异常学习和皮质纹状体可塑性中的作用

Jessica L. Koranda[1], *Jeff A. Beeler*[2]

1. Department of Neurobiology, University of Chicago, Chicago, IL, United States
2. Department of Psychology, Queens College and the Graduate Center, CUNY, Flushing, NY, United States

缩略语

AMPAR	AMPA 谷氨酸受体	**LTP**	长期增强
cNIC	慢性烟碱	**MSN**	中棘神经元
HFS	高频刺激	**NMDAR**	NMDA 谷氨酸受体
L-DOPA	左旋多巴	**NR2B**	NMDA 谷氨酸受体的2B 亚基
LDR	长期反应	**PD**	帕金森病
LTD	长期抑制		

23.1 引言

基底神经节通过皮质-基底神经节-皮质重入回路影响皮质的活动。多巴胺功能的改变会改变该回路，这种改变与产生帕金森病（PD）和与药物成瘾相关的行为强迫的关键特征有关。多巴胺信号可以响应环境中持续的刺激而改变皮质纹状体传递。然而，多巴胺在调节皮质纹状体突触的突触可塑性方面也起着关键作用（Augustin et al. 2014; Kreitzer, Malenka, 2008; Lovinger, 2010），允许经验依赖性修正-学习会发生在皮质-基底神经节环路中，来纠正未来的行为。慢性烟碱暴露（如在吸烟中发生）会诱发多种神经和生理适应，并带来无数的功能和行为后果。在本章中，我们着重讨论在PD和成瘾的情况下，慢性烟碱引起的皮质纹状体可塑性调节的变化。

23.2 帕金森病、烟碱和神经保护

帕金森病是由黑质致密部（SNc）中多巴胺（DA）神经元的进行性变性引起的，以运动障碍为特征。用左旋多巴代替多巴胺治疗仍是主要的治疗手段。在疾病进展的早期，左旋多巴治疗可以有效地改善运动症状，但不能防止退化，并在后期变得不那么有效，这强调了新疗法的必要性，特别是神经保护策略。

流行病学研究已发现吸烟与PD发病率呈反比关系。这种降低的风险可跨烟碱产品转化，涉及烟碱而不是卷烟烟雾中的其他成分（Chen et al. 2010; Van Der Mark et al. 2014）。PD 风险降低与持续时间（吸烟年数）而非数量（重度吸烟者与轻度吸烟者）的相关性更大。停止吸烟后，PD 风险逐渐恢复正常，这表明假定的烟碱诱导的神经适应阻止了进行性神经退行性过程。

尚不清楚烟碱是如何降低PD风险的。在细胞培养中进行的研究表明，烟碱可以保护细胞免

受损伤，如氧化应激和兴奋性刺激（Jin, Gao, Flagg, Deng, 2004），但在动物研究中却更加自相矛盾。在报道保护作用的研究中，慢性烟碱剂量依赖性地保留纹状体多巴胺活性的生化标记物，通常不保留SNc中酪氨酸羟化酶免疫反应纤维或细胞的数量（Huang, Lin et al. 2009）。烟碱治疗不能改善已存在黑质纹状体损伤的动物的多巴胺能的完整性（Huang, Lin et al. 2009），这表明烟碱可以减轻神经支配的功能性后果。

尽管烟碱具有明显的神经保护特性，但对烟碱治疗帕金森病的临床研究仍未得出结论。这种差异可能是由于治疗时间的不同而引起的。烟碱能改善运动症状，烟碱治疗持续2周至1年（Hanagasi et al. 2007; Kelton et al. 2000），而研究报告中的症状没有变化或恶化（Vieregge et al. 2001），烟碱治疗是急性的，仅限于几天。Kelton等（2000）发现，烟碱治疗中止后，运动症状改善持续1个月。烟碱停药后这种效果的持久性以及观察到的吸烟年数与PD发病率降低程度呈反比关系，表明慢性烟碱（cNIC）会引起进行性神经适应性疾病的发生和逐渐减少。

23.3 异常的运动学习假说

尽管多巴胺去神经支配改变了皮质纹状体的可塑性，但这对PD的影响尚不清楚。在间接途径的中棘神经元（MSNs）中，多巴胺的消耗或阻断会削弱长期抑郁（LTD），并可在通常诱发LTD的条件下（高频刺激）诱发异常的长期增强（LTP）（Calabresi et al. 1997; Kreitzer, Malenka, 2007; Shen et al. 2008）。间接途径中的皮质纹状体LTD通过选择性地减少基底神经节对皮质活动的抑制而促进运动（Kreitzer, Malenka, 2008）。通常会产生LTD的不适当的LTP会产生相反的效果：突触编码运动抑制而不是促进抑制，这是一种我们称之为异常学习的突触可塑性病理生理学（图23.1; Beeler, 2011; Beeler et al. 2010, 2012; Beeler, Petzinger, Jakowec, 2013; Zhuang, Mazzoni, Kang, 2013）。由异常学习引起的不适当抑制专门针对应促进的皮质传入活动：本质上，通过揭示终身学习的运动技能，将可塑性转化为运动，加速功能退化。

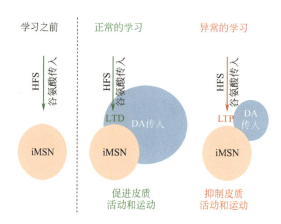

图23.1 异常运动学习假说

高传入神经活动结合多巴胺能刺激诱导间接通路MSN皮质纹状体突触的抑制，促进运动和适当行为的选择。在多巴胺阻断或去神经的情况下，皮质传入的HFS诱导增强，抑制运动并产生不适应的异常运动学习。

为了在实验上将多巴胺对突触可塑性和学习（影响未来行为）的影响与其对突触传递（调节当前行为）的影响分离出来，我们在加速旋转体的多相变化中采用了多巴胺的可逆性阻断作用,这是一项评估运动表现和学习的小鼠行为任务(图23.2)。在第1阶段,小鼠在接受多巴胺D_1和D_2拮抗剂(对照和盐水)混合液的情况下接受5~7d的训练。至少休息72h后,在第2阶段("恢复阶段")为小鼠提供其他无药品训练。

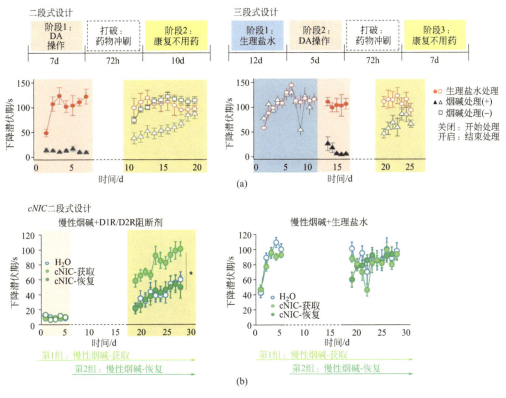

图23.2 cNIC减轻了异常学习

(a) D_1(SCH23390,0.10mg/kg)和D_2(伊替必利,0.16mg/kg)多巴胺拮抗剂,用于在两相(左)或三相(右)设计中诱导多巴胺阻滞。在多巴胺阻滞下进行旋转训练后,经验依赖的异常学习表现为恢复过程中渐近性能的时间增加。
(b) 在多巴胺阻滞下进行旋转训练之前(而非之后)的cNIC(100μg/mL,饮用水中)减少了异常运动学习(左)。在正常的多巴胺下,cNIC不会改变学习(右)。数据表示为平均下降延迟±SEM。图经Koranda等(2016)《神经科学杂志》许可改编。

在第2阶段无药物状态下的性能受损反映出在多巴胺拮抗剂的影响下发生的学习。如预期的那样,用多巴胺拮抗剂治疗会损害第1阶段的性能。但是,用拮抗剂治疗的小鼠在无药物恢复阶段(第2阶段)继续表现出受损的性能。这些小鼠的恢复非常缓慢,需要一周以上的时间才能获得渐近性能,这通常是由幼稚小鼠在训练后2~3d内获得的[图23.2(a)]。在第2阶段(恢复过程),性能受损不是残留的药理作用,因为小鼠接受了相同的多巴胺拮抗剂治疗,但是在没有旋转脚架训练的情况下将其放在笼中,也没有随后的损伤[图23.2(a)]。因此,多巴胺拮抗后的性能受损取决于经验,表明学习过程。我们将这些结果解释为在多巴胺拮抗作用下的初始训练期间发生的异常学习。一旦就位,先前的异常学习会干扰适当的重新学习,并且性能的提高比初始的天真学习要慢得多。在单独测试D_1和D_2受体拮抗剂时,D_1阻滞尽管会损害性能,但对后续恢复没有影响,而仅D_2阻滞则有影响,这表明异常学习是间接途径特有的。此任务的三个阶段的版本测试了既定运动技能中的异常学习:首先对小鼠进行渐近性能训练,然后在第2阶段对小鼠进行多巴胺拮抗剂训练,随后进行无药物恢复(第3阶段)[图23.2(a)]。

在缺乏Pitx3转录因子的小鼠中也观察到类似的运动学习的分解。这些小鼠的黑质纹状体多巴胺神经元选择性丢失，导致背侧纹状体多巴胺减少90%（Beeler et al. 2009）。Pitx3小鼠无法学习旋转任务，除非使用L-DOPA治疗，它可以恢复正常的运动学习。停用L-DOPA治疗后，随后的性能不会立即受到损害，而是会逐渐下降。这不是L-DOPA的残留效应，因为停药之间的间隔可以延长至2周，且结果相同。L-DOPA停用后的性能下降取决于经验。这些结果使我们提出，对L-DOPA了解甚少但临床上关键的长期反应（LDR）可能源于皮质纹状体可塑性失调和异常学习的纠正（Beeler, 2011; Beeler et al. 2010, 2012; Zhuang et al. 2013），解释了其在初始治疗期间的逐渐发作和停药后的逐渐下降。我们假设针对性异常学习可能代表PD中的神经保护策略：通过保护已建立的技能和终身学习，功能恶化的速度可能会减慢。

23.4　烟碱减轻了多巴胺缺乏引起的异常运动学习

我们假设cNIC诱导神经适应、减少与多巴胺损失相关的异常学习，这可能有助于其对帕金森病的假定保护作用（Koranda et al. 2016）。在饮用水中给予小鼠cNIC 2周，然后用上述多巴胺拮抗剂进行旋转训练。cNIC剂量依赖性地减少由多巴胺拮抗剂［图23.2（b）］或单独由D_{2R}拮抗剂诱导的异常运动学习。相比之下，在异常学习后产生的cNIC并不促进恢复［图23.2（b）］，这表明cNIC减少了多巴胺阻滞下产生的异常学习，但不促进随后的"再学习"。此外，如果在第2阶段给予急性注射，这并不能缓解异常学习和恶化的恢复（Koranda et al. 2016）。

表明这种益处来自cNIC诱导的神经适应，随着时间的推移而发展，以应对长期暴露于烟碱。这种cNIC诱导的神经适应可能涉及含有烟碱乙酰胆碱受体的β2亚基的慢性脱敏和/或功能降低，因为缺乏β2亚基的小鼠，包括多巴胺细胞的选择性缺失，也表现出异常学习的减少（Koranda et al. 2016）。

这些结果表明，cNIC可以防止因多巴胺信号丢失而引起的异常学习。我们认为，这诱导了一种类似LDR的神经保护治疗效果。在渐进式去神经支配的过程中，这种效应可能会减缓支持行为的突触连接的逐渐解除，进而减缓与渐进式多巴胺去神经支配相关的功能下降。这种假定的保护作用存在的时间越长，一个人吸烟的时间越长，减缓吸烟过程的累积效益就越大。因为cNIC实际上减少了多巴胺的功能（Koranda et al. 2014; Perez et al. 2012），神经保护适应可能出现在多巴胺信号的下游。我们的研究表明，cNIC可以抵消皮质纹状体可塑性的失调和与多巴胺去神经支配相关的异常学习。

23.5　烟碱成瘾和异常学习

戒烟被普遍认为是非常困难的，长期成功率很低。困难来自导致复发的持续渴望。这种渴望会持续很长一段时间，有时是几年。虽然人们可能认为，渴望会随着时间的推移而减少，但有证据表明，在戒烟后的几个月中，渴望实际上会增加，这种现象被称为潜伏期（Li, Caprioli, Marchant, 2015）。这些渴望归因于药物使用期间的药物强化联想学习，该学习将无数刺激、活动和状态（如压力）与强迫使用联系起来。尚不清楚的是，为什么这种学习如此显著地抵抗灭绝；也就是说，在突触生理学水平上，尚不清楚是什么使得代表特定学习的突触连接比其他"正常"突触更能抵抗变化。一种可能性是慢性烟碱和其他滥用药物诱导神经适应，改变突触可塑性的机制，包括突触可塑性的调节。也就是说，烟碱可能诱导异常的突触可塑性：其本身并未受损，但发生了改变,使得获得新的学习和修正已建立的学习与长期暴露于药物之前的操作不同。

23.6 烟碱诱导的沉默突触和皮质纹状体可塑性的改变

反复使用可卡因和阿片类药物可在纹状体中棘细胞中诱导沉默突触（Graziane et al. 2016; Huang, Parameswaran, et al. 2009）。沉默突触只含NMDA谷氨酸受体,不含AMPARs。因此,NMDARs中的Mg^{2+}阻断阻止了静息电位下的快速谷氨酸能传递,使这些突触"沉默"。在早期发育中很常见,突触连接过度表达,然后被选择或修剪,成年动物中基本不存在沉默突触（Hanse, Seth, Riebe, 2013）,但有一些例外。值得注意的是,MSNs上的沉默突触在成年后仍然存在,占正常健康小鼠兴奋性突触的5%～15%（Brown et al. 2011; Huang, Parameswaran et al. 2009; Koya et al. 2012; Whitaker et al. 2015; Xia, Meyers, Beeler, 2017）。虽然这些残留的沉默突触在成年人MSNs中的功能作用尚不清楚,但可卡因和阿片类药物可显著增加其患病率（35%～55%）的发现导致了"返老还童假说",该假说认为这些沉默突触是被滥用药物"劫持"的回路重构的底物（Dong, Nestler, 2014）,很像滥用药物"劫持奖励系统"的观点。

最近的一项研究（Xia et al. 2017）证明cNIC也增加了MSNs中的沉默突触［图23.3（a）］。可卡因和阿片类药物通过不同的机制分别不同地增加了直接和间接途径MSNs中的沉默突触。可卡因上调NR2B NMDA亚基,通过重新产生沉默突触来增加沉默突触。阿片类药物通过从已建立的突触中去除AMPARs来增加沉默突触。我们已经证明,cNIC像阿片类药物一样,通过NR2b介导的机制（如可卡因）增加间接途径中的沉默突触,但我们尚未评估其对直接途径的影响。已经研究了沉默突触和药物相关行为之间的联系（Brown et al. 2011; Koya et al. 2012; Lee et al. 2013; Ma et al. 2014; Whitaker et al. 2015）,特别证明了沉默突触与孵化有关（Lee et al. 2013; Ma et al. 2014）。然而,这种关系是复杂的,因为在停药后,某些区域激活的沉默突触的复位减少了孵化,但在其他区域却增加了孵化（Ma et al. 2014）。这些数据表明,沉默突触本身并不介导特定的行为效应,而是反映了突触可塑性的变化,其中行为后果是区域依赖性的。

cNIC如何改变皮质纹状体的可塑性? 我们测试了饮用水中含有cNIC（100μg/mL）的小鼠

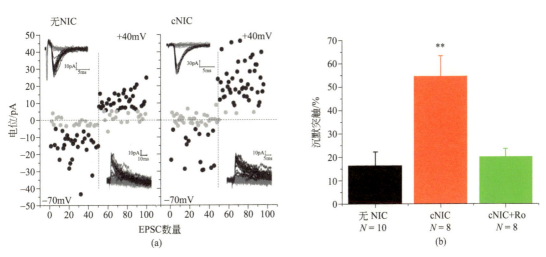

图23.3

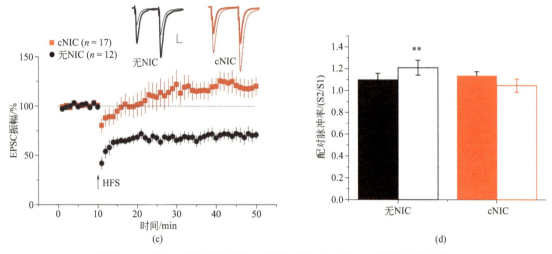

图 23.3　cNIC 在间接途径 MSNs 中增加沉默突触并逆转皮质纹状体的可塑性

（a）最小刺激试验，评估间接途径MSNs中沉默突触的患病率，比较cNIC处理的小鼠和对照组小鼠。与−70mV相比，在保持电位为+40mV时，失败（灰色圆圈）减少，这反映了沉默突触的存在，因为在+40mV时，NMDARs的mg^{2+}阻断被解除，允许仅NMDA的突触发挥作用。插图：所有细胞的痕迹，黑色代表成功，灰色代表失败。（b）cNIC增加沉默突触（红条），这依赖于NR2B亚基，因为增加的成功率被NR2B选择性拮抗剂阻断。（c）用膜片钳记录用慢性烟碱治疗的小鼠（红色）或对照组（黑色）的间接途径MSNs。在HFS（箭头）之后，对照小鼠表现出突触抑制，而cNIC处理的小鼠表现出增强。（d）HFS前后的配对脉冲率。对照组小鼠表现出预期的配对脉冲易化，表明发生了突触前抑制，而cNIC处理的小鼠则没有，这与突触后增强位点一致。数据表示为平均值±SEM。图经Xia等（2017）《神经精神药理学》改编。

的间接MSN的高频刺激（HFS）。正常情况下，HFS在间接途径兴奋性突触处诱导LTD，这对于选择性降低基底神经节对皮层活动的抑制以促进行为至关重要。在用cNIC处理的小鼠中，HFS反而诱导LTP，逆转了可塑性的正常方向［图23.3（b）］。这种皮质纹状体可塑性的改变伴随着NR2B富集的NMDAR电流的整体增加，并伴随着沉默突触的显著增加。因此，暴露于cNIC会诱导神经适应，从而改变间接途径中皮质纹状体突触可塑性的调节。

23.7　慢性烟碱难题

cNIC揭示了两种非常不同的现象，一种是积极的，一种是消极的。一方面，cNIC提供了某种形式的神经保护，降低了帕金森病的风险，尽管如何降低风险尚不清楚。另一方面，cNIC会导致上瘾，并且通过吸烟成为可预防死亡的主要原因。这两种现象都可能涉及烟碱诱导的皮质纹状体可塑性的神经适应。如果是这样的话，我们可能会认为在间接途径MSNs中cNIC抑制LTP而促进LTD。然而，我们观察到的恰恰相反：cNIC本身似乎在间接途径中逆转了皮质纹状体的可塑性，这被假设为cNIC明显减少异常学习的原因。这只是加剧了先前的悖论，即已知cNIC会削弱多巴胺功能（Koranda et al. 2014; Perez et al. 2012），在某种程度上保护了多巴胺的渐进性损失。

23.8　慢性烟碱和突触稳定性：最初的假设

沉默突触可以很容易地通过插入AMPARs而不被激活。一旦被激活，这些未沉默的突触可以稳定并保持为正常的功能性突触，也可以重新沉默并可能移除（Hanse et al. 2013）。细胞中沉默突触的普遍存在是由于新的沉默突触的产生与它们作为功能性突触的激活、选择和稳定和/或它们在重新定位时的去除之间的动态平衡。因此，沉默突触发生率的增加可能是由于产生率的增加、利用率的降低（选择/稳定）或去除率的降低（图23.4）。

在用cNIC处理的小鼠的膜片钳切片记录中，我们观察到间接途径MSNs中反向的皮质纹状体可塑性 [图23.3（b）]，其中这些细胞在HFS后表达LTP而不是LTD。然而，"长期增强"是在切片记录的时间范围内定义的（45～50min）；这种增强作用在活体动物身上持续几天、几周还是几年尚不清楚。假设吸烟导致的cNIC引起了类似的变化，这将反驳这种LTP是稳定和持久的假设。多年来，高频皮层传入到间接通路的增强会显著增加对皮层活动的抑制性调节，而传入活动通常由LTD促进。也就是说，吸烟会导致异常学习，在这种情况下，人们可能会出现帕金森病症状。吸烟者不仅不会出现帕金森病样症状，而且患帕金森病的风险也降低了。另一种解释是，在cNIC处理的小鼠中观察到的HFS-LTP不是稳定的，而是短暂的（图23.4）。在这种情况下，在cNIC（可能还有其他滥用药物）中观察到的沉默突触的增加可能是由于未能通过选择和稳定适当地利用这种基质进行可塑性，可能还与未能在未沉默时去除沉默突触从而允许它们积累有关。因此，细胞将维持一个大的沉默突触池，导致在激活时产生明显的LTP，即未沉默，但这种可塑性是不稳定的，很容易随着那些激活的突触再次返回沉默突触池而重新减弱。最终结果将是可塑性和回路重塑的基质增加，沉默突触增加，但功能减少。简而言之，我们假设沉默突触的增加反映了沉默突触利用的损伤。

这并不是说cNIC会导致明显的学习障碍，因为它不会。接触cNIC的小鼠表现出正常的运动学习（Koranda et al. 2016）。相反，我们建议，当新学习和回路重塑被允许时，cNIC会增加严格性或阈值调节，有效保护已建立的先前学习，减少（但不是消除）新学习。文献中将沉默突触与孵化联系起来的一个难题是，旨在促进新学习的底物似乎处于休眠状态，并在未沉默时编码先前的学习（即药物渴求）（如，Lee et al. 2013）。一种可能性是，除了未能利用沉默突触之外，去除这些突触的能力也随之受损。也就是说，虽然通常有一个过程可以去除未被选择的未沉默的突触，从而有效地修剪不需要的连接，但cNIC（和其他滥用药物）可能会阻止这种去除，从而创建一个"鬼"连接网络，在未沉默和稳定（一种在禁欲时可能恢复的能力）时，编码应该被修剪的

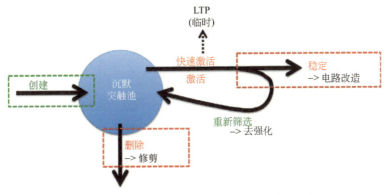

图 23.4　决定沉默突触的发生率/池的循环过程示意图

增加沉默突触发生率的机制用绿色标出，包括（1）通过将NMDARs插入新的位点或通过从现有突触中去除AMPARs来产生，（2）通过去除最近插入的AMPARs来重新定位激活的（未沉默的）沉默突触。减少沉默突触池的机制用红色标出，包括（1）通过AMPAR插入（激活）和随后的稳定解除沉默，或（2）完全去除沉默突触。当未被沉默时，这些突触有助于突触增强。激活的沉默突触可以稳定下来，随后被修饰，有助于回路重塑，或者被重新沉默，导致电位下降。沉默突触的去除反映了一个修剪和选择的过程。在沉默突触的生命周期中，慢性烟碱可能改变可用突触池的点，用虚线框表示，包括改变新的沉默突触的产生速度、改变激活的沉默突触的选择和稳定与抑制的调节以及调节沉默突触的去除和修剪。

先前连接（与药物相关刺激相关的先前连接）。激活的沉默突触的这种不稳定性可能促进帕金森病cNIC神经保护的一个方面。如果多巴胺去神经支配诱导适应不良的突触可塑性，即异常学习，那么受损的新（异常）学习的选择和稳定可能是有益的，并且减缓已建立的学习和技能的功能退化，否则这些功能退化可能随着进行性去神经支配而发生。

术语解释

- 皮质-基底神经节重入回路：皮质密集地投射到纹状体，这是基底神经节的主要输入，再向回投射到皮质，构成重入回路，允许基底神经节调节皮质活动。
- 直接/间接途径：基底神经节中的主要途径。直接途径通过去抑制促进了皮质活性和运动，而间接途径抑制了皮质活性。孵化：在戒断后对药物的渴望随时间而增加的现象。
- 长期反应（LDR）：左旋多巴（L-DOPA）治疗可引起与血液中L-DOPA不对应的症状的逐步改善，在剂量之间的"低谷"期间，并在停用L-DOPA后持续改善，尽管没有药物。
- 长期增强/抑制（LTP/LTD）：突触功效的增加/减少会在将来增加/减少神经元对相同刺激的反应。
- 中棘神经元（MSN）：纹状体的投射神经元由直接和间接途径MSNs组成，以蛋白质表达（包括多巴胺D_1和D_2受体的表达）区分。

沉默突触的关键事实

- 沉默突触包含NMDA但不包含AMPA受体，并且在静息膜电位下对谷氨酸无反应。
- 在早期发育过程中，沉默突触在大脑中广泛表达，它以一种依赖于经验的方式修剪，与发育的关键时期有关。
- 在20世纪90年代，在海马中发现沉默突触是建立突触后长期增强位点的重要一步。
- 沉默突触在某些神经元群体（包括纹状体）中持续存在，而在成年人中不多见。
- 滥用药物会增加纹状体中棘神经元中沉默突触的表达，并与渴望的孵化有关。

要点总结

- 本章重点介绍慢性烟碱和皮质纹状体的可塑性。
- 多巴胺信号的缺失会引起皮质纹状体可塑性的异常，从而导致异常的学习，这可能导致帕金森病的功能恶化。
- 吸烟降低了患帕金森病的风险，尽管如何降低尚不清楚。慢性烟碱可以减轻与多巴胺阻滞有关的异常学习，提示这可能是烟碱神经保护的机制。
- 慢性烟碱上调沉默通路的中棘神经元的沉默突触，并改变皮质纹状体可塑性的方向。
- 我们假设由慢性烟碱引起的沉默突触增加反映了该底物用于回路修饰的利用率降低，从而降低了可塑性。此外，这通过保护既定的药物强化学习来降低行为灵活性，同时通过减少异常学习而对帕金森病产生积极影响。

参考文献

Augustin, S.M., Beeler J. A., McGehee, D.S., Zhang, X. (2014). Cyclic AMP and afferent activity govern bidirectional synaptic plasticity in Striatopallidal neurous. The Journal of Neuro science, 34, 6692-6699.

Beeler, J. A. (2011). Preservation of function in Parkinson's disease: what's learning got to do with it?Brain Research, 1423, 9 6-113.

Beeler, J. A.; Cao, Z. F. H.; Kheirbek, M. A.; Ding, Y.; Koranda, J.; Murakami, M. et al. (2010). Dopamine-dependent motor learning insight into Levodopa's long-duration response. Annals of Neurology, 67, 639-647.

Beeler, J. A.; Cao, Z. F. H.; Kheirbek, M. A.; Zhuang, X. (2009). Loss of cocaine locomotor response in Pitx3-deficient mice lacking a nigros triatal pathway. Neuropsychopharmacology, 34, 1149-1161.

Beeler, J. A.; Frank, M. J.; McDaid, J.; Alexander, E.; Turkson, S.; Sol Bernandez, M. et al. (2012). A role for dopamine-mediated learning in the pathophysiology and treatment of Parkinson's disease. Cell Reports, 2, 1747-1761.

Beeler, J. A.; Petzinger, G.; Jakowec, M. W. (2013). The enemy within: propagation of aberrant corticostriatal learning to cortical function in Parkinson's disease. Frontiers in Neurology, 4, 134.

Brown, T. E.; Lee, B. R.; Mu, P.; Ferguson, D.; Dietz, D.; Ohnishi, Y. N. et al. (2011). A silent synapse-based mechanism for cocaine-induced locomotor sensitization. The Journal of Neuroscience, 31, 8163-8174.

Calabresi, P.; Saiardi, A.; Pisani, A.; Baik, J.; Centonze, D.; Mercuri, N. B. et al. (1997). Abnormal synaptic plasticity in the striatum of mice lacking dopamine D_2 receptors. The Journal of Neuroscience, 17, 4536-4544.

Chen, H.; Huang, X.; Guo, X.; Mailman, R. B.; Park, Y.; Kamel, F. et al. (2010). Smoking duration, intensity, and risk of Parkinson disease. Neurology, 74, 878-884.

Dong, Y.; Nestler, E. J. (2014). The neural rejuvenation hypothesis of cocaine addiction. Trends in Pharmacological Sciences, 35, 374-383.

Graziane, N. M.; Sun, S.; Wright, W. J.; Jang, D.; Liu, Z.; Huang, Y. H. et al. (2016). Opposing mechanisms mediate morphine- and cocaine induced generation of silent synapses. Nature Neuroscience, 19, 915-925.

Hanagasi, H. A.; Lees, A.; Johnson, J. O.; Singleton, A.; Emre, M. (2007). Smoking-responsive juvenile-onset Parkinsonism. Movement Disor-ders: Official Journal of the Movement Disorder Society, 22, 115-119.

Hanse, E.; Seth, H.; Riebe, I. (2013). AMPA-silent synapses in brain development and pathology. Nature Reviews. Neuroscience, 14, 839-850.

Huang, L. Z.; Parameswaran, N.; Bordia, T.; Michael McIntosh, J.; Quik, M. (2009). Nicotine is neuroprotective when administered before but not after nigrostriatal damage in rats and monkeys. Journal of Neurochemistry, 109, 826-837.

Huang, Y. H.; Lin, Y.; Mu, P.; Lee, B. R.; Brown, T. E.; Wayman, G. et al. (2009). In vivo cocaine experience generates silent synapses. Neuron, 63, 40-47.

Jin, Z.; Gao, F.; Flagg, T.; Deng, X. (2004). Nicotine induces multi-site phosphorylation of bad in association with suppression of apoptosis. The Journal of Biological Chemistry, 279, 23837-23844.

Kelton, M. C.; Kahn, H. J.; Conrath, C. L.; Newhouse, P. A. (2000). The effects of nicotine on Parkinson's disease. Brain and Cognition, 43, 274-282.

Koranda, J. L.; Cone, J. J.; McGehee, D. S.; Roitman, M. F.; Beeler, J. A.; Zhuang, X. (2014). Nicotinic receptors regulate the dynamic range of dopamine release in vivo. Journal of Neurophysiology, 111, 103-111.

Koranda, J. L.; Krok, A. C.; Xu, J.; Contractor, A.; McGehee, D. S.; Beeler, J. A. et al. (2016). Chronic nicotine mitigates aberrant inhibitory motor learning induced by motor experience under dopamine deficiency. The Journal of Neuroscience, 36, 5228-5240.

Koya, E.; Cruz, F. C.; Ator, R.; Golden, S. A.; Hoffman, A. F.; Lupica, C. R. et al. (2012). Silent synapses in selectively activated nucleus accumbens neurons following cocaine sensitization. Nature Neuroscience, 15, 1556-1562.

Kreitzer, A. C.; Malenka, R. C. (2007). Endocannabinoid-mediated rescue of striatal LTD and motor deficits in Parkinson's disease models. Nature, 445, 643-647.

Kreitzer, A. C.; Malenka, R. C. (2008). Striatal plasticity and basal ganglia circuit function. Neuron, 60, 543-554.

Lee, B. R.; Ma, Y. -Y.; Huang, Y. H.; Wang, X.; Otaka, M.; Ishikawa, M. et al. (2013). Maturation of silent synapses in amygdala-accumbens projection contributes to incubation of cocaine craving. Nature Neu- roscience, 16, 1644-1651.

Li, X.; Caprioli, D.; Marchant, N. J. (2015). Recent updates on incubation of drug craving: a mini-review: updates: incubation of craving. Addiction Biology, 20, 872-876.

Lovinger, D. M. (2010). Neurotransmitter roles in synaptic modulation, plasticity and learning in the dorsal striatum. Neuropharmacology, 58, 951-961.

Ma, Y. -Y.; Lee, B. R.; Wang, X.; Guo, C.; Liu, L.; Cui, R. et al. (2014). Bidirectional modulation of incubation of cocaine craving by silent synapse-based remodeling of prefrontal cortex to accumbens projec-tions. Neuron, 83, 1453-1467.

Perez, X. A.; Ly, J.; McIntosh, J. M.; Quik, M. (2012). Long-term nicotine exposure depresses dopamine release in nonhuman primate nucleus accumbens. The Journal of Pharmacology and Experimental Therapeutics, 342, 335-344.

Shen, W.; Flajolet, M.; Greengard, P.; Surmeier, D. J. (2008). Dichotomous dopaminergic control of striatal synaptic plasticity. Science, 321, 848-851.

Van Der Mark, M.; Nijssen, P. C.; Vlaanderen, J.; Huss, A.; Mulleners, W. M.; Sas, A. M. et al. (2014). A case-control study of the protective effect of alcohol, coffee, and cigarette consumption on Parkinson disease risk: time-since-cessation modifies the effect of tobacco smoking. PLoS One, 9, e95297.

Vieregge, A.; Sieberer, M.; Jacobs, H.; Hagenah, J. M.; Vieregge, P. (2001). Transdermal nicotine in PD: a randomized, double-blind, placebo-controlled study. Neurology, 57, 1032-1035.

Whitaker, L. R.; Carneiro de Oliveira, P. E.; McPherson, K. B.; Fallon, R. V.; Planeta, C. S.; Bonci, A. et al. (2015). Associative learning drives the formation of silent synapses in neuronal ensembles of the nucleus accumbens. Biological Psychiatry, 80, 246-256.

Xia, J.; Meyers, A. M.; Beeler, J. A. (2017). Chronic nicotine alters corticostriatal plasticity in the Striatopallidal pathway mediated by NR2B-containing silent synapses. Neuropsychopharmacology. https://doi.org/10.1038/npp.2017.87(Epub ahead of print).

Zhuang, X., Mazzoni, P., Kang, U.J. (2013). The role of neuroplasticity in dopaminergic therapy for Parkinson disease. Nature Reviews. Neurology, 9, 248-256.

24
产前烟碱暴露及其对后代行为的影响

Tursun Alkam[1,2], *Toshitaka Nabeshima*[1,3,4]

1. Japanese Drug Organization of Appropriate Use and Research, Nagoya, Japan
2. Department of Basic Medical Sciences, College of Osteopathic Medicine of the Pacific, Western University of Health Sciences, Pomona, CA, United States
3. Advanced Diagnostic System Research Laboratory, Graduate School of Health Sciences, Fujita Health University, Toyoake, Japan
4. Aino University, Ibaraki, Japan

缩略语

5-CSRT 任务	5-选择序列反应时间任务	**nAChR**	烟碱乙酰胆碱受体
5-HT	5-羟色胺	**NAergic**	去甲肾上腺素能
5-HT-ergic	5-羟色胺能	**NRT**	烟碱替代疗法
ACh	乙酰胆碱	**NSF 测试**	新奇抑制摄食测试
ADHD	注意缺陷多动障碍	**OBA 测试**	基于对象的注意力测试
CA 测试	悬崖回避测试	**OF 测试**	旷场测试
DA	多巴胺	**PNE**	产前烟碱暴露
EPM 测试	高架十字迷宫测试	**PPI 测试**	前脉冲抑制测试
LDB 测试	明暗箱测试	**SN 测试**	社会新奇测试
LDT	背外侧被盖核	**SS 任务**	停止信号任务
MBB 测试	大理石掩埋性能测试	**TBFC 测试**	双瓶自由选择测试
mPFC	内侧前额叶皮层	**Y-M 测试**	Y 型迷宫测试
NA	去甲肾上腺素		

24.1 引言

怀孕期间吸烟对后代的总体质量有显著的不利影响。流行病学研究和临床调查报告表明，怀孕期间吸烟的女性所生的孩子患有神经行为障碍，如持续性焦虑、学习障碍、决策障碍、冲动行为、躁动不安、注意缺陷多动障碍（ADHD）和成瘾（图24.1）（Abbott, Winzer-Serhan, 2012; Clifford, Lang, Chen, 2012; De Genna et al. 2016; Fitzpatrick, Barnett, Pagani, 2014; Garcia-Rill et al. 2007; Thapar et al. 2003）。在烟草烟雾中的多种成分中，烟碱扩散到吸烟母亲的肺部血管中，并随着血液循环迅速流向大脑，在那里烟碱结合并刺激nAChR。刺激神经元中的nAChR导致钠或钙的大量流入，从而触发神经元中细胞内钙的最终增加，并导致与愉悦感和对烟碱的依赖有关的神经递质的释放，这是烟草成瘾的原因。尽管孕妇知道烟草烟雾中含有许多对胎儿有害的有毒物质，但由于烟碱成瘾，她们无法轻易戒烟。为了减少对烟草中烟碱的渴望并帮助戒烟，将烟碱替代疗法（NRT）与认知行为疗法结合用于怀孕期间的戒烟（Osadchy, Kazmin, Koren, 2009）。但是，无论是通过吸烟还是通过使用NRT，烟碱都会进入母亲的血液，很容易穿透血液-胎盘屏障，在发育中的胎儿大脑中与nAChR相互作用，通过影响神经发生和突触形成而干扰大脑的正常功能发育，并导致神经递质信号的长期异常（Dempsey, Benowitz, 2001; Slotkin, 1998）。

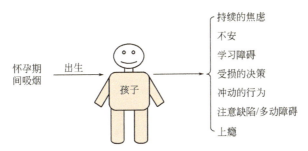

图 24.1　怀孕期间吸烟的女性所生孩子的行为

24.2　产前烟碱暴露

动物模型的报告表明，产前烟碱暴露（PNE）损害了发育中的大脑中关键神经通路的发育，并导致情绪和认知行为异常，这种异常在怀孕期间吸烟的女性所生的后代中尤为明显。这些研究大多数是在啮齿动物（小鼠和大鼠）中进行的，它们的胚胎发育与人类有许多相似之处，但也有一些重要的区别。啮齿动物的整个妊娠期在发育上仅相当于人类妊娠的前三个月和后三个月（图24.2）（Cross, Linker, Leslie, 2017; Dwyer et al. 2008）。在前三个月末出现nAChRs之后的第二个三个月中，发生了许多关键的大脑发育事件，如神经发生和早期突触形成（Cross et al. 2017; Dwyer et al. 2008）。小鼠出生后的前两周相当于人类发育的前三个月，其大脑在第一周达到结构成熟阶段（Cross et al. 2017; Dwyer et al. 2008）。nAChRs最早在妊娠第10天出现在小鼠大脑皮层中（Atluri et al. 2001），而在前三个月末出现在人类大脑中（Cross et al. 2017; Dwyer et al. 2008）。nAChR通过调节神经发生和突触形成在大脑发育的许多方面起着至关重要的作用，这取决于它们的区域表达和其亚基组成的药理学。nAChR在神经发育中的动态作用始终由内源性神经递质乙酰胆碱（ACh）驱动。胎儿神经发育过程中的烟碱暴露会夸大ACh的作用或干扰nAChR的调节作用，并影响关键神经递质信号的时机和强度，这些信号是为确保众多神经回路和途径正常发育所必需的（Pauly, Slotkin, 2008）。在评估PNE的动物模型时，要考虑的因素是给药途径、烟碱剂量和暴露时间（Slotkin, 1998）。在PNE的动物研究中，在白天的光亮阶段应用母体多次注射或在一天的整个24小时内皮下植入渗透性微型泵，或通过饮用水给予烟碱以模拟吸烟的时间间隔药代动力学（Alkam et al. 2013; Alkam et al. 2013; Slotkin, 1998）。一些在啮齿动物上进行的PNE

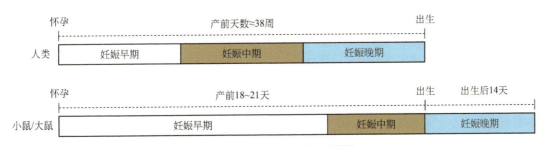

图 24.2　人类和啮齿动物的产前期

研究更倾向于在产后早期通过母体哺乳增加产后烟碱的暴露，以模拟人类妊娠中所有三个月的烟碱暴露。在各种PNE动物模型中，无论烟碱剂量、给药途径、发作时间和暴露时间的选择是否一致，所有报道均支持PNE引起后代行为异常的观点。

24.3 对后代行为的影响

与PNE对后代行为影响有关的现有研究为PNE的行为神经毒性提供了系统的理解（图24.3）。由于特定大脑区域中功能性nAChR或不同浓度的烟碱本身的可用性，PNE在胎儿大脑发育的不同时间窗口中的行为影响可能有所不同。

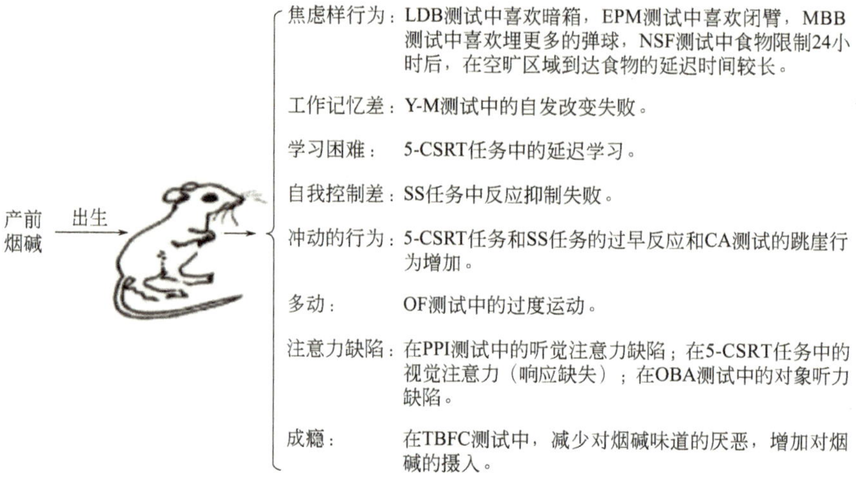

产前烟碱 → 出生 →

焦虑样行为：LDB测试中喜欢暗箱，EPM测试中喜欢闭臂，MBB测试中喜欢埋更多的弹球，NSF测试中食物限制24小时后，在空旷区域到达食物的延迟时间较长。

工作记忆差：Y-M测试中的自发改变失败。

学习困难：5-CSRT任务中的延迟学习。

自我控制差：SS任务中反应抑制失败。

冲动的行为：5-CSRT任务和SS任务的过早反应和CA测试的跳崖行为增加。

多动：OF测试中的过度运动。

注意力缺陷：在PPI测试中的听觉注意力缺陷；在5-CSRT任务中的视觉注意力（响应缺失）；在OBA测试中的对象听力缺陷。

成瘾：在TBFC测试中，减少对烟碱味道的厌恶，增加对烟碱的摄入。

图 24.3　产前烟碱暴露引起的啮齿动物后代的行为变化

24.4 情绪行为

使用明暗箱测试（LDB测试）、新奇抑制摄食测试（NSF测试）、社会新奇测试（SN测试）、高架十字迷宫测试（EPM测试）、悬崖回避测试（CA测试）、5-选择序列反应时间任务（5-CSRT任务）和停止信号任务（SS任务）来调查情绪行为。

在LDB测试中，PNE小鼠在似乎更安全的暗盒中的时间比在看起来不安全的明亮的盒子中的时间更长，这是一种类似焦虑的行为指标（Alkam, Kim, Hiramatsu, et al. 2013）。在LDB测试中，孕晚期和哺乳期母体烟碱暴露同样会增加大鼠后代的焦虑样行为（Lee, Chung, Noh, 2016）。在MBB测试中，PNE小鼠比对照组的雄性小鼠掩埋更多的大理石（陌生的发光物体）（Alkam, Kim, Hiramatsu, et al. 2013; Aoyama et al. 2016）。在EPM测试中，PNE小鼠在张开的双臂中比在隐藏闭合的手臂中花费更多时间探究，并且进入闭合的手臂的次数更多，这两者都表明存在焦虑样行为（Alkam, Kim, Hiramatsu et al. 2013; Hall et al. 2016; Parameshwaran et al. 2012）。在SN测试中，PNE小鼠更喜欢与固定的熟悉小鼠待在一起，而不是与固定的陌生小鼠待在一起，同时显示出更愿意独自待在空的房间中（Alkam, Kim, Hiramatsu et al. 2013）。在同一项研究中，在NSF测试中，使用PNE的食物受限的饥饿小鼠在24h内在露天场所开始进食的潜伏期延长。在CA测试中，PNE小鼠比对照小鼠明显更早地跳出平台，这是冲动行为的迹象（Alkam et al. 2017; Zhu et al. 2017）。PNE使大鼠冲动，这是通过对5-CSRT任务和SS任务中以有序和可预测的顺序呈现的视觉刺激做出更早反应来表明的（Bryden et al. 2016; Schneider et al. 2011）。

PNE大鼠显示出更多的过早反应，这些过早反应是在试验开始后但在有序和可预测的序列中出现视觉刺激之前发生的反应以及遗漏错误。响应时间更长，以及5-CSRT任务中学习延迟的准确性较低，并表明PNE对注意力、抑制性控制或晚年学习的重要方面具有直接影响（Schneider et al. 2011）。

PNE会导致胆碱乙酰转移酶大量缺乏，该酶存在于轴突突触前末端，并催化后代大脑皮层中兴奋性神经递质ACh的合成（Slotkin et al. 2007）。PNE会破坏大脑皮层的5-羟色胺（5-HT）投射（Xu et al. 2001），并降低5-HT的转化率，同时增加5-HT转运蛋白的密度（Muneoka et al. 1997; Muneoka et al. 2001）。5-HT通过其各种受体介导兴奋性和抑制性神经传递，并作为情绪调节的神经生物学基础。PNE还减少了$5-HT_{1A}$受体的结合，而$5-HT_2$受体的结合在后代的大脑皮层中显示出明显的总体增加（Slotkin et al. 2007）。微透析研究表明，突触后刺激$5-HT_{1A}$受体可以增加清醒大鼠大脑各个区域（包括海马和额叶皮层）的去甲肾上腺素（NA）的释放和转换（Done, Sharp, 1994; Hajos-Korcsok, McQuade, Sharp, 1999; Suzuki et al. 1995）。$5-HT_{1A}$受体水平的降低可能会导致NA转换的减少。有趣的是，PNE降低了额叶皮层中NA的含量和周转率（Alkam, Kim, Mamiya et al. 2013; Ribary, Lichtensteiger, 1989）。PNE破坏了内侧前额叶皮层（mPFC）神经元的发射，这些神经元携带与反应方向和冲突监测有关的信号（Bryden et al. 2016）。这些信号转导的减少可能是PNE后代行为改变的原因。

24.5 认知行为

认知行为通过Y型迷宫测试（Y-M测试）、基于对象的注意力测试（OBA测试）、前脉冲抑制测试（PPI测试）、旷场测试（OF测试）、5-选择序列反应时间任务（5-CSRT任务）和停止信号任务（SS任务）进行评估。

在小鼠的Y-M测试中，PNE会降低自发性交替行为（一种短期工作记忆的量度）（Alkam, Kim, Mamiya et al. 2013; Parameshwaran et al. 2012）。在OBA测试中，PNE小鼠对测试前不久呈现给它们的"熟悉的物体"的熟悉度降低，这表明PNE小鼠对细节不专心（Alkam, Kim, Mamiya et al. 2013）。当通过PPI测试研究感觉运动门控的注意过程时，PNE小鼠和大鼠的感觉运动处理受到损害（Alkam et al. 2017; Alkam, Kim, Mamiya, et al. 2013; Lacy, Mactutus, Harrod, 2011）。在OF测试中，PNE可增加小鼠和大鼠的自发运动能力（Schneider et al. 2012; Zhu et al. 2012）。PNE使大鼠在"停止"试验中减少了自我抑制，在此期间，大鼠必须停止SS任务中已经开始的反应（Bryden et al. 2016）。PNE大鼠显示出更多的过早反应，这些过早反应是在试验开始后但在有序和可预测的序列中出现视觉刺激之前发生的反应以及遗漏错误。响应时间更长，以及5-CSRT任务中学习延迟的准确性较低，并表明PNE对注意力、抑制性控制或晚年学习的重要方面具有直接影响（Schneider et al. 2011）。这些由PNE诱发的行为异常模仿ADHD样的行为。

尽管ADHD的确切病因尚不清楚，但是多巴胺能（DA能）和NA能传递的缺陷都被认为是ADHD症状的原因（Halperin et al. 1997; Shaywitz, Cohen, Bowers Jr., 1977; Shekim et al. 1987; Shekim et al. 1983）。PNE会降低小鼠后代PFC中多巴胺（DA）的含量及其释放和周转率（Alkam et al. 2017; Alkam, Kim, Mamiya et al. 2013; Zhu et al. 2012; Zhu et al. 2014）。PNE还破坏了DA能和NA能的

传递以及整个皮层的树突形态和突触连接性（Muhammad et al. 2012; Mychasiuk et al. 2013; Seidler et al. 1992; Zhu et al. 2012）。PNE 减少了 mPFC 中酪氨酸羟化酶阳性静脉曲张的数量，其中发生了 NA 和 DA 的合成、释放和再摄取（Alkam et al. 2017）。通过增加突触 DA 和 NA 的药物进行急性治疗，可减轻 PNE 诱导的 ADHD 样行为缺陷（Alkam et al. 2017; Zhu et al. 2017）。综上所述，这些发现支持以下观点：PNE 通过破坏 NA 能和 DA 能神经递质系统诱导小鼠后代的行为异常。

24.6 成瘾行为

PNE 是在晚年阶段发展成对烟碱成瘾的危险因素（Christensen et al. 2015）。PNE 增加了产后早期和青春期大鼠对烟碱气味的偏好（Mantella et al. 2013）。在 TBFC 测试中，PNE 会诱导对烟碱溶液的厌恶降低，并增加了青春期大鼠的烟碱消耗（Schneider et al. 2012）。PNE 大鼠还表现出烟碱和其他滥用物质的消耗量显著增加，而其食物、摄食量或体重没有变化（Chang et al. 2013）。PNE 诱导胆碱能背外侧被盖核（LDT）发生变化，该变化主要参与对动机刺激的反应以及与药物成瘾相关的行为的发展（Christensen et al. 2015; McNair, Kohlmeier, 2015）。PNE 改变了 LDT 中的谷氨酸信号，并且 PNE 增加了具有 PNE 和更大幅度的兴奋性突触后电流的年轻小鼠大脑中 LDT 细胞中的钙浓度（Christensen et al. 2015; McNair, Kohlmeier, 2015）。这些报告支持 PNE 诱导对烟碱的渴望反应，并可能在以后的生活中成瘾。

24.7 结论

在动物模型中进行 PNE 研究的行为发现与在怀孕期间吸烟的母亲所生的孩子中观察到的症状一致。当前可获得的报告提供了足够的证据来支持 PNE 对后代的情绪、认知和成瘾行为的不利影响（图 24.3）并解释其潜在机制（图 24.4）。这些发现敦促人们认真考虑在怀孕期间通过包括 NRT 在内的任何方式进行烟碱暴露。

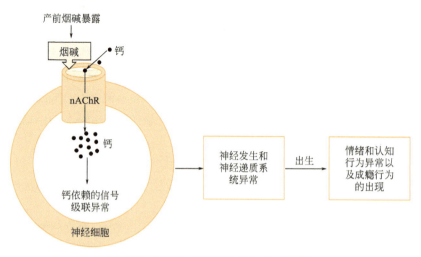

图 24.4 产前烟碱暴露行为改变的可能机制

如本章所述，产前烟碱暴露会损害神经递质系统，包括乙酰胆碱能、多巴胺能、5-羟色胺能和去甲肾上腺素能神经递质系统。有关产前烟碱暴露对神经发生的损害，请参阅"产前烟碱暴露和神经前体细胞"章节。

术语解释	
	■ 5-选择序列反应时间任务：此任务使用视觉辨别力和冲动控制性能来衡量啮齿动物的注意力表现，以响应基于操作的任务中的视觉刺激。注意力不集中的啮齿动物会表现出对短时间视觉刺激的反应缺失。冲动的啮齿动物会在给予视觉刺激之前表现出过早的反应。
	■ 悬崖回避测试：该测试评估了啮齿动物对悬崖跳跃行为的渴望，而没有考虑受伤的危险。具有冲动行为的啮齿动物立即跳下悬崖。
	■ 高架十字迷宫测试：该测试可以选择在开放的无保护臂或从地面升高的封闭的受保护臂中测量啮齿类动物花费的时间和进入次数。焦虑的啮齿动物通常倾向于避开开放区域，而倾向于封闭的"安全"空间。
	■ 明暗箱测试：该测试利用了啮齿动物探索新环境的自然趋势。在此测试中，评估焦虑相关行为的关键措施反映在光（无保护的）盒中和暗（受保护的）盒中所花费的时间上。焦虑的啮齿动物更喜欢深色（受保护的）隔室。
	■ 新奇抑制摄食测试：该测试衡量啮齿动物避开新颖开放区域的情况，因为在开放区域它们可能更容易被捕食。受食物限制的饥饿的啮齿动物通常表现出更长的等待时间（由于对安全性确认的研究时间较长），因此无法进入新颖的开放区域。
	■ 基于对象的注意力测试：该测试利用了老鼠探索新对象的自然趋势。在此任务中，将老鼠暴露于五个对象中3min（训练期）。然后，在短暂的间隔后，将老鼠暴露于两个对象中，其中包括在一个训练中出现的"熟悉的对象"和一个新颖的对象。注意力不足的老鼠会将新颖的对象和"熟悉的对象"探索为新颖的对象。
	■ 旷场测试：在此测试中，将啮齿动物放在露天的盒子或笼子中，并在平行于地面的位置放置光束运动传感器。动物的一举一动都会破坏光束。多动的动物在测试期间会破坏更多的光束。
	■ 前脉冲抑制测试：该测试测量在很短的间隔（如30～500ms）后，对弱刺激（前脉冲）之后的强刺激（脉冲）的惊吓反应的衰减。据认为，前脉冲激活了抑制惊吓反应的注意前门控机制。注意力不集中的啮齿动物表现出减弱的前脉冲抑制能力。
	■ 停止信号任务：此任务测量受试者抑制其已启动的反应（对刺激）的能力。抑制反应是执行控制的一个标志。目标导向行为受损的受试者对学习的刺激没有立即反应抑制作用。
	■ 大理石掩埋测试：该测试是检查小鼠的恐惧症、焦虑症和强迫行为的有用方法。患有任何这些情绪障碍的老鼠都倾向于掩埋更多的大理石。
	■ 双瓶自由选择测试：在此测试中，啮齿动物可以接近笼中的两个饮水瓶。一瓶装有烟碱溶液（加有n%蔗糖），另一瓶装有n%蔗糖溶液。瓶子的位置每天交替。每天测量每种溶液的体积，以获取动物对任何溶液的偏好。成瘾的啮齿动物表现出对烟碱溶液的偏好，并且会饮用更多。
	■ Y型迷宫测试：该测试利用啮齿动物的自然趋势来交替探索新的空间，并评估自发交替行为，这是啮齿动物空间工作记忆的一个指标。工作记忆差的啮齿动物倾向于重复"访问"刚刚退出的（Y型迷宫的）手臂，而不是交替"访问"迷宫的另一手臂。
怀孕期间烟碱替代疗法的关键事实	■ 为了减少对烟草的渴望并帮助普通人群戒烟，已开发出烟碱替代疗法（NRT）。
	■ NRT与认知行为疗法相结合被认为是在怀孕期间实现戒烟的最有效策略，尽管就烟碱暴露而言，它与PNE相当。
	■ 尽管在妊娠期进行NRT可以提高戒烟率，但是NRT和安慰剂的疗效相似。
	■ 使用动物模型进行的临床前研究提供了有关PNE不安全性的足够数据，这与人类妊娠期间的NRT相当。
	■ 需要进行安慰剂随机对照临床试验，以研究NRT在人类妊娠戒烟中是否安全。

要点总结
- 怀孕期间吸烟对大脑发育的有害影响正成为日益重要的公共卫生问题。
- 怀孕期间吸烟的母亲所生的孩子患有神经行为异常。
- 烟碱是烟草中使人们吸烟的主要化合物。
- 正在使用烟碱替代疗法作为怀孕期间戒烟的辅助手段。
- 产前烟碱暴露对胎儿脑功能发育有害,并导致后代行为异常。
- 产前烟碱暴露会引起后代神经递质系统的长期异常。

参考文献

Abbott, L. C.; Winzer-Serhan, U. H. (2012). Smoking during pregnancy: lessons learned from epidemiological studies and experimental studies using animal models. Critical Reviews in Toxicology, 42(4), 279-303.

Alkam, T.; Kim, H. C.; Hiramatsu, M.; Mamiya, T.; Aoyama, Y.; Nitta, A. et al. (2013). Evaluation of emotional behaviors in young offspring of C57BL/6J mice after gestational and/or perinatal exposure to nicotine in six different time-windows. Behavioural Brain Research, 239, 80-89.

Alkam, T.; Kim, H. C.; Mamiya, T.; Yamada, K.; Hiramatsu, M.; Nabeshima, T. (2013). Evaluation of cognitive behaviors in young off spring of C57BL/6J mice after gestational nicotine exposure during different time-windows. Psychopharmacology, 230(3), 451-463.

Alkam, T.; Mamiya, T.; Kimura, N.; Yoshida, A.; Kihara, D.; Tsunoda, Y. et al. (2017). Prenatal nicotine exposure decreases the release of dopamine in the medial frontal cortex and induces atomoxetine responsive neurobehavioral deficits in mice. Psychopharmacology, 234(12), 1853-1869.

Aoyama, Y.; Toriumi, K.; Mouri, A.; Hattori, T.; Ueda, E.; Shimato, A. et al. (2016). Prenatal nicotine exposure impairs the proliferation of neuronal progenitors, leading to fewer glutamatergic neurons in the medial prefrontal cortex. Neuropsychopharmacology, 41(2), 578-589.

Atluri, P.; Fleck, M. W.; Shen, Q.; Mah, S. J.; Stadfelt, D.; Barnes, W. et al. (2001). Functional nicotinic acetylcholine receptor expression in stem and progenitor cells of the early embryonic mouse cerebral cortex. Developmental Biology, 240(1), 143-156.

Bryden, D. W.; Burton, A. C.; Barnett, B. R.; Cohen, V. J.; Hearn, T. N.; Jones, E. A. et al. (2016). Prenatal nicotine exposure impairs executive control signals in medial prefrontal cortex. Neuropsychopharmacology, 41(3), 716-725.

Chang, G. Q.; Karatayev, O.; Leibowitz, S. F. (2013). Prenatal exposure to nicotine stimulates neurogenesis of orexigenic peptide-expressing neurons in hypothalamus and amygdala. The Journal of Neuroscience, 33(34), 13600-13611.

Christensen, M. H.; Nielsen, M. L.; Kohlmeier, K. A. (2015). Electrophysiological changes in laterodorsal tegmental neurons associated with prenatal nicotine exposure: implications for heightened susceptibility to addict to drugs of abuse. Journal of Developmental Origins of Health and Disease, 6(3), 182-200.

Clifford, A.; Lang, L.; Chen, R. (2012). Effects of maternal cigarette smoking during pregnancy on cognitive parameters of children and young adults: a literature review. Neurotoxicology and Teratology, 34(6), 560-570.

Cross, S. J.; Linker, K. E.; Leslie, F. M. (2017). Sex-dependent effects of nicotine on the developing brain. Journal of Neuroscience Research, 95(1-2), 422-436.

De Genna, N. M.; Goldschmidt, L.; Day, N. L.; Cornelius, M. D. (2016). Prenatal and postnatal maternal trajectories of cigarette use predict adolescent cigarette use. Nicotine, Tobacco Research, 18(5), 988-992.

Dempsey, D. A.; Benowitz, N. L. (2001). Risks and benefits of nicotine to aid smoking cessation in pregnancy. Drug Safety, 24(4), 277-322.

Done, C. J.; Sharp, T. (1994). Biochemical evidence for the regulation of central noradrenergic activity by 5-HT1A and 5-HT2 receptors: microdialysis studies in the awake and anaesthetized rat. Neuropharmacology, 33(3-4), 411-421.

Dwyer, J. B.; Broide, R. S.; Leslie, F. M. (2008). Nicotine and brain development. Birth Defects Research. Part C, Embryo Today, 84(1), 30-44.

Fitzpatrick, C.; Barnett, T. A.; Pagani, L. S. (2014). Parental bad habits breed bad behaviors in youth: exposure to gestational smoke and child impulsivity. International Journal of Psychophysiology, 93(1), 17-21.

Garcia-Rill, E.; Buchanan, R.; McKeon, K.; Skinner, R. D.; Wallace, T. (2007). Smoking during pregnancy: postnatal effects on arousal and attentional brain systems. Neurotoxicology, 28(5), 915-923.

Hajos-Korcsok, E.; McQuade, R.; Sharp, T. (1999). Influence of 5-HT1A receptors on central noradrenergic activity: microdialysis studies using (+/−)-MDL 73005EF and its enantiomers. Neuropharmacology, 38(2), 299-306.

Hall, B. J.; Cauley, M.; Burke, D. A.; Kiany, A.; Slotkin, T. A.; Levin, E. D. (2016). Cognitive and behavioral impairments evoked by low-level exposure to tobacco smoke components: comparison with nicotine alone. Toxicological Sciences, 151(2), 236-244.

Halperin, J. M.; Newcorn, J. H.; Koda, V. H.; Pick, L.; McKay, K. E.; Knott, P. (1997). Noradrenergic mechanisms in ADHD children with and without reading disabilities: a replication and extension. Journal of the American Academy of Child and Adolescent Psychiatry, 36(12), 1688-1697.

Lacy, R. T.; Mactutus, C. F.; Harrod, S. B. (2011). Prenatal IV nicotine exposure produces a sex difference in sensorimotor gating of the auditory startle reflex in adult rats. International Journal of Developmental Neuroscience, 29(2), 153-161.

Lee, H.; Chung, S.; Noh, J. (2016). Maternal nicotine exposure during late gestation and lactation increases anxiety-like and impulsive decision-making behavior in adolescent offspring of rat. Toxicology Research, 32(4), 275-280.

Mantella, N. M.; Kent, P. F.; Youngentob, S. L. (2013). Fetal nicotine exposure increases preference for nicotine odor in early postnatal and adolescent, but not adult, rats. PLoS One, 8(12), e84989.

McNair, L. F.; Kohlmeier, K. A. (2015). Prenatal nicotine is associated with reduced AMPA and NMDA receptor-mediated rises in calcium within the laterodorsal tegmentum: a pontine nucleus involved in addiction processes. Journal of Developmental Origins of Health and Disease, 6(3), 225-241.

Muhammad, A.; Mychasiuk, R.; Nakahashi, A.; Hossain, S. R.; Gibb, R.; Kolb, B. (2012). Prenatal nicotine exposure alters neuroanatomical organization of the developing brain. Synapse, 66(11), 950-954.

Muneoka, K.; Ogawa, T.; Kamei, K.; Mimura, Y.; Kato, H.; Takigawa, M. (2001). Nicotine exposure during pregnancy is a factor which influences serotonin transporter density in the rat brain. European Journal of Pharmacology, 411(3), 279-282.

Muneoka, K.; Ogawa, T.; Kamei, K.; Muraoka, S.; Tomiyoshi, R.; Mimura, Y. et al. (1997). Prenatal nicotine exposure affects the development of the central serotonergic system as well as the dopaminergic system in rat offspring: involvement of route of drug administrations. Brain Research Developmental Brain Research, 102(1), 117-126.

Mychasiuk, R.; Muhammad, A.; Gibb, R.; Kolb, B. (2013). Long-term alterations to dendritic morphology and spine density associated with prenatal exposure to nicotine. Brain Research, 1499, 53-60.

Osadchy, A.; Kazmin, A.; Koren, G. (2009). Nicotine replacement therapy during pregnancy: recommended or not recommended? Journal of Obstetrics and Gynaecology Canada, 31(8), 744-747.

Parameshwaran, K.; Buabeid, M. A.; Karuppagounder, S. S.; Uthayathas, S.; Thiruchelvam, K.; Shonesy, B. et al. (2012). Developmental nicotine exposure induced alterations in behavior and glutamate receptor function in hippocampus. Cellular and Molecular Life Sciences, 69(5), 829-841.

Pauly, J. R.; Slotkin, T. A. (2008). Maternal tobacco smoking, nicotine replacement and neurobehavioural development. Acta Paediatrica, 97 (10), 1331-1337.

Ribary, U.; Lichtensteiger, W. (1989). Effects of acute and chronic prenatal nicotine treatment on central catecholamine systems of male and female rat fetuses and offspring. The Journal of Pharmacology and Experimental Therapeutics, 248(2), 786-792.

Schneider, T.; Bizarro, L.; Asherson, P. J.; Stolerman, I. P. (2012). Hyperactivity, increased nicotine consumption and impaired performance in the five-choice serial reaction time task in adolescent rats prenatally exposed to nicotine. Psychopharmacology, 223(4), 401-415.

Schneider, T.; Ilott, N.; Brolese, G.; Bizarro, L.; Asherson, P. J.; Stolerman, I. P. (2011). Prenatal exposure to nicotine impairs performance of the 5-choice serial reaction time task in adult rats. Neuropsychopharmacology, 36(5), 1114-1125.

Seidler, F. J.; Levin, E. D.; Lappi, S. E.; Slotkin, T. A. (1992). Fetal nicotine exposure ablates the ability of postnatal nicotine challenge to release norepinephrine from rat brain regions. Brain Research. Developmental Brain Research, 69(2), 288-291.

Shaywitz, B. A.; Cohen, D. J.; Bowers, M. B.; Jr. (1977). CSF monoamine metabolites in children with minimal brain dysfunction: evidence for alteration of brain dopamine. A preliminary report. TheJournal of Pediatrics, 90(1), 67-71.

Shekim, W. O.; Javaid, J.; Davis, J. M.; Bylund, D. B. (1983). Urinary MHPG and HVA excretion in boys with attention deficit disorder and hyperactivity treated with d-amphetamine. Biological Psychiatry, 18(6), 707-714.

Shekim, W. O.; Sinclair, E.; Glaser, R.; Horwitz, E.; Javaid, J.; Bylund, D. B. (1987). Norepinephrine and dopamine metabolites and educational variables in boys with attention deficit disorder and hyperactivity. Journal of Child Neurology, 2(1), 50-56.

Slotkin, T. A. (1998). Fetal nicotine or cocaine exposure: which one is worse?The Journal of Pharmacology and Experimental Therapeutics, 285(3), 931-945.

Slotkin, T. A.; MacKillop, E. A.; Rudder, C. L.; Ryde, I. T.; Tate, C. A.; Seidler, F. J. (2007). Permanent, sex-selective effects of prenatal or adolescent nicotine exposure, separately or sequentially, in rat brain regions: indices of cholinergic and serotonergic synaptic function, cell signaling, and neural cell number and size at 6 months of age. Neuropsychopharmacology, 32(5), 1082-1097.

Suzuki, M.; Matsuda, T.; Asano, S.; Somboonthum, P.; Takuma, K.; Baba, A. (1995). Increase of noradrenaline release in the hypothalamus of freely moving rat by postsynaptic 5-hydroxytryptamine1A receptor activation. British Journal of Pharmacology, 115(4), 703-711.

Thapar, A.; Fowler, T.; Rice, F.; Scourfield, J.; van den Bree, M.; Thomas, H. et al. (2003). Maternal smoking during pregnancy and attention deficit hyperactivity disorder symptoms in offspring. The American Journal of Psychiatry, 160(11), 1985-1989.

Xu, Z.; Seidler, F. J.; Ali, S. F.; Slikker, W.; Jr.; Slotkin, T. A. (2001). Fetal and adolescent nicotine administration: effects on CNS serotonergic systems. Brain Research, 914(1-2), 166-178.

Zhu, J.; Fan, F.; McCarthy, D. M.; Zhang, L.; Cannon, E. N.; Spencer, T. J. et al. (2017). A prenatal nicotine exposure mouse model of methylphenidate responsive ADHD-associated cognitive phenotypes. International Journal of Developmental Neuroscience, 58, 26-34.

Zhu, J.; Lee, K. P.; Spencer, T. J.; Biederman, J.; Bhide, P. G. (2014). Transgenerational transmission of hyperactivity in a mouse model of ADHD. The Journal of Neuroscience, 34(8), 2768-2773.

Zhu, J.; Zhang, X.; Xu, Y.; Spencer, T. J.; Biederman, J.; Bhide, P. G. (2012). Prenatal nicotine exposure mouse model showing hyperactivity, reduced cingulate cortex volume, reduced dopamine turnover, and responsiveness to oral methylphenidate treatment. The Journal of Neuroscience, 32(27), 9410-9418.

25
以吸烟为重点的物质使用渴望障碍

Stephen J. Wilson [1], *Michael A. Sayette* [2]

1. Department of Psychology, The Pennsylvania State University, University Park, PA, United States
2. Department of Psychology, University of Pittsburgh, Pittsburgh, PA, United States

缩略语

fMRI 功能磁共振成像

25.1 引言

渴望已成为成瘾领域中研究最深入、争议最大的构造之一。这种强调反映了广泛的共识，即渴望是药物成瘾的临床重要特征（Tiffany, Wray, 2012）。特别地，有关吸烟的研究已经大量记录了渴望与物质使用之间的联系（Ferguson, Shiffman, 2009），这仍然是世界上主要的可预防死亡原因之一（Reitsma et al. 2017）。尽管渴望与吸烟之间关系的确切性质仍然是研究和持续辩论的活跃领域（如Sayette, Tiffany, 2013; Wray, Gass, Tiffany, 2013），但多项研究的结果表明，渴望破坏了尝试戒烟（如Allen et al. 2008; Bagot, Heishman, Moolchan, 2007; Killen, Fortmann, 1997; Shiffman et al. 1996）。急性渴望事件是由特定情况或刺激（如暴露于卷烟提示）触发的冲动迅速而强烈地增加，可能对行为产生特别显著的影响（Ferguson, Shiffman, 2009）。本章简要概述了与渴望在物质使用中的作用有关的精选问题和观察，重点是对卷烟和吸烟行为的渴望。我们首先考虑了渴望与欲望之间的联系，并质疑渴望表现为线性还是非线性现象，这是在成瘾领域内尚未解决的基本问题。然后，我们简要地介绍了渴望对自我调节的影响，研究表明渴望导致认知过程的转变，从而增加了药物使用的可能性。最后，我们讨论了使用脑成像方法研究渴望的日益普遍的方法，以及神经成像和行为方法在促进渴望科学方面的补充作用。

25.2 渴望的构造

药物渴望是一种假设性的构造，可以用来解释观察结果和推进有关吸烟及其他形式药物使用的研究（Sayette, 2016）。因此，至关重要的是，必须认真地定义渴望并将其有意义地与一个连贯的理论框架内的可观察变量联系起来（Cronbach, Meehl, 1955）。然而，这已被证明是一个挑战，因为成瘾理论家一直在努力定义和概念化渴望。尽管人们普遍认为，最好将渴望概念化为寻求、获得和使用药物的动机不断增强的状态（Tiffany, 1990），但仍有许多定义和概念问题尚未解决（Sayette et al. 2000）。一个尚未解决的、具有重大影响的问题涉及到渴望是否应该被概念化为可以沿着欲望的连续性来衡量的一种连续现象，或者是否应该将渴望视为一种本质上与不太强烈的欲望不同的渴望状态（Abrams, 2000; Kozlowski, Wilkinson, 1987; Sayette et al. 2000）。在经典文献中，成瘾研究人员通常将渴望评估为一个连续的变量，其强度范围从不存在/低到高，并且渴望和期望这两个术语经常互换使用。但是，从概念和临床的角度来看，最好将渴望视为一种结构，该结构的核心不仅代表了对使用药物的任何渴望，而且特别代表了对使用药物的强烈或极端的渴望。正如我们在其他地方提到的（Wilson, Sayette, 2015），Nora Volkow和George Koob等主要成瘾研究者已经认识到渴望的"压倒性"和"强烈性"，认为这种敏锐的经历反映了导致药物摄入的"不可阻挡的力量"，并代表了成瘾的核心特征（George, Koob, 2013; Volkow et al. 2010）。最新版的《精神疾病诊断与统计手册》（DSM-5；American Psychiatric Association, 2013；第483页）也强调了对渴望的渗透性和对使用药物的明显渴望具有临床意义的观念。渴望被添加在DSM-5中，作为药物使用障碍的标准之一，手册将其定义为"强烈的欲望或冲动"，如果曾经有过，他们应该通过"询问[个人]"来评估强烈渴望使用这种药物，以至于他们再也没有想到其他任何东西。因此，似乎可以在概念上、临床上和诊断上区分渴望和弱至中度的欲望状态，尽管在涉及操纵和评估渴望的研究中很少做出这种区分。

25.3 渴望、认知和自我调节

尽管人们一直不确定渴望的概念和界限，但仍有令人信服的证据表明它是具有临床意义的构造（Sayette, 2016; Tiffany, Wray, 2012）。除此之外，人们发现渴望会改变认知过程，这被认为有助于药物使用和复发（Sayette, Creswell, 2016）。例如，使用多种方法的研究结果表明，渴望需要非自动（能力有限）的认知处理资源（Tiffany, 1990; Waters, Sayette, 2006）。换句话说，渴望可能会"占用"精神资源，如主动维护工作记忆中的信息所需的精神资源。此外，通过选择性注意环境中的相关刺激物（如人行道上的烟头）和积极阐述与吸毒渴望相关的思想，维持与渴望相关的表征可能导致越来越多的类似信息进入工作记忆的内容。吸毒欲望（Kavanagh, Andrade, May, 2005）。最近的发现表明，渴望也干扰了这些效应发生时对它们的识别能力，因此这些效应对认知过程的影响可能会加剧（Sayette et al. 2010）。一种方法已被证明对研究渴望对认知过程的影响特别有用，它涉及通过结合急性药物剥夺和高度显著的药物提示来产生强烈的（"被激起的"）渴望（Sayette, Tiffany, 2013）。例如，一项研究使用此策略，通过比较峰值渴望状态和低渴望控制状态，研究渴望对吸烟者产生和评估吸烟相关信息的方式，在低渴望控制状态下，参与者最近吸烟并暴露于中性线索（Sayette, Hufford, 1997）。在峰值渴望的情况下，参与者产生了一系列吸烟特征，这些特征相对于他们不渴望的时候是有积极倾向的，即峰值渴望与产生的积极而非消极特征的数量显著增加相关。除了影响与药物有关的信息的产生外，渴望似乎也改变了这种药物的评价。在两项研究中，与低渴望状态的吸烟者相比，处于高渴望状态的吸烟者倾向于判断积极吸烟的可能性更大，而不是消极吸烟后果（Sayette et al. 2005; Sayette et al. 2001）。这些发现表明，渴望可能导致对药物使用的预期结果的期望发生变化，从而使积极的结果比消极的结果更显著和更可能。渴望似乎对非药物激励措施的估值产生了钝化效应，这可能会使情况更加复杂（Piper, 2015; Wilson, Delgado et al. 2014）。不难想象，认知过程中的这些变化会如何导致药物使用。例如，渴望吸烟并将要复发的吸烟者可能会专注于吸烟的感知收益（如卷烟的味道如何），而低估了潜在的负面后果（如与吸烟有关的疾病导致死亡的可能性），在那一刻，吸烟的决定可能显得很合理。渴望似乎也以可能有助于维持戒烟者的药物使用和自我调节失败的方式影响时间认知。也就是说，处于渴望状态的吸烟者比没有渴望的吸烟者描述时间流逝更慢（Klein, Corwin, Stine, 2003; Sayette et al. 2005）。此外，吸烟者渴望达到峰值的状态是，如果他们不吸烟，他们的冲动会随着时间的推移而稳步上升，从而增加了人们对卷烟使用的感觉（甚至是必要的），以缓解这种不愉快的状态（Sayette et al. 2005）。重要的是，这种预期是不准确的，因为无论是否吸烟，渴望往往会在短时间内自然消散（Marlatt, 1985; Niaura et al. 1999）。总而言之，有越来越多的证据表明，渴望会以增加药物使用和复发可能性的方式影响认知过程（Baker, Morse, Sherman, 1986）。在渴望状态下，药物使用者可能更容易注意到周围环境中与药物有关的线索，反过来，他们可能认为使用行为更具吸引力，而与非药物活动有关的线索则比在中立状态下吸引力更弱。此外，时间感知的改变可能会阻碍尝试抵抗这种吸引力。认知变化过程中的这些变化不太可能是渴望与药物使用之间潜在联系的详尽组合。这些变化是渴望的体现还是仅仅渴望的效果取决于个人的概念化（Sayette et al. 2000）。无论如何，这些变化都突出了在衡量对药物使用的态度时仔细考虑评估环境的重要性。例如，得知吸烟者对吸烟持负面看法并极有戒烟意愿的治疗提供者，可能会惊讶地发现该吸烟者在几天后复发。但是，很显然，如果在渴望状态下对吸烟者进行评估，吸烟者容易对戒烟产生矛盾心理。这种动机上的转变可能会破坏戒烟尝试，因为在高风险的情况下，决心戒烟的人只需要一瞬间的软弱就可以重新考虑并恢复吸烟（Sayette, Creswell, 2016）。未来研究的一个重要目标是表征药物渴望影响认知过程和后续决策的各种方式。

25.4 渴望的神经生物学和行为学研究的整合使用

功能性脑成像技术［尤其是功能磁共振成像（fMRI）］已成为检查渴望的一种越来越普遍的方法，导致近年来此类研究的数量急剧增加（Wilson, 2015）。功能性脑成像方法使研究人员能够在旨在刺激药物渴望的条件下测量大脑活动。在相对较短的时间内，该领域已经超越了专注于将大脑对药物相关线索的反应集中化的领域，并越来越多地解决与神经生物学和渴望有关的更细微的问题（Ekhtiari et al. 2016, 第7章）正如其他地方所回顾的那样，这项工作带来了挑战和机遇（Sayette, Wilson, 2015）。

可以说，许多研究都太快采用从行为文献中诱发渴望的方法，而这些方法可能不适合神经成像研究。由于大多数脑成像方法的信噪比低（Culham, 2006），研究经常采用重复出现的设计，这些设计旨在激发渴望，通常散布着表面上中性的设计，以引起欲望的最小变化。根据测量和统计的基本概念（Nunnally, 1978），这种方法的基本原理是，随着呈现出每种类型的更多刺激并将响应平均化，估计的对渴望相关与中性提示的大脑反应的可靠性增加。每个条件下的试验或障碍。虽然从心理学角度来看很合理，但许多研究使用的快速多重演示设计可能并不是与渴望响应的典型时间过程的最佳匹配，后者渴望持续几分钟（Heishman et al. 2010）。神经成像研究中经常使用的交错式设计的另一个潜在缺点是，与渴望相关线索相关的大脑活动可能会延续并与随后的对照试验/阻滞过程中测得的信号混淆，从而降低了检测条件之间差异的能力（Franklin et al. 2011; Wilson et al. 2007）。更普遍的担忧是，一些试图评估渴望的神经成像研究已经检查了轻度的欲望状态，这可能对相关结果的性质和解释产生重要影响（Wilson, Sayette, 2015）。尽管存在这些挑战，但对大脑活动模式的神经成像研究与渴望和体验的调节有关，有可能导致重要的科学进步，并为新一代行为研究提供信息。确实，神经成像方法可以作为对涉及测量主观反应和行为的方法的宝贵补充（Berkman, Falk, Lieberman, 2011; Wilson, Smyth, MacLean, 2014）。通过这种方式，使用行为和神经成像方法获得的见解可以进入一个研究周期，在这个周期中，新的想法随着时间的推移而产生、测试和完善。例如，一项行为研究表明，使用药物的机会会极大地影响人们的渴望（Wertz, Sayette, 2011）。这项行为研究被用来帮助整理以前不一致的渴望的神经成像研究的结果（Wilson, Sayette, Fiez, 2004），随后进行了实证研究，确定了与不同情境相关的独特神经模式。毒品使用机会的术语（Wilson, Sayette, Fiez, 2012）。未来将脑成像与其他评估行为的方法（如生态瞬时评估和情感面部表情编码）结合起来的研究，可能会导致人们对渴望的理解进一步提高。

25.5 结论

显然，尽管没有解决概念和方法上的问题，但渴望仍然是成瘾研究和治疗中的主要内容。在临床环境中，可以通过自我报告轻松、可靠地评估药物使用者所经历的渴望。类似地，存在在受控实验室条件下诱发强渴望状态的方法，以便可以检查与渴望相关的响应以及对决策和行为的后续影响。尽管如此，尽管人们普遍认为渴望是一种在临床和概念上有意义的概念，但仍需要更多的研究来更好地理解这种复杂的、多模式的经历（Abrams, 2000; Sayette et al. 2000）。先前的研究强调了渴望强度的潜在重要性，还需要进行其他研究来确定温和和强烈的使用欲望之间的区别是渴望连续体上的两点，还是根本不同的经历。还需要更多的工作来表征将渴望与行为和信息联系起来的机制，这对于改善成瘾的治疗特别有用。本章概述了为什么渴望会促进复发的一些解释，包括它对处理与药物和非药物相关的信息以及时间认知的影响。这些可能仅代表渴望与药物使用之间联系的过程的一个子集，并且可能通过不断的实验研究发现其他机制。鉴于实施起来很容易，自我报告措施可能会继续在渴望研究中发挥重要作用，尽管这也是该领域继续优先发展和完善非语言评估渴望的方法的优先事项。为此，神经成像方法已被证明在测量非语言渴望反应方面特别有价值。如本章中提供的示例所示，脑成像方法可以创新的方式与先进的行为方法和发现相结合，为增进我们对渴望与物质使用之间联系的理解提供了巨大的希望。这种综合工作的结果还将有助于完善旨在减少渴望以促进行为改变的干预措施。

术语解释

- 渴望：通常将其概念化为寻求、获取和使用药物的动机不断增强的一种状态，并就是否应将渴望视为一种极端的向往状态（本质上与较不强烈的欲望有所区别）进行辩论。
- 提示反应性范例：将药物使用者暴露于药物提示中，以引起和测量一个或多个响应系统中的伴随变化（如自我报告的冲动和认知任务表现）。
- 功能磁共振成像：功能神经成像的一种类型，涉及测量与血流变化相关的信号，这些信号随神经活动的变化而发生。
- 功能性神经成像：一组非侵入性地测量与神经活动相关的直接或间接信号的方法。
- 自我调节：改变或超越自己的反应的能力。

功能性脑成像的关键事实

- 功能性脑成像方法使研究人员能够研究人类执行各种任务时大脑的工作方式。
- 功能磁共振成像（fMRI）是当前使用最广泛的功能性脑成像技术。
- 功能磁共振成像和其他功能性脑成像方法的可用性有助于刺激科学的新跨学科领域，如认知神经科学和社会神经科学。

要点总结

- 渴望是成瘾研究领域中的一个核心结构。
- 虽然通常将渴望概念化为寻求、获取和使用药物的动机不断增强的一种状态，但有关该结构的许多定义和概念问题仍未解决。
- 一个重要的悬而未决的问题涉及欲望与渴望之间的关联以及轻度和强烈欲望在数量上与质量上的不同程度。
- 尽管在渴望的概念和界限方面仍存在不确定性，但有充分的证据表明这是一种具有临床意义的构造。
- 研究表明，渴望以各种可能改变药物使用和复发的方式改变认知过程。
- 功能性脑成像方法已成为检验渴望对认知和行为的影响的越来越普遍的方法。
- 需要进一步的研究，特别是将多种方法整合在一起的跨学科工作，以加深我们对渴望与物质使用之间联系的理解。

参考文献

Abrams, D. B. (2000). Transdisciplinary concepts and measures of craving: commentary and future directions. Addiction, 95(8s2), 237-246.

Allen, S. S.; Bade, T.; Hatsukami, D.; Center, B. (2008). Craving, withdrawal, and smoking urges on days immediately prior to smokingrelapse. Nicotine, Tobacco Research, 10(1), 35-45.

American Psychiatric Association (2013). Diagnostic and statistical manual of mental disorders (DSM-5®). Arlington, VA: American Psychiatric Publishing.

Bagot, K. S.; Heishman, S. J.; Moolchan, E. T. (2007). Tobacco craving predicts lapse to smoking among adolescent smokers in cessation treatment. Nicotine, Tobacco Research, 9(6), 647-652.

Baker, T. B.; Morse, E.; Sherman, J. E. (1986). The motivation to use drugs: a psychobiological analysis of urges. Nebraska Symposium on Motivation, 34, 257-323.

Berkman, E. T.; Falk, E. B.; Lieberman, M. D. (2011). In the trenches of real-world self-control: neural correlates of breaking the link between craving and smoking. Psychological Science, 22(4), 498-506.

Cronbach, L. J.; Meehl, P. E. (1955). Construct validity in psychological tests. Psychological Bulletin, 52(4), 281. Culham, J. C. (2006). Functional neuroimaging: experimental design and analysis. Cambridge, MA: MIT Press.

Ekhtiari, H.; Nasseri, P.; Yavari, F.; Mokri, A.; Monterosso, J. (2016). Neuroscience of drug craving for addiction medicine: from circuits to therapies. In: H. Ekhtiari, M. Paulus (Eds.), Progress in brain research, Vol. 223 (pp. 115-141). Cambridge. MA: Elsevier.

Ferguson, S. G.; Shiffman, S. (2009). The relevance and treatment of cue-induced cravings in tobacco dependence. Journal of Substance Abuse Treatment, 36(3), 235-243.

Franklin, T. R.; Wang, Z.; Suh, J. J.; Hazan, R.; Cruz, J.; Li, Y. et al. (2011). Effects of varenicline on smoking cue-triggered neural and craving responses. Archives of General Psychiatry, 68(5), 516-526.

George, O.; Koob, G. F. (2013). Control of craving by the prefrontal cortex. Proceedings of the National Academy of Sciences, 110(11), 4165-4166.

Heishman, S. J.; Lee, D. C.; Taylor, R. C.; Singleton, E. G. (2010). Prolonged duration of craving, mood, and autonomic responses elicited by cues and imagery in smokers: effects of tobacco deprivationand sex. Experimental and Clinical Psychopharmacology, 18(3), 245-256.

Kavanagh, D. J.; Andrade, J.; May, J. (2005). Imaginary relish and exquisite torture: the elaborated intrusion theory of desire. Psychological Review, 112(2), 446.

Killen, J. D.; Fortmann, S. P. (1997). Craving is associated with smoking relapse: findings from three prospective studies. Experimental and Clinical Psychopharmacology, 5(2), 137-142.

Klein, L.; Corwin, E.; Stine, M. (2003). Smoking abstinence impairs time estimation accuracy in cigarette smokers. Psychopharmacology Bulletin, 37(1), 90-95.

Kozlowski, L. T.; Wilkinson, D. A. (1987). Use and misuse of the concept of craving by alcohol, tobacco, and drug researchers. Addiction, 82(1), 31-36.

Marlatt, G. A. (1985). Cognitive factors in the relapse process. In G. A. Marlatt, J. R. Gordon (Eds.), Relapse prevention: Maintenance strategies in the treatment of addictive behaviors (pp. 128-200). New York: Guilford.

Niaura, R.; Abrams, D. B.; Shadel, W. G.; Rohsenow, D. J.; Monti, P. M.; Sirota, A. D. (1999). Cue exposure treatment for smoking relapseprevention: a controlled clinical trial. Addiction, 94(5), 685-695.

Nunnally, J. C. (1978). Psychometric theory(2nd ed.). New York: McGraw-Hill.

Piper, M. E. (2015). Withdrawal: expanding a key addiction construct. Nicotine, Tobacco Research, 17(12), 1405-1415.

Reitsma, M. B.; Fullman, N.; Ng, M.; Salama, J. S.; Abajobir, A.; Abate, K. H. et al. (2017). Smoking prevalence and attributable disease burden in 195 countries and territories, 1990-2015: a systematic analysis from the Global Burden of Disease Study 2015. The Lancet, 389 (10082), 1885-1906.

Sayette, M. A. (2016). The role of craving in substance use disorders: theoretical and methodological issues. Annual Review of Clinical Psychology, 12(1), 407-433.

Sayette, M. A.; Creswell, K. G. (2016). Self-regulatory failure and addiction. Handbook of self-regulation: Research, theory, and applications, Vol. 3 (pp. 571-590). New York: Guilford Press.

Sayette, M. A.; Hufford, M. R. (1997). Effects of smoking urge on generation of smoking-related information. Journal of Applied Social Psychology, 27(16), 1395-1405.

Sayette, M. A.; Loewenstein, G.; Kirchner, T. R.; Travis, T. (2005). Effects of smoking urge on temporal cognition. Psychology of Addictive Behaviors, 19(1), 88.

Sayette, M. A.; Martin, C. S.; Wertz, J. M.; Shiffman, S.; Perrott, M. A. (2001). A multi-dimensional analysis of cue-elicited craving in heavy smokers and tobacco chippers. Addiction, 96(10), 1419-1432.

Sayette, M. A.; Schooler, J. W.; Reichle, E. D. (2010). Out for a smoke: the impact of cigarette craving on zoning out during reading. Psychological Science, 21(1), 26-30.

Sayette, M. A.; Shiffman, S.; Tiffany, S. T.; Niaura, R. S.; Martin, C. S.; Schadel, W. G. (2000). The measurement of drug craving. Addiction, 95(8s2), 189-210.

Sayette, M. A.; Tiffany, S. T. (2013). Peak provoked craving: an alternative to smoking cue-reactivity. Addiction, 108(6), 1019-1025.

Sayette, M. A.; Wilson, S. J. (2015). The measurement of craving and desires. In W. Hofmann, L. Nordgren (Eds.), The psychology of desire (pp. 104-126). New York: Guilford.

Shiffman, S.; Paty, J. A.; Gnys, M.; Kassel, J. A.; Hickcox, M. (1996). First lapses to smoking: within-subjects analysis of real-time reports. Journal of Consulting and Clinical Psychology, 64(2), 366-379.

Tiffany, S. T. (1990). A cognitive model of drug urges and drug-use behavior: role of automatic and nonautomatic processes. Psychological Review, 97(2), 147.

Tiffany, S. T.; Wray, J. M. (2012). The clinical significance of drug craving. Annals of the New York Academy of Sciences, 1248(1), 1-17.

Volkow, N. D.; Wang, G. J.; Fowler, J. S.; Tomasi, D.; Telang, F.; Baler, R. (2010). Addiction: decreased reward sensitivity and increased expectation sensitivity conspire to overwhelm the brain's control circuit. BioEssays, 32(9), 748-755.

Waters, A. J.; Sayette, M. A. (2006). Implicit cognition and tobacco addiction. InHandbook of implicit cognition and addiction (pp. 309-338). London: SAGE.

Wertz, J. M.; Sayette, M. A. (2001). A review of the effects of perceived drug use opportunity on self-reported urge. Experimental and Clinical Psychopharmacology, 9(1), 3.

Wilson, S. J. (Ed.). (2015). The Wiley handbook on the cognitive neuroscience of addiction. Chichester, UK: John Wiley, Sons, Ltd.

Wilson, S. J.; Delgado, M. R.; McKee, S. A.; Grigson, P. S.; MacLean, R. R.; Nichols, T. T. et al. (2014). Weak ventral striatal responses to monetary outcomes predict an unwillingness to resist cigarette smoking. Cognitive, Affective, Behavioral Neuroscience, 14(4), 1196-1207.

Wilson, S. J.; Sayette, M. A. (2015). Neuroimaging craving: urge intensity matters. Addiction, 110(2), 195-203. https://doi. org/10. 1111/add. 12676.

Wilson, S. J.; Sayette, M. A.; Fiez, J. A. (2004). Prefrontal responses to drug cues: a neurocognitive analysis. Nature Neuroscience, 7(3), 211-214.

Wilson, S. J.; Sayette, M. A.; Fiez, J. A. (2012). Quitting-unmotivated and quitting-motivated cigarette smokers exhibit different patterns of cue-elicited brain activation when anticipating an opportunity to smoke. Journal of Abnormal Psychology, 121(1), 198-211.

Wilson, S. J.; Sayette, M. A.; Fiez, J. A.; Brough, E. (2007). Carry-over effects of smoking cue exposure on working memory performance. Nicotine, Tobacco Research, 9(5), 613-619.

Wilson, S. J.; Smyth, J. M.; MacLean, R. R. (2014). Integrating ecological momentary assessment and functional brain imaging methods: new avenues for studying and treating tobacco dependence. Nicotine, Tobacco Research, 16(Suppl. 2), S102-S110.

Wray, J. M.; Gass, J. C.; Tiffany, S. T. (2013). A systematic review of the relationships between craving and smoking cessation. Nicotine, Tobacco Research, 15(7), 1167-1182.

26
运动对渴望和戒断症状的急性影响

Wuyou Sui, Scott Rollo, Harry Prapavessis

Faculty of Health Sciences, School of Kinesiology, The University of Western Ontario, London, ON, Canada

缩略语

DtS	吸烟渴望	**SJWS**	Shiffman-Jarvik 戒断量表
HR$_{max}$	最大心率	**SoD**	吸烟渴望的强度
MPSS	情绪和身体症状量表	**TWS**	烟草戒断症状
NRT	烟碱替代疗法		
PA	体力活动		
RPE	感知劳累等级		

本章将首先总结急性运动对吸烟的影响，特别是运动对渴望和烟草戒断症状（TWS）的急性影响。本章还将深入研究产生这些作用的机制，并提出将急性运动作为治疗/干预措施的临床建议。

26.1 渴望

所有吸烟者，无论他们是否尝试戒烟，都会经历某种形式的渴望或吸烟渴望。这些渴望本质上是偶发性的、强烈的、断断续续的或习惯性的，并且常常是由线索或环境引起的（Shiffman, 2000）。渴望也可能表现为背景渴望，这种渴望由于长期渴望吸烟而持续一整天。在那些对烟碱依赖性较高的人群中，两种渴望都倾向于表现出更多的症状（Dunbar et al. 2014）。渴望强度可以通过多种方式进行评估：自我报告问卷、提示性反应、注意偏见或功能磁共振成像。其中，主要使用自我报告问卷，以测量吸烟渴望（DtS; Tiffany, Drobes, 1991）或吸烟渴望的强度（SoD; West, Hajek, 2004）。

药理疗法［即烟碱替代疗法（NRT）］是缓解渴望的标准疗法。NRT 与大脑中的烟碱乙酰胆碱受体结合，取代了卷烟中的烟碱。NRT 可以通过多种方式给药：口香糖、含片、口服喷雾剂或贴剂。烟碱口香糖、含片和喷雾剂可相对较快地向人体提供一定剂量的烟碱，因此，它们在遏制突发性渴望方面更有效。相比之下，贴片在抑制背景渴望方面更有效；烟碱的释放时间较长。总的来说，NRT 对缓解急性渴望是有效的（Kotlyar et al. 2007）。

26.1.1 急性运动对渴望的影响

单次运动会显著并立即降低暂时戒烟者和戒烟者的渴望水平。运动的有益效果在急性运动期间和之后最明显，并且可以持续至运动后 30min（Ussher et al. 2009）。急性运动的渴望减少效果与 NRT 辅助设备相当或更高（Haasova et al. 2013）。此外，急性运动可提供渴望缓解的速度可能比NRT快，NRT可能需要30min才能获得最大缓解（Hansson et al. 2012）。锻炼的多功能性和成本效益意味着消除了诸如财务负担或NRT可用性之类的障碍。渴望减少的强度的确因许多因素而异：强度、持续时间、运动类型以及压力源的存在；确定急性运动对渴望的有效性时，必须考虑同时进行治疗（图26.1～图26.3）。

运动强度。运动强度的作用已在轻度、中度和剧烈强度的方案中进行了考查。尽管三种强度都可以有效减少渴望，但是中等强度则要有效得多。剧烈运动似乎并没有比中度运动明显减少更多的渴望（Haasova et al. 2014）。一些研究表明，剧烈运动可能会对情绪产生负面影响（Everson et al. 2008）。从临床角度来看，中等强度对运动者来说更容易，这可能会增加锻炼的依从性和乐趣。

运动时间。运动时间对减少渴望有影响。中等时间（10min）和长时间（15min以上）的急性运动可显著缓解暂时戒烟者的渴望（Haasova et al. 2014）。持续时间越长，表示渴望量的减少幅度越大；但是，从临床角度来看，中等持续时间的运动可能足以缓解渴望（见图26.4）。

运动类型。某些类型的运动对渴望有更明显的影响。有氧运动也同样会减弱渴望的强度。等距运动也被证明可以减少暂时戒烟者的渴望，尽管其程度远低于有氧运动（Haasova et al. 2014）。瑜伽也可以显著减少渴望（Elibero et al. 2011）。虽然进行了简单的研究，但阻力训练并未显示出

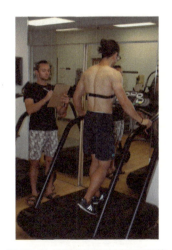

图26.1 典型的有氧运动干预设施

研究人员正在监视受试者的感知劳累等级（RPE）和心率，以维持特定强度。

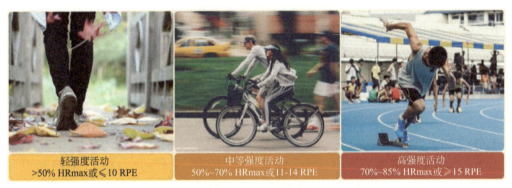

图26.2 运动强度的分类

该图分别通过步行、骑自行车和短跑的示例描述了轻度、中度和剧烈强度运动的标志性措施。该图尚未发布；该图通过stocksnap.io和CC0的使用许可。

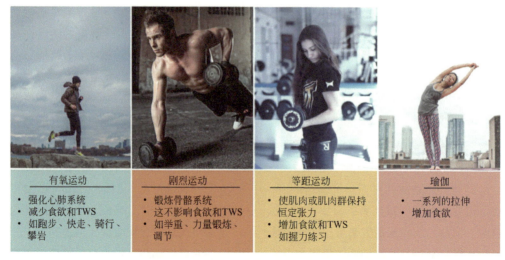

图 26.3　运动类型的分类及其对渴望/戒断症状的影响

该图总结了特定运动类型/方式对渴望和烟草戒断症状（TWS）的影响。该图尚未发布；该图通过stocksnap.io和CC0的使用许可。

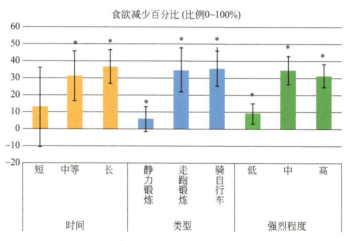

图 26.4　与运动参数有关的渴望减少百分比

条形表示与特定运动参数相关的渴望的平均减少。星号表示显著性（$P<0.05$）。该图改编自Haasova等（2014）的数据。该图尚未发布。

明显的渴望减少（Ho et al. 2014）。需要对阻力训练和渴望进行进一步的研究。种类繁多的运动证明了其作为一种疗法的应用：方便、快捷、具有与NRT相似或更好的效果。

压力源的存在。其他吸烟者的存在、吸烟用具、认知压力或吸烟行为的诱因都可能使吸烟者的渴望程度达到峰值。鉴于这些环境诱因的普遍性，"提示引起的渴望"（Taylor, Katomeri, 2007）对那些希望避免复发的人构成了严重威胁。在运动后30min出现压力源时，运动仍然可以降低渴望的水平（最多8%）（Taylor, Katomeri, 2007）。然而，这种连续施加压力的方法在生态学上不如同时施加压力的方法有效。Fong等（2014）发现，在同时承受急性运动的压力下，运动后的SoD仍显著降低了37%，这证明了运动对渴望的普遍影响。然而，研究人员没有报告两组之间初次抽气时间的差异，这表明并发压力可能会限制运动对运动后渴望的影响。

并行治疗。急性运动可产生与NRT相似的渴望减少，因此已详细研究了急性运动和NRT或其他疗法的潜在综合作用。与单独使用NRT相比，急性运动与NRT结合可以显著减少渴望。

在暂时戒烟者中，将NRT与15min的急性运动相结合，至少在运动后40min内表现出更大的持续减少的渴望（Tritter, Fitzgeorge, Prapavessis, 2015）。即使在目前使用NRT的戒烟尝试者中，急性运动也可以维持其减少渴望的累加性。有趣的是，剧烈运动能够保持一致的减少效果，即使NRT的剂量在戒烟方案中减少（21mg→14mg→7mg）（图26.5；Harper et al. 2012）。从理论上讲，运动的累加作用是由于体育活动而发生的，烟碱通过单独的机制使人们的渴望得到缓解。

即使在NRT戒烟计划中，背景渴望可能在个人的渴望中扮演更重要的角色，急性运动也会显著缓解渴望的程度（图26.5；Harper et al. 2012）。急性运动是一种有效的方法，可以立即减少吸烟者在同时或即将发生的压力刺激下的渴望水平升高。

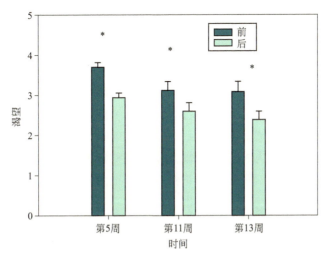

图26.5　在戒烟计划中经过一轮急性运动后的渴望水平

该图表示在戒烟计划中进行一轮急性运动前后的渴望程度。第5周、第11周和第13周分别代表戒烟后的第1周、第7周和第9周。星号表示显著性（$P<0.05$）。根据Harper等（2012）的数据改编。该图尚未发布。

行为疗法和急性运动也被作为一种减少渴望的并行模型进行了简要研究。将自我调节策略与急性运动相结合似乎不会影响运动后的DtS（Hatzigeorgiadis et al. 2016）。然而，对不同行为模型的进一步探索和联合干预的交付是一个成熟的研究途径。

特殊人群。对暂时戒烟的孕妇的研究表明，孕妇对急性运动的反应与正常人群相似。锻炼20min后，轻度至中度强度的运动会引起运动后立即减少的渴望，运动后10min的渴望水平显著持续降低（Prapavessis et al. 2014）。

研究人员研究了在短暂禁欲的青少年中进行10min中等强度的运动对渴望的影响，发现运动期间或运动后DtS并未降低（Everson et al. 2006）。这些结果暗示与成年人相比，青少年对运动的反应不同，并激发了该领域的未来研究。由于缺乏其他特殊人群（如老年人、肥胖成年人和患病人群）的证据，需要研究更专业的急性运动范例。

26.1.2　临床重要性

急性运动可在运动后最多30min为吸烟者提供即时和持续的渴望缓解。具体来说，进行10min以上的中等强度的有氧运动可以最大限度地减少渴望，对于新手锻炼者可能更可持续。运动类型的多功能性可以方便地缓解渴望。不论吸烟状况如何，急性运动都能带来与NRT相似的缓解作用，并且两者结合时可以累加减少渴望。仅有限的证据表明这些影响可以在特殊人群中复制。总体而言，急性运动应作为单一疗法或与NRT并用，以抑制渴望。

26.2 烟草戒断症状

戒烟会导致焦虑、压力、烦躁、注意力不集中和睡眠障碍。这些烟草戒断症状（TWS）对可能想要戒烟的吸烟者构成了挑战。此外，吸烟后不久即可缓解这些症状，从而促进了进一步的吸烟行为。有效的TWS管理可以减少吸烟者中有害的吸烟行为，并可以通过预防复发来提高成功戒烟的概率。

可靠地表示各种TWS非常重要。情绪和身体症状量表（MPSS; West, Hajek, 2004）是一份经过验证的五点自我报告调查问卷，用于评估抑郁、焦虑、烦躁、心神不定、饥饿、集中注意力、夜间睡眠和身体症状（如单项量表的口腔溃疡、便秘和咳嗽/喉咙痛）。另一种常用的问卷是Shiffman-Jarvik戒断量表（SJWS; Shiffman, Jarvik, 1976），用于评估渴望（五项）、心理症状（五项）、身体症状（三项）、镇静（单项）和食欲（单项）。尽管MPSS和SJWS是针对TWS的有效措施，但它们是自我报告的问卷，无法捕获认知变量（如注意力、记忆力或执行功能）的客观差异。因此，可以使用特定的认知测试来测试认知能力。常见的测试包括Stroop任务（注意力；Homack, Riccio, 2004）和n-back测试（工作记忆；Kirchner, 1958）。

26.2.1 急性运动对TWS的影响

急性运动已对许多TWS产生积极影响。烦躁、抑郁、紧张、心神不定、注意力不集中和压力（Roberts et al. 2012; Taylor et al. 2007）以及心理症状和镇静作用（Harper et al. 2012），在急性运动后都显示出显著减少。与渴望类似，在运动过程中和运动刚结束后，运动减少TWS的效力最大。这些影响是在步行、骑自行车和等距运动期间引起的，表明不同类型的运动可以引起类似的反应。如果吸烟者可以从多种锻炼中选择，坚持锻炼可能更为可行，尽管还需要进一步研究阻力训练、瑜伽和其他替代锻炼的效果（图26.6）。

运动强度也对TWS起作用。运动对TWS的影响主要是采用中等强度的方案进行的。有证据表明，在剧烈运动中，TWS可能会增加，但运动后症状会减轻（Everson et al. 2008）。有趣的是，参加戒烟计划时似乎没有剧烈运动的负面影响。Harper等（2012）发现，在运动辅助性NRT戒烟计划的第11周（即戒烟后第7周），剧烈运动可改善心理和镇静戒断症状。

在同时存在压力源的情况下，进行中度强度的急性运动也可能会使TWS衰减。Fong等（2014）发现应激源后，仅运动组的心理戒断症状显著减少。这些结果令人鼓舞，因为在体验TWS的情况下，暴露于线索和触发因素是更有效的外部情景。

早期证据也暗示了认知特征可能对暂时戒烟者的急性运动产生积极影响。Guirguis等（2016）通过比较急性运动状况和烟碱（NRT）状况通过n-back任务检查了工作记忆。结果表明，运动在改善工作记忆方面与烟碱同样有效，甚至更好。我们实验室目前正在研究在吸烟者中应用这种范例的未来工作。

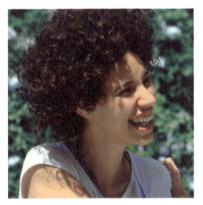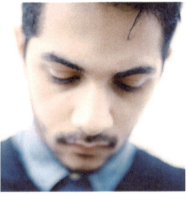

图 26.6 积极和消极影响的表现

影响是情感的体验。积极影响是积极情绪的体验；消极影响是消极情绪的体验。该图尚未发布；该图通过stocksnap.io和CC0的使用许可。

26.2.2 临床重要性

综合考虑，中等强度的急性运动似乎可以有效减轻许多TWS（如易怒、压力和抑郁），即使同时存在压力源也是如此。戒烟初期，剧烈运动可能会对TWS产生不利影响。

26.3 机制

人们对运动作用于渴望和TWS的确切机制尚不十分了解。从生理学/心理生物学的角度来看，皮质醇、心率变异性、儿茶酚胺以及大脑的奖励和视觉空间区域的激活转移受到了一些研究的关注，但是结果是模棱两可的和/或有待再现（如Janse Van Rensburg, et al. 2012; Roberts et al. 2015）。从心理学的角度来看，预期和分散注意力的假设尚未得到支持（Daniel, Cropley, Fife-Schaw, 2007）。目前，情感仍然是调节运动与渴望之间关系的最广泛研究的心理机制之一（Haasova et al. 2014; Roberts et al. 2012）。不幸的是，只有少数研究发现了对调节的支持（Janse Van Rensburg, et al. 2013; Tart et al. 2010; Taylor et al. 2006）。Janse Van Rensburg等（2013）表明，运动通过积极影响减少了渴望，而Tart等（2010）和Taylor等（2006）发现，运动通过消极影响减少了渴望。支持情感调节假设的研究数量少的原因包括情感的可衡量维度不一致、样本能力不足、统计调节方法不健全以及设计欠佳（即非随机对照试验）。针对这些问题，De Jesus和Prapavessis（2017）探索了积极和消极影响作为运动-渴望关系的一种机制。结果令人鼓舞，因为积极和消极的影响都被认为是有效的媒介。推测了这种调节作用的多种原因：运动可以抵消渴望和TWS带来的消极影响；通过运动产生积极影响而释放多巴胺可能会模仿与烟碱渴望相关的奖励途径；和/或改善的情绪可能会改善通常由于心理困扰/压力而失去的自我调节力（De Jesus, Prapavessis, 2017）。这一发现引起了人们的注意，将急性运动干预措施设计为既有趣又通用，并最大限度地减少不适和消极影响。值得注意的是，所有提议的运动与烟碱关系的机制都依赖于烟碱（即烟碱乙酰胆碱受体）机制所独有的途径，这支持运动与NRT结合作为戒烟疗法的累加作用。

不仅仅是NRT，NRT与令人愉悦且可行的急性运动结合使用，可能会增加吸烟者戒烟的概率。未来研究运动受情感影响的确切方法和比例以及其他机制的潜在作用，需要进一步探索。

26.4 急性运动的临床重要性摘要

急性运动对渴望和TWS的积极影响是显而易见的。应该将运动作为减少烟碱渴望的有效疗法。中度强度运动或更长时间（10min以上）的适度体力活动（11～13 RPE或40%～60%最大心率）被证明是最有效的减少渴望的方法。更高的强度似乎并不能为渴望或TWS带来更多好处。当前的证据表明，情感是急性范例中运动的一种可能机制，因此，应量身定制运动干预措施，以改善积极影响并减少消极影响。尽管确切的运动机制尚有争议，但它可能是在与烟碱不同的途径下运作的，因此与NRT搭配使用时，可以累加减少渴望。总体而言，急性运动是减少从事暂时或实际戒烟尝试的烟民渴望的有效手段。

术语解释	
	■ 急性运动：一次运动。强度、持续时间和/或运动类型的范围。
	■ 有氧运动：一类主要挑战心肺系统运动的运动。包括步行，骑自行车，跑步和游泳等活动。
	■ 影响：情感的体验。可以进一步分为积极或消极影响——个人分别经历积极或消极情绪的方式。
	■ 运动持续时间：一轮运动的时间长度。在本综述中，一轮运动的持续时间将分为短（5min）、中（10min）和长（>15min）。
	■ 运动：身体活动的一个子类别。旨在改善身体健康和/或心理健康程度的结构性和有目的的活动。有目的的运动通常以中等到重度强度（MVPA）进行，持续时间>10min。
	■ 运动频率：从一次急性运动到每周多次进行更规律的运动。
	■ 最大心率（HR_{max}）：一个人通过体育锻炼可以获得的最大预测心率。通常以220减去年龄计算。
	■ 运动强度：运动期间所需的运动水平。可以客观地（如心率监测器）或主观地（自我报告的运动量表）进行测量。通常分为轻度（<50% HR_{max}）、中度（50%～70% HR_{max}）和剧烈（70%～85% HR_{max}）强度。
	■ 等距运动：一类涉及肌肉/肌肉群的静态、持续收缩的运动。可以使用握把、阻力带或举重来执行。
	■ 体力活动（PA）：通过骨骼肌收缩引起的身体运动，导致能量消耗。
	■ 缺乏体育锻炼：该术语描述无法达到建议的体育锻炼水平的那些人。
	■ 感知劳累等级（RPE）：个人在一轮运动中瞬间感觉到的主观感觉努力；自我报告的瞬时运动强度的量度。
	■ 阻力训练：一类主要挑战肌肉骨骼系统的运动。包括举重、锻炼等活动。
	■ 运动类型：进行运动的方式。包含各种运动形式，如有氧运动、阻力运动、等距运动。

体力活动和锻炼的关键事实	
	■ 缺乏运动是全球第四大死亡原因。
	■ 研究人员评估了缺乏运动的风险与吸烟或肥胖的风险相似（Lee et al. 2012）。
	■ 体育锻炼的长期益处包括降低体重增加和肥胖的风险、降低冠心病的风险、降低罹患2型糖尿病的风险以及降低阿尔茨海默病和痴呆症的发病率。
	■ 一次中等强度到剧烈强度的运动可以增加循环免疫和炎症标记物（Brown et al. 2015），增强许多认知过程（Tomporowski, 2003），减少与压力相关的血压反应（Hamer, Taylor, Steptoe, 2006），改善代谢指标（Dunstan et al. 2012）。

- 有四个用于分类和规定运动的参数：频率、强度、时间（持续时间）和活动类型（方式）。这些术语共同构成了FITT原则，经常在规定运动的研究人员和卫生保健专业人员中使用（Bushman, 2017）。
- 要想在大多数国家（如加拿大和美国）进行体育锻炼，个人必须每周积累150min的中度强度运动，并进行10min以上的锻炼。

点总结

- 本章重点介绍运动对渴望和烟草戒断症状的急性影响。
- 急性运动是指单次运动，从轻度到剧烈运动，持续时间小于5min到大于15min，并通过多种方式（如有氧运动、阻力和伸展）完成。
- 急性运动可在运动后长达30min的时间内为吸烟者提供即时和持续的渴望缓解，特别是中度强度的运动或更长时间（10min以上）的适度体力活动［11～13级的感知劳累等级（RPE）或40%～60%最大心率（HR_{max}）］已被证明是减少渴望的最有效方法。
- 与烟碱替代疗法（NRT）结合使用时，运动也可提供累加作用。
- 即使在同时存在压力源的情况下，进行中度强度的急性运动似乎也能有效减轻许多烟草戒断症状（TWS；如易怒、压力和抑郁）。
- 戒烟初期，剧烈运动可能会对TWS产生不利影响。
- 目前，情感似乎是运动-渴望关系的最佳支持机制。
- 运动是减少烟碱渴望的有效疗法，因此应开具处方。

参考文献

Brown, W. M. C.; Davison, G. W.; McClean, C. M.; Murphy, M. H. (2015). A systematic review of the acute effects of exercise on immune and inflammatory indices in untrained adults. Sports Medicine: Open, 1(1), 35.

Bushman, B. (2017). In B. Bushman (Ed.), ACSM's complete guide to fitness, health(2nd ed.). Champaign, IL: Human Kinetics.

Daniel, J. Z.; Cropley, M.; Fife-Schaw, C. (2007). Acute exercise effectson smoking withdrawal symptoms and desire to smoke are not related to expectation. Psychopharmacology, 195(1), 125-129.

De Jesus, S.; Prapavessis, H. (2017). Cortisol and affect mechanisms through which acute exercise attenuates cigarette cravings during a temporary quit attempt. Unpublished work.

Dunbar, M. S.; Shiffman, S.; Kirchner, T. R.; Tindle, H. A.; Scholl, S. M. (2014). Nicotine dependence, "background" and cue-induced craving and smoking in the laboratory. Drug and Alcohol Dependence, 142, 197 203.

Dunstan, D. W.; Kingwell, B. A.; Larsen, R.; Healy, G. N.; Cerin, E.; Hamilton, M. T. et al. (2012). Breaking up prolonged sitting reduces postprandial glucose and insulin responses. Diabetes Care.

Elibero, A.; Janse Van Rensburg, K.; Drobes, D. J. (2011). Acute effects of aerobic exercise and hatha yoga on craving to smoke. Nicotine, Tobacco Research, 13(11), 1140-1148.

Everson, E. S.; Daley, A. J.; Ussher, M. (2006). Does exercise have an acute effect on desire to smoke, mood and withdrawal symptoms in abstaining adolescent smokers? Addictive Behaviors, 31(9), 1547-1558.

Everson, E. S.; Daley, A. J.; Ussher, M. (2008). The effects of moderate and vigorous exercise on desire to smoke, withdrawal symptoms and mood in abstaining young adult smokers. Mental Health and Physical Activity, 1(1), 26-31.

Fong, A. J.; De Jesus, S.; Bray, S. R.; Prapavessis, H. (2014). Effect of exercise on cigarette cravings and ad libitum smoking following concurrent stressors. Addictive Behaviors, 39(10), 1516-1521.

Guirguis, S.; Sui, W.; Prapavessis, H. (2016). The acute effects of nicotine and exercise on working memory in non-smokers. Unpublished work.

Haasova, M.; Warren, F. C.; Ussher, M.; Janse Van Rensburg, K.; Faulkner, G.; Cropley, M. et al. (2013). The acute effects of physical activity on cigarette cravings: systematic review and meta-analysis with individual participant data. Addiction, 108(1), 26-37.

Haasova, M.; Warren, F. C.; Ussher, M.; Janse Van Rensburg, K.; Faulkner, G.; Cropley, M. et al. (2014). The acute effects of physical activity on cigarette cravings: exploration of potential moderators, mediators and physical activity attributes using individual participant data (IPD) meta-analyses. Psychopharmacology, 231(7), 1267-1275.

Hamer, M.; Taylor, A.; Steptoe, A. (2006). The effect of acute aerobic exercise on stress related blood pressure responses: a systematic review and meta-analysis. Biological Psychology, 71(2), 183-190.

Hansson, A.; Hajek, P.; Perfekt, R.; Kraiczi, H. (2012). Effects of nicotine mouth spray on urges to smoke, a randomised clinical trial. BMJ Open, 2(5). e001618.

Harper, T.; Fitzgeorge, L.; Tritter, A.; Prapavessis, H. (2012). Acute exercise effects on craving and withdrawal symptoms among women attempting to quit smoking using nicotine replacement therapy. Journal of Smoking Cessation, 1-8.

Hatzigeorgiadis, A.; Pappa, V.; Tsiami, A.; Tzatzaki, T.; Georgakouli, K.; Zourbanos, N. et al. (2016). Self-regulation strategies may enhance the acute effect of exercise on smoking delay. Addictive Behaviors, 57, 35-37.

Ho, J. Y.; Kraemer, W. J.; Volek, J. S.; Vingren, J. L.; Fragala, M. S.; Flanagan, S. D. et al. (2014). Effects of resistance exercise on the HPA axis response to psychological stress during short-term smoking abstinence in men. Addictive Behaviors, 39(3), 695-698.

Homack, S.; Riccio, C. A. (2004). A meta-analysis of the sensitivity and specificity of the Stroop Color and Word Test with children. Archive of Clinical Neuropsychology, 19(6), 725-743.

Janse Van Rensburg, K.; Elibero, A.; Kilpatrick, M.; Drobes, D. J. (2013). Impact of aerobic exercise intensity on craving and reactivity to smoking cues. Experimental and Clinical Psychopharmacology, 21(3), 196-203.

Janse Van Rensburg, K.; Taylor, A.; Benattayallah, A.; Hodgson, T. (2012). The effects of exercise on cigarette cravings and brain activation in response to smoking-related images. Psychopharmacology, 221(4), 659-666.

Kirchner, W. K. (1958). Age differences in short-term retention of rapidly changing information. Journal of Experimental Psychology, 55(4), 352-358.

Kotlyar, M.; Mendoza-Baumgart, M. I.; Li, Z. -Z.; Pentel, P. R.; Barnett, B. C.; Feuer, R. M. et al. (2007). Nicotine pharmacokinetics and subjective effects of three potential reduced exposure products, moist snuff and nicotine lozenge. Tobacco Control, 16(2), 138-142.

Lee, I. -M.; Shiroma, E. J.; Lobelo, F.; Puska, P.; Blair, S. N.; Katzmarzyk, P. T. et al. (2012). Impact of physical inactivity on the World's Major Non-Communicable Diseases. The Lancet, 380 (9838), 219-229.

Prapavessis, H.; De Jesus, S.; Harper, T.; Cramp, A.; Fitzgeorge, L.; Mottola, M. F. et al. (2014). The effects of acute exercise on tobacco cravings and withdrawal symptoms in temporary abstinent pregnant smokers. Addictive Behaviors, 39(3), 703-708.

Roberts, V.; Gant, N.; Sollers, J. J.; Bullen, C.; Jiang, Y.; Maddison, R. (2015). Effects of exercise on the desire to smoke and physiological responses to temporary smoking abstinence: a crossover trial. Psychopharmacology, 232(6), 1071-1081.

Roberts, V.; Maddison, R.; Simpson, C.; Bullen, C.; Prapavessis, H. (2012). The acute effects of exercise on cigarette cravings, withdrawal symptoms, affect, and smoking behaviour: systematic review update and meta-analysis. Psychopharmacology, 222(1), 1-15.

Shiffman, S. (2000). Comments on craving. Addiction, 95(8s2), 171-175. https://doi.org/10.1046/j.1360-0443.95.8s2.6.x.

Shiffman, S. M.; Jarvik, M. E. (1976). Smoking withdrawal symptoms in two weeks of abstinence. Psychopharmacology, 50(1), 35-39.

Tart, C. D.; Leyro, T. M.; Richter, A.; Zvolensky, M. J.; Rosenfield, D.; Smits, J. A. J. (2010). Negative affect as a mediator of the relationship between vigorous-intensity exercise and smoking. Addictive Behaviors, 35(6), 580-585.

Taylor, A.; Katomeri, M. (2007). Walking reduces cue-elicited cigarette cravings and withdrawal symptoms, and delays ad libitum smoking. Nicotine, Tobacco Research, 9(11), 1183-1190.

Taylor, A.; Katomeri, M.; Ussher, M. (2006). Effects of walking on cigarette cravings and affect in the context of Nesbitt's paradox and the Circumplex model. Journal of Sport, Exercise Psychology, 28.

Taylor, A. H.; Ussher, M. H.; Faulkner, G. (2007). The acute effects of exercise on cigarette cravings, withdrawal symptoms, affect, and smoking behaviour: a systematic review. Addiction, 102, 534-543.

Tiffany, S. T.; Drobes, D. J. (1991). The development and initial validation of a questionnaire on smoking urges. British Journal of Addiction, 86(11), 1467-1476.

Tomporowski, P. D. (2003). Effects of acute bouts of exercise on cognition. Acta Psychologica, 112(3), 297-324.

Tritter, A.; Fitzgeorge, L.; Prapavessis, H. (2015). The effect of acute exercise on cigarette cravings while using a nicotine lozenge. Psychopharmacology, 232(14), 2531-2539.

Ussher, M.; Cropley, M.; Playle, S.; Mohidin, R.; West, R. (2009). Effect of isometric exercise and body scanning on cigarette cravings and withdrawal symptoms. Addiction, 104(7), 1251-1257.

West, R.; Hajek, P. (2004). Evaluation of the mood and physical symptoms scale (MPSS) to assess cigarette withdrawal. Psychopharmacology, 177(1-2), 195-199.

27

CRF2 受体激动剂和烟碱戒断

Zsolt Bagosi

Department of Pathophysiology, Faculty of Medicine, University of Szeged, Szeged, Hungary

缩略语

ACTH	促肾上腺皮质激素	**HPA 轴**	下丘脑 - 垂体 - 肾上腺轴
AVP	精氨酸加压素	**icv**	脑室内
CFLP	Carworth Farm Lane-Petter	**ip**	腹膜内
CNS	中枢神经系统	**SNS**	交感神经系统
CRF	促肾上腺皮质激素释放因子	**Ucn1**	尿皮质素 1
CRF1	促肾上腺皮质激素释放因子受体 1 型	**Ucn2**	尿皮质素 2
CRF2	促肾上腺皮质激素释放因子受体 2 型	**Ucn3**	尿皮质素 3
CRF-BP	促肾上腺皮质激素释放因子结合蛋白		

促肾上腺皮质激素释放因子（CRF）和尿皮质素是哺乳动物CRF肽家族的成员，具有相似的生化结构，但具有不同的解剖分布、生理功能和药理学特征（Fekete, Zorrilla, 2007; Suda et al. 2004）。

CRF是一种41氨基酸的哺乳动物神经肽，与鱼的同源尿素显示54%的相似性，与青蛙的同源鼠尾草素显示48%的相似性（Vale et al. 1981）。CRF在下丘脑室旁核和杏仁核中央核中合成，从中调节对压力的神经内分泌，自主神经和行为反应（Bale, Lee, Vale, 2002; Bale, Vale, 2004）。神经内分泌反应以下丘脑 - 垂体 - 肾上腺（HPA）轴的激活为代表，并由心室旁CRF介导，与协同的精氨酸加压素（AVP）一起刺激垂体前叶释放促肾上腺皮质激素（ACTH）。随后从肾上腺皮质释放糖皮质激素（Bale et al. 2002; Bale, Vale, 2004）。自主神经反应以交感神经系统（SNS）的激活为代表，并由杏仁核CRF介导，杏仁核CRF刺激蓝斑释放儿茶酚，进而刺激肾上腺髓质释放儿茶酚胺（Bale et al. 2002; Bale, Vale, 2004）。因此，CRF不仅起下丘脑神经激素的作用，还起下丘脑外神经递质的作用，调节对应激的行为反应，表现为运动能力增强，食物和水摄入减少等（Bale et al. 2002; Bale, Vale, 2004）。

尿皮质素 1（Ucn1）是一种40个氨基酸的神经肽，与鱼的硬骨鱼紧张肽有63%的相似性，与人CRF有着45%的相似性，由此衍生出尿皮质素的名字（Vaughan et al. 1995）。Ucn1主要在爱丁格 - 韦斯特法尔核和尾外侧投射到脊髓和外侧中隔的上橄榄上合成（Reul, Holsboer, 2002）。尽管这些大脑区域具有动眼、瞳孔和听觉功能，但与CRF相比，Ucn1更能调节神经内分泌和对压力的行为反应，是一种较弱的运动激活剂和较强的食物和水摄入抑制剂（Skelton, Owens, Nemeroff, 2000）。

CRF和Ucn1的作用由两个不同的G蛋白偶联受体CRF1和CRF2介导（Chang et al. 1993; Lovenberg et al. 1995），并受CRF结合蛋白质（CRF-BP）抑制（Behan, Cepoi et al. 1996; Behan,

DeSouza, et al. 1996）。CRF优先通过CRF1起作用，与CRF1的亲和力比对CRF2的亲和力高15倍，而Ucn1通过两个CRF受体发挥同等作用，与CRF1结合的亲和力是CRF本身的7倍（Reul, Holsboer, 2002）。在中枢神经系统（CNS）中，CRF1大量分布在大脑皮层、小脑、杏仁核和垂体前叶（Valdez et al. 2002）。

尿皮质素2（Ucn2），在人类中也称为顶压素相关肽，是一种38个氨基酸的神经肽，与CRF有34%的同一性（Reyes et al. 2001）。Ucn2的表达出现在室旁核、视上核、下丘脑弓状核、蓝斑核和参与神经内分泌控制、食物摄入、水摄入和自主控制的脑区，但Ucn2的投射尚不清楚。Ucn2被证明具有轻度的运动抑制和延迟抗焦虑样作用（Valdez et al. 2002）。

尿皮质素3（Ucn3），在人类中也称为顶压素，是另一种38个氨基酸的神经肽，与CRF具有36%的同一性（Lewis et al. 2001）。Ucn3的表达发现于下丘脑穹窿周围区、杏仁核内侧核和终纹床核，它们与下丘脑室旁核和外侧隔相邻或向其突出，是参与压力应对的脑区（Reul, Holsboer, 2002）。与Ucn2相比，Ucn3被证明具有更强的急性运动抑制和抗焦虑样作用（Valdez et al. 2003）。

Ucn2和Ucn3的作用仅由CRF2介导，两者对CRF2的亲和力比CRF1高1000倍以上（Reul, Holsboer, 2002）。因此，它们被认为是CRF2的选择性激动剂。CRF2集中位于大脑皮层下区域：外侧隔、下丘脑、杏仁核和海马（Dautzenberg, Hauger, 2002; Van Pett et al. 2000）。

中枢给药CRF和Un1诱导HPA轴的激活，这反映在小鼠和大鼠血浆皮质酮浓度的升高以及焦虑和抑郁样行为（Bagosi et al. 2014; Spina et al. 1996, 2002; Tanaka, Telegdy, 2008）。相比之下，Ucn2和Ucn3的中枢给药在啮齿动物中产生抗焦虑和抗抑郁作用（Inoue et al. 2003; Tanaka, Telegdy, 2008; Valdez et al. 2002, 2003）。据此假设，在生理条件下，慢性肾功能衰竭会启动应激反应，激活垂体前叶的CRF1，而尿皮质素会终止这些反应，激活下丘脑室旁核的CRF 2（Bale et al. 2002; Bale, Vale, 2004）。过度应激可能会导致大脑皮层和杏仁核中的CRF/CRF1系统的病理刺激，而不是侧隔和海马的尿皮质素/CRF2系统的病理刺激，从而导致HPA轴的过度活跃、焦虑和抑郁（Bale et al. 2002; Bale, Vale, 2004）。然而，尿皮质素/CRF2系统在调节HPA轴中的生理作用仍存在争议，因为对小鼠和大鼠的研究导致了矛盾的结果（Bagosi et al. 2013; Jamieson et al. 2006; Maruyama et al. 2007; Pelleymounter et al. 2004）。然而，最近的一个假设质疑了CRF1和CRF2的双重和互补作用，并表明压力会在大脑区域和神经元群体中以特定的方式招募CRF系统（Janssen, Kozicz, 2013）。

除了应激反应的调节外，慢性肾功能衰竭和尿皮质素也与烟碱成瘾有关（Bruijnzeel, Gold, 2005; Sarnyai et al. 2001）。受CRF1和CRF2在中枢神经系统中发挥（主要）拮抗作用的原始假设的启发，我们最近的研究旨在研究通过中枢给药Ucn2和Ucn3激活CRF2是否会减轻小鼠在慢性烟碱治疗和随后的急性戒断期间出现的焦虑和抑郁样状态（Bagosi et al. 2016）。

为此，将72只雄性CFLP小鼠进行腹腔注射烟碱或盐水溶液的处理7d，每天4次，然后停药1d。在最后一次腹腔注射后12h或24h，进行单次侧脑室注射Ucn2、Ucn3或盐水溶液。30min后，分别在高架十字迷宫试验（见"高架十字迷宫试验的关键因素"）和强迫游泳试验（见"强迫游泳试验的关键因素"）中评估小鼠的焦虑和抑郁症状。焦虑和抑郁状态通常与HPA轴的过度活跃有关；因此，5min后，也通过化学荧光测定法测定血浆皮质酮浓度（见"化学荧光测定法的关键事实"）。

一半小鼠在第8天（最后一次腹腔注射后12h）进行实验，另一半小鼠在第9天（最后一次腹腔注射后24h）进行实验（Bagosi et al. 2016）。

在第8天，烟碱处理的小鼠表现出焦虑和抑郁的迹象，血浆皮质酮浓度显著增加（Bagosi et al.2016）。实际上，在高架十字迷宫测试中，与盐水对照组相比，烟碱处理小鼠的张开双臂次数和张开时间显著减少，而总进入次数没有明显变化。用尿皮质素处理这些小鼠后，前两个参数增加或标准化（图27.1）。此外，在强迫游泳测试中，烟碱处理后，小鼠用于攀爬和游泳的时间显著减少，而这些参数在尿皮质素处理后下降得更多，但与盐水处理的小鼠相比，烟碱处理的小鼠一动不动的时间没有显著变化（图27.2）。烟碱戒断12h后的大多数行为变化不显著，并伴有轻微但不显著的血浆皮质酮浓度升高，尿皮质素处理后显著降低（图27.3）。

根据三项观察结果，先前的研究已经表明CRF和CRF样肽可促进烟碱的急性、慢性和戒断作用（Bruijnzeel, Gold, 2005; Sarnyai et al. 2001）。

第一，烟碱的急性给药引起HPA轴的剂量依赖性激活，这反映在人的唾液皮质醇与小鼠和大鼠的血浆皮质酮的积累上，这似乎是由下丘脑CRF启动的（Bruijnzeel, Gold, 2005; Sarnyai et al. 2001）。尽管单次进食后可能会出现这种作用的快速脱敏，以及反复进食后可能出现耐受性下降，但长期服用烟碱常常会导致糖皮质素浓度升高（Bruijnzeel, Gold, 2005; Sarnyai et al. 2001）。

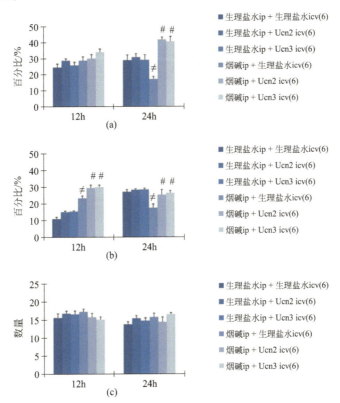

图 27.1　暴露于慢性烟碱治疗和急性烟碱戒断的小鼠中的 Ucn2 和 Ucn3 的作用，并在高架十字迷宫试验中进行研究

（a）进入公开比赛的数量/参赛总数量；（b）在公开比赛中花费的时间/总时间；（c）参赛总数量

值表示为平均值±SEM，$P<0.05$，有显著统计学差异。烟碱ip+生理盐水icv与生理盐水ip+生理盐水icv的差异为≠烟碱ip+Ucn2或Ucn3 icv与烟碱ip+生理盐水icv的差异#。缩略语：icv，脑室内；ip，腹膜内；Ucn2，尿皮质素2；Ucn3，尿皮质素3。

改编自Bagosi等（2016），获Elsevier许可。

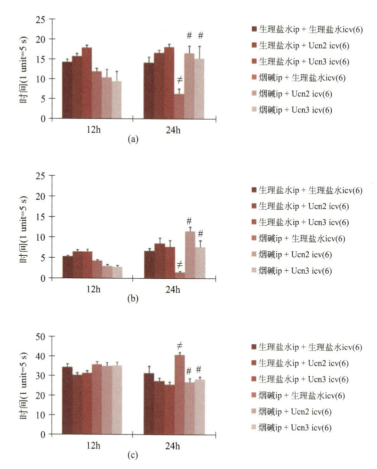

图 27.2 暴露于慢性烟碱治疗和急性烟碱戒断的小鼠中的 Ucn2 和 Ucn3 的作用,并在强迫游泳试验中进行研究

(a)攀爬活动;(b)游泳活动;(c)不动

值表示为平均值±SEM,$P<0.05$,有显著统计学差异。烟碱ip+生理盐水icv 与生理盐水ip+生理盐水icv 的差异为≠,烟碱 ip+Ucn2 或 Ucn3 icv 与烟碱ip+生理盐水icv 的差异为#。缩略语:icv,脑室内;ip,腹膜内;Ucn2,尿皮质素2;Ucn3,尿皮质素3。改编自 Bagosi 等(2016),经 Elsevier 许可。

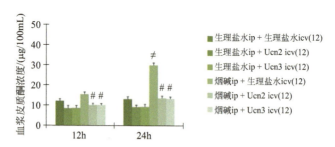

图 27.3 Ucn2 和 Ucn3 对暴露于慢性烟碱治疗和急性烟碱戒断的小鼠通过化学荧光法测定的血浆皮质酮浓度的影响

值表示为平均值±SEM;$P<0.05$,有显著统计学差异。烟碱ip+生理盐水icv 与生理盐水ip+生理盐水ic 的差异为≠,烟碱ip+Ucn2 或 Ucn3 icv 与烟碱ip+生理盐水icv 的差异为≠。缩略语:icv,脑室内;ip,腹膜内;Ucn2,尿皮质素2;Ucn3,尿皮质素3。改编自 Bagosi 等(2016),并得到 Elsevier 的许可。

第二,急性烟碱戒断会在人和啮齿动物中引起一组类似于压力反应的症状,并且似乎由下丘脑 CRF 介导(Bruijnzeel, Gold, 2005; Sarnyai et al. 2001)。这种烟碱戒断综合征由身体和情感两部分组成,在烟碱停用后的几小时内出现,几天或几周内消失(Kenny, Markou, 2001; Markou,

2008; Wonnacott et al. 2005)。人类的身体症状包括心动过缓、胃肠道不适和食欲增加；在啮齿动物中，它们对应于腹部收缩、面部束缚、眨眼、上睑下垂和喘息、尝试逃避、舔脚、生殖器梳理、划痕和打哈欠（Kenny, Markou, 2001; Markou, 2008; Wonnacott et al. 2005）。人类的情感症状包括渴望、焦虑、沮丧、烦躁不安和难以集中注意力。在啮齿动物中，它们与快感缺乏症（对奖励刺激的兴趣或愉悦度降低）和条件厌恶（与环境暗示相关的厌恶动机状态）相关（Kenny, Markou, 2001; Markou, 2008; Wonnacott et al. 2005）。

第三，在长期烟碱戒断过程中暴露于压力下会增加人类吸烟复发和啮齿类动物烟碱自我管理的脆弱性（Bruijnzeel, Gold, 2005; Sarnyai et al. 2001）。急性戒断期间出现的负面情感状态可能在长期戒断期间持续存在，避免这种情绪状态在复发中起着至关重要的作用，从而在维持烟碱成瘾中起着重要作用（Kenny, Markou, 2001; Markou, 2008; Wonnacott et al. 2005）。

此外，最近的研究表明，烟碱戒断综合征的情感和身体成分分别由CRF1和CRF2介导（Bruijnzeel, 2012; Bruijnzeel et al. 2012; Bruijnzeel, Gold, 2005; Bruijnzeel, Prado, Isaac, 2009; Bruijnzeel et al. 2007; George et al. 2007; Kamdi et al. 2009; Marcinkiewcz et al. 2009）。几项研究报道称，选择性CRF1拮抗剂的使用可防止烟碱戒断期间观察到的烦躁不安和奖励不足（Bruijnzeel et al. 2012; Marcinkiewcz et al. 2009）。另一项研究指出，非选择性CRF2激动剂（如CRF和Ucn1）的使用可防止烟碱戒断期间的食欲亢进和体重增加（Kamdi et al. 2009）。但是，我们的研究首次证明脑室内使用Ucn2和Ucn3可以改善在慢性烟碱治疗和随后的急性戒断期间出现的焦虑和抑郁样状态，这表明选择性CRF2激动剂可以成为烟碱治疗的潜在候选药物（Bagosi et al. 2016）。为了更好地了解其生理和药理作用，未来的研究应在特定的大脑区域（例如，下丘脑和室间隔的脑室旁核）注入这些肽，其中CRF2与Ucn2神经元共定位，并且Ucn3的轴突投影神经元（Reul, Holsboer, 2002; Van Pett et al. 2000）。

术语解释

- **急性烟碱戒断**：反复接触烟碱后突然停止；在啮齿类动物中，它可以是自发的，也可以是通过烟碱乙酰胆碱或阿片受体拮抗剂的给药而引起的，可能在烟碱停止后持续2～3h至2～3d。

- **焦虑症**：一种病理状态，其特征在于对各种主题、事件或活动过度担心。在啮齿动物中，可以通过野外探索试验、高架迷宫试验、明暗探索试验、社交互动试验等进行研究。

- **CFLP小鼠**：一种杂种小鼠，通常用于遗传、毒理学和药理研究；CFLP一词来自Carworth Farms和Lane-Petter公司。

- **长期服用烟碱**：反复接触烟碱；在啮齿动物中，可以通过饮水摄入，蒸气吸入，微型渗透泵，静脉、皮下或腹膜内注射可能需要7～270d。

- **促肾上腺皮质激素释放因子（CRF）**：也称为促肾上腺皮质激素释放激素。不仅是一种下丘脑神经激素，还是一种下丘脑外神经递质，介导对压力的神经内分泌、自主神经和行为反应。

- **抑郁症**：一种以情绪低落，对日常活动的乐趣或兴趣减弱为特征的病理状态；在啮齿动物中，可以通过强迫游泳测试、尾部悬吊测试、性欲减退测试、条件性位置偏爱测试等进行研究。

- **下丘脑-垂体-肾上腺（HPA）轴**：一种神经内分泌系统，以下丘脑室旁核中CRF的释放为代表，与协同AVP一起刺激垂体前叶释放ACTH，随后释放糖皮质激素从肾上腺皮质。

- **尿皮质素（Ucn1、Ucn2和Ucn3）**：CRF样神经肽，与CRF相比具有相似的氨基酸结构，但药理特性不同。

| 高架迷宫测试的关键事实 | ■ 高架迷宫测试是一种经过Pellow等（1985）验证的方法，用于研究啮齿动物的焦虑样行为和抗焦虑药的功效。
■ 该设备由一个加高形的木制平台组成，该平台距离地面40cm，由四个30cm×5cm的相对臂组成。相对的两个臂被15cm高的侧壁和端壁包围（封闭的臂），而另两个臂则没有壁（开放的臂）。
■ 将每只鼠标放在迷宫的中央区域（5cm×5cm）中，面对一只张开的手臂，坐在离迷宫中心1m处的观察者评估它们的行为。
■ 在5分钟的时间段内，记录以下参数：（a）进入开放臂的次数与进入总次数的比，（b）处于开放臂的时间与总时间的比值，以及（c）进入的总次数（进入手臂的定义为该动物四只脚全部进入该手臂）。
■ 测试的原理是开放臂更容易引起恐惧，开放臂与闭合臂所花费的时间之比，或进入开放臂或闭合臂的时间之比，反映了闭合臂的相对安全性与开放臂的相对危险性之比。以上几点列出了用于评估啮齿动物焦虑样症状的高架迷宫测试的关键事实。 |
|---|---|
| 强迫游泳试验的关键事实 | ■ 强迫游泳试验是Porsolt等（1977）发明的一种方法，用于研究啮齿动物中的抑郁样行为和药物的抗抑郁特性。
■ 该设备由一个高度为40cm，直径为12cm的有机玻璃圆柱体组成，其中装有1.5L水，温度保持在（25±1）℃，位于桌子上。
■ 将每只老鼠单独丢入水中，并由距桌子1m远的观察者评估其行为。
■ 在5分钟的时间内，记录以下参数，并以时间单位（1个时间单位为5s）表示：（a）攀爬活动（小鼠攀爬时企图逃避圆柱的时间）等，（b）游泳活动（小鼠在水中游泳的时间，试图停留在水面的时间），以及（c）固定性（小鼠前爪一起在水面上直立的时间）。
■ 测试的原理是，在无法逃脱的情况下，动物迅速变得不动，漂浮在直立的位置，只做很小的动作即可使头保持在水面之上。同时，他们试图通过攀爬或游泳逃脱圆柱的尝试最终可能会减少或停止。
■ 以上几点列出了强迫游泳试验的主要事实，该试验用于调查啮齿类动物的抑郁样症状。 |
| 化学荧光测定法的关键事实 | ■ 化学荧光测定法是Zenker和Bernstein（1958）描述的方法，并由Purves和Sirett（1965）进行了修改，用于确定血浆皮质酮浓度。
■ 该测定基于以下原理：可以用二氯甲烷从啮齿动物的血浆中提取疏水性皮质酮，并用硫酸和乙醇的荧光混合物进行测定。
■ 使用的化学物质是肝素、蒸馏水、皮质酮标准品、二氯甲烷、硫酸和乙醇。
■ 使用的设备是Hitachi 204-A荧光分光光度计，设置为激发波长456nm和发射波长515nm。
■ 血浆皮质酮浓度是根据标准值计算得出的，以μg/100mL为单位。
■ 以上几点列出了用于确定血浆皮质酮浓度的化学荧光测定法的关键事实。 |
| 要点总结 | ■ 促肾上腺皮质激素释放因子（CRF）和尿皮质素（Ucn1、Ucn2和Ucn3）属于哺乳动物CRF肽家族。
■ CRF和Ucn1与两个CRF受体（CRF1和CRF2）结合，而Ucn2和Ucn3选择性与CRF2结合。
■ 除了调节应激反应外，CRF和尿皮质素还与烟碱成瘾有关。 |

- Ucn2和Ucn3减轻了在慢性烟碱治疗期间和随后的急性戒断期间出现的焦虑和抑郁样状态。
- 因此，选择性CRF2激动剂可能是烟碱戒断治疗的潜在候选者。

参考文献

Bagosi, Z.; Csabafi, K.; Palotai, M.; Jaszberenyi, M.; Foldesi, I.; Gardi, J. et al. (2013). The interaction of urocortin II and urocortin III with amygdalar and hypothalamic cotricotropin-releasing factor (CRF)-reflections on the regulation of the hypothalamic-pituitary-adrenal (HPA) axis. Neuropeptides, 47(5), 333-338

Bagosi, Z.; Csabafi, K.; Palotai, M.; Jaszberenyi, M.; Foldesi, I.; Gardi, J. et al. (2014). The effect of urocortin I on the hypothalamic ACTH secretagogues and its impact on the hypothalamic-pituitary-adrenal axis. Neuropeptides, 48(1), 15-20.

Bagosi, Z.; Palotai, M.; Simon, B.; Bokor, P.; Buzas, A.; Balango, B. et al. (2016). Selective CRF2 receptor agonists ameliorate the anxiety- and depression-like state developed during chronic nicotine treatment and consequent acute withdrawal in mice. Brain Research, 1652, 21-29.

Bale, T. L.; Lee, K. F.; Vale, W. W. (2002). The role of corticotropin releasing factor receptors in stress and anxiety. Integrative and Comparative Biology, 42(3), 552-555.

Bale, T. L.; Vale, W. W. (2004). CRF and CRF receptors: role in stress responsivity and other behaviors. Annual Review of Pharmacology and Toxicology, 44, 525-557.

Behan, D. P.; Cepoi, D.; Fischer, W. H.; Park, M.; Sutton, S.; Lowry, P. J. et al. (1996). Characterization of a sheep brain corticotropin releasing factor binding protein. Brain Research, 709(2), 265-274.

Behan, D. P.; De Souza, E. B.; Potter, E.; Sawchenko, P.; Lowry, P. J.; Vale, W. W. (1996). Modulatory actions of corticotropin-releasing factor-binding protein. Annals of the New York Academy of Sciences, 780, 81-95.

Bruijnzeel, A. W. (2012). Tobacco addiction and the dysregulation of brain stress systems. Neuroscience and Biobehavioral Reviews, 36(5), 1418-1441.

Bruijnzeel, A. W.; Ford, J.; Rogers, J. A.; Scheick, S.; Ji, Y.; Bishnoi, M. et al. (2012). Blockade of CRF1 receptors in the central nucleus of the amygdala attenuates the dysphoria associated with nicotine withdrawal in rats. Pharmacology, Biochemistry, and Behavior, 101(1), 62-68.

Bruijnzeel, A. W.; Gold, M. S. (2005). The role of corticotropin- releasing factor-like peptides in cannabis, nicotine, and alcohol dependence. Brain Research. Brain Research Reviews, 49(3), 505-528.

Bruijnzeel, A. W.; Prado, M.; Isaac, S. (2009). Corticotropin-releasing factor-1 receptor activation mediates nicotine withdrawal-induced deficit in brain reward function and stress-induced relapse. Biological Psychiatry, 66(2), 110-117.

Bruijnzeel, A. W.; Zislis, G.; Wilson, C.; Gold, M. S. (2007). Antagonism of CRF receptors prevents the deficit in brain reward function associated with precipitated nicotine withdrawal in rats. Neuropsychopharmacology, 32(4), 955-963.

Chang, C. P.; Pearse, R. V.; II, O'Connell, S.; Rosenfeld, M. G. (1993). Identification of a seven transmembrane helix receptor for corticotropin-releasing factor and sauvagine in mammalian brain. Neuron, 11(6), 1187-1195.

Dautzenberg, F. M.; Hauger, R. L. (2002). The CRF peptide family and their receptors: yet more partners discovered. Trends in Pharmacological Sciences, 23(2), 71-77.

Fekete, E. M.; Zorrilla, E. P. (2007). Physiology, pharmacology, and therapeutic relevance of urocortins in mammals: ancient CRF paralogs. Frontiers in Neuroendocrinology, 28(1), 1-27.

George, O.; Ghozland, S.; Azar, M. R.; Cottone, P.; Zorrilla, E. P.; Parsons, L. H. et al. (2007). CRF-CRF1 system activation mediates withdrawal-induced increases in nicotine self-administration in nicotine-dependent rats. Proceedings of the National Academy of Sciences of the United States of America, 104(43), 17198-17203.

Hsu, S. Y.; Hsueh, A. J. (2001). Human stresscopin and stresscopin related peptide are selective ligands for the type 2 corticotropin-releasing hormone receptor. Nature Medicine, 7(5), 605-611.

Inoue, K.; Valdez, G. R.; Reyes, T. M.; Reinhardt, L. E.; Tabarin, A.; Rivier, J. et al. (2003). Human urocortin II, a selective agonist for the type 2 corticotropin-releasing factor receptor, decreases feeding and drinking in the rat. The Journal of Pharmacology and ExperimentalTherapeutics, 305(1), 385-393.

Jamieson, P. M.; Li, C.; Kukura, C.; Vaughan, J.; Vale, W. (2006). Urocortin 3 modulates the neuroendocrine stress response and is regulated in rat amygdala and hypothalamus by stress and glucocorticoids. Endocrinology, 147(10), 4578-4588.

Janssen, D.; Kozicz, T. (2013). Is it really a matter of simple dualism? Corticotropin-releasing factor receptors in body and mental health. Front Endocrinol (Lausanne), 4, 28.

Kamdi, S. P.; Nakhate, K. T.; Dandekar, M. P.; Kokare, D. M.; Subhedar, N. K. (2009). Participation of corticotropin-releasing factor type 2 receptors in the acute, chronic and withdrawal actions of nicotine associated with feeding behavior in rats. Appetite, 53(3), 354-362.

Kenny, P. J.; Markou, A. (2001). Neurobiology of the nicotine withdrawal syndrome. Pharmacology, Biochemistry, and Behavior, 70(4), 531-549.

Lewis, K.; Li, C.; Perrin, M. H.; Blount, A.; Kunitake, K.; Donaldson, C. et al. (2001). Identification of urocortin III, an additional member of the corticotropin-releasing factor (CRF) family with high affinity for the CRF2 receptor. Proceedings of the National Academy of Sciences of the United States of America, 98(13), 7570-7575.

Lovenberg, T. W.; Liaw, C. W.; Grigoriadis, D. E.; Clevenger, W.; Chalmers, D. T.; De Souza, E. B. et al. (1995). Cloning and characterization of a functionally distinct corticotropin-releasing factor receptor subtype from rat brain. Proceedings of the National Academy of Sciences of the United

States of America, 92(3), 836-840.

Marcinkiewcz, C. A.; Prado, M. M.; Isaac, S. K.; Marshall, A.; Rylkova, D.; Bruijnzeel, A. W. (2009). Corticotropin-releasing factor within the central nucleus of the amygdala and the nucleus accumbens shell mediates the negative affective state of nicotine withdrawal in rats. Neuropsychopharmacology, 34(7), 1743-1752.

Markou, A. (2008). Review. Neurobiology of nicotine dependence. Philosophical Transactions of the Royal Society of London. Series B, Biological Sciences, 363(1507), 3159-3168.

Maruyama, H.; Makino, S.; Noguchi, T.; Nishioka, T.; Hashimoto, K. (2007). Central type 2 corticotropin-releasing hormone receptor mediates hypothalamic-pituitary-adrenocortical axis activation in the rat. Neuroendocrinology, 86(1), 1-16.

Pelleymounter, M. A.; Joppa, M.; Ling, N.; Foster, A. C. (2004). Behavioral and neuroendocrine effects of the selective CRF2 receptor agonists urocortin II and urocortin III. Peptides, 25(4), 659-666.

Pellow, S.; Chopin, P.; File, S. E.; Briley, M. (1985). Validation of open:closed arm entries in an elevated plus-maze as a measure of anxiety in the rat. Journal of Neuroscience Methods, 14(3), 149-167.

Porsolt, R. D.; Bertin, A.; Jalfre, M. (1977). Behavioral despair in mice: a primary screening test for antidepressants. Archives Internationales de Pharmacodynamie et de Thérapie, 229(2), 327-336.

Purves, H. D.; Sirett, N. E. (1965). Assay of corticotrophin in dexamethasone-treated rats. Endocrinology, 77(2), 366-374.

Reul, J. M.; Holsboer, F. (2002). Corticotropin-releasing factor receptors 1 and 2 in anxiety and depression. Current Opinion in Pharmacology, 2(1), 23-33.

Reyes, T. M.; Lewis, K.; Perrin, M. H.; Kunitake, K. S.; Vaughan, J.; Arias, C. A. et al. (2001). Urocortin II: a member of the corticotropin-releasing factor (CRF) neuropeptide family that isselectively bound by type 2 CRF receptors. Proceedings of the National Academy of Sciences of the United States of America, 98(5), 2843-2848.

Sarnyai, Z.; Shaham, Y.; Heinrichs, S. C. (2001). The role of corticotropin-releasing factor in drug addiction. Pharmacological Reviews, 53(2), 209-243.

Skelton, K. H.; Owens, M. J.; Nemeroff, C. B. (2000). The neurobiology of urocortin. Regulatory Peptides, 93(1-3), 85-92.

Spina, M. G.; Merlo-Pich, E.; Akwa, Y.; Balducci, C.; Basso, A. M.; Zorrilla, E. P. et al. (2002). Time-dependent induction of anxiogenic-like effects after central infusion of urocortin or corticotropin-releasing factor in the rat. Psychopharmacology, 160(2), 113-121.

Spina, M.; Merlo-Pich, E.; Chan, R. K.; Basso, A. M.; Rivier, J.; Vale, W. et al. (1996). Appetite-suppressing effects of urocortin, a CRF-related neuropeptide. Science, 273(5281), 1561-1564.

Suda, T.; Kageyama, K.; Sakihara, S.; Nigawara, T. (2004). Physiological roles of urocortins, human homologues of fish urotensin I, and their receptors. Peptides, 25(10), 1689-1701.

Tanaka, M.; Telegdy, G. (2008). Antidepressant-like effects of the CRF family peptides, urocortin 1, urocortin 2 and urocortin 3 in a modified forced swimming test in mice. Brain Research Bulletin, 75(5), 509-512.

Valdez, G. R.; Inoue, K.; Koob, G. F.; Rivier, J.; Vale, W.; Zorrilla, E. P. (2002). Human urocortin II: mild locomotor suppressive and delayed anxiolytic-like effects of a novel corticotropin-releasing factor related peptide. Brain Research, 943(1), 142-150.

Valdez, G. R.; Zorrilla, E. P.; Rivier, J.; Vale, W. W.; Koob, G. F. (2003). Locomotor suppressive and anxiolytic-like effects of urocortin 3, a highly selective type 2 corticotropin-releasing factor agonist. Brain Research, 980(2), 206-212.

Vale, W.; Spiess, J.; Rivier, C.; Rivier, J. (1981). Characterization of a 41-residue ovine hypothalamic peptide that stimulates secretion of corticotropin and beta-endorphin. Science, 213(4514), 1394-1397.

Van Pett, K.; Viau, V.; Bittencourt, J. C.; Chan, R. K.; Li, H. Y.; Arias, C. et al. (2000). Distribution of mRNAs encoding CRF receptors in brain and pituitary of rat and mouse. The Journal of Comparative Neurology, 428(2), 191-212.

Vaughan, J.; Donaldson, C.; Bittencourt, J.; Perrin, M. H.; Lewis, K.; Sutton, S. et al. (1995). Urocortin, a mammalian neuropeptide related to fish urotensin I and to corticotropin-releasing factor. Nature, 378(6554), 287-292.

Wonnacott, S.; Sidhpura, N.; Balfour, D. J. (2005). Nicotine: from molecular mechanisms to behaviour. Current Opinion in Pharmacology, 5(1), 53-59.

Zenker, N.; Bernstein, D. E. (1958). The estimation of small amounts ofcorticosterone in rat plasma. The Journal of Biological Chemistry, 231 (2), 695-70.

28
精神错乱和烟碱戒断

Kataria Dinesh, Goel Ankit, Tiwari Sucheta, Kukreti Prerna

Department of Psychiatry, Lady Hardinge Medical College, New Delhi, India

缩略语

CRF	促肾上腺皮质激素释放因子	**ICU**	重症监护病房
DSM-5	《精神疾病诊断和统计手册》(第5版)	**NMDA**	N-甲基-D-天冬氨酸
EEG	脑电图	**NRT**	烟碱替代疗法
GABA	γ-氨基丁酸	**REM**	快速眼动
HPA轴	下丘脑-垂体-肾上腺轴		

28.1 引言

烟草使用失调构成了世界范围内的主要健康危害。吸烟是世界上最常见的成瘾行为,烟碱是烟草的主要成分,导致依赖性的发展(Benowitz, 2009; Hatsukami, Stead, Gupta, 2008)。停止吸烟可能会引起令人不快的烟碱戒断综合征。烟碱戒断的症状包括沮丧、易怒、愤怒、焦虑、情绪低落、失眠和躁动不安。这些症状在戒烟的7天内达到顶峰,可能持续约2~4周(Awissi et al. 2013)。

精神错乱是一种临床综合征,其特征是注意力和认知发生急性改变(美国精神病学协会,2013;世界卫生组织,1992)。精神错乱的临床表现是多变的,其核心症状包括时间、地点或人的定向障碍、工作记忆障碍;精神运动障碍;以及睡眠觉醒周期受到干扰(WHO, 1992)。它常见于重症患者,据报道发病率为15%~80% (Ely et al. 2004; Jacobi et al. 2002)。根据唤醒和精神运动行为,精神错乱可分为三种亚型。多动症的精神错乱的特点是躁动、定向障碍和幻觉,而多动性精神错乱以嗜睡、镇静和混乱为主。第三个子类型是具有组合特征的混合类型(Lipowski, 1983)。

戒断某些精神活性物质导致的精神错乱是众所周知的现象(WHO, 1992)。然而,仅在最近十年中,才开始出现烟碱戒断导致精神错乱的证据(Brody, 2006; Kukreti, Garg, Gautam, 2015)。药物戒断精神错乱会引起不良后果,包括发病率增加、死亡率增加、住院时间延长和经济负担增加(Dubos et al. 1996; Inouye et al. 1998)。

28.2 烟碱作为精神错乱的危险因素:理论上的概念

DSM-5已将精神错乱描述为注意力、意识和认知障碍,包括记忆力减退(American Psychiatric Association, 2013)。烟碱戒断性精神错乱的特征是精神错乱、躁动、精神运动活动增加和易怒,类似于多动性精神错乱的特征(Park, Kim, Yoon, 2016)。很少有作者报道烟碱戒断期间注意力不集中和工作记忆障碍(Brody, 2006; Heishman, 1998)。

与烟草使用有关的功能性脑成像显示，烟碱可通过前额叶和上肢边缘的皮质-基底神经节丘回路增强神经传递（Brody，2006）。事实证明，这可以提高任务唤醒和维持注意力的性能。

烟碱戒断的总持续时间似乎在2～4周之间，峰值在2周以下（Hughes，2007）。愤怒/刺激在第一周达到高峰，可能持续长达4周。戒断的前3天精神错乱状增加，总持续时间为2周。烟碱戒断开始后的前几天，在烟碱戒断中出现精神错乱特征，尤其是活动过度的精神错乱，并可能持续长达2～4周（Papaioannou et al. 2005; Vandrey et al. 2008）。

有证据表明，烟碱对吸烟者和不吸烟者记忆力和注意力的影响可能会有所不同。难以集中注意力在2～3天达到高峰，持续3～4周。烟碱给药后，吸烟者和不吸烟者的认知记忆均得到改善，但注意力的改善仅在戒烟者中显著（Heishman 1998）。这种神经元适应也可能导致戒断状态下的注意力缺陷。

精神错乱和烟碱戒断均以睡眠障碍为特征。在精神错乱中，失眠是严重的，睡眠-觉醒周期有时会逆转，晚上症状会加重。尽管烟碱戒断中的睡眠障碍不那么严重，但烟碱戒断中睡眠的碎片化增加（Hughes，2007）。这可能导致REM睡眠频率增加，并增加对梦的记忆，表明这两种情况下可能存在影响睡眠障碍的共同神经系统因素。在清醒状态下，生动的、令人不安的梦可能会以幻觉的形式持续存在（American Psychiatric Association, 2013; Webster, Holroyd, 2000）。因此，从现象学上看，精神错乱和烟碱戒断几乎没有这两种状态的共同特征（表28.1）。

表28.1 烟碱戒断和精神错乱的共同特征

・躁动	・不安
・烦躁	・注意障碍
・混乱	・睡眠障碍

28.3 烟碱戒断和精神错乱之间的神经生物学联系

下面讨论了可以介导烟碱戒断性精神错乱的各种神经生物学机制（图28.1和表28.2）。

28.3.1 胆碱能系统失调

乙酰胆碱介导皮层唤醒、注意过程、学习、记忆、REM睡眠诱导、行为运动成分、情绪思维、知觉和方向。因此，撤除胆碱能刺激会导致注意力和记忆力被干扰、过度活跃和脑电节律的减慢，这也是精神错乱的经典表现（Trzepacz，2000）。乙酰胆碱缺乏状态容易患上精神错乱（Hshieh et al. 2008）。

烟碱通过与nAChR复合物结合而产生其中枢和外周作用。整个中脑边缘途径［包括腹侧被盖区（VTA）、前额叶皮层、杏仁核、中隔区和伏隔核］存在各种nAChR α和β亚基组合，尤其是α4β2亚型。这些受体是潜在的结合位点，烟碱可通过这些结合位点激活这些结构中的神经元，以刺激几种神经递质的释放（Marks et al. 1992; Picciotto et al. 2000; Sargent, 1993）。动物研究表明，中枢和外周胆碱能神经系统在调节烟碱戒断症状中均起着作用（Malin et al. 1997）。烟碱的突然戒断导致丘脑皮质通路的胆碱能输入减少，从而影响注意力、机敏性和警惕性（Dani, Heinemann, 1996）。戒断引起的这种低胆碱能状态可能与精神错乱的发展有关。

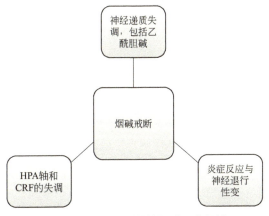

图 28.1 烟碱戒断精神错乱的可能机制

表 28.2 各种神经递质在烟碱戒断精神错乱中的作用

神经递质	在烟碱戒断精神错乱中的作用
乙酰胆碱（抑制）	记忆和注意力受到干扰，过度活跃，脑电图节律减慢
多巴胺（释放/脱敏）	神经过度兴奋
GABA（释放/脱敏）	由于神经元兴奋抑制脱敏，GABA 功能正常
谷氨酸（释放/脱敏）	惊吓反应，神经元兴奋，焦虑的急性症状
5-羟色胺（抑制）	休克反应，低活性焦虑

28.3.2 其他神经递质的失调

烟碱还通过在最初的 nAChR 刺激后释放的多种其他神经递质（包括多巴胺、谷氨酸和 5-羟色胺）介导其作用（Watkins, Koob, Markou, 2000）。烟碱对注意力的影响可通过直接刺激烟碱乙酰胆碱受体或通过增加基底神经节中的多巴胺和抑制单胺氧化酶来实现（Vandrey et al. 2008）。慢性烟碱暴露会导致杏仁核和伏核中胞外多巴胺水平下降，突然戒断与 GABA 能神经元脱敏有关（Fung et al. 1996; Hildebrand et al. 1997）。因此，在戒断状态下对多巴胺释放的抑制作用丧失在临床上可表现为过度活跃的精神错乱（Zhu, Chiappinelli, 1999）。一部分谷氨酸能受体会增强听觉惊吓反应，这是与烟碱戒断有关的对环境刺激反应性的量度（Wiley, 1998）。烟碱给药激活突触位于谷氨酸能末端上的 nAChR，并导致诱发的谷氨酸释放增加（Gray et al. 1996）。反过来，谷氨酸通过 NMDA 受体的兴奋作用，增加了腹侧被盖多巴胺能神经元的突发性放电，导致伏隔核中多巴胺的释放。这会导致严重的精神错乱。可以看出，通过使用 NMDA 受体拮抗剂可以逆转这些作用（Shoaib et al. 1994; Watkins et al. 2000）。如何将其与烟碱戒断联系起来尚待阐明，但谷氨酰胺受体的脱敏可能是造成这种情况的原因。

28.3.3 中脑血清素能功能的下降

烟碱刺激位于正中沟核中体树突区域的 nAChR，并且前脑的终末区域促进 5-羟色胺的释放。有人提出，烟碱戒断期间惊吓反应的增加是由于突触血清素的可用性降低，这对惊吓反应有抑制作用（Geyer et al. 1980）。在烟碱戒断状态下，缺乏烟碱与突触后5-HT1A血清素能受体上调共同导致血清素能系统功能低下，可以推测其会导致机能减退的精神错乱状态（Hughes et al. 1991）。

28.3.4 下丘脑（HPA）和促肾上腺皮质激素释放因子失调

烟碱的给药抑制了促肾上腺皮质激素释放因子（CRF）的功能，而戒断状态与功能升高有关（George et al. 2007; Watkins et al. 2000），从而解释了烟碱的免疫抑制作用。CRF是已知的具有促炎作用（Agelaki et al. 2002）。精神错乱和痴呆患者的炎症标志物均升高，表明它们位于同一连续体的两端，可能是离散实体（Simone,Tan,2011）。

因此，急性烟碱戒断也可能与由于CRF激活引起的循环皮质酮增加有关，这反过来可能影响HPA轴，以与其他主要药物滥用如乙醇和大麻素戒断状态相同的方式促进精神错乱的发展（Epping-Jordan et al. 1998）。

28.3.5 神经元炎症和精神错乱易感性增加

精神错乱的发展甚至与很小的神经元损伤有关，van Gool等（2010）认为，长期使用烟碱与炎症细胞因子导致的基底神经节胆碱能神经元的神经退行性变有关。另一篇综述提出，烟碱可能具有抗炎作用，可能是通过CRF抑制作用介导的，如前所述（George et al. 2007; Piao et al. 2009; Watkins et al. 2000）。这是为什么吸烟似乎可以预防神经退行性疾病（例如阿尔茨海默氏病）的推定原因。因此，炎症标志物的失调也可能导致精神错乱（表28.3）。

表28.3 炎症标志物在烟碱戒断精神错乱中的作用

CRF作用和介质	在烟碱戒断精神错乱中的作用
烟碱戒断期间CRF水平增加	促进促炎状态导致焦虑 循环皮质酮增加
炎性细胞因子	基底神经节胆碱能神经元的神经变性

28.4 临床证据

已经发表了ICU场所烟碱戒断精神错乱的病例报告，其他合并症未对此进行解释（Kukreti et al. 2015; Mayer et al. 2001），并在给予烟碱替代后完全解决。尽管报告的病例还有其他重大的医学和精神病合并症，但他们对常规干预措施没有反应，而精神错乱对烟碱替代的反应表明，烟碱可能在这些特定患者亚组的精神错乱发展中发挥作用。一项对ICU患者发生精神错乱的危险因素进行的前瞻性研究发现，重度吸烟史（每天超过10支卷烟）和以往任何水平的吸烟史都是发生精神错乱的重要危险因素，与其他风险因素无关（Van Rompaey et al. 2009）。一项回顾性病例对照研究比较了在ICU环境中吸烟者与戒烟者之间的关系，发现突然停止烟碱摄入者中发生精神错乱的概率明显更高（Park et al. 2016）。另一项研究发现与烟碱戒断有关的躁动在统计学上显著增加，但精神错乱没有统计学意义的增加（Lucidarme et al. 2010）。

根据这些临床经验，对于在ICU设置中接受烟碱依赖的患者，建议使用客观量表评估烟碱戒断。尽管个别研究表明烟碱戒断和精神错乱可能存在普遍联系，但一项全面的系统综述报告了不确定的结果（Hsieh et al. 2013）。这篇综述推荐了对未来的研究，这些研究应统一定义暴露和结果变量，具有更大的样本量和方法上的严谨性，以建立结论性联系。此外，大多数研究都将吸烟作为烟碱暴露的唯一形式，但对无烟烟草没有评论（表28.4）。

表28.4 烟碱戒断精神错乱的临床证据

参考文献	研究类型	在烟碱戒断精神错乱中的作用
Van Rompaey et al. (2009)	系统综述	每天吸烟10支与ICU患者精神错乱的发生显著相关
Park et al. (2016)	双盲病例对照研究	发现在ICU环境中突然停止烟碱摄入的患者患上多动性精神错乱的概率显著增加
Lucidarme et al. (2010)	部分交叉显著性研究	研究发现，危重病患者烟碱戒断与躁动有统计学意义的增加，但与精神错乱无关
Kukreti et al. (2015)	病例报告	如果及时诊断，烟碱戒断可能是精神错乱的可治疗原因
Mayer et al. (2001)	病例报告	烟碱戒断可能是急性脑损伤患者精神错乱的一个未被充分认识的原因
Hsieh et al. (2013)	系统综述	将烟碱戒断与精神错乱联系起来的证据尚不确定

28.5 精神错乱中的烟碱替代疗法

个别病例报告提到了在出现精神错乱的慢性吸烟者中使用烟碱替代疗法的有希望的结果，但临床试验表明结果不一（表28.5）。

在对六项研究（Kowalski et al. 2016）的综述中，有一项研究未发现与使用NRT相关的结果有任何差异。其中三项研究实际上发现，使用NRT会增加躁动和精神错乱，另外两项发现烟碱戒断症状有所减轻。但是，该综述中仅一项研究是随机双盲病例对照研究（Pathak et al. 2013）。

该研究报道了接受NRT的ICU患者使用呼吸机的天数减少，但结果无统计学意义。同样，另一项研究报道了住院的吸烟者在戒烟后2～10天内出现躁动性精神错乱。使用NRT后，这种问题要么完全解决，要么显示出明显的改善（Mayer et al. 2001）。

与上述发现相反，一项回顾性病例对照研究对90例病例（在接受ICU入院的最初24小时内接受NRT的吸烟者）和90例对照例（未接受NRT的吸烟者）进行了总结，得出结论：NRT与医院死亡率增加相关。这是一个值得注意的发现，但由于是在单一中心进行的回顾性研究，很难建立任何确凿的证据（Lee, Afessa, 2007）。

另一项研究引起了人们对使用NRT的担忧，因为据报道，接受NRT的接受心脏手术的患者死亡率显著增加（Paciullo et al. 2009）。但是，由于它仅包括心脏病患者，因此烟碱的有害心血管作用可能有助于这些发现。因此，在将NRT视为治疗精神错乱的合法方法之前，必须严格研究导致NRT症状改善和恶化的因素。

注意研究使用的是NRT的异构模式。结果好坏参半；但是，有必要考虑的是，在ICU环境中，透烟碱贴剂似乎是最可行和最有效的模式或NRT，特别是在这类患者感觉改变和警觉性降低的背景下。其次，还应考虑其他现有的合并疾病，例如，使用烟碱会使整体医学状况恶化的心血管疾病。NRT在重度吸烟者的精神错乱管理中的作用很有趣，但目前尚无研究领域。NRT在重度吸烟者的精神错乱管理中很有作用，但临床研究值得谨慎考虑，烟碱戒断可能是重度吸烟者发生精神错乱的可能病因。

表28.5 在精神错乱中使用烟碱替代疗法的临床证据

参考文献	研究类型	在烟碱戒断精神错乱中的作用
Kowalski et al.（2016）	系统综述	NRT在ICU精神错乱管理中的非结论性证据
Pathak et al.（2013）	双盲病例对照研究	需要NRT的患者使用呼吸机的天数和ICU住院天数减少（但结果无统计学意义）
Mayer et al.（2001）	病例报告	使用NRT后，脑损伤患者的烟碱戒断性精神错乱症状完全缓解或明显改善
Lee, Afessa（2007）	回顾性病例对照研究	NRT与医院死亡率增加相关
Paciullo et al.（2009）	回顾性配对队列试验研究	接受NRT的心脏手术患者死亡率显著增加

28.6 结论

烟碱成瘾是一种正在迅速发展的流行病，危害人类健康。它通常与严重的合并精神病和医疗疾病有关。临床医生在诊断和管理烟碱依赖及相关健康危害方面极为敏感，但对烟碱戒断评估和治疗仍缺乏敏感性。

烟碱戒断精神错乱的理论基础确实存在；然而，临床研究仍然存在方法上的局限性，无法建立结论性的联系。但是，越来越多的证据表明，烟碱戒断可以有多种表现形式，从轻微的易怒和焦虑到精神错乱的严重表现，特别是在患有医学疾病的重度吸烟者中。

烟碱戒断常常没有引起注意，烟碱戒断与精神错乱在日常护理中不存在差异。因此，有必要提高所有卫生专业人员对烟碱使用和戒断的积极筛查的敏感性。特别是在有大量烟碱使用史的危重患者中，应始终牢记烟碱戒断可能会引起躁动和精神错乱。

需要进一步的研究来阐明烟碱戒断性精神错乱的最终神经生物学基础，并为在这种情况下使用NRT制定系统指南。

术语解释

- 精神错乱：一种精神状态改变的急性综合征，其特征是注意力、定向和其他高级心理功能的快速起伏波动。根据精神运动的活动，可能是（a）活动性moto精神错乱：表现为精神活动活跃，表现为躁动和焦虑，还可能出现妄想和幻觉的"阳性症状"，以及（b）活动性表现为嗜睡、运动缓慢和反应迟缓，表现为精神运动活动减少。依赖性慢性经常复发和缓解的疾病，其特征是尽管有不利后果，但仍反复沉迷于某种行为。神经递质的失调由于异常合成，释放，再摄取或受体活性，突触间隙中神经递质的上调或下调。
- 下丘脑-垂体-肾上腺轴：下丘脑，垂体和肾上腺之间的神经内分泌轴，介导人体对压力的反应，包括物质戒断状态的压力。
- 神经适应过程：通过进行必要的改变以使其能够正常运行，人体适应体内化学物质的存在。
- 神经变性：神经元发生生理或结构损伤的过程。
- 神经递质：神经系统内的化学物质，有助于传导神经冲动。由于突触前神经元所携带的电脉冲的作用，这些物质在突触内释放（神经元之间或神经元与另一种结构之间的空间），并作用于特定的突触后受体，从而成功地将冲动从一个神经元传递到另一个神经元。

- 烟碱替代疗法：涉及通过多种途径以无烟形式输送烟碱的医学治疗。可提供贴剂、口香糖、锭剂和鼻内喷雾剂。
- 奖赏环路：将大脑腹侧被盖区与腹侧纹状体连接起来的大脑中的多巴胺能途径。也称为中脑边缘途径。负责由食物、水、性和精神活性物质等介导的愉悦、动机和欲望。
- 戒断：当某人对某种物质有依赖性的物质的摄入量减少或停止时，就会出现一系列症状。

- 烟碱戒断包括沮丧、烦躁、焦虑、情绪低落、失眠和躁动。
- 这些症状在戒烟的7天内达到高峰，可能持续2～4周。
- 尤其是在ICU中，突然停止烟碱摄入也可能导致精神错乱，尤其是活动过度的精神错乱。
- 在这类患者中用烟碱替代可能被证明对治疗精神错乱有用。

- 本章重点介绍烟碱戒断引起的精神错乱。
- 在病例对照研究和病例报告方面存在临床证据，支持烟碱戒断与精神错乱相关联的观点。
- 在精神错乱中使用烟碱替代疗法（NRT）显示出好坏参半。
- 我们认为，对于精神错乱患者，应始终评估烟碱的使用，将其作为可能的病因。
- 因此，我们强烈建议将来进行更多研究，以更好地了解烟碱戒断与精神错乱之间的联系。

参考文献

Agelaki, S.; Tsatsanis, C.; Gravanis, A.; Margioris, A. N. (2002). Corticotropin-releasing hormone augments proinflammatory cytokine production from macrophages in vitro and in lipopolysaccharide-induced endotoxin shock in mice. Infection and Immunity, 70(11), 6068-6074.

American Psychiatric Association & DSM-5 Task Force (2013). Diagnostic and statistical manual of mental disorders: DSM-5. Washington, DC: American Psychiatric Association.

Awissi, D. -K.; Lebrun, G.; Fagnan, M.; Skrobik, Y.; Regroupement deSoins Critiques, Réseau de Soins Respiratoires, Québec (2013). Alcohol, nicotine, and iatrogenic withdrawals in the ICU. Critical Care Medicine, 41(9 Suppl. 1), S57-S68.

Benowitz, N. L. (2009). Pharmacology of nicotine: addiction, smoking-induced disease, and therapeutics. Annual Review of Pharmacology and Toxicology, 49, 57-71.

Brody, A. L. (2006). Functional brain imaging of tobacco use and dependence. Journal of Psychiatric Research, 40(5), 404-418.

Dani, J. A. & Heinemann, S. (1996). Molecular and cellular aspects of nicotine abuse. Neuron, 16(5), 905-908.

Dubos, G.; Gonthier, R.; Simeone, I.; Camus, V.; Schwed, P.; Cadec, B. et al. (1996). Confusion syndromes in hospitalized aged patients: polymorphism of symptoms and course. Prospective study of 183 patients. La Revue De Medecine Interne, 17(12), 979-986.

Ely, E. W.; Shintani, A.; Truman, B.; Speroff, T.; Gordon, S. M.; Harrell, F. E.; Jr. et al. (2004). Delirium as a predictor of mortality in mechanically ventilated patients in the intensive care unit. JAMA, 291(14), 1753-1762.

Epping-Jordan, M. P.; Watkins, S. S.; Koob, G. F.; Markou, A. (1998). Dramatic decreases in brain reward function during nicotine withdrawal. Nature, 393(6680), 76-79.

Fung, Y. K.; Schmid, M. J.; Anderson, T. M.; Lau, Y. -S. (1996). Effects of nicotine withdrawal on central dopaminergic systems. Pharmacology Biochemistry and Behavior, 53(3), 635-640.

George, O.; Ghozland, S.; Azar, M. R.; Cottone, P.; Zorrilla, E. P.; Parsons, L. H. et al. (2007). CRF-CRF1 system activation mediates withdrawal-induced increases in nicotine self-administration in nicotine-dependent rats. Proceedings of the National Academy of 226 28. Delirium and Nicotine withdrawal Sciences of the United States of America, 104(43), 17198-17203.

Geyer, M. A.; Petersen, L. R.; Rose, G. J. (1980). Effects of serotonergiclesions on investigatory responding by rats in a holeboard. Behavioraland Neural Biology, 30(2), 160-177.

Gray, R.; Rajan, A. S.; Radcliffe, K. A.; Yakehiro, M.; Dani, J. A. (1996). Hippocampal synaptic transmission enhanced by low concentrations of nicotine. Nature, 383(6602), 713-716.

Hatsukami, D. K.; Stead, L. F.; Gupta, P. C. (2008). Tobacco addiction. Lancet (London, England), 371(9629), 2027-2038.

Heishman, S. J. (1998). What aspects of human performance aretruly enhanced by nicotine? Addiction (Abingdon, England), 93(3), 317-320.

Hildebrand, B. E.; Nomikos, G. G.; Bondjers, C.; Nisell, M.; Svensson, T. H. (1997). Behavioral manifestations of the nicotineabstinence syndrome in the rat: peripheral versus central mechanisms. Psychopharmacology, 129(4), 348-356.

Hshieh, T. T.; Fong, T. G.; Marcantonio, E. R.; Inouye, S. K. (2008). Cholinergic deficiency hypothesis in delirium: a synthesis of currentevidence. The Journals of Gerontology Series A, Biological Sciences andMedical Sciences, 63(7), 764-772.

Hsieh, S. J.; Shum, M.; Lee, A. N.; Hasselmark, F.; Gong, M. N. (2013). Cigarette smoking as a risk factor for delirium in hospitalized andintensive care unit patients. A systematic review. Annals of theAmerican Thoracic Society, 10(5), 496-503.

Hughes, J. R. (2007). Effects of abstinence from tobacco: etiology, animalmodels, epidemiology, and significance: a subjective review. Nicotine, Tobacco Research, 9(3), 329-339.

Hughes, J. R.; Gust, S. W.; Skoog, K.; Keenan, R. M.; Fenwick, J. W. (1991). Symptoms of tobacco withdrawal. A replication andextension. Archives of General Psychiatry, 48(1), 52-59.

Inouye, S. K.; Rushing, J. T.; Foreman, M. D.; Palmer, R. M.; Pompei, P. (1998). Does delirium contribute to poor hospital out-comes? A three-site epidemiologic study. Journal of General InternalMedicine, 13(4), 234-242.

Jacobi, J.; Fraser, G. L.; Coursin, D. B.; Riker, R. R.; Fontaine, D.; Wittbrodt, E. T. et al. (2002). Clinical practice guidelines for thesustained use of sedatives and analgesics in the critically ill adult. Critical Care Medicine, 30(1), 119-141.

Kowalski, M.; Udy, A. A.; McRobbie, H. J.; Dooley, M. J. (2016). Nicotine replacement therapy for agitation and delirium manage-ment in the intensive care unit: a systematic review of the literature. Journal of Intensive Care, 4, 69.

Kukreti, P.; Garg, A.; Gautam, P. (2015). Delirium: nicotine withdrawal as a rare etiology. Delhi Psychiatry Journal, 18(1), 210-211.

Lee, A. H.; Afessa, B. (2007). The association of nicotinereplacement therapy with mortality in a medical intensive care unit. Critical Care Medicine, 35(6), 1517-1521.

Lipowski, Z. J. (1983). Transient cognitive disorders (delirium, acuteconfusional states) in the elderly. In Psychosomatic medicine and liaisonpsychiatry (pp. 289-306). Boston, MA: Springer.

Lucidarme, O.; Seguin, A.; Daubin, C.; Ramakers, M.; Terzi, N.; Beck, P. et al. (2010). Nicotine withdrawal and agitation in ventilated critically ill patients. Critical Care, 14(2), R58.

Malin, D. H.; Lake, J. R.; Schopen, C. K.; Kirk, J. W.; Sailer, E. E.; Lawless, B. A. et al. (1997). Nicotine abstinence syndrome precipitated by central but not peripheral hexamethonium. PharmacologyBiochemistry and Behavior, 58(3), 695-699.

Marks, M. J.; Pauly, J. R.; Gross, S. D.; Deneris, E. S.; Hermans-Borgmeyer, I.; Heinemann, S. F. et al. (1992). Nicotine bindingand nicotinic receptor subunit RNA after chronic nicotine treatment. The Journal of Neuroscience, 12(7), 2765-2784.

Mayer, S. A.; Chong, J. Y.; Ridgway, E.; Min, K. C.; Commichau, C.; Bernardini, G. L. (2001). Delirium from nicotine withdrawal inneuro-ICU patients. Neurology, 57(3), 551-553.

Paciullo, C. A.; Short, M. R.; Steinke, D. T.; Jennings, H. R. (2009). Impact of nicotine replacement therapy on postoperative mortalityfollowing coronary artery bypass graft surgery. The Annals ofPharmacotherapy, 43(7), 1197-1202.

Papaioannou, A.; Fraidakis, O.; Michaloudis, D.; Balalis, C.; Askitopoulou, H. (2005). The impact of the type of anaesthesia oncognitive status and delirium during the first postoperativedays in elderly patients. European Journal of Anaesthesiology, 22(7), 492-499.

Park, H.; Kim, K. W.; Yoon, I. -Y. (2016). Smoking cessation and therisk of hyperactive delirium in hospitalized patients: a retrospectivestudy. Canadian Journal of Psychiatry Revue Canadienne de Psychiatrie, 61(10), 643-651.

Pathak, V.; Rendon, I. S. H.; Lupu, R.; Tactuk, N.; Olutade, T.; Durham, C. et al. (2013). Outcome of nicotine replacement therapyin patients admitted to ICU: a randomized controlled double-blindprospective pilot study. Respiratory Care, 58(10), 1625-1629.

Piao, W. -H.; Campagnolo, D.; Dayao, C.; Lukas, R. J.; Wu, J.; Shi, F. -D. (2009). Nicotine and inflammatory neurological disorders. Acta Pharmacologica Sinica, 30(6), 715-722.

Picciotto, M. R.; Caldarone, B. J.; King, S. L.; Zachariou, V. (2000). Nicotinic receptors in the brain. Links between molecular biology and behavior. Neuropsychopharmacology, 22(5), 451-465.

Sargent, P. B. (1993). The diversity of neuronal nicotinic acetylcholine receptors. Annual Review of Neuroscience, 16, 403-443.

Shoaib, M.; Benwell, M. E. M.; Akbar, M. T.; Stolerman, I. P.; Balfour, D. J. K. (1994). Behavioural and neurochemical adaptationsto nicotine in rats: influence of NMDA antagonists. British Journal ofharmacology, 111(4), 1073-1080.

Simone, M. J.; Tan, Z. S. (2011). The role of inflammation in the pathogenesis of delirium and dementia in older adults: a review. CNS Neuroscience, Therapeutics, 17(5), 506-513.

Trzepacz, P. T. (2000). Is there a final common neural pathwayin delirium? Focus on acetylcholine and dopamine. Seminars in Clinical Neuropsychiatry, 5(2), 132-148.

van Gool, W. A.; van de Beek, D.; Eikelenboom, P. (2010). Systemic infection and delirium: when cytokines and acetylcholine collide. Lancet (London, England), 375(9716), 773-775.

Van Rompaey, B.; Elseviers, M. M.; Schuurmans, M. J.; Shortridge Baggett, L. M.; Truijen, S.; Bossaert, L. (2009). Risk factors for delirium in intensive care patients: a prospective cohort study. CriticalCare, 13(3), R77.

Vandrey, R. G.; Budney, A. J.; Hughes, J. R.; Liguori, A. (2008). A within-subject comparison of withdrawal symptoms during abstinence from cannabis, tobacco, and both substances. Drug and AlcoholDependence, 92(1-3), 48-54.

Watkins, S. S.; Koob, G. F.; Markou, A. (2000). Neural mechanisms underlying nicotine addiction: acute positive reinforcement and withdrawal. Nicotine, Tobacco Research, 2(1), 19-37.

Webster, R.; Holroyd, S. (2000). Prevalence of psychotic symptoms indelirium. Psychosomatics, 41(6), 519-522.

Wiley, J. L. (1998). Nitric oxide synthase inhibitors attenuate phencyclidine-induced disruption of prepulse inhibition. Neuropsychopharmacology, 19(1), 86-94.

World Health Organisation (1992). The ICD-10 classification of mental and behavioural disorders: Clinical descriptions and diagnostic guidelines.

Zhu, P. J.; Chiappinelli, V. A. (1999). Nicotine modulates evoked GABAergic transmission inthe brain. Journal of Neurophysiology, 82(6), 3041-3045.

29
术后烟碱戒断

Paul Zammit

Department of Geriatrics, Karen Grech Hospital, Pieta, Malta

缩略语

CAM	意识模糊评估法	ITU	强化治疗病房
CAM-ICU	重症监护评估法	NuDesc	护理焦虑症筛查量表
DSI	焦虑症状访谈	POD	术后焦虑症
ICDSC	重症监护焦虑症筛查量表		

29.1 引言

早在公元一世纪,"焦虑症"一词就被首先描述为医学术语解释,用于描述发烧或头部外伤期间发生的精神障碍。焦虑症是常见的临床综合征,尤其是在老年人中,以注意力不集中和急性认知功能障碍为特征。此后出现了各种各样的术语解释来描述焦虑症。这些术语解释包括"急性精神错乱状态""急性脑综合征""急性脑供血不足"和"毒性代谢性脑病",但"焦虑症"仍应用作该综合征的标准术语解释。随着时间的推移,焦虑症一词已经演变成描述一种短暂的、可逆的综合征,它既是急性的,也是波动的,会在医疗条件下发生(Fong, Tulebaev, Inouye, 2009)。

临床经验和循证研究表明,焦虑症可以成为慢性或导致永久性后遗症。在老年人中,焦虑可能会是引发或导致一系列事件的关键组成部分,导致功能下降、丧失独立性、制度化,最终死亡。焦虑症影响了14%~56%住院老年患者。在美国,每年住院的65岁以上的1250万患者中,至少有20%因焦虑症而在住院期间出现并发症(Inouye, 1998)。

29.2 术后麻醉性焦虑症

60岁以上的人数正在呈指数增长,并且在接下来的10~20年中还将继续增长。因此,那些需要手术的人的数量也会增加。外科研究表明,47%的患者出现术后焦虑症(POD),更常见于老年人。更重要的是,POD与发病率、死亡率、住院时间和护理之家的安置相关(Noimark, 2009)。由于每位患者发作的医疗保健费用的大幅增加,医疗服务也面临负担。

POD与麻醉苏醒的时间无关。根据定义尽管可能有其他因素,但POD患者没有可识别的病因。这些病人通常在术后立即痊愈,在麻醉后的护理单元中也可能是清醒的。但是,在此初始时间间隔之后,患者会出现经典的精神波动状态。这种情况最常见于术后第1天和第3天之间。一些术后患者可能会住在强化治疗病房(ITU)中。然而,焦虑症一词(以前称为精神病)可能包括内科和外科患者(Brauer et al. 2000)。由于两组患者的入院特征可能不同,POD患者可能与焦虑症患者不同。根据定义，因急性医学适应症住院的患者通常病情很重，可能会加重慢性病。大多数外科手术是择期的，在入院前已对患者病情进行了控制，以确保其身体状况最佳。内科患者通常不进行手术以及相关的麻醉和镇痛药，但会导致POD（Deiner, Silverstein, 2009）。

29.3 发病机理

人们提出了许多假说来解释术后焦虑症的发病机理（Lipowski, 1987）。有人认为，当大脑的氧化代谢下降时，大脑内的神经递质（例如乙酰胆碱）的水平会下降，从而导致精神障碍。研究表明，脑乙酰胆碱合成对缺氧敏感。此外，还观察到术后意识模糊和抗胆碱能药物活性之间存在关联（Hshiehet al. 2008）。第二个假设表明，由于手术或麻醉的压力导致血清皮质醇水平升高可能是造成术后混乱的原因（MacLullich et al. 2008）。体外循环性精神病的发病机理也归因于体外循环后色氨酸的利用率降低（Parikh, Chung, 1995）。

29.4 术后焦虑症的原因

焦虑症通常是生理压力（例如手术）和诱发患者危险因素的结果。术后诱发因素可能有便秘、尿潴留药物（见下文）、感染、电解质异常和环境原因。有关更多的焦虑症原因，请参见表29.1。当怀疑有焦虑症诊断时，需要进行标准检查以排除焦虑症的有机或可识别原因。评估的第一步是完整的病史和体格检查，并进行焦虑症的认知评估。如前所述，可以借助筛查工具对患者进行焦虑症评估。

表29.1 术后焦虑症的危险因素

・年龄大于60岁	・贫血
・痴呆	・缺氧
・多种并发症	・营养不足
・听力或视力问题	・脱水
・髋部骨折入院	・电解质异常，如高钠血症或低钠血症
・急性感染的存在	・功能状态差
・疼痛控制不足	・不活动或活动受限
・抑郁症	・多药，特别是使用精神药物（苯二氮䓬类药物、抗胆碱能药物、抗组胺药物和抗精神病药物）
・酒精滥用	
・睡眠不足或障碍	・有尿潴留或便秘的风险
・肾功能衰竭	・插入导尿管

29.5 临床表现

POD的表现是多种多样的，并且与这种情况相关的迹象多种多样（MacLullich et al. 2008）。《精神障碍诊断与统计手册》第5版（American Psychiatric Association, 2013）的焦虑症诊断标准如下：

① 注意障碍（即引导、集中、维持和转移注意力的能力降低）。

② 认知变化（例如，记忆力减退、神志不清、语言障碍和知觉障碍）不能由先前存在、已建立或正在发展的痴呆症更好地解释。

③ 干扰会在短时间内（通常是数小时到数天）发展，并且在一天中会有所波动。

④ 从病史，体格检查或实验室检查结果中可以看出，干扰是由一般医学状况、醉酒物质、

药物使用或多种原因引起的直接生理后果引起的。

术后焦虑症的各种临床表现见表29.2。

表29.2 焦虑相关症状

·警惕性水平的变化：困倦或警惕性降低（低活跃性焦虑症）或警惕性增加伴有高度警觉（高活跃性焦虑） ·麻醉延迟苏醒 ·认知功能的突然变化（在数小时或数天内混乱加剧）。这些问题可能包括注意力问题、难以集中注意力、新的记忆问题、和新的定向障碍 ·难以跟踪对话和遵循简单的指示 ·思考和讲话更加混乱、难以理解、缓慢或快速 ·快速变化的情绪，变得容易易怒、流泪、异常地拒绝参与术后护理	·产生新的偏执狂思想、想法或妄想（即固定的错误信念） ·新的知觉障碍（如错觉和幻觉） ·运动功能的改变，包括运动减慢或减少，无目的的烦躁不安或坐立不安，以及在保持姿势（如坐着或站着）方面出现新的困难 ·睡眠/觉醒周期紊乱，如白天睡觉和/或夜间清醒和活跃 ·食欲下降 ·新发大小便失禁 ·几分钟到几小时内的波动症状和/或觉醒水平

29.6 诊断

多项研究表明，护士和医生不能根据他们的床边评估准确诊断焦虑症，包括在ITU、医疗和外科病房（Spronk et al. 2009）。非专业床边人员使用的用于焦虑症检测的筛查工具或简要仪器很多。其中包括意识模糊评估方法（CAM）、焦虑症症状访谈（DSI）和护理焦虑症筛查量表（NuDesc）。在ITU设置中，重症监护室的意识模糊评估方法（CAM-ICU）或重症监护焦虑症检查表（ICDSC）更为合适。这些诊断测试差异很大，并取决于使用它们的患者人群。因此，有证据表明，对患者进行焦虑症筛查时，应培训多学科保健专业人员，并使用已根据参考标准进行验证的筛查仪器（美国老年医学会，2015）。由于药物引起的焦虑症很常见，因此复查治疗很重要。镇静催眠药、抗胆碱能药物和哌替啶对老年人术后焦虑症的风险有显著影响（Marcantonio et al. 1994）。已经证明，药物本身或这些类别中的药物是老年患者发生焦虑症的概率的两倍以上。苯海拉明可将老年人焦虑症的概率提高至2.3（95% CI: 1.4～3.6）（Agostini, Leo-Summers, Inouye, 2001）。哌替啶与50岁以上成年人焦虑症相关，比值比为2.7（95% CI: 1.3～5.5），而苯二氮䓬类比值比升高3.0（95% CI: 1.3～6.8）。改善老年人用药安全性的临床指南建议避免使用容易增加焦虑症风险或严重程度的药物。麻醉在焦虑症发展中的作用尚不清楚。最近的荟萃分析得出的结论是，与区域麻醉相比，全身麻醉具有更高的发生术后认知功能障碍的风险（Vijayakumar et al. 2014）。需要对患者出现物质问题（例如酒精滥用）的可能性进行仔细的审查，因为撤回该药物需要特殊的治疗。常规血液检查包括全血细胞计数、电解质、葡萄糖和可疑感染源的化粪筛查。神经成像如脑部计算机断层扫描等神经影像检查仅限于最近跌倒或头部受伤、使用抗凝药、局灶性神经系统体征或发烧而无其他解释的患者（Inouye et al. 2014）。

29.7 术后患者的烟碱戒断

烟碱是鼻烟的主要生物碱，其成瘾力很大。它被迅速吸收并到达大脑，导致各种神经递质的释放。伏隔核介导的多巴胺能系统的刺激解释了烟碱的成瘾性（Adinoff, 2004）。烟碱的摄入会导致愉悦、焦虑减轻、执行任务的能力增强、记忆力增强、情绪调节和肌肉放松（Knott et al. 2011）。

依赖吸烟者的烟碱含量低会引起戒断症状，包括愤怒、易怒、焦虑、失眠、注意力不集中、嗜睡、疲倦、饥饿、体重增加、心神不定、焦虑不安、情绪低落，以及很少出现焦虑症（Hughes, 2006）。这些症状在最初的24小时内开始出现，在1～2周内达到最大值，通常在1个月后消失（Talwar et al. 2004）。烟碱戒断综合征的发生频率很难预测，但可能被低估了。该综合征已经在一些病例报告中进行了描述（Kallel et al. 2012; Miranda et al. 2005; Zammit et al. 2015）。急性烟碱在ITU设定的脑后损伤中，急性焦虑症的发作被认为是戒断的原因。在重症监护中，美国神经重症监护小组公布了一系列的5例病例（Mayer et al. 2001）。这些患者包括中风和脑膜出血患者，他们在戒烟后2～10天出现躁动和意识混乱。在所有5例中，建立了21mg/24h的烟碱贴片，导致情况迅速改善。对于收入ITU的吸烟患者，由于戒烟是完全和突然的，很可能发生烟碱戒断综合征。

在外科和ITU中，也有关于吸烟患者焦虑症的研究，但结果相矛盾。Hsieh等（2013）对这方面的14项研究进行了系统的综述。它指出了现有文献中的一些不足之处，这些不足可以解释调查结果的不确定性。首先，现有文献受到对主动吸烟状况的次优评估的限制。一些研究没有使用经过验证的量表。也有一些研究对焦虑症的潜在混杂因素（例如先前存在的认知障碍和抑郁症）进行了不完全的调整。这种系统的审查也有一些局限性。结论是，住院和危重病人中吸烟者和焦虑症的患病率很高，因此需要进行一项研究来仔细、果断地确定这种关联是否存在。这将具有重大的潜在预防和治疗意义。它还得出结论，未来对吸烟者焦虑的研究应专门研究这种关联，并应使用吸烟的生化测量来客观地量化吸烟行为。

29.8 烟碱戒断的诊断

怀疑是烟碱戒断，重要的是要排除其他引起焦虑症的原因，例如感染、代谢紊乱、神经病理学和其他如前所述的可能的病理。预防措施包括感官增强、活动能力增强、认知取向、疼痛控制、足够的液体摄入、优化睡眠质量、药物复查以及每日的多学科复查，其中包括老年患者的老年医学。焦虑教育是预防和治疗老年人术后焦虑症的重要组成部分。教育内容应基于对焦虑的认识、筛查工具、结果、危险因素以及预防和管理的非药物和药物方法。当教育与强化、强化活动、同伴支持、一对一互动和反馈相结合时，是最有效的（American Geriatrics Society, 2015）。

29.9 治疗

具体治疗方法是使用20mg的烟碱贴剂，如果无反应则增加至每天30 mg（Miranda et al. 2005）。如果使用这种药物可以快速消灭焦虑症，则可通过使用烟碱透皮贴剂（构成诊断测试和治疗手段）来促进该综合征的诊断。烟碱贴片与严重的心血管并发症如心肌梗死和脑出血有关（Ottervanger et al. 1995）。尽管没有大量的随机对照研究可以证明这一点，但在进行冠状动脉手术的患者中应注意这一点。

对于躁动不安的患者，滴定剂量的抗精神病药，尤其是氟哌啶醇，可能会有所帮助（Robinson, Eiseman, 2008）。抗精神病药的潜在益处是降低焦虑症的严重程度，尽管临床试验结果不一致。与抗精神病药物相关的各种潜在危害，例如嗜睡、尿液滞留、便秘和抗精神病药物恶性综合征，仅举几例。没有证据表明抗精神病药物的治疗对没有躁动的患者有好处。当有可能造成实质伤害时，抗精神病药物的使用应保留给急性躁动的短期治疗，即：用于治疗具有严重威胁患者或他人安全的躁动等行为的老年外科患者术后焦虑症（American Geriatrics Society, 2015）。目前没有证据支持常规使用苯二氮䓬类药物治疗焦虑，有大量证据表明苯二氮䓬类药物促进焦虑（Zaal et al. 2015）。

非药物干预对烟碱戒断并发焦虑症的管理是重要的，特别是对老年人。这些干预措施包括环境（没有过多、不足或模棱两可的感觉输入；药物不中断睡眠；一次提供一种刺激或任务）、方向（房间应该有时钟、日历和日程安排表；评估对眼镜、助听器和口译员的需求）、治疗活动（避免身体束缚，允许活动并鼓励自我护理和个人活动）、视力/听力优化、沟通（清晰、缓慢、简单、重复、面对病人、热情、坚定的善意、称呼病人的名字、认同自我、鼓励表达）、充实口腔容量、增强睡眠和熟悉医院环境（来自家中的物品、相同工作人员、家属与患者住在一起，以及对熟悉区域的讨论）（Hipp, Ely, 2012）。这些介入项目认识和处理的多因素性质已经在减少焦虑方面取得了成功。

29.10 结论

POD是一种重要且往往未被认识的并发症，对个人和卫生保健组织都有重要影响。烟碱戒断是术后焦虑症的罕见原因。临床诊断是排除其他更常见的原因，可通过烟碱替代治疗。术后焦虑症的最佳治疗可降低老年术后患者这种并发症的发生率、持续时间和副作用。

术语解释
- 焦虑症：焦虑症是一种严重的精神错乱和大脑功能快速变化的状况。焦虑症本身并不是疾病，而是可能由疾病或其他临床过程引起的一系列症状。也可称为"急性精神错乱状态"或"急性脑综合征"。
- 多学科护理：多学科护理是指来自具有不同但互补的技能、知识和经验的各个学科的专业人员共同努力，以提供全面的医疗保健，旨在为患者的生理和心理需求及其职业提供最佳的结果。
- 老年人：通常根据年龄范围、社会角色变化和功能能力变化等一系列特征来定义该队列。在西方国家，通常将年龄定义为与有偿工作退休和领取养老金有关，年龄为60岁或65岁。
- 术后时期：这是指手术后的时期。它从患者从麻醉中出来开始，一直持续到麻醉的急性影响和手术程序解决所需的时间。
- 戒断状态：一组戒断或减轻严重程度的症状，通常在长时间和/或大剂量服用后，停止或减少使用重复服用的精神活性物质而出现。

术后焦虑症关键事实
- 这可能发生在术后不久的时期。
- 在老年人和有多种合并症的人中更常见。
- 与显著的发病率和死亡率有关。
- 原因可能是多因素的，包括感染、心脏和药物管理或戒断。
- 管理通过多学科方法进行，涉及预防措施、病因治疗和非药物干预。

要点总结
- POD是术后干预的常见并发症，并伴有明显的发病率和死亡率。
- 烟碱戒断是引起POD的众多原因之一，在术后即刻突然戒烟的患者中应怀疑烟碱戒断。
- 表现可能较轻，出现焦虑等症状，或更严重的症状包括嗜睡、躁动和全天波动。

- 通过排除焦虑症的其他代谢原因（例如感染、尿液潴留和电解质紊乱）来诊断烟碱戒断。
- 烟碱戒断的调查与焦虑症的调查相似，涉及常规血液检查，很少进行影像学检查以排除症状的其他原因。
- 诊断后的治疗采用多学科方法，涉及通过烟碱贴片和非药物干预来替代烟碱。

参考文献

Adinoff, B. (2004). Neurobiologic processes in drug reward and addiction. Harvard Review of Psychiatry, 12(6), 305-320.

Agostini, J. V.; Leo-Summers, L. S.; Inouye, S. K. (2001). Cognitive and other adverse effects of diphenhydramine use in hospitalized older patients. Archives of Internal Medicine, 161, 2091-2097.

American Geriatrics Society. (2015). Postoperative delirium in older adults: best practice statement from the American Geriatrics Society. Journal of the American College of Surgeons, 220(2), 136-148. e1.

American Psychiatric Association. (2013). Diagnostic and statistical manual of mental disorders (5th ed.). Washington, DC: American Psychiatric Association.

Brauer, C.; Morrison, R. S.; Silberzweig, S. B.; Siu, A. L. (2000). The cause of delirium in patients with hip fracture. Archives of Internal Medicine, 160(12), 1856-1860.

Deiner, S.; Silverstein, J. H. (2009). Postoperative delirium and cognitive dysfunction. British Journal of Anaesthesia, 103 (Suppl. 1), i41-i46.

Fong, T. G.; Tulebaev, S.; Inouye, S. (2009). Delirium in elderly adults: diagnosis, prevention and treatment. Nature Reviews. Neurology, 5(4), 210-220.

Hipp, D. M.; Ely, E. W. (2012). Pharmacological and nonpharmacological management of delirium in critically ill patients. Neurotherapeutics, 9(1), 158-175.

Hshieh, T. T.; Fong, T. G.; Marcantonio, E. R.; Inouye, K. S. (2008). Cholinergic deficiency hypothesis in delirium: A synthesis of currentevidence. The Journals of Gerontology. Series A, Biological Sciences and Medical Sciences, 63(7), 764-772.

Hsieh, S. J.; Andrew, M. S.; Lee, N.; Hasselmark, F.; Gong, M. N. (2013). Cigarette smoking as a risk factor for delirium in hospitalized and intensive care unit patients. A systematic review. Annals of the American Thoracic Society, 10(5), 496-503.

Hughes, J. R. (2006). Clinical significance of tobacco withdrawal. Nicotine, Tobacco Research, 8, 153-156.

Inouye, S. K. (1998). Delirium in hospitalized older patients: recognition and risk factors. Journal of Geriatric Psychiatry and Neurology, 11, 118-125.

Inouye, S. K.; Westendorp, R. G.; Saczynski, J. S. (2014). Delirium ineldery people. Lancet, 383, 911-922.

Kallel, S.; Ellouze, M.; Triki, Z.; Karoui, A. (2012). Le syndrome de sevrage nicotine après chirurgie cardiaque: à propos d'un cas. ThePan African Medical Journal, 13, 10 [in French].

Knott, V.; Heenan, A.; Shah, D.; Bolton, K.; Fisher, D.; Villeneuve, C. (2011). Electrophysiological evidence of nicotine's distracter-filtering properties in non-smokers. Journal of Psychopharmacology, 25(2), 239-248.

Lipowski, Z. J. (1987). Delirium (acute confusional states). JAMA, 258, 1789-1792.

MacLullich, A. M. J.; Ferguson, K. J.; Miller, T.; de Rooij, S. E. J. A.; Cunningham, C. (2008). Unravelling the pathophysiology of delirium: a focus on the role of aberrant stress responses. Journal of PsychosomaticResearch, 65, 229-238.

Marcantonio, E. R.; Juarez, G.; Goldman, L.; Mangione, C. M.; Ludwig, L. E.; Lind, L. et al. (1994). The relationship of postoperativedelirium with psychoactive medications. JAMA, 272(19), 1518-1522.

Mayer, S. A.; Chong, J. Y.; Ridgway, E.; Min, K. C.; Commichau, C.; Bernardini, G. L. (2001). Delirium from nicotine withdrawal inneuro-ICU patients. Neurology, 57(3), 551-553.

Miranda, M.; Slachevsky, A.; Venegas, P. (2005). Delirium from nicotine withdrawal in a post-operative adult patient. Revista Medica de Chile, 133, 385-386 [in Spanish].

Noimark, D. (2009). Predicting the onset of delirium in the postoperative patient. Age Ageing, 38(4), 368-373.

Ottervanger, J. P.; Festen, J. M.; de Vries, A. G.; Stricker, B. H. (1995). Acute myocardial infarction while using the nicotine patch. Chest, 107(6), 1765-1766.

Parikh, S. S.; Chung, F. (1995). Postoperative delirium in the elderly. Anesthesia and Analgesia, 80(6), 1223-1232.

Robinson, T.; Eiseman, B. (2008). Postoperative delirium in the elderly:diagnosis and management. Clinical Interventions in Aging, 3(2), 351-355.

Spronk, P. E.; Riekerk, B.; Hofhuis, J.; Rommes, J. H. (2009). Occurrenceof delirium is severely underestimated in the ICU during daily care. Intensive Care Medicine, 35(7), 1276-1280.

Talwar, A.; Jain, M.; Vijayan, V. (2004). Pharmacotherapy of tobacco dependence. Medical Clinics of North America, 88, 1517-1534.

Vijayakumar, B.; Elango, P.; Ganessan, R. (2014). Post-operative deliriumin elderly patients. Indian Journal of Anaesthesia, 58(3), 251-256.

Zaal, I. J.; Devlin, J. W.; Hazelbag, M.; Klein Klouwenberg, P. M.; van derKooi, A. W.; Ong, D. S. et al. (2015). Benzodiazepine-associated deliriumin critically ill adults. Intensive Care Medicine, 41(12), 2130-2137.

Zammit, P.; Cordina, J.; Vassallo, M.; Dalli, S. (2015). Post-operative nicotine withdrawal in an elderly patient. European Geriatric Medicine, 6(6), 607-608.

30
烟碱和 α3β2 神经烟碱乙酰胆碱受体

Doris Clark Jackson, Sterling N. Sudweeks

Brigham Young University, Physiology and Developmental Biology, Provo, UT, United States

缩略语

ACh	乙酰胆碱	**nAChR**	烟碱乙酰胆碱受体
EC_{50}	有效浓度为50%活性	**SNP**	单核苷酸多态性
HEK-293	人胚肾细胞	**VTA**	腹侧被盖区
M1-M4	M1-M4跨膜区域		

30.1 引言

烟碱乙酰胆碱受体（nAChR）是五聚体、配体门控离子通道，在神经和神经肌肉接头处均有发现。每个亚基由四个跨膜区域（M1～M4）组成，细胞内的M3-M4环是亚基之间最不保守的区域。每个亚基的M2构成了受体的孔（图30.1）。nAChR具有阳离子选择性，某些亚型对钙离子具有渗透性（α3β2具有一定的渗透性，α5的加入显著增加了Ca^{2+}的渗透性）。当突触前发现这些受体时，Ca^{2+}渗透性nAChR在促进甚至独立刺激其他神经递质（如多巴胺）释放方面发挥着独特的作用。在神经肌肉连接处发现的nAChR由5个不同的亚基（α1、β1、γ、δ和ε）组成。神经元烟碱乙酰胆碱受体可以是同源的，也可以是异源的。然而，只有α7和α9亚基可以形成同源受体。大多数神经元nAChR由α和β亚基［α2、α3α4、α5（必须有一个额外的α亚基）、α6、α7、α8、α9、α10、β2、β3和β4］组成。最常见的异源nAChR具有两个α2和三个β（α*₂β*₃）或三个α和两个β2（α*₃β*₂）。最具特征的nAChR亚型是同源α7和α4β2。我们已经确定了至少两种亚型的α3β2 nAChR（图30.2），并将详细说明α3β2 nAChR在烟碱上瘾症中可能发挥的作用。

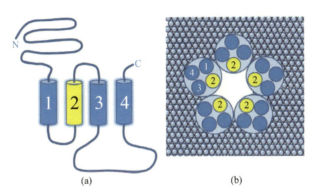

图 30.1 nAChR亚基和嵌入式组件

(a) 每个烟碱乙酰胆碱受体（nAChR）亚基包含四个跨膜区域。跨膜区3和4之间的细胞内环（M3-M4）是nAChR亚基之间变化最大的；(b) 五个单元（通常是αs和βs的组合）形成一个功能性受体，M2形成通道孔隙

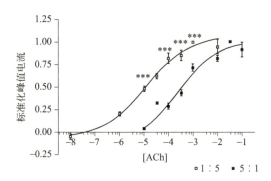

图 30.2　ACh 的剂量－响应曲线区分出了不同的类型

在以 1：5 和 5：1 的比例向爪蟾卵母细胞中注射 3 个和 2 个 mRNA 后，会产生两种不同的烟碱乙酰胆碱受体（nAChR）。β 和 α 表达导致更多乙酰胆碱（ACh）敏感 α3β2 亚型 [EC_{50}=（12.2±1.7）μmol/L；n_H=0.49±0.13（R^2=0.74）]（n=14，4 个重复，删除 1 个异常值），而多 β 和 α 表达导致少 ACh-敏感 α3β2 亚型 [EC_{50}=（263.8±1.6）μmol/L；n_H=0.55±0.15（R^2=0.77）]（n=12，4 个重复，删除 2 个异常值）。单因素方差分析导致显著性差异（$F_{[15, 258]}$=54.644；＊＊＊$P<0.001$）。数据代表平均值±SEM。

30.2　分亚型的烟碱敏感性

α3β2 nAChR 是烟碱贴片最不敏感的 nAChR 亚型之一，仅是烟碱贴片的一部分（Gerzanich et al. 1998; Olale et al. 1997; Wang et al. 1996, 1998）。传统上，只有 α4β2 nAChR 被认为是高亲和力烟碱贴片结合位点。然而，α4β2 nAChR 仅代表 90% 的高亲和力烟碱结合位点。α 和 β 亚基都有助于烟碱亲和力和效力。经证明，与 β4 亚基相比，β2 亚基具有更强的烟碱结合亲和力，更容易脱敏（Fenster et al. 1997; Parker, Beck, Luetje, 1998），而 α3* 受体比 β4* 受体的脱敏程度更低（Fenster et al. 1997）。同样地，在 α3β2 中加入 α5 亚基显著提高了烟碱效率（Wang et al. 1996, 1998）。然而，这不大可能是因为烟碱亲和力的变化，而是通道门控的变化（Wang et al. 1998）。α5 亚基最可能的位置不会改变结合位点，而是会影响通道内衬（Wang et al. 1996）。

M1 氨基酸的差异（224 和 226）解释了 β2 亚基比 β4 亚基对烟碱的亲和力高（Rush, et al. 2002）。M1（图 30.1）解释了 α3* 和 α4* nAChR 亚型烟碱结合亲和力的差异（Rush et al. 2002）。即使 α3 比 β4 具有更大的结合亲和力，但 α3β2 nAChR 仅具有部分效力。Rush 等（2002）提出了在 α3β2 nAChR 上烟碱的部分激动剂活性的几种机制。一种机制可能是烟碱结合不能有效地将通道转换到开放状态，另一机制可能是烟碱与结合位点的结合较弱。Kuryatov 等（2000）表明，当使用由 α4β2 结合位点与 α3β2 通道组成的嵌合场时，烟碱充当部分激动剂；而当使用 α3β2 结合位点与 α4β2 通道烟碱，有充分的功效。他们的结论是，α3β2 nAChR 在用烟碱激活时存在通道阻塞。Rush 等（2002）的一项研究支持了这一观点，即烟碱可能通过与一个低亲和力的结合位点结合，从而阻塞通道。然而，通道阻塞所需的烟碱浓度比吸烟者预期的要大（Benowitz et al. 1990）。此外，当将一种 α6 亚基并入到 α3β2 nAChR 中时，烟碱具有 100% 的功效（Kuryatov et al. 2000）。因此，通道块可能需要多个 α3β2 接口（Rush et al. 2002）。

30.3　烟碱诱导的向上调节

像其他 nAChR 亚型一样，在烟碱暴露下，α3β2 nAChR 上调。在大鼠、小鼠和死后的人脑中观察到 nAChR 的普遍上调（Breese et al. 1997; Perry, Davila-Garcia, Stockmeier, Kellar, 1999; Yates et al. 1995)。像烟碱结合亲和力一样，亚基组成影响烟碱诱导的不同阶段的上调。例如，含有 β2* nAChR 比含有 β4* 的 nAChR 具有更大的烟碱诱导的上调率（Gahring et al. 2008; Wang et al. 1998）。然而，Meyer 等（2001）在加入 β4 后并没有表现出上调的变化。当比较 α3β2、α4β2 和 α6β2 nAChR，α3β2 受体需要最高的烟碱浓度才能上调，大约比 α4β2 的上调快 10 倍，但略慢于 α6β2 nAChR 的上调（Walsh et al. 2008）。因此，在最初的烟碱接触中，该药物的作用可能不大，但在烟碱水平较高的慢性接触中，其作用更为显著。

在人胚胎肾细胞（HEK-293）和人神经母细胞瘤 SH-SY5Y 中，以及在死后大脑中证实的神经元中，都出现了烟碱水平的上调，表明上调依赖于受体而不是神经元细胞过程的反应（Wang et al. 1998）。然而，Wang 等（1998）在非洲爪蟾卵母细胞中并没有发现上调。X. laevis 卵母细胞可能没有像缔合蛋白那样的细胞机制来允许上调。尽管如此，人类细胞系和神经元与人类生理的关系比卵母细胞更直接。在解释有关卵母细胞 nAChR 上调的数据时，应该考虑到这一点。

上调可能是转录前和后。在 HEK-293 细胞（tsA201）中，慢性烟碱暴露 [上调，EC_{50} =（2±0.3）μmol/L；烟碱激活，EC_{50} =（70±6）μmol/L] 导致 α3β2 nAChR（以及 α3β2α5）增加 24 倍。最初暴露于烟碱后 15min 就观察到上调，但随着暴露时间延长，上调趋势继续增加（Wang et al. 1998）。值得注意的是，与 α3β2 受体激活所需的烟碱水平相比，上调所需的烟碱浓度低得多，生理上更类似于吸烟者的血清烟碱水平。这种变化被记录为细胞表面表达的增加和 nAChRs 总数的增加。上调几乎是立即开始的，这可能意味着组装增加和集会的增加。

此外，随着受体膜整合的增加，内质网减缓了 α3β2 nAChR 的降解，从而导致受体整体表达的增加。具体而言，Rezvani 等（2009）研究表明，烟碱可以通过部分抑制泛素蛋白酶体系统来阻止蛋白质降解。注意，慢性烟碱暴露在人类神经母细胞瘤 SH-SY5Y 细胞系导致 α3β2 只增长了 6 倍 nAChR。然而，这只是受体数量的增加，而不是膜的整合。有趣的是，慢性烟碱暴露在 HEK-293 和人神经母细胞瘤 SH-SY5Y 中，并没有引起 α3β4 或 α3β4α5 的上调（Wang et al. 1998）。

此外，温度和促炎细胞因子可以影响烟碱诱导的上调，这有助于分析和解释翻译和转录阶段的结果，TNF-α 可以引起 α3β2 上调的增加，尽管其程度小于 α4β2 和 α4β4 的增加（Gahring et al. 2008）。吸烟引起的炎症会进一步加重吸烟的影响。总的来说，降低温度会减少受体的更替，这可能会影响上调的结果，给出一个错误的高结果（Devreotes, Fambrough, 1975; Paulson, Claudio, 1990）。对于 α4β2 nAChR，降低温度至 29℃ 或 30℃ 可显著增加细胞表面表达（Cooper et al. 1999）。考虑到吸烟会导致皮肤温度下降 1.5℃，这是一个有趣的效应（Benowitz et al. 2006）。

上调也可以通过改变磷酸化而受到影响。例如，肌肉 nAChR 是通过 cAMP 和蛋白激酶 A 上调的。这种机制可以提高组装效率并防止降解（Green et al. 1991）。Wang 等（1998）表明，蛋白激酶抑制剂 H-7 可以阻断至少 50% 烟碱诱导的 HEK-293 细胞内的（tsA201）α3β2 nAChR 的上调。因此，在烟碱上调的细胞过程中有许多可能的因素，包括亚单位组成、细胞表达系统、温度、细胞因子和磷酸化。

30.4 位置

当考虑到的位置的 α3β2 nAChR，限制子单元是 α3。至少在中枢神经系统中，比比皆是，但在外周神经系统中也很容易发现（图 30.3; Hill Jr et al. 1993）。在大鼠和小鼠中，在丘脑、内侧缰核、上丘和松果体中发现了3亚基（图30.4; Cimino et al. 1992）。在更有限的表达模式下，α3更有可能是α3β2表达中的限制性亚基（图30.5）。β2敲除小鼠不自我给药烟碱，中边缘神经元不释放多巴胺以响应烟碱几乎消除成瘾（Picciotto et al. 1998），而α3敲除小鼠会导致多个自主系统问题（Xu et al. 1999）。

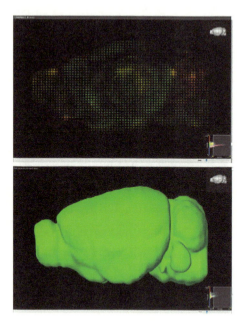

图 30.3　小鼠脑内 β2 nAChR 的表达

热图（红色高，蓝色低）详细描述了小鼠大脑中无处不在的β2亚基的表达。表达谱量化如图30.5所示。图片来自经许可的艾伦大脑图谱，http://mouse.brain map.org/experiment/show/2098。

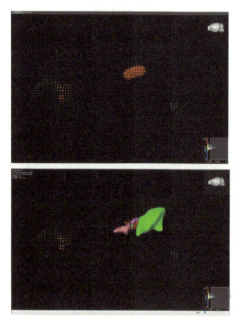

图 30.4　小鼠脑内 α3 nAChR 的表达

热图（红色高，蓝色低）详细描述了小鼠大脑中有限的α3亚基的表达。外侧缰核（粉红色）、橄榄核（紫色）和上丘（绿色）。图片来自经许可的艾伦大脑图谱，http://mouse.brain map.org/experiment/show/69734723。

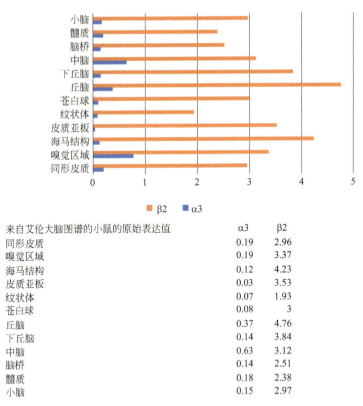

图 30.5　艾伦大脑图谱小鼠原始表达值

小鼠（C57BL/6J）脑区含有β2和α3亚基的相对表达谱。结果是使用反义原位杂交的成年（56d）雄性小鼠。如前所述，在分析的所有区域中，β2亚基的表达均高于α3。数据来自经许可的艾伦大脑图谱。

除了这些位置，猕猴（食蟹猴）还在海马体识别出了3个亚基（Cimino et al. 1992）。考虑到人类和非人灵长类动物之间的高度保护，这种差异在将研究成果转化为人类研究中可能很重要（Shorey-Kendrick, 2015）。此外，α3β2 nAChR M.束状神经细胞和人体组织中都发现了高水平的交感神经和副交感神经神经节中的-3mRNA亚基（Ciminoet al. 1992）。α3亚基的位置可能决定中枢神经系统中α3β2 nAChR的存在，β2亚基可能决定外周神经系统中α3β2的表达。

在中枢神经系统中，α3β2 nAChR影响纹状体多巴胺释放和最终成瘾效果（Picciotto et al. 1998）。然而，在外周神经系统中，α3β4 nAChR比α3β2 nAChR贡献更大（Covernton et al. 1994）。然而，α3亚基仍然是外周神经系统的主要亚基。因此，α3β2 nAChR在自主生理烟碱反应中，可能具有更大的作用。

中脑（上丘）的多巴胺神经元可能参与烟碱自我给药所需的身体运动。阻断多巴胺受体可以防止烟碱的自我给药（Corrigall, Coen, 1991）。α3β2 nAChR在上丘中高表达，可能影响多巴胺释放，并间接影响烟碱的自我给药。

此外，通过高亲和力烟碱和n-金环蛇毒素结合，在腹侧被盖区（VTA）和伏隔核中鉴定了α3和β2 mRNA亚基（Azam et al. 2002）。在VTA中，并没有认为α3β2 nAChR是最重要的导致烟碱上瘾的因素，但考虑到其在烟碱暴露后的上调和烟碱亲和力的增加，与前两者相比，其可能在不同的成瘾阶段起作用（Azam et al. 2002）。

在伏隔核突触前多巴胺能神经元上使用^{125}I-nBgt或^{125}I-α-芋螺毒素MII标记的nAChR进行放

射自显影和实验。虽然α-芋螺毒素MII最初被认为是α3β2特异性的,但后来证明它也能结合α6* nAChR(Kuryatov et al. 2000; Parker et al. 2004)。因此,含α3和α6的nAChR之一/两者都可能有助于伏隔核多巴胺的释放。此外,α3亚基在缰核中具有相对较高的水平(图30.4),因此可能在该途径中另外介导多巴胺释放,并有助于烟碱成瘾状态。

30.5 烟碱的生理效应

Wang等(1998)研究了在HEK 293细胞中以1:1 α3-β2比例表达α3β2 nAChR的烟碱剂量-反应曲线。其烟碱的$EC_{50}=(70\pm26)\mu mol/L$,这比吸烟者血液中的烟碱水平要高。典型吸烟者的烟碱血清浓度为$0.2\mu mol/L$(Benowitz et al. 1990)。因此,α3β2 nAChR可能在初始烟碱成瘾中没有作用。然而,考虑到α3β2 nAChR在烟碱暴露后的高表达,α3β2 nAChR可能在维持成瘾中起重要作用。α4β2 nAChR对烟碱高度敏感,可能在初始成瘾中发挥重要作用。在典型的烟碱血清水平下,α4β2 nAChR会像α3β2 nAChR一样被上调,但它们也会几乎完全脱敏。然而,α3β2 nAChR(非特定化学计量)不容易脱敏,在吸烟者中可能保持正常功能,因为在吸烟者的正常血清烟碱水平下,它们仍有80%的活性(Fenster et al. 1997; Olale et al. 1997; Picciotto et al. 1998)。α3β2 nAChR可能比α4β2 nAChR在烟碱成瘾的大脑中对乙酰胆碱(ACh)介导的信号传导作用更大(Olale et al. 1997; Wang et al. 1998)。此外,其上调或缺乏可能在大脑区域之间有所不同,就像细胞系之间存在差异(HEK-293、神经母细胞瘤和卵母细胞)(Wang et al. 1998)。考虑到大脑区域比其他区域受到的影响更大,这种上调的可能性和可能性可能会影响行为。然而,这些基因在α3β2 nAChR特异性亚型上的上调研究均未见报道。与其他nAChR亚型一样,我们的初步数据显示,不同化学计量数的α3β2 nAChR在烟碱亲和力和功效上存在差异。

α3 nAChR是目前自主神经系统中数量最多的亚基。虽然在自主神经节中主要的nAChR是α3β4(Vernallis et al. 1993),但α3β2可能也在信号传导和烟碱反应中发挥重要作用。烟碱对自主神经系统有许多影响,包括心率增加、心肌收缩力增加、呼吸增强、动脉收缩、出汗、恶心、腹泻和血压升高(Haass, Kübler, 1997)。

30.6 α3亚基的变异

α3 nAChR亚基具有单核苷酸变异(rs3743078、rs6495308、rs1051730),与烟碱渴望增加、吸烟增加或烟碱相关行为增加有关(Shmulewitz et al. 2016; Wu et al. 2015)。Nees等(2013)得出结论,在α3基因上发现的单核苷酸多态性(SNP)rs578776与吸烟风险增加有关,因为它抑制了前扣带皮层的奖励反应。其中几个多态性包含在与烟碱依赖相关的α5-α3-β4亚基之间的基因簇中。Polina等(2014)的一项研究表明,α3基因的两个多态性(rs578776和rs3743078)与多动症患者的吸烟风险增加有关,但对非多动症人群的吸烟具有保护作用。

此外,在α3 nAChR亚基中发现了多个多态性(rs578776、rs938682、rs6495309和rs3743073),增加了肺癌的易感性(Qu et al. 2016; Shen et al. 2012; Xiao et al. 2014)。另外两个α3 nAChR亚基的多态性(rs8042059和rs7177514)可能仅通过吸烟行为间接增加肺癌易感性(Zhou et al. 2015)。SNP rs12910984、rs6495309和rs1051730已被证明与慢性阻塞性肺病风险增加相关

（Kaur-Knudsen et al. 2012; Kim et al. 2013; Yang et al. 2012）。SNP rs6495308 已被发现与高血压风险增加相关（Wu et al. 2015）。α3 亚基 rs8042374 a SNP 与腺癌风险增加相关（He et al. 2014）。

30.7 治疗的含义

如前所述，α3 亚基的变异可能影响成瘾的可能性和烟碱相关疾病的可能性，甚至有助于预测对治疗的反应。通过识别和描述这些变异在不同人群中的影响，烟碱成瘾治疗可能被证明是更个性化和更有效的。我们仍处于 α3β2 nAChR 及其与烟碱成瘾的关系的初步研究阶段，但有证据表明，通过靶向 α3β2，考虑到 α3 亚基的位置，我们可能能够抵消烟碱的自主效应。此外，考虑到 α3β2 nAChR 的位置和功能，针对 α3β2 nAChR 的药物治疗方法可能会改变与成瘾相关的多巴胺释放，从而使烟碱的愉悦感降低。最后，由于促炎细胞因子导致 α3β2 nAChR 和其他亚型的上调，在开发联合治疗方案时应考虑使用抗炎药物或饮食。

30.8 总结

综上所述，α3β2 nAChR 可能在中枢和外周神经系统烟碱反应中均发挥作用。α3β2 nAChR 在接触烟碱时上调，并且有许多变异，可影响烟碱的成瘾和疾病效应。

术语解释

- **亲和力**：是指受体激活所需的浓度。较高的烟碱亲和力意味着激活所需的烟碱浓度较小，而较低的烟碱亲和力意味着激活所需的烟碱浓度较大。
- **功效**：在此背景下，烟碱诱导的上调是指烟碱暴露后 nAChR 表达数量的增加。上调可能改变细胞对慢性烟碱暴露的反应。
- **烟碱诱导的上调**：是指暴露于烟碱后 nAChRs 表达数量的增加。上调可能改变细胞对慢性烟碱暴露的反应。
- **烟碱乙酰胆碱受体（nAChR）**：一种传导正离子导致电势变化的神经递质受体。这种电势的变化可能会引起神经元或其他细胞类型之间的细胞间通信。
- **跨膜区**：nAChR 蛋白跨膜的区域。跨膜区大部分是疏水的，有助于形成通道孔隙。nAChR 亚基有四个跨膜区。
- **变异**：是亚基蛋白质的微小差异。这些差异可能是由于基因序列或蛋白质生产的变化。

神经元烟碱乙酰胆碱受体的关键事实

- 神经元烟碱乙酰胆碱受体（nAChR）是一种五聚体、配体门控的离子通道，由内源性神经递质乙酰胆碱或外源性化学物质烟碱激活。
- 大多数神经元 nAChR 由 α 亚基和 β 亚基组成。
- 神经元 nAChR 是阳离子选择性的，具有钙离子（Ca^{2+}）渗透性的特定亚型。
- 神经元 nAChR 可定位于突触前、突触后、末梢，甚至非神经元细胞上。
- 根据位置和 Ca^{2+} 渗透性，特定的亚型可以诱导神经递质释放。
- 烟碱可上调和脱敏许多亚型的神经元 nAChR。
- nAChR 亚基变异可能改变烟碱敏感性或对烟碱的生理反应。

要点总结
- α3β2神经元烟碱乙酰胆碱受体（nAChR）及其与烟碱和烟碱成瘾的关系
- α3β2神经元nAChR仅是部分烟碱激动剂，与其他亚型相比，需要更高的烟碱浓度才能激活。
- α3β2神经元nAChR的表达明显高于α4β2 nAChR。
- 在烟碱浓度下，α3β2神经元nAChR仍有80%的活性，这使其他nAChR亚型脱敏。
- α3亚基是自主神经节中最显著的nAChR亚型。
- 烟碱影响自主神经系统的许多方面，包括心率、血压和消化。
- α3亚基的位置可能决定了α3β2 nAChR在中枢神经系统中的存在，而β2亚基的位置可能决定了α3β2 nAChR在自主神经节中的存在。
- α3亚基的若干变体增加了烟碱成瘾的可能性和/或对与烟碱有关的疾病的易感性。

参考文献

Azam, L.; Winzer-Serhan, U. H.; Chen, Y.; Leslie, F. M. (2002). Expression of neuronalnicotinic acetylcholine receptor subunit mRNAs within midbrain dopamine neurons. The Journal of Comparative Neurology, 444, 260-274.

Benowitz, N. L.; Jacob, P.; III, Herrera, B. (2006). Nicotine intake and dose response when smoking reduced nicotine content cigarettes. Clinical Pharmacology and Therapeutics, 80, 703-714.

Benowitz, N.; Porchet, H.; Jacob, P. (1990). In S. Wonnacott, M. Russell, I. Stolerman (Eds.), Nicotine psychopharmacology (pp. 112-157). Oxford, England: Oxford University.

Breese, C. R.; Marks, M. J.; Logel, J.; Adams, C. E.; Sullivan, B.; Collins, A. C. et al. (1997). Effect of smoking history on [3H]nicotine binding inhuman postmortem brain. The Journal of Pharmacology and Experimental Therapeutics, 282, 7-13.

Cimino, M.; Marini, P.; Fornasari, D.; Cattabeni, F.; Clementi, F. (1992). Distribution of nicotinic receptors in cynomolgus monkey brain. Neuroscience, 51, 77-86.

Cooper, S. T.; Harkness, P. C.; Baker, E. R.; Millar, N. S. (1999). Upregulation of cell-surface alpha4beta2 neuronal nicotinic receptors by lower temperature and expression of chimeric subunits. The Journal of Biological Chemistry, 274, 27145-27152.

Corrigall, W. A.; Coen, K. M. (1991). Selective dopamine antagonists reduce nicotine self-administration. Psychopharmacology, 104, 171-176.

Covernton, P. J.; Kojima, H.; Sivilotti, L. G.; Gibb, A. J.; Colquhoun, D. (1994). Comparison of neuronal nicotinic receptors in rat sympathetic neurones with subunit pairs expressed in Xenopusoocytes. The Journal of Physiology, 481(Pt1), 27-34.

Devreotes, P. N.; Fambrough, D. M. (1975). Acetylcholine receptor turnover in membranes of developing muscle fibers. The Journal of Cell Biology, 65, 335-358.

Fenster, C. P.; Rains, M. F.; Noerager, B.; Quick, M. W.; Lester, R. A. (1997). Influence of subunit composition on desensitization of neuronal acetylcholine receptors at low concentrations of nicotine. The Journal of Neuroscience, 17, 5747-5759.

Gahring, L. C.; Osborne-Hereford, A. V.; Vasquez-Opazo, G. A.; Rogers, S. W. (2008). Tumor necrosis factor alpha enhances nicotinicreceptor up-regulation via a p38MAPK-dependent pathway. The Journal of Biological Chemistry, 283, 693-699.

Gerzanich, V.; Wang, F.; Kuryatov, A.; Lindstrom, J. (1998). Alpha 5 subunit alters desensitization pharmacology Ca^{2+} permeability and Ca^{2+} modulation of human neuronal alpha 3 nicotinic receptors. The Journal of Pharmacology and Experimental Therapeutics, 286, 311-320.

Green, W. N.; Ross, A. F.; Claudio, T. (1991). Acetylcholine receptor assembly is stimulated by phosphorylation of its gamma subunit. Neuron, 7, 659-666.

Haass, M.; K€ubler, W. (1997). Nicotine and sympathetic neurotransmission. Cardiovascular Drugs and Therapy, 10, 657-665.

He, P.; Yang, X. X.; He, X. Q.; Chen, J.; Li, F. X.; Gu, X. et al. (2014). CHRNA3 polymorphism modifies lung adenocarcinoma risk in the Chinese Han population. International Journal of Molecular Sciences, 15, 5446-5457.

Hill, J. A.; Jr.; Zoli, M.; Bourgeois, J. P.; Changeux, J. P. (1993). Immunocytochemical localization of a neuronal nicotinic receptor: the beta 2-subunit. The Journal of Neuroscience, 13(4), 1551-1568.

Kaur-Knudsen, D.; Nordestgaard, B. G.; Bojesen, S. E. (2012). CHRNA3 genotype, nicotine dependence, lung function and disease in the general population. The European Respiratory Journal, 40, 1538-1544.

Kim, W. J.; Oh, Y. M.; Kim, T. H.; Lee, J. H.; Kim, E. K.; Lee, J. H. et al. (2013). CHRNA3 variant for lung cancer is associated with chronic obstructive pulmonary disease in Korea. Respiration, 86, 117-122.

Kuryatov, A.; Olale, F.; Cooper, J.; Choi, C.; Lindstrom, J. (2000). Human alpha6 AChR subtypes: subunit composition, assembly and pharmacological responses. Neuropharmacology, 39, 2570-2590.

Meyer, E. L.; Xiao, Y.; Kellar, K. J. (2001). Agonist regulation of rat alpha 3 beta 4 nicotinic acetylcholine receptors stably expressed in human embryonic kidney 293 cells. Molecular Pharmacology, 60, 568-576.

Nees, F.; Witt, S. H.; Lourdusamy, A.; Vollst€adt-Klein, S.; Steiner, S.; Poustka, L. et al. (2013). Genetic risk for nicotine dependence in the cholinergic system and activation of the brain reward system in healthy adolescents. Neuropsychopharmacology, 38(11), 2081-2089.

Olale, F.; Gerzanich, V.; Kuryatov, A.; Wang, F.; Lindstrom, J. (1997). Chronic nicotine exposure differentially affects the function of human alpha3, alpha4, and alpha7 neuronal nicotinic receptor subtypes. The Journal of Pharmacology and Experimental Therapeutics, 283, 675-683.

Parker, M. J.; Beck, A.; Luetje, C. W. (1998). Neuronal nicotinic receptor beta2 and beta4 subunits confer large differences in agonist binding affinity. Molecular Pharmacology, 54(6), 1132-1139.

Parker, S. L.; Fu, Y.; McAllen, K.; Luo, J.; McIntosh, J. M.; Lindstrom, J. M. et al. (2004). Upregulation of brain nicotinic acetylcholine receptors in the rat during long-term self-administration of nicotine: disproportionate increase of the alpha6 subunit. Molecular Pharmacology, 65, 611-622.

Paulson, H. L.; Claudio, T. (1990). Temperature-sensitive expression of all-Torpedo and Torpedorat hybrid AChR in mammalian muscle cells. The Journal of Cell Biology, 110, 1705-1717.

Perry, D. C.; Davila-Garcia, M. I.; Stockmeier, C. A.; Kellar, K. J. (1999). Increased nicotinic receptors in brains from smokers: membrane binding and autoradiography studies. The Journal of Pharmacology and Experimental Therapeutics, 289, 1545-1552.

Picciotto, M. R.; Zoli, M.; Rimondini, R.; Lena, C.; Marubio, L. M.; Pich, E. M. et al. (1998). Acetylcholine receptors containing the beta2 subunit are involved in the reinforcing properties of nicotine. Nature, 391, 173-177.

Polina, E. R.; Rovaris, D. L.; de Azeredo, L. A.; Mota, N. R.; Vitola, E. S.; Silva, K. L. et al. (2014). ADHD diagnosis may influence the association between polymorphisms in nicotinic acetylcholine receptor genes and tobacco smoking. Neuro Molecular Medicine, 16, 389-397.

Qu, X.; Wang, K.; Dong, W.; Shen, H.; Wang, Y.; Liu, Q. et al. (2016). Association between two CHRNA3 variants and susceptibility of lung cancer: a meta-analysis. Scientific Reports, 6, 20149.

Rezvani, K.; Teng, Y.; Pan, Y.; Dani, J. A.; Lindstrom, J.; García Gras, E. A. et al. (2009). UBXD4, a UBX-containing protein, regulates the cell surface number and stability of alpha3-containing nicotinic acetylcholine receptors. The Journal of Neuroscience, 29(21), 6883-6896.

Rush, R.; Kuryatov, A.; Nelson, M. E.; Lindstrom, J. (2002). First andsecond transmembrane segments of alpha3, alpha4, beta2, and beta4 nicotinic acetylcholine receptor subunits influence the efficacy and potency of nicotine. Molecular Pharmacology, 61, 1416-1422.

Shen, B.; Shi, M. Q.; Zheng, M. Q.; Hu, S. N.; Chen, J.; Feng, J. F. (2012). Correlation between polymorphisms of nicotine acetylcholine acceptor subunit CHRNA3 and lung cancer susceptibility. Molecular Medicine Reports, 6, 1389-1392.

Shmulewitz, D.; Meyers, J. L.; Wall, M. M.; Aharonovich, E.; Frisch, A.; Spivak, B. et al. (2016). CHRNA5/A3/B4 variant rs3743078 and nicotine-related phenotypes: indirect effects through nicotine craving. Journal of Studies on Alcohol and Drugs, 77(2), 227-237.

Shorey-Kendrick, L. E.; Ford, M. M.; Allen, D. C.; Kuryatov, A.; Lindstrom, J.; Wilhelm, L. et al. (2015). Nicotinic receptors in nonhuman primates: Analysis of genetic and functional conservation with humans. Neuropharmacology, 96(Pt B), 163-173.

Vernallis, A. B.; Conroy, W. G.; Berg, D. K. (1993). Neurons assemble acetylcholine receptors with as many as three kinds of subunits while maintaining subunit segregation among receptor subtypes. Neuron, 10(3), 451-464.

Walsh, H.; Govind, A. P.; Mastro, R.; Hoda, J. C.; Bertrand, D.; Vallejo, Y. et al. (2008). Upregulation of nicotinic receptors by nicotine varies with receptor subtype. The Journal of Biological Chemistry, 283, 6022-6032.

Wang, F.; Gerzanich, V.; Wells, G. B.; Anand, R.; Peng, X.; Keyser, K. et al. (1996). Assembly of human neuronal nicotinic receptor alpha5 subunits with alpha3, beta2 and beta4 subunits. The Journal of Biological Chemistry, 271, 17656-17665.

Wang, F.; Nelson, M. E.; Kuryatov, A.; Olale, F.; Cooper, J.; Keyser, K. et al. (1998). Chronic nicotine treatment up-regulates human alpha3 beta2 but not alpha3 beta4 acetylcholine receptors stably transfectedin human embryonic kidney cells. The Journal of Biological Chemistry, 273, 28721-28732.

Wu, X. Y.; Zhou, S. Y.; Niu, Z. Z.; Liu, T.; Xie, C. B.; Chen, W. Q. (2015). CHRNA3 rs6495308 genotype as an effect modifier of the association between daily cigarette consumption and hypertension in Chinese male smokers. International Journal of Environmental Research and Public Health, 12, 4156-4169.

Xiao, M.; Chen, L.; Wu, X.; Wen, F. (2014). The association between the rs6495309 polymorphism in CHRNA3 gene and lung cancer risk in Chinese: a meta-analysis. Scientific Reports, 4, 6372.

Xu, W.; Orr-Urtreger, A.; Nigro, F.; Gelber, S.; Sutcliffe, C. B.; Armstrong, D. et al. (1999). Multiorgan autonomic dysfunction in mice lacking the beta2 and the beta4 subunits of neuronal nicotinic acetylcholine receptors. The Journal of Neuroscience, 19, 9298-9305.

Yang, L.; Qiu, F.; Lu, X.; Huang, D.; Ma, G.; Guo, Y. (2012). Functional polymorphisms of CHRNA3 predict risks of chronic obstructive pulmonary disease and lung cancer in Chinese. PLoS ONE, 7(10). e46071.

Yates, S. L.; Bencherif, M.; Fluhler, E. N.; Lippiello, P. M. (1995). Upregulation of nicotinic acetylcholine receptors following chronic exposure of rats to mainstream cigarette smoke or alpha 4 beta 2receptors to nicotine. Biochemical Pharmacology, 50, 2001-2008.

Zhou, W.; Geng, T.; Wang, H.; Xun, X.; Feng, T.; Zou, H. et al. (2015). CHRNA3 genetic polymorphism and the risk of lung cancer in the Chinese Han smoking population. Tumour Biology, 36, 4987-4992.

31
烟碱成瘾和 α4β2* 烟碱乙酰胆碱受体

John J. Maurer[1,2], *Heath D. Schmidt*[2,3]

1. Pharmacology Graduate Group, Perelman School of Medicine, University of Pennsylvania, Philadelphia, PA, United States
2. Department of Biobehavioral Health Sciences, School of Nursing, University of Pennsylvania, Philadelphia, PA, United States
3. Department of Psychiatry, Perelman School of Medicine, University of Pennsylvania, Philadelphia, PA, United States

缩略语

dFBr	去甲酰氟溴胺	**nAChR**	烟碱乙酰胆碱受体
DhβE	二氢-*β*-刺桐啶碱	**PAM**	正变构调节剂
NAcc	伏隔核	**VTA**	腹侧被盖区

31.1 引言

烟草和大多数电子烟中主要的精神活性化合物是烟碱,它在烟碱乙酰胆碱受体(nAChR)上起非选择性激动剂的作用。神经元nAChR是五聚体配体离子通道,可以是由α(α2~α6)和β(β2~β4)亚基的各种组合组成的异聚蛋白复合物,也可以是由α7亚基组成的同聚蛋白复合物。单个nAChR的化学计量关系赋予每种受体亚型不同的药代动力学特性(Le Novere, Corringer, Changeux, 2002)。

神经元nAChR最丰富的亚型是由α4和β2子基组成(α4β2* nAChR,其中星号表示nAChR包含指定的亚基,但确切的化学计量数仍然保留)(Flores et al. 1992)。在全脑均有表达包括中脑边缘的多巴胺系统,这是一个神经元网络,调节所有主要的药物滥用的强化和奖励效应(Tuesta, Fowler, Kenny, 2011)。烟碱对腹侧被盖区(VTA)多巴胺神经元的刺激作用向伏隔核(NAcc)传递阳性信号,介导了烟碱的强化作用(Corrigall, Franklin, Coen, Clarke, 1992)。事实上,直接将烟碱注入VTA会增加NAcc中多巴胺的释放(Ferrari, Le Novere et al. 2002)。烟碱激活中伏隔核多巴胺投射的能力是复杂的,依赖于VTA多巴胺和GABA神经元上表达的α4β2* nAChR(Mameli-Engvall et al. 2006)(图31.1)。

值得注意的是,谷氨酸在大脑中的传递在尼古丁成瘾中也起着关键作用(Li et al. 2014)。具体来说,烟碱激活突触前7 nAChRs,增加腹侧被盖区谷氨酸的释放,刺激中脑多巴胺神经元(Mansvelder, McGehee, 2000)(图31.1)。烟碱的增强作用是通过实验动物和人类使用药物自给药模式来测量的(O'Dell, Khroyan, 2009)。在所有烟碱成瘾动物模型中,烟碱的自给药程度最高,主要是因为它模拟了人类主动吸烟(O'Dell, Khroyan, 2009)。因此,药物自给药模式是主要研究啮齿类动物主动吸烟和寻找烟碱的神经机制的重要组成部分(Rose, Corrigall, 1997; Tuesta et al.

2011）。在人类受试者的烟碱自给药研究中通常调查吸烟行为，但大多数对啮齿动物的烟碱自给药研究涉及在操作反应（例如，按压杠杆或戳鼻）后立即进行静脉注射。使用静脉内自给药主要是因为这一途径模拟了动脉烟碱的快速上升和烟碱快速分布到大脑的过程，这是通过人体典型的肺部途径暴露的（Gourlay, Benowitz, 1997）。自服用烟碱的动物血浆烟碱水平与人类吸烟者相似，进一步验证了这一烟碱成瘾动物模型（Shoaib, Stolerman, 1999）。此外，啮齿类动物自服用烟碱再现了在人类吸烟者中观察到的一些神经元适应。例如，在自服用烟碱的啮齿动物（Gaimarri et al. 2007）和吸烟的人类（Staley et al.2006）的大脑中，α4和β2 nAChR亚基的表达增加。此外，与改变烟碱自给药和戒烟药物的有效性相关的预测效度似乎相对较高（Lerman et al. 2007）。

吸烟复发的典型模型是在动物中使用自给药/消失/恢复范式。同样的刺激（例如，压力、再次暴露于与药物相关的线索，以及再次暴露于烟碱本身）在人类戒断期间导致吸烟复发，也可以用来恢复啮齿动物寻找烟碱的行为（Stoker, Markou, 2015）。在烟碱自给药消失后，全身烟碱注射和/或之前与烟碱服用配对的线索恢复了啮齿类动物在缺乏烟碱强化时的操作反应（Stoker, Markou, 2015）。烟碱恢复模型作为体内药物筛查的有效性似乎有利于吸烟复发（Epstein et al. 2006）。

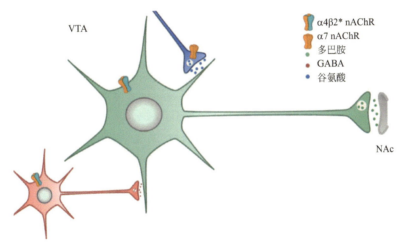

图 31.1　烟碱激活了 α4 β2* 和 α7 nAChR

烟碱还能激活VTA中GABA能神经元突触上表达的α4β2* nAChR。此外，烟碱激活VTA谷氨酸末端的突触前α7 nAChR。由于α4β2* nAChR对GABA中间神经元脱敏快，烟碱对VTA多巴胺细胞放电的影响主要是由于α4β2* nAChR对多巴胺神经元的激活和增强了VTA谷氨酸信号通路。

在此，我们讨论了α4β2* nAChR在烟碱增强作用中的作用。具体来说，我们回顾了支持α4β2* nAChR在烟碱自给药和烟碱寻求行为恢复中发挥关键作用的文献。

31.2　α4β2* nAChR在烟碱自给药和恢复中的作用

α4β2* nAChR拮抗剂已被证明可减弱啮齿动物的烟碱摄入和寻找。Corrigall和Coen首次证明，全身灌注非竞争性和非选择性的nAChR拮抗剂美加明减少了大鼠自愿烟碱摄入（Corrigall, Coen, 1989）。这些结果被许多实验室重复，清楚地表明烟碱的强化作用是由nAChR的激活介导的。与这些结果一致的是，甲胺降低了烟碱恢复，这表明对nAChR的药物抑制可能会减少戒烟者的吸烟复发（Liu et al. 2007）。在此基础上，对甲胺作为一种抗吸烟药物进行了研究。临床试验表明，甲胺在减少吸烟行为和促进戒烟方面有一定的功效（Tennant Jr. et al. 1984）。然而，不良反应限制了甲胺在人类中的临床应用（Tennant Jr. et al. 1984）。

亚型选择性nAChR拮抗剂的发展为研究单个nAChR亚型在烟碱强化中的作用提供了机会。全身给药二氢-β-刺桐啶碱（DhβE），一种竞争性的nAChR拮抗剂，对α4β2* nAChR具有中度选择性（Williams, Robinson, 1984），可减少大鼠烟碱自给药（Watkins et al. 1999）。与这些效应相一致的是，直接向VTA中注入DHβE可减少自愿烟碱摄入，表明VTA中α4β2* nAChR在烟碱强化中发挥关键作用（Corrigall et al. 1994）。综上所述，这些发现提供了强有力的药理学证据，支持α4β2* nAChR在烟碱摄入和烟碱寻求行为中的作用。

31.3 含β2的nAChR在烟碱自给药中的作用

基因工程小鼠的发展允许在体内研究单个nAChR亚基在动物烟碱成瘾模型中的功能作用。与野生型对照组相比，缺乏β2 nAChR亚基的突变小鼠，烟碱给药后，VTA多巴胺神经元的基础放电率、烟碱诱发的多巴胺细胞放电和NAcc中细胞外多巴胺的释放都降低了（Mameli-Engvall et al.2006; Picciotto et al. 1998; Zhou, Liang, Dani, 2001）。关于主动给药，β2基因敲除小鼠不会主动去获取烟碱（Epping-Jordan et al. 1999; Orejarena et al. 2012; Picciotto et al. 1998）。此外，与野生型小鼠不同，β2基因敲除小鼠不会将烟碱直接注入VTA，这表明VTA中含有β2的nAChR是烟碱的正增强作用所必需的（Besson et al. 2006）。重要的是，病毒介导的VTA中β2亚基的再表达恢复了NAcc中烟碱诱发的多巴胺释放和烟碱自给药（Maskos et al. 2005; Orejarena et al. 2012; Pons et al. 2008）。总的来说，这些发现支持了含有β2的nAChR在烟碱强化中的关键作用，并表明这种受体群体是烟碱自给药所必需的。

31.4 含α4的nAChR在烟碱自给药中的作用

与β2基因敲除小鼠类似，缺乏α4 nAChR亚基的突变小鼠也未能显示NAc中烟碱诱发的多巴胺释放增加（Marubio et al. 2003）。此外，含有α4的nAChR对烟碱诱导的VTA多巴胺神经元的突发放电是必需的（Exley et al. 2011）。由于α4β2* nAChR在VTA中大量表达（Klink et al. 2001），以及来自β2基因敲除小鼠的发现表明，α4β2* nAChR对烟碱成瘾至关重要。然而，在烟碱自给药中检测含α4的nAChR的研究是混合的。一份初步报告表明，缺乏α4亚基的突变小鼠在一次操作试验期间未能获得烟碱自给药（Pons et al. 2008）。病毒介导的这些基因敲除小鼠VTA中α4亚基的再表达恢复了烟碱的自给药，这表明含有α4的nAChR在烟碱强化中起着重要作用（Pons et al. 2008）。相比之下，最近的一项研究表明，α4亚基的组成性敲除对反复烟碱自我给药没有影响，说明含有α4的nAChR不参与烟碱摄入（Cahir et al. 2011）。这些不一致的发现可能是由于研究方法上的差异。在Pons等（2008）最初的研究中，小鼠在一个单一的烟碱自给药测试过程中受到限制，以保存其尾静脉中植入的临时导管。这是一个重大的困惑，因为约束会使小鼠被迫朝向操纵杆，并且只允许一次自给药试验。Cahir等（2011）的研究使用了一种更传统的药物自给药模式，即小鼠通过留置颈静脉导管自给药烟碱，这允许重复测试。表达突变α4亚基的转基因小鼠也被开发出来，以研究含有α4的nAChR在烟碱成瘾中的作用。第一只α4转基因小鼠是通过单点突变产生的，在α4亚基的假定成孔结构域内，氨基酸残基9处的亮氨酸被丙氨酸（L9A）取代，使含α4的nAChR对烟碱过敏（Tapper et al. 2004）。这些转基因小鼠在阈下剂量下对烟碱的奖赏效应具有更高的敏感性，从而在野生型小鼠中产生增强效应（Tapper et al. 2004）。开发了第二线超敏α4转基因小鼠，其中α4亚基中氨基酸残基248处的丝氨酸被苯丙氨酸（S248F）取代（Cahir et al. 2011）。与野生型小鼠相比，这些转基因小鼠在较低的烟碱剂量下自给予更多烟碱。（Cahir et al. 2011）。最后，最近的一项研究表明，成年小鼠VTA中α4亚基的条件性缺失增加了相对高剂量烟碱的自给药，这表明含α4的nAChR可能会介导较高单位剂量烟碱的厌恶效应（Peng et al. 2017）。总的来说，这些研究表明，在自愿服用烟碱的过程中，含α4的nAChR具有复杂的调节作用。

31.5 α4β2* nAChR部分激动剂在烟碱自给药和恢复中的作用

基于α4β2* nAChR在调节烟碱强化中的作用，它们被确定为开发戒烟药物疗法的分子靶点。nAChR激动剂替代烟碱的强化作用，缓解与烟碱戒断相关的一些不良症状，并且通常耐受性良好（Dwoskin et al. 2009）。虽然烟碱替代疗法一直是戒烟药物疗法的主流，但α4β2* nAChR的部分激动剂作为治疗吸烟复发的潜在疗法已越来越受到关注。与完全激动剂相比，部分激动剂产生的nAChR刺激低于最大值，因此替代烟碱的强化作用，滥用可能性较小。nAChR的部分激动剂也起到拮抗剂的作用，因为它们减少了烟碱强化和大脑中烟碱释放的神经递质（Dwoskin et al. 2009）。

基于其作为α4β2* nAChR部分激动剂的功能，伐伦克林被合理设计为一种戒烟药物（Coe et al. 2005）。作为一种部分激动剂，伐伦克林可单独增加NAcc中的多巴胺释放（最大烟碱反应的60%），并减少NAcc中烟碱诱发的多巴胺释放（Coe et al. 2005）。在缺乏β2亚基的突变小鼠中没有这些作用，这表明伐伦克林对烟碱强化的作用是通过激活大脑中含有β2的nAChR来介导的（Reprant et al. 2010）。在药物鉴别研究中，伐伦克林完全替代烟碱，并减弱了啮齿类动物自服用烟碱的能力（Coe et al. 2005; Le Foll et al. 2012; O'Connor et al. 2010）。此外，伐伦克林减弱了烟碱寻求行为的恢复（Le Foll et al. 2012; O'Connor et al. 2010），这表明伐伦克林可能减少人类吸烟者的吸烟复发。与这些临床前研究结果一致，临床试验表明，与安慰剂治疗的对照组相比，使用伐伦克林治疗的吸烟者的戒断率更高（Gonzales et al. 2006）。尽管有这些结果，伐伦克林在促进长期禁欲方面的效果并不明显（Cahill et al. 2014）。

此外，不良反应限制了患者的依从性（Gonzales et al. 2006）。伐伦克林也作为α7 nAChR的全激动剂和α3β4* 与α6* nAChR的部分激动剂，这可能是其副作用的原因（Mihalak et al. 2006）。最近，人们将伐伦克林与烟碱替代法进行了比较。在戒烟方面，发现两种疗法之间没有区别，这就提出了伐伦克林相对有效性的质疑（Baker et al. 2016）。

伐伦克林和烟碱增加了大脑中α4β2* nAChR的表达，被认为是有助于持续吸烟行为和吸烟复发（Hussmann et al. 2012）。因此，最近的研究主要集中在开发不增加大脑中nAChR表达的α4β2* nAChR的部分激动剂上。沙氮替丁-A被设计为一种部分激动剂，与伐伦克林相比，它对α4β2* nAChR具有更高的亲和力和选择性（Xiao et al. 2006）。沙氮替丁-A已被证明可以减少烟碱的自给药（Levin et al. 2010）。重要的是，与烟碱和伐伦克林相反，沙氮替丁-A不会增加大脑中nAChR的表达（Hussmann et al. 2012）。如果α4β2* nAChR表达增加是一种神经适应性反应，促进了吸烟复发并限制了伐伦克林的戒烟效果，那么不增加α4β2* nAChR表达的部分激动剂如沙氮替丁-A可能是更有效的戒烟药物。不幸的是，老鼠会自服用沙氮替丁-A，这表明人类有滥用的倾向（Paterson et al. 2010）。因此，沙氮替丁-A还没有在临床试验中进行测试。最近已经开发出更有效的沙氮替丁-A类似物，包括VMY-2-95，用于戒烟（Yenugonda et al. 2013）。反复给药VMY-2-95会减少大鼠的烟碱自给药（Rezvani et al.2017; Yenugonda et al. 2013）。VMY-2-95跨越血脑屏障，具有较长的半衰期，并且可以口服，使其成为临床试验的良好候选药物（Kong et al. 2015）。然而，目前尚不清楚VMY-2-95是否有滥用倾向，或是否增加了大脑中α4β2* nAChR的表达。研究人员继续扩大这些研究，并发现α4β2* nAChR的新型部分激动剂，可能防止吸烟渴望和复发（Lee et al. 2014）。

31.6　α4β2* nAChR在烟碱成瘾和恢复中的正变构调节作用

另一种开发新型戒烟药物的方法集中在α4β2* nAChR的正变构调节剂（PAM）上。PAM与nAChR结合的变构位点不同于烟碱的正构体结合位点。因此，PAM在没有乙酰胆碱或烟碱的情况下具有较低的内在活性（Uteshev, 2014）。通过提高受体活性和烟碱诱导通道打开的概率，PAM可以实质上增加和延长α4β2* nAChR对烟草烟雾中烟碱的反应（Williams et al. 2011）。基于这一独特的药理作用机制，α4β2* nAChR的PAM可通过增强单位剂量较低烟碱的强化作用，减少烟碱的消耗量，类似于高剂量的烟碱（Maurer et al. 2017）。事实上，一个新兴的文献支持这一假设。α4β2* nAChR的PAM包括去甲酰氟溴胺（dFBr）和加兰他敏（也作为胆碱酯酶抑制剂）减少了烟碱自给药和烟碱恢复（Hopkins et al. 2012; Liu, 2013）。与它们的作用机制相一致，α4β2* nAChR的PAM自身不产生增强作用，也不产生类似烟碱的歧视刺激效应，表明人类滥用倾向的可能性较低（Liu, 2013; Mohler et al. 2014）。这些临床前研究是最近一项转化研究的基础，该研究表明加兰他敏治疗后吸烟者烟碱摄入量减少（Ashare et al. 2016）。这一临床试验具有挑衅性，因为它表明α4β2* nAChR的PAM可能有利于人类戒烟。

虽然dFBr和加兰他敏选择性地与α4β2* nAChR结合，但它们不能区分由不同比例的α4β2亚基组成的α4β2* nAChR亚型（Williams et al. 2011）。α4β2* nAChR组合成两个化学计量和功能上不同的组合，以α4：β2亚基比为特征（图31.2）。2(α4)3(β2)和3(α4)2(β2) nAChR亚型分别代表对乙酰胆碱高灵敏度或低灵敏度的通道（Moroni et al. 2006）。烟碱和伐伦克林可以结合并激活α4β2 nAChR高敏感性和低敏感性群体，尽管二者具有不同的效力和结合亲和力（Moroni et al. 2006）。虽然这些发现与烟碱和伐伦克林治疗效果的相关性尚不清楚，但它提出了一个有趣的可能性，即仅针对高或低敏感性α4β2 nAChR的化合物可能是更有效的抗吸烟药物。最近，选择性地结合低敏感性3(α4)2(β2) nAChR的PAM已被识别，并首次有机会识别3(α4)2(β2) nAChR亚型在烟碱成瘾中的精确作用（Grupe et al. 2013; Timmermann et al. 2012）。NS9283，一种低敏感性3(α4)2(β2) nAChR的化学计量学选择性PAM，可减弱大鼠烟碱自给药和恢复（Maurer et al. 2017）。NS9283本身并不支持自给药行为（Maurer et al. 2017），也不会产生类似于烟碱的主观效应（Mohler et al. 2014），这表明在人类中没有潜在的滥用倾向。这些结果提出了一个有趣的可能性，即靶向低敏感性 3(α4)2(β2) nAChR 的 PAM 可能会减少人类的慢性吸烟行为和复发。

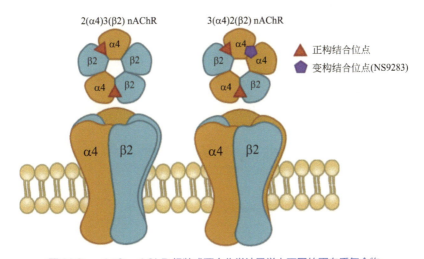

图 31.2　α4 β2* nAChR 组装成两个化学计量学上不同的蛋白质复合物

其特征为 α4：β2 亚基比针对一个人群的 α4β2 nAChR 可能对戒烟治疗更有效。

31.7　对治疗和结论的影响

大量证据清楚地表明，α4β2* nAChR 在烟碱强化中发挥了重要作用，并支持药物发现方法，旨在识别针对 α4β2* nAChR 的戒烟新药物疗法。由于 α4β2* nAChR 的部分激动剂已被证明对吸烟复发有中等疗效，最近的方法集中于 α4β2* nAChR 的 PAMs 和化学计量选择性 α4β2 nAChR 化合物。进一步了解特定 α4β2 nAChR 群体在烟碱成瘾中的作用将有助于开发更有效的药物。准确定义 α4β2 nAChR 在促进烟碱介导行为的神经回路中表达的化学计量将是改进现有靶向 α4β2* nAChR 的药物的关键。

术语解释

- **自给药实验**：当配对或有条件地注入一种正增强的药物时，动物将完成一个操作反应（即杠杆按压）。一种药物的增强功效可以通过这种自愿服药的模型来确定。
- **中脑边缘多巴胺系统**：中脑边缘多巴胺系统是药物滥用的首要目标。这个系统起源于腹侧背盖区（VTA）产生多巴胺的神经元，这些神经元投射到包括伏隔核在内的前脑区域。一般来说，所有滥用的药物都会激活中脑边缘多巴胺系统，从而增加伏隔核中的多巴胺信号。
- **受体亚基和亚型**：nAChR 是一种蛋白质复合物，由五个不同的亚基包围一个中央孔。nAChR 的亚基组成各不相同，导致许多不同的受体亚型。由于每个 nAChR 亚型都有不同的特性，因此确定每个 nAChR 亚型在烟碱成瘾中的作用是很有意义的。
- **药物寻求行为**：吸烟复发的恢复可以用恢复范式在实验动物中建模。受试者获得稳定的烟碱自给药后，停止服用烟碱。在这段戒断期间，寻求烟碱的行为可以由促使人类吸烟复发的相同刺激引起（即再次暴露于烟碱和/或与自愿吸烟有关的条件提示）。
- **化学计量数**：受体复合物中亚基的确切数目（或比例）称为受体的化学计量数。例如，α4β2* nAChR 由 5 个不同组合的 α 和 β 亚基组成。确切的组合，无论是 3α-2β 与 2α-3β 的比值，都赋予不同的药代动力学特性和功能。

烟碱自给药的关键事实

- 实验室的动物包括非人类的灵长类动物、狗和啮齿类动物可以自给药。
- 静脉注射烟碱是最常见的自给药途径。然而，一些研究调查了自给药的烟碱在饮用水，吸入烟碱/烟草蒸气，或直接注入大脑。
- 自给药烟碱的动机是通过渐进比率强化计划来研究的。简单地说，随后每一次注入烟碱的反应需求都呈指数增长。最终，动物放弃了，而这个断点被用来衡量服用药物的动机，或者动物为了获得药物奖励愿意付出多大的努力。
- 当获得一定剂量的烟碱时，啮齿动物会根据倒"U"形剂量反应曲线自行给药烟碱。剂量-反应曲线的形状反映了烟碱的竞争性奖励（上升肢）和厌恶（下降肢）特性。
- 烟碱自给药被认为是一种可靠的、与自愿吸食烟碱相似的模式，因为它模拟了人类烟碱消费的行为（自愿吸食）和生理（维持稳定的烟碱血浆水平）两个方面。

要点总结

- α4β2* nAChR在烟碱成瘾中扮演重要角色。
- 烟碱的增强作用主要是由大脑中的α4β2* nAChR介导的。α4β2* nAChR在全脑表达，包括中脑边缘多巴胺系统。
- 在啮齿类动物和人类中，部分受体激动剂能减弱烟碱的自愿吸收，但在促进长期戒烟方面效果不明显。
- 开发新型戒烟药物的新方法主要集中在α4β2* nAChR的正变构调节剂（PAM）和针对α4β2 nAChR亚型的化学计量选择性化合物。

参考文献

Ashare, R. L.; Kimmey, B. A.; Rupprecht, L. E.; Bowers, M. E.; Hayes, M. R.; Schmidt, H. D. (2016). Repeated administration of an acetylcholinesterase inhibitor attenuates nicotine taking in rats and smoking behavior in human smokers. Translational Psychiatry, 6, e713.

Baker, T. B.; Piper, M. E.; Stein, J. H.; Smith, S. S.; Bolt, D. M.; Fraser, D. L. et al. (2016). Effects of nicotine patch vs varenicline vs combination nicotine replacement therapy on smoking cessation at 26 weeks: a randomized clinical trial. JAMA, 315(4), 371-379.

Besson, M.; David, V.; Suarez, S.; Cormier, A.; Cazala, P.; Changeux, J. P. et al. (2006). Genetic dissociation of two behaviors associated with nicotine addiction: beta-2 containing nicotinic receptors are involved in nicotine reinforcement but not in withdrawal syndrome. Psychopharmacology, 187(2), 189-199.

Cahill, K.; Stevens, S.; Lancaster, T. (2014). Pharmacological treatments for smoking cessation. JAMA, 311(2), 193-194.

Cahir, E.; Pillidge, K.; Drago, J.; Lawrence, A. J. (2011). The necessity of alpha4* nicotinic receptors in nicotine-driven behaviors: dissociation between reinforcing and motor effects of nicotine. Neuropsychopharmacology, 36(7), 1505-1517.

Coe, J. W.; Brooks, P. R.; Vetelino, M. G.; Wirtz, M. C.; Arnold, E. P.; Huang, J. et al. (2005). Varenicline: an alpha4beta2 nicotinic receptor partial agonist for smoking cessation. Journal of Medicinal Chemistry, 48(10), 3474-3477.

Corrigall, W. A.; Coen, K. M. (1989). Nicotine maintains robust self-administration in rats on a limited-access schedule. Psychopharmacology, 99(4), 473-478.

Corrigall, W. A.; Coen, K. M.; Adamson, K. L. (1994). Self-administered nicotine activates the mesolimbic dopamine system through the ventral tegmental area. Brain Research, 653(1-2), 278-284.

Corrigall, W. A.; Franklin, K. B.; Coen, K. M.; Clarke, P. B. (1992). The mesolimbic dopaminergic system is implicated in the reinforcing effects of nicotine. Psychopharmacology, 107(2-3), 285-289.

Dwoskin, L. P.; Pivavarchyk, M.; Joyce, B. M.; Neugebauer, N. M.; Zheng, G.; Zhang, Z. et al. (2009). Targeting reward-relevant nicotinic receptors in the discovery of novel pharmacotherapeutic agents to treat tobacco dependence. Nebraska Symposium on Motivation, 55, 31-63.

Epping-Jordan, M. P.; Picciotto, M. R.; Changeux, J. P.; Pich, E. M. (1999). Assessment of nicotinic acetylcholine receptor subunit contributions to nicotine self-administration in mutant mice. Psychopharmacology, 147(1), 25-26.

Epstein, D. H.; Preston, K. L.; Stewart, J.; Shaham, Y. (2006). Toward a model of drug relapse: an assessment of the validity of the reinstatement procedure. Psychopharmacology, 189(1), 1-16.

Exley, R.; Maubourguet, N.; David, V.; Eddine, R.; Evrard, A.; Pons, S. et al. (2011). Distinct contributions of nicotinic acetylcholine receptor subunit alpha4 and subunit alpha6 to the reinforcing effects of nicotine. Proceedings of the National Academy of Sciences of the United States of America, 108(18), 7577-7582.

Ferrari, R.; Le Novere, N.; Picciotto, M. R.; Changeux, J. P.; Zoli, M. (2002). Acute and long-term changes in the mesolimbic dopamine pathway after systemic or local single nicotine injections. The European Journal of Neuroscience, 15(11), 1810-1818.

Flores, C. M.; Rogers, S. W.; Pabreza, L. A.; Wolfe, B. B.; Kellar, K. J. (1992). A subtype of nicotinic cholinergic receptor in rat brainis composed of alpha 4 and beta 2 subunits and is up-regulatedby chronic nicotine treatment. Molecular Pharmacology, 41(1), 31-37.

Gaimarri, A.; Moretti, M.; Riganti, L.; Zanardi, A.; Clementi, F.; Gotti, C. (2007). Regulation of neuronal nicotinic receptor traffic and expression. Brain Research Reviews, 55(1), 134-143.

Gonzales, D.; Rennard, S. I.; Nides, M.; Oncken, C.; Azoulay, S.; Billing, C. B. et al. (2006). Varenicline, an alpha4beta2 nicotinic acetylcholine receptor partial agonist, vs sustained-release bupropion and placebo for smoking cessation: a randomized controlled trial. JAMA, 296(1), 47-55.

Gourlay, S. G.; Benowitz, N. L. (1997). Arteriovenous differences in plasma concentration of nicotine and catecholamines and related cardiovascular effects after smoking, nicotine nasal spray, and intravenous nicotine. Clinical Pharmacology and Therapeutics, 62(4), 453-463.

Grupe, M.; Jensen, A. A.; Ahring, P. K.; Christensen, J. K.; Grunnet, M. (2013). Unravelling the mechanism of action ofNS9283, a positive allosteric modulator of (alpha4)3(beta2)2 nicotinic ACh receptors. British Journal of Pharmacology, 168(8), 2000-2010.

Hopkins, T. J.; Rupprecht, L. E.; Hayes, M. R.; Blendy, J. A.; Schmidt, H. D. (2012). Galantamine, an acetylcholinesterase inhibitorand positive allosteric modulator of nicotinic acetylcholine receptors, attenuates nicotine taking and seeking in rats. Neuropsychopharmacology, 37(10), 2310-2321.

Hussmann, G. P.; Turner, J. R.; Lomazzo, E.; Venkatesh, R.; Cousins, V.; Xiao, Y. et al. (2012). Chronic sazetidine-A at behaviorally active doses does not increase nicotinic cholinergic receptors in rodent brain. The Journal of Pharmacology and Experimental Therapeutics 343(2), 441-450.

Klink, R.; de Kerchove d'Exaerde, A.; Zoli, M.; Changeux, J. P. (2001). Molecular and physiological diversity of nicotinic acetylcholine receptors in the midbrain dopaminergic nuclei. The Journal of Neuroscience, 21(5), 1452-1463.

Kong, H.; Song, J. K.; Yenugonda, V. M.; Zhang, L.; Shuo, T.; Cheema, A. K. et al. (2015). Preclinical studies of the potent and selective nicotinic alpha4beta2 receptor ligand VMY-2-95. Molecular Pharmaceutics, 12(2), 393-402.

Le Foll, B.; Chakraborty-Chatterjee, M.; Lev-Ran, S.; Barnes, C. Pushparaj, A.; Gamaleddin, I. et al. (2012). Varenicline decreases nicotine self-administration and cue-induced reinstatement of nicotine-seeking behaviour in rats when a long pretreatment time is used. The International Journal of Neuropsychopharmacology, 15(9), 1265-1274.

Le Novere, N.; Corringer, P. J.; Changeux, J. P. (2002). The diversity ofsubunit composition in nAChRs: evolutionary origins, physiologicand pharmacologic consequences. Journal of Neurobiology, 53(4), 447-456.

Lee, A. M.; Arreola, A. C.; Kimmey, B. A.; Schmidt, H. D. (2014). Administration of the nicotinic acetylcholine receptor agonistsABT-089 and ABT-107 attenuates the reinstatement of nicotine-seeking behavior in rats. Behavioural Brain Research, 274, 168-175.

Lerman, C.; LeSage, M. G.; Perkins, K. A.; O'Malley, S. S.; Siegel, S. J.; Benowitz, N. L. et al. (2007). Translational research in medication development for nicotine dependence. Nature Reviews. Drug Discovery, 6(9), 746-762.

Levin, E. D.; Rezvani, A. H.; Xiao, Y.; Slade, S.; Cauley, M.; Wells, C. et al. (2010). Sazetidine-A, a selective alpha4beta2 nicotinic receptor desensitizing agent and partial agonist, reduces nicotine self-administration in rats. The Journal of Pharmacology and Experimental Therapeutics, 332(3), 933-939.

Li, X.; Semenova, S.; D'Souza, M. S.; Stoker, A. K.; Markou, A. (2014). Involvement of glutamatergic and GABAergic systems in nicotine dependence: Implications for novel pharmacotherapies for smoking cessation. Neuropharmacology, 76(Pt B), 554-565.

Liu, X. (2013). Positive allosteric modulation of alpha4beta2 nicotinic acetylcholine receptors as a new approach to smoking reduction: evidence from a rat model of nicotine self-administration. Psychopharmacology, 230(2), 203-213.

Liu, X.; Palmatier, M. I.; Caggiula, A. R.; Donny, E. C.; Sved, A. F. (2007). Reinforcement enhancing effect of nicotine and its attenuation by nicotinic antagonists in rats. Psychopharmacology, 194(4), 463-473.

Mameli-Engvall, M.; Evrard, A.; Pons, S.; Maskos, U.; Svensson, T. H.; Changeux, J. P. et al. (2006). Hierarchical control of dopamine neuron-firing patterns by nicotinic receptors. Neuron, 50(6), 911-921.

Mansvelder, H. D.; McGehee, D. S. (2000). Long-term potentiation ofexcitatory inputs to brain reward areas by nicotine. Neuron, 27(2), 349-357.

Marubio, L. M.; Gardier, A. M.; Durier, S.; David, D.; Klink, R.; ArroyoJimenez, M. M. et al. (2003). Effects of nicotine in the dopaminergic system of mice lacking the alpha4 subunit of neuronal nicotinic acetylcholine receptors. The European Journal of Neuroscience, 17(7), 1329-1337.

Maskos, U.; Molles, B. E.; Pons, S.; Besson, M.; Guiard, B. P.; Guilloux, J. P. et al. (2005). Nicotine reinforcement and cognition restored by targeted expression of nicotinic receptors. Nature, 436(7047), 103-107.

Maurer, J. J.; Sandager-Nielsen, K.; Schmidt, H. D. (2017). Attenuationof nicotine taking and seeking in rats by the stoichiometry-selective alpha4beta2 nicotinic acetylcholine receptor positive allosteric modulator NS9283. Psychopharmacology, 234(3), 475-484.

Mihalak, K. B.; Carroll, F. I.; Luetje, C. W. (2006). Varenicline is a partial agonist at alpha4beta2 and a full agonist at alpha7 neuronal nicotinic receptors. Molecular Pharmacology, 70(3), 801-805.

Mohler, E. G.; Franklin, S. R.; Rueter, L. E. (2014). Discriminativestimulus effects of NS9283, a nicotinic alpha4beta2* positive allosteric modulator, in nicotine-discriminating rats. Psychopharmacology, 231(1), 67-74.

Moroni, M.; Zwart, R.; Sher, E.; Cassels, B. K.; Bermudez, I. (2006). Alpha4beta2 nicotinic receptors with high and low acetylcholine sensitivity: pharmacology, stoichiometry, and sensitivity to long-termexposure to nicotine. Molecular Pharmacology, 70(2), 755-768.

O'Connor, E. C.; Parker, D.; Rollema, H.; Mead, A. N. (2010). Thealpha4beta2 nicotinic acetylcholine-receptor partial agonist varenicline inhibits both nicotine self-administration following repeated dosing and reinstatement of nicotine seeking in rats. Psychopharmacology, 208(3), 365-376.

O'Dell, L. E.; Khroyan, T. V. (2009). Rodent models of nicotine reward:what do they tell us about tobacco abuse in humans? Pharmacology, Biochemistry, and Behavior, 91(4), 481-488.

Orejarena, M. J.; Herrera-Solis, A.; Pons, S.; Maskos, U.; Maldonado, R.; Robledo, P. (2012). Selective re-expression of beta2 nicotinic acetylcholine receptor subunits in the ventral tegmental area of the mouse restores intravenous nicotine self-administration. Neuropharmacology, 63(2), 235-241.

Paterson, N. E.; Min, W.; Hackett, A.; Lowe, D.; Hanania, T.; Caldarone, B. et al. (2010). The high-affinity nAChR partial agonists varenicline and sazetidine-A exhibit reinforcing properties in rats. Progress in Neuro-Psychopharmacology, Biological Psychiatry, 34(8), 1455-1464.

Peng, C.; Engle, S. E.; Yan, Y.; Weera, M. M.; Berry, J. N.; Arvin, M. C. et al. (2017). Altered nicotine reward-associated behavior following alpha4 nAChR subunit deletion in ventral midbrain. PLoS ONE, 12(7). e0182142.

Picciotto, M. R.; Zoli, M.; Rimondini, R.; Lena, C.; Marubio, L. M.; Pich, E. M. et al. (1998). Acetylcholine receptors containing the β2 subunit are involved in the reinforcing properties of nicotine. Nature, 391(6663), 173-177.

Pons, S.; Fattore, L.; Cossu, G.; Tolu, S.; Porcu, E.; McIntosh, J. M. et al. (2008). Crucial role of alpha4 and alpha6 nicotinic acetylcholine receptor subunits from ventral tegmental area in systemic nicotine self-administration. The Journal of Neuroscience, 28(47), 12318-12327.

Reperant, C.; Pons, S.; Dufour, E.; Rollema, H.; Gardier, A. M.; Maskos, U. (2010). Effect of the alpha4beta2* nicotinic acetylcholinereceptor partial agonist varenicline on dopamine release in β2knock-out mice with selective re-expression of the beta2 subunit inthe ventral tegmental area. Neuropharmacology, 58(2), 346-350.

Rezvani, A. H.; Slade, S.; Wells, C.; Yenugonda, V. M.; Liu, Y.; Brown, M. L. et al. (2017). Differential efficacies of the nicotinic α4β2 desensitizing agents in reducing nicotine self-administration infemale rats. Psychopharmacology, 234(17), 2517-2523.

Rose, J. E.; Corrigall, W. A. (1997). Nicotine self-administration in animals and humans: similarities and differences. Psychopharmacology, 130(1), 28-40.

Shoaib, M.; Stolerman, I. P. (1999). Plasma nicotine and cotinine levels following intravenous nicotine self-administration in rats. Psychopharmacology, 143(3), 318-321.

Staley, J. K.; Krishnan-Sarin, S.; Cosgrove, K. P.; Krantzler, E.; Frohlich, E.; Perry, E. et al. (2006). Human tobacco smokers in early abstinence have higher levels of beta2* nicotinic acetylcholine receptors than nonsmokers. The Journal of Neuroscience, 26(34), 8707-8714.

Stoker, A. K.; Markou, A. (2015). Neurobiological bases of cue- and nicotine-induced reinstatement of nicotine seeking: implications for the development of smoking cessation medications. Current Topics in Behavioral Neurosciences, 24, 125-154.

Tapper, A. R.; McKinney, S. L.; Nashmi, R.; Schwarz, J.; Deshpande, P.; Labarca, C. et al. (2004). Nicotine activation of alpha4* receptors:sufficient for reward, tolerance, and sensitization. Science, 306(5698), 1029-1032.

Tennant, F. S.; Jr.; Tarver, A. L.; Rawson, R. A. (1984). Clinical evaluation of mecamylamine for withdrawal from nicotine dependence. NIDA Research Monograph, 49, 239-246.

Timmermann, D. B.; Sandager-Nielsen, K.; Dyhring, T.; Smith, M.; Jacobsen, A. M.; Nielsen, E. O. et al. (2012). Augmentation of cognitive function by NS9283, a stoichiometry-dependent positive allosteric modulator of alpha2- and alpha4-containing nicotinic acetylcholine receptors. British Journal of Pharmacology, 167(1), 164-182.

Tuesta, L. M.; Fowler, C. D.; Kenny, P. J. (2011). Recent advances inunderstanding nicotinic receptor signaling mechanisms that regulatedrug self-administration behavior. Biochemical Pharmacology, 82(8), 984-995.

Uteshev, V. V. (2014). The therapeutic promise of positive allosteric modulation of nicotinic receptors. European Journal of Pharmacology, 727, 181-185.

Watkins, S. S.; Epping-Jordan, M. P.; Koob, G. F.; Markou, A. (1999). Blockade of nicotine self-administration with nicotinic antagonists in rats. Pharmacology, Biochemistry, and Behavior, 62(4), 743-751.

Williams, M.; Robinson, J. L. (1984). Binding of the nicotinic cholinergic antagonist, dihydro-beta-erythroidine, to rat brain tissue. The Journal of Neuroscience, 4(12), 2906-2911.

Williams, D. K.; Wang, J.; Papke, R. L. (2011). Positive allosteric modulators as an approach to nicotinic acetylcholine receptor-targeted therapeutics: advantages and limitations. Biochemical Pharmacology, 82(8), 915-930.

Xiao, Y.; Fan, H.; Musachio, J. L.; Wei, Z. L.; Chellappan, S. K.; Kozikowski, A. P. et al. (2006). Sazetidine-A, a novel ligand that desensitizes alpha4beta2 nicotinic acetylcholine receptors without activating them. Molecular Pharmacology, 70(4), 1454-1460.

Yenugonda, V. M.; Xiao, Y.; Levin, E. D.; Rezvani, A. H.; Tran, T.; AlMuhtasib, N. et al. (2013). Design, synthesis and discovery of picomolar selective alpha4beta2 nicotinic acetylcholine receptor ligands. Journal of Medicinal Chemistry, 56(21), 8404-8421.

Zhou, F. M.; Liang, Y.; Dani, J. A. (2001). Endogenous nicotinic cholinergic activity regulates dopamine release in the striatum. Nature Neuroscience, 4(12), 1224-1229.

32

α3β4 烟碱乙酰胆碱受体和 P 物质在烟碱致敏中的作用

Branden Eggan[1], Sarah McCallum[2]

1. Department of Liberal Arts and Science, Maria College, Albany, NY, United States
2. Department of Neuroscience and Experimental Therapeutics, Albany Medical College, Albany, NY, United States

缩略语

ACh	乙酰胆碱	NAcc	伏隔核
ChAT	胆碱乙酰转移酶	NK1R	神经激肽-1受体
IPN	脚间核	VTA	腹侧被盖区
MHb	内侧缰核		

32.1 引言

α3β4 nAChR 是烟碱受体的一个亚型，在感觉神经节、自主神经节以及大脑的内侧缰核和脚间核均有密集表达。虽然α4β2 nAChR 在大脑的多巴胺奖励通路中密集表达，并已被证明直接调节烟碱成瘾和依赖（Epping-Jordan et al. 1999; Tapper et al. 2004），但包括α3β4 nAChR 在内的其他烟碱受体的作用研究还很少。人类基因组研究显示，编码α3β4 nAChR基因突变的个体不仅更有可能吸食烟碱，而且在生命早期就开始吸食烟碱（Liu et al. 2010; Schlaepfer et al. 2008）；受体亚型并不在中脑边缘通路中表达；相反，它们在被称为MHb-IPN通路的"替代奖励通路"中密集表达（Sutherland, Nakajima, 1981）。最近的动物研究主要集中在缰核nAChR在调节烟碱厌恶和戒断中的作用，而较少强调它们对烟碱奖励效应的贡献（Antolin-Fontes et al. 2015）。

32.2 MHb中α3β4 nAChR的表达

α3β4 nAChR主要表达在MHb的腹侧2/3处，这与乙酰胆碱转移酶的表达有关（ChAT; Conteablile et al. 1987; Quick et al. 1999），提示这些受体可能位于MHb内含乙酰胆碱（ACh）神经元的突触后。研究表明，ACh神经元上的α3β4 nAChR支配着MHb的功能（Quick et al.1999）。在IPN中，α3β4 nAChR位于MHb投射的ACh神经元的突触前（Grady et al. 2009）。突触体研究表明，加入α3β4 nAChR拮抗剂可减弱Ca^{2+}介导的ACh释放（Grady et al. 2001）。这些受体也可表达在IPN的GABA能中间神经元上（Lena et al. 1993），提示在MHb-IPN通讯中ACh释放的调节也可能有另一种贡献（Lena et al. 1993）。

32.3 烟碱成瘾动物模型中的α3β4 nAChR

烟碱成瘾的动物模型也证明了MHb和IPN α3β4 nAChR的重要作用。虽然MHb和IPN神经元富含含有α2～α6和β2～β4亚基的nAChR，但只有α3β4*和α3β3β4*亚型刺激才会导致随后在IPN释放ACh（Grady et al. 2009）。α5亚基与α3和β4形成功能性异构体（Groot-Kormelink et al. 2001），当被激活时，会导致IPN中谷氨酸的释放（Fowler et al. 2011）。这种谷氨酸很可能与MHb神经元中的ACh共同释放（Ren et al. 2011），并导致IPN中神经元的激活。最近，越来越多的证据支持MHb-IPN α3β4*（可能与α5）nAChR介导烟碱成瘾的负奖励成分的理论。α5 nAChR亚基的缺失降低了人们对高浓度烟碱的厌恶，这种效应被α5 nAChR亚基在MHb中的重新表达逆转（Fowler et al. 2011）。

在过表达β4受体的转基因小鼠模型中，增加α3β4* nAChR水平增强了对烟碱的厌恶，这被α5 nAChR亚基对MHb的表达逆转（Frahm et al. 2011）。此外，β4和α5 nAChR基因敲除小鼠的烟碱戒断迹象减少（Salas et al. 2004；Salas et al. 2009）。

CHRNA4/A3/B4基因组簇的转基因过表达导致β4*受体结合的显著增加和烟碱自给药的增加（Grego et al. 2012）。同时，MHb内注射α3β4* nAChR拮抗剂18-甲氧基冠醚可减少烟碱自给药和急性烟碱诱导的伏隔多巴胺增加（Glick et al. 2011；McCallum et al. 2012）。烟碱自给药也被全身注射α3β4* nAChR拮抗剂AT-1001所阻断（Toll et al. 2012），这表明这些受体的独特之处在于它们在烟碱成瘾的积极和消极奖励成分中发挥作用。

32.4 烟碱敏化：成瘾研究中的一个重要模型

烟碱敏化是成瘾研究中的一个重要模型，敏化发生在药物成瘾的初始组成部分，即偶然吸毒开始升级为寻求毒品和强迫吸毒行为（Koob, LeMoal, 1997）。任何精神刺激药物，包括烟碱，都会产生致敏反应。这一现象可以分为两个主要组成部分：归纳和表达（DiFranza, Wellman, 2007）。诱导性是从第一次使用药物开始发展起来的，但因为它强烈地依赖于药物使用的频率和剂量。在动物模型和人类中，药物表达的速度不同。致敏作用的独特之处在于它是药物使用的持久影响。对烟碱的敏感化反应可以在最后一次药物暴露后的几个月内被看到，因此，可能是复发的一个重要因素（Miller et al. 2001）。烟碱敏化模型对成瘾研究至关重要，因为它们最能反映成瘾行为初期的神经变化，而不是传统上在疾病完全显现后测量的效果。中脑边缘奖励通路中多巴胺传递的改变似乎是致敏行为的基础，特别是腹侧被盖区的神经适应（Nisell et al. 1996；Saal et al. 2003）。除了复发，在致敏过程中发生的大脑变化可能是许多吸烟者传统上看到的药物寻求的基础，特别是在戒烟期之后（Steketee, Kalivas, 2011）。

32.5 烟碱敏化的动物模型

实验上，烟碱敏化可以通过两种不同的模型来测量：行为敏化和神经化学敏化。早期的大鼠烟碱敏化模型显示，5天的烟碱注射足以诱导对烟碱的行为和神经化学敏化（Benwell, Balfour, 1992）。图32.1（a）显示了实验中使用的传统敏化模型。在这个模型中，致敏治疗组的动物每天接受一次特定剂量的烟碱挑战。对照组同时运行，以确认治疗药物对致敏反应的影响确实是由于致敏反应本身的影响，而不仅仅是整体运动或多巴胺的释放。对照组包括每天接受一次生理盐水注射的赋形剂组和急性组，接受四次生理盐水注射，然后进行为期5天的单次烟碱注射。

图32.1（b）说明了行为敏化的诱导，致敏的动物仅在烟碱攻击后30分钟的光电池活动室中

测量到的活动计数明显更高（在光电池活动室中测量的烟碱攻击后30分钟的活动计数）。对烟碱的反应很难研究。治疗的效果既可以通过诱导（在烟碱刺激的5天过程中），也可以在表达（5天的运动活动计数）上进行衡量。

神经化学敏感度可以通过体内微透析，通过测定烟碱给药后伏隔核中多巴胺的释放来测量。由于实验装置的技术性，每天很难监测多巴胺的释放，所以传统上使用表达（5天烟碱挑战）数据来分析治疗药物对神经化学敏化的影响。图32.1（c）示，在烟碱刺激5天后，致敏的多巴胺释放显著高于急性组和赋形剂对照组。

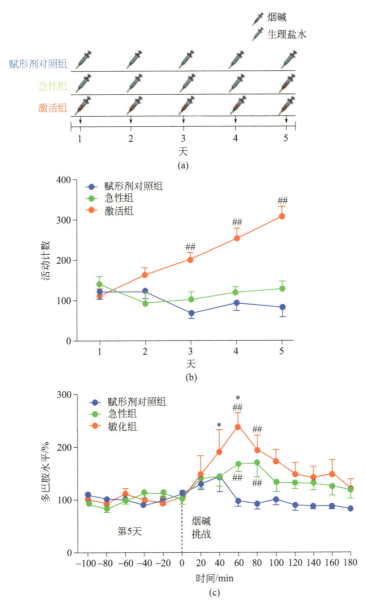

图32.1 烟碱致敏给药方案以及剂量的行为和神经化学结果

（a）传统的烟碱实验剂量方案，以引起过敏和适当的控制。每天注射一次，疗程为5天；（b）由光电池活动室测量的自由活动动物的每日活动计数增加，反映出运动敏感化；（c）神经化学敏化，通过体内微透析测量，烟碱治疗5天后伏隔区多巴胺释放增加。来自Eggan和McCallum的数据，未发布。

32.6　α3β4 nAChR在烟碱致敏中的作用

在我们实验室的一组实验中，研究了MHb α3β4 nAChR拮抗剂对烟碱运动敏化的诱导（发育）和表达（表现）的影响（Eggan, McCallum, 2016）。这些研究使用18-甲氧基冠状病毒啶、抗成瘾药物的同源物伊博格碱和非竞争性α3β4 nAChR拮抗剂（$IC_{50} = 0.75\mu mol/L$; Kuehne et al. 2003）。结果表明，烟碱给药前每日给予α3β4 nAChR拮抗剂，其增加的活动计数或运动敏化显著降低，说明α3β4 nAChR拮抗剂减弱了致敏的诱导。由于在中枢神经系统中，α3β4 nAChR主要集中在MHb，而在大脑其他区域不密集表达，推测这种作用集中于药物在该区域的作用。在致敏表达方面，从行为学和神经化学两个方面观察了α3β4 nAChR拮抗剂对MHb的影响。在对烟碱敏感的动物中，当MHbα3β4 nAChR通过MHb全身阻断或经MHb内阻断时，敏化的运动效应显著降低。同样地，当非竞争性的α3β4 nAChR和α-芋螺毒素AuIB（$IC_{50} = 0.75\mu mol/L$; Luo et al. 1998）注射到MHb中时，运动敏感化也被减弱。这些数据支持α3β4 nAChR的定位和作用主要在MHb，而不是进入大脑区域。在一个新的研究范式中，MHb α3β4 nAChR拮抗剂对致敏表达的影响相似，直接给予α3β4 nAChR拮抗剂可显著降低烟碱致敏后累积多巴胺的增加（Eggan, McCallum,2017）。综上所述，这些数据表明MHb α3β4 nAChR受体在介导烟碱的致敏反应中起着重要作用。此外，当其他药物（包括其他烟碱受体拮抗剂、谷氨酸调节剂和神经激肽-1拮抗剂）在MHb中测试时，对致敏反应没有结果（Eggan, McCallum, 2017），这表明这是MHb中α3β4 nAChR的选择性作用，与核内的其他信号无关。

32.7　MHb的下游靶点

MHb仅通过反屈肌束将传出纤维发送到脚间核（IPN）（Herkenham, Nauta, 1977）。虽然IPN的特征不如MHb，但它含有来自MHb和突触前nAChR的丰富的胆碱能纤维，包括α3β4 nAChR（Grady et al. 2009）。除了IPN的胆碱能群体外，IPN还含有丰富的P物质阳性纤维（Nakaya et al. 1994）和P物质受体，即神经激肽-1受体（NK1R; Yip, Chahl, 2001）。这一群体可能在MHb-IPN通讯中发挥作用，因为ACh和P物质是在卷束中发现的两种主要递质系统（Cuello et al. 1978）。NK1R位于大脑的许多区域，这些区域与情感行为的调节有关。这些区域包括杏仁核、纹状体、中缝核、海马体、MHb-IPN通路，以及其他几个单胺能脑干区（Quirion et al. 1983; Yip, Chahl, 2001）。其他大脑区域，包括蓝斑、下丘脑、中脑、基底节和背侧被盖区也富含NK1R（Maeno et al. 1993）。虽然在中脑边缘奖赏通路中存在NK1R，但在VTA的胞体中P物质的表达很少，这表明中脑边缘多巴胺通路中的P物质信号来自NAcc和VTA（Lessard et al. 2009）。富含P物质胞体的大脑区域包括新皮质、海马体、尾壳核、下丘脑、MHb、IPN、上丘、中央灰质和中缝核团（Warden, Young, 1988）。

32.8　P物质作为一种共同的神经递质

传统的神经肽，包括P物质，通常被包裹在神经元内，与常见的神经递质一起释放在一个囊泡中。双重免疫荧光研究表明，在大脑的几个区域，P物质的免疫反应与ChAT的表达几乎完全重叠，这支持了这些递质共同释放的观点。基底节及邻近基底前脑区几乎所有ChAT阳性神经元均显示P物质免疫反应阳性（Chen et al. 2001），提示P物质直接调节含ACh神经元的活动。此外，免疫组织化学实验还表明，P物质与30%～70%的5-羟色胺能神经元（Thor, Helke, 1989）、15%～30%的背根神经节谷氨酸神经元（Battaglia, Rustioni, 1988）和3%的GABA能视网膜神经节细胞（Caruso et al. 1990）共存，再次支持P物质与其他递质系统的共同释放。

32.9　NK1R在成瘾和烟碱敏化中的作用

P物质影响成瘾表型的确切机制尚不清楚。关于P物质在中脑边缘奖赏通路中的作用，将P物质直接注入VTA可引起VTA多巴胺神经元的激活（Stinus et al. 1978），这表明P物质具有直接调节中脑边缘奖赏通路的能力。此外，VTA中的NK1R激动剂引起NAc随后的多巴胺释放，而VTA中的NK1R拮抗剂导致NAcc多巴胺能细胞放电减少（Minabe et al. 1996）。含有P物质的VTA传入纤维的确切输入或存在尚不清楚。有关P物质传递在成瘾中的作用的研究有限。研究表明，随着NK1R的全球缺失和全身性的NK1R阻断，吗啡奖励显著减少（Murtra et al. 2000; Ripley et al. 2002）。同样，酒精的奖励效应在NK1R基因整体敲除中（George et al. 2008）和当NK1R拮抗剂被脑室注射以靶向CNS NK1R时都降低了。在可卡因方面，全身性NK1R拮抗导致伏隔多巴胺在受到急性可卡因刺激时反应迟钝（Loonam et al. 2003）。

32.10　NK1受体在烟碱敏化中的作用

P物质在烟碱成瘾中的作用除了一组致敏研究外，还没有受到关注。结果表明，当竞争性NK1R拮抗剂依洛匹坦（K_i=1.6～34nm；Margolis, Obach, 2003）全身应用时，对运动敏感化没有影响（Eggan, McCallum，未发表的数据）。有趣的是，虽然MHb中NK1R的阻断对致敏没有影响，但如果依洛匹坦直接应用于IPN，行为和神经化学敏感性均显著减弱（Eggan, McCallum, 2017）。这些数据表明，IPN NK1R在介导这种基于奖赏的成瘾成分中发挥了重要作用，并首次表明这些受体在介导对烟碱的任何反应中发挥了关键作用。

32.11　MHb-IPN通路调节烟碱敏化的神经回路

尚不清楚MHb-IPN通路是如何调节致敏反应的，但对这个问题的进一步研究可能会为大脑中的成瘾信号提供新的见解。如果切断反屈肌，IPN内ACh几乎完全丢失，但P物质只有少量丢失（Artymyshyn,Murray,1985）。这些数据表明，IPN的P物质传入可能起源于MHb以外的核。在所有已发现的IPN传入神经元中，隔核和背外侧被盖核（LDTg）是仅有的两个含有P物质和ACh的细胞体（Baker et al. 1991; Brownstein et al. 1976; Conteablile, FlumerFeel, 1981; Perry, Kella, 1995）。由于P物质在其他脑区与ACh共传递，以及MHb-IPN通路的神经化学特性，ACh很可能是MHb以外的P物质的IPN传入共递质（Chen et al. 2001）。我们通过免疫组织化学分析更密切地研究了这种可能性。在一系列实验中（Eggan,McCallum，未发表的数据），将荧光金逆行染料注入IPN，并允许10天后运输到传入细胞体。大脑切片以确定传入连通性，这些区域与P物质或ACh神经元标记物ChAT并列标记。隔核和背外侧被盖核（LDTg）是有希望的分析目标，因为它们以前发现含有ACh和P物质的细胞体，但我们发现这些细胞体只与荧光金在LDTg中共存（图32.2）。这些数据是初步的，虽然它们支持LDTg P物质在介导烟碱致敏反应中发挥重要作用的可能性。有必要进行进一步的研究，以确定这一潜在靶点的作用，并进一步了解MHb-IPN对中脑边缘奖赏通路的调节，以及这些受体和大脑区域在烟碱敏化反应中所起的作用（图32.3）。

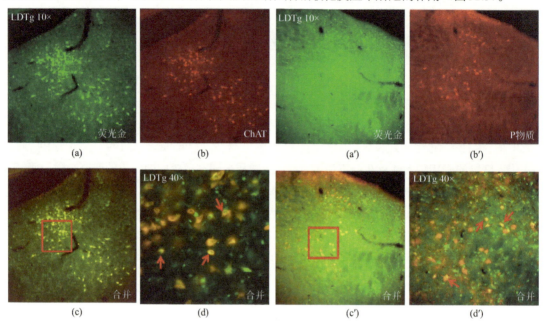

图 32.2 在 LDTg 中使用 ACh 和 P 物质标记的荧光金标记

图32.2 荧光金与乙酰胆碱和P物质标记物在LDTg中的协同标记

左图：（a）10天前单次IPN荧光金注射后LDTg中荧光金标记的细胞体。（b）在LDTg中ChAT标记的细胞体。（c）荧光金和ChAT在10倍放大。（d）荧光金和ChAT在40倍放大显示LDTg细胞体的合作标记。右图：（a′）10天前单次IPN荧光金注射后LDTg中荧光金标记的细胞体。（b′）LDTg中P物质标记的细胞体。（c′）荧光金与P物质在10倍放大。（d′）荧光金和P物质在40倍放大显示LDTg细胞体的合作标记。图片来自Eggan, McCallum，未发表。

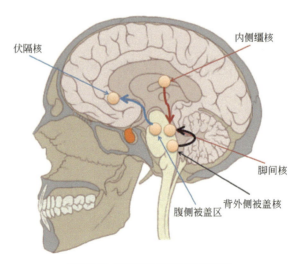

图 32.3 相关结构的神经解剖位置

中脑边缘奖赏通路（蓝色；多巴胺能）、MHb-IPN通路（红色；胆碱能和P物质能）以及LDTg-IPN连接性（黑色；未知）的神经解剖学定位。

| 术语解释 | - **行为敏化**：由于反复接触精神刺激剂药物而导致的运动活动的增加。表现为明显高于单一心理刺激挑战的敏化反应。
- **荧光金**：一种神经元逆行示踪剂，实验上用来显示连接到目标注射部位的传入纤维和细胞体。
- **体内微透析**：是一种实验技术，当动物自由活动时，它可以采样和收集目标脑区细胞外空间的内容，并允许分析收集的样本中的特定成分。
- **诱导敏化的发育或习得阶段**：神经化学敏化随后伏隔区多巴胺释放增加，这是反复接触精神刺激性药物造成的。
- **光电池活动室**：一种实验装置，用于通过测量自由移动的动物交叉光束的光束断裂量来测试开阔场地的活动能力。 |

| 核-脚间通路的键事实 | - 缰核在拉丁语中的意思是"小缰绳"，根据它的形状，它是一个小型但复杂的进化保守的上皮结构，位于第三脑室的外侧。
- 缰核分为内侧缰核和外侧缰核两部分，它们在神经解剖学和神经化学上都截然不同。
- 内侧缰核被认为与调节压力、抑郁、记忆，以及最近的烟碱成瘾有关。
- 脚间核是内侧缰核的主要输出，顾名思义，它位于大脑脚之间。
- 脚间核在大脑的许多区域都有强直抑制性，并被认为在快速眼动睡眠的调节中发挥着重要作用。
- 内侧缰核-脚间核通路与多巴胺能纹状体和边缘前脑具有独特的传入和传出联系，使该通路成为这些脑区之间串扰的重要调节器。
- 内侧缰核-脚间核通路与厌恶情绪状态、动机以及最重要的成瘾有关。
- 内侧缰核-脚间核通路为自己赢得了大脑中"替代奖赏通路"的称号。 |

| 要点总结 | - 内侧缰核-脚间核通路与成瘾的多种因素有关，包括烟碱成瘾。
- 内侧缰核和脚间核之间的联系主要是通过神经递质乙酰胆碱和P物质实现的。
- 内侧缰核和脚间核富含α3β4烟碱型乙酰胆碱受体。在内侧缰核-脚间核通路之外，这些受体在任何脑区都不密集表达。
- 药理学阻断内侧缰核α3β4烟碱型乙酰胆碱受体显著降低行为和神经化学对烟碱的敏感度。阻断脚间核α3、β4烟碱型乙酰胆碱受体对致敏反应无影响。
- 内侧缰核和脚间核富含神经激肽-1受体和P物质胞体。
- 通过药物阻断脚间核神经激肽-1受体，可以显著降低行为和神经化学对烟碱的敏感度。阻断内侧缰核的神经激肽-1受体对致敏反应无影响。
- 内侧缰核对脚间核的乙酰胆碱投射几乎全部贡献，但只占P物质投射的一小部分。
- 其他大脑区域，如背外侧被盖核，同时含有P物质和乙酰胆碱，这使它们可能是脚间核P物质的贡献者。 |

参考文献

Antolin-Fontes, B.; Ables, J. L.; Gorlich, A.; Ibanez-Tallon, I. (2015). The habenulo-interpeduncular pathway in nicotine aversion and withdrawal. Neuropharmacology, 96, 213-222.

Artymyshyn, R.; Murray, M. (1985). Substance P in the interpeduncu-lar nucleus of the rat: Normal distribution and the effects of deafferentation.

Journal of Comparative Neurology, 231, 78-90.

Baker, K. G.; Halliday, G. M.; Hornung, J. P.; Geffen, L. B.; Cotton, R. G.; Tork, I. (1991). Distribution, morphology and number of monoamine-synthesizing and substance-P containing neurons in the human dorsal raphe nucleus. Neuroscience, 42, 757-775.

Battaglia, G.; Rustioni, A. (1988). Coexistence of glutamate and substance P in dorsal root ganglion neurons of rat and monkey. Journal of Comparative Neurology, 277, 302-312.

Benwell, M. E.; Balfour, D. J. (1992). The effects of acute and repeated nicotine treatment on nucleus accumbens dopamine and locomotor activity. British Journal of Pharmacology, 105, 849-856.

Brownstein, M. J.; Mroz, E. A.; Kizer, J. S.; Palkovits, M.; Leeman, S. E. (1976). Regional distribution of substance P in the brain of the rat. Brain Research, 116, 299-305.

Caruso, D. M.; Owczarzak, M. T.; Pourcho, R. G. (1990). Colocalization of substance P and GABA in retinal ganglion cells: a computerassisted visualization. Visual Neuroscience, 5, 389-394.

Chen, L. W.; Wei, L. C.; Liu, H. L.; Chan, Y. S. (2001). Cholinergic neurons expressing substance P receptor (NK1) in the basal forebrain of the rat: a double immunocytochemical study. Brain Research, 904, 161-166.

Contestabile, A.; Flumerfelt, B. A. (1981). Afferent connections of the interpeduncular nucleus and the topographical organization of the habenulo-interpeduncular pathway: an HRP study in the rat. Journal of Comparative Neurology, 169, 253-270.

Contestabile, A.; Villani, L.; Fasolo, A.; Franzoni, M. F.; Gribaudo, L.; Oktedalen, O. et al. (1987). Topography of cholinergic and substance P pathways in the habenulo-interpeduncular system of the rat. An immunocytochemical and microchemical approach. Neuroscience, 21, 253-270.

Cuello, A. C.; Emson, P. C.; Paxinos, G.; Jessell, T. (1978). Substance P containing and cholinergic projections from the habenula. Brain Research, 149, 413-429.

DiFranza, J. R.; Wellman, R. J. (2007). Sensitization to nicotine: how the animal literature might inform future human research. Nicotine, Tobacco Research, 9, 9-20.

Dwoskin, L. P.; Crooks, P. A.; Teng, L.; Green, T. A.; Bardo, M. T. (1999). Acute and chronic effects of nornicotine on locomotor activity in rats: altered response to nicotine. Psychopharmacology, 145, 442-451.

Eggan, B. L.; McCallum, S. E. (2016). 18-Methoxycoronaridine acts in the medial habenula to attenuate behavioral and neurochemical sen- sitization to nicotine. Behavioural Brain Research, 307, 186-193.

Eggan, B. L.; McCallum, S. E. (2017). α3β4 nicotinic acetylcholine receptors in the medial habenula and substance P transmission in the interpeduncular nucleus modulate nicotine sensitization. Behavioral Brain Research, 316, 94-103.

Epping-Jordan, M. P.; Picciotto, M. R.; Changeux, J. P.; Pich, E. M. (1999). Assessment of nicotinic acetylcholine receptor subunit contributions to nicotine self-administration in mutant mice. Psycho-pharmacology (Berlin), 147, 25-26.

Fowler, C. D.; Lu, Q.; Johnson, P. M.; Marks, M. J.; Kenny, P. J. (2011). Habenular α5 nicotinic receptor signaling controls nicotine intake. Nature, 471, 597-601.

Fowler, C. D.; Tuesta, L.; Kenny, P. J. (2011). Role of α5* nicotinic acetylcholine receptors in the effects of acute and chronic nicotine treatment on brain reward function in mice. Psychopharmacology, 229, 503-513.

Frahm, S.; Slimak, M. A.; Ferrarese, L.; Santos-Torres, J.; Antolin-f, B.; Auer, S. et al. (2011). Aversion to nicotine is regulated by the balanced activity of β4 and α5 nicotinic receptor subunits in the medialhabenula. Neuron, 70, 522-535.

Gallego, X.; Molas, S.; Amador-Arjona, A.; Marks, M. J.; Robles, N.; Murta, P. et al. (2012). Overexpression of the CHRNA5/A3/B4 genomic cluster in mice increases the sensitivity to nicotine and modifies its reinforcing effects. Amino Acids, 44, 897-909.

George, D. T.; Gilman, J.; Hersh, J.; Thorsell, A.; Herion, D.; Geyer, C. et al. (2008). Neurokinin 1 receptor antagonism as a possible therapy for alcoholism. Science, 319, 1535-1539.

Glick, S. D.; Sell, E. M.; McCallum, S. E.; Maisonneuve, I. M. (2011). Brain regions mediating α3β4 nicotinic antagonist effects of 18-MC on nicotine self-administration. European Journal of Pharmacology, 699, 71-75.

Grady, S. R.; Meinerz, N. M.; Cao, J.; Reynolds, A. M.; Piccioto, M. R.; Changeux, J. P. et al. (2001). Nicotinic agonists stimulate acetylcholine release from mouse interpeduncular nucleus: a function mediated by a different nAChR than dopamine release from striatum. Journal of Neurochemistry, 76, 258-268.

Grady, S. R.; Moretti, M.; Zoli, M.; Marks, M. J.; Zanardi, A.; Pucci, L. et al. (2009). Rodent habenulo-interpeduncular pathway expresses a large variety of uncommon nAChR subtypes, but only the α3β4* and α3β3β4* subtypes mediate acetylcholine release. Journal of Neu-roscience, 29, 2272-2282.

Groot-Kormelink, P. J.; Boorman, J. P.; Sivilotti, L. G. (2001). Formation of functional α3β4α5 human neuronal nicotinic receptors in Xenopus oocytes: a reporter mutation approach. British Journal of Pharmacology, 134, 789-796.

Herkenham, M.; Nauta, W. J. H. (1977). Afferent connections of the habenular nuclei in the rat. A horseradish peroxidase study, with a note on the fiber-of-passage problem. Journal of Comparative Neurology, 173, 277-299.

Koob, G. F.; LeMoal, M. L. (1997). Drug abuse: hedonic homeostatic dysregulation. Science, 278, 52-58.

Kuehne, M. E.; He, L.; Joikel, P. A.; Pace, C. J.; Fleck, M. W.; Maisonneuve, I. M. et al. (2003). Synthesis and biological evaluation of 18-methoxycoronaridine congeners. Potential antiaddiction agents. Journal of Medicinal Chemistry, 46, 2716-2730.

Lena, C.; Changeux, J. P.; Mulle, C. (1993). Evidence for "preterminal"nicotinic receptors on GABAergic axons in the rat interpeduncular nucleus. Journal of Neuroscience, 13, 2680-2688.

Lessard, A.; Savard, M.; Gobeil, F.; Pierce, J. P.; Pickel, V. M. (2009). The neurokinin-3 (NK3) and the neurokinin-1 (NK1) receptors are differentially targeted to mesocortical and mesolimbic projection neurons, and to neuronal nuclei in the rat ventral tegmental area. Synapse, 63, 484-501.

Liu, J. Z.; Tozzi, F.; Waterworth, D. M. et al. (2010). Meta-analysis and imputation refines the association of 15q25 with smoking quantity. Nature

Genetics, 42, 436-440.

Loonam, T. M.; Noailles, P. A.; Yu, J.; Zhu, J. P.; Angulo, J. A. (2003). Substance P and cholecystokinin regulate neurochemical responses to cocaine and methamphetamine in the striatum. Life Sciences, 73, 727-739.

Luo, S.; Kulak, J. M.; Cartier, G. E.; Jacobsen, R. B.; Yoshikami, D.; Olivera, B. M. et al. (1998). α-Conotoxin AuIB selectively blocks α3β4 nicotinic acetylcholine receptors and nicotine-evoked norepinephrine release. Journal of Neuroscience, 18, 8571-8579.

Maeno, H.; Kiyama, H.; Tohyama, M. (1993). Distribution of the substance P receptor (NK-1 receptor) in the central nervous system. Molecular Brain Research, 18, 43-58.

Margolis, J. M.; Obach, R. S. (2003). Impact of nonspecific binding to microsomes and phospholipid on the inhibition of cytochrome P4502D6: implications for relating in vitro inhibition data to in vivo drug interactions. Drug Metabolism and Disposition, 31, 606-611.

McCallum, S. E.; Cowe, M. A.; Lewis, S. W.; Glick, S. D. (2012). α3β4 nicotinic acetylcholine receptors in the medial habenula modulate the mesolimbic dopaminergic response to acute nicotine in vivo. Neuropharmacology, 63, 434-440.

Miller, D. K.; Wilkins, L. H.; Bardo, M. T.; Crooks, P. A.; Dwoskin, L. B. (2001). Once weekly administration of nicotine produces longlasting locomotor sensitization in rats via a nicotinic receptor-mediated mechanism. Journal of Psychopharmacology, 156, 469-476.

Minabe, Y.; Emori, K.; Toor, A.; Stutzman, G. E.; Ashby, C. R. (1996). The effect of acute and chronic administration of CP 96, 345, a selective neurokinin1 antagonist, on midbrain dopamine neurons in the rat. Synapse, 22, 35-45.

Murtra, P.; Sheasby, A. M.; Hunt, S. P.; De Felipe, C. (2000). Rewarding effects of opiates are absent in mice lacking the receptor for substance P. Nature, 405, 180-183.

Nakaya, Y.; Kaneko, T.; Shigemoto, R.; Shigetada, N.; Mizuno, N. (1994). Immunohisotchemical localization of substance P receptor in the central nervous system of the adult rat. Journal of Comparative Neurology, 347, 249-274.

Nisell, M.; Nomikos, G. G.; Hertel, P.; Panagis, G.; Svensson, T. H. (1996). Condition-independent sensitization of locomotor stimulation and mesocortical dopamine release following chronic nicotine treatment in the rat. Synapse, 22, 369-381.

Perry, D. C.; Kellar, K. J. (1995). [^{3}H] Epibatidine labels nicotinic receptors in rat brain: an autoradiographic study. Journal of Pharmacology and Experimental Therapeutics, 276, 1030-1034.

Quick, M. W.; Ceballos, M. R.; Kasten, M.; McIntosh, M. J.; Lester, R. A. (1999). α3β4 subunit-containing nicotinic receptors dominate function in the medial habenula neurons. Neuropharmacology, 38, 769-783.

Quirion, R.; Shults, C. W.; Moody, T. W.; Pert, C. B.; Chase, T. N.; O'Donohue, T. L. (1983). Autoradiographic distribution of substance P receptors in the rat central nervous system. Nature, 303, 714-716.

Ren, J.; Qin, C.; Hu, F.; Tan, J.; Qui, L.; Zhao, S. et al. (2011). Habenula"cholinergic" neurons corelease glutamate and acetylcholine and activate postsynaptic neurons via distinct transmission modes. Neuron, 69, 445-452.

Ripley, T. L.; Gadd, C. A.; De Felipe, C.; Hunt, S. P.; Stephens, D. N. (2002). Lack of self administration and behavioral sensitization to morphine, but not cocaine, in mice lacking NK1 receptors. Neuropharmacology, 43, 1258-1268.

Saal, D.; Dong, Y.; Bonci, A.; Malenka, R. C. (2003). Drugs of abuse and stress trigger a common synaptic adaptation in dopamine neurons. Neuron, 37, 577-582.

Salas, R.; Pieri, F.; De Biasi, M. (2004). Decreased signs of nicotine withdrawal in mice null for the beta4 nicotinic acetylcholine receptor subunit. Journal of Neuroscience, 24, 10035-10039.

Salas, R.; Sturm, R.; Boutler, J.; De Biasi, M. (2009). Nicotinic receptors in the habenulo-interpeduncular system are necessary for nicotine withdrawal in mice. Journal of Neuroscience, 29, 4934-4938.

Schlaepfer, I. R.; Hoft, N. R.; Collins, A. C.; Corley, R. P.; Hewitt, J. K.; Hopfer, C. J. et al. (2008). The CHRNA5/A3/B4 gene cluster variability as an important determinant of early alcohol and tobacco initiation in young adults. Biological Psychiatry, 63, 1039-1046.

Steketee, J. D.; Kalivas, P. W. (2011). Drug wanting: behavioral sensitization and relapse to drug-seeking behavior. Pharmacology Review, 63, 348-365.

Stinus, L.; Kelley, A. E.; Iversen, S. D. (1978). Increased spontaneous activity following substance P infusion into A10 dopaminergic area. Nature, 276, 616-618.

Sutherland, R. J.; Nakajima, S. (1981). Self-stimulation of the habenular complex in the rat. Journal of Comparative and Physiological Psychology, 95, 781-791.

Tapper, A. R.; McKinney, S. L.; Dashmi, R.; Schwarz, J.; Deshpande, P.; Labarca, C. et al. (2004). Nicotine activation of α4* receptors: sufficient for reward, tolerance, and sensitization. Science, 306, 1029-1032.

Thor, K. B.; Helke, C. J. (1989). Serotonin and substance P colocalization in the medullary projections to the nucleus tractus solitaries: dual-colour immunohistochemistry combined with retrograde tracing. Journal of Chemical Neuroanatomy, 2, 139-148.

Toll, L.; Zaveri, N. T.; Polgar, W. E.; Jiang, F.; Khroyan, T. V.; Zhou, W. et al. (2012). AT-1001: a high affinity and selective α3β4 nicotinic acetylcholine receptor antagonist blocks nicotine self-administration in rats. Neuropsychopharmacology, 37, 1367-1376.

Warden, M. K.; Young, W. S. (1988). Distribution of cells containing mRNAs encoding substance P and neurokinin B in the rat central nervous system. Journal of Comparative Neurology, 272, 90-113.

Yip, J.; Chahl, L. A. (2001). Localization of NK1 and NK3 receptors in Guinea-pig brain. Regulatory Peptides, 98, 55-62.

33
靶向烟碱型乙酰胆碱受体治疗疼痛

Deniz Bagdas[1], S.Lauren Kyte[2], Wisam Toma[1], M.Sibel Gurun[2], M.Imad Damaj[1]

1. Department of Pharmacology, Toxicology, Virginia Commonwealth University, Richmond, VA, United States
2. Department of Pharmacology, Faculty of Medicine, Uludag University, Bursa, Turkey

缩略语

ACh	乙酰胆碱	**nAChR**	烟碱乙酰胆碱受体
ago-PAM	变构激动剂-阳性变构调节剂	**PAM**	正变构调节剂

33.1 烟碱乙酰胆碱受体药物简介

目前，非甾体类消炎药和阿片类药物仍然是疼痛治疗药物的最常见形式，其次是抗抑郁药和抗癫痫药。但是，这些药物要么效力不足，要么会引起不良反应。这些药物对于几种类型的慢性疼痛（例如神经性疼痛）也不太有效（Woolf, 2010）。因此，迫切需要用于控制疼痛的新型治疗药物。nAChR是提出的减轻疼痛的新靶标之一。

这些受体是五聚体配体门控离子通道的Cys环超家族的成员，该通道由围绕离子孔的五个亚基组成。它们参与了整个外周和中枢神经系统中乙酰胆碱（ACh）介导的信号转导。此外，nAChR在疼痛和几种烟碱诱发的反应中起重要作用（Decker et al. 2004）。

迄今为止，已经鉴定出nAChR的12种神经元亚基（$\alpha2 \sim \alpha10$和$\beta2 \sim \beta4$）。nAChRs可以异源形式出现，包括α和β亚基的各种组合，或同分异构形式，其中nAChR仅表达α亚基。最普遍的nAChR亚型是异源$\alpha4\beta2^*$和同源$\alpha7$受体（*表示这些nAChR也可以包含其他α和β亚基，Gotti et al. 2006年进行了综述）。除ACh外，nAChR还对几种类型的配体产生反应，例如激动剂、拮抗剂和变构调节剂。当激动剂与其正构结合位点结合时，它将稳定开放状态和脱敏状态。当通道被激动剂打开时，它允许钠离子和钙离子进入细胞，而钾离子退出（图33.1）。

在没有内源性或外源性激动剂的情况下，正变构调节剂（PAM）是一类新型的nAChR配体，在与正构结合位点不同的位点与nAChR结合而不激活受体（图33.2）。但是，它们通过增加激动剂的效价、功效和/或nAChR的开放性来增强激动剂诱导的应答（Williams et al. 2011）。虽然PAM的增强作用是由于它们具有防止受体脱敏和延长突触传递的能力而引起的，但正构激动剂却恰恰相反，从而使它们的整体疗效较差。PAM主要分为Ⅰ型和Ⅱ型。Ⅰ型PAM可以增加激动剂反应，而对nAChR的脱敏作用几乎没有或没有影响，而Ⅱ型PAM可以增加激动剂反应并延缓激动剂的脱敏率，如针对α7 nAChR的PAM所见（Williams et al. 2011）。

另一类新的选择性nAChR配体由沉默激动剂组成，它们具有以非常低的效率与受体结合的独特能力，但它们不引起电流，而是稳定了与脱敏相关的非导电状态（图33.1）。因此，仅这些配体就能调节信号转导（Chojnacka et al. 2013）。

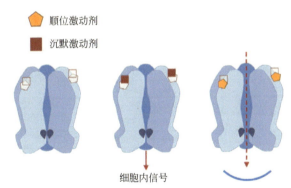

图 33.1 正构激动剂与正构结合位点结合,打开离子通道并激活受体,而沉默激动剂与沉默激动剂结合位点结合,不激活受体。沉默激动剂通过未知的细胞内机制引起其作用

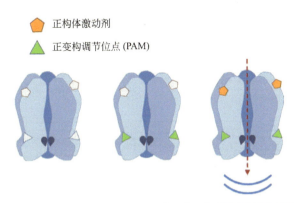

图 33.2 PAM 结合到正变构调节位点(▲),但不激活受体。在正构体激动剂 [与正构体结合位点(⬠)结合] 存在的情况下,PAM 可增强激动剂的作用

33.2 疼痛调节中的α4β2* nAChR

除了在烟草中增强烟碱的作用外,它还对人类和啮齿类动物具有显著的止痛作用,尤其是通过在疼痛传递途径中表达的α4β2* nAChR 来缓解疼痛(参见综述 Damaj et al. 2014)。在转基因小鼠中已经表明,在急性疼痛试验中,α4 或 β2 nAChR 亚基的缺失降低了对烟碱类化合物抗伤害感受作用的敏感性(Marubio et al. 1999)。但是,烟碱的半衰期短和有害的副作用限制了它的使用。然而,烟碱提供的抗伤害感受仍可洞悉疼痛中α4β2* nAChR 的基本机制,并有助于治疗性α4β2* 配体的发展。据报道,在各种啮齿动物疼痛模型中,各种α4β2* 激动剂具有抗伤害作用(表33.1)。

表33.1 α4、β2* nAchR配体对不同疼痛动物模型的疗效

成分	配体类型	动物模型/测定	动物	响应	参考文献
烟碱	兴奋剂	悬尾	小鼠	镇痛	Damaj et al. (1998)
		热板	大鼠	镇痛	Boyce et al. (2000)
		CCI	小鼠	逆转机械异常性疼痛	Bagdas et al. (2017) Bagdas, AlSharari et al. (2015)

成分	配体类型	动物模型/测定	动物	响应	参考文献
地棘蛙素	兴奋剂	热板	小鼠	镇痛	Badio, Daly (1994)
			大鼠	镇痛	Boyce et al. (2000)
		悬尾	小鼠	镇痛	Damaj et al. (1998)
		福尔马林	小鼠	镇痛	Curzon et al. (1998)
		CIIP	大鼠	↓热痛觉过敏	Lawand, Lu, Westlund (1999)
		CFA	大鼠	逆转炎症和神经性痛觉过敏	Kesingland et al. (2000)
		PSNL	大鼠	逆转炎症和神经性痛觉过敏	Kesingland et al. (2000)
ABT-594	兴奋剂	热板	大鼠	镇痛	Boyce et al. (2000)
		悬尾		镇痛	Kesingland et al. (2000)
		CFA		逆转炎症和神经性痛觉过敏	
		PSNL			
		CIIP	大鼠	↓热痛觉过敏、机械异常性疼痛和骨关节炎疼痛	Zhu et al. (2011)
		爪子皮肤切口			
		单碘乙酸引起的关节炎			
		SNL	大鼠	↓机械性异常性疼痛和痛觉过敏	Bannon et al. (1998)
		糖尿病性神经病			
		长春新碱诱导的CIPN		↓机械性异常性疼痛	Lynch, Wade, Mikusa, Decker, Honore (2005)
NS3956	兴奋剂	福尔马林	大鼠	镇痛	Rode et al. (2012)
5-Iodo-A-85380	兴奋剂	哈格里夫	大鼠	镇痛	Rueter, Meyer, Decker (2000)
沙氮替丁-A	部分激动剂	悬发, 热板	小鼠	无影响	AlSharari et al. (2012)
		福尔马林		镇痛	
		福尔马林	小鼠	镇痛	Bagdas, AlSharari et al. (2015)
伐伦克林	部分激动剂	悬尾, 热板	小鼠	无影响	AlSharari et al. (2012)
		福尔马林	小鼠	镇痛	Bagdas, AlSharari et al. (2015)
NS9283	Ⅱ型 PAM	福尔马林	大鼠	NS3956的增强镇痛作用	Rode et al. (2012)
		CIIP	大鼠	ABT-594的增强镇痛作用	Zhu et al. (2011)
		爪子皮肤切口			
		单碘乙酸引起的关节炎			
		SNL	大鼠	结合ABT-594逆转机械异常性疼痛	Lee et al. (2011)
去甲酰氟溴明	Ⅱ型 PAM	CCI	小鼠	烟碱增强的抗痛觉过敏作用	Bagdas et al. (2017)

注：CCI，慢性缩窄性神经损伤；CFA，完全弗氏佐剂；CIIP，角叉菜胶炎性疼痛；CIPN，化疗诱导的周围神经病变；PAM，正变构调节剂；PSNL，部分坐骨神经结扎；SNL，脊神经结扎。（↓）减少。

重要的化合物之一是地棘蛙素，它是多种nAChR的有效激动剂。尽管地棘蛙素具有很强的抗伤害作用，但作用时间却很短（Bannon et al. 1998; Curzon et al. 1998）。另一个重要的化合物是ABT-594，它是第一种证明具有可治疗人类糖尿病性神经病的功效的物质。但是，ABT-594会产生副作用，例如恶心、头晕、呕吐、异常的梦境和乏力等（Rowbotham et al. 2009）。

α5烟碱亚基是辅助亚基，仅在与主要亚基（例如α3或α4）和一个互补亚基（β2或β4；例如α4β2α5、α3β2α5或α3β4α5受体）共表达时才能形成功能性受体（Lindstrom, Whiteaker et al. 2007）。在疼痛动物模型中，α5亚基极大地影响了烟碱对nAChR功能的调控。例如，已提出α5 nAChR亚基在神经性疼痛中伤害性信息处理中的可能作用（Vincler, Eisenach, 2004）。我们还报道了在小鼠中α5 nAChR亚基的缺失会影响慢性疼痛模型中伤害感受行为的发展和强度。此外，在α5亚基敲除小鼠中烟碱的抗伤害感受特性降低或不存在（Bagdas et al. 2015）。

在福尔马林试验中，两个α4β2部分激动剂沙氮替丁-A和伐伦克林均具有抗伤害感受特性（AlSharari et al. 2012），但沙氮替丁-A的作用依赖于α5亚基，而伐伦克林并非如此（Bagdas, AlSharari, et al. 2015）。尽管α4β2*激动剂由于在不同nAChR亚型中相对较低的功能选择性而受到限制（Zhang et al. 2012），但α4β2* PAM可以增强烟碱激动剂的性能。例如，NS9283在啮齿动物的疼痛模型中增强了ABT594和NS3956的抗伤害感受作用（表33.1）。此外，α4β2* PAM去甲酰氟溴明与烟碱的结合可增强神经性疼痛行为的逆转而无运动障碍，从而确认了镇痛活性和不良反应的解除（Bagdas et al. 2017）。由于在上述研究中NS9283和去甲酰基氟嘧啶单独缺乏活性，因此表明在神经性疼痛中不存在β2* nAChR介导的内源性抗伤害性胆碱能基调。这与α7 nAChR PAM相反，后者在临床前模型中单独给药时显示出活性（见下文）。

33.3 nAChR在痛觉调节中的作用

大量研究表明，α7 nAChR亚型的激活在疼痛控制中具有潜在的作用（表33.2）。α7 nAChR已被证明在痛觉传导通路中分布着大量的神经细胞和非神经细胞，特别是免疫细胞（Corradi, Bouzat, 2016; Khan et al. 2003）。α7 nAChR下调细胞因子的产生和相关的炎症反应，使其成为胆碱能抗炎途径的重要组成部分，胆碱能抗炎途径被定义为通过迷走神经传递的抑制细胞因子释放的神经信号（Pavlov et al. 2009）。例如，α7 nAChR基因敲除小鼠的关节炎发病率和严重程度显著增加（van Maanen et al. 2010）。此外，与野生型小鼠相比，在α7基因敲除小鼠中观察到与足底完全弗氏佐剂注射相关的水肿、痛觉过敏和异常性疼痛显著增加（AlSharari et al. 2013）。此外，研究表明，选择性的α7 nAChR激动剂胆碱和PHA-543613显著减少了福尔马林试验中舔爪子的时间（Freitas et al. 2013; Freitas et al. 2013）。据报道，II型PAM PNU-120596可以逆转神经病理性疼痛模型中的机械性痛觉过敏（Freitas et al. 2013）。另一种II型PAM，3-呋喃-2-基-N-对甲苯基丙烯酰胺，逆转了慢性疼痛模型中的机械性超敏和热痛觉过敏（Bagdas, Targowska-Duda, et al. 2015）。GAT107是一种新的α7选择性双重变构激动剂-PAM（ago-PAM；图33.3），显示出抗炎和抗伤害作用（Bagdas et al. 2016）。此外，沉默激动剂NS6740减少了福尔马林试验中舔爪子的时间，并通过一种未知的信号机制减轻了神经病理性疼痛模型中的机械性痛觉异常（Papke et al. 2015）。此外，这些化合物有效地减少了醋酸诱导的条件性位置厌恶（Bagdas et al. 2016; Bagdas, Targowska-Duda, et al. 2015; Papke et al. 2015）。最后，我们最近证实了α7 nAChR和核过氧化物酶体增殖物激活受体类型α之间的体内串扰；在福尔马林试验中，α7 nAChR被选择性完全激活剂（即pNU282987）激活可能导致内源性过氧化物酶体增殖物激活受体类型α音调增加，介导所观察到的抗伤害效应（Donvito et al. 2017）。

表33.2 α7 nAChR配体对不同疼痛动物模型的疗效

成分	配体类型	动物模型/测定	动物	响应	参考文献
胆碱	兴奋剂	悬尾	小鼠	镇痛	Damaj, Meyer, Martin (2000)
		福尔马林		镇痛	Freitas, Negus et al. (2013)
		切口术后疼痛		↓热痛觉过敏和机械异常性疼痛	Rowley, McKinstry, Greenidge, Smith, Flood (2010)
PNU-282987	兴奋剂	福尔马林	小鼠	镇痛	Donvito et al. (2017)

续表

成分	配体类型	动物模型/测定	动物	响应	参考文献
PHA-543613	兴奋剂	福尔马林	大鼠	通过中枢介导机制镇痛	Umana, Daniele, Miller, Gallagher, Brown (2017)
NS6740	沉默激动剂	福尔马林	小鼠	镇痛	Papke et al. (2015)
		CCI		↓机械性异常性疼痛	
		CPA		逆转 CPA	
PNU-120596	Ⅱ型 PAM	悬尾，热板	小鼠	无影响	Freitas, Negus et al. (2013)
		福尔马林		PHA-543613 的单独镇痛作用和增强作用	Freitas, Carroll, Damaj (2013)
					Freitas, Ghosh et al. (2013)
		CIIP		↓热痛觉过敏	
		CCI		↓热痛觉过敏和机械异常性疼痛	
3-呋喃-2-基-N-对甲苯基丙烯酰胺	Ⅱ型 PAM	CIIP	小鼠	↓胆碱的机械异常性疼痛和增强的抗异常性疼痛作用	Bagdas, Targowska-Duda et al. (2015)
		CFA		↓热痛觉过敏	
		CCI		↓机械性异常性疼痛	
		CPA		逆转 CPA	
GAT107	Ago-PAM（变构激动剂和Ⅱ型 PAM）	悬尾，热板	小鼠	无影响	Bagdas et al. (2016)
		福尔马林		镇痛	
		CFA	小鼠	↓热痛觉过敏	
		LPS	小鼠	↓机械性痛觉异常	
		酸致伸展	小鼠	↓伸展	
		CCI	小鼠	↓机械性痛觉异常	
		CPA	小鼠	逆转 CPA	

注：CCI，慢性缩窄性神经损伤；CFA，完全弗氏佐剂；CIIP，角叉菜胶炎性疼痛；CPA，条件性位置厌恶；LPS，脂多糖；PAM，正变构调节剂。（↓）减少。

尽管经典的观点认为 α7 nAChR 是同分异构体，但新的证据表明存在异构体 α7 nAChR，它与 β2 亚基共同组装（见综述 Wu et al. 2016）。然而，α7β2 nAChR 在痛觉调制中的作用尚不清楚。

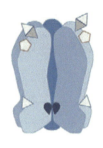

- 顺位激动剂
- 正变构调节剂
- 别构和正变构激动剂 (ago-PAM)

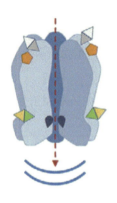
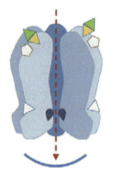
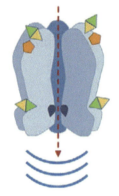

图 33.3　ago-PAM 可以通过与直接变构激活结合位点（◆）结合而自行激活受体。ago-PAM 能与正变构调节位点（▶）结合，并能增强正构体激动剂的作用，而正构体激动剂又能与正构结合位点（●）结合

33.4 α9/α9α10 nAChR在痛觉调制中的作用

α9 nAChR亚基可以与其他α9亚基组装成同戊异构体，与α10 nAChR亚基组装成异戊异构体，形成功能性nAChR。α9和α10亚基都在外周神经系统中表达，但在大脑中不表达（见综述Gotti et al. 2006）。与其他nAChR一样，α9α10受体被ACh激活；然而，烟碱通过抑制ACh诱发的电流而起到拮抗剂的作用（Elgoyhen et al.2001;Elgoyhen et al. 1994）。

一类有望用于nAChR介导的疼痛治疗的药物是α-芋螺毒素家族（表33.3），它由从圆锥海螺毒液中分离出来的短肽组成，其中一些是α9α10 nAChR(McIntosh et al. 2009; Napier et al. 2012)。α-芋螺毒素RgIA是哺乳动物中最具选择性的α9α10拮抗剂（McIntosh et al. 2009），已被证明可以逆转神经病理性疼痛模型中的机械性痛觉过敏和痛觉过敏（Di Cesare Mannelli et al. 2014; Vcler et al. 2006）；然而，该药物在人类α9α10 nAChR中的效力要低300倍（Azam, McIntosh, 2012）。类似的化合物RgIA4对大鼠和人的α9α10 nAChR都有很高的亲和力，并已被证明可以预防草酸铂诱导的神经病理性疼痛（Romero et al. 2017）。另一种令人感兴趣的α-芋螺毒素是Vc1.1，它成功地通过了临床试验的第一阶段，但在体外数据表明Vc1.1对人α9α10 nAChR的选择性低于大鼠之后，它没有继续超过2A阶段（Azam, McIntosh, 2012）。此外，研究表明，选择性的α9α10拮抗剂ZZ1-61c，烟碱的异氮杂芳季铵类似物，与长春新碱联合使用或与之后使用时，可以预防和逆转化疗引起的机械性痛觉过敏（Wala et al. 2012）。ZZ1-61c与其他α9α10拮抗剂联用时，这种作用不是一过性的，表明急性给药引起持久的生理变化。

表33.3 α9α10 nAchR配体对不同疼痛动物模型的疗效

混合物	配体类型	动物模型	动物	应答	参考文献
RgIA	拮抗剂	CCI	大鼠	预防和逆转机械性痛觉超敏	Di Cesare Mannelli et al.（2014）
		CCI		逆转机械性痛觉过敏	Vincler et al.（2006）
RgIA4	拮抗剂	奥沙利铂诱导的CIPN	大鼠	预防冷性痛觉超敏和机械性痛觉过敏	Romero et al.（2017）
Vc1.1	拮抗剂	CCI, PSNL	大鼠	逆转机械性痛觉过敏	Satkunanathan et al.（2005）
ZZ1-61c	拮抗剂	长春新碱诱导的CIPN	大鼠	预防/逆转机械性痛觉超敏	Wala et al.（2012）

注：CCI，慢性缩窄性神经损伤；CIPN，化疗所致周围神经病变；PSNL，部分坐骨神经结扎术。

33.5 结论

在疼痛和炎症动物模型中，nAChR激动剂、沉默激动剂、PAM、AGO-PAM和拮抗剂的不断发现和表征为以这些受体为靶点开发替代止痛药创造了新的机会。为了促进这一过程，未来的药物开发将集中于确定nAChR介导的负责抗伤害感受和神经保护的机制，目标不仅是缓解疼痛，而且还可以防止慢性疼痛状态的启动和/或进展。

术语解释

- 激动剂：一种能与受体的正构体结合，从而改变受体状态并产生生理反应的药物（Neubig et al. 2003）。
- 触摸痛：由通常不会引起疼痛的刺激引起的痛觉过敏性疼痛（Merskey, Bogduk, 1994）。
- 变构激动剂阳性变构调节剂：与两个变构位点结合的配体，一个位于胞外区，另一个位于跨膜区，以诱导和增强受体激活（Papke et al. 2017）。
- 止痛：通常是疼痛的刺激后没有疼痛（Merskey, Bogduk, 1994）。
- 拮抗剂：一种阻断激动剂作用的药物（Neubig et al. 2003）。
- 痛觉过敏：会加剧通常会引起疼痛的刺激引起的疼痛（Merskey, Bogduk, 1994）。
- 伤害性刺激：伤害性刺激的编码和传输（Merskey, Bogduk, 1994）。
- 疼痛：对实际或可能的身体伤害做出的不愉快的感觉和情绪反应（Bonica, 1979）。
- 正变构调节剂：一种药物，能与受体的变构位点结合，在正构激动剂存在的情况下增强激活（Papke et al. 2017）。
- 沉默激动剂：一种药物，能与受体的正构体结合，引起与脱敏、不传导状态相关的构象变化（Papke et al. 2015）。

NAChR 及其配体的关键事实

- 烟碱在α7和α4β2* nAChR 上是激动剂，但在α9α10 nAChR 上是拮抗剂。
- 激动剂结合后，α7 nAChR 开放后迅速脱敏。
- nAChR 激动剂诱导孔道开放和阳离子通量。
- 虽然沉默激动剂不允许 nAChR 开放，但它们诱导了介导下游信号的构象变化。
- PAM 与 nAChR 的跨膜调控位点结合，而 ago-PAM 既可与该位点结合，也可与胞外结构域结合。

要点总结

- 本章重点研究用于治疗疼痛的 nAChR 配体。
- α4β2* nAChR 激动剂可缓解各种伤害性测试中的疼痛，如急性和慢性疼痛。
- α7 nAChR 的静默激动剂 PAM 和 ago-PAM 可减少慢性疼痛行为，但对急性疼痛敏感性没有影响。
- 在临床前疼痛模型中，α4β2* PAM 单独使用时缺乏活性，但α7 PAM 能够单独产生抗伤害效应。
- α9α10 nAChR 的拮抗剂可以减轻神经病理性疼痛行为。

致谢

鉴于参考文献的局限性，我们很抱歉没有引用一些原创作品。

参考文献

AlSharari, S. D.; Carroll, F. I.; McIntosh, J. M.; Damaj, M. I. (2012). The Antinociceptive effects of nicotinic partial agonists varenicline and sazetidine-A in murine acute and tonic pain models. Journal of Pharmacology and Experimental Therapeutics, 342(3), 742-749.

AlSharari, S. D.; Freitas, K.; Damaj, M. I. (2013). Functional role of alpha7 nicotinic receptor in chronic neuropathic and inflammatory pain: studies in transgenic mice. Biochemical Pharmacology, 86(8), 1201-1207.

Azam, L.; McIntosh, J. M. (2012). Molecular basis for the differential sensitivity of rat and human α9α10 nAChRs to α-conotoxin RgIA. Journal of Neurochemistry, 122(6), 1137-1144.

Badio, B.; Daly, J. W. (1994). Epibatidine, a potent analgetic and nicotinic agonist. Molecular Pharmacology, 45(4), 563-569.

Bagdas, D.; AlSharari, S. D.; Freitas, K.; Tracy, M.; Damaj, M. I. (2015). The role of alpha5 nicotinic acetylcholine receptors in mouse models of chronic inflammatory and neuropathic pain. Biochemical Pharmacology, 97(4), 590-600.

Bagdas, D.; Ergun, D.; Jackson, A.; Toma, W.; Schulte, M. K.; Damaj, M. I. (2017). Allosteric modulation of α4β2* nicotinic acetylcholine receptors: desformylflustrabromine potentiates antiallodynic response of nicotine in a mouse model of neuropathic pain. European Journal of Pain, 1-10.

Bagdas, D.; Targowska-Duda, K. M.; López, J. J.; Perez, E. G.; Arias, H. R.; Damaj, M. I. (2015). The antinociceptive and anti-inflammatory properties of 3-furan-2-yl-N-p-tolyl-acrylamide, a positive allosteric modulator of α7 nicotinic acetylcholine receptors in mice. Anesthesia, Analgesia, 121(5), 1369-1377.

Bagdas, D.; Wilkerson, J. L.; Kulkarni, A.; Toma, W.; AlSharari, S.; Gul, Z. et al. (2016). The α7 nicotinic receptor dual allosteric agonist and positive allosteric modulator GAT107 reverses nociception in mouse models of inflammatory and neuropathic pain. British Journal of Pharmacology.

Bannon, A. W.; Decker, M. W.; Kim, D. J. B.; Campbell, J. E.; Arneric, S. P. (1998). ABT-594, a novel cholinergic channel modulator, is efficacious in nerve ligation and diabetic neuropathy models of neuropathic pain. Brain Research, 801(1-2), 158-163.

Bonica, J. J. (1979). The need of a taxonomy. Pain 6(3), 247-248.

Boyce, S.; Webb, J. K.; Shepheard, S. L.; Russell, M. G. N.; Hill, R. G.; Rupniak, N. M. J. (2000). Analgesic and toxic effects of ABT-594 resemble epibatidine and nicotine in rats. Pain, 85(3), 443-450.

Brown, R. W. B.; Collins, A. C.; Lindstrom, J. M.; Whiteaker, P. (2007). Nicotinic alpha5 subunit deletion locally reduces high-affinity agonist activation without altering nicotinic receptor numbers. Journal of Neurochemistry.

Chojnacka, K.; Papke, R. L.; Horenstein, N. A. (2013). Synthesis and evaluation of a conditionally-silent agonist for theα7 nicotinic acetylcholine receptor. Bioorganic, Medicinal Chemistry Letters, 23(14), 4145-4149.

Corradi, J.; Bouzat, C. (2016). Understanding the bases of function and modulation of α7 nicotinic receptors: implications for drug discovery. Molecular Pharmacology, 288-299.

Curzon, P.; Nikkel, A. L.; Bannon, A. W.; Arneric, S. P.; Decker, M. W. (1998). Differences between the antinociceptive effects of the cholinergic channel activators A-85380 and (+/-)-epibatidine in rats. The Journal of Pharmacology and Experimental Therapeutics, 287(3), 847-853.

Damaj, M. I.; Fei-Yin, M.; Dukat, M.; Glassco, W.; Glennon, R. A.; Martin, B. R. (1998). Antinociceptive responses to nicotinic acetylcholine receptor ligands after systemic and intrathecal administration in mice. The Journal of Pharmacology and Experimental Therapeutics, 284(3), 1058-1065.

Damaj, M. I.; Freitas, K.; Bagdas, D.; Flood, P. (2014). Nicotinic receptors as targets for novel analgesics and anti-inflammatory drugs. In:R. A. J. Lester (Ed.), Nicotinic receptors (pp. 239-254). Vol. 11 (pp. 239-254). New York: Springer.

Damaj, M. I.; Meyer, E. M.; Martin, B. R. (2000). The antinociceptive effects of alpha7 nicotinic agonists in an acute pain model. Neuropharmacology, 39(13), 2785-2791.

Decker, M. W.; Rueter, L. E.; Bitner, R. S. (2004). Nicotinic acetylcholine receptor agonists: a potential new class of analgesics. Current Topics in Medicinal Chemistry, 4(3), 369-384.

Di Cesare Mannelli, L.; Cinci, L.; Micheli, L.; Zanardelli, M.; Pacini, A.; McIntosh, J. M. et al. (2014). α-Conotoxin RgIA protects against the development of nerve injury-induced chronic pain and prevents both neuronal and glial derangement. Pain, 155(10), 1986-1995.

Donvito, G.; Bagdas, D.; Toma, W.; Rahimpour, E.; Jackson, A.; Meade, J. A. et al. (2017). The interaction between alpha 7 nicotinic acetylcholine receptor and nuclear peroxisome proliferator-activated receptor-α represents a new antinociceptive signaling pathway in mice. Experimental Neurology, 295, 194-201.

Elgoyhen, A. B.; Johnson, D. S.; Boulter, J.; Vetter, D. E.; Heinemann, S. (1994). α9: an acetylcholine receptor with novel phar-macological properties expressed in rat cochlear hair cells. Cell, 79(4), 705-715.

Elgoyhen, A. B.; Vetter, D. E.; Katz, E.; Rothlin, C. V.; Heinemann, S. F.; Boulter, J. (2001). Alpha10: a determinant of nicotinic cholinergic receptor function in mammalian vestibular and cochlear mechanosensory hair cells. Proceedings of the National Academy of Sciences ofthe United States of America, 98(6), 3501-3506.

Freitas, K.; Carroll, F. I.; Damaj, M. I. (2013). The antinociceptive effects of nicotinic receptors α7-positive allosteric modulators in murine acute and tonic pain models. The Journal of Pharmacology and Experimental Therapeutics, 344(1), 264-275.

Freitas, K.; Ghosh, S.; Ivy Carroll, F.; Lichtman, A. H.; ImadDamaj, M. (2013). Effects of alpha 7 positive allosteric modulators in murine inflammatory and chronic neuropathic pain models. Neuropharmacology, 65, 156-164.

Freitas, K.; Negus, S.; Carroll, F. I.; Damaj, M. I. (2013). In vivo pharmacological interactions between a type II positive allosteric modulator of α7 nicotinic ACh receptors and nicotinic agonists in a murine tonic pain model. British Journal of Pharmacology, 169(3), 567-579.

Gotti, C.; Zoli, M.; Clementi, F. (2006). Brain nicotinic acetylcholine receptors: native subtypes and their relevance. Trends in Pharmacological Sciences, 27(9), 482-491.

Kesingland, A. C.; Gentry, C. T.; Panesar, M. S.; Bowes, M. A.; Vernier, J. M.; Cube, R. et al. (2000). Analgesic profile of the nicotinic acetylcholine receptor agonists, (+)-epibatidine and ABT-594 in models of persistent inflammatory and neuropathic pain. Pain, 86(1-2), 113-118.

Khan, I.; Osaka, H.; Stanislaus, S.; Calvo, R. M.; Deerinck, T.; Yaksh, T. L. et al. (2003). Nicotinic acetylcholine receptor distribution in relation to spinal neurotransmission pathways. Journal of Comparative Neurology, 467(1), 44-59.

Lawand, N. B.; Lu, Y.; Westlund, K. N. (1999). Nicotinic cholinergic receptors: potential targets for inflammatory pain relief. Pain, 80(1-2), 291-299.

Lee, C. H.; Zhu, C.; Malysz, J.; Campbell, T.; Shaughnessy, T.; Honore, P. et al. (2011). α4β2 neuronal nicotinic receptor positive allosteric modulation: an approach for improving the therapeutic index of α4β2 nAChR agonists in pain. Biochemical Pharmacology, 82(8), 959-966.

Lynch, J. J.; Wade, C. L.; Mikusa, J. P.; Decker, M. W.; Honore, P. (2005). ABT-594 (a nicotinic acetylcholine agonist): antiallodynia in a rat chemotherapy-induced pain model. European Journal of Pharmacology, 509(1), 43-48.

Marubio, L. M.; del Mar Arroyo-Jimenez, M.; Cordero-Erausquin, M.; Léna, C.; Le Novère, N.; de Kerchove d'Exaerde, M. et al. (1999). Reduced antinociception in mice lacking neuronal nicotinic receptor subunits. Nature, 398(6730), 805-810.

McIntosh, J. M.; Absalom, N.; Chebib, M.; Elgoyhen, A. B.; Vincler, M. (2009). Alpha9 nicotinic acetylcholine receptors and the treatment of pain. Biochemical Pharmacology, 78(7), 693-702.

Merskey, H.; Bogduk, N. (1994). Classification of chronic pain. IASP Pain Terminology.

Napier, I. A.; Klimis, H.; Rycroft, B. K.; Jin, A. H.; Alewood, P. F.; Motin, L. et al. (2012). Intrathecal α-conotoxins Vc1. 1, AuIB and MII acting on distinct nicotinic receptor subtypes reverse signs of neuropathic pain. Neuropharmacology, 62(7), 2201-2206.

Neubig, R. R.; Spedding, M.; Kenakin, T.; Christopoulos, A. (2003). International Union of Pharmacology Committee on Receptor Nomenclature and Drug Classification. XXXVIII. Update on terms and symbols in quantitative pharmacology. Pharmacological Reviews, 55(4), 597-606.

Papke, R. L.; Bagdas, D.; Kulkarni, A. R.; Gould, T.; AlSharari, S. D.; Thakur, G. A. et al. (2015). The analgesic-like properties of the alpha7 nAChR silent agonist NS6740 is associated with non-conducting conformations of the receptor. Neuropharmacology, 91, 34-42.

Papke, R. L.; Stokes, C.; Damaj, M. I.; Thakur, G. A.; Manther, K.; Treinin, M. et al. (2017). Persistent activation of α7 nicotinic ACh receptors associated with stable induction of different desensitized states. British Journal of Pharmacology, 1-17.

Pavlov, V. A.; Parrish, W. R.; Rosas-Ballina, M.; Ochani, M.; Puerta, M.; Ochani, K. et al. (2009). Brain acetylcholinesterase activity controls systemic cytokine levels through the cholinergic anti-inflammatory pathway. Brain, Behavior, and Immunity, 23(1), 41-45.

Rode, F.; Munro, G.; Holst, D.; Nielsen, E.; Troelsen, K. B.; Timmermann, D. B. et al. (2012). Positive allosteric modulation of α4β2 nAChR agonist induced behaviour. Brain Research, 1458, 67-75.

Romero, H. K.; Christensen, S. B.; Di Cesare Mannelli, L.; Gajewiak, J.; Ramachandra, R.; Elmslie, K. S. et al. (2017). Inhibition of α9α10 nicotinic acetylcholine receptors prevents chemotherapy-induced neuropathic pain. Proceedings of the National Academy of Sciences.

Rowbotham, M. C.; Rachel Duan, W.; Thomas, J.; Nothaft, W.; Backonja, M. M. (2009). A randomized, double-blind, placebo-controlled trial evaluating the efficacy and safety of ABT-594 in patients with diabetic peripheral neuropathic pain. Pain, 146(3), 245-252.

Rowley, T. J.; McKinstry, A.; Greenidge, E.; Smith, W.; Flood, P. (2010). Antinociceptive and anti-inflammatory effects of choline in a mouse model of postoperative pain. British Journal of Anaesthesia, 105(2), 201-207.

Rueter, L. E.; Meyer, M. D.; Decker, M. W. (2000). Spinal mechanisms underlying A-85380-induced effects on acute thermal pain. Brain Research, 872(1-2), 93-101.

Satkunanathan, N.; Livett, B.; Gayler, K.; Sandall, D.; Down, J.; Khalil, Z. (2005). Alpha-conotoxin Vc1. 1 alleviates neuropathic pain and accelerates functional recovery of injured neurones. Brain Research, 1059(2), 149-158.

Umana, I. C.; Daniele, C. A.; Miller, B. A.; Gallagher, K.; Brown, M. A. (2017). Nicotinic modulation of descending pain control circuitry. Pain, 158, 1938-1950.

van Maanen, M. A.; Stoof, S. P.; LaRosa, G. J.; Vervoordeldonk, M. J.; Tak, P. P. (2010). Role of the cholinergic nervous system in rheuma-toid arthritis: aggravation of arthritis in nicotinic acetylcholine receptor α7 subunit gene knockout mice. Annals of the Rheumatic Diseases, 69(9), 1717-1723.

Vincler, M.; Eisenach, J. C. (2004). Plasticity of spinal nicotinic acetyl-choline receptors following spinal nerve ligation. Neuroscience Research, 48(2), 139-145.

Vincler, M.; Wittenauer, S.; Parker, R.; Ellison, M.; Olivera, B. M.; McIntosh, J. M. (2006). Molecular mechanism for analgesia involving specific antagonism of α9α10 nicotinic acetylcholine receptors. Pro-ceedings of the National Academy of Sciences, 103(47), 17880-17884.

Wala, E. P.; Crooks, P. A.; McIntosh, J. M.; Holtman, J. R. (2012). Novel small molecule α9α10 nicotinic receptor antagonist prevents and reverses chemotherapy-evoked neuropathic pain in rats. Anesthesia and Analgesia, 115(3), 713-720.

Williams, D. K.; Wang, J.; Papke, R. L. (2011). Positive allosteric mod-ulators as an approach to nicotinic acetylcholine receptor-targeted therapeutics: advantages and limitations. Biochemical Pharmacology, 82(8), 915-930.

Woolf, C. J. (2010). Overcoming obstacles to developing new analgesics. Nature Medicine, 16(11), 1241-1247.

Wu, J.; Liu, Q.; Tang, P.; Mikkelsen, J. D.; Shen, J.; Whiteaker, P. et al. (2016). Heteromeric α7β2 nicotinic acetylcholine receptors in the brain. Trends in Pharmacological Sciences, 37(7), 562-574.

Zhang, J.; Xiao, Y. D.; Jordan, K. G.; Hammond, P. S.; Van Dyke, K. M.; Mazurov, A. A. et al. (2012). Analgesic effects mediated by neuronal nicotinic acetylcholine receptor agonists: correlation with desensitization of α4β2* receptors. European Journal of Pharmaceutical Sciences, 47(5), 813-823.

Zhu, C. Z.; Chin, C. -L.; Rustay, N. R.; Zhong, C.; Mikusa, J.; Chandran, P. et al. (2011). Potentiation of analgesic efficacy but not side effects: co-administration of an α4β2 neuronal nicotinic acetylcholine receptor agonist and its positive allosteric modulator in experimental models of pain in rats. Biochemical Pharmacology, 82(8), 967-976.

34
肌肉型烟碱受体的药理作用

Armando Alberola-Die, Raúl Cobo, Isabel Ivorra, Andrés Morales

Division of Physiology, Department of Physiology, Genetics and Microbiology, Universidad de Alicante（Spain），Alicante, Spain

缩略语

A	激动剂	ICD	胞内结构域
ACh	乙酰胆碱	LGIC	配体门控离子通道
AM	变构调节剂	$nAChR_m$	肌肉型烟碱乙酰胆碱受体
CCh	氨基甲酰胆碱	NAM	负变构调节剂
CI	竞争性抑制剂	NCI	非竞争性抑制剂
ECD	胞外结构域	NMJ	神经肌肉接头
epp	终板电位	PAM	正变构调节剂
FCS	快通道综合征	SCS	慢通道综合征
I_{ACh}	由Ach引起的膜电流	TMD	跨膜结构域

34.1 引言

一个多世纪以来，一些最杰出的神经科学家（其中许多是诺贝尔奖获得者）一直致力于破译突触传递的机制。为此，运动神经和横纹肌纤维之间的突触，即神经肌肉接头（NMJ）成为最有用的模型之一。在NMJ，肌肉型烟碱乙酰胆碱受体（nAChRm）是位于自身肌肉纤维中的关键成分。很可能，第一个涉及钠离子通道阻滞剂的药理学研究是在19世纪由C. Bernard进行的，他发现治愈的青蛙在神经刺激后骨骼肌缺乏收缩。后来，Langley（1905）发现烟碱，一种烟草叶中的生物碱，诱导家禽肌肉的有效收缩，这种收缩被箭毒抑制；他的结论是"肌肉含有一些与烟碱和箭毒结合的辅助物质"。然后，Dale等（1936）表明，即使是在通过治疗防止肌肉收缩的情况下，刺激灌注的随意肌中的运动神经元纤维会诱导静脉液中ACh的出现。此后不久，Eccles等（1941）通过细胞外记终板电位（epps）探索了神经肌肉传递，并测试了抗胆碱酯酶药物毒扁豆碱对它们的作用。随后，Katz的小组通过用细胞内微电极记录肌纤维详细研究了epps的特征，为突触传递奠定了基础（图34.1）。此外，他们在NMJ用装有乙酰胆碱的微管通过离子电渗法精确释放乙酰胆碱。通过这种局部乙酰胆碱的应用，他们可以模拟神经刺激对肌肉的影响（Del Castillo, Katz, 1955），并绘制了肌纤维上$nAChR_m$的分布图，这使他们能够检测连接和连接外受体（Miledi, 1960）。

由于几个里程碑，在分子水平上对$nAChR_m$的结构和功能特性有更深入的了解已成为可能：①Neher和Sakmann（1976）引入了膜片钳技术，该技术能够记录单个$nAChR_m$的活性。②Miledi等（1971）利用放射性标记的α-银环蛇毒素（银环蛇毒的一种成分，可特异性地和不可逆地阻断乙酰胆碱对NMJ的去极化作用）对来自鱼雷真鲷的氯化钠进行生化纯化（Lee,

Tseng, 1966)。随后, 纯化的钠离子交换膜在人工脂质基质中进行功能性重组, 从而可以详细研究无细胞模型中的活性, 如脂质双层 (Nelsonet al. 1980) 或宿主细胞 [如非洲爪蟾卵母细胞, 在其微移植后 (Morales et al. 1995)]。③随着分子生物学技术的进步, 可以解决α亚基序列 (Noda et al. 1982) 和后来的cDNA克隆编码为其他nAChR$_m$子单元 (Changeux, Edelstein, 2005), 这为揭示nAChR$_m$关键结构残基的功能作用的诱变实验铺平了道路。④高分辨率电子显微镜, 在其中nAChR$_m$被密集地填充, 能够开发nAChR$_m$结构的原子尺度模型 (Unwin, 2005), 这已经成为在硅研究的nAChR功能和调制的关键工具。

34.2 钠离子通道的整体结构和功能

钠离子通道是一种配体门控离子通道 (LGIC), 属于受体的Cys环亚家族, 参与快速突触传递。它们都有一个五聚体结构, 每个亚基有四个跨膜 (M1-M4) 疏水区 (TMD), 两个半胱氨酸残基之间有一个二硫键, 在胞外侧形成一个由13个氨基酸组成的独特环。来自成年脊椎动物的nAChR$_m$由2α1、1β1、1δ和1ε亚基组成, 它们是与鱼类的nAChR的ε亚基 (连接型) 相当的γ亚基。在胚胎和连接外 (图34.1) nAChR$_m$s中, ε亚基被不同的γ亚基取代。nAChR$_m$组合亚基的这种异质性是相关的, 因为至少它部分地决定了它们的功能和药理特性 (见下文)。nAChR$_m$的高分辨率电子显微镜图像的结构模型显示它的五个亚基围绕一个中心轴排列构成通道孔, 细胞外和细胞内结构域 (分别为ECD和ICD) 从膜双层突出 [Unwin, 2005; 图34.2 (a_1) 和 (a_2)]。通道孔由每个亚基的M2片段 (通道内环) 排列, 而M4片段构成最外环, 直接与双层脂质相互作用 [见图34.2 (a_2)]。在电子捕获检测器中, nAChR$_m$有两个配体结合 (正交) 位点, 分别位于α-γ (或α-ε) 和α-δ界面 [图34.2 (a_1)]。nAChR$_m$是变构蛋白, 可能至少采用三种不同的可相互转换的构象状态 [Albuquerque et al. 2009; Bouzat, Sine, 2017; Changeux, 2012; 图34.2 (b)]。在没有

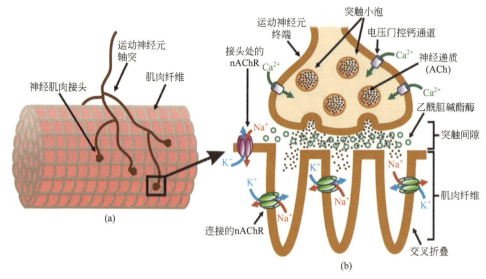

图34.1 神经肌肉接头处的突触传递方案 (NMJ)

(a) 在NMJ, 一个运动神经元轴突分支并终止于它控制的每条肌肉纤维的表面; (b) 所示NMJ区域的放大图, 显示突触前神经末梢含有乙酰胆碱囊泡和参与递质释放的电压依赖性Ca^{2+}通道。乙酰胆碱释放到突触间隙, 富含乙酰胆碱酯酶, 最终到达含有大量 (高达20.000/μm^2) 连接nAChR$_m$的交叉折叠。罕见的连接外 (胎儿亚型) 钠离子通道超出了这个突触区域。

激动剂的情况下,位于膜深处的疏水通道门关闭,钠通道处于静止状态。当乙酰胆碱或其他激动剂如氨基甲酰胆碱（CCh）结合到立体位置时,钠通道迅速激活（在微秒范围内）,通道打开,主要允许钠离子和钾离子通过膜,产生离子电流[见图34.2（c_1）和（c_2）]。$nAChR_m$长时间暴露于ACh会引发构象变化被称为脱敏状态的转变（Thesleff, 1955）,其特征是对激动剂亲和力增强的非传导构象。最有可能的是,有几种中间脱敏状态,每种状态都有自己的动力学特征,但总体脱敏率明显取决于激动剂浓度,当乙酰胆碱浓度升高时,脱敏率会增加[图34.2（c_2）]。

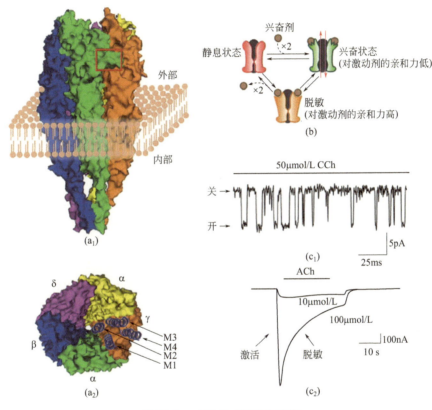

图 34.2 $nAChR_m$ 的结构与功能

34.3 $nAChR_m$的调制机制

$nAChR_m$是相关的治疗靶点,因为它们的功能障碍与导致运动活动受损的几个病理生理过程的发生有关,就像在各种先天性肌无力综合征中所发生的那样（Kalamida et al. 2007）。因此,了解这些受体受不同分子调控的机制并解开它们的特定结合位点（Chatzidaki, Millar, 2015）,以开发新的治疗药物是很重要的。

在过去的几十年里,研究表明,许多具有不同化学结构的分子通过与$nAChR_m$受体的不同区域结合来调节$nAChR_m$的功能,因此,它们通过不同的机制发挥作用：

（1）竞争性　由结合到立体结合位点的分子介导（图34.3；位点1）,干扰激动剂-受体的相互作用（参见表34.1的例子）。这些分子中的许多也可以作为完全或部分激动剂。所有这些分子的药理学特征表现为剂量反应曲线的右移[图34.4（a_2）和（b）]。

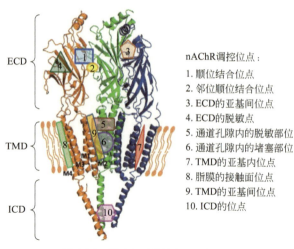

图 34.3 钠离子通道的主要调节位点

所有 nAChR、胞外（ECD）、跨膜（TMD）和胞内（ICD），三个结构域都有相应的调控位点。
主要的调节位点显示在 nAChRs 结构上［与图 34.2（a）中的模板相同］，并总结在右侧。

（2）空间位阻 由与①靠近空间位阻的残基相互作用的分子引发以阻碍/限制激动剂结合到立体位的方式结合位点（图 34.3，位点 2；表 34.1）和②当受体处于活性状态时，位于通道孔中的残基，充当开放通道阻断剂（图 34.3，位点 6）。空间阻断剂引起非竞争性抑制［NCI；图 34.4（a_2）和（b）］；然而，开放通道阻断剂不断地与它们的相互作用位点结合和分离，导致动态阻断，这在记录单通道电流时观察到"闪烁"（Neher, Steinbach, 1978）。通常，开放通道阻断是由生理酸碱度下的带电分子施加的，如他克林、塞来膦酸钠或氟西汀（表 34.1），它们的阻断程度在很大程度上取决于细胞膜电位［图 34.4（a_1）和（a_2）］。

（3）变构 在不同于原构位点的位点相互作用并改变钠离子通道功能活性的分子。它们被分类为阴性变构调节剂或正变构调节剂，无论它们分别降低还是增强钠通道功能。这些调节剂可以通过结合不同的 nAChR$_m$ 位置起作用：

① ECD 作用调节剂。这些分子结合位于 ECD 的残基，因此，它们可以作用于静止状态的 nAChR$_m$ 触发构象变化，从而阻碍或促进 nAChR$_m$ 的开放（图 34.3；位点 3）或改变其脱敏作用［图 34.3，位点 4；图 34.4（a_3），表 34.1］。作用于这些位点的纳米粒不会显著改变剂量-反应曲线，通常表现为 NCI 效应，导致封闭通道阻断［图 34.4（a_2）和（b）］。然而，当与激动剂合用时，它们中的一些表现出"明显的竞争性"药理学特征，剂量-反应曲线略微向右偏移［图 34.4（a_2）和（b）］。当不结盟运动主要引发封闭通道封锁，但也引发开放通道封锁时，情况就是如此。因此，乙酰胆碱浓度越高，打开的钠通道就越多，因此停留在静息状态的就越少状态，并易于在孔外发生阻滞作用。因此，乙酰胆碱浓度的增加将降低抑制程度，类似于利多卡因的竞争性抑制机制（Alberrola-Die et al. 2011；表 34.1）。

② TMD 作用调节剂。它们大多是疏水性分子，与位于 M1-M4 片段的亚基腔内（图 34.3，位点 7）或亚基间裂缝（图 34.3，位点 9；表 34.1）的残基结合。此外，这些疏水分子可以通过膜扩散，并与位于脂质-蛋白质界面的氨基酸相互作用（Barrantes, 2004；图 34.3，位点 8）。此外，一些 TMD 调制器可以通过与位于细胞外侧特定位置的离子通道中的残基相互作用来修饰 nAChR$_m$ 脱敏（Arias, 2010；图 34.3，位点 5）。

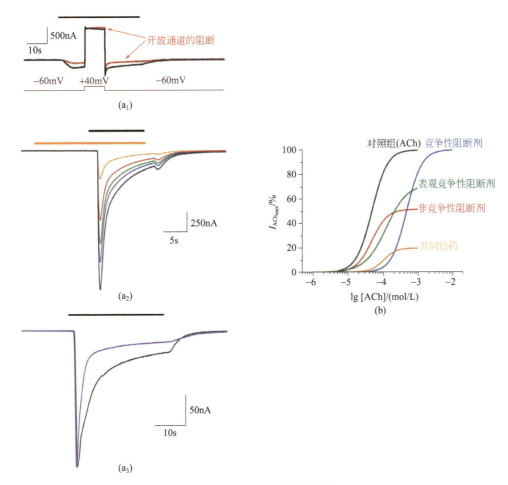

图 34.4 nAChR$_m$ 封闭的机制

(a)记录说明了 nAChR$_m$ 封闭的不同机制:(a$_1$)电压依赖性(开放通道)阻断,通常由结合在通道孔内的带电分子引起。在 60mV 时(棕色迹线表示施加的电压电位),阻断剂减少(比较空白和红色记录),但阻断在 +40mV 时消失。(a$_2$)非竞争性阻断剂,在其 IC$_{50}$ 时,将对照 IACh(黑色记录)减少到一半(红色记录);竞争性(蓝色记录)和表观竞争性(绿色记录)阻断剂根据乙酰胆碱浓度降低抗胆碱酯酶活性;预给药后与激动剂共同给药时,同时作为封闭和开放通道阻滞剂的分子会引起更大和复杂的抑制作用(橙色记录)。(a$_3$)当乙酰胆碱与调节剂(紫色记录)共同使用时,改变乙酰胆碱的呈现率,由乙酰胆碱(黑色记录)引起的呈现显著增强。(b)乙酰胆碱单独(黑色)或与通过不同机制起作用的调节化合物一起引起的剂量-反应曲线模型:非竞争性方式(红色曲线),例如,当药物结合到通道孔中时;当分子在立体位置相互作用时的竞争方式(蓝色曲线);由通过开放和封闭通道阻断作用的分子引发的表观竞争机制(绿色曲线)(详见正文);最后,某些分子在不同的位置与钠离子交换膜相互作用,导致大而复杂的抑制(橙色曲线)。

③ ICD 作用调节剂。这些分子通过结合细胞内残基来修饰钠通道功能(图 34.3,位点 10)。至少,其中一些通过间接途径改变脱敏作用,包括细胞内信号分子的产生,使 nAChR$_m$ 上的 ICD 残基磷酸化(Ochoa et al. 1989)。

表 34.1 调节 nAChR$_m$ 的功能选定分子

类别	分子作用	结合位点	效价	参考文献
肌肉松弛剂	琥珀酰胆碱	A; (NCI)/1, 5, 6	EC$_{50}$=10.8 μmol/L IC$_{50}$=126 μmol/L	Jonsson et al. (2006)
	巴夫龙	CI/1	IC$_{50}$=15 nmol/L	Liu, Dilger (2009)

34 肌肉型烟碱受体的药理作用

续表

类别	分子作用	结合位点	效价	参考文献
乙酰胆碱酯酶抑制剂	他克林	NAM (NCI)/3, 6	$IC_{50}=1.6 \sim 4.6 \mu mol/L$	Prince, Pennington, Sine (2002)
	艾宙酚	NAM (NCI)/3, 6	$IC_{50}=10 \mu mol/L$	Olivera-Bravo, Ivorra, Morales (2007)
	毒扁豆碱	PAM; NAM/2, 3	$IC_{50}=10 mmol/L$	Hamouda, Kimm, Cohen (2013)
	加兰他敏	PAM; NAM/2, 3	$IC_{50}=2.8 mmol/L$	Hamouda et al. (2013)
阳离子	Ca^{2+}	NAM/4	$0.1 \sim 1 mmol/L$ 范围	Ochoa et al. (1989)
	Zn^{2+}	PAM/3	测试浓度=$200 \mu mol/L$	García-Colunga, Vázquez-Gómez, Miledi (2004)
内源性分子	孕酮	NAM (NCI)/3, 7, 8, 9	$IC_{50}=1.0 \sim 6.1 \mu mol/L$	Ke, Lukas (1996)
	雌二醇	NAM (NCI)/3, 7, 8, 9	$IC_{50}=20 \sim 56 \mu mol/L$	Ke, Lukas (1996)
	皮质甾酮	NAM (NCI)/3, 7, 8, 9	$IC_{50}=30 \sim 92.1 \mu mol/L$	Ke, Lukas (1996)
	胆固醇	AM/7, 8, 9		Barrantes (2004)
	P物质	NAM (NCI)/5		Arias (1997)
	5-羟色胺	NAM (NCI)/6		Arias (1997)
	脂肪酸	NAM (NCI)/8, 9		Barrantes (2004)
	蛋白激酶A	NAM (NCI)/10		Hoffman, Ravindran, Huganir (1994)
	蛋白激酶C	NAM (NCI)/10		Ochoa et al. (1989)
抗疟药	阿的平	NAM (NCI)/8, 9	$10 \sim 100 \mu mol/L$	Arias (1997), Kaldany, Karlin (1983)
	奎宁	NAM (NCI)/3, 6	$50 \mu mol/L$	Sieb, Milone, Engel (1996)
抗生素	庆大霉素	NAM (NCI, CI)/1, 4	$IC_{50}=25 \mu mol/L$	Amici, Eusebi, Miledi (2005)
	青霉素	NAM (NCI, CI)/1, 6	$IC_{50}=0.71 mmol/L$	Schlesinger, Krampfl, Haeseler, Dengler, Bufler (2004)
抗精神病药物	氯丙嗪	NAM (NCI)/4, 6	$IC_{50}>300 nmol/L$	Changeux, Edelstein (2005)
	氟西汀	NAM (NCI)/3, 5	测试浓度=$2 \mu mol/L$	García-Colunga, Awad, Miledi (1997)
	安非他酮	NAM (NCI)/3, 4, 5, 6	$IC_{50}=0.40 \sim 40.1 \mu mol/L$	Arias et al. (2009)
	丙咪嗪	NAM (NCI)/5	$K_i=0.85 \sim 3.8 \mu mol/L$	Sanghvi et al. (2008)
全麻药	丙酚	NAM (NCI)/5, 6, 7, 9	$IC_{50}=40 \sim 125 \mu mol/L$	Jayakar, Dailey, Eckenhoff, Cohen (2013)
	异氟烷	NAM (NCI)/5, 6	$K_d=0.36 mmol/L$	Arias, Bhumireddy (2005)
	氯胺酮	NAM (NCI, CI)/2, 5, 6	$K_d=2 \mu mol/L$	Scheller et al. (1996)
	戊巴比妥	NAM (NCI, CI)/1, 2, 6	$K_d=15 \sim 30 \mu mol/L$	Krampfl, Schlesinger, Dengler, Bufler (2000)
局部麻醉剂	普鲁卡因	NAM (NCI)/6, 8	$K_d=690 \sim 790 \mu mol/L$	Arias, Bhumireddy (2005)
	利多卡因	NAM (NCI)/3, 4, 7, 9, 5, 6	$IC_{50}=70 \mu mol/L$	Alberola-Die et al. (2011)
	普罗地芬	NAM (NCI, CI)/1, 3, 4	$IC_{50}=19 \mu mol/L$	Spitzmaul, Gumilar, Dilger, Spitzmaul et al. (2009)
	解痉素	NAM (NCI)/4, 5	$IC_{50}=15 \mu mol/L$	Spitzmaul et al. (2009)
毒素	类毒素A	A/1	$EC_{50}=50 nmol/L$	Wonnacott, Barik (2007)

续表

类别	分子作用	结合位点	效价	参考文献
毒素	新热带蛙毒素	NAM (NCI)/4, 6	K_i=0.1～1μmol/L	Changeux, Edelstein (2005)
	筒箭毒碱	CI/1	IC_{50}=50～100nmol/L	Arias (1997), Wonnacott, Barik (2007)
	α-银环蛇神经毒素	CI/1	测试浓度=0.01～10nmol/L	Wonnacott, Barik (2007)
	α-芋螺毒素	CI/1	K_d=0.1～1nmol/L	Wonnacott, Barik (2007)
	烟碱	A/1	ED_{20}=20μmol/L	Wonnacott, Barik (2007)
	地棘蛙素	A/1	测试浓度=2～300μmol/L	Prince, Sine (1998)
	马钱子碱	NCI/3	IC_{50}=7.3μmol/L	García-Colunga, Miledi (1999)
其他胺/铵化合物	美加明	NCI/5, 6	1～10μmol/L至100μmol/L	Varanda et al. (1985)
	四乙基铵盐	A; NAM (CI)/1, 3, 6	IC_{50}=2～3mmol/L	Akk, Steinbach (2003)
	二乙胺	NAM/2、3、6、7	IC_{50}=70μmol/L	Alberola Die, Fernándezballester, González Ros, Ivorra, Morales (2016a)
	2,6-二甲基苯胺	NAM/4,9,5,6	IC_{50}=2.1mmol/L	Alberola-Die, Fernández-Ballester, González-Ros, Ivorra, Morales (2016b)

由于许多配体的化学结构中存在不同的官能团，并非所有上述作用机制都是相互排斥的。实际上，单个分子可以结合到不同的甚至更远的位点，产生复杂的药理学特征，这取决于应用方式和所用调节剂的浓度。此外，$nAChR_m$调节剂可以通过两种不同的非排他性途径获得它们的结合位点（Hille, 1977；图34.5）：首先是亲水途径，由极性配体使用，与位于ECD或通道孔的残基相互作用（图34.5，红色箭头），其次是疏水途径，随后是非极性和亲脂性分子在不同TMD区域（包括脂

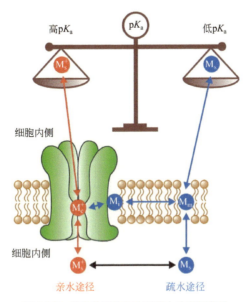

图34.5 药物作用的亲水和疏水途径示意图

许多调节$nAChR_m$的分子是两亲性的；因此，介质中存在带电和不带电的形式。带电（质子化）分子主要通过亲水途径（红色箭头）到达其结合位点，而不带电形式主要遵循疏水途径（蓝色箭头）。每种形式的比例取决于分子pK_a和介质的酸碱度；在该方案中，天平"感知"分子pK_a，随着粒子数的增加，带电分子的百分比增加。

质蛋白界面）和ICD（图34.5，蓝色箭头）结合nAChR$_m$残基。每个分子作用于nAChR$_m$的路径主要取决于调节剂的pK_a和受体环境的酸碱度，因为两者都决定分子质子化。许多两亲性分子，如局部麻醉剂利多卡因，在生理pH值下被部分质子化，因此，它们可以通过两种途径到达结合位点。

34.4 不同治疗药物对nAChR$_m$功能的调节

关于nAChR$_m$的功能调节，应考虑NMJ的三个特点：①存在两种在胎儿和成人生活中差异表达的nAChR$_m$。结合型和结外型nAChR$_m$在功能和药理特性上都不同。因此，结合型表现出较大的通道电导和较短的平均开放时间（Katz, Miledi, 1972; Neher, Sakmann, 1976），而且，结合型则表现出较快的脱敏（Morales, Sumikawa, 1992）。此外，由于αA-芋螺毒素OIVB与连接亚型的亲和力几乎降低了2000倍，因此它选择性地被从暗圆锥蛇毒中提纯的OIVB阻断（Teichert et al. 2005）。②epps振幅大，为信号传输提供了很高的安全系数，使NMJ成为一个单一的突触。③nAChR$_m$直接暴露在循环化合物（包括毒素）中，而神经元nAChR则受到血-脑或血-神经屏障的部分保护。值得注意的是，大量的非均相分子，其中许多是两亲性的，与nAChR相互作用，调节其功能。其中有内源性分子（包括激素）和许多临床上常用的化合物，如肌肉松弛剂、乙酰胆碱酯酶抑制剂、抗生素、抗疟药、抗精神病药物以及局部和全身麻醉药，其中许多作用在微摩尔范围（表34.1）。此外，大量毒素、胺/铵化合物和其他分子作为NAM或PAM对nAChR$_m$具有强大的作用。更重要的是，某些分子对钠离子交换膜的作用明显依赖于浓度，很可能是因为它们作用于几个具有不同亲和力的调节位点，因此，它们可以引起不同的，甚至是拮抗的效应。

34.5 未来展望

为了更好地理解调节剂作用于nAChR$_m$的确切机制，还需要对nAChR$_m$的变构调节进行进一步的研究。这些知识与减少/预防不同治疗分子引发的某些副作用相关。例如，地塞米松因其免疫抑制作用而被广泛用于改善重症肌无力患者；然而，起初，这种合成糖皮质激素可能会抑制肾上腺皮质激素释放激素，导致患者症状恶化。此外，这些研究为开发新的治疗分子奠定了基础，这些分子更熟练且副作用更少，可用于治疗与脑钠肽代谢综合征功能障碍相关的病理生理过程。

术语解释

- 乙酰胆碱激活电流：（I_{ACh}）由ACh引起的离子膜电流，作用于nAChR$_m$。
- 乙酰胆碱酯酶：酯酶位于切割ACh的突触间隙中。与nAChR$_m$正构位点外结合并改变其功能的变构调节剂分子。根据它们分别降低还是增强nAChR$_m$的性能，将它们分为负或正变构调节剂。
- 闭路阻滞剂：防止受体被激动剂激活。稳定暴露于激动剂时，nAChR$_m$受体的脱敏作用降低。配体门控离子通道（LGIC）受体膜离子通道被特定的配体激活，参与快速的突触传递。
- 肌肉型烟碱样受体：（nAChR$_m$）由ACh激活的异源五聚体（2α1、1β1、1ε和1δ亚基）膜蛋白，存在于成人或胎儿神经肌肉接头（突触型）、突触外或神经支配的肌肉中（由γ而不是ε亚基组成）。
- 重症肌无力：可由不同的nAChR$_m$功能障碍引起。明渠阻滞剂分子结合到孔隙中，堵塞明渠。正激动剂结合位点的正构结合位点，以激活受体。

- Thesleff（1955）首先对nAChR$_m$进行了描述。
- 稳定暴露于激动剂时，nAChR$_m$切换为高亲和力配体结合状态，该状态为不导电（闭合状态）。
- ACh和一些部分激动剂引起nAChR$_m$脱敏，其随着激动剂浓度的增加而增加。
- 并非所有LGIC都会降低灵敏度。nAChR脱敏的速率在很大程度上取决于亚基的组成。
- nAChR$_m$至少有两个脱敏状态，它们具有自己的动力学常数。
- 脱敏剂引起的nAChR$_m$恢复可能会在激动剂退出后持续数秒甚至数分钟。
- nAChR$_m$调节剂通过作用于细胞外、跨膜或细胞内基因座来影响脱敏率。
- 一些阴性的变构调节剂会增加nAChR$_m$脱敏，而某些阳性的变构调节剂会降低甚至阻止它。
- 一些先天性肌无力综合征会改变nAChR$_m$脱敏。

- 大多数nAChR$_m$功能障碍会导致肌无力，即肌肉无力。
- 一些毒素（α-真菌毒素和α-芋螺毒素）或生物碱（D-微管尿素）作用于nAChR，导致严重的肌无力甚至瘫痪。
- 肌无力可能由一种或几种nAChR$_m$亚基的遗传改变（通常引起慢通道或快速通道综合征）或突触后nAChR$_m$的数量减少（重症肌无力）或释放的ACh量的自身免疫性降低（Lambert-Eaton综合征）引起。
- 与慢通道综合征（SCS）相关的肌肉无力是由长时间的突触后去极化引起的，这是由延迟的通道关闭，降低的脱敏作用或对ACh的亲和力引起的。
- 某些nAChR$_m$（氟西汀和奎尼丁）的开放通道阻滞剂可缓解由于SCS引起的肌无力，而胆碱酯酶抑制剂会加剧肌无力（RodríguezCruz, Palace, Beeson, 2014）。
- 由于亚基突变引起通道开放缓慢、开放通道可能性降低、开放停留时间较短、脱敏性增强或ACh结合亲和力降低，患有快速通道综合征（FCS）的重症肌无力患者的终板电位降低。
- 抗胆碱酯酶药物（吡啶斯的明）可减轻FCS和重症肌无力症状。
- K$^+$通道阻滞剂3,4-二氨基吡啶可用于治疗FCS和Lambert-Eaton综合征引起的肌无力。

- 一生中肌肉烟碱型乙酰胆碱受体（nAChR$_m$）的两种亚型差异表达。
- nAChR$_m$是神经肌肉连接处突触传递的关键元素。
- 多种化合物（包括内源性分子和广泛使用的治疗药物）与nAChR$_m$相互作用。
- nAChR$_m$可以通过竞争、空间和变构机制进行调节。
- 单个分子可能通过不同的机制以及与不同基因座的结合来调节nAChR$_m$。
- 变构调节剂可以降低或增强nAChR$_m$活性。
- 更好地了解nAChR$_m$的调节将有助于开发新的治疗分子，以治疗nAChR$_m$功能障碍引起的疾病。

致谢

R.C.在阿利坎特大学获得准博士奖学金（FPUUA36）。

参考文献

Akk, G.; Steinbach, J. H. (2003). Activation and block of mouse muscle-type nicotinic receptors by tetraethylammonium. The Journal of Physiology, 551(1), 155-168.

Alberola-Die, A.; Fernández-Ballester, G.; González-Ros, J. M.; Ivorra, I.; Morales, A. (2016a). Muscle-type nicotinic receptor blockade by diethylamine, the hydrophilic moiety of lidocaine. Frontiers in Molecular Neuroscience, 9, 12.

Alberola-Die, A.; Fernández-Ballester, G.; González-Ros, J. M.; Ivorra, I.; Morales, A. (2016b). Muscle-type nicotinic receptor modulation by 2,6-dimethylaniline, a molecule resembling the hydrophobic moiety of lidocaine. Frontiers in Molecular Neuroscience, 9, 127.

Alberola-Die, A.; Martinez-Pinna, J.; González-Ros, J. M.; Ivorra, I.; Morales, A. (2011). Multiple inhibitory actions of lidocaine on Torpedo nicotinic acetylcholine receptors transplanted to Xenopus oocytes. Journal of Neurochemistry, 117(6), 1009-1019.

Albuquerque, E. X.; Pereira, E. F.; Alkondon, M.; Rogers, S. W. (2009).Mammalian nicotinic acetylcholine receptors: from structure to function. Physiological Reviews, 89(1), 73-120.

Amici, M.; Eusebi, F.; Miledi, R. (2005). Effects of the antibiotic gentamicin on nicotinic acetylcholine receptors. Neuropharmacology, 49(5), 627-637.

Arias, H. R. (1997). Topology of ligand binding sites on the nicotinic acetylcholine receptor. Brain Research Reviews, 25(2), 133-191.

Arias, H. R. (2010). Positive and negative modulation of nicotinic receptors. Advances in Protein Chemistry and Structural Biology, 80, 153-203.

Arias, H. R.; Bhumireddy, P. (2005). Anesthetics as chemical tools tostudy the structure and function of nicotinic acetylcholine receptors.Current Protein, Peptide Science, 6(5), 451-472.

Arias, H. R.; Gumilar, F.; Rosenberg, A.; Targowska-Duda, K. M.; Feuerbach, D.; Jozwiak, K. et al. (2009). Interaction of bupropion with muscle-type nicotinic acetylcholine receptors in different conformational states. Biochemistry, 48(21), 4506-4518.

Barrantes, F. J. (2004). Structural basis for lipid modulation of nicotinic acetylcholine receptor function. Brain Research Reviews, 47(1-3), 71-95.

Bouzat, C.; Sine, S. M. (2017). Nicotinic acetylcholine receptors at the single-channel level. British Journal of Pharmacology.https://doi.org/10.1111/bph.13770.

Changeux, J. P. (2012). The nicotinic acetylcholine receptor: the founding father of the pentameric ligand-gated ion channel superfamily. The Journal of Biological Chemistry, 287(48), 40207-40215.

Changeux, J. P.; Edelstein, S. J. (2005). Nicotinic acetylcholine receptors:From molecular biology to cognition. New York: Odile Jacob Publishing Corporation.

Chatzidaki, A.; Millar, N. S. (2015). Allosteric modulation of nicotinic acetylcholine receptors. Biochemical Pharmacology, 97(4), 408-417.

Dale, H. H.; Feldberg, W.; Vogt, M. (1936). Release of acetylcholine at voluntary motor nerve endings.The Journal of Physiology, 86.

Del Castillo, J.; Katz, B. (1955). On the localization of acetylcholine receptors. The Journal of Physiology, 128(1), 157-181.

Eccles, J. C.; Katz, B.; Kuffler, S. W. (1941). Nature of the "end-plate potential"in curarized muscle.Journal of Neurophysiology, 4(5), 362-387.

García-Colunga, J.; Awad, J. N.; Miledi, R. (1997). Blockage of muscle and neuronal nicotinic acetylcholine receptors by fluoxetine (Prozac). Proceedings of the National Academy of Sciences of theUnited States of America, 94(5), 2041-2044.

García-Colunga, J.; Miledi, R. (1999). Modulation of nicotinic acetylcholine receptors by strychnine. Proceedings of the National Academy of Sciences of the United States of America, 96(7), 4113-4118.

García-Colunga, J.; Vázquez-Gómez, E.; Miledi, R. (2004). Combined actions of zinc and fluoxetine on nicotinic acetylcholine receptors.The Pharmacogenomics Journal, 4(6), 388-393.

Hamouda, A. K.; Kimm, T.; Cohen, J. B. (2013). Physostigmine and galanthamine bind in the presence of agonist at the canonical and non-canonical subunit interfaces of a nicotinic acetylcholine receptor.The Journal of Neuroscience, 33(2), 485-494.

Hille, H. R. (1977). Local anesthetics: hydrophilic and hydrophobic pathways for the drug-receptor reaction. The Journal of General Physiology, 69(4), 497-515.

Hoffman, P. W.; Ravindran, A.; Huganir, R. L. (1994). Role of phosphorylation in desensitization of acetylcholine receptors expressedin Xenopus oocytes. The Journal of Neuroscience, 14(7), 4185-4195.

Jayakar, S. S.; Dailey, W. P.; Eckenhoff, R. G.; Cohen, J. B. (2013).Identification of propofol binding sites in a nicotinic acetylcholine receptor with a photoreactive propofol analog. The Journal of Biological Chemistry, 288(9), 6178-6189.

Jonsson, M.; Dabrowski, M.; Gurley, D. A.; Larsson, O.; Johnson, E. C.; Fredholm, B. B. et al. (2006). Activation and inhibition of human muscular and neuronal nicotinic acetylcholine receptors by succinylcholine. Anesthesiology, 104, 724-733.

Kalamida, D.; Poulas, K.; Avramopoulou, V.; Fostieri, E.; Lagoumintzis, G.; Lazaridis, K. et al. (2007). Muscle and neuronal nicotinic acetylcholine receptors. Structure, function and pathogenicity. The FEBS Journal, 274(15), 3799-3845.

Kaldany, R. R.; Karlin, A. (1983). Reaction of quinacrine mustard withthe acetylcholine receptor from Torpedo californica. The Journal of Biological Chemistry, 258(10), 6232-6242.

Katz, B.; Miledi, R. (1972). The statistical nature of the acetylcholine potential and its molecular components. The Journal of Physiology, 224(3), 665-699.

Ke, L.; Lukas, R. J. (1996). Effects of steroid exposure on ligand bindingand functional activities of diverse nicotinic acetylcholine receptor subtypes. Journal of Neurochemistry, 67(3), 1100-1112.

Krampfl, K.; Schlesinger, F.; Dengler, R.; Bufler, J. (2000). Pentobarbital has curare-like effects on adult-type nicotinic acetylcholine receptor channel currents. Anesthesia and Analgesia, 90(4), 970-974.

Langley, J. N. (1905). On the reaction of cells and of nerve-endings to certain poisons, chiefly as regards the reaction of striated muscle to nicotine and to curari. The Journal of Physiology, 33(4-5), 374-413.

Lee, C. Y.; Tseng, L. F. (1966). Distribution of Bungarus multicinctus venom following envenomation. Toxicon, 3(4), 281-290.

Liu, M.; Dilger, J. P. (2009). Site selectivity of competitive antagonists for the mouse adult muscle nicotinic acetylcholine receptor. Molecular Pharmacology, 75(1), 166-173.

Miledi, R. (1960). Junctional and extra-junctional acetylcholine receptors in skeletal muscle fibres. The Journal of Physiology, 151(1), 24-30.

Miledi, R.; Molinoff, P.; Potter, L. T. (1971). Isolation of the cholinergic receptor protein of Torpedoelectric tissue.Nature, 229(5286), 554-557.

Morales, A.; Aleu, J.; Ivorra, I.; Ferragut, J. A.; González-Ros, J. M.; Miledi, R. (1995). Incorporation of reconstituted acetylcholine receptors from Torpedo into the Xenopus oocyte membrane. Proceedings of the National Academy of Sciences of the United States of America, 92(18), 8468-8472.

Morales, A.; Sumikawa, K. (1992). Desensitization of junctional and extrajunctional nicotinic ACh receptors expressed in Xenopus oocytes. Brain Research Molecular Brain Research, 16(3-4), 323-329.

Neher, E.; Sakmann, B. (1976). Noise analysis of drug induced voltage clamp currents in denervated frog muscle fibres. The Journal of Physiology, 258(3), 705-729.

Neher, E.; Steinbach, J. H. (1978). Local anaesthetics transiently block currents through single acetylcholine-receptor channels. The Journal of Physiology, 277, 153-176.

Nelson, N.; Anholt, R.; Lindstrom, J.; Montal, M. (1980). Reconstitution of purified acetylcholine receptors with functional ion channels in planar lipid bilayers. Proceedings of the National Academy of Sciences of the United States of America, 77(5), 3057-3061.

Noda, M.; Takahasi, H.; Tanabe, T.; Toyosato, M.; Furutani, Y.; Hirose, T. et al. (1982). Primary structure of α-subunit precursor of Torpedo californica acetylcholine receptor deduced from cDNA sequence. Nature, 299(5886), 793-797.

Ochoa, E. L.; Chattopadhyay, A.; McNamee, M. G. (1989). Desensitization of the nicotinic acetylcholine receptor. Molecular mechanisms and effect of modulators. Cellular and Molecular Neurobiology, 9(2), 141-178.

Olivera-Bravo, S.; Ivorra, I.; Morales, A. (2007). Diverse inhibitory actions of quaternary ammonium cholinesterase inhibitors on Torpedo nicotinic ACh receptors transplanted to Xenopus oocytes. British Journal of Pharmacology, 151(8), 1280-1292.

Prince, R. J.; Pennington, R. A.; Sine, S. M. (2002). Mechanism of tacrine block at adult human muscle nicotinic acetylcholine receptors.The Journal of General Physiology, 120(3), 369-393.

Prince, R. J.; Sine, S. M. (1998). Epibatidine activates muscle acetylcholine receptors with unique site selectivity. Biophysical Journal, 75(4), 1817-1827.

Rodríguez Cruz, P. M.; Palace, J.; Beeson, D. J. (2014). Inherited disorders of the neuromuscular junction: an update. Journal of Neurology, 261(11), 2234-2243.

Sanghvi, M.; Hamouda, A. K.; Jozwiak, K.; Blanton, M. P.; Trudell, J. R.; Arias, H. R. (2008). Identifying the binding site(s) for antidepressants on the Torpedo nicotinic acetylcholine receptor: [^{3}H]2-azidoimipramine photolabeling and molecular dynamics studies. Biochimica et Biophysica Acta, 1778(12), 2690-2699.

Scheller, M.; Bufler, J.; Hertle, I.; Schneck, H. J.; Franke, C.; Kochs, E. (1996). Ketamine blocks currents through mammalian nicotinic acetylcholine receptor channels by interaction with both the open and the closed state. Anesthesia and Analgesia, 83(4), 830-836.

Schlesinger, F.; Krampfl, K.; Haeseler, G.; Dengler, R.; Bufler, J. (2004).Competitive and open channel block of recombinant nAChR channels by different antibiotics. Neuromuscular Disorders, 14(5), 307-312.

Sieb, J. P.; Milone, M.; Engel, A. G. (1996). Effects of the quinoline derivatives quinine, quinidine, and chloroquine on neuromuscular transmission. Brain Research, 712(2), 179-189.

Spitzmaul, G.; Gumilar, F.; Dilger, J. P.; Bouzat, C. (2009). The local anaesthetics proadifen and adiphenine inhibit nicotinic receptors by different molecular mechanisms. British Journal of Pharmacology, 157(5), 804-817.

Teichert, R. W.; Rivier, J.; Torres, J.; Dykert, J.; Miller, C.; Olivera, B.M. (2005). A uniquely selective inhibitor of the mammalian fetal neuromuscular nicotinic acetylcholine receptor. The Journal of Neuroscience, 25(3), 732-736.

Thesleff, S. (1955). The mode of neuromuscular block caused by acetylcholine, nicotine, decamethonium and succinylcholine. Acta Physiologica Scandinavica, 34(2-3), 218-231.

Unwin, N. (2005). Refined structure of the nicotinic acetylcholine receptor at 4 Å resolution. Journal of Molecular Biology, 346(4), 967-989.

Varanda, W. A.; Aracava, Y.; Sherby, S. M.; VanMeter, W. G.; Eldefrawi, M.E.; Albuquerque, E. X. (1985). The acetylcholine receptor of the neuromuscular junction recognizes mecamylamine as a noncompetitiveantagonist. Molecular Pharmacology, 28(2), 128-137.

Wonnacott, S.; Barik, J. (2007). Nicotinic ACh receptors.Tocris Reviews, 28, Tocris Cookson.

35
阿片类药物受体参与烟碱相关的强化和愉悦

Ari P. Kirshenbaum

Department of Psychology, Neuroscience Program, Saint Michael's College, Colchester, VT, United States

缩略语

ACCx	前扣带皮层	NAcc	伏隔核
AL	垂体前叶	nAChR	烟碱型乙酰胆碱受体
AON	前嗅核	NRT	烟碱替代疗法
ARC	下丘脑弓状核	OR	阿片受体
BLA	基底外侧核，杏仁核	pCREB	磷酸化反应元件结合蛋白
BNST	终纹床核	PET	正电子发射断层扫描
CeA	中央核，杏仁核	PFC	前额叶皮层
CPP	条件性位置偏爱	PiR	梨状皮质
CPu	尾状核	POA	视前区
DMH	下丘脑背侧内侧核	PR	累进比率
DMR	中缝背核	PVN	下丘脑室旁核
DOR	δ-阿片受体	RM	大中缝
FR	固定比率	RN	红核
Fr, Pr, T和OCx	额叶、顶叶、颞叶和枕叶皮层	S_D	歧视性刺激
ICSS	颅内自我刺激	SON	视上结核
KOR	κ-阿片受体	VL, VM	丘脑腹外侧和内侧
MOR	μ-阿片受体	VTA	腹侧被盖区

35.1 引言

药物试验和随后的自给药可以被认为是由于这些物质对由奖励引起的基本满足感的影响而得到加强的（Castro, Berridge, 2014），因此推测阿片系统在所有药物依赖中无处不在的作用可能是合情合理的，这一假设也得到了相当大的支持（Le Merrer et al. 2009; Shippenberg et al. 2008; Trigo et al. 2010; 综述）。本章讨论的主要主题是受试者参与烟碱产生的快感体验的程度。与这个话题相关的是烟碱参与的阿片受体如何改变和强化有关的动机过程。

探究烟碱对奖励过程的最初影响必须包括在内，以此作为理解烟草依赖的神经生物学的一种手段。积极的强化和满足感是相关的，但不是相同的，这种区别在烟碱相关的阿片受体参与的数据中得到了很好的证明。简而言之，烟碱通过阿片受体激活所激发的快感并不能表征烟草产品的滥用倾向。烟碱激活的阿片受体改变一般奖励相关学习的方式，以及习惯性吸烟如何导致阿片系统失调，从而导致戒断（Berrendero et al. 2010; Pomerleau, 1998; Watkins et al. 2000），让我们更接近于更全面的特征。在这篇简短的综述中，没有研究长期烟碱暴露（即烟草依赖）导致的神经适应性改变；这些都在其他地方进行了全面的回顾（例如，Norman, D'Souza, 2017）。

重要的综述（Berrendero et al., 2010; Hadjiconstantinou, Neff, 2011）表明，烟碱和阿片受体在与强化有关的细胞通路中是紧密相连的；许多富含阿片受体的通路与动机和情感有关（Shippenberg et al. 2008）的中皮质多巴胺能通路（例如：Tanda, Di Chiara, 1998）相关。有证据表明，μ-阿片受体是烟碱反应的主要因素；δ-阿片受体激活在烟碱奖励相关反应中的确切作用因实验范式而异。κ-阿片受体的参与与烟碱的奖励效应无关，但κ-阿片受体的参与可能与戒断最为相关。阿片受体的激活与烟碱暴露导致的多肽释放相关；参见表35.1和图35.1。

表35.1 与烟碱相关的内源性阿片系统

受体	μ-阿片受体	δ-阿片受体	κ-阿片受体
亲和力最高的配体/肽	β-内啡肽	脑啡肽	强啡呔
前体细胞	阿黑皮素	脑啡肽原	前强啡肽
位置	纹状体，伏隔核，下丘脑，前额叶皮质	纹状体，尾状核，海马体，伏隔核	纹状体，尾状核，伏隔核
干预系统	多巴胺促肾上腺皮质激素释放因子	多巴胺和谷氨酸	多巴胺和谷氨酸

注：该表信息来源于Berrendero et al.（2010, 2012）、Hadjiconstantinou and Neff（2011）、Norman and D'Souza（2017）、Pomerleau（1998）、Trigo et al.（2010）。

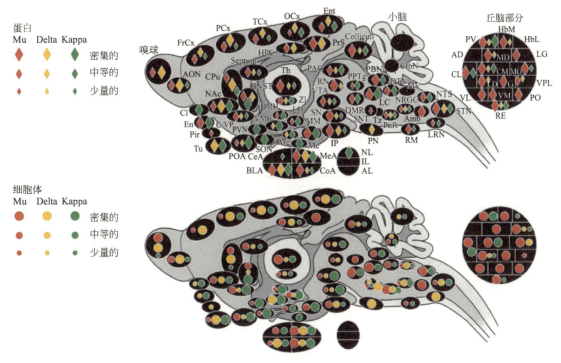

图35.1 阿片受体在大鼠脑内的分布

大鼠脑内阿片受体和含阿片受体胞体的分布。这一受版权保护的数字得到了Le Merrer等（2009）的许可。

35.2 问题的核心：烟碱的内感受

烟碱产生的内感刺激（Bevins, Besheer, 2014）可能与阿片受体激活有关，享乐内感可以用喜欢药物而不是想要药物（Castro, Berridge, 2014）来描述。在烟碱的感觉方面，Duke 等（2015）发现，以双盲方式口服烟碱的不吸烟者报告了积极的愉悦体验。此外，吸烟增加了对幸福和感官体验的享受的评价，并增强了对各种非烟碱奖励的反应（Perkins et al. 2015; Rukstalis et al. 2005）。

在未经治疗的情况下，对吸烟者的神经药理学研究表明，在许多情况下，阿片受体的拮抗作用降低了吸烟的欲望，减少了从吸烟中获得的快感，并减少了对含烟碱香烟和去烟碱香烟的选择；表35.2中King和Meyer（2000）发现纳曲酮降低了吸烟的欲望和吸烟的快感，尽管阿片受体的阻断也会产生轻微的不适感觉。Rukstails等（2005）发现，与去烟碱香烟相比，纳曲酮减少了对含烟碱香烟的选择，减弱了由于烟碱传递而产生的渴求缓解，并降低了含烟碱香烟诱导的快感程度，尽管后者的发现低于统计学意义的标准门槛。阿片受体已被证明会引起戒断症状和对烟草的渴望（Krishnan-Sarin, Rosen, O'Malley, 1999），并与外部应激源相互作用，从而增加吸烟欲望和由压力造成的负面影响（Hutchison et al. 1996）。这些之后的发现表明，当烟碱起到负面强化（即逃避压力）的作用时，阿片受体就参与了这一过程。值得注重的是，阿片受体拮抗剂的结果并不是普遍肯定的；一些研究表明没有任何效果（表35.2）。此外，对非选择性阿片受体拮抗剂（纳曲酮或纳洛酮）的任何研究结果的警告是，它们已被证明在体外影响烟碱型乙酰胆碱受体（Almeida et al. 2000; Tomé et al. 2001），因此它们对烟碱的享乐反应的影响可能是通过阿片受体外周的受体相互作用完成的。

表35.2 烟碱主观影响的实验室人类行为药理学，非治疗研究

参考文献	阿片类拮抗剂	结果
Brauer, Behm, Westman, Patel, Rose（1999）	纳曲酮与非甾体抗炎药	与不含烟碱的香烟相比，它改变了烟碱香烟产生的清醒状态，并破坏了烟碱贴片产生的渴望缓解的情绪，即在实验室外略减少吸烟
Epstein, King（2004）	纳曲酮	减少了在实验室吸烟的数量，减少了积极情绪，但增加了负面情绪和镇静；女性戒烟增加，但男性没有
Gorelick, Rose, Jarvik（1989）	10mg 纳洛酮	减少吸烟次数，对吸烟产生的主观评分没有影响
Hutchison et al.（1999）	纳曲酮与非甾体抗炎药	与接受NRT和安慰剂组有关的对吸烟相关线索的反应性降低
Hutchison et al.（1996）*	纳曲酮	压力，加上阿片类药物的阻滞，增加了香烟的压力
Karras, Kane（1980）	10mg 纳洛酮	减少吸烟和香烟需求
King, Meyer（2000）	纳曲酮	减少吸烟，香烟的需求和快感
Knott, Fisher（2007）	纳曲酮	烟碱口香糖引起的警觉性和愉悦程度降低；介导了θ和α2，但不影响烟碱引起的增量波变化；烟碱对戒断症状没有效果
Krishnan-Sarin et al.（1999）	0.8～3.2mg/70kg 纳洛酮	吸烟者和不吸烟者出现戒断症状和皮质醇增加

续表

参考文献	阿片类拮抗剂	结果
Lee et al.（2005）*	25～50mg纳曲酮	提示引起的渴求降低，但催乳素、皮质醇和促肾上腺皮质激素升高；β-内啡肽或强啡肽A没有变化
Nemeth-Coslett, Griffiths（1986）	0.06～4.0mg纳洛酮	对吸烟行为没有影响；镇静作用增强
Roche et al.（2010）	纳曲酮	吸烟增强纳曲酮诱导的促肾上腺皮质激素和皮质醇增加
Rohsenow et al.（2007）	纳曲酮与非甾体抗炎药	对烟雾的线索反应减弱，对非线索反应没有影响
Rukstalis et al.（2005）*	纳曲酮	与不含烟碱的香烟相比，含烟碱香烟的选择减少了；吸烟欲望降低了，但这两种香烟的满意度都没有显著影响
Sutherland, Stapelton, Russell, Feyerabend（1995）	50mg和100mg纳曲酮	对主观满意度或吸烟行为没有影响，但减少了警觉感，感觉难以戒除和渴望，并增加了负面情绪

注：表中列出的研究是双盲的，需要隔夜禁食，*表示例外；除非另有说明，纳曲酮的剂量为50mg。

表35.3 用正电子发射断层扫描（PET）和MOR放射性配基[^{11}C]卡芬太尼研究阿片类药物对烟碱的反应

参考文献	结果
Kuwabara et al. (2014)	烟碱引起的左侧额叶改变与主观愉悦相关
Falcone et al. (2012)	过夜戒烟引起的杏仁核差异，吸烟对杏仁核、VTA、岛叶、尾状核、丘脑或ACCx无影响
Nuechterlein, Ni, Domino, Zubeita (2016)	与戒烟者相比，非吸烟者的基底节和丘脑对烟碱的激活作用更强；在吸烟者中，NAcc和杏仁核的双侧激活与OPRM1基因型的确定有关
Ray et al. (2011)	OPRM1 A118G等位基因携带者的偏侧化差异：杏仁核、尾状核、ACCx和丘脑激活
Scott, Domino, Heitzeg, Koeppe, Ni (2007)	ACCx活性降低，VTA活性增加，杏仁核和丘脑局部半球激活；这些发现与烟碱减少烟草欲望有关
Weerts et al. (2013)	OPRM1 A118G等位基因基因型与全球MOR差异相对应；烟碱不在本研究中使用

注：表35.3中列出的成像研究使用正电子发射断层扫描（PET）和MOR放射性配体[^{11}C]卡芬太尼。

35.3 临床前证据：烟碱内感

关于烟碱内感的非人类研究分为两种模式，即条件性位置偏爱（CPP）和药物歧视。在CPP中，烟碱与环境背景有关，在缺乏烟碱的情况下，环境背景起到条件性增强剂的作用，运动到以前与烟碱相关的区域表示CPP。吗啡阻断干扰烟碱诱导的小鼠CPP并阻断烟碱诱发的脑奖励区pCREB阳性细胞的变化（VTA, NAcc; Walters, Cleck, Kuo, Blendy, 2005）。此外，缺乏β-内啡肽基因（Trigo et al. 2010）和MOR和DOR基因敲除（分别见：Berrendero, Kieffer, Maldonado, 2002; Berrendero et al. 2012）的小鼠对烟碱诱导的CPP不太敏感，这表明这些受体高度参与内感。

关于ORs和烟碱作为歧视性刺激（S_D）的能力，证据尚不确定。在药物辨别中，受试者被注射烟碱，然后被训练成"左转"（例如，在"T"字形迷宫或两个选项的杠杆按压中），以体验强化事件。与药物训练混杂在一起的是盐水训练课程，在这些课程中，受试者被强化为"向右走"。

因此，烟碱的内感刺激起到了标示强化方向的作用。在测试过程中，给出一种不同的药物，然后评估这种新药替代烟碱的程度。在老鼠和猴子身上，吗啡不是不能替代烟碱（Romano et al. 1981; Takada et al. 1988），就是不能完全替代烟碱（Moerke et al. 2017）。没有理由期望烟碱激活ORs的程度与纯阿片类激动剂相同，因此吗啡可能会产生与烟碱不同的主观体验，而接受吗啡S_D训练的大鼠很容易辨别烟碱（Romano et al. 1981）。因此，使用OR激动剂替代品的解释存在固有的问题，但人们可以推测剂量很重要，烟碱的程度也是如此，因为与药物相关的内感会随着随后的暴露而改变（Paulus, Tapert, Schulteis, 2009）。此外，阿片类激动剂的一般减速作用使这项工作充满混乱。OR拮抗剂联合给药对烟碱S_D的影响有限。Romano等（1981）研究发现，共同使用2.0mg/kg纳洛酮不能破坏0.4mg/kg烟碱的S_D质量，但单次给药并不确定。在最近一项使用相关巴甫洛夫目标跟踪程序的研究中，Palmatier等（2004）研究发现，纳洛酮（0.5～6.0mg/kg）剂量依赖性地减弱了烟碱引发"接近"反应的能力，这些大鼠接受了将食物递送与烟碱联系在一起的训练。

35.4 烟碱作为增强剂

烟碱自给药与OR激活有关（表35.4）。Ismayilova和Shoaib（2010）研究发现，纳洛酮呈剂量依赖性地减少烟碱自给药，但不影响食物强化。在大多数情况下，选择性更强的拮抗剂会减少大鼠的烟碱自给药，但对DOR和KOR-选择性拮抗剂无效（表35.4）。然而，已经在小鼠身上发现了DOR选择性拮抗或基因敲除对烟碱自给药的干扰（Berrendero et al. 2012）。KOR的作用方式可能与OR不同；例如，KOR选择性激动剂在一定剂量下会破坏烟碱的强化，但最低剂量的激动剂会略微增加烟碱的自给药（Ismayilova, Shoaib, 2010）。其他人（Liu, Jernigan, 2011）没有发现KOR拮抗改变烟碱自给药的证据，所以目前KOR对烟碱自给药的贡献似乎可以忽略不计。

OR拮抗剂对烟碱自给药的影响可能与改变享乐反应或破坏烟碱的激励价值有关。因此，消退和消退后恢复的反应对于分析阿片受体拮抗剂对烟碱增强的影响具有重要意义。Liu等（2009）研究发现，急性或重复使用纳曲酮都不会减少烟碱自给药；然而，纳曲酮显著抑制线索维持水平的消退反应，并减少线索诱导的恢复。Liu等（2009）的结论是，纳曲酮减弱了烟碱相关的动机线索，因此可能与烟碱依赖的治疗有关，因为它可能会减轻线索引发的复发。一系列人类行为药理学研究（表35.2，例如，Hutchison et al. 1999）表明，OR阻断可以影响烟碱相关线索促使烟碱自给药的有效性；因此，OR参与了烟碱上下文中关于强化的学习。

表35.4 啮齿动物烟碱自给药研究

参考文献	阿片类拮抗剂	每次输注烟碱	结论
Berrendero et al. (2012)	DOR选择性；2.5和5.0纳曲啶	0.015和0.03；FR1, PR	FR剂量依赖性递减；PR断点上的剂量非依赖性递减
	DOR淘汰赛		与未经修饰的野生型小鼠相比减少
Corrigall, Coen (1991)	0.1～10纳洛酮	0.03；FR5	无效
Corrigall, Coen, Adamson, Chow, Zhang (2000)	MOR选择性激动剂；静脉曲张输注0.005～0.05μg DAMGO	0.01～0.03；FR5	低剂量烟碱剂量依赖性减少；高剂量无效
DeNoble, Mele (2006)	0.7、1.5和3.0纳洛酮	0.032；FR1	无效

参考文献	阿片类拮抗剂	每次输注烟碱	结论
Liu, Jernigan (2011)	MOR 选择性；5.0 和 15.0 纳洛嗪	0.03; FR5	依赖剂量的减量；对食物强化没有影响
	DOR 选择性；0.5 和 5.0 纳曲啶		无效
	KOR 选择性；0.25 和 1.0 的 5-胍基三萘啶		无效
Liu et al. (2009)	0.25～2.0 纳曲酮	0.03; FR5	没有影响，但增加了对灭绝的反应，减少了线索诱导的恢复
Ismayilova, Shoaib (2010)	0.3、1.0 和 3.0 纳洛酮	0.03; FR3	所有剂量都减少了；对食物强化没有影响
	DOR 选择性；0.3、1.0 和 3.0 纳曲啶		无效
	KOR 选择性激动型*；0.3、1.0 和 3.0 的 U50488		只有最高剂量的剂量才有小幅下降

注：表中列出的研究涉及烟碱自给药，并列出了每次烟碱输注的固定比率（FR）要求；剂量以mg/kg为单位，所有药物都是拮抗剂（见标记"*"的例外情况）。有一次，使用了累进比率（PR）加固计划。

35.5 烟碱诱导的奖励敏感性

十多年的研究表明，烟碱可以提高在烟碱存在下的增强剂的功效（Donny, Caggiula, Weaver, Levin, Sved, 2011, 综述）。当使用累进比率（PR）计划来评估烟碱对大鼠蔗糖强化的影响时，烟碱的给药呈剂量依赖性地增加了为蔗糖工作所花费的努力（Kirshenbaum et al. 2015; Palmatier et al. 2008）。增强剂不是刺激物，而是参与反应的机会（Allison,1993），烟碱增强了这些作用；重要的是，增强效应包含了一系列增强剂，而不仅仅是吃东西（Kirshenbaum et al. 2015; Perkins et al. 2015）。当与烟碱联合应用时，纳洛酮干扰烟碱对蔗糖强化的促进作用，但在没有烟碱的情况下，纳洛酮本身并不影响蔗糖强化（Kirshenbaum, Suhaka, Phillips, Voltolini de Souza Pinto, 2016）。这一结果和其他研究结果（Ismayilova, Shoaib, 2010; Liu, Jernigan, 2011）表明，一定剂量的阿片拮抗剂对大鼠体内烟碱相关强化的影响是特定的。烟碱的强化增强效应的临床意义尚不清楚，但在人类吸烟者中存在一些证据（Perkins et al.2015）；OR拮抗是否否定了人类的强化增强仍有待测试。

烟碱增强可能与大脑奖励敏感度的改变有关。急性烟碱降低大鼠的颅内自我刺激（ICSS）阈值（HustonLyons, Kornetsky,1992），这一效应已成为理解药物如何成为强化剂的神经生物学的金标准。在阻断其他滥用药物（例如D-苯异丙胺）的阈值降低作用的剂量中，与纳洛酮的ORs拮抗作用不能阻止烟碱的阈值降低影响（Esposito, Perry, Kornetsky, 1980）。虽然纳洛酮干扰烟碱强化增强，但它不改变烟碱诱导的ICSS阈值的降低。

ICSS文献中第二个同样可靠的发现是，当长期烟碱暴露被烟碱拮抗剂（甲基胺）终止或阻止时，阈值急剧上升（Watkins, Stinus, Koob, Markou, 2000）。烟碱戒断引起的大脑奖励脱敏在其他范例中也得到了证实。例如，Pergadia等（2014）为老鼠提供了一项关于食物强化的概率同时选择测试，然后让它们长期接触烟碱。停止烟碱摄入后，大鼠对强化的概率变得不敏感。当人类吸烟者被给予类似的任务（为了钱）时，他们在戒烟过程中对不同的增强剂概率也变得不敏感了（Pergadia et al. 2014）。综上所述，ICSS 阈值增加，Pergadia 等（2014）和其他人（Kirshenbaum et al. 2015, 2016）的研究结果表明，烟碱停用会产生增强剂不敏感；然而，在人类中，奖励反应的变化是不一致的（Hughes et al. 2017），可能与快感缺乏有关，也可能与此无关。

纳洛酮（>1.0mg/kg）剂量依赖性地诱导长期烟碱治疗大鼠 ICSS 阈值显著升高（Watkins, Stinus et al. 2000）。一个重要的条件是，尽管烟碱和盐水预处理的大鼠之间存在细微的差异，但纳洛酮在剂量超过 2.0mg/kg 的盐水预处理的动物中也提高了 ICSS 阈值。由于组间差异不显著，作者（Watkins, Koob et al. 2000; Watkins, Stinus et al. 2000）不能肯定阿片系统控制烟碱依赖的大脑奖励敏感性。其他研究人员发现，仅纳洛酮（高达 16mg/kg）不能改变 ICSS（Esposito et al. 1980），因此关于 OR 本身的阻断存在重要的不一致。此外，纳洛酮可阻止烟碱增强强化作用，但不能阻止烟碱停药的奖励脱敏效应（Kirshenbaum et al. 2016）。这些结果一致表明，大脑奖赏不敏感与 ORs 的拮抗作用无关。

35.6 进入临床：阿片类拮抗剂和烟草依赖

长期接触烟碱导致 OR 改变，这对烟草依赖有重要影响。例如，受 ORs 支配的疼痛敏感性会因长期接触烟碱而改变（见综述：Yoon, Lane, Weaver, 2015）。这些 OR 调整超出了本章的范围，但简要地说，临床研究结果表明阿片类拮抗剂与 NRT 联合使用的疗效不高。在目标戒烟日期之前给予患者纳曲酮可以产生比安慰剂更好的结果（King, Cao, Zhang, Rueger, 2013），并且与 NRT 联合使用可以减少复发（Krishnan-Sarin, Meandzija, O'Malley, 2003），临床文献中有足够的负面研究结果或小影响，足以证明对阿片类拮抗剂是否是有效治疗的怀疑（David et al. 2014）。然而，许多与 OR 系统有理论关联的变量可能有助于解决不一致的发现；负面情绪（Walsh, Epstein, Munisamy, King, 2008）、性别（King et al. 2012; Roche, Childs, Epstein, King, 2010）和 OPRM1 基因多态性（Ray et al. 2006）可能是可以用于提高阿片类拮抗剂疗效的重要变量（Norman, D'Souza, 2017）。

术语解释	■ 条件性强化物：由于与主要增强剂相关而起到增强剂作用的事件。
	■ 辨别性刺激：指导行为的事件；在毒品辨别的情况下，这些事件是由药物管理产生的内部事件。
	■ 享乐的：主观的感觉、愉悦或满足。
	■ 内感作用：影响行为的内部事件，在这种情况下，刺激是由烟碱注射引起的。
	■ 中皮层多巴胺能通路：涉及 VTA、杏仁核、海马区、NAcc 区和 PFC 区神经元的大脑奖赏回路。
	■ 阿片受体：由内源性配体激活的受体，通常参与伤害性感受和奖励。
	■ 巴甫洛夫趋近行为：当烟碱与食物联系在一起时，烟碱的摄入会刺激啮齿类动物寻找食物。
ORs 的关键事实	■ 纯阿片类激动剂（如海洛因）激活 OR 可产生享乐性感觉，而如纳洛酮等 OR 拮抗剂可逆转这一效应。
	■ OPMR1 基因多态性或 OR 表达的遗传易感性与多种药物依赖相关。

要点总结

- 自给药、CPP和药物鉴别是传统上用于阿片类药物滥用责任的临床前鉴定的行为分析方法。
- 滥用药物产生的ICSS阈值改变支持了OR作用的化学物质改变大脑奖励敏感性的理论。
- 烟碱的使用会加重慢性疼痛。
- 阿片类药物滥用者吸烟的可能性更大。
- 阿片类药物参与人类对烟碱的享乐反应的证据是确凿的,但这种影响的大小并不一致,也没有人们预期的那么强烈。
- 结合研究工具和技术,如阿片类拮抗剂、[^{11}C]卡芬太尼和OPMR1基因分型,可能会解决有关烟碱享乐反应的不一致问题。
- 阿片受体阻滞剂很大程度上干扰了大鼠的烟碱自给药,并对烟碱依赖者的香烟选择、线索反应性和吸烟行为有一定的影响。
- 对条件性位置偏爱和巴甫洛夫接近行为的研究可靠地表明,阿片类拮抗剂可以干扰烟碱的内感刺激,但当烟碱在药物辨别中充当S_D时,阿片类药物参与的证据是否定的或缺乏的。
- 阿片类拮抗剂治疗烟草依赖的临床结果是多种多样的,几个患者因素的异质性可能导致研究结果的不一致。

参考文献

Allison, J. (1993). Response deprivation, reinforcement, and economics. Journal of the Experimental Analysis of Behavior, 60(1), 129-140.

Almeida, L. E.; Pereira, E. F.; Alkondon, M.; Fawcett, W. P.; Randall, W. R.; Albuquerque, E. X. (2000). The opioid antagonist naltrexone inhibits activity and alters expression of alpha7 and alpha4beta2 nicotinic receptors in hippocampal neurons: implications for smoking cessation programs. Neuropharmacology, 39(13), 2740-2755.

Berrendero, F.; Kieffer, B. L.; Maldonado, R. (2002). Attenuation of nicotine-induced antinociception, rewarding effects, and dependence in mu-opioid receptor knock-out mice. The Journal of Neuroscience, 22(24), 10935-10940.

Berrendero, F.; Plaza-Zabala, A.; Galeote, L.; Flores, Á.; Bura, S. A.; Kieffer, B. L. et al. (2012). Influence of δ-opioid receptors in the behavioral effects of nicotine. Neuropsychopharmacology, 37(10), 2332-2344.

Berrendero, F.; Robledo, P.; Trigo, J. M.; Martín-García, E.; Maldonado, R. (2010). Neurobiological mechanisms involved in nicotine dependence and reward: participation of the endogenous opioid system. Neuroscience and Biobehavioral Reviews, 35, 220-231.

Bevins, R. A.; Besheer, J. (2014). Interoception and learning: import to understanding and treating diseases and psychopathologies. ACS Chemical Neuroscience, 5(8), 624-631.

Brauer, L. J.; Behm, F. M.; Westman, E. C.; Patel, P.; Rose, J. E. (1999). Naltrexone blockade of nicotine effects in cigarette smokers. Psychopharmacology, 143, 339-346.

Castro, D. C.; Berridge, K. C. (2014). Advances in the neurobiological bases for food 'liking' versus 'wanting'. Physiology, Behavior, 136, 22-30.

Corrigall, W. A.; Coen, K. M. (1991). Opiate antagonists reduce cocaine but not nicotine self-administration. Psychopharmacology, 104, 167-170.

Corrigall, W. A.; Coen, K. M.; Adamson, K. L.; Chow, B. L. C.; Zhang, J. (2000). Response of nicotine self-administration in the rat to manipulations of mu-opioid and γ-aminobutyric acid receptors in the ventral tegmental area. Psychopharmacology, 149, 107-114.

David, S. P.; Chu, I. M.; Lancaster, T.; Stead, L. F.; Evins, A. E.; Prochaska, J. J. (2014). Systematic review and meta-analysis of opioid antagonists for smoking cessation. BMJ Open, 4(3)e004393.

DeNoble, V. J.; Mele, P. C. (2006). Intravenous nicotine self-administration in rats: Effects of mecamylamine, hexamethonium and nalaxone. Psychopharmacology, 136, 8 3-90.

Donny, E. C.; Caggiula, A. R.; Weaver, M. T.; Levin, M. E.; Sved, A. F. (2011). The reinforcement-enhancing effects of nicotine: implications for the relationship between smoking, eating and weight. Physiology, Behavior, 104(1), 143-148.

Duke, A. N.; Johnson, M. W.; Reissig, C. J.; Griffiths, R. R. (2015). Nicotine reinforcement in never-smokers. Psychopharmacology, 232(23), 4243-4252.

Epstein, A. M.; King, A. C. (2004). Naltrexone attenuates acute acute cigarette smoking behavior. Pharmacology Biochemistry and Behavior, 77, 2 9-37.

Esposito, R. U.; Perry, W.; Kornetsky, C. (1980). Effects of d-amphetamine and naloxone on brain stimulation reward. Psychopharmacology, 69(2), 187-191.

Falcone, M.; Gold, A. B.; Wileyto, E. P.; Ray, R.; Ruparel, K.; Newberg, A. et al. (2012). μ-Opioid receptor availability in the amygdala is associated with smoking for negative affect relief. Psychopharmacology, 222(4), 701-708.

Gorelick, D. A.; Rose, J.; Jarvik, M. E. (1989). Effect of naloxone on cigarette smoking. Journal of Substance Abuse, 1, 153-159.

Hadjiconstantinou, M.; Neff, N. (2011). Nicotine and endogenous opioids: neurochemical and pharmacological evidence. Neuropharmacology, 60, 1209-1220.

Hughes, J. R.; Budney, A. J.; Muellers, S. R.; Lee, D. C.; Callas, P. W.; Sigmon, S. C. et al. (2017). Does tobacco abstinence decrease reward sensitivity? A human laboratory test. Nicotine, Tobacco Research, 19(6), 677-685.

Huston-Lyons, D.; Kornetsky, C. (1992). Effects of nicotine on the threshold for rewarding brain stimulation in rats. Pharmacology, Biochemistry, and Behavior, 41(4), 755-759.

Hutchison, K. E.; Collins, F. R.; Tassey, J.; Rosenberg, E. (1996). Stress, naltrexone, and the reinforcement value of nicotine. Experimental and Clinical Psychopharmacology, 4(4), 431-437.

Hutchison, K. E.; Monti, P. M.; Rohsenow, D. J.; Swift, R. M.; Colby, S. M.; Gnys, M. et al. (1999). Effects of naltrexone with nicotine replacement on smoking cue reactivity: preliminary results. Psychopharmacology, 142(2), 139-143.

Ismayilova, N.; Shoaib, M. (2010). Alteration of intravenous nicotine self-administration by opioid receptor agonist and antagonists in rats. Psychopharmacology, 210(2), 211-220.

Karras, A.; Kane, J. M. (1980). Naloxone reduces cigarette smoking. Life Sciences, 27, 1541-1545.

King, A. C.; Cao, D.; O'Malley, S. S.; Kranzler, H. R.; Cai, X.; deWit, H. et al. (2012). Effects of naltrexone on smoking cessation outcomes and weight gain in nicotine-dependent men and women. Journal of Clinical Psychopharmacology, 32(5), 630-636.

King, A.; Cao, D.; Zhang, L.; Rueger, S. Y. (2013). Effects of the opioid receptor antagonist naltrexone on smoking and related behaviors in smokers preparing to quit: a randomized controlled trial. Addiction, 108(10), 1836-1844.

King, A. C.; Meyer, P. J. (2000). Naltrexone alteration of acute smoking response in nicotine-dependent subjects. Pharmacology, Biochemistry, and Behavior, 66(3), 563-572.

Kirshenbaum, A.; Green, J.; Fay, M.; Parks, A.; Phillips, J.; Stone, J. et al. (2015). Reinforcer devaluation as a consequence of acute nicotine exposure and withdrawal. Psychopharmacology, 232(9), 1583-1594.

Kirshenbaum, A. P.; Suhaka, J. A.; Phillips, J. L.; Voltolini de Souza Pinto, M. (2016). Nicotine enhancement and reinforcer devaluation: interaction with opioid receptors. Pharmacology, Biochemistry, and Behavior, 150-151, 1-7.

Knott, V. J.; Fisher, D. J. (2007). Naltrexone alteration of nicotine-induced EEG and mood activation response in tobacco-deprived cigarette smokers. Experimental, Clinical Psychopharmacology, 15, 368-381.

Krishnan-Sarin, S.; Meandzija, B.; O'Malley, S. (2003). Naltrexone and nicotine patch smoking cessation: a preliminary study. Nicotine, Tobacco Research, 5(6), 851-857.

Krishnan-Sarin, S.; Rosen, M. I.; O'Malley, S. S. (1999). Naloxone challenge in smokers. Preliminary evidence of an opioid component in nicotine dependence. Archives of General Psychiatry, 56(7), 663-668.

Kuwabara, H.; Heishman, S. J.; Brasic, J. R.; Contoreggi, C.; Cascella, N.; Mackowick, K. M. et al. (2014). Mu opioid receptor binding correlates with nicotine dependence and reward in smokers. PLoSONE, 9(12), e113694.

Lee, Y. S.; Joe, K. H.; Sohn, I. K.; Na, C.; Kee, B. S.; Chae, S. L. (2005). Changes of smoking behavior and serum adrenocorticotropic hormone, cortisol, prolactin, and endogenous opioid levels in nicotine dependence after naltrexone treatment. Progress in Neuro-Psychopharmacology, Biological Psychiatry, 29, 639-647.

Le Merrer, J.; Becker, J. J.; Befort, K.; Kieffer, B. L. (2009). Reward processing by the opioid system in the brain. Physiological Reviews, 89(4), 1379-1412.

Liu, X.; Jernigan, C. (2011). Activation of the opioid μ1, but not δ or κ, receptors is required for nicotine reinforcement in a rat model of drug self-administration. Progress in Neuro-Psychopharmacology, Biological Psychiatry, 35(1), 146-153.

Liu, X.; Palmatier, M.; Caggiula, A.; Sved, A.; Donny, E.; Gharib, M. et al. (2009). Naltrexone attenuation of conditioned but not primary reinforcement of nicotine in rats. Psychopharmacology, 202(4), 589-598.

Moerke, M. J.; Zhu, A. X.; Tyndale, R. F.; Javors, M. A.; McMahon, L. R. (2017). The discriminative stimulus effects of i. v. nicotine in rhesus monkeys: pharmacokinetics and apparent pA2 analysis with dihydro-β-erythroidine. Neuropharmacology, 116, 9-17.

Nemeth-Coslett, R.; Griffiths, R. R. (1986). Naloxone does not affect cigarette smoking. Psychopharmacology, 89, 261-264.

Norman, H.; D'Souza, M. S. (2017). Endogenous opioid system: a promising target for future smoking cessation medications. Psychopharmacology, 234(9-10), 1371-1394.

Nuechterlein, E. B.; Ni, L.; Domino, E.; Zubeita, J. -K. (2016). Nicotine-specific and non-specific effects of cigarette smoking on endogenous opioid mechanisms. Progress in Neuro-Psychopharmacology, Biological Psychiatry, 69, 69-77.

Palmatier, M. I.; Coddington, S. B.; Liu, X.; Donny, E. C.; Caggiula, A. R.; Sved, A. F. (2008). The motivation to obtain nicotine-conditioned reinforcers depends on nicotine dose. Neuropharmacology, 55, 1425-1430.

Palmatier, M. I.; Peterson, J. L.; Wilkinson, J. L.; Bevins, R. A. (2004). Nicotine serves as a feature-positive modulator of Pavlovian appetitive conditioning in rats. Behavioural Pharmacology, 15(3), 183-194.

Paulus, M. P.; Tapert, S. F.; Schulteis, G. (2009). The role of interoception and alliesthesia in addiction. Pharmacology, Biochemistry, and Behavior, 94(1), 1-7.

Pergadia, M. L.; Der-Avakian, A.; D'Souza, M. S.; Madden, P. F.; Heath, A. C.; Shiffman, S. et al. (2014). Association between nicotine withdrawal and reward responsiveness in humans and rats. JAMA Psychiatry, 71(11), 1238-1245.

Perkins, K. A.; Karelitz, J. L.; Michael, V. C. (2015). Reinforcement enhancing effects of acute nicotine via electronic cigarettes. Drug and Alcohol Dependence, 153, 104-108.

Pomerleau, O. F. (1998). Endogenous opioids and smoking: a review of progress and problems. Psychoneuroendocrinology, 23(2), 115-130.

Ray, R.; Jepson, C.; Patterson, F.; Strasser, A.; Rukstalis, M.; Perkins, K. et al. (2006). Association of OPRM1 A118G variant with relative reinforcing value of nicotine. Psychopharmacology, 188, 355-363.

Ray, R.; Ruparel, K.; Newberg, A.; Wileyto, E. P.; Loughead, J. W.; Divgi, C. et al. (2011). Human mu opioid receptor (OPRM1 A118G) polymorphism is associated with brain mu-opioid receptor binding potential in smokers. Proceedings of the National Academy of Sciences of the United States of America, 108(22), 9268-9273.

Roche, D. O.; Childs, E.; Epstein, A. M.; King, A. C. (2010). Acute HPA axis response to naltrexone differs in female vs. male smokers. Psychoneuroendocrinology, 35(4), 596-606.

Rohsenow, D. J.; Monti, P. M.; Hutchison, K. E.; Swift, R. M.; MacKinnon, S. V.; Sirota, A. D. et al. (2007). High-dose transdermal nicotine with naltrexone: Effect on nicotine withdrawal, urges, smoking, and effects of smoking. Experimental, Clinical Psychophar-macology, 15, 81-92.

Romano, C.; Goldstein, A.; Jewell, N. P. (1981). Characterization of the receptor mediating the nicotine discriminative stimulus. Psychopharmacology, 74(4), 310-315.

Rukstalis, M.; Jepson, C.; Strasser, A.; Lynch, K. G.; Perkins, K.; Patterson, F. et al. (2005). Naltrexone reduces the relative reinforcing value of nicotine in a cigarette smoking choice paradigm. Psychopharmacology, 180(1), 41-48.

Scott, D. J.; Domino, E. F.; Heitzeg, M. M.; Koeppe, R. A.; Ni, L. (2007). Smoking modulation of mu-opioid and dopamine receptor D2 receptor-mediated neurotransmission in humans. Neuropsychopharmacology, 32, 450-457.

Shippenberg, T. S.; LeFevour, A.; Chefer, V. I. (2008). Targeting endogenous mu- and delta-opioid receptor systems for the treatment of drug addiction. CNS, Neurological Disorders Drug Targets, 7(5), 442-453.

Sutherland, G.; Stapelton, J. A.; Russell, M. A.; Feyerabend, C. (1995). Naltrexone, smoking behavior, and cigarette withdrawal. Psychopharmacology, 120, 418-425.

Takada, K.; Hagen, T. J.; Cook, J. M.; Goldberg, S. R.; Katz, J. L. (1988). Discriminative stimulus effects of intravenous nicotine in squirrel monkeys. Pharmacology, Biochemistry, and Behavior, 30(1), 243-247.

Tanda, G.; Di Chiara, G. (1998). A dopamine-mu1 opioid link in the rat ventral tegmentum shared by palatable food (Fonzies) and non-psychostimulant drugs of abuse. The European Journal of Neuroscience, 10(3), 1179-1187.

Tomé, A. R.; Izaguirre, V.; Rosário, L. M.; Ceña, V.; González-García, C. (2001). Naloxone inhibits nicotine-induced receptor current and catecholamine secretion in bovine chromaffin cells. Brain Research, 903(1-2), 62-65.

Trigo, J. M.; Martin-García, E.; Berrendero, F.; Robledo, P.; Maldonado, R. (2010). The endogenous opioid system: a common substrate in drug addiction. Drug and Alcohol Dependence, 108(3), 183-194.

Walsh, Z.; Epstein, A.; Munisamy, G.; King, A. (2008). The impact of depressive symptoms on the efficacy of naltrexone in smoking cessation. Journal of Addictive Diseases, 27(1), 65-72.

Walters, C. L.; Cleck, J. N.; Kuo, Y.; Blendy, J. A. (2005). Mu-opioid receptor and CREB activation are required for nicotine reward. Neuron, 46(6), 933-943.

Watkins, S. S.; Koob, G. F.; Markou, A. (2000). Neural mechanisms underlying nicotine addiction: acute positive reinforcement and withdrawal. Nicotine, Tobacco Research, 2(1), 19-37.

Watkins, S. S.; Stinus, L.; Koob, G. F.; Markou, A. (2000). Reward and somatic changes during precipitated nicotine withdrawal in rats: centrally and peripherally mediated effects. The Journal of Pharmacology and Experimental Therapeutics, 292(3), 1053-1064.

Weerts, E. M.; McCaul, M. E.; Kuwabara, H.; Yang, X.; Xu, X. Dannals, R. F. et al. (2013). Influence of OPMR1 Asn40Asp variant (A118G) on [11C] carfentanil binding potential: preliminary findings in human subjects. International Journal of Neuropsychopharmacology, 16, 47-53.

Yoon, J. H.; Lane, S. D.; Weaver, M. F. (2015). Opioid analgesics and nicotine: more than blowing smoke. Journal of Pain, Palliative Care Pharmacotherapy, 29(3), 281-289.

36
烟碱诱导的诱发效应：年龄、性别、抗氧化剂预防的影响

Danielle Macedo, Adriano José Maia Chaves Filho, Patrícia Xavier Lima Gomes, Lia Lira Olivier Sanders, David Freitas de Lucena

Department of Physiology and Pharmacology, Drug Research and Development Centre, Faculty of Medicine, Federal University of Ceara, Fortaleza, Brazil

缩略语

BDNF	脑源性神经营养因子	**NAC**	N-乙酰半胱氨酸
CREB	cAMP反应元件结合蛋白	**nAChR**	烟碱乙酰胆碱受体
ERKs	细胞外信号调节激酶	**NMDAR**	N-甲基-D-天冬氨酸受体
GABA	γ-氨基丁酸	**PTZ**	戊四唑
GSH	还原型谷胱甘肽	**SOD**	超氧化物歧化酶

36.1 引言

诱发反应是一种与进行性癫痫有关的突触可塑性的模型（Bertram, 2007; Pinel, Rovner, 1978），并且与应激相关疾病（如焦虑症、抑郁症、药物滥用和躁郁症）中自发出现的症状有关（Post, 2007）。人们很早就认识到，反复使用中枢神经系统兴奋剂，如可卡因，会引发诱发反应（Post, Kopanda, 1976），但直到最近十年，才出现烟碱引发的诱发反应的特征（Bastlund, Berry, Watson, 2005）。烟碱是一种精神活性药物，根据特定的实验方案，它可以引起刺激性（多动）或抑制性（镇静）行为效应（Clarke, Kumar, 1983）。除了烟草的主要成分烟碱外，吸烟还提供了许多具有前惊厥的（如烟碱和一氧化碳）或抗惊厥的（如硒、锌和丙酮）药物（Rong, Frontera, Benbadis, 2014）。高剂量的烟碱会引起癫痫发作，这是这种药物中毒（过量）在人体内的症状之一。先前的一项研究表明，与不吸烟者相比，吸烟者患癫痫的风险增加了一倍，过去的吸烟者患癫痫的风险有所增加，但未达到统计学意义（Dworetzky et al. 2010）。如上所述，吸烟有几种与癫痫发作风险增加有关的因素。因此，有关吸烟的研究不能直接暗示烟碱是烟草中与癫痫风险有关的成分。与吸烟相关的一些并发症会增加癫痫发作的风险，这是其他混杂因素。因此，很难去确定烟碱对与吸烟相关的癫痫发作的影响。关于吸烟和癫痫发作这一主题的一篇最新综述得出的结论是，对吸烟和癫痫发作之间关系的调查提出了更多的问题，而不是提供了答案（Rong et al. 2014）。

因此，为了更好地评估烟碱在癫痫发作中的作用，证据必须来自临床前的研究或使用烟碱贴片或电子烟治疗的患者的临床研究。到目前为止，关于烟碱贴片诱导癫痫发作的证据很少。相反，烟碱贴片已被用来治疗某些类型的癫痫，例如与烟碱型乙酰胆碱受体突变相关的癫痫（Sieciechowicz, Kohrman, 2015）。关于电子烟，据报道，一名儿童被烟碱浓度为1.8%（18mg/mL）

的再补充烟油毒死。这名儿童出现了胆碱能危机，并伴有中枢神经毒性的迹象，可能包括运动失调和癫痫发作。作者呼吁人们注意由于电子烟的日益使用而可能致命的婴幼儿液态烟碱中毒（Bassett, Osterhoudt, Brabazon, 2014）。

来自临床前研究的证据表明，烟碱可以引发与癫痫发作相关的相反作用，从保护作用到诱发惊厥作用不等。该作用是剂量依赖性的，即低剂量的烟碱是不惊厥的，而高剂量的是引发惊厥的。烟碱的前惊厥作用通过假定的烟碱型乙酰胆碱受体的刺激，例如α7受体，以及谷氨酸的释放和N-甲基-D-天冬氨酸受体（NMDAR）的刺激的介导，导致一氧化氮的形成和癫痫发作（Damaj, Glassco, Dukat, Martin, 1999）。

尽管研究烟碱诱发的诱发反应对于更好地理解烟碱长期作用所涉及的神经可塑性机制的重要性，但迄今为止，有关该主题的信息很少。

本章回顾了有关烟碱诱发反应的现有文献，年龄和性别对其发展的影响以及抗氧化剂在预防诱发反应发展中的作用。

36.2 诱发反应及其与癫痫发作和神经精神疾病的关系

小小的电刺激如果反复使用，最终会引起癫痫发作，导致完全性惊厥，这种现象称为诱发反应。诱发反应作为局部癫痫模型的发现是偶然的。通过检查杏仁核复合体（情绪、情绪行为和动机综合中心）的电刺激对学习的影响，Graham Goddard注意到，多次重复刺激后，他的许多老鼠都出现了癫痫发作（Goddard, McIntyre, Leech, 1969）。Goddard意识到，大脑在不断刺激下不断变化，这种变化构成了一种可塑性，可以为癫痫病提供有用的神经模型。后来，他详细描述了诱发反应的过程，他将诱发过程划分为五个不同的行为阶段，从伴随面部自动症的运动停止（阶段1）到伴有前肢阵挛和后肢紧张的完全诱发的癫痫发作，并通过翻身和两足不稳定来确定（阶段5）（Racine, 1972）。

除了电刺激，诱发反应也可能是由化合物引起的，如可卡因（Itzhak, 1996）和戊四唑（PTZ）（Zhu et al. 2015），以及环境因素，如情绪压力（表36.1）。

应激相关障碍（如焦虑、抑郁、物质使用和躁郁症）中观察到的症状的自发表现似乎与诱发机制有关。重要的是，这些精神疾病在杏仁核内呈现出结构和功能的变化（Trevor, 2012）。在这些疾病中，主要生活压力的暴露从最初的发作转变为随后的复发；例如，与再次住院的狂躁症患者相比，首次住院的狂躁症患者在入院前一个月经历入院前事件的可能性要大得多（平均压力评分明显要高）（Ambelas, 1987）。因此，有一个命题一直在人类身上持续研究，但是由于方法学问题尚未完全阐明，那就是，尽管连续的情感发作似乎与压力源联系较少，或者最终可能是自主发生的，但主要的生活压力是诱导情感发作开始和复发所必需的（Bender, Alloy, 2011）。

诱发反应引起的变化会持续很长一段时间，通常被认为是半永久性的（Dennison, Campbell Teskey, Cain, 1995）。基于这种观察，如上所述，这个模型可以概念化出现反复和周期性症状的一系列神经精神障碍的一般机制（Post, 2007）。根据诱发机制参与神经精神障碍的一些证据，基于其抗诱发作用，抗惊厥药物已被成功地用于治疗其中一些障碍，例如丙戊酸盐用于治疗双向情感障碍。

诱发反应的发展涉及依赖活动的功能可塑性，随着这个过程，即时基因（如 c-Fos）和后期效应基因（包括神经肽和神经营养因子）及其他基因的时空诱导，涉及神经递质的合成和释放（更多详细信息，请阅读 Post, 2007）。引发现象最深入的机制是 NMDARs，神经营养因子[例如脑源性神经营养因子（BDNF）]和氧化失衡的改变（Kaminski et al. 2011; Zhu et al. 2015）（图 36.1）。

表 36.1 与实验诱发反应发展相关的主要刺激

刺激类型		当前强度或剂量	暴露时间	参考文献
电刺激	杏仁核	60Hz，一组 1 ms 双相方波脉冲，在 500μA 时输出	至少七次刺激	Hosford et al. (1995)
	角膜	3mA（持续时间 3s）	10～12d	Potschka, Löscher (1999)
化学刺激	戊四唑	35mg/kg	13d（平均）	Dhir (2012)
	可卡因	35mg/kg	10d	Itzhak (1996)
	荷苞牡丹碱	3.5mg/kg	28d	Nutt, Cowen, Batts, Grahame-Smith, Green (1982)
	苦味毒	5mg/kg	5d	Nutt et al. (1982)
环境刺激	心理压力	—	出生后第 2～14d 的早期生活压力	Kumar et al. (2011)

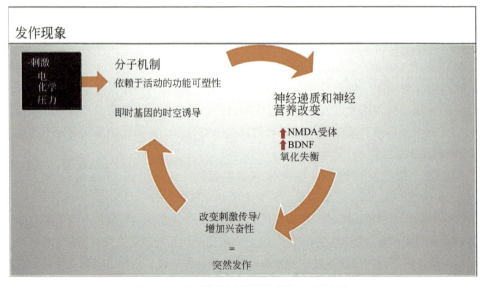

图 36.1 与诱发反应的发展有关的一系列事件

不同类型的刺激，如电、化学和压力，都能引发诱发反应。每种刺激都会触发与基因诱导相关的分子机制，进而可能改变受体和神经营养因子（如 BDNF）的表达，导致氧化失衡。总之，这些改变增加了神经元的兴奋性，导致癫痫的发生。一旦诱发反应发生，即使在没有初始刺激的情况下，这个循环过程也会导致癫痫的自发复发。（D. Macedo, 2017 提供）。

36.3 烟碱诱发反应

烟碱能够引发诱发反应的第一个证据来自 Bastlund 等（2005）的研究。这些作者进行了一项优雅的研究，他们将公认的 γ-氨基丁酸（GABA）拮抗剂（颞叶癫痫模型）诱发模型与新提出的烟碱诱发模型进行了比较。此外，他们在这些模型中验证了抗惊厥药物的保护作用，并通过

c-Fos 的测定评估了几个脑区的神经元过度活动。为诱导烟碱诱发反应,雄性成年小鼠每工作日腹腔注射2.3mg/kg,连续2周,隔日(周一、周三、周五)腹腔注射37mg/kg的PTZ,连续3周。此外,他们还对烟碱3.3mg/kg和PTZ 70mg/kg诱导的急性癫痫发作进行了治疗。

Bastlund等(2005)的研究表明,与PTZ诱发的癫痫相比,从测试的抗惊厥药物,即左乙拉西坦、盐酸噻加宾和苯妥英钠来看,左乙拉西坦的效力大约是后者的10倍,而盐酸噻加宾对烟碱诱发的癫痫同样有效。分析立即早期基因*c-Fos*时,该基因在细胞内钙水平升高后在神经元中诱导,这些作者在烟碱诱发的动物中观察到*c-Fos*免疫反应模式,与用PTZ获得的动物不同。烟碱诱发小鼠黑质致密部、内侧缰核内侧和外侧*c-Fos*免疫反应增强。另一方面,PTZ诱发的动物杏仁皮质和梨状皮质(即边缘结构)*c-Fos*免疫反应增强。值得一提的是,内侧缰核高表达α6、α4、β2、β2和β4亚基,这意味着烟碱诱发可以改变这些亚基,但还需要进一步证实。

其他一些机制,虽然还没有被研究,但可能与烟碱引发的诱发的发展有关。事实上,在其他诱发模型中存在的谷氨酸和多巴胺能神经传递的改变应该被研究,以便更好地理解烟碱诱发发生和发展的机制(图36.2)。

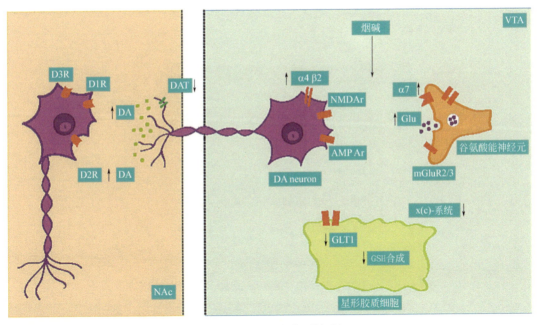

图36.2 烟碱诱发的可能机制

在边缘脑区(腹侧被盖区),烟碱直接刺激多巴胺能神经元的α4β2 nAChR,诱导其去极化,并通过投射到伏核的囊泡释放多巴胺。烟碱也作用于谷氨酸能神经元表达的α7 nAChR,导致谷氨酸的突触释放。这可以激活突触后离子型谷氨酸受体AMPA和NMDA,从而促进多巴胺能神经元的去极化和维持增加的多巴胺能张力。烟碱还可以抑制谷氨酸转运蛋白1(GLT1)等神经胶质转运蛋白对谷氨酸的摄取,从而导致谷氨酸能传递方式的改变和致离子受体过度激活。(A. J. M. Chaves Filho, 2017提供)。

总之,Bastlund等(2005)的研究结果发现,与PTZ诱导的诱发不同,烟碱诱发模型表现出较少的边缘激活,并且在检测左乙拉西坦的抗惊厥作用方面更敏感,左乙拉西坦是一种具有独特作用机制的药物。到目前为止,初步研究结果表明,左乙拉西坦可能对酒精依赖和共发性焦虑症患者的酒精使用和焦虑症状有有益的影响(Mariani, Levin, 2008)。因此,确定该药物治疗烟碱依赖的效果还需要进一步研究。

36.3.1 性别和年龄的影响

最近，我们的研究小组发现，与雄性大鼠相比，雌性青春期大鼠对烟碱诱发的发展具有明显的敏感性。在我们的实验条件下，雌性青春期大鼠在工作日注射烟碱2mg/kg，出现完全诱发发作的平均时间为19天，而在青春期周围的雄性大鼠，观察到诱发发作的平均时间为24天（图36.3）（Gomes et al. 2013）。另一方面，在成年期间，雄性和雌性的诱发反应发展时间是相同的，为19天（未公布的数据）。

在之前的报告中（Gomes et al. 2013），我们表明氧化改变是烟碱诱发发展过程中的性别差异的基础。在这方面，雌性青少年期烟碱诱发的大鼠在大脑区域、海马体和纹状体中呈现低水平的还原型谷胱甘肽（GSH）（主要的内源性抗氧化剂），并伴随额叶前皮层和纹状体中的超氧化物歧化酶（SOD）水平降低，以及前额叶皮层、海马体和纹状体中脂质过氧化的增加。相反，雄性大鼠只在海马体出现低水平的GSH（图36.3）。在这项研究中，与性别偏见改变相关的主要大脑区域是纹状体。

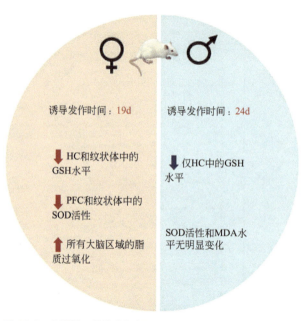

图36.3　在雄性和雌性动物中观察到的烟碱诱导诱发的差异综述

在Gomes等（2013）进行的这项研究中，雌性青春期动物诱发发育的中位数为19天，而雄性大鼠则延长至24天，表明雌性动物更容易发生诱发。观察到，与雄性相比，雌性大鼠大脑区域的氧化促进剂状态揭示了性别偏向的氧化改变。缩写：GSH，还原型谷胱甘肽；HC，海马体；MDA，丙二醛；SOD，超氧化物歧化酶（P.X.L. Gomes, 2017 提供）。

与我们之前关于烟碱诱发的动物中的纹状体性别偏见改变的结果一致，我们研究组未发表的数据显示，在雌性青春期烟碱诱发大鼠的纹状体中，NMDARs的磷酸化NR1亚基和磷酸化CREB转录因子（cAMP反应元件结合蛋白）的表达增加（图36.4）。

事实上，滥用药物引起的行为改变与纹状体转录和神经营养因子的异常有关。转录因子CREB活性的变化与精神运动敏感化记忆功能和精神刺激剂诱导的寻药行为有关。因此，我们推测，在雌性烟碱诱发的动物中，NMDARs的激活可以介导强烈的钙离子内流到纹状体细胞，导致细胞外信号调节激酶（ERKs）1和2的激活，从而使CREB因子磷酸化。值得注意的是，CREB参与长期形式的突触可塑性，并调节神经元的内在兴奋性（Benito, Barco, 2010），

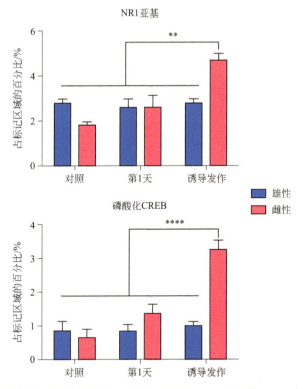

图 36.4 青春期大鼠纹状体 NMDAR 亚基 NR1 和磷酸化 CREB 在烟碱诱发过程中的免疫表达

大鼠在工作日注射烟碱 2mg/kg，在注射烟碱的第一天和诱导发作的当天（雌性第 19 天，雄性第 24 天）解剖摘除纹状体。对照组注射生理盐水。免疫荧光技术检测 NMDAR 亚基 NR1 和磷酸化 CREB 的免疫表达。条形表示平均值±平均值的标准误差（SEM）。数据分析采用双因素方差分析，然后进行 Tukey 后检验。我们观察到雌性烟碱诱发动物的 NR1 亚基和磷酸化 CREB 的水平显著升高（**$P<0.01$）和磷酸化 CREB（****$P<0.0001$）。资料来源：来自作者数据库的未发表的数据。

因此与药物滥用敏感性的发展有关（Guerriero et al. 2005）。值得一提的是，我们还观察到在青春期动物中，雄性烟碱诱发大鼠的 BDNF 水平降低，而雌性大鼠的 BDNF 水平较高（数据未显示）。综上所述，这些结果指向烟碱诱发的雌性青春期动物的大脑氧化失衡和类学习机制的激活。这一机制已经被认为与压力和可卡因诱导的行为敏感化过程有关（见综述：Kalivas, Stewart, 1991）。

36.3.2 通过使用抗氧化剂进行预防

在我们的第一项研究中，我们证明了口服维生素 E 200mg/kg 和 400mg/kg 可以阻止雄性和雌性青春期大鼠烟碱诱发的发展。之所以决定使用这种抗氧化剂，是因为研究结果显示，烟碱诱发的大鼠大脑区域的脂质过氧化增加（Gomes et al. 2013）。阻止脂质过氧化自由基（LOO·）和终止脂质过氧化链式反应是维生素 E 的主要抗氧化机制（Nimse, Pal, 2015）。

由于我们还观察到雌性烟碱诱发大鼠脑区 GSH 水平的降低（Gomes et al. 2013），我们决定测试 N-乙酰半胱氨酸（NAC）作为预防诱发的策略（Okamura et al. 2016）。值得注意的是，NAC 是半胱氨酸的前体，半胱氨酸是谷胱甘肽合成的关键决定因素之一（Lu, 2013）。270mg/kg NAC 预防雌性青春期大鼠烟碱诱发癫痫的发生发展（Okamura et al. 2016）。

近年来，越来越多的证据表明 NAC 可能用于治疗神经精神障碍。一些研究报告称，NAC 对情感性（Berk et al. 2011）和物质使用障碍（包括烟碱依赖）有很好的疗效（Schmaal et al. 2011）。NAC治疗精神障碍的普遍性很耐人寻味，可能与它在几个途径上的作用有关，如氧化应激、炎症、线粒体功能障碍和神经递质失衡（Dean, Giorlando, Berk, 2011）。

N-乙酰半胱氨酸可以减弱可卡因和烟碱等精神刺激剂引起的药物寻找行为。这些作用与减少兴奋性神经递质谷氨酸的囊泡运输（Moussawi et al. 2009），恢复谷氨酸稳态有关。

因此，NAC可直接或间接调节谷氨酸能神经递质，进而调节多巴胺能神经递质。考虑到谷氨酸和多巴胺能通路以及氧化应激在几种神经精神疾病中的作用，人们可以推测NAC的广泛治疗作用是通过它对这些靶点的作用来实现的（图36.5）。最后，NAC可能代表着一种新的有前途和安全的策略，作为药物使用障碍的附加疗法，其假定的神经生物学机制包括"诱发"过程。

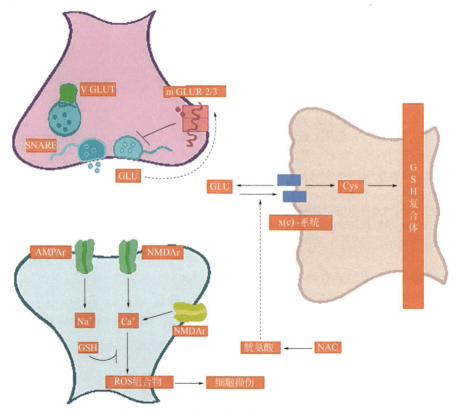

图36.5 N-乙酰半胱氨酸预防烟碱诱发的机制

N-乙酰半胱氨酸被代谢成半胱氨酸。半胱氨酸通过半胱氨酸-谷氨酸逆向转运蛋白[x(c)-系统]转运到细胞内。在细胞内，半胱氨酸被还原为半胱氨酸以合成谷胱甘肽。当x(c)-系统内化半胱氨酸时，它通过非囊泡途径将谷氨酸转移到胞外介质。谷氨酸的这种释放优先激活突触前代谢性谷氨酸受体2/3(mGluR2/3)，该受体负性调节这种神经递质的囊泡释放。这一机制阻止了谷氨酸离子亲电受体AMPA和NMDA的激活及其相关的兴奋性毒性过程，并降低了活性氧(ROS)水平，提高了细胞存活率（A.J.M. Chaves Filho, 2017提供）

36.4 结论与展望

目前的综述表明，烟碱诱导的诱发已成为研究烟碱重复暴露引起的长期神经可塑性改变的有用工具。尽管烟碱诱发很重要，但目前对它的研究还很少。到目前为止，有证据表明，与雄性大鼠相比，青春期雌性大鼠对诱发的易感性增加。大脑氧化、谷氨酸能和神经营养机制是性别偏见结果的基础。成年后，这种易感性似乎是一样的（Gomes et al. 2013）。

基于烟碱诱发动物体内存在的氧化改变，使用抗氧化剂策略，如维生素E和NAC，可以有效地防止诱发的发生。

此外，鉴于诱发机制参与了几种神经精神疾病的进展过程，该模型与筛选新的抗诱发药物有关，以提高这些疾病的治疗水平，特别是那些与烟碱使用相关的疾病。

术语解释

- **胆碱能危象**：过度刺激胆碱能受体，导致过度流涎、抽筋、腹泻和视力模糊等症状，并伴有或不伴有癫痫等中枢神经系统症状。
- **吸烟相关并发症**：在医学上，共病一词指的是两种或两种以上疾病共存。第一种疾病的存在或暴露于风险因素会增加第二种疾病发生的可能性。吸烟是一个危险因素，会增加中风、缺氧、感染和炎症的风险，这些都是与吸烟有关的共病。
- **电子烟**：用来模拟吸烟感觉的手持电子设备。与含有烟碱和大量有害化合物的烟草不同，电子烟的成分主要是烟碱，含量从低（6mg）到超高（24mg）不等。
- **癫痫产生**：癫痫发作一种渐进的过程，通过这个过程，先前正常的大脑向产生支持慢性癫痫发作的异常电活动的方向发展。
- **引火物**：指的是容易诱发的物质，就像一个小火花会诱发一团火焰，最终会成长为熊熊燃烧的篝火。生物学中的这个术语指的是反复暴露在低强度刺激（如杏仁核电刺激）下而引发的行为改变（如癫痫发作）。
- **神经可塑性**：这个术语与大脑形成和重组突触连接的能力有关。神经可塑性涉及生理过程，如记忆的形成，以及损伤后的大脑重组。
- **神经精神障碍**：精神障碍与影响情绪、认知和行为的大脑功能改变有关的精神障碍。神经精神障碍的例子有情绪障碍（例如，双相情感障碍和严重抑郁症）、精神分裂症和自闭症谱系障碍。
- **氧化应激**：产生更多的活性氧（自由基）或/和抗氧化剂防御能力降低，从而损害细胞功能的一种状态。
- **青春期**：啮齿动物的青春期是与人类青春期有关的发育期。它发生在最早检测到的日间促性腺激素循环（大约出生后第28天）和生殖成熟（大约出生后38～42d）之间。
- **拉辛诱发级数**：由拉辛开发的一种量表，用于评估癫痫啮齿动物模型的癫痫发作强度。该量表分为五类，分别为"嘴巴和面部运动"（阶段1）、"点头"（阶段2）、"前肢阵挛"（阶段3）、以举起为特征的发作（阶段4）和以"全面"发作为特征的发作（阶段5）。

诱发模型的关键事实

- 电、化学和心理压力等刺激会引发诱发。
- 诱发模型概念化了进行性癫痫的神经适应机制。
- 诱发机制与神经精神疾病的复发和周期性症状有关。
- NMDAR、神经营养因子和氧化失衡的变化与诱发的发生有关。
- 抗诱导药物是治疗情感性精神障碍的有效药物。

烟碱诱发的关键因素

- 烟碱诱发是在过去的十年中被证明的。
- 烟碱诱发导致黑质致密部和内侧缰核内侧和外侧的神经元过度活跃。
- 抗惊厥药物左乙拉西坦可有效预防烟碱诱发。

- 性别影响青春期前动物诱发的发育，雌性更容易受到影响。
- 氧化、谷氨酸能和嗜神经性改变是诱发发育过程中性别差异的基础。
- 在成年动物中，没有观察到性别对烟碱诱发发展的影响。
- 抗氧化剂，如维生素E和N-乙酰半胱氨酸，可以抑制烟碱诱发的发展。

要点总结
- 诱发是研究长效神经可塑性的一个模型。
- 诱发机制与癫痫的发生和神经精神障碍（如情感障碍和物质使用障碍）症状的自发表现有关。
- 诱发模型似乎是研究烟碱重复给药引发神经可塑性机制的重要途径。
- 诱发有助于了解烟碱引起的神经精神症状和脑结构改变。
- 烟碱诱发的研究具有为治疗药物开发开发合适靶点的前景。

参考文献

Ambelas, A. (1987). Life events and mania. A special relationship? British Journal of Psychiatry, 150, 235-240.

Bassett, R. A.; Osterhoudt, K.; Brabazon, T. (2014). Nicotine poisoning in an infant. New England Journal of Medicine, 370(23), 2249-2250.

Bastlund, J. F.; Berry, D.; Watson, W. P. (2005). Pharmacological and histological characterisation of nicotine-kindled seizures in mice. Neuropharmacology, 48(7), 975-983.

Bender, R. E.; Alloy, L. B. (2011). Life stress and kindling in bipolar disorder: review of the evidence and integration with emerging biopsychosocial theories. Clinical Psychology Review, 31(3), 383-398.

Benito, E.; Barco, A. (2010). CREB's control of intrinsic and synaptic plasticity: implications for CREB-dependent memory models. Trends in Neurosciences, 33(5), 230-240.

Berk, M.; Munib, A.; Dean, O.; Malhi, G. S.; Kohlmann, K.; Schapkaitz, I. et al. (2011). Qualitative methods in early-phase drug trials: broadening the scope of data and methods from an RCT of N-acetylcysteine in schizophrenia. The Journal of Clinical Psychiatry, 72(7), 909-913.

Bertram, E. (2007). The relevance of kindling for human epilepsy. Epilepsia, 48(s2), 65-74. https:/ /doi. org/10. 1111/j. 1528-1167. 2007. 01068. x.

Clarke, P. B. S.; Kumar, R. (1983). The effects of nicotine on locomotor activity in non-tolerant and tolerant rats. British Journal of Pharmacology, 78(2), 329-337.

Damaj, M. I.; Glassco, W.; Dukat, M.; Martin, B. R. (1999). Pharmacological characterization of nicotine-induced seizures in mice. The Journal of Pharmacology and Experimental Therapeutics, 291(3), 1284-1291.

Dean, O.; Giorlando, F.; Berk, M. (2011). N-acetylcysteine in psychiatry: current therapeutic evidence and potential mechanisms of action. Journal of Psychiatry, Neuroscience: JPN, 36(2), 78-86.

Dennison, Z.; Campbell Teskey, G.; Cain, D. P. (1995). Persistence of kindling: effect of partial kindling, retention interval, kindling site, and stimulation parameters. Epilepsy Research, 21(3), 171-182.

Dhir, A. (2012). Pentylenetetrazol (PTZ) kindling model of epilepsy. Current Protocols in Neuroscience, 58, 9.37.1-9.37.12.

Dworetzky, B. A.; Bromfield, E. B.; Townsend, M. K.; Kang, J. H. (2010). A prospective study of smoking, caffeine, and alcohol as risk factors for seizures or epilepsy in young adult women: data from the Nurses' Health Study II. Epilepsia, 51(2), 198-205.

Goddard, G. V.; McIntyre, D. C.; Leech, C. K. (1969). A permanent change in brain function resulting from daily electrical stimulation. Experimental Neurology, 25(3), 295-330.

Gomes, P. X. L.; De Oliveira, G. V.; De Araújo, F. Y. R.; De Barros Viana, G. S.; De Sousa, F. C. F.; Hyphantis, T. N. et al. (2013). Differences in vulnerability to nicotine-induced kindling between female and male periadolescent rats. Psychopharmacology, 225(1),https:/ / doi. org/10. 1007/s00213-012-2799-5.

Guerriero, R. M.; Rajadhyaksha, A.; Crozatier, C.; Giros, B.; Nosten-Bertrand, M.; Kosofsky, B. E. (2005). Augmented constitutive CREB expression in the nucleus accumbens and striatum may contribute to the altered behavioral response to cocaine of adult mice exposed to cocaine in utero. Developmental Neuroscience, 27(2-4), 235-248.

Hosford, D. A.; Simonato, M.; Cao, Z.; Garcia-Cairasco, N.; Silver, J. M.; Butler, L. et al. (1995). Differences in the anatomic distribution of immediate-early gene expression in amygdala and angular bundle kindling development. The Journal of Neuroscience_ The Official Journal of the Society for Neuroscience, 15(3 Pt 2), 2513-2523.

Itzhak, Y. (1996). Attenuation of cocaine kindling by 7-nitroindazole, an inhibitor of brain nitric oxide synthase. Neuropharmacology, 35(8), 1065-1073.

Kalivas, P. W.; Stewart, J. (1991). Dopamine transmission in the initiation and expression of drug-induced and stress-induced sensitization of motor-activity. Brain Research Reviews, 16(3), 223-244.

Kaminski, R. M.; Núñez-Taltavull, J. F.; Budziszewska, B.; Lasoń, W.; Gasior, M.; Zapata, A. et al. (2011). Effects of cocaine-kindling on the expression of NMDA receptors and glutamate levels in mouse brain. Neurochemical Research, 36(1), 146-152.

Kumar, G.; Jones, N. C.; Morris, M. J.; Rees, S.; O'Brien, T. J.; Salzberg, M. R. (2011). Early life stress enhancement of limbic epilep togenesis in adult rats: Mechanistic insights. M. Avoli (Ed.), PLoSOne, 6(9), e24033.

Lu, S. C. (2013). Glutathione synthesis. Biochimica et Biophysica Acta, 1830 (5), 3143-3153. https://doi.org/10.1016/j.bbagen.2012.09.008.

Mariani, J. J.; Levin, F. R. (2008). Levetiracetam for the treatment of co-occurring alcohol dependence and anxiety: case series and review. The American Journal of Drug and Alcohol Abuse, 34(6), 683-691.

Moussawi, K.; Pacchioni, A.; Moran, M.; Olive, M. F.; Gass, J. T.; Lavin, A. et al. (2009). N-acetylcysteine reverses cocaine-induced metaplasticity. Nature Neuroscience, 12(2), 182-189.

Nimse, S. B.; Pal, D. (2015). Free radicals, natural antioxidants, and their reaction mechanisms. RSC Advances, 5(35), 27986-28006.

Nutt, D. J.; Cowen, P. J.; Batts, C. C.; Grahame-Smith, D. G.; Green, A. R. (1982). Repeated administration of subconvulsant doses of GABA antagonist drugs—I. Effect on seizure threshold (kindling). Psychopharmacology (Berlin), 76(1), 84-87.

Okamura, A. M. N. C.; Gomes, P. X. L.; de Oliveira, G. V.; Araújo, F. Y. R. D.; Tomaz, V. S.; Chaves Filho, A. J. M. et al. (2016). *N*-acetylcysteine attenuates nicotine-induced kindling in female periadolescent rats. Progress in Neuro-Psychopharmacology and Biological Psychiatry, 67, https://doi.org/10.1016/j.pnpbp.2016.01.010.

Pinel, J. P. J.; Rovner, L. I. (1978). Experimental epileptogenesis kindling-induced epilepsy in rats. Experimental Neurology, 58(2), 190-202.

Post, R. M. (2007). Kindling and sensitization as models for affective episode recurrence, cyclicity, and tolerance phenomena. Neuroscience and Biobehavioral Reviews, 31, 858-873.

Post, R. M.; Kopanda, R. T. (1976). Cocaine, kindling, and psychosis. American Journal of Psychiatry, 133(6), 627-634.

Potschka, H.; Löscher, W. (1999). Corneal kindling in mice: Behavioral and pharmacological differences to conventional kindling. Epilepsy Research, 37(2), 109-120.

Racine, R. J. (1972). Modification of seizure activity by electrical stimulation. II. Motor seizure. Electroencephalography and Clinical Neurophysiology, 32(3), 281-294.

Rong, L.; Frontera, A. T.; Benbadis, S. R. (2014). Tobacco smoking, epilepsy, and seizures. Epilepsy, Behavior, 31, 210-218. https://doi.org/10.1016/j.yebeh.2013.11.022.

Schmaal, L.; Berk, L.; Hulstijn, K. P.; Cousijn, J.; Wiers, R. W.; van den Brink, W. (2011). Efficacy of N-acetylcysteine in the treatment of nicotine dependence: a double-blind placebo-controlled pilot study. European Addiction Research, 17(4), 211-216.

Sieciechowicz, D.; Kohrman, M. (2015). Transdermal nicotine patch as a novel treatment for epilepsy associated with a mutation in the nicotinic acetylcholine receptor (S35.002). Neurology, 84(14 Suppl).

Trevor, H. (2012). Amygdalar models of neurological and neuropsychiatric disorders. In The amygdala—A discrete multitasking manager. InTech https://doi.org/10.5772/50244.

Zhu, X.; Dong, J.; Shen, K.; Bai, Y.; Zhang, Y.; Lv, X. et al. (2015). NMDA receptor NR2B subunits contribute to PTZ-kindling-induced hippocampal astrocytosis and oxidative stress. Brain Research Bulletin, 114, 70-78.

37

烟碱奖励和戒烟：CB1 受体的作用

S. Tannous, S. Caille

Aquitaine Institute for Cognitive and Integrative Neuroscience, University of Bordeaux, CNRS UMR5287, Bordeaux, France

缩略语

2-AG	2-花生四烯酸甘油酯	IM	肌肉注射
AEA	大麻素	IP	腹腔注射
BLA	杏仁基底外侧核	IV	静脉注射
BNST	终纹床核	IVSA	静脉自给药
CB1	大麻素1型受体	LTP	长时程增强
CPA	条件性位置厌恶	MAGL	单酰甘油脂肪酶
CPP	条件性位置偏好	NAcc	伏隔核
D9-THC	δ-9-四氢大麻酚	PFC	前额叶皮层
DA	多巴胺	VTA	腹侧被盖区
FAAH	脂肪酰胺水解酶		

37.1 引言

37.1.1 烟碱成瘾

就全球健康而言，吸烟是最可预防的死亡原因。现在，人们普遍认为烟碱是烟草的实际成瘾性化合物，尽管有负面后果，但反复使用烟碱仍会导致强迫寻求和使用药物，在试图戒烟的人中，约有80%的人会在戒烟后出现戒断症状和复发。此外，吸烟行为不是减少的甚至是增加的成瘾，因为现在通过电子烟设备消耗了汽化的烟碱。事实上，自2010年以来，全球电子烟使用者的数量一直在持续增加，其中大多数是前吸烟者（世界卫生组织）。总之，无论烟碱的消费途径是什么，这些数据都强调，如果我们想要解决这一公共健康问题，了解烟碱成瘾机制是多么重要。尽管已经进行了大量的研究来开发治疗工具，但目前可用的针对烟碱成瘾的临床治疗在一年的治疗后成功率非常低（Cahill, Stevens, Perera, Lancaster, 2013）。

烟碱和滥用药物一样，通过增加腹侧被盖区多巴胺能神经元（"奖赏系统"）的神经元活动来促进奖励和学习。烟碱通过靶向和刺激烟碱型乙酰胆碱受体（配体门控离子通道），更具体地说是定位和刺激位于伏隔核内的异构体α4β2和同构体α7亚型，增加伏隔核和前额叶皮层的多巴胺（DA）释放。相反，烟碱戒断降低了大脑奖励系统的敏感性（Kenny, Markou, 2005），并降低了伏隔核内细胞外DA的水平（Zhang et al. 2012），导致与烟碱戒断和抑郁行为相关的烦躁状态。

37.1.2 如何探究烟碱成瘾行为？

药物开发的一个陷阱可能是，动物模型不能模拟烟碱依赖和戒烟的所有方面，但现有的模型在测量成瘾过程的几个行为参数方面仍然有效。此外，使用这些范例有助于深入研究烟碱的欲望和奖励效应所涉及的几种神经机制。两种主要模式中的第一种是静脉注射烟碱自给药，动物在静脉注射烟碱的过程中，特别是通过瞄准一个主动的动作，通过静脉注射烟碱，与传递提示灯相关，以促进联想学习。它可以量化吸毒和寻找毒品的行为。第二种模式是烟碱诱导的条件性位置偏爱，即动物被条件化地将烟碱的摄入与特定的环境联系起来，测试包括允许没有药物的动物返回或避免之前与烟碱相关的环境。烟碱的食欲效应将促使大鼠"更喜欢"与药物相关的环境，而不是与盐水相关的环境。此外，在一段时间内通过重复注射或皮下渗透性微泵长期给药烟碱后，戒断综合征和戒断神经底桩已被广泛研究。自发的和拮抗剂催促的药物戒断都会导致维持寻药行为的消极动机状态和包括几个不同强度的躯体症状的戒断综合征。在烟碱戒断综合征期间观察到的躯体体征如下：身体颤抖、脸颊颤抖、逃跑尝试、眨眼、喘息、舔生殖器、摇头、上睑下垂、牙齿颤抖、扭动和打哈欠（见综述，Kenny, Markou, 2001）。总之，这些动物模型已经证实了几种"经典"治疗工具的使用，如烟碱受体激动剂药理学与烟碱替代疗法（NRT），烟碱受体部分激动剂药理学与伐伦克林（商标为Champix），或去甲肾上腺素/多巴胺能受体间接激动剂药物疗法，如安非他酮（商标为Zyban）（Anthenelli et al. 2016; Cahill et al. 2013）。它还带来了最近烟碱成瘾药物开发的努力。

37.2 CB1受体直接药物治疗

最有前途的药物疗法之一涉及到内源性大麻系统的几个关键成员。鉴定中枢的 $\it\Delta$-9-四氢大麻酚（大麻的活性成分），结合其靶点，发现了第一个内源性受体：大麻素1型受体（CB1）。随后，CB1受体的两个主要内源性配体——烷基酰胺（AEA）和2-花生四烯酸甘油酯（2AG）及其相关的降解酶——脂肪酸水解酶（FAAH）和单酰甘油脂肪酶（MAGL）分别被分离出来。这些CB1受体是动物和人类大脑中含量最丰富的G蛋白偶联受体，参与广泛的生理功能。它们的定位表明，它们在大脑结构如基底节、小脑和海马体中的密度很高，在大脑奖励结构中的密度也较低。有强有力的证据表明，CB1受体大多是突触前受体，它们可以通过这些受体控制神经递质的释放。在这些发现之后不久，强有力的证据承认CB1受体在调节自然和药理奖励的积极强化效应中起着关键作用。随后，一种选择性的CB1受体拮抗剂被建议作为治疗肥胖症的药物疗法。与此同时，利莫那班（SR141716A，商标为AComplia）也被用于治疗烟碱成瘾，因为一项开创性的临床前研究显示，CB1受体敲除可以阻断烟碱的渴求特性。这种化合物是一个很有前途的候选药物，因为它还可能帮助吸烟者调节与戒烟尝试相关的体重增加。因此，急性注射利莫那班已经在几种烟碱成瘾相关行为上进行了测试，并证明了CB1受体在静脉注射范式中控制烟碱诱导的条件性位置偏爱、烟碱摄取和烟碱寻找行为（Cohen et al. 2005; Forget et al. 2005; Simonnet et al. 2013）。令人惊讶的是，急性利莫那班对甲氨基甲酰胺诱导的烟碱依赖动物戒断体征的减弱没有贡献。最后，CB1受体似乎参与烟碱诱导的NAcc中DA的释放（Cohen et al. 2002）。总之，就选择性CB1受体拮抗剂在烟碱成瘾治疗中的潜在应用而言，这些结果是非常有希望的。不幸的是，长期使用CB1

受体拮抗剂伴随有引起焦虑和抑郁的副作用（Cahill, Ussher, 2011）。因此，利莫那班和他拉那班（另一种CB1受体拮抗剂）的开发在2008年停止，因为它们与精神障碍（Rigotti et al., 2009）和不可接受的副作用有关。在这里，我们回顾了CB1受体信号在烟碱诱导的奖励、寻求和戒断中的功能作用的最新证据，包括最新的内源性大麻素药理工具的介绍（见表37.1和表37.2）。关于CB1受体和内源性大麻素参与烟碱成瘾过程的早期发现的更广泛的内容已经在别处进行了回顾（Gamaleddin et al. 2015）。

表37.1 直接或间接靶向CB1受体药物对烟碱奖励和烟碱寻求行为的影响

CB1r依赖药理学	给药途径	行为效应	参考文献
SR141716A	腹腔注射	减少静脉自给药	De Vries, de Vries, Janssen, Schoffelmeer (2005)
	肌肉注射	减少药物寻找；减少条件性位置偏好	Le Foll, Goldberg (2004), Cohen et al. (2005) Merritt et al. (2008), Schindler et al. (2016)
	伏隔核壳	减少药物寻找	Kodas, Cohen, Louis, Griebel (2007)
	杏仁基底外侧核	自发活动无影响	
	前额叶皮层		
AM 251	腹侧被盖区	减少静脉自给药	Simonnet et al. (2013)
	伏隔核	静脉自给药无影响	Hashemizadeh, Sardari, Rezayof (2014)
	杏仁基底外侧核	减少条件性位置偏好	
	静脉注射	减少静脉注射在终纹床核诱导的长时间增强	Reisiger et al. (2014)
	终纹床核		
	腹腔注射	减少静脉注射	Shoaib (2008)
	静脉注射	减少药物寻找	Simonnet et al. (2013)
AM4113	腹腔注射	减少静脉注射和冲动	Gueye et al. (2016)
	肌肉注射	减少药物和压力诱导的寻求 减少VTA多巴胺神经元的活动	Schindler et al. (2016)
URB597	腹腔注射	减少或增加条件性位置偏好	Merritt et al. (2008)
	静脉注射	减少静脉注射；减少药物寻找	Scherma et al. (2008) Justinova et al. (2015)
URB694	静脉注射	减少静脉注射；减少药物寻求	Justinova et al. (2015)
JZL184	腹腔注射	静脉注射无影响；增加线索诱导的寻求	Trigo, Le Foll (2016)
AM404	腹腔注射	减少条件性位置偏好和寻求；减少烟碱诱导的NAC壳中的DA	Scherma et al. (2012)
WIN55, 212-2	腹腔注射	增加静脉注射和冲动；增加药物寻求	Gamaleddin et al. (2012)

注：内源性大麻素药理对烟碱食欲相关行为的影响。效果可以增加、减少或保持不变（无修改）。根据抑制/激活CB1受体的能力对化合物进行排序。首先是反向激动剂（SR141716A和AM251），然后是中性拮抗剂（AM4113）；其次是FAAH抑制剂（URB597和URB694）、MAGL抑制剂（JZL184）或AEA转运蛋白抑制剂（AM404），最后是CB1受体激动剂WIN55、212-2。

表37.2 靶向CB1受体药物对戒断行为的影响

CB1受体依赖药理学	给药途径	行为效应	参考文献
SR141716A	腹腔注射	躯体戒断症状减少；退缩记忆障碍增加	Merritt et al. (2008) Saravia et al. (2017)
URB597	腹腔注射	戒断引起的焦虑减弱；戒断增强或减弱	Cippitelli et al. (2011) Merritt et al. (2008)

续表

CB1受体依赖药理学	给药途径	行为效应	参考文献
O7460	腹腔注射	戒断记忆损伤减弱； 躯体戒断严重程度增强	Saravia et al. (2017)
JZL184	腹腔注射	认知缺陷无影响； 戒断严重程度减弱	Saravia et al. (2017) Muldoon et al. (2015)
D9-THC	腹腔注射	退缩迹象减弱； 尾壳核和齿状回的c-Fos减弱	Balerio, Aso, Berrendero, Murtra, Maldonado (2004)

注：内源性大麻素药理对烟碱戒断行为的影响。效果可以增加、减少或保持不变（无修改）。根据抑制/激活CB1受体的能力对化合物进行排序。首先是反向激动剂（SR141716A），然后是FAAH抑制剂（URB597），然后是2-AG生物合成酶抑制剂（O7460）和MAGL抑制剂（JZL184），最后是CB1受体激动剂D9-THC。

37.3　CB1受体间接药物治疗

另一种帮助戒烟的策略是通过使用内源性大麻素降解酶的抑制剂来恢复内源性大麻素系统的平衡。实际上，这一假设是，如果靶向CB1受体可以阻止烟碱奖赏，这表明内源性大麻素与烟碱成瘾的诱导或表达密切相关。此外，内源性大麻素系统与应激反应有关，因为研究表明，在应激过程中，内源性大麻素被吸收，以减缓皮质酮的升高，减轻焦虑和抑郁样行为（Patel et al. 2017）。因此，考虑到烟碱的戒断会引起负面的情绪状态，这些额外的治疗特性进一步支持了FAAH/MAGL抑制剂的有益用途。针对JZL184抑制单酰甘油脂肪酶的研究很少。而Muldoon等（2015）表明MAGL基因缺失或联合使用JZL184可以减少烟碱戒断综合征，另一项研究表明JZL184可以增强提示诱导的烟碱复发（Trigo, Le Foll, 2016）。总而言之，这些数据表明2-AG主要参与了复杂的过程。另一方面，对FAAH抑制剂URB597进行了几项研究。研究表明，急性URB597降低了啮齿动物的烟碱奖励特性（Scherma et al. 2008），减少了烟碱静脉注射自给药和烟碱寻求的获得（Forget et al. 2009; Forget et al. 2016），并改善了烟碱戒断诱导的情感症状，但不是躯体症状（Cippitelli et al. 2011; Merritt et al. 2008）。此外，抑制FAAH似乎可以阻止烟碱诱导的NAcc细胞外多巴胺的升高（Scherma et al. 2008）。因此，抑制FAAH似乎是治疗烟碱成瘾的最佳药物。

37.4　CB1靶向药物治疗的急性与慢性对照研究

重要的是，大多数研究都检查了这些药物疗法的急性使用，往往忽略了这样一个事实，即戒烟药物通常是在达到长期戒断（至少6个月）的结果之前给予的（见表37.3）。然而，在临床和临床前环境中使用利莫那班慢性治疗的条件下，已经证明发生了严重的不良反应（Beyer et al. 2010; Cahill, Ussher, 2011; O'Brien et al. 2013），并且已经做出了停用利莫那班的决定。最近开发的一种中性CB1受体拮抗剂AM4113（Gueye et al. 2016）为帮助戒烟的治疗干预开辟了新的前景。事实上，它减弱了在递进强化计划下自行静脉注射烟碱的大鼠的动机；它还减少了由线索、压力或药物启动诱导的烟碱寻求行为。此外，在长期接触后，它似乎显示出更好的精神耐受性。在长期使用JZL184或URB597治疗烟碱成瘾之前，还没有进行过研究，直到最近我们研究了长期戒断期间慢性FAAH抑制对烟碱依赖大鼠的影响（Simonnet et al. 2017）。在我们的条件下，大鼠首先被暴露在长时间的烟碱静脉注射中，这使动物对烟碱产生依赖，如烟碱停药后戒断所致的快感缺乏。然后，我们试图评估URB597对烟碱戒断大鼠和对照组大鼠的慢性治疗效果。我们的假设是，通过恢复AEA基调，URB597将防止烟碱戒断期间出现负面情绪相关症状，并成为戒烟治疗的良好候选者。与预期相反，我们的结果显示URB597会导致持续性的快感缺乏和严重的抑郁样行为和生物标志物（Simonnet et al. 2017）。总而言之，这些新数据表明，长期服用URB597可能有更多的CB1受体拮抗剂的作用，促进相同类型的情感副作用。因此，为了检验我们的新假设，我们检查了几个大脑区域的CB1受体结合和功能，包括缰核，这是基于它与烟碱成瘾和抑郁症状的关系（Baldwin, Alanis, Salas, 2011; Fowler, Kenny, 2014）。实际上，我们证实慢性URB597不仅没有恢复内源性大麻素的平衡，反而特异性地降低了烟碱戒断大鼠缰核中CB1受体的密度和活性。去除CB1受体介导的抑制可能是导致抑郁样症状出现的原因之一（Lecca et al. 2016; Simonnet et al. 2017）。

由于不了解针对内源性大麻素的长期治疗后发生的神经适应，严重阻碍了它的治疗应用。因此，我们在这里简要介绍了与烟碱成瘾慢性治疗相关的内源性大麻素药理学，强调了这样一个事实，即目前的动物和人类实验室模型的预测性临床有效性有限，往往忽略了这些药物的长期使用（见表37.3）。

表37.3　CB1直接药理和间接药理急、慢性用药的关键事实

烟碱被动给药和静脉给药增加了几个大脑结构中细胞外的内源性大麻素水平，包括奖励通路的区域（VTA、NAC、PFC等）
急性给予CB1受体间接激动剂，如降解酶抑制剂化合物，可促进对烟碱成瘾过程的抑制控制，与急性给予CB1受体拮抗剂类似（见表37.1和表37.2）
临床前研究表明，在啮齿动物中长期服用利莫那班（Beyer et al. 2010）或FAAH抑制剂会导致认知障碍和抑郁样行为（Basavarajappa et al. 2014; Ceci et al. 2014; Wu et al. 2014）
然而，在最近的研究被报道之前，内源性大麻素药理学从未在药物戒断动物身上进行过慢性治疗（Gueye et al. 2016; Simonnet et al. 2017）
研究表明，小剂量URB597 [0.3mg/(kg·d)] 延长对烟碱戒断大鼠的FAAH抑制作用，不仅不能改善戒断症状，反而会加重戒断症状。它增加了抑郁样症状和应激诱导的血浆皮质酮升高（图37.1和图37.2）
行为和生理抑郁生物标记物都与缰核CB1受体密度和活性的改变相关（图37.3）

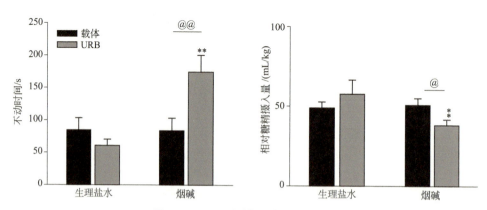

图37.1　FAAH抑制和抑郁状行为症状

慢性URB597对长期戒酒抑郁样症状的影响。左侧面板，在戒断第38天的强迫游泳试验中测量不动时间（s）。右侧面板，在戒断第41天测量相对糖精摄入量（mL/kg）。生理盐水与烟碱自给药暴露大鼠，载体（Veh，黑条）-URB597（URB，灰条）处理大鼠。来自Simonnet等(2017)，获得了出版商许可。

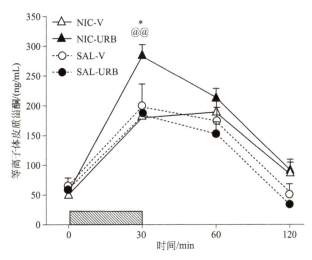

图 37.2　FAAH 对应激诱导的血浆皮质酮升高的抑制作用，皮质酮是抑郁症的生物标志物

烟碱戒断期间慢性URB597对血浆皮质酮水平的影响。在第44天测定应激后0min、30min、60min和120min（条纹条表示束缚30min）的血浆皮质酮浓度。生理盐水与烟碱自给药暴露大鼠,Vehicle（V，白色符号）-vs URB597（URB，黑色符号）处理大鼠。

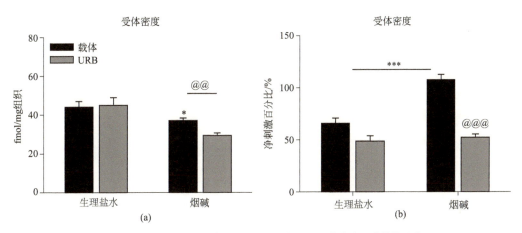

图 37.3　烟碱戒断过程中抑制 FAAH 对 CB1 受体密度和功能的影响

缰核放射自显影中CB1受体结合和CP55,940刺激的[35S]GTPgS结合。(a) CB1受体密度以"fmol/mg组织"表示；(b) CB1受体功能以"净刺激百分比"表示。生理盐水（SAL）与烟碱（NIC）自给药暴露大鼠。Vehicle（Veh，黑条）-vs URB597（URB，灰条）-处理组大鼠。

术语解释

- 戒断：成瘾过程的这一部分描述了一个没有停止吸烟行为的戒断过程。

- 大麻素1型受体：大麻素1型（Cannabinoid type 1, CB1）受体是Gi/o蛋白偶联受体，主要定位于轴突末端。因此，内源性配体或外源性配体如 δ-9- 四氢大麻酚激活CB1受体，可显著抑制神经递质向突触的释放。

- 条件性位置偏好/厌恶：作为一种行为的临床前和非手术过程，范式用于探索烟碱/烟碱戒断的正/负特性。起初，动物被允许探索所有的环境。然后，烟碱或烟碱戒断效应与特定环境有关。在实验过程中，如果有积极的条件性记忆，动物会花更多的时间在药物相关记忆室；如果有厌恶的条件性记忆，动物会避开与退出相关记忆室。

- 依赖：病理体内平衡状态，指神经适应发展以补偿慢性药物使用，通常称为身体依赖。心理依赖是指导致强迫性药物使用的精神状态。

- 内源性大麻素系统：内源性大麻素系统（endocannabinoid system, ECS）是一种神经调节脂质系统，是包括奖励控制在内的多种生理过程所必需的。该系统包括大麻素受体（CB1和CB2）；内源性配体，如丙烯酰胺（AEA）和2-花生四烯酸甘油酯（2-AG）；其降解酶分别为脂肪酸酰胺水解酶（FAAH）和单酰基甘油脂肪酶（MAGL）。
- 静脉自给药：允许动物自给药的操作行为，在实验室中用于评估其对药物上瘾的可能性。烟碱的自给药通常与提示光传递有关，这是药物传递的信号。强劲的自给药表明烟碱的奖赏效应。它允许在固定比率强化时间表下测量烟碱消耗，并且允许在渐进比率强化时间表下检查烟碱的动机（比率工作量/奖励中断点）。
- 复发/觅药：这是人类药物复发的动物模型。用来指自给药行为在消失或戒断后恢复的术语，也称为"寻求毒品"行为。恢复可以由药物本身的剂量、线索或与药物可用性相关的环境或应激源引起。
- 戒断综合征：戒断后的身体和情感上的消极状态，这是由于药物依赖过程中"对手"过程的暴露而引起的。这些症状是这种药特有的。通过药物停止（自发综合征）或使用选择性烟碱拮抗剂（如甲胺），可在动物体内诱发烟碱戒断。在啮齿类动物中，烟碱的戒断涉及了一种生理成分，包括爪和身体颤抖、摇头、后退、跳跃、卷曲和上睑下垂，以及一种消极的情感成分，包括焦虑和抑郁类行为。

类似抑郁行为的关键事实

- 到目前为止，对于抑郁症的具体啮齿动物模型还没有达成一致。因此，处理这个问题的行为研究是在谈论"类似抑郁"的行为。
- 它收集了一些行为测试，在这些测试中，我们对大多数活动的兴趣或乐趣降低（快感缺乏），体重显著变化，睡眠变化，绝望行为，高压力反应/易怒情绪。
- 甜味溶液的摄入量减少反映了快感缺乏。
- 在强迫游泳测试中，不动的增加反映了行为上的绝望。
- 应激反应越高，皮质酮（一种抑郁的生物标志物）水平越高。

要点总结

- 在人类中，30%尝试吸烟的人会患上烟碱上瘾。
- 临床上有效的戒烟治疗很少，主要是由卫生组织开出的瓦伦尼克林、安非他酮和烟碱替代疗法。
- 开发治疗烟碱依赖的新药物疗法的挑战仍然存在。
- 内源性大麻素系统，特别是针对CB1受体的分子，开启了新的治疗机会。
- 然而，慢性使用内源性大麻素药物治疗提出了几个问题，需要进一步研究，以完善其治疗用途。

参考文献

Anthenelli, R. M.; Benowitz, N. L.; West, R.; St Aubin, L.; McRae, T.; Lawrence, D. et al. (2016). Neuropsychiatric safety and efficacy of varenicline, bupropion, and nicotine patch in smokers with and without psychiatric disorders (EAGLES): a double-blind, randomised, placebo-controlled clinical trial. Lancet, 387(10037), 2507-2520.

Baldwin, P. R.; Alanis, R.; Salas, R. (2011). The role of the habenula in nicotine addiction. Journal of Addiction Research, Therapy, S1(2).

Balerio, G. N.; Aso, E.; Berrendero, F.; Murtra, P.; Maldonado, R. (2004). Delta9-tetrahydrocannabinol decreases somatic and motivational manifestations of nicotine withdrawal in mice. The European Journal of Neuroscience, 20(10), 2737-2748.

Basavarajappa, B. S.; Nagre, N. N.; Xie, S.; Subbanna, S. (2014). Elevation of endogenous anandamide impairs LTP, learning, and memory through CB1 receptor signaling in mice. Hippocampus, 24(7), 808-818.

Beyer, C. E.; Dwyer, J. M.; Piesla, M. J.; Platt, B. J.; Shen, R.; Rahman, Z. et al. (2010). Depression-like phenotype following chronic CB1 receptor antagonism. Neurobiology of Disease, 39(2), 148-155.

Cahill, K.; Stevens, S.; Perera, R.; Lancaster, T. (2013). Pharmacological interventions for smoking cessation: an overview and network metaanalysis.

Cochrane Database of Systematic Reviews, 5, CD009329.

Cahill, K.; Ussher, M. H. (2011). Cannabinoid type 1 receptor antagonists for smoking cessation. Cochrane Database of Systematic Reviews, 3, CD005353.

Ceci, C.; Mela, V.; Macri, S.; Marco, E. M.; Viveros, M. P.; Laviola, G. (2014). Prenatal corticosterone and adolescent URB597 administration modulate emotionality and CB1 receptor expression in mice. Psychopharmacology, 231(10), 2131-2144.

Cippitelli, A.; Astarita, G.; Duranti, A.; Caprioli, G.; Ubaldi, M.; Stopponi, S. et al. (2011). Endocannabinoid regulation of acute and protracted nicotine withdrawal: effect of FAAH inhibition. PLoS ONE, 6(11), e28142.

Cohen, C.; Perrault, G.; Griebel, G.; Soubrie, P. (2005). Nicotine-associated cues maintain nicotine-seeking behavior in rats several weeks after nicotine withdrawal: reversal by the cannabinoid (CB1) receptor antagonist, rimonabant (SR141716). Neuropsychopharmacology, 30(1), 145-155.

Cohen, C.; Perrault, G.; Voltz, C.; Steinberg, R.; Soubrie, P. (2002). SR141716, a central cannabinoid (CB(1)) receptor antagonist, blocks the motivational and dopamine-releasing effects of nicotine in rats. Behavioural Pharmacology, 13(5-6), 451-463.

De Vries, T. J.; de Vries, W.; Janssen, M. C.; Schoffelmeer, A. N. (2005). Suppression of conditioned nicotine and sucrose seeking by the cannabinoid-1 receptor antagonist SR141716A. Behavioural Brain Research, 161(1), 164-168.

Forget, B.; Coen, K. M.; Le Foll, B. (2009). Inhibition of fatty acid amide hydrolase reduces reinstatement of nicotine seeking but not break point for nicotine self-administration-comparison with CB(1) receptor blockade. Psychopharmacology.

Forget, B.; Guranda, M.; Gamaleddin, I.; Goldberg, S. R.; Le Foll, B. (2016). Attenuation of cue-induced reinstatement of nicotine seeking by URB597 through cannabinoid CB1 receptor in rats. Psychopharmacology, 233(10), 1823-1828.

Forget, B.; Hamon, M.; Thiebot, M. H. (2005). Cannabinoid CB1 receptors are involved in motivational effects of nicotine in rats. Psychopharmacology, 181(4), 722-734.

Fowler, C. D.; Kenny, P. J. (2014). Nicotine aversion: neurobiological mechanisms and relevance to tobacco dependence vulnerability. Neuropharmacology, 76(Pt B), 533-544.

Gamaleddin, I. H.; Trigo, J. M.; Gueye, A. B.; Zvonok, A.; Makriyannis, A.; Goldberg, S. R. et al. (2015). Role of the endogenous cannabinoid system in nicotine addiction: novel insights. Frontiers in Psychiatry, 6, 41.

Gamaleddin, I.; Wertheim, C.; Zhu, A. Z.; Coen, K. M.; Vemuri, K.; Makryannis, A. et al. (2012). Cannabinoid receptor stimulation increases motivation for nicotine and nicotine seeking. Addiction Biology, 17(1), 47-61.

Gueye, A. B.; Pryslawsky, Y.; Trigo, J. M.; Poulia, N.; Delis, F.; Antoniou, K. et al. (2016). The CB1 neutral antagonist AM4113 retains the therapeutic efficacy of the inverse agonist rimonabant for nicotine dependence and weight loss with better psychiatric tolerability. The International Journal of Neuropsychopharmacology, 19(12).

Hashemizadeh, S.; Sardari, M.; Rezayof, A. (2014). Basolateral amygdala CB1 cannabinoid receptors mediate nicotine-induced place preference. Progress in Neuro-Psychopharmacology, Biological Psychiatry, 51, 65-71.

Justinova, Z.; Panlilio, L. V.; Moreno-Sanz, G.; Redhi, G. H.; Auber, A.; Secci, M. E. et al. (2015). Effects of fatty acid amide hydrolase (FAAH) inhibitors in non-human primate models of nicotine reward and relapse. Neuropsychopharmacology, 40(9), 2185-2197.

Kenny, P. J.; Markou, A. (2001). Neurobiology of the nicotine withdrawal syndrome. Pharmacology, Biochemistry, and Behavior, 70(4), 531-549.

Kenny, P. J.; Markou, A. (2005). Conditioned nicotine withdrawal profoundly decreases the activity of brain reward systems. The Journal of Neuroscience, 25(26), 6208-6212.

Kodas, E.; Cohen, C.; Louis, C.; Griebel, G. (2007). Cortico-limbic circuitry for conditioned nicotine-seeking behavior in rats involves endocannabinoid signaling. Psychopharmacology, 194(2), 161-171.

Le Foll, B.; Goldberg, S. R. (2004). Rimonabant, a CB1 antagonist, blocks nicotine-conditioned place preferences. NeuroReport, 15(13), 2139-2143.

Lecca, S.; Pelosi, A.; Tchenio, A.; Moutkine, I.; Lujan, R.; Herve, D. et al. (2016). Rescue of GABAB and GIRK function in the lateral habenula by protein phosphatase 2A inhibition ameliorates depression-like phenotypes in mice. Nature Medicine, 22(3), 254-261.

Merritt, L. L.; Martin, B. R.; Walters, C.; Lichtman, A. H.; Damaj, M. I. (2008). The endogenous cannabinoid system modulates nicotine reward and dependence. The Journal of Pharmacology and Experimental Therapeutics, 326(2), 483-492.

Muldoon, P. P.; Chen, J.; Harenza, J. L.; Abdullah, R. A.; Sim-Selley, L. J.; Cravatt, B. F. et al. (2015). Inhibition of monoacylglycerol lipase reduces nicotine withdrawal. British Journal of Pharmacology, 172(3), 869-882.

O'Brien, L. D.; Wills, K. L.; Segsworth, B.; Dashney, B.; Rock, E. M.; Limebeer, C. L. et al. (2013). Effect of chronic exposure to rimonabant and phytocannabinoids on anxiety-like behavior and saccharin palatability. Pharmacology, Biochemistry, and Behavior, 103(3), 597-602.

Patel, S.; Hill, M. N.; Cheer, J. F.; Wotjak, C. T.; Holmes, A. (2017). The endocannabinoid system as a target for novel anxiolytic drugs. Neuroscience, Biobehavioral Reviews, 76(Pt A), 56-66.

Reisiger, A. R.; Kaufling, J.; Manzoni, O.; Cador, M.; Georges, F.; Caille, S. (2014). Nicotine self-administration induces CB1-dependent LTP in the bed nucleus of the stria terminalis. The Journal of Neuroscience, 34(12), 4285-4292.

Rigotti, N. A.; Gonzales, D.; Dale, L. C.; Lawrence, D.; Chang, Y.; CIRRUS Study Group. (2009). A randomized controlled trial of adding the nicotine patch to rimonabant for smoking cessation: efficacy, safety and weight gain. Addiction, 104(2), 266-276.

Saravia, R.; Flores, A.; Plaza-Zabala, A.; Busquets-Garcia, A.; Pastor, A.; de la Torre, R. et al. (2017). CB1 cannabinoid receptors mediate cognitive deficits and structural plasticity changes during nicotine withdrawal. Biological Psychiatry, 81(7), 625-634.

Scherma, M.; Justinova, Z.; Zanettini, C.; Panlilio, L. V.; Mascia, P.; Fadda, P. et al. (2012). The anandamide transport inhibitor AM404 reduces the rewarding effects of nicotine and nicotine-induced dopamine elevations in the nucleus accumbens shell in rats. British Journal of Pharmacology, 165(8), 2539-2548.

Scherma, M.; Panlilio, L. V.; Fadda, P.; Fattore, L.; Gamaleddin, I.; Le Foll, B. et al. (2008). Inhibition of anandamide hydrolysis by cyclohexyl carbamic acid 30-carbamoyl-3-yl ester (URB597) reverses abuse-related behavioral and neurochemical effects of nicotine in rats. The Journal of

Pharmacology and Experimental Therapeutics, 327(2), 482-490.

Schindler, C. W.; Redhi, G. H.; Vemuri, K.; Makriyannis, A.; Le Foll, B.; Bergman, J. et al. (2016). Blockade of nicotine and cannabinoid reinforcement and relapse by a cannabinoid CB1-receptor neutral antagonist AM4113 and inverse agonist rimonabant in squirrel monkeys. Neuropsychopharmacology, 41(9), 2283-2293.

Shoaib, M. (2008). The cannabinoid antagonist AM251 attenuates nicotine self-administration and nicotine-seeking behaviour in rats. Neuropharmacology, 54(2), 438-444.

Simonnet, A.; Cador, M.; Caille, S. (2013). Nicotine reinforcement is reduced by cannabinoid CB1 receptor blockade in the ventral tegmental area. Addiction Biology, 18(6), 930-936.

Simonnet, A.; Zamberletti, E.; Cador, M.; Rubino, T.; Caille, S. (2017). Chronic FAAH inhibition during nicotine abstinence alters habenular CB1 receptor activity and precipitates depressive-like behaviors. Neuropharmacology, 113(Pt A), 252-259.

Trigo, J. M.; Le Foll, B. (2016). Inhibition of monoacylglycerol lipase (MAGL) enhances cue-induced reinstatement of nicotine-seeking behavior in mice. Psychopharmacology, 233(10), 1815-1822.

Wu, C. S.; Morgan, D.; Jew, C. P.; Haskins, C.; Andrews, M. J.; Leishman, E. et al. (2014). Long-term consequences of perinatal fatty acid amino hydrolase inhibition. British Journal of Pharmacology, 171(6), 1420-1434.

Zhang, L.; Dong, Y.; Doyon, W. M.; Dani, J. A. (2012). Withdrawal from chronic nicotine exposure alters dopamine signaling dynamics in the nucleus accumbens. Biological Psychiatry, 71(3), 184-191.

38

烟碱和其他烟碱乙酰胆碱受体激动剂的认知增强作用的治疗潜力

Britta Hahn

University of Maryland School of Medicine, Maryland Psychiatric Research Center, Baltimore, MD, United States

大量的实验室证据表明，典型的烟碱乙酰胆碱受体（nAChR）兴奋剂烟碱可以促进认知表现，特别是注意力过程（Hahn, 2015; Heishman, Kleykamp, Singleton, 2010）。并不是所有的报道都是积极的，观察到的影响往往是小规模到中等规模（Heishman et al. 2010）；然而，对于以认知缺陷和烟碱乙酰胆碱受体（nAChR）功能低下为特征的疾病，如轻度认知障碍、阿尔茨海默病（AD）和精神分裂症，预计会有更深远的好处（Adams, Stevens, 2007; Kendziorra et al. 2011）。到目前为止，已经开发了一系列对nAChR亚型具有更高选择性的新型激动剂，并已进入临床试验阶段，用于治疗上述疾病的认知障碍（Haydar, Dunlop, 2010）。然而，尽管经过了二十多年的药物开发努力，被测试的化合物的认知益处一直很小，临床意义也不确定。到目前为止，还没有nAChR配体获得FDA批准用于治疗认知障碍。本章讨论了造成这一令人失望的趋势的可能原因和潜在的未来战略。

38.1 目标是哪些nAChR亚型？

作为认知增强剂的新型nAChR激动剂的开发针对的是nAChR的α4β2*和α7亚型（Gundisch, Eibl, 2011; Wallace et al. 2011）。这是大脑中表达最丰富和最广泛的两种nAChR亚型，几乎没有系统不受影响（Gotti et al. 2007; Seguela et al. 1993）。因此，虽然与非选择性nAChR激动剂烟碱相比，这些化合物的外周副作用可以减少（并且已经被观察到），但保留认知益处的潜力很低，中枢介导的有害影响较低，例如，与奖励处理或依赖有关的副作用。

基本的问题是，对nAChR激动剂的认知增强效应起关键作用的大脑系统在很大程度上是未知的。来自临床前和人类fMRI研究的证据表明，去甲肾上腺素能和谷氨酸能神经元以及额顶和默认网络区域的调节可能是重要的（例如：Hahn et al. 2007; Hahn, Stolerman, 2005; Lawrence, Ross, Stein, 2002; Quarta et al. 2007; Sutherland et al. 2015），但更多的研究是有必要的。由于目标系统的不确定性，用于选择性调制相关系统的目标nAChR亚型也是未知的。由于有证据表明，中脑边缘多巴胺系统在烟碱的积极增强效应中起核心作用，因此对该系统的调节亚型进行了深入的研究（Exley et al. 2008; Gotti et al. 2010）。对烟碱认知增强作用的核心靶系统的了解将导致对调节这些系统的nAChR亚型的类似详细分析，并将药物开发引导到更有选择性表达的亚型，从而实现更窄的效应谱。因此，药物开发工作的重点可能集中在两个表达最广泛的nAChR亚型上，这可能反映了对相关靶系统的严重缺乏了解。

在α4β2*选择性和α7选择性nAChR激动剂（Haydar, Dunlop, 2010）中都观察到了较小的益处，这一事实表明，作用于多种nAChR亚型的化合物可能会有更大的疗效。例如，针对与精神分裂症相关的认知缺陷的nAChR激动剂的开发主要集中在α7亚型上，其基础是精神分裂症患者及其亲属的感觉门控缺陷和精神分裂症本身的诊断与α7亚基基因附近的多态性有关（Freedman et al. 1997; Leonard et al. 2002; Martin, Kem, Freedman, 2004）。然而，精神分裂症中α7和α4β2 nAChR结合位点均减少（Martin et al. 2004），α5亚基基因的多态性也与精神分裂症的诊断有关（Hong et al. 2011）。关键的挑战将是找到nAChR亚基活动的正确组合，以最大限度地提高相对于不期待的大脑系统调节的可取程度。这只能通过选择性nAChR配体的组合来实现，这些配体使大脑的大部分区域不受影响。

38.2 药物过量?

临床前研究表明烟碱和其他nAChR激动剂的认知增强作用呈倒U形剂量反应功能（Bushnell et al. 1997; Hahn et al. 2003; Hahn et al. 2002; Levin, 1992; McGaughy et al. 1999）。其原因可能不仅与大剂量的厌恶效应有关（Perkins et al. 1994; Stolerman, 1999），还与nAChR的药理学特性有关，nAChR的主要信号机制似乎涉及对乙酰胆碱和非突触弥漫性容量传递引起的乙酰胆碱和胆碱浓度持续升高的反应（Dani, Bertrand, 2007）。因为随着激动剂浓度的增加，nAChR脱敏变得越来越快和持久，当浓度低于其EC_{50}时，受体反应最大（Mike et al. 2000）。的确，在持续的平衡条件下，低浓度而不是高浓度的激动剂可以引起稳定状态的nAChR激活（Papke et al. 2011）。

在一项早期的人类Ⅰ期试验中，两种剂量的部分α7 nAChR激动剂DMXB-A在精神分裂症患者身上进行了测试，较小的剂量往往在认知电池中有更显著的急性益处（Olincy et al. 2006），这与临床前文献一致。在该化合物的后续Ⅱ期试验中，测试了相同剂量一天两次，发现两种剂量对认知功能的益处相当小，但较大剂量的不良反应更大（Freedman et al. 2008）。图38.1描绘了认知益处与不良反应之间的假设剂量-反应关系。在用于认知增强的nAChR激动剂的开发中，早期药物开发的决策过程可能是一种不适应的策略，在这种过程中，为了证明疗效，选择的剂量往往接近符合安全标准的最大剂量。

nAChR正变构调节剂（PAM）的发展与nAChR的调控策略是一致的，nAChR的调控策略更

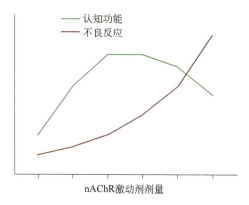

图38.1 nAChR激动剂的认知增强效应与其不良反应之间的假设剂量－反应关系
将剂量增加到超过最佳浓度可能会增加不良反应，而不会带来任何进一步的认知益处。

为微妙，并考虑了受体的内源性生理参数。PAM本身并不激活nAChR，但通过与第二个调节位点结合来促进激动剂诱导的反应（Schrattenholz et al. 1996; Williams et al. 2011）。通过放大预先存在的信号，但不影响休眠受体，PAM可以增强烟碱基调，同时避免了天然电路的动态变化。将非常小剂量的nAChR激动剂与nAChR PAM相结合可能是另一种卓有成效的途径。鉴于两个复合类都可以实现nAChR亚型选择性，组合策略在针对正确的nAChR亚型同时也可能实现更大的灵活性和微调。例如，特定nAChR亚型的选择性调制可以通过将针对一组nAChR亚型选择性的nAChR激动剂的亚阈值剂量与针对不同亚型组选择性但与目标亚型上的第一组重叠的PAM的亚阈剂量相结合来实现（图38.2）。

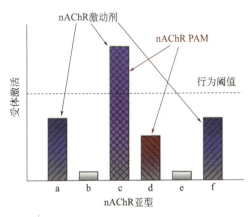

图 38.2　nAChR 激动剂与 PAM 联合应用策略

低剂量的激动剂作用于nAChR亚型的一个子集，而低剂量的PAM作用于另一个部分重叠的子集，这两种药物的结合可能有助于产生更窄的期望行为效果。

38.3　没有免费午餐这回事？

当面临基于nAChR的药理学策略是否可以实现长期认知增强的问题时，也许最大的不确定性是神经适应性变化是否会抵消相对于药物前基线的益处。烟碱文献表明，在这方面需要谨慎。烟碱的提高成绩的效果可以在不吸烟的人身上表现出来，但在评估强迫戒烟的吸烟者的研究中更可靠（Foulds et al. 1996; Heishman et al. 1994）。这表明，戒断诱导的缺陷的逆转在很大程度上有助于长期接触烟碱的个人受益。事实上，集中注意力困难是超过65%的戒烟者的主要抱怨问题（Ward, Swan, Jack, 2001），也是烟碱戒断的诊断标准之一（American Psychiatric Association, 2013）。

从药物开发的角度来看，与nAChR激动剂停药相关的认知损害的神经机制并不比药物诱导的认知益处的机制重要。长期暴露于nAChR激动剂的神经适应可发生在nAChR激活（或脱敏）下游很远的地方，并可能出现在次级神经递质系统中（例如：Avila-Ruiz et al. 2014; Rademacher et al. 2016）。然而，在吸烟或长期烟碱暴露的实验背景下，可能研究最多的神经适应是nAChR上调（例如：Colombo et al. 2013; Cosgrove et al. 2009），很可能是慢性nAChR脱敏的结果（Fenster et al. 1999）。一项对小鼠的研究报告称，慢性烟碱暴露后持续的海马体nAChR上调与戒断诱导的记忆力障碍的时间进程平行（Gould et al. 2012）。然而，除此之外，人们对戒断导致认知缺陷的神经基础知之甚少。

对于化合物和给药方案，要想产生相对于药物前基线的长期益处，它们必须没有神经适应，这些神经适应会导致不使用药物的认知表现向负面方向转变。因此，了解这些机制将有利于药物开发，因为新化合物可以在临床试验阶段之前很久就被筛选出这些特性。关于到目前为止已经进入临床试验阶段的新型nAChR激动剂，作者并不知道这种潜在的基线改变已经被解决了，例如，在洗脱后不久获得随访结果测量，并将治疗前后的差异与安慰剂治疗的时间对照进行比较。可以想象，与安慰剂组相比，治疗阶段后期较低的基线是缺乏疗效的原因（图38.3）。换句话说，虽然被测试的化合物仍可能产生显著的改善，但这些益处可能发生在受损的基线上，并不代表与治疗开始前相比的净效益。

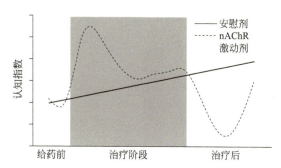

图38.3 nAChR激动剂在慢性治疗和冲洗期的假想时间进程

反适应基线改变可能会使最初的药物暴露所带来的认知益处化为乌有。这种转变将表现为药物冲洗后的缺陷。结果测量通常在冲刷前的治疗阶段之前和结束时进行。因此，在没有后续评估的情况下，没有或最低限度的疗效与这里描述的情景是难以区分的。

38.4 天真的前提？

认知能力取决于不同的神经元群体、电路和结构之间复杂和正确的时间相互作用。因此，认知加工缺陷可能来源于大量的潜在来源。即使在有证据表明nAChR功能低下的疾病（如阿尔茨海默病和精神分裂症）中，也存在广泛的潜在神经病理学（例如：Bakhshi, Chance, 2015; Elahi, Miller, 2017; Lodge, Grace, 2011），这表明纠正nAChR激活水平低不太可能实质性地纠正认知缺陷。其他受损的组件可能会继续阻碍神经元顺畅而高效的发条。

另一种更普遍地质疑药物疗法治疗潜力的思路是，与中枢神经系统障碍相关的认知缺陷是一种慢性的、可能自我延续的现象。认知缺陷预计会减少认知投入，这种使用的减少很可能会导致进一步的认知下降，在生理水平上伴随着神经元连接的丧失和回路调谐的衰退，类似于感觉剥夺后的初级感觉皮质（例如：Kral et al. 2017）。在这种背景下，通过对nAChR（或任何其他系统）激活水平的急剧优化来立即显著改善认知缺陷，似乎是一种天真的期望。

然而，正是在自我永续的背景下，nAChR激动剂在治疗认知障碍方面的潜力可能存在。nAChR激动剂的存在带来的轻微的功能增强，无论是由于感觉处理的增强、警觉性，还是更高的注意力或助记功能，可能会在几个月或几年内微妙地增加认知处理资源的投入，如果持续下去，这可能有助于防止进一步的下降，甚至导致渐进的改善。如上所述，这将需要相对于药物前基线持续的药物效应。到目前为止，进行的临床试验可能持续时间太短，无法测试这种现象。

nAChR激动剂可能有益于认知缺陷治疗的另一种方式是作为认知训练干预的增强工具

（Hahn, Gold, Buchanan, 2013）。在阿尔茨海默病和精神分裂症等疾病中，训练导致的认知改善往往具有低到中等的效果（Hill et al. 2017; McGurk et al. 2007）。这些干预措施有效的时间要求可能会限制它们的临床适用性；然而，增强和加快训练效果的手段可能会增强它们的可行性和临床意义。在训练时使用药剂可以优化训练效果的神经环境。使用这种方法，治疗的成功将在药物清除系统很长一段时间后表现为增强的效果。除了潜在的更持久的好处外，另一个好处是药物暴露的时间从根本上被缩短了，从而最大限度地减少了反适应神经适应的可能性。在这种情况下，只要药物作用显现的窗口与认知训练的信息处理挑战反复结合，短的半衰期甚至会是一个更好的特性。

nAChR 激动剂可能是促进经验依赖性改变的候选药物。烟碱促进早期感觉过程（Fisher et al. 2010; Knott et al. 2010; Phillips et al. 2007），对于选择性 α7 的 nAChR 激动剂也是如此（Martin, Freedman, 2007）。更准确的感官表征可能会为更高的功能形成更好的构建块，更有效的感官处理可能会释放资源，使训练挑战能够在更高的难度水平上得到满足。此外，nAChR 激动剂在训练过程中对警觉性和注意力的急剧促进（Newhouse, Potter, Singh, 2004）可能会使参与者更深入地参与训练，并可能使参与者在任务中停留更长的时间。最后，nAChR 的激活通过不同的细胞机制在大脑中诱导了持久的可塑性变化（Buccafusco, Letchworth, Bencherif, Lippiello, 2005; Castner et al. 2011; Hasselmo, 2006）。值得注意的是，研究表明烟碱可以促进长时程增强（LTP）的诱导（Kenney, Gould, 2008; Matsuyama et al. 2000）。通过增强神经可塑性，nAChR 激动剂可能通过训练促进学习、记忆和技能发展。事实上，有证据表明，胆碱能系统对于与运动技能学习相关的皮质可塑性至关重要（Conner et al. 2003）。

38.5 结论

在许多方面，用于治疗认知缺陷的 nAChR 激动剂的开发似乎已经超前了。缺乏对关键靶系统的了解可能促使人们把注意力集中在大脑中最广泛表达的两个 nAChR 亚型上。剂量的选择倾向于忽略 nAChR 剂量反应动力学的临床前和体外数据。神经适应和戒断诱发缺陷的机制在很大程度上是未知的，在药物开发和临床试验设计中也很少被考虑，这两个现象都是长期服用烟碱的众所周知的现象。最后，作为一种目标结果，认知功能可能需要更长期的方法，可能需要整合额外的干预措施。nAChR 激动剂作为认知增强剂的临床试验结果令人失望，这可能表明，与其把孩子和洗澡水一起倒掉，不如是时候重新制定策略了。

术语解释

- 依赖经验的变化：生物与环境的相互作用所带来的神经元功能的长期变化。
- 倒 U 型剂量-效应函数：一种现象，即上升的剂量仅在特定剂量前才与更大的药物效应有关，超过该剂量后，进一步的剂量增加将导致更小的效应。
- nAChR 脱敏：暴露于 nAChR 激动剂后 nAChR 反应减弱。
- nAChR 亚型：每个 nAChR 由五个亚基组成。不同的 nAChR 亚基可以不同的组合方式结合，形成具有不同药理性质和受体动力学的 nAChR。
- 神经可塑性：神经元根据它们参与的程度或类型改变它们的反应或连通性的能力。
- 神经适应：随着药物的频繁使用，神经元的活动将机械地调整以保持体内平衡。这通常导致对药物作用的耐受性，而当药物不存在时则是与这些作用相反的状态。

- 非突触弥漫性容积传递：神经递质在远离靶点的地方释放信号，并广泛地通过细胞外液扩散。
- 受体音调：在更广泛的时间尺度上的激活水平。
- 次级神经递质系统：药物不直接作用的系统，但由药物直接改变的系统调节。
- 持续均衡：一种相互对立的过程平衡的状态，例如吸收与消除或受体激活与脱敏，维持当前状态。

烟碱激动剂治疗认知缺陷的关键事实

- 使用烟碱受体激动剂治疗认知障碍的想法可以追溯到40多年前。
- 作为认知增强剂的烟碱激动剂的开发始于20世纪90年代初。
- 除了烟碱和伐伦克林，已经测试了20多种不同的烟碱激动剂在临床人群中增强认知能力的潜力。
- 超过100个测试新型烟碱激动剂作为认知增强剂的临床试验已经发布。
- 到目前为止，还没有一种烟碱化合物被FDA批准用于治疗认知缺陷。

要点总结

- nAChR激动剂的发展并没有导致任何新的治疗认知缺陷的方法。
- 关键的靶标系统，因此最有希望作为靶标的nAChR亚型，在很大程度上是未知的。
- nAChR激动剂的认知增强作用遵循倒U形的剂量-反应函数；因此，大剂量的选择可能掩盖了有益的效果。
- 慢性暴露引起的抗适应神经变化可能是缺乏净疗效的原因，但这些神经适应在很大程度上未被研究，因此在药物开发中未被考虑。
- 与疾病状态相关的广泛的潜在神经病理学和认知缺陷的慢性本质可能需要长时间的治疗和综合认知训练干预。

参考文献

Adams, C. E.; Stevens, K. E. (2007). Evidence for a role of nicotinic acetylcholine receptors in schizophrenia. Frontiers in Bioscience, 12, 4755-4772.

American Psychiatric Association. (2013). Diagnostic and statistical manual of mental disorders (5th ed.). Washington, DC/London, England: American Psychiatric Publishing.

Avila-Ruiz, T.; Carranza, V.; Gustavo, L. L.; Limon, D. I.; Martinez, I.; Flores, G. et al. (2014). Chronic administration of nicotine enhances NMDA-activated currents in the prefrontal cortex and core part of the nucleus accumbens of rats. Synapse, 68(6), 248-256.

Bakhshi, K.; Chance, S. A. (2015). The neuropathology of schizophrenia: a selective review of past studies and emerging themes in brain structure and cytoarchitecture. Neuroscience, 303, 82-102.

Buccafusco, J. J.; Letchworth, S. R.; Bencherif, M.; Lippiello, P. M. (2005). Long-lasting cognitive improvement with nicotinic receptor agonists: mechanisms of pharmacokinetic-pharmacodynamic discordance. Trends in Pharmacological Sciences, 26(7), 352-360.

Bushnell, P. J.; Oshiro, W. M.; Padnos, B. K. (1997). Detection of visual signals by rats: effects of chlordiazepoxide and cholinergic and adrenergic drugs on sustained attention. Psychopharmacology, 134 (3), 230-241.

Castner, S. A.; Smagin, G. N.; Piser, T. M.; Wang, Y.; Smith, J. S.; Christian, E. P. et al. (2011). Immediate and sustained improvements in working memory after selective stimulation of alpha 7 nicotinic acetylcholine receptors. Biological Psychiatry, 69(1), 12-18.

Colombo, S. F.; Mazzo, F.; Pistillo, F.; Gotti, C. (2013). Biogenesis, trafficking and up-regulation of nicotinic ACh receptors. Biochemical Pharmacology, 86(8), 1063-1073.

Conner, J. M.; Culberson, A.; Packowski, C.; Chiba, A. A.; Tuszynski, M. H. (2003). Lesions of the basal forebrain cholinergic system impair task acquisition and abolish cortical plasticity associated with motor skill learning. Neuron, 38(5), 819-829.

Cosgrove, K. P.; Batis, J.; Bois, F.; Maciejewski, P. K.; Esterlis, I.; Kloczynski, T. et al. (2009). Beta2-nicotinic acetylcholine receptor availability during acute and prolonged abstinence from tobacco smoking. Archives of General Psychiatry, 66(6), 666-676.

Dani, J. A.; Bertrand, D. (2007). Nicotinic acetylcholine receptors and nicotinic cholinergic mechanisms of the central nervous system. Annual Review of Pharmacology and Toxicology, 47, 699-729.

Elahi, F. M.; Miller, B. L. (2017). A clinicopathological approach to the diagnosis of dementia. Nature Reviews. Neurology, 13(8), 457-476.

Exley, R.; Clements, M. A.; Hartung, H.; McIntosh, J. M.; Cragg, S. J. (2008). Alpha 6-containing nicotinic acetylcholine receptors dominate the nicotine control of dopamine neurotransmission in nucleus accumbens. Neuropsychopharmacology, 33(9), 2158-2166.

Fenster, C. P.; Whitworth, T. L.; Sheffield, E. B.; Quick, M. W.; Lester, R. A. (1999). Upregulation of surface alpha4beta2 nicotinic receptors is initiated by receptor desensitization after chronic exposure to nicotine. The Journal of Neuroscience, 19(12), 4804-4814.

Fisher, D. J.; Scott, T. L.; Shah, D. K.; Prise, S.; Thompson, M.; Knott, V. J. (2010). Light up and see: enhancement of the visual mismatch negativity (vMMN) by nicotine. Brain Research, 1313, 162-171.

Foulds, J.; Stapleton, J.; Swettenham, J.; Bell, N.; McSorley, K.; Russell, M. A. (1996). Cognitive performance effects of subcutaneous nicotine in smokers and never-smokers. Psychopharmacology, 127(1), 31-38.

Freedman, R.; Coon, H.; Myles Worsley, M.; Orr Urtreger, A.; Olincy, A.; Davis, A. et al. (1997). Linkage of a neurophysiological deficit in schizophrenia to a chromosome 15 locus. Proceedings of the National Academy of Sciences of the United States of America, 94(2), 587-592.

Freedman, R.; Olincy, A.; Buchanan, R. W.; Harris, J. G.; Gold, J. M.; Johnson, L. et al. (2008). Initial phase 2 trial of a nicotinic agonist in schizophrenia. The American Journal of Psychiatry, 165(8), 1040-1047.

Gotti, C.; Guiducci, S.; Tedesco, V.; Corbioli, S.; Zanetti, L.; Moretti, M. et al. (2010). Nicotinic acetylcholine receptors in the mesolimbic pathway: primary role of ventral tegmental area alpha 6 beta 2*receptors in mediating systemic nicotine effects on dopamine release, locomotion, and reinforcement. Journal of Neuroscience, 30 (15), 5311-5325.

Gotti, C.; Moretti, M.; Gaimarri, A.; Zanardi, A.; Clementi, F.; Zoli, M. (2007). Heterogeneity and complexity of native brain nicotinic receptors. Biochemical Pharmacology, 74(8), 1102-1111.

Gould, T. J.; Portugal, G. S.; Andre, J. M.; Tadman, M. P.; Marks, M. J.; Kenney, J. W. et al. (2012). The duration of nicotine withdrawal-associated deficits in contextual fear conditioning parallels changes in hippocampal high affinity nicotinic acetylcholine receptor upregulation. Neuropharmacology, 62(5-6), 2118-2125.

Gundisch, D.; Eibl, C. (2011). Nicotinic acetylcholine receptor ligands, a patent review (2006-2011). Expert Opinion on Therapeutic Patents, 21 (12), 1867-1896.

Hahn, B. (2015). Nicotinic receptors and attention. Current Topics in Behavioral Neurosciences, 23, 103-135.

Hahn, B.; Gold, J. M.; Buchanan, R. W. (2013). The potential of nicotinic enhancement of cognitive remediation training in schizophrenia. Neuropharmacology, 64, 185-190.

Hahn, B.; Ross, T. J.; Yang, Y.; Kim, I.; Huestis, M. A.; Stein, E. A. (2007). Nicotine enhances visuospatial attention by deactivating areas of the resting brain default network. The Journal of Neuroscience, 27(13), 3477-3489.

Hahn, B.; Sharples, C. G.; Wonnacott, S.; Shoaib, M.; Stolerman, I. P. (2003). Attentional effects of nicotinic agonists in rats. Neuropharmacology, 44(8), 1054-1067.

Hahn, B.; Shoaib, M.; Stolerman, I. P. (2002). Nicotine-induced enhancement of attention in the five-choice serial reaction time task: the influence of task-demands. Psychopharmacology, 162(2), 129-137.

Hahn, B.; Stolerman, I. P. (2005). Modulation of nicotine-induced attentional enhancement in rats by adrenoceptor antagonists. Psychopharmacology, 177(4), 438-447.

Hasselmo, M. E. (2006). The role of acetylcholine in learning and memory. Current Opinion in Neurobiology, 16(6), 710-715.

Haydar, S. N.; Dunlop, J. (2010). Neuronal nicotinic acetylcholine receptors - targets for the development of drugs to treat cognitive impairment associated with schizophrenia and Alzheimer's disease. Current Topics in Medicinal Chemistry, 10(2), 144-152.

Heishman, S. J.; Kleykamp, B. A.; Singleton, E. G. (2010). Metaanalysis of the acute effects of nicotine and smoking on human performance. Psychopharmacology, 210(4), 453-469.

Heishman, S. J.; Taylor, R. C.; Henningfield, J. E. (1994). Nicotine and smoking: a review of effects on human performance. Experimental and Clinical Psychopharmacology, 2(4), 345-395.

Hill, N. T.; Mowszowski, L.; Naismith, S. L.; Chadwick, V. L.; Valenzuela, M.; Lampit, A. (2017). Computerized cognitive training in older adults with mild cognitive impairment or dementia: a systematic review and meta-analysis. The American Journal of Psychiatry, 174(4), 329-340.

Hong, L. E.; Yang, X.; Wonodi, I.; Hodgkinson, C. A.; Goldman, D.; Stine, O. C. et al. (2011). A CHRNA5 allele related to nicotine addiction and schizophrenia. Genes, Brain, and Behavior, 10(5), 530-535.

Kendziorra, K.; Wolf, H.; Meyer, P. M.; Barthel, H.; Hesse, S.; Becker, G. A. et al. (2011). Decreased cerebral α4β2* nicotinic acetylcholine receptor availability in patients with mild cognitive impairment and Alzheimer's disease assessed with positron emission tomography. European Journal of Nuclear Medicine and Molecular Imaging, 38, 515-525.

Kenney, J. W.; Gould, T. J. (2008). Modulation of hippocampus-dependent learning and synaptic plasticity by nicotine. Molecular Neurobiology, 38(1), 101-121.

Knott, V. J.; Fisher, D. J.; Millar, A. M. (2010). Differential effects of nicotine on P50 amplitude, its gating, and their neural sources in low and high suppressors. Neuroscience, 170(3), 816-826.

Kral, A.; Yusuf, P. A.; Land, R. (2017). Higher-order auditory areas in congenital deafness: top-down interactions and corticocortical decoupling. Hearing Research, 343, 50-63.

Lawrence, N. S.; Ross, T. J.; Stein, E. A. (2002). Cognitive mechanisms of nicotine on visual attention. Neuron, 36(3), 539-548.

Leonard, S.; Gault, J.; Hopkins, J.; Logel, J.; Vianzon, R.; Short, M. et al. (2002). Association of promoter variants in the alpha 7 nicotinic acetylcholine receptor subunit gene with an inhibitory deficit found in schizophrenia. Archives of General Psychiatry, 59(12), 1085-1096.

Levin, E. D. (1992). Nicotinic systems and cognitive function. Psychopharmacology, 108(4), 417-431.

Lodge, D. J.; Grace, A. A. (2011). Hippocampal dysregulation of dopamine system function and the pathophysiology of schizophrenia. Trends in Pharmacological Sciences, 32(9), 507-513.

Martin, L. F.; Freedman, R. (2007). Schizophrenia and the alpha 7 nicotinic acetylcholine receptor. Integrating the Neurobiology of Schizophrenia,

78, 225-246.

Martin, L. F.; Kem, W. R.; Freedman, R. (2004). Alpha-7 nicotinic receptor agonists: potential new candidates for the treatment of schizophrenia. Psychopharmacology, 174(1), 54-64.

Matsuyama, S.; Matsumoto, A.; Enomoto, T.; Nishizaki, T. (2000). Activation of nicotinic acetylcholine receptors induces long-term potentiation in vivo in the intact mouse dentate gyrus. The European Journal of Neuroscience, 12(10), 3741-3747.

McGaughy, J.; Decker, M. W.; Sarter, M. (1999). Enhancement of sustained attention performance by the nicotinic acetylcholine receptor agonist ABT-418 in intact but not basal forebrain-lesioned rats. Psychopharmacology, 144(2), 175-182.

McGurk, S. R.; Twamley, E. W.; Sitzer, D. I.; McHugo, G. J.; Mueser, K. T. (2007). A meta-analysis of cognitive remediation in schizophrenia. The American Journal of Psychiatry, 164(12), 1791-1802.

Mike, A.; Castro, N. G.; Albuquerque, E. X. (2000). Choline and acetylcholine have similar kinetic properties of activation and desensitization on the alpha7 nicotinic receptors in rat hippocampal neurons. Brain Research, 882(1-2), 155-168.

Newhouse, P. A.; Potter, A.; Singh, A. (2004). Effects of nicotinic stimulation on cognitive performance. Current Opinion in Pharmacology, 4(1), 36-46.

Olincy, A.; Harris, J. G.; Johnson, L. L.; Pender, V.; Kongs, S.; Allensworth, D. et al. (2006). Proof-of-concept trial of an alpha7 nicotinic agonist in schizophrenia. Archives of General Psychiatry, 63(6), 630-638.

Papke, R. L.; Trocme-Thibierge, C.; Guendisch, D.; Abdullah, S.; Rubaiy, A. A.; Bloom, S. A. (2011). Electrophysiological perspectives on the therapeutic use of nicotinic acetylcholine receptor partial agonists. Journal of Pharmacology and Experimental Therapeutics, 337 (2), 367-379.

Perkins, K. A.; Grobe, J. E.; Fonte, C.; Goettler, J.; Caggiula, A. R.; Reynolds, W. A. et al. (1994). Chronic and acute tolerance to subjective, behavioral and cardiovascular effects of nicotine in humans. The Journal of Pharmacology and Experimental Therapeutics, 270(2), 628-638.

Phillips, J. M.; Ehrlichman, R. S.; Siegel, S. J. (2007). Mecamylamine blocks nicotine-induced enhancement of the P20 auditory eventrelated potential and evoked gamma. Neuroscience, 144(4), 1314-1323.

Quarta, D.; Naylor, C. G.; Morris, H. V.; Patel, S.; Genn, R. F.; Stolerman, I. P. (2007). Different effects of ionotropic and metabotropic glutamate receptor antagonists on attention and the attentional properties of nicotine. Neuropharmacology, 53(3), 421-430.

Rademacher, L.; Prinz, S.; Winz, O.; Henkel, K.; Dietrich, C. A.; Schmaljohann, J. et al. (2016). Effects of smoking cessation on presynaptic dopamine function of addicted male smokers. Biological Psychiatry, 80(3), 198-206.

Schrattenholz, A.; Pereira, E. F.; Roth, U.; Weber, K. H.; Albuquerque, E. X.; Maelicke, A. (1996). Agonist responses of neuronal nicotinic acetylcholine receptors are potentiated by a novel class of allosterically acting ligands. Molecular Pharmacology, 49(1), 1-6.

Seguela, P.; Wadiche, J.; Dineley-Miller, K.; Dani, J. A.; Patrick, J. W. (1993). Molecular cloning, functional properties, and distribution of rat brain alpha 7: a nicotinic cation channel highly permeable to calcium. The Journal of Neuroscience, 13(2), 596-604.

Stolerman, I. P. (1999). Inter-species consistency in the behavioural pharmacology of nicotine dependence. Behavioural Pharmacology, 10(6-7), 559-580.

Sutherland, M. T.; Ray, K. L.; Riedel, M. C.; Yanes, J. A.; Stein, E. A.; Laird, A. R. (2015). Neurobiological impact of nicotinic acetylcholine receptor agonists: an activation likelihood estimation meta-analysis of pharmacologic neuroimaging studies. Biological Psychiatry, 78(10), 711-720.

Wallace, T. L.; Ballard, T. M.; Pouzet, B.; Riedel, W. J.; Wettstein, J. G. (2011). Drug targets for cognitive enhancement in neuropsychiatric disorders. Pharmacology Biochemistry and Behavior, 99(2), 130-145.

Ward, M. M.; Swan, G. E.; Jack, L. M. (2001). Self-reported abstinence effects in the first month after smoking cessation. Addictive Behaviors, 26(3), 311-327.

Williams, D. K.; Wang, J. Y.; Papke, R. L. (2011). Positive allosteric modulators as an approach to nicotinic acetylcholine receptor-targeted therapeutics: advantages and limitations. Biochemical Pharmacology, 82(8), 915-930.

39
烟碱和多巴胺 DA_1 受体药理学

Agnieszka Michalak, Barbara Budzyńska

Department of Pharmacology and Pharmacodynamics, Medical University of Lublin, Lublin, Poland

缩略语

AC	腺苷酸环化酶	IP3	三磷酸肌醇
CaMKII	Ca^{2+}/钙调蛋白依赖性蛋白激酶Ⅱ	LTP	长时程增强
cAMP	环磷酸腺苷	MEK	MAPK/ERK 激酶
CaN	钙调神经磷酸酶	mRNA	信使核糖核酸
CNS	中枢神经系统	NAcc	伏隔核
CPA	条件性位置厌恶	nAChR	烟碱型乙酰胆碱受体
CPP	条件性位置偏爱	NK1	神经激肽受体 1
CREB	cAMP 反应元件结合蛋白	NMDA	N-甲基-D-天冬氨酸受体
DA	多巴胺	PKA	蛋白激酶 A
DA_1	多巴胺能 1 型受体	PKC	蛋白激酶 C
DAG	二酰基甘油	PLC	磷脂酶 C
DARPP-32	多巴胺和 cAMP 调节的磷蛋白，32kDa	PP1	蛋白磷酸酶-1
DARPP-32-P	磷酸化多巴胺和 cAMP 调节的磷蛋白	sc	皮下地
DRD1	多巴胺 DA1 受体基因	SN	黑质
ERK	细胞外信号调节激酶	SP	P 物质
GP	苍白球	SPLI	P 物质样免疫反应
IA	抑制性回避	VTA	腹侧被盖区
ip	腹膜内		

39.1 引言

39.1.1 多巴胺 DA_1 受体的定位和信号转导

多巴胺（DA）受体分为两类 G 蛋白偶联受体，DA_1 和 DA_2 样受体。DA_1 样受体亚家族包括 DA_1 和 DA_5 亚型，DA_2 样受体亚家族包括 DA_2、DA_3 和 DA_4 受体（图 39.1）。DA_1 受体是中枢神经系统（CNS）中最常见的 DA 受体亚型，其密度水平随脑结构的不同而不同。DA_1 在黑质纹状体、中脑边缘和中皮质通路中的表达水平最高，特别是在背侧纹状体、杏仁核、伏隔核（NAcc）、黑质（SN）、额叶皮层和嗅球等区域，而 DA_1 在小脑、海马体、丘脑和下丘脑中的表达水平较低（Beaulieu, Gainetdinov, 2011）。DA_1 受体的分布与其功能相对应。DA_1 受体参与学习和记忆，它们在运动控制中起着重要作用，它们的激活对奖赏机制至关重要（图 39.2 和图 39.3）。此外，DA_1 受体的异常也会导致精神障碍，如帕金森病（PD）、精神分裂症或亨廷顿病（Beaulieu, Gainetdinov, 2011; Komatsu, 2015）。

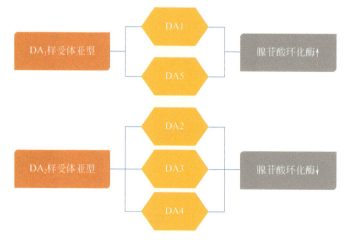

图 39.1　DA_1 受体亚型及其对腺苷酸环化酶的影响

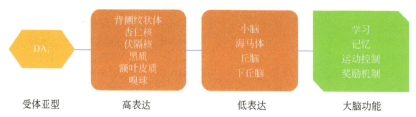

图 39.2　DA_1 受体的定位、表达和脑功能

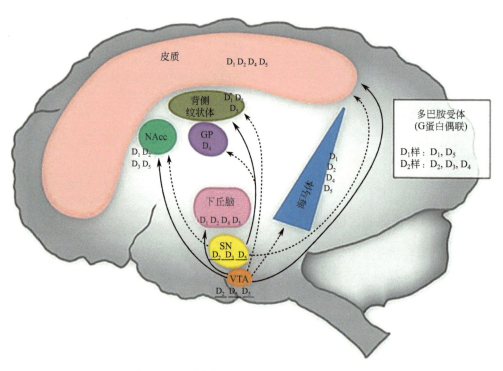

图 39.3　人脑中多巴胺能受体的表达和多巴胺投射

来自 SN 的 DA 神经元不仅主要投射到背侧纹状体，还投射到皮层、GP 和伏隔核。VTA 内 DA 神经元的轴突主要投射到伏隔核和皮质，以及背侧纹状体、海马体和下丘脑。文中描述了 DA_1 受体在大脑中的定位。带下划线的是自体感受器。Brichta, Greengard, Flajolet (2013)。

DA₁受体主要与G蛋白的Gα_s和Gα_olf亚型偶联，激活腺苷酸环化酶（AC），刺激环磷酸腺苷（CAMP）的产生，激活蛋白激酶A（PKA）。PKA磷酸化多巴胺和cAMP调节的磷酸蛋白32 kDa（DARPP-32），导致蛋白磷酸酶-1（PP1）失活，从而阻止其对MAPK/ERK激酶（MEK）的抑制作用。它可以激活细胞外信号调节激酶（ERK）和ERK介导的cAMP反应元件结合蛋白（CREB）磷酸化（Beaulieu, Gainetdinov, 2011; Hisahara, Shimohama, 2011）。DARPP-32的激活可以被用于NMDA受体刺激而激活的钙调神经磷酸酶（CaN）等所抵消（Svenningsson et al. 2004）。DA₁受体也可能与磷脂酶C相连的Gα_q偶联。激活PLC会导致二酰基甘油（DAG）和三磷酸肌醇（IP3）的增加。DAG激活蛋白激酶C（PKC），而IP3增加内质网钙（Ca²⁺）的动员，激活CaMKⅡ（Ca²⁺/钙调蛋白依赖的蛋白激酶Ⅱ）。PKC和CaMKⅡ均可诱导CREB相关基因转录（Beaulieu, Gainetdinov, 2011; Hisahara, Shimohama, 2011）（图39.4）。

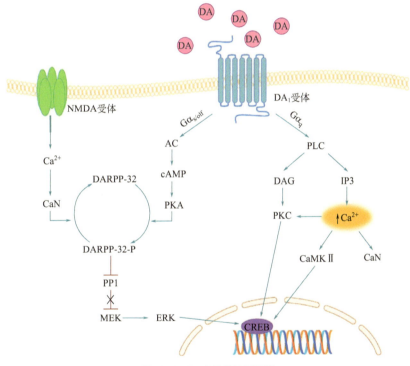

图39.4 D₁介导的信号通路

DA与DA₁受体结合可激活Gα_s/olf/PKA/DARPP-32和Gα_q/PLC信号转导通路。蓝色箭头表示激活，而T形箭头表示抑制。用DARPP-32-P灭活PP1可以消除PP1对MEK的抑制作用（未发表，作者：Agnieszka Michalak）。

39.1.2 烟碱和DA₁受体——分子洞察力

许多报道认为DA₁受体与烟碱的作用密切相关，烟碱通过烟碱乙酰胆碱受体（nAChR）间接刺激DA₁受体，增加DA的释放。最有可能的是，nAChR的两个亚型，α4β2和α7，对烟碱/DA₁的相互作用至关重要。推测烟碱对DA₁受体的间接激活与刺激多巴胺能终末的α4β2 nAChR和谷氨酸能终末的α7 nAChR有关，谷氨酸能终末负责调节黑质纹状体通路中的多巴胺能传递（Hamada et al. 2005）。有趣的是，烟碱以一种频率依赖的方式调节DA的释放，至少部分地依赖于DA₁受体。结果表明，烟碱可减弱低频电场刺激（1或5个10Hz脉冲）诱发的纹状体DA释放，但增强高频（5个100Hz脉冲）刺激引起的DA外流。为探讨其作用机制，我们同时使用了DA_1受体激动剂（SKF-38393）和拮抗剂（SCH-23390）。虽然这两种配体都不影响烟碱对5个10Hz和100Hz脉冲诱发的DA释放的影响，但它们都阻断了烟碱对10Hz刺激的一个脉冲触发的DA释放的抑制作用（Goutier et al. 2016）。

39.1.2.1 PKA/DARPP-32/PP1 信号级联

烟碱通过激活α4β2和α7 nAChR介导DA的释放，从而导致DA_1受体的激活和$G\alpha_{s/olf}$/PKA/DARPP-32信号级联的激活。在DARPP-32之后，磷酸化可能发生在其不同的位点，对PP1活性有不同的调节作用。Thr34位的DARPP-32磷酸化是PP1失活所必需的，而Thr75位的DARPP-32磷酸化导致PKA失活，从而抑制信号转导。此外，当DARPP-32在Ser97位同时磷酸化时，PKA对Thr34位的DARPP-32的磷酸化程度可以增加，而在Ser130位的DARPP-32的磷酸化降低了CaN对Thr34的去磷酸化。研究发现，高浓度烟碱（100μmol/L）通过增加DARPP-32在Ser97和Ser130的磷酸化和降低Thr75-DARPP-32的磷酸化状态，促进PKA/DARPP-32/PP1级联反应（Hamada et al. 2005）。此外，Abdolahi等（2010）揭示了在戒毒期间，寻求烟碱的增加与PKA/DARPP-32信号的增强有关，这是由于在戒毒7天时，岛叶皮质中Thr34-DARPP-32的磷酸化增加和NAcc中Thr75-DARPP-32的磷酸化水平降低。

39.1.2.2 遗传背景

强有力的数据表明，烟碱依赖与DA_1受体基因（DRD_1）之间存在显著的联系。研究发现，亚慢性烟碱暴露 [0.4mg/（kg·d），皮下注射，15天] 可增加大鼠前额叶皮层DRD_1 mRNA的表达，这可能与组蛋白H4乙酰化水平升高有关（Gozen et al. 2013）。此外，研究还表明，一次烟碱注射可提高青春期预先暴露于烟碱的大鼠NAcc壳中DRD_1 mRNA的水平（Wheeler et al. 2013）。在人类吸烟者中，DRD_1和烟碱依赖之间的显著关联已被证实。此外，rs686（位于DRD_1启动子区域的单核苷酸多态性）的遗传变异被发现是导致这种关联的一个位点，microRNA在其对DRD_1表达的影响中起着重要作用（Huang, Li, 2009）。

39.2 DA1受体与烟碱的行为效应

39.2.1 激励效果

有充分的证据表明DA_1受体在烟碱的厌恶和增强效应中起作用。结果表明，DA_1受体定位于接受胆碱能输入的奖励相关脑区。由于神经生物学的最新发展集中在大脑中DA的外流，因此出现了有趣的信息。结果表明，多巴胺能神经元释放DA有两种方式：时相释放和紧张性释放。大而快的DA时相释放主要激活DA_1受体，而紧张性释放DA主要激活DA_2受体（Floresco et al. 2003）。此外，提示-奖励联想和激励性显著的获得是由阶段性活动介导的，而反应抑制和行为灵活性则是由紧张性活动促进的（Grieder et al. 2012）。因此，多巴胺能系统的激活被认为在烟碱的厌恶和奖励效应中起着关键作用。

自治范式：许多研究表明，DA_1受体在烟碱自给药消失后线索诱导的烟碱寻找行为的恢复中起作用。首先，值得一提的是，烟碱会唤起寻找行为；例如，在自我管理范式中观察到，在没有接触烟碱的情况下，这种行为可以在几天后消失。然而，烟碱相关的线索在没有药物的情况下，即使在几个月后，也可以在广泛的测试后保持反应。研究表明，环境信号在烟碱自给药的获得中起着关键作用（Caggiula et al. 2001），而多巴胺能系统对这种作用至关重要（Bossert et al. 2007）。Liu等（2010）评价了DA_1受体在烟碱相关线索条件性刺激特性恢复中的重要作用。在这项研究中，大鼠接受了烟碱（30d，0.03 mg/kg/次输液）的自给药训练，并提供了光/音提示。在停止后，通过引入两个杠杆和光来恢复这种反应。为探讨DA_1受体在线索诱导的烟碱寻找行为恢复中的作用，腹腔注射DA_1拮抗剂SCH-23390（5μg/kg、10μg/kg和30μg/kg）。研究表明，最高剂量的SCH-23390减少了先前与烟碱传递相关的照明信号引起的烟碱寻找行为。综上所述，这些结果表明，刺激DA_1受体介导了烟碱暗示的条件性动机。同样，Guy和Fletcher（2014）发现，SCH-23390阻断DA_1受体可降低条件性刺激引起的杠杆按压反应，并削弱急性给予烟碱以增加这种反应的能力。

DA_1受体在烟碱强化中的作用已被Hall等（2015）在自我管理范式中证实。向NAcc、顶叶联合皮质、前扣带回皮质注入SCH-23390（每侧1～4μg）可减少烟碱自给药。这些结果证实了DA_1受体在烟碱成瘾中的关键作用，并勾勒出这种联系的神经解剖学图谱。此外，SCH-23390阻断DA_1受体可降低烟碱对大鼠的增强作用，且不依赖于性别（Barrett et al. 2017）。

条件性地点偏爱/厌恶范式：Laviolette等（2008）在条件性位置偏爱（CPP）/条件性位置厌恶（CPA）范式中评估了位于NAcc不同区域的DA_1受体在烟碱强化和厌恶效应中的作用。值得一提的是，NAcc是对滥用药物的动机性影响至关重要的区域之一。NAcc包括核心和外壳两个区域（Zahm, 1999）。几条证据表明，NAcc外壳通过空间/上下文线索参与控制精神活性物质和药物寻找行为的奖赏效应，而NAcc核心对于离散线索很重要（Bossert et al. 2007; Chaudhri et al. 2010）。在CPP实验中，将DA_1拮抗剂注入NAcc壳内可减弱烟碱诱导的CPP的获得（Spina, Fenu, Longoni, Rivas, Di Chiara, 2006）。小剂量烟碱（0.008.5nmol/0.5μL）或sc（0.8mg/kg）均可引起CPA，而向NAcc壳内微量注射SCH-23390（1μg/0.5μL）不能改变这种厌恶。同时，在NAcc注射SCH-23390的动物在给予相同剂量的烟碱时表现出强烈的位置偏爱，从而将CPA转换为CPP。将中性剂量（0.8nmol/0.5μL）的烟碱与SCH-23390（1μg/0.5μL）共同注入NAcc壳内，不能引起烟碱偶联环境的厌恶或偏好。然而，在NAcc核心注射SCH-23390的动物在与次奖励剂量的烟碱联合给药时表现出强烈的位置偏爱。此外，停止长期接触烟碱可以降低啮齿类动物纹状体中DA的水平（Rada et al. 2001）。研究表明，抑制NAcc外壳中的DA_1受体可以阻止烟碱的戒断，而SCH-23390注入NAcc核心后，这种作用不明显（Laviolette et al. 2008）。因此，位于NAcc核心区的DA_1受体参与了烟碱厌恶转换为奖赏和增强烟碱的作用，而位于NAcc壳层的DA_1受体在烟碱戒断过程中起着重要作用。

此外，Grieder等（2012）的研究表明，DA_1受体的激活和抑制都减弱了在非依赖小鼠急性给予烟碱后观察到的厌恶动机反应。对烟碱依赖和烟碱戒断的啮齿动物没有影响。这些结果表明DA_1受体只在烟碱的急性厌恶效应中起重要作用。有趣的是，进行辨别性刺激试验的实验表明，DA_1拮抗剂SCH-23390减弱了烟碱的辨别性刺激效应（Corrigall, Coen, 1994），而DA_1受体激动剂SKF82958在这一范例中取代了烟碱（Gasior et al. 1999）。上述结果明确地证实了DA_1受体在烟碱奖赏效应中的作用。

戒断：为评价DA_1受体在烟碱戒断后1d（9mg/kg/d，7d渗透压小泵给药）缓解自发戒断症状中的作用,给予$DA_{1/5}$激动剂SKF81297。结果表明,SKF81297在0.32 mg/kg剂量下激活DA_1样受体可减少牙齿颤抖/咀嚼,对湿狗抖动无影响。由于DA_2受体的激活降低了上述两种躯体戒断症状,作者建议应考虑使用DA_2而不是DA_1激动剂来治疗烟碱依赖的躯体症状(Ohmura et al. 2011)。这些研究与Grieder等(2012)和Laviolette等(2008)进行的前述实验一起,未能清楚地表明DA_1受体参与烟碱戒断。因此,这件事还需要进一步调查。

对运动效应的敏化:行为致敏是指药物在反复、间歇给药后活性增强(Vanderschuren, Kalivas, 2000)。烟碱注射(5d,0.4mg/kg,sc)可引起啮齿类动物运动活动增强,提示存在突触神经可塑性。在休息5天(激发剂量)后最后一次注射后,这一效应明显增强,这表明烟碱诱导的运动敏感化的发展。肌注DA_1拮抗剂SCH-23390(0.03mg/kg,ip)后,对烟碱运动敏感型小鼠的运动活动有明显的抑制作用。因此,烟碱诱导的行为敏化与由DA_1受体激活引起的cAMP依赖的信号级联反应的激活有关(Goutier, Lowry, McCreary, O'Connor, 2015)。

39.2.2 其他烟碱—DA_1受体集体

记忆、焦虑和神经元重塑:在抑制回避(IA)辨别任务中,涉及NAcc中DA_1受体的多巴胺能传递也参与了烟碱对记忆恢复的改善作用。烟碱本身可以改善被吗啡损害的IA记忆的恢复。NAcc内注射DA_1受体拮抗剂(SCH-23390)本身对记忆提取没有影响,但在全身注射烟碱之前给药,可阻止烟碱诱导的记忆提取的恢复。提示烟碱可能通过与DA_1受体相互作用而影响IA记忆的恢复(Azizbeigi et al. 2011)。众所周知,急性接触烟碱会引起焦虑,Zarrindast等(2013)也证实了这一点。他们表明,向中央杏仁核注射烟碱(1μg/只)可以产生焦虑效应,在高架加迷宫测试中,观察到的焦虑效应是张开双臂和进入张开双臂所花费的时间减少。有趣的是,每只大鼠静脉注射SCH-23390 0.25μg可减弱烟碱的焦虑效应。这表明DA_1受体在烟碱的焦虑性作用机制中也起着重要作用。最后,烟碱诱导的青春期神经元重塑依赖于DA_1受体。大多数吸烟者在青春期开始吸烟(NIDA, 2012)。因此,追切需要评估烟碱对大脑发育的影响。烟碱诱导的树突重塑在青少年的NAcc壳中高度表达(McDonald et al. 2007)。出生后28~42d可观察到新的树突和棘突的形成,并持续21d。烟碱与DA_1受体拮抗剂SCH-23390联合应用可阻断这种对树突的重塑效应。因此,可以认为多巴胺能系统在烟碱诱导的青春期神经适应性改变中起关键作用(Ehlinger et al. 2016)。

烟碱、DA_1受体与神经肽:神经肽与药物滥用的病理相关,主要是通过影响多巴胺能神经传递。P物质(SP)是一种神经肽,它影响边缘和锥体外区的多巴胺能神经传递,可能在药物依赖的发生和维持中起作用。研究表明,SP通过激活神经激肽受体1(NK1)发挥作用,因为阿片类药物在NK1基因敲除小鼠中不产生奖励效应,无论是在CPP模式还是自给药模式下。此外,SP还参与阿片类药物戒断后的戒断综合征(Murtra et al. 2000)。Alburges等(2009)研究了烟碱对SP水平的影响及其与SP/DA_1受体的相互作用。他们发现,每天重复注射烟碱4.0mg/kg(每2小时注射5次)会降低边缘系统和基底节中SP样免疫反应(SPLI)的组织水平,这反映了SP的释放和周转增加。SPLI水平在末次注射后持续12~18h,48h后基本消失。有趣的是,用DA_1受体拮抗剂(SCH-23390)预处理可以消除烟碱引起的VTA的SPLI水平的改变,但不能抑制SN的SPLI水平。因此,可以认为DA_1受体阻断等机制介导了烟碱诱导的中脑边缘通路中SP的改变。

烟碱在药物治疗中的作用—DA_1受体的作用:长期以来,人们一直认为黑质多巴胺能神经元的丢失是帕金森病发病的基础。此外，研究还发现，吸烟者患帕金森病的风险较低，另外，烟碱可以缓解帕金森病患者的运动功能障碍。在6-羟基多巴胺诱导的帕金森病大鼠模型中，长期摄入烟碱（15～30mg/L，27周）可增强纹状体DA_1受体的活性。因此，可以认为，通过改变多巴胺能平衡暴露于烟碱可能有助于缓解帕金森病症状（García-Montes et al. 2012）。

此外，还对烟碱对链脲佐菌素诱导的糖尿病大鼠的兴奋作用机制进行了评估。链脲佐菌素是一种对产生胰岛素的胰岛β细胞有毒性的物质。有充分的证据表明，中脑边缘系统的活动仍然受到胰岛素的影响。胰岛素受体定位于NAc和VTA。已有研究表明，胰岛素受体的激活对奖励反应有负向的调节作用（Figlewicz et al. 2003）。流行病学研究表明，糖尿病患者吸烟的倾向增加。在自给药模式下，发现链脲佐菌素诱导的糖尿病大鼠对烟碱的欲望增强。实验大鼠NAcc内DA转运体水平升高，DA_1受体表达减少。因此，可以得出结论，链脲佐菌素处理的啮齿动物NAcc中多巴胺能神经传递的减少增加了烟碱的自给药（O'Dell et al. 2014）。

术语解释

- **行为敏感化**：一种现象，包括对反复间歇性接触刺激（如滥用药物）的行为反应增强。
- **条件性位置厌恶**：一种简单的非侵入性技术，基于巴甫洛夫条件反射，动物学会避开以前伴随着厌恶刺激的隔间。
- **条件性位置偏爱**：一种经典的巴甫洛夫条件反射。滥用药物具有增强作用，可以提供无条件的刺激。他们的管理与一定的环境相结合，使这种环境获得了回报属性，从而成为一种条件性刺激。
- **自给药**：操作性条件作用的一种形式，动物做出努力，例如，按下杠杆，以提供一定剂量的药物。

烟碱与D1受体联系的关键事实

- 烟碱通过激活α4β2和α7烟碱型乙酰胆碱受体介导多巴胺的释放，从而导致多巴胺能1型受体的激活和$Gα_{s/olf}$/PKA/DARPP-32信号级联的激活。
- rs686是多巴胺1型受体基因与烟碱依赖相关的致病基因。
- 多巴胺能1型受体参与烟碱的奖励和厌恶作用。然而，关于多巴胺能1型受体参与烟碱戒断的证据是相互矛盾的。
- 烟碱通过增加多巴胺能1型受体的活性来减轻帕金森氏症的症状。
- 烟碱通过多巴胺能1型受体依赖机制诱导青春期树突重塑。
- 多巴胺能1型受体在烟碱诱导的焦虑和记忆过程中起重要作用。
- 糖尿病啮齿动物伏隔核多巴胺能神经传递减少，烟碱自给药增加。

要点总结

- 本章的目的是总结有关多巴胺能1型受体对烟碱影响的研究结果。
- 多巴胺能1型受体定位于奖励相关的脑区，如中脑边缘和中皮质通路，特别是纹状体、杏仁核、伏隔核、黑质、额叶皮层和嗅球等也接受胆碱能输入的区域。中脑边缘系统仍然受肽（即胰岛素）的影响。
- 烟碱依赖和多巴胺能1型之间有显著的联系。
- 多巴胺能1型受体在记忆和焦虑过程中起关键作用，并导致帕金森氏症、精神分裂症或亨廷顿病等精神障碍。

- 实验数据表明，P物质对边缘和锥体外区多巴胺能神经传递有影响，可能在药物依赖的形成和维持中起作用。
- 烟碱诱导发育中大脑的树突重塑。

参考文献

Abdolahi, A.; Acosta, G.; Breslin, F. J.; Hemby, S. E.; Lynch, W. J. (2010). Incubation of nicotine seeking is associated with enhanced protein kinase A-regulated signaling of dopamine- and cAMP-regulated phosphoprotein of 32 kDa in the insular cortex. European Journal of Neuroscience, 31(4), 733-741.

Alburges, M. E.; Frankel, P. S.; Hoonakker, A. J.; Hanson, G. R. (2009). Responses of limbic and extrapyramidal substance P systems to nicotine treatment. Psychopharmacology, 201(4), 517-527.

Azizbeigi, R.; Ahmadi, S.; Babapour, V.; Rezayof, A.; Zarrindast, M. R. (2011). Nicotine restores morphine-induced memory deficit through the D1 and D2 dopamine receptor mechanisms in the nucleus accumbens. Journal of Psychopharmacology, 25(8), 1126-1133.

Barrett, S. T.; Geary, T. N.; Steiner, A. N.; Bevins, R. A. (2017). Sex differences and the role of dopamine receptors in the reward-enhancing effects of nicotine and bupropion. Psychopharmacology, 234(2), 187-198.

Beaulieu, J. M.; Gainetdinov, R. R. (2011). The physiology, signaling, and pharmacology of dopamine receptors. Pharmacological Reviews, 63(1), 182-217.

Bossert, J. M.; Poles, G. C.; Wihbey, K. A.; Koya, E.; Shaham, Y. (2007). Differential effects of blockade of dopamine D1-family receptors in nucleus accumbens core or shell on reinstatement of heroin seeking induced by contextual and discrete cues. Journal of Neuroscience, 27, 12655-12663.

Brichta, L.; Greengard, P.; Flajolet, M. (2013). Advances in the pharmacological treatment of Parkinson's disease: targeting neurotransmitter systems. Trends in Neurosciences, 36(9), 543-554.

Caggiula, A. R.; Donny, E. C.; White, A. R.; Chaudhri, N.; Booth, S.; Gharib, M. A. et al. (2001). Cue dependency of nicotine self-administration and smoking. Pharmacology, Biochemistry and Behavior, 70(4), 515-530.

Chaudhri, N.; Sahuque, L. L.; Schairer, W. W.; Janak, P. H. (2010). Separable roles of the nucleus accumbens core and shell in context- and cue-induced alcohol-seeking. Neuropsychopharmacology, 35, 783-791.

Corrigall, W. A.; Coen, K. M. (1994). Dopamine mechanisms play at best a small role in the nicotine discriminative stimulus. Pharmacology, Biochemistry and Behavior, 48(3), 817-820.

Ehlinger, D. G.; Bergstrom, H. C.; Burke, J. C.; Fernandez, G. M.; McDonald, C. G.; Smith, R. F. (2016). Adolescent nicotine-induced dendrite remodeling in the nucleus accumbens is rapid, persistent, and D1-dopamine receptor dependent. Brain Structure and Function, 221(1), 133-145.

Figlewicz, D. P.; Evans, S. B.; Murphy, J.; Hoen, M.; Baskin, D. G. (2003). Expression of receptors for insulin and leptin in the ventral tegmental area/substantia nigra (VTA/SN) of the rat. Brain Research, 964, 107-115.

Floresco, S. B.; West, A. R.; Ash, B.; Moore, H.; Grace, A. A. (2003). Afferent modulation of dopamine neuron firing differentially regulates tonic and phasic dopamine transmission. Nature Neuroscience, 6, 968-973.

García-Montes, J. R.; Boronat-García, A.; López-Colomé, A. M.; Bargas, J.; Guerra-Crespo, M.; Drucker-Colín, R. (2012). Is nicotine protective against Parkinson's disease? An experimental analysis. CNS, Neurological Disorders: Drug Targets, 11(7), 897-906.

Gasior, M.; Shoaib, M.; Yasar, S.; Jaszyna, M.; Goldberg, S. R. (1999). Acquisition of nicotine discrimination and discriminative stimulus effects of nicotine in rats chronically exposed to caffeine. Journal of Pharmacology and Experimental Therapeutics, 288(3), 1053-1073.

Goutier, W.; Lowry, J. P.; McCreary, A. C.; O'Connor, J. J. (2015). Frequency-dependent modulation of dopamine release by nicotine and dopamine D1 receptor ligands: an in vitro fast cyclic voltammetry study in rat striatum. Neurochemical Research, 41(9), 945-950.

Goutier, W.; O'Connor, J. J.; Lowry, J. P.; McCreary, A. C. (2016). The effect of nicotine induced behavioral sensitization on dopamine D1 receptor pharmacology: an in vivo and ex vivo study in the rat. European Neuropsychopharmacology, 25(6), 933-943.

Gozen, O.; Balkan, B.; Yildirim, E.; Koylu, E. O.; Pogun, S. (2013). The epigenetic effect of nicotine on dopamine D1 receptor expression in rat prefrontal cortex. Synapse, 67(9), 545-552.

Grieder, T. E.; George, O.; Tan, H.; George, S. R.; Le Foll, B.; Laviolette, S. R. et al. (2012). Phasic D1 and tonic D2 dopamine receptor signaling double dissociate the motivational effects of acute nicotine and chronic nicotine withdrawal. Proceedings of the National Academy of Sciences of the United States of America, 109(8), 3101-3106.

Guy, E. G.; Fletcher, P. J. (2014). Responding for a conditioned reinforcer, and its enhancement by nicotine, is blocked by dopamine receptor antagonists and a 5-HT(2C) receptor agonist but not by a 5-HT(2A) receptor antagonist. Pharmacology, Biochemistry, and Behavior, 125, 4 0-47.

Hall, B. J.; Slade, S.; Allenby, C.; Kutlu, M. G.; Levin, E. D. (2015). Neuro-anatomic mapping of dopamine D1 receptor involvement in nicotine self-administration in rats. Neuropharmacology, 99, 689-695.

Hamada, M.; Hendrick, J. P.; Ryan, G. R.; Kuroiwa, M.; Higashi, H.; Tanaka, M. et al. (2005). Nicotine regulates DARPP-32 (dopamine-and cAMP-regulated phosphoprotein of 32 kDa) phosphorylation at multiple sites in neostriatal neurons. Journal of Pharmacology and Experimental Therapeutics, 315(2), 872-878.

Hisahara, S.; Shimohama, S. (2011). Dopamine receptors and Parkinson's disease. International Journal of Medicinal Chemistry. https://doi.org/10.1155/2011/403039.

Huang, W.; Li, M. D. (2009). Differential allelic expression of dopamine D1 receptor gene (DRD1) is modulated by microRNA miR504. Biological

Psychiatry, 65(8), 702-705.

Komatsu, H. (2015). Novel therapeutic GPCRs for psychiatric disorders. International Journal of Molecular Sciences, 16(6), 14109-141021.

Laviolette, S. R.; Lauzon, N. M.; Bishop, S. F.; Sun, N.; Tan, H. (2008). Dopamine signaling through D1-like versus D2-like receptors in the nucleus accumbens core versus shell differentially modulates nicotine reward sensitivity. Journal of Neuroscience, 28(32), 8025-8033.

Liu, X.; Jernigen, C.; Gharib, M.; Booth, S.; Caggiula, A. R.; Sved, A. F. (2010). Effects of dopamine antagonists on drug cue-induced reinstatement of nicotine-seeking behavior in rats. Behavioral Pharmacology, 21(2), 153-160.

McDonald, C. G.; Eppolito, A. K.; Brielmaier, J. M.; Smith, L. N.; Bergstrom, H. C.; Lawhead, M. R. et al. (2007). Evidence for elevated nicotine-induced structural plasticity in nucleus accumbens of adolescent rats. Brain Research, 1151, 211-218.

Murtra, P.; Sheasby, A. M.; Hunt, S. P.; De Felipe, C. (2000). Rewarding effects of opiates are absent in mice lacking the receptor for substance P. Nature, 405, 180-183.

National Institute on Drug Abuse (2012). Research report series: Tobacco addiction. Washington: Department of Health and Human Services (US) [NIH Pub No. 12-4342].

O'Dell, L. E.; Natividad, L. A.; Pipkin, J. A.; Roman, F.; Torres, I.; Jurado, J. et al. (2014). Enhanced nicotine self-administration and suppressed dopaminergic systems in a rat model of diabetes. Addiction Biology, 19(6), 1006-1019.

Ohmura, Y.; Jutkiewicz, E. M.; Zhang, A.; Domino, E. F. (2011). Dopamine D1/5 and D2/3 agonists differentially attenuate somatic signs of nicotine withdrawal in rats. Pharmacology Biochemistry and Behavior, 99(4), 552-556.

Rada, P.; Jensen, K.; Hoebel, B. G. (2001). Effects of nicotine and mecamylamine induced withdrawal on extracellular dopamine and acetylcholine in the rat nucleus accumbens. Psychopharmacology, 157, 105-110.

Spina, L.; Fenu, S.; Longoni, R.; Rivas, E.; Di Chiara, G. (2006). Nicotine-conditioned single-trial place preference: selective role of nucleus accumbens shell dopamine D1 receptors in acquisition. Psychopharmacology, 184(3-4), 447-455.

Svenningsson, P.; Nishi, A.; Fisone, G.; Girault, J. A.; Nairn, A. C.; Greengard, P. (2004). DARPP-32: an integrator of neurotransmission. Annual Review of Pharmacology and Toxicology, 44, 269-296.

Vanderschuren, L. J.; Kalivas, P. W. (2000). Alterations in dopaminergic and glutamatergic transmission in the induction and expression of behavioral sensitization: a critical review of preclinical studies. Psychopharmacology, 151(2-3), 99-120.

Wheeler, T. L.; Smith, L. N.; Bachus, S. E.; McDonald, C. G.; Fryxell, K. J.; Smith, R. F. (2013). Low-dose adolescent nicotine and methylphenidate have additive effects on adult behavior and neurochemistry. Pharmacology Biochemistry and Behavior, 103(4), 723-734.

Zahm, D. S. (1999). Functional-anatomical implications of the nucleus accumbens core and shell subterritories. Annals of the New York Academy of Sciences, 877, 113-128.

Zarrindast, M. R.; Eslahi, N.; Rezayof, A.; Rostami, P.; Zahmatkesh, M. (2013). Modulation of ventral tegmental area dopamine receptors inhibit nicotine-induced anxiogenic-like behavior in the central amygdala. Progress in Neuro-Psychopharmacology and Biological Psychiatry, 41, 11-17.

40
烟碱奖励背景下的大脑基因表达：对胆碱能基因的关注

Mark D. Namba[1], *Gregory L. Powell*[1], *Armani P. Del Franco*[2], *Julianna G. Goenaga*[1], *Cassandra D. Gipson*[1]

1. Department of Psychology, Arizona State University, Tempe, AZ, United States
2. Department of Neuroscience, University of Minnesota, Minneapolis, MN, United States

缩略语

GWAS	全基因组关联研究	**ND**	烟碱依赖
KO	敲除	**SNP**	单核苷酸多态性
nAChR	烟碱型乙酰胆碱受体		

40.1 引言

遗传学研究的进展极大地提高了我们对吸烟行为病因的认识。一些研究发现烟碱依赖（ND）的遗传率约为50%（Rose et al. 2009），这些基因贡献者受到社会经济、文化和其他环境的影响（Mackillop et al. 2010）。重要的是，烟草使用开始背后的基因贡献似乎与其持久性背后的基因贡献不同（Morley et al. 2007），这突出了基因在获得和维持吸烟习惯中发挥的动态作用。药物的反复使用通常被认为是多基因相互作用的结果。许多临床和临床前研究检测了烟碱成瘾易感性的遗传因素，揭示了多种神经递质、神经调节剂和代谢系统中的几个变异，它们与烟碱的获得、维持和复发有关（Mackillop et al. 2010）。特别是，几个胆碱能基因的遗传变异与大量吸烟有关，而不吸烟的人患ND的遗传风险较低（Belsky et al. 2013）。在这一章中，我们将简要讨论检查烟草使用的胆碱能基因靶点的临床和临床前研究，必要时找出文献中的空白。此外，我们还将讨论其他值得进一步研究的潜在基因靶点。最后，我们将解决在临床环境中应用这些知识的潜在挑战和重要考虑因素。

40.2 烟碱成瘾患者胆碱能基因变异的临床检测

临床数据强调了一些基因簇作为烟碱依赖媒介的重要性。其中，胆碱能基因是烟碱有益特性的主要驱动力，可能是促进烟碱停止使用的治疗的有益靶点。正如Bühler及其同事所回顾的那样，文献中发现的与烟碱相关表型相关的大多数单核苷酸多态性（SNPs）都涉及烟碱型乙酰胆碱受体（nAChR）基因（Bühler et al. 2015）。众所周知，烟碱主要通过激活腹侧被盖区（VTA）和伏隔核（NAcc）等区域的nAChR（包括α4β2和α7）来发挥奖赏和增强作用（Laviolette, van der Kooy, 2004）。nAChRs的基因变异是临床和临床前研究之间最一致的翻译发现，与对烟碱的依赖和肺癌易感性等合并症显著相关（Li, Burmeister, 2009）。此外，不同的nAChR亚型具有不同的脱敏特性，基于c的受体快速脱敏，而基于α4β2的受体对烟碱的亲和力增强，并且结合烟碱的时间更长（Quick, Lester, 2002; α4β2和α7结构见图40.1）。这些nAChR亚型的潜在遗传变异或不同人群亚型的差异表达将影响受体的功能和对长期烟碱暴露的反应。因此，检查nAChR表达的遗传异质性是至关重要的，因为它与ND有关。编码α4亚基的CHRNA4已被证明与多种种族（主要是欧洲裔美国人和非裔美国人样本）以及男性和女性的ND检测结果有显著的相关性（Feng et al. 2004; Hutchison et al. 2007; Li et al. 2005）。最近，一项对两个独立的纵向家庭研究进行的荟萃分析发现，CHRNA4 SNP与ND之间存在中度关联（Kamens et al. 2013）。其他研究没有报道CHRNB2（编码β2亚基）与ND之间的关联（Feng et al. 2004; Li et al. 2005; Silverman et al. 2000）；然而，CHRNB2变异体的作用可能取决于CHRNA4的变异体（Li, Burmeister, 2009; Li, Lou, et al. 2008）。

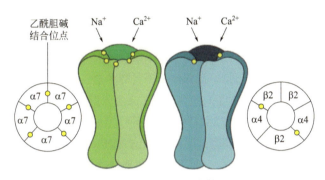

图40.1　nAChR结构

同构体α7（绿色）和异构体α4β2（蓝色）nAChR的遗传变异与ND相关。α7和α4β2都有钙通道，这可能是这些受体改变不同脑区和细胞类型的细胞信号的一个可能机制。

全基因组关联研究（GWAS）（图40.2）显示，位于15号染色体（15q25.1）上的CHRNA5-CHRNA3-CHRNB4基因位点的变异与ND和疾病易感性都有关（图40.3）。例如，Saccone和他的同事发现CHRNB3和CHRNA5中的SNP与ND相关，揭示了潜在的遗传风险位点（Saccone et al. 2006）。其他研究也支持这样的发现，该基因簇之间的遗传变异不仅与ND有关（Berrettini et al. 2008; Bierut et al. 2008），而且还与肺癌和其他心肺疾病有关（Thorgeirsson et al. 2008）。

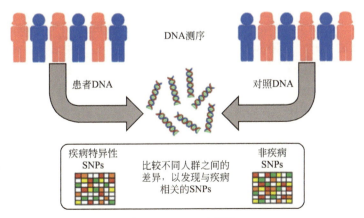

图40.2　GWAS综述

来自疾病易感个体和健康对照的DNA被测序，并在整个基因组中比较与感兴趣疾病相关的特定SNP的群体差异。

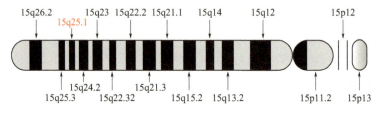

图 40.3　15 号染色体示意图

CHRNA5-CHRNA3-CHRNB4 基因位点位于 15q25.1（红色加亮），与 ND 和疾病易感性相关。

最近一项对 *CHRNA5-CHRNA3-CHRNB4* 基因簇的研究发现，在不吸烟的青少年中，*CHRNA3* SNP rs578776 与基于奖励的任务中前扣带回（ACC）的钝性激活有关，这可能是奖励处理改变和 ND 易感性增加的潜在原因（Nees et al. 2013）。ACC 参与几个更高级别的执行功能，如奖励处理、冲动控制和决策。此外，在青少年中，在 CHRNA5 含有功能性 SNP 的个体中，同伴对 ND 的影响较小，而总体而言，*CHRNA5*、*CHRNA3*、*CHRNB3* 和 *CHRND* 中的四个特定 SNP 与 ND 相关（Johnson et al. 2010）。最近对两个物质依赖性 GWAS 数据集的路径分析在基因本体（GO）术语中发现了胆碱能受体，此外还有感觉知觉、核糖体和视黄醇术语（Harari et al. 2012），加强了 nAChR 基因表达变异与 ND 的关联。胆碱乙酰转移酶（ChAT）的遗传变异研究也揭示了对戒烟和 ND 的重要影响。特别是，ChAT SNP 的一个子集与 8 周替代疗法和咨询治疗方案后的戒烟成功显著相关（Ray et al. 2010），而在欧洲裔美国人和非洲裔美国人的样本中，其他 SNP 与 ND 相关（Wei et al. 2010）。

这些遗传学研究提供了令人信服的证据，表明胆碱能基因与 ND 和疾病易感性有关。然而，值得注意的是，nAChR 还介导了炎症（Bencherif, 2009）和疼痛（Decker, Meyer, Sullivan, 2001）等生理机制，并参与了其他神经精神疾病，如焦虑和抑郁（Picciotto, Brunzell, Caldarone, 2002）。这些神经精神疾病通常是并存的，可能会加重 ND。因此，胆碱能基因变异的临床相关性应该在 ND 以外的更广泛的疾病状态的背景下进行全面的检查。

40.3　检测烟碱成瘾患者胆碱能基因变异的临床前模型

药理学和遗传学方法已经揭示了关于这些亚基在调节烟碱的奖励和增强特性中的作用的重要信息。早期的研究表明，烟碱系统是认知功能的关键调节器（Levin, 2002），β2 nAChR 亚基的基因缺失介导了联想学习过程和烟碱诱导的下丘脑室旁核释放多巴胺（Picciotto et al. 1995, 1998）。一些 nAChR 亚基（α3、α5、α6 和 β4）在室旁核的多巴胺能神经元中表达，化学消融后这些亚基的 mRNA 信号消失（Charpantier et al. 1998）。Klink 等（2001）发现，几乎所有的室旁核细胞都含有 α4 和 β2 亚基的 mRNA。本研究还观察到 α5、α6、α7 和 β3 mRNA 在下丘脑室旁核的 P 能和 GABA 能细胞中的差异表达。直到最近，阐明 nAChR 亚基在调节烟碱增强效应中的作用的证据仅限于 β2 亚基（Epping-Jordan et al. 1999; Picciotto et al. 1998）。然而，一项使用病毒在基因敲除（KO）小鼠中重新表达（或"拯救"）β2 的研究发现，被拯救的 β2 KO 小鼠在暴露于烟碱的情况下，NA 中的多巴胺释放增加，与野生型小鼠相似。在类似于野生型的 Y 迷宫中，获救的 β2 KO 小鼠更喜欢烟碱配对的手臂，而 β2 KO 小鼠则没有表现出这样的神经行为特征（Maskos et al. 2005）。目前，研究脑内 nAChR 的新基因技术正在实施中，例如 Cre-Lox（或 FLP-FRT）重组酶技术（图 40.4）（Fowler, Kenny, 2012; Hernandez et al. 2014; Ngolab et al. 2015）。

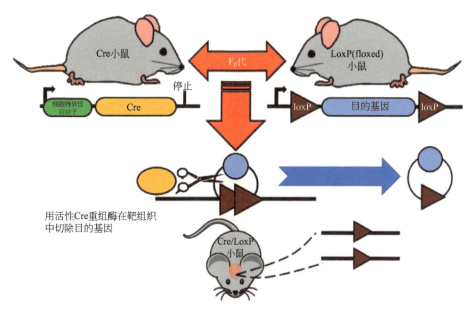

图 40.4　Cre-Lox 条件性基因敲除概述

Cre 小鼠与 loxP（"Floxed"）小鼠杂交，部分后代表达活性 Cre 重组酶，目的基因在靶组织中被活性 Cre 切除。

如前所述，编码 α5 nAChR 亚基的 *CHRNA5* 的遗传变异与 ND 有关。最近的研究表明，含有 α5 的 nAChR 可能参与了烟碱摄取的调节，也可能介导了烟碱的厌恶。在一项研究中，含有 α5 零突变的小鼠表现出烟碱摄入量增加，这一效应可以通过在内侧缰核重新表达 *CHRNA5* 来挽救（Fowler et al. 2011）。这项研究还表明，敲除 MHb 中的 α5 不会改变烟碱奖励，但在较高烟碱剂量时确实降低了颅内自我刺激阈值，这表明 MHb α5 调节对烟碱消费的抑制控制（Fowler et al. 2011）。同样，最近的一项研究发现，在非烟碱依赖的小鼠中，α5 的缺失（α5-/-），在较低的非激励性剂量下增强烟碱奖励，并消除对较高剂量烟碱的条件性味觉回避（Grieder et al. 2017）。此外，本研究还表明烟碱依赖的 α5-/- 小鼠对烟碱戒断没有表现出厌恶的条件性反应，这些效应与多巴胺受体拮抗剂所观察到的相似（Grieder et al. 2017）。烟碱戒断症状导致吸烟者的高复发率（Benowitz, 2009），从 MHb 到脚间核（IPN）的投射可能介导这些症状（Gorlich et al. 2013; Zhao-Shea et al. 2015）。最近的研究表明，病毒上调 MHb 胆碱能神经元的 α4 功能会增加烟碱戒断小鼠的焦虑样行为（Pang et al. 2016）。因此，这种特殊的 nAChR 亚基的遗传变异可能导致烟碱依赖和复发易感性（McClure-Begley et al. 2014）。图 40.5 提供了与 ND 相关的缰核回路和相关的 nAChR 亚基的非穷尽示意图。

40.4　ND 的其他潜在基因

目前的戒烟治疗主要用于取代烟碱对 nAChRs 的刺激，以减轻对药物的渴求，而不会产生有益的效果（Nides, 2008）。例如，伐伦克林（Chantix®）是 α4β2 的部分激动剂和 α7 nAChR 的完全激动剂，在帮助个人戒烟方面显示出一定的临床疗效（Kasza et al. 2015; McClure et al. 2013）。无论如何，即使对于接受替代治疗的个体来说，高复发率仍然存在（Leshner, Stapleton, 1997），这突显了对 ND 易感性背后的遗传易感性进行更全面了解的必要性。表 40.1 总结了可能与 ND 易感性和复发易感性有关的非胆碱能基因靶点。

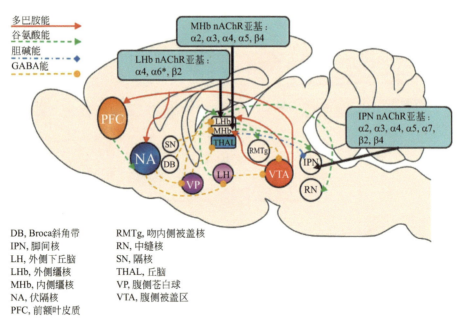

图 40.5 ND 患者缰核回路与 nAChR 亚基分布

遗传学研究揭示了缰核和 IPN 中与 ND 相关的几个 nAChR 亚基。外侧缰核（LHb）分别接受来自腹侧苍白球（VP）和外侧下丘脑（LH）的抑制性和兴奋性输入，以及来自其他皮质和皮质下结构（未示出）的兴奋性输入。MHb 主要接受隔核（SN）和 Broca 斜角带（DB）的抑制性输入。LHb 被厌恶刺激激活，通过吻内侧被盖核（RMTg）的兴奋性投射间接对 VTA 实施抑制性控制，从而调节烟碱摄入量。除了 α4 和 β2 亚基外，α6* nAChR 还能增强 LHb 活性，并可能调节烟碱厌恶或奖励。IPN 接收来自 MHb 的兴奋性投射，并通过 α5* nAChRs 调节烟碱的消耗。沿 MHb-IPN 通路的 β4 亚基也调节烟碱的厌恶和摄取。

表 40.1 ND 潜在的其他潜在基因靶点

基因	功能	参考文献
DBH	多巴胺 β- 羟化酶—催化多巴胺转化为去甲肾上腺素	McKinney et al. (2000)
COMT	儿茶酚 -O- 甲基转移酶—催化降解儿茶酚胺和其他具有儿茶酚结构的化合物	Beuten et al. (2006)
DRD2/3/4	多巴胺 D_2、D_3、D_4（G_i 偶联）受体—抑制腺苷酸环化酶（AC）和环磷酸腺苷（cAMP）	Vandenbergh et al. (2007) David, Munafò (2008)
OPRM1	$μ_1$- 阿片受体（G_i 偶联）—抑制 AC 和 cAMP	Kuwabara et al. (2014)
SLC6A4	5- 羟色胺转运体（5-HTT）—介导突触前 5- 羟色胺再摄取	Herman, Balogh (2012)
GABBR1/2	$GABA_{B1}$ 和 $GABA_{B2}$（$G_{i/o}$ 偶联）受体—抑制 AC 和 cAMP 并激活 K^+ 通道	Cui et al.(2012)
CNR1	大麻素受体 1 型（$G_{i/o}$ 偶联）—抑制 AC 和 cAMP 并增加丝裂原活化蛋白激酶	Chen et al. (2008)
BDNF	脑源性神经营养因子—神经营养生长因子在海马、皮质和基底前脑高表达	Jamal, Van der Does, Elzinga, Molendijk, Penninx (2015)

40.5 结论

在过去的几十年里，科学家们在阐明 ND 发生和维持的遗传病因方面取得了很大进展。与 ND 相关的胆碱能底物中的遗传变异是文献中最一致的发现，尽管其他非胆碱能基因靶点也可能与 ND 相关。毫无疑问，这些基因研究有可能指导促进戒烟和长期戒烟的治疗策略的发展。然而，值得注意的是，ND与其他神经精神疾病（Grant et al. 2004）高度并存，许多基因变异并不能单独预测ND易感性。胆碱能系统在中枢和外周神经组织中广泛表达，因此对其他神经递质系统起着调节作用。因此，胆碱能底物的遗传变异可能不是ND所特有的。ND的遗传风险还受到发育和环境的影响，给定单倍型的ND的表型表达可能取决于诸如发病年龄、压力和情绪状态等因素（Baker et al. 2009; Mackillop et al. 2010）。此外，与ND相关的基因变异也可能受到压力、发育中的烟碱暴露、既往药物使用和许多其他因素的表观遗传修饰的影响（Renthal, Nestler, 2008; Volkow, 2011）。很可能是这些并发症导致了人类基因研究之间的不一致。然而，了解ND和复发易感性背后的遗传机制将有助于指导未来开发新的治疗策略，更好地促进戒烟和长期戒烟。

术语解释

- 胆碱乙酰转移酶：一种转移酶，用来合成乙酰胆碱。
- 表观遗传学：研究在不改变遗传密码的情况下对基因表达进行的环境修饰的研究。
- 病因：一种疾病或状况的起因、一组起因或起因方式。
- 基因簇：一组邻近的基因，编码相似的多肽和功能。
- 基因型：个体携带的一个或一组基因。
- 单体型：一组倾向于一起遗传的遗传变异。
- 基因敲除：不表达目标基因的动物（通常是老鼠）。
- 表型：某一特定特征或特征的表现。
- 单核苷酸多态性：DNA序列中单个碱基对的变异。
- 野生型：表达感兴趣基因的动物。

基因技术在床前/临床模型中的关键事实

- GWAS检查整个基因组中的遗传变异，以将遗传特征与人类的某些疾病联系起来。
- 通常，GWAS侧重于特定SNP与身体疾病特征之间的关联。病例对照设计是最常见的GWAS类型（图40.2）。等位基因频率被用作对照组和疾病组之间的衡量标准。
- Cre-Lox重组酶系统使研究人员能够对动物模型中的基因表达进行时间和细胞类型特异性的控制（Nagy，2000），这与传统的基因敲除方法不同，它在整个发育过程中保持目标基因的内源性活性；Cre-Lox重组涉及由loxP"侧翼"的DNA序列的缺失、倒置或移位，这取决于lox位点的方向性和方向。

要点总结

- 胆碱能基因的遗传多态性是烟碱依赖（ND）发生和维持的潜在危险因素。
- 胆碱能基因是ND易感性和治疗的潜在生物标志物。
- *CHRNA4*（编码α4 nAChR亚基）的多态性与ND有显著的相关性。
- *CHRNA5-CHRNA3-CHRNB4*基因位点与ND易感性相关。
- 聚集在胆碱乙酰转移酶（ChAT）周围的单核苷酸多态性（SNPs）与烟碱的成功持续使用密切相关。
- 胆碱能基因与其他精神疾病相关，说明了与ND共病的重要神经生物学基础。
- 非胆碱能基因的遗传变异也可能与ND有关。
- ND的遗传风险受发育和环境因素的影响。
- 胆碱能基因的表观遗传修饰可以解释人类遗传学研究之间的不一致。

参考文献

Baker, T. B.; Weiss, R. B.; Bolt, D.; von Niederhausern, A.; Fiore, M. C.; Dunn, D. M. et al. (2009). Human neuronal acetylcholine receptor A5-A3-B4 haplotypes are associated with multiple nicotine dependence phenotypes. Nicotine, Tobacco Research, 11(7), 785-796.

Belsky, D. W.; Moffitt, T. E.; Baker, T. B.; Biddle, A. K.; Evans, J. P.; Harrington, H. et al. (2013). Polygenic risk and the developmental progression to heavy, persistent smoking and nicotine dependence: evidence from a 4-decade longitudinal study. JAMA Psychiatry, 70 (5), 534-542.

Bencherif, M. (2009). Neuronal nicotinic receptors as novel targets for inflammation and neuroprotection: mechanistic considerations and clinical relevance. Acta Pharmacologica Sinica, 30(6), 702-714.

Benowitz, N. L. (2009). Pharmacology of nicotine: addiction, smoking-induced disease, and therapeutics. Annual Review of Pharmacology and Toxicology, 49(1), 57-71.

Berrettini, W.; Yuan, X.; Tozzi, F.; Song, K.; Francks, C.; Chilcoat, H. et al. (2008). α-5/α-3 nicotinic receptor subunit alleles increase risk for heavy smoking. Molecular Psychiatry, 13(4), 368-373.

Beuten, J.; Payne, T. J.; Ma, J. Z.; Li, M. D. (2006). Significant association of catechol-O-methyltransferase (COMT) haplotypes with nicotine dependence in male and female smokers of two ethnic populations. Neuropsychopharmacology, 31(3), 675-684.

Bierut, L. J.; Stitzel, J. A.; Wang, J. C.; Hinrichs, A. L.; Grucza, R. A.; Xuei, X. et al. (2008). Variants in nicotinic receptors and risk for nicotine dependence. The American Journal of Psychiatry, 165(9), 1163-1171.

Bühler, K. M.; Giné, E.; Echeverry-Alzate, V.; Calleja-Conde, J.; De Fonseca, F. R.; López-Moreno, J. A. (2015). Common single nucleotide variants underlying drug addiction: more than a decade of research. Addiction Biology 20(5), 845-871.

Charpantier, E.; Barnéoud, P.; Moser, P.; Besnard, F.; Sgard, F. (1998). Nicotinic acetylcholine subunit mRNA expression in dopaminergic neurons of the rat substantia nigra and ventral tegmental area. NeuroReport, 9(13), 3097-3101.

Chen, X.; Williamson, V. S.; An, S.; Hettema, J. M.; Aggen, S. H.; Neale, M. C. et al. (2008). Cannabinoid receptor 1 gene association with nicotine dependence. Archives of General Psychiatry, 65(7), 816-824.

Cui, W. -Y.; Seneviratne, C.; Gu, J.; Li, M. D. (2012). Genetics of GABAergic signaling in nicotine and alcohol dependence. Human Genetics, 131(6), 843-855.

David, S. P.; Munafò, M. R. (2008). Genetic variation in the dopamine pathway and smoking cessation. Pharmacogenomics, 9(9), 1307-1321.

Decker, M. W.; Meyer, M. D.; Sullivan, J. P. (2001). The therapeutic potential of nicotinic acetylcholine receptor agonists for pain control. Expert Opinion on Investigational Drugs, 10(10), 1819-1830.

Epping-Jordan, M. P.; Picciotto, M. R.; Changeux, J. P.; Pich, E. M. (1999). Assessment of nicotinic acetylcholine receptor subunit contributions to nicotine self-administration in mutant mice. Psychopharmacology, 147(1), 25-26.

Feng, Y.; Niu, T.; Xing, H.; Xu, X.; Chen, C.; Peng, S. et al. (2004). A common haplotype of the nicotine acetylcholine receptor alpha 4 subunit gene is associated with vulnerability to nicotine addiction in men. The American Journal of Human Genetics, 75(1), 112-121.

Fowler, C. D.; Kenny, P. J. (2012). Utility of genetically modified mice for understanding the neurobiology of substance use disorders. Human Genetics, 131(6), 941-957.

Fowler, C. D.; Lu, Q.; Johnson, P. M.; Marks, M. J.; Kenny, P. J. (2011). Habenular α5 nicotinic receptor subunit signalling controls nicotine intake. Nature, 471(7340), 597-601.

Gorlich, A.; Antolin-Fontes, B.; Ables, J. L.; Frahm, S.; Slimak, M. A.; Dougherty, J. D. et al. (2013). Reexposure to nicotine during withdrawal increases the pacemaking activity of cholinergic habenular neurons. Proceedings of the National Academy of Sciences, 110(42), 17077-17082.

Grant, B. F.; Hasin, D. S.; Chou, S. P.; Stinson, F. S.; Dawson, D. A. (2004). Nicotine dependence and psychiatric disorders in the United States. Archives of General Psychiatry, 61(11), 1107.

Grieder, T. E.; George, O.; Yee, M.; Bergamini, M. A.; Chwalek, M.; Maal-Bared, G. et al. (2017). Deletion of α5 nicotine receptor subunits abolishes nicotinic aversive motivational effects in a manner that phenocopies dopamine receptor antagonism. European Journal of Neuroscience, 46(1), 1673-1681.

Harari, O.; Wang, J. -C.; Bucholz, K.; Edenberg, H. J.; Heath, A.; Martin, N. G. et al. (2012). Pathway analysis of smoking quantity in multiple GWAS identifies cholinergic and sensory pathways. PLoS ONE, 7(12), e50913.

Herman, A. I.; Balogh, K. N. (2012). Polymorphisms of the serotonin transporter and receptor genes: Susceptibility to substance abuse. Substance Abuse and Rehabilitation, 3(1), 49-57.

Hernandez, C. M.; Cortez, I.; Gu, Z.; Colón-Sáez, J. O.; Lamb, P. W.; Wakamiya, M. et al. (2014). Research tool: validation of floxed α7 nicotinic acetylcholine receptor conditional knockout mice using in vitro and in vivo approaches. The Journal of Physiology, 592(15), 3201-3214.

Hutchison, K. E.; Allen, D. L.; Filbey, F. M.; Jepson, C.; Lerman, C.; Benowitz, N. L. et al. (2007). CHRNA4 and tobacco dependence: from gene regulation to treatment outcome. Archives of General Psychiatry, 64(9), 1078.

Jamal, M.; Van der Does, W.; Elzinga, B. M.; Molendijk, M. L.; Penninx, B. W. J. H. (2015). Association between smoking, nicotine dependence, and BDNF Val66Met polymorphism with BDNF concentrations in serum. Nicotine, Tobacco Research, 17 (3), 323-329.

Johnson, E. O.; Chen, L. -S.; Breslau, N.; Hatsukami, D.; Robbins, T.; Saccone, N. L. et al. (2010). Peer smoking and the nicotinic receptor genes: an examination of genetic and environmental risks for nicotine dependence. Addiction, 105(11), 2014-2022.

Kamens, H. M.; Corley, R. P.; McQueen, M. B.; Stallings, M. C.; Hopfer, C. J.; Crowley, T. J. et al. (2013). Nominal association with CHRNA4 variants and nicotine dependence. Genes, Brain and Behavior, 12(3), 297-304.

Kasza, K. A.; Cummings, K. M.; Carpenter, M. J.; Cornelius, M. E.; Hyland, A. J.; Fong, G. T. (2015). Use of stop-smoking medications in the United States before and after the introduction of varenicline. Addiction (Abingdon, England), 110(2), 346-355.

Klink, R.; de Kerchove d'Exaerde, A.; Zoli, M.; Changeux, J. P. (2001). Molecular and physiological diversity of nicotinic acetylcholine receptors in the midbrain dopaminergic nuclei. The Journal of Neuroscience, 21(5), 1452-1463.

Kuwabara, H.; Heishman, S. J.; Brasic, J. R.; Contoreggi, C.; Cascella, N.; Mackowick, K. M. et al. (2014). Mu opioid receptor binding correlates with nicotine dependence and reward in smokers. PLoS ONE, 9(12), e113694.

Laviolette, S. R.; van der Kooy, D. (2004). The neurobiology of nicotine addiction: bridging the gap from molecules to behaviour. Nature Reviews Neuroscience, 5(1), 55-65.

Leshner, A. I.; Stapleton, J. A. (1997). Addiction is a brain disease, and it matters. Science (New York, NY), 278(5335), 45-47.

Levin, E. D. (2002). Nicotinic receptor subtypes and cognitive function. Journal of Neurobiology, 53(4), 633-640.

Li, M. D.; Beuten, J.; Ma, J. Z.; Payne, T. J.; Lou, X.-Y.; Garcia, V. et al. (2005). Ethnic- and gender-specific association of the nicotinic acetylcholine receptor alpha4 subunit gene (CHRNA4) with nicotine dependence. Human Molecular Genetics, 14(9), 1211-1219.

Li, M. D.; Burmeister, M. (2009). New insights into the genetics of addiction. Nature Reviews Genetics, 10(4), 225-231.

Li, M. D.; Lou, X. Y.; Chen, G.; Ma, J. Z.; Elston, R. C. (2008). Gene-gene interactions among CHRNA4, CHRNB2, BDNF, and NTRK2 in nicotine dependence. Biological Psychiatry, 64(11), 951-957.

Mackillop, J.; Obasi, E.; Amlung, M. T.; McGeary, J. E.; Knopik, V. S. (2010). The role of genetics in nicotine dependence: mapping the pathways from genome to syndrome. Current Cardiovascular Risk Reports, 4(6), 446-453.

Maskos, U.; Molles, B. E.; Pons, S.; Besson, M.; Guiard, B. P.; Guilloux, J.-P. et al. (2005). Nicotine reinforcement and cognition restored by targeted expression of nicotinic receptors. Nature, 436(7047), 103-107.

McClure, E. A.; Vandrey, R. G.; Johnson, M. W.; Stitzer, M. L. (2013). Effects of varenicline on abstinence and smoking reward following a programmed lapse. Nicotine, Tobacco Research, 15(1), 139-148.

McClure-Begley, T. D.; Papke, R. L.; Stone, K. L.; Stokes, C.; Levy, A. D.; Gelernter, J. et al. (2014). Rare human nicotinic acetylcholine receptor 4 subunit (CHRNA4) variants affect expression and function of high-affinity nicotinic acetylcholine receptors. Journal of Pharmacology and Experimental Therapeutics, 348(3), 410-420.

McKinney, E. F.; Walton, R. T.; Yudkin, P.; Fuller, A.; Haldar, N. A.; Mant, D. et al. (2000). Association between polymorphisms in dopamine metabolic enzymes and tobacco consumption in smokers. Pharmacogenetics, 10(6), 483-491.

Morley, K. I.; Lynskey, M. T.; Madden, P. A.; Treloar, S. A.; Heath, A. C.; Martin, N. G. (2007). Exploring the inter-relationship of smoking age-at-onset, cigarette consumption and smoking persistence: genes or environment? Psychological Medicine, 37(9), 1357.

Nagy, A. (2000). Cre recombinase: the universal reagent for genome tailoring. Genesis, 26(2), 99-109.

Nees, F.; Witt, S. H.; Lourdusamy, A.; Vollstädt-Klein, S.; Steiner, S.; Poustka, L. et al. (2013). Genetic risk for nicotine dependence in the cholinergic system and activation of the brain reward system in healthy adolescents. Neuropsychopharmacology, 38(11), 2081-2089.

Ngolab, J.; Liu, L.; Zhao-Shea, R.; Gao, G.; Gardner, P. D.; Tapper, A. R. (2015). Functional upregulation of α4* nicotinic acetylcholine receptors in VTA GABAergic neurons increases sensitivity to nicotine reward. The Journal of Neuroscience, 35(22), 8570-8578.

Nides, M. (2008). Update on pharmacologic options for smoking cessation treatment. The American Journal of Medicine, 121(4), S20-S31.

Pang, X.; Liu, L.; Ngolab, J.; Zhao-Shea, R.; McIntosh, J. M.; Gardner, P. D. et al. (2016). Habenula cholinergic neurons regulate anxiety during nicotine withdrawal via nicotinic acetylcholine receptors. Neuropharmacology, 107, 294-304.

Picciotto, M. R.; Brunzell, D. H.; Caldarone, B. J. (2002). Effect of nicotine and nicotinic receptors on anxiety and depression. NeuroReport, 13(9), 1097-1106.

Picciotto, M. R.; Zoli, M.; Léna, C.; Bessis, A.; Lallemand, Y.; LeNovère, N. et al. (1995). Abnormal avoidance learning in mice lacking functional high-affinity nicotine receptor in the brain. Nature, 374(6517), 65-67.

Picciotto, M. R.; Zoli, M.; Rimondini, R.; Léna, C.; Marubio, L. M.; Pich, E. M. et al. (1998). Acetylcholine receptors containing the beta2 subunit are involved in the reinforcing properties of nicotine. Nature, 391(6663), 173-177.

Quick, M. W.; Lester, R. A. (2002). Desensitization of neuronal nicotinic receptors. Journal of Neurobiology, 53(4), 457-478.

Ray, R.; Mitra, N.; Baldwin, D.; Guo, M.; Patterson, F.; Heitjan, D. F. et al. (2010). Convergent evidence that choline acetyltransferase gene variation is associated with prospective smoking cessation and nicotine dependence. Neuropsychopharmacology, 35(6), 1374-1382.

Renthal, W.; Nestler, E. J. (2008). Epigenetic mechanisms in drug addiction. Trends in Molecular Medicine, 14(8), 341-350.

Rose, R. J.; Broms, U.; Korhonen, T.; Dick, D. M.; Kaprio, J. (2009). Genetics of smoking behavior. In Handbook of behavior genetics (pp. 411-432). New York, NY: Springer New York.

Saccone, S. F.; Hinrichs, A. L.; Saccone, N. L.; Chase, G. A.; Konvicka, K.; Madden, P. A. F. et al. (2006). Cholinergic nicotinic receptor genes implicated in a nicotine dependence association study targeting 348 candidate genes with 3713 SNPs. Human Molecular Genetics, 16(1), 36-49.

Silverman, M. A.; Neale, M. C.; Sullivan, P. F.; Harris-Kerr, C.; Wormley, B.; Sadek, H. et al. (2000). Haplotypes of four novel single nucleotide polymorphisms in the nicotinic acetylcholine receptor β2-subunit (CHRNB2) gene show no association with smoking initiation or nicotine dependence. American Journal of Medical Genetics, 96(5), 646-653.

Thorgeirsson, T. E.; Geller, F.; Sulem, P.; Rafnar, T.; Wiste, A.; Magnusson, K. P. et al. (2008). A variant associated with nicotine dependence, lung cancer and peripheral arterial disease. Nature, 452 (7187), 638-642.

Vandenbergh, D. J.; O'Connor, R. J.; Grant, M. D.; Jefferson, A. L.; Vogler, G. P.; Strasser, A. A. et al. (2007). Dopamine receptor genes (DRD2, DRD3 and DRD4) and gene-gene interactions associated with smoking-related behaviors. Addiction Biology, 12(1), 106-116.

Volkow, N. D. (2011). Epigenetics of nicotine: another nail in the coughing. Science Translational Medicine, 3(107), 107ps43.

Wei, J.; Ma, J. Z.; Payne, T. J.; Cui, W.; Ray, R.; Mitra, N. et al. (2010). Replication and extension of association of choline acetyltransferase with nicotine dependence in European and African American smokers. Human Genetics, 127(6), 691-698.

Zhao-Shea, R.; DeGroot, S. R.; Liu, L.; Vallaster, M.; Pang, X.; Su, Q. et al. (2015). Increased CRF signalling in a ventral tegmental area-interpeduncular nucleus-medial habenula circuit induces anxiety during nicotine withdrawal. Nature Communications, 6, 6770.

41
HIV 感染者与吸烟：关注烟碱对大脑的影响

Manuel Delgado-Vélez, José A. Lasalde-Dominicci

Department of Biology, University of Puerto Rico and the Clinical Bioreagent Center,
Molecular Sciences Research Center, San Juan, Puerto Rico

缩略语

AIDS	获得性免疫缺陷综合征	gp120	包膜糖蛋白 GP120
ANI	无症状性神经认知功能障碍	HAD	HIV 相关性痴呆
BBB	血脑屏障	HAND	HIV 相关性神经认知障碍
CCR5	C-C 趋化因子受体 5 型	HIV	人类免疫缺陷病毒
CDC	疾病控制和预防中心	MND	轻度神经认知障碍
CNS	中枢神经系统	nAChR	烟碱乙酰胆碱受体
CXCR4	C-X-C 趋化因子受体 4 型	PAM	正变构调节剂

41.1 引言

根据世界卫生组织（WHO）的数据，2015 年，全球约有 11 亿人吸烟。据估计，吸烟习惯每年造成约 600 万人死亡，其中约 89 万人死于二手烟（CDC, 2017; WHO, 2017）。此外，据推测，到 2030 年，烟草烟雾将导致全球约 800 万人死亡（CDC, 2017）。虽然香烟中最广为人知的成分是烟碱，但它们含有无数的有害化合物，包括一氧化碳、甲苯、焦油、镍和许多其他代表严重威胁健康的成分。即使对那些没有患病或感染的人来说，吸烟也是有害的。然而，在患有免疫功能受损疾病的人中，吸烟会显著降低他们有效对抗病原体的能力。艾滋病病毒感染提供了一个典型的例子，说明了在免疫功能受损的疾病状态下吸烟的有害影响。

在 HIV 感染者中，吸烟率高于正常人群。从烟雾中获得的烟碱与中枢神经系统（CNS）中的烟碱型乙酰胆碱受体（nAChR）相互作用，从而触发多巴胺释放，产生愉悦的效果，强化有害的吸烟习惯。烟碱是烟草烟雾中令人上瘾的成分，是 HIV 感染者的主要健康负担，因为它不仅会促进依赖性和成瘾，还会加速 HIV 相关性神经认知障碍（HAND）的出现。此外，吸烟与发展为获得性免疫缺陷综合征（AIDS）有关。烟碱的消费有多种认知影响，但总体而言，这些影响的天平倾向于弊大于利。

HIV 感染的特点是 CD4+ 表达细胞的生产性感染。然而，虽然神经元不表达 CD4，但一些神经元亚群确实表达 HIV 辅助受体（CXCR4 和 CCR5），它们与 HIV 可溶性病毒毒素（如 gp120）相互作用，从而触发信号转导通路。随着时间的推移，持续的慢性病毒感染会破坏免疫细胞，特别是 CD4+T 淋巴细胞，促使免疫缺陷的免疫系统出现，无法有效地对抗外来入侵者。更糟糕的是，在这种免疫受损的情况下，吸烟/烟碱的加入进一步降低了免疫系统对抗外来入侵者的能力，并使其复杂化。吸烟和烟碱对 HIV 感染有一系列影响，如病毒复制增加（Abbud, Finegan, Guay,

Rich, 1995; Rock et al. 2008)、巨噬细胞吞噬功能受损和T淋巴细胞功能调节。

41.2 吸烟产生的烟碱与大脑烟碱型乙酰胆碱受体

通常情况下，烟碱是直接从吸烟中获得的。烟碱为3-（1-甲基-2-吡咯烷基）吡啶，是一种挥发性生物碱，分子量为162.23g/mol。此外，它也是烟草中的主要精神活性成分，其吸收和肾脏排泄高度依赖于pH。在高pH（碱性）下，烟碱处于非电离状态，这与烟碱更容易通过脂蛋白膜的能力有关（CDC, 2010）。当吸入香烟烟雾时，25%的烟碱在大约7秒内到达大脑，大约是静脉给药时的两倍。虽然一些吸入的烟碱在肺部代谢，但80%～90%的烟碱在肝脏代谢，少量在肾脏代谢。烟碱的消除半衰期因人而异，但通常接近2小时（Benowitz,1988），吸烟者血液中烟碱的平均浓度为203nmol/L，范围为25～444nmol/L（Russell et al.1980）。在中枢神经系统，脑脊液研究显示烟碱浓度在37nmol/L～1.3μmol/L，而可替宁浓度范围为155nmol/L～2.6μmol/L（Malkawi et al. 2009）。可替宁是烟碱的主要氧化代谢物，代表烟碱消费或接触的标志。实际上，从感染艾滋病毒的轻/中度吸烟者和重度吸烟者中回收的血清样本中可替宁的定量中位数分别为2.1μmol/L和2.8μmol/L。此外，在轻度/中度（2.5μmol/L）和重度吸烟（3.6μmol/L）习惯的艾滋病毒感染静脉注射吸毒者中，观察到平均可替宁值更高（Marshall et al. 2011），这表明吸烟率更高。因此，感染艾滋病毒的吸毒者不太可能有无法检测到的病毒载量，并且经常患有影响抗逆转录病毒治疗和戒烟药物依从性的心理社会合并症（例如，抑郁和情绪障碍）（图41.1）。

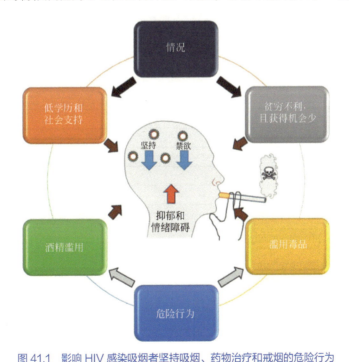

图 41.1　影响 HIV 感染吸烟者坚持吸烟、药物治疗和戒烟的危险行为
感染艾滋病病毒的吸烟者对戒烟疗法的依从性和戒烟率都很低，这两者都与危险行为有关。

如前所述，烟碱迅速到达中枢神经系统。烟碱的主要作用部位是大脑中的nAChR。这些跨膜蛋白是五聚体配体门控离子传导通道，对内源性激动剂（如乙酰胆碱和胆碱）或外源性物质

（如烟碱）开放。在大脑中，烟碱的存在和规律的摄入诱导了几种nAChR的上调，包括与烟碱成瘾有关的异构体α4β2 nAChR、α3β2 nAChR、α6β2 nAChR和同分异构体α7 nAChR（Govind et al. 2009）。事实上，对于α4β2，长期烟碱暴露导致受体脱敏和上调，这被认为在烟碱强化导致成瘾的过程中起着关键作用。因此，烟碱暴露增强了突触强度，并产生了对腹侧被盖区多巴胺能神经元的兴奋性突触的长期增强（Mansvelder, McGehee, 2000），从而加强了突触联系，使成瘾持续下去。

41.3　HIV感染吸烟者的戒烟努力

烟草烟雾中烟碱的成瘾特性使人很难戒烟。到目前为止，几种戒烟药物已经在HIV感染者身上进行了测试，结果显示戒烟率有限（Calvo-Sánchez, Martinez, 2015）（表41.1）。在这一人群中，低依从性戒烟药物治疗和低戒烟率是典型的（表41.1），并且与严重威胁健康的危险行为有关（图41.1）。测试的主要药理学策略包括烟碱替代疗法、安非他酮和瓦伦尼克林，并辅之以非药物干预方法，如动机咨询、动机干预、自助和行为支持（表41.1）。目前，正在进行六项临床试验，重点是艾滋病毒感染的吸烟者戒烟。这些试验涉及使用药理学和非药理学干预方法来增加戒烟效果（表41.2）。值得注意的是，其中三项试验使用了之前测试过的相同药物，安非他酮和伐伦克林（表41.2）。因此，需要更多的药物来治疗这些想戒烟、迫切需要增加抗逆转录病毒治疗依从性的人群。

表41.1　HIV感染吸烟者的戒烟研究

设计	处理方式	戒烟率/%
NR	NRT，心理咨询，技能培训	50
NR	NRT，激励性咨询，日志	22
NR	心理咨询，NRT	38
NR	安非他酮	38
NR	心理咨询，自助材料，NRT，手机干预，日常护理	10.3
NR	心理咨询，安非他酮，伐伦克林，或NRT	25
NR	伐伦克林	24
R	NRT，自助	22
R	NRT，激励性干预	9
NR	伐伦克林	42
R	心理咨询，NRT 计算机干预，NRT 自助，NRT	25.6 20.4 19.7
NR	量身定做的团体咨询，NRT	10
RS	NRT，伐伦克林，行为支持	13
S	伐伦克林，面对面咨询	15① 18②

① 由意向治疗分析确定。
② 由改良的意向治疗分析确定。
注：NR，非随机化的；R，随机的；NRT，烟碱替代疗法；RS，回顾研究。
使用药物疗法进行研究的描述。
摘自Calvo-Sánchez, Martinez (2015)。

表41.2 针对HIV感染吸烟者的正在进行的戒烟临床试验

研究标题	处理方式	研究类型	阶段	登记量
对艾滋病病毒携带者妇女的戒烟干预	行为疗法：认知，行为疗法	介入性	N/A	50
艾滋病病毒携带者戒烟的故事叙事性沟通干预	组合产品：讲故事叙事干预	介入性	阶段1	50
艾滋病病毒携带者/艾滋病患者的戒烟	药物疗法：安非他酮 行为疗法：简短咨询，高额奖金应急管理，受监督的戒烟支持，奖励戒酒应急管理，低强度奖品应急管理	介入性	N/A	400
HIV阳性吸烟者的斑贴研究干预	其他疗法：综合疗法，标准护理干预	介入性	阶段4	600
优化HIV/AIDS吸烟者的戒烟方式	药物疗法：伐伦克林，安慰剂 行为疗法：积极无烟和标准护理	介入性	阶段3	300
吸烟和戒烟对全身和气道免疫激活的影响	行为疗法：心理咨询 药物疗法：戒烟药物	介入性	N/A	120

注：N/A，不详。
目前的临床试验测试艾滋病病毒感染吸烟者的药理和/或行为方法。
2018年3月24日，国家卫生研究院、国家医学图书馆（ClinicalTrials.gov）汇编的数据。

41.4　HIV感染者对吸烟的依赖性和流行率

与未感染的人相比，感染HIV-1的人更容易依赖烟碱，戒烟的可能性更小。最近的一项戒烟研究发现，83%的接受戒烟药物（烟碱替代疗法、伐伦克林、安非他酮和/或联合治疗）的患者在至少一次或多次随访中没有坚持戒烟治疗（Chew et al. 2014）。重要的是，吸烟依赖和危险行为（如冲动）密切相关。因此，感染艾滋病病毒的强效吸烟者对烟碱的依赖程度高于专有注射者或专有强效吸烟者（Hershberger et al. 2004）。值得注意的是，在越南进行的一项确定吸烟是否影响抗逆转录病毒治疗依从性的横断面研究中，在接受检查的患者中发现了较高的依从性，那些烟碱依赖程度较高的患者更有可能不坚持抗逆转录病毒治疗（Nguyen et al. 2016）。

几项研究已经证实，HIV-1阳性个体的吸烟流行率是HIV-1阴性人群的三到四倍（Manda et al. 2010），吸烟者占受感染者的40%～84%（Browning et al. 2013）。吸烟对艾滋病病毒感染者的影响是毁灭性的。在丹麦感染艾滋病病毒的队列中，研究表明，吸烟和不吸烟显著减少了12.3年的寿命；在艾滋病不吸烟者和普通不吸烟者的对照组中，寿命年损失的数字是5.1；在吸烟和不吸烟的对照组中，这一数字是3.6（Helleberg et al. 2013）（图41.2）。因此，艾滋病病毒感染者因吸烟而损失的寿命比因艾滋病病毒感染而损失的寿命更多。与此一致的是，众所周知，HIV-1阳性人群与烟草相关的发病率和死亡率更高，吸烟已成为HIV携带者中的头号杀手（Stanton et al. 2015）。人口统计学研究还表明，烟草使用和艾滋病毒感染之间存在正相关关系。对卢旺达（Chao et al. 1994）和海地（Boulos et al. 1990）孕妇进行的横断面调查（控制了许多危险因素）发现，吸烟增加了艾滋病毒血清转换率。此外，一项对美国同性恋男性进行风险调整的队列研究还发现，吸烟与艾滋病病毒感染之间存在正相关（Burns et al. 1991）。除了这些研究，越来越多的证据表明，吸烟与艾滋病（Zhao et al. 2010）和HIV相关性痴呆（HAD）进展更快有关（Manda et al. 2010）。

因此，HIV感染和吸烟对这一人群来说是致命的组合，因为它促进了危险行为，可能导致非法药物使用，未能坚持抗逆转录病毒治疗，并已发展起来。

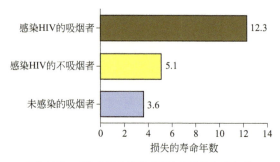

图41.2　感染艾滋病毒的吸烟者损失的寿命年数

艾滋病病毒感染的吸烟者因吸烟而损失的寿命比因艾滋病病毒而损失的寿命更多。感染艾滋病病毒的吸烟者失去的寿命是不吸烟对照组的两倍多。对照研究来自哥本哈根总人口研究。Helleberg et al.（2013）。

41.5　吸烟和烟碱对HIV感染者的影响

HIV感染者患有神经系统并发症，尽管有效的药物病毒抑制，可接受的CD4+细胞计数，并且没有症状，但这些并发症仍然存在。详细而全面的神经学研究已将患者的神经症状定性并归类为HAND症状（表41.3）。这一人群的HAND患病率为20%～69%不等（Carroll, Brew, 2017），包括无症状性神经认知障碍（ANI）、HIV相关的轻度神经认知障碍（MND）和HIV相关性痴呆（HAD），其中HAD是神经认知恶化的最严重形式（Antinori et al. 2007）（表 41.3）。如前所述，与未感染HIV的吸烟者相比，吸烟者在工作记忆、处理速度和个体内变异性方面的表现更差，这就证明了吸烟会加速HAND的现象（Harrison et al. 2017）。重要的是，最近的一项研究确定了烟碱和HIV协同作用对突触可塑性基因表达和脊柱密度进行负面调节的独特联系，这可能导致吸烟者HAND的风险增加（Atluri et al. 2014）。此外，众所周知，烟碱损害了体外和体内研究确定的血脑屏障（BBB）的完整性（Hawkins et al. 2004; Manda et al. 2010），从而促进了艾滋病毒感染的巨噬细胞招募到中枢神经系统，并加速了HAND的出现（图41.3）。

表41.3　HAND分类

HAND阶段	描述和特点
ANI[①]	认知功能获得性损害，至少涉及两个能力领域。这种损害不会干扰日常功能，也不符合精神错乱或痴呆症的标准
MND[①]	这种认知障碍会对日常功能（工作、家庭生活和社会活动）产生明显的干扰。 认知障碍的模式不符合精神错乱的标准（例如，意识模糊不是一个突出的特征）
HAD	明显的获得性认知功能损害，至少涉及两个能力领域；通常，这种损害涉及多个领域，特别是在学习新信息、信息处理速度减慢和注意力/注意力缺陷方面。HAD对日常运作产生了明显的干扰

① 神经心理学评估必须至少考察以下能力：言语/语言、注意力/工作记忆、抽象/执行、记忆（学习、回忆）、信息处理速度和感觉-知觉-运动技能。

注：HIV感染者HAND的分类和诊断标准。

改编自 Ramachandran, V.S. (Eds.). (2002). Grant I: The neurocognitive complications of HIV infection. In Encyclopedia of the human brain (pp. 475-489). San Diego: Academic Press.

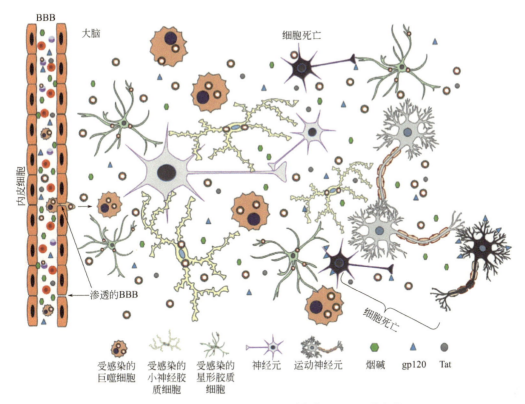

图 41.3 艾滋病病毒、其成分和烟碱有助于 HAND 的出现

循环中的 HIV 病毒毒素和烟碱能渗透血脑屏障，促进受感染的巨噬细胞进入大脑。一旦到达那里，HIV 病毒粒子感染星形胶质细胞和小胶质细胞，可溶性 gp120 和 Tat 促进神经元死亡，从而促进 HAND 的出现。

一旦进入大脑，HIV 就会感染小胶质细胞和星形胶质细胞。星形胶质细胞对血脑屏障的形成、建立和维持至关重要。然而，一旦星形胶质细胞被感染，中枢神经系统中病毒成分（例如 gp120）和细胞因子的存在，加上病毒毒素（例如 Tat）的全身循环，会损害血脑屏障的完整性，从而促进新感染的巨噬细胞的渗透，最终造成更高的神经元损伤（图 41.3）。此外，在烟碱的存在下，神经元的损伤会加剧，因为烟碱也会渗透到血脑屏障中，这也有助于 HAND 的发育（图 41.3）。就神经元而言，它们也暴露在 HIV 感染的吸烟者体内的 HIV、病毒蛋白和烟碱中。在大鼠中的现有研究表明，病毒蛋白（如 Tat）可影响中皮质边缘多巴胺系统，改变 cAMP 反应元件结合蛋白和细胞外信号调节激酶信号（Midde et al. 2011），该神经回路由表达 α4β2 烟碱型乙酰胆碱受体的烟碱反应多巴胺能神经元组成。值得注意的是，烟碱激活 α4β2 烟碱型乙酰胆碱受体可增加多巴胺能神经元的放电频率，提升前额叶皮层和伏隔核中的多巴胺水平，从而提供快感。此外，α4β2 烟碱型乙酰胆碱受体的激活介导烟碱奖励和焦虑缓解（McGranahan et al. 2011），这加强了吸烟习惯并使成瘾持续。

吸烟不仅会影响艾滋病病毒感染者的中枢神经系统，还会影响他们的免疫系统。据报道，烟草的核素可以促进体外感染的肺泡巨噬细胞和小胶质细胞（脑巨噬细胞）中 HIV-1 的产生，因为它以 TGF-β1 依赖的方式增强了 HIV-1 的水平（Abbud et al. 1995），据报道，烟草的核素可以促进体外感染的肺泡巨噬细胞和小胶质细胞（脑巨噬细胞）中 HIV-1 的产生（Rock et al. 2008）。有趣的是，在 T 淋巴细胞中，烟草烟雾提取物增加了 HIV 的传染性和不依赖烟碱和一氧化碳的病毒产量。这是通过上调已知能够增强艾滋病病毒感染或保护艾滋病病毒本身的基因，以及下调几个与细胞防御和抗原呈递有关的基因来实现的（Zhao et al. 2010）。这表明烟碱的增强前病毒效应是细胞依赖的，吸烟的其他成分也可以促进这些患者中HIV的增殖。总体而言，吸烟和烟碱会影响中枢神经系统，并加剧HIV感染者的HIV感染。

另一方面，无论是在体外还是在体内，烟碱和吸烟都与α7烟碱型乙酰胆碱受体上调有关。事实上，在感染艾滋病病毒的吸烟者中，他们的单核细胞上调了α7 nAChR。此外，单核细胞、T淋巴细胞和单核细胞来源的巨噬细胞的α7 nAChR表达上调，尽管处于吸烟状态。

41.6 艾滋病病毒感染吸烟者认知状况调查

吸烟影响HIV感染者的认知。现有的少数几项调查吸烟对艾滋病病毒感染吸烟者的影响的研究得出了相互矛盾的结果。在吸烟的HIV感染的酗酒者中进行的第一项这样的研究发现，吸烟给接受检查的患者的神经生物学和神经认知造成了额外的负担，导致吸烟者的认知表现比不吸烟者更差（Durazzo et al. 2007）。第二项研究是一项观察性横断面研究，显示吸烟史与HIV血清阳性妇女较好的额叶/执行认知域表现以及较差的病毒免疫状况相关（Wojna et al. 2007）。类似地，使用HIV-1转基因大鼠对神经结构的评估表明，烟碱"纠正"了前额叶皮层、背侧纹状体和海马体因HIV-1感染而改变的几条通路（Cao et al. 2013）。相比之下，对正在接受HIV感染治疗的患者的第三项研究结果表明，目前吸烟与学习、记忆和全球认知功能呈负相关。这些作者的结论是，吸烟可能只是反映了一种普遍的倾向，即更广泛的缺陷和共病，而不是直接影响认知功能（Bryant et al. 2013）。最后，最近的一项研究报告说，感染艾滋病病毒的长期吸烟者表现出冲动、抑郁和认知功能障碍（Chang et al. 2017）（图41.1）。这些研究之间的差异可能是由于患者群体的性别和种族差异，烟碱浓度测定的固有困难，以及吸烟频率和吸烟类型所致。综上所述，关于HIV环境下吸烟的一般结论（Evans, Drobes, 2009; Wojna et al. 2007）与烟碱在精神分裂症、注意力缺陷多动障碍和阿尔茨海默病患者中的认知增强作用形成了鲜明对比（Jasinska et al. 2014）。烟碱，而不是吸烟，开启了使用胆碱能激动剂、正变构调节剂（PAMs）或拮抗剂来治疗HIV引起的神经缺陷的可能性。

术语解释
- 获得性免疫缺陷综合征（AIDS）：由艾滋病病毒引起的免疫系统疾病。
- 血脑屏障：保护神经组织免受循环毒素的伤害，并允许水、气体和营养物质通过。
- 中枢神经系统：由大脑和脊髓组成的系统。
- 胆碱能激动剂：刺激或激活烟碱型乙酰胆碱受体的药物。
- 胆碱能抑制剂：抑制或阻断烟碱型乙酰胆碱受体的药物。
- 脱敏：当配体门控受体反复或长期暴露在配体中，促进其反应性降低并导致非导电状态时，就会发生这种情况。
- HAND：这个术语用来描述与HIV感染相关的无数神经认知功能障碍。
- HIV：一种逆转录病毒，优先感染和破坏表达表面受体CD4的细胞，包括T淋巴细胞。

- HIV相关性痴呆（HAD）：艾滋病病毒感染者所遭受的最严重的认知障碍形式，出现在中枢神经系统的艾滋病病毒感染和炎症中。
- 长时程增强：指突触兴奋性突触后电位幅度的持续增加，通常由短暂的高频传入刺激引起。
- 正变构调节剂：胆碱能增强剂，拯救脱敏的烟碱型乙酰胆碱受体。
- 上调：细胞内烟碱型乙酰胆碱受体数量的增加。
- 腹侧被盖区：一种由多巴胺能神经元组成的结构，位于中脑内，将神经束延伸到边缘和皮质区域。
- α4β2 nAChR：一种由五个亚基组成的异构型烟碱乙酰胆碱受体，主要在哺乳动物的大脑中表达，对烟碱有很高的亲和力。
- α7 nAChR：一种同源烟碱乙酰胆碱受体，由神经细胞和免疫细胞表达的五个亚基组成。

HAND的关键事实

- 自从第一份报告显示艾滋病病毒相关的神经系统并发症以来，已经过去了近30年。
- 最严重的HAND和HAD的发生率相对较低（2%～4%），但较轻的形式在无艾滋病的HIV感染者中为30%，在HIV感染者中为50%。
- 在接受抗逆转录病毒治疗或接受早期治疗（病毒抑制）的患者中，HAND感染率为20%～69%。
- 临床研究人员一致认为，使用神经心理学方法可以准确识别中度到重度HAND疾病；然而，区分MND和ANI是具有挑战性的，他们更喜欢报告MND和HAD。
- 排除ANI的诊断是一个令人担忧的问题，因为这种轻微的HAND水平预示着更多的认知能力下降。
- 最近的证据表明，抗逆转录病毒药物马拉韦罗改善了病毒学抑制的HIV感染者的神经认知能力。

烟碱诱导的α4β2 nAChR上调的关键事实

- 烟碱一旦摄入，就会到达大脑，并与基础的α4β2 nAChR相互作用，促进变化。已提出三种机制来解释烟碱诱导的上调。
- 机制1：α4β2 nAChR数目增加。这种机制包括减少表面周转，增加组装和成熟，增加向细胞表面的运输，以及减慢亚基的降解。
- 机制2：烟碱诱导的化学计量学改变，包括亚基的改变，而不增加α4β2 nAChR的数量。
- 机制3：烟碱诱导的上调可通过构象改变而不改变α4β2 nAChR的数量。
- 烟碱暴露后受体脱敏启动了α4β2 nAChR的上调。

要点总结

- 本章重点讨论吸烟和烟碱消费对HIV感染者的影响。
- 艾滋病病毒感染者的吸烟率比非感染者高出三到四倍。
- 烟碱迅速扩散到大脑，激活、脱敏和/或上调nAChR，如α4β2 nAChR和α7 nAChR。
- 艾滋病病毒感染者患有被称为HAND的神经损伤。
- HAND患病率相对较高（20%～69%），包括ANI、MND和HAD。
- 虽然已经发现了一些认知上的好处，但吸烟和烟碱会加速HAND的出现。
- 吸烟和烟碱会加剧艾滋病。
- 胆碱能激动剂、PAMs和拮抗剂可作为治疗吸烟和手部疾病的选择。

参考文献

Abbud, R. A.; Finegan, C. K.; Guay, L. A.; Rich, E. A. (1995). Enhanced production of human immunodeficiency virus type 1 by in vitro-infected alveolar macrophages from otherwise healthy cigarette smokers. The Journal of Infectious Diseases, 172, 859-863.

Antinori, A.; Arendt, G.; Becker, J. T.; Brew, B. J.; Byrd, D. A.; Cherner, M. et al. (2007). Updated research nosology for HIV-associated neurocognitive disorders. Neurology, 69, 1789-1799.

Atluri, V. S. R.; Pilakka-Kanthikeel, S.; Samikkannu, T.; Sagar, V.; Kurapati, K. R. V.; Saxena, S. K. et al. (2014). Vorinostat positively regulates synaptic plasticity genes expression and spine density in HIV infected neurons: role of nicotine in progression of HIV-associated neurocognitive disorder. Molecular Brain, 7, 37.

Benowitz, N. L. (1988). Nicotine and smokeless tobacco. CA: A Cancer Journal for Clinicians, 38, 244-247.

Boulos, R.; Halsey, N. A.; Holt, E.; Ruff, A.; Brutus, J. R.; Quinn, T. C. et al. (1990). HIV-1 in Haitian women 1982-1988. The Cite Soleil/JHU AIDS Project Team. Journal of Acquired Immune Deficiency Syndrome, 3, 721-728.

Browning, K. K.; Wewers, M. E.; Ferketich, A. K.; Diaz, P. (2013). Tobacco use and cessation in HIV-infected individuals. Clinics in Chest Medicine, 34, 181-190.

Bryant, V. E.; Kahler, C. W.; Devlin, K. N.; Monti, P. M.; Cohen, R. A. (2013). The effects of cigarette smoking on learning and memory performance among people living with HIV/AIDS. AIDS Care, 25, 1308-1316.

Burns, D. N.; Kramer, A.; Yellin, F.; Fuchs, D.; Wachter, H.; DiGioia, R. A. et al. (1991). Cigarette smoking: a modifier of human immunodeficiency virus type 1 infection? Journal of Acquired Immune Deficiency Syndromes, 4, 7 6-83.

Calvo-Sánchez, M.; Martinez, E. (2015). How to address smoking cessation in HIV patients. HIV Medicine, 16, 201-210.

Cao, J.; Wang, S.; Wang, J.; Cui, W.; Nesil, T.; Vigorito, M. et al. (2013). RNA deep sequencing analysis reveals that nicotine restores impaired gene expression by viral proteins in the brains of HIV-1 transgenic rats. PLoS One, 8, e68517.

Carroll, A.; Brew, B. (2017). HIV-associated neurocognitive disorders: recent advances in pathogenesis, biomarkers, and treatment. F1000Research, 6.

CDC (2017) Announcement: World No Tobacco Day. (2017). MMWR Morb. Mortal. Wkly. Rep. 66, 545.

CDC, National Center for Chronic Disease Prevention and Health Promotion (US), Office on Smoking and Health (US)(2010) Nicotine addiction: past and present. Centers for Disease Control and Prevention (US).

Chang, L.; Lim, A.; Lau, E.; Alicata, D. (2017). Chronic tobacco-smoking on psychopathological symptoms, impulsivity and cognitive deficits in HIV-infected individuals. Journal of Neuroimmune Pharmacology: The Official Journal of Society on NeuroImmune Pharmacology, 12, 389-401.

Chao, A.; Bulterys, M.; Musanganire, F.; Habimana, P.; Nawrocki, P.; Taylor, E. et al. (1994). Risk factors associated with prevalent HIV-1 infection among pregnant women in Rwanda. National University of Rwanda-Johns Hopkins University AIDS Research Team. International of Journal of Epidemiology, 23, 371-380.

Chew, D.; Steinberg, M. B.; Thomas, P.; Swaminathan, S.; Hodder, S. L. (2014). Evaluation of a smoking cessation program for HIV infected individuals in an urban HIV clinic: challenges and lessons learned. AIDS Research and Treatment, 2014.

Durazzo, T. C.; Rothlind, J. C.; Cardenas, V. A.; Studholme, C.; Weiner, M. W.; Meyerhoff, D. J. (2007). Chronic cigarette smoking and heavy drinking in human immunodeficiency virus: consequences for neurocognition and brain morphology. Alcohol Fayetteville N, 41, 489-501.

Evans, D. E.; Drobes, D. J. (2009). Nicotine self-medication of cognitive-attentional processing. Addiction Biology, 14, 32-42.

Govind, A. P.; Vezina, P.; Green, W. N. (2009). Nicotine-induced upregulation of nicotinic receptors: underlying mechanisms and relevance to nicotine addiction. Biochemical Pharmacology, 78, 756-765.

Harrison, J. D.; Dochney, J. A.; Blazekovic, S.; Leone, F.; Metzger, D.; Frank, I. et al. (2017). The nature and consequences of cognitive deficits among tobacco smokers with HIV: a comparison to tobacco smokers without HIV. Journal of Neurovirology, 23, 550-557.

Hawkins, B. T.; Abbruscato, T. J.; Egleton, R. D.; Brown, R. C.; Huber, J. D.; Campos, C. R. et al. (2004). Nicotine increases in vivo blood-brain barrier permeability and alters cerebral microvascular tight junction protein distribution. Brain Research, 1027, 48-58.

Helleberg, M.; Afzal, S.; Kronborg, G.; Larsen, C. S.; Pedersen, G.; Pedersen, C. et al. (2013). Mortality attributable to smoking among HIV-1-infected individuals: a nationwide, population-based cohort study. Clinical Infectious Diseases, 56, 727-734.

Hershberger, S. L.; Fisher, D. G.; Reynolds, G. L.; Klahn, J. A.; Wood, M. M. (2004). Nicotine dependence and HIV risk behaviors among illicit drug users. Addictive Behaviors, 29, 623-625.

Jasinska, A. J.; Zorick, T.; Brody, A. L.; Stein, E. A. (2014). Dual role of nicotine in addiction and cognition: a review of neuroimaging studies in humans. Neuropharmacology, 84, 111-122.

Malkawi, A. H.; Al-Ghananeem, A. M.; de Leon, J.; Crooks, P. A. (2009). Nicotine exposure can be detected in cerebrospinal fluid of active and passive smokers. Journal of Pharmaceutical and Biomedical Analysis, 49, 129-132.

Manda, V. K.; Mittapalli, R. K.; Geldenhuys, W. J.; Lockman, P. R. (2010). Chronic exposure to nicotine and saquinavir decreases endothelial Notch-4 expression and disrupts blood-brain barrier integrity. Journal of Neurochemistry, 115, 515-525.

Mansvelder, H. D.; McGehee, D. S. (2000). Long-term potentiation of excitatory inputs to brain reward areas by nicotine. Neuron, 27, 349-357.

Marshall, M. M.; Kirk, G. D.; Caporaso, N. E.; McCormack, M. C.; Merlo, C. A.; Hague, J. C. et al. (2011). Tobacco use and nicotine dependence among HIV-infected and uninfected injection drug users. Addictive Behaviors, 36, 61-67.

McGranahan, T. M.; Patzlaff, N. E.; Grady, S. R.; Heinemann, S. F.; Booker, T. K. (2011). alpha4beta2 nicotinic acetylcholine receptors on dopaminergic neurons mediate nicotine reward and anxiety relief. Journal of Neuroscience: The Official Journal of the Society for Neuroscience, 31, 10891-10902.

Midde, N. M.; Gomez, A. M.; Harrod, S. B.; Zhu, J. (2011). Genetically expressed HIV-1 viral proteins attenuate nicotine-induced behavioral sensitization and alter mesocorticolimbic ERK and CREB signaling in rats. Pharmacology, Biochemistry, and Behavior, 98, 587-597.

Nguyen, N. T. P.; Tran, B. X.; Hwang, L. Y.; Markham, C. M.; Swartz, M. D.; Vidrine, J. I. et al. (2016). Effects of cigarette smoking and nicotine dependence on adherence to antiretroviral therapy among HIV-positive patients in Vietnam. AIDS Care, 28, 359-364.

Rock, R. B.; Gekker, G.; Aravalli, R. N.; Hu, S.; Sheng, W. S.; Peterson, P. K. (2008). Potentiation of HIV-1 expression in microglial cells by nicotine: Involvement of transforming growth factor-beta 1. Journal of Neuroimmune Pharmacology: An Official Journal of Society Neuroimmune Pharmacology, 3, 143-149.

Russell, M. A.; Jarvis, M.; Iyer, R.; Feyerabend, C. (1980). Relation of nicotine yield of cigarettes to blood nicotine concentrations in smokers. British Medical Journal, 280, 972-976.

Stanton, C. A.; Papandonatos, G. D.; Shuter, J.; Bicki, A.; Lloyd-Richardson, E. E.; de Dios, M. A. et al. (2015). Outcomes of a tailored intervention for cigarette smoking cessation among Latinos living with HIV/AIDS. Nicotine, Tobacco Research: The Official Journal of the Society for Research on Nicotine and Tobacco, 17, 975-982.

WHO. (2017). WHO j tobacco [WWW document]. WHO, URL(2017). http:// www. who. int/mediacentre/factsheets/fs339/en/.

Wojna, V.; Robles, L.; Skolasky, R. L.; Mayo, R.; Selnes, O.; de la Torre, T. et al. (2007). Associations of cigarette smoking with viral immune and cognitive function in human immunodeficiency virus-seropositive women. Journal of Neurovirology, 13, 561-568.

Zhao, L.; Li, F.; Zhang, Y.; Elbourkadi, N.; Wang, Z.; Yu, C. et al. (2010). Mechanisms and genes involved in enhancement of HIV infectivity by tobacco smoke. Toxicology, 278, 242-248.

42
肾素 - 血管紧张素系统基因与烟碱依赖

Sergej Nadalin[1], *Hrvoje Jakovac*[2]

1. Department of Biology and Medical Genetics, School of Medicine, University of Rijeka, Rijeka, Croatia
2. Department of Physiology, Immunology and Pathophysiology, School of Medicine, University of Rijeka, Rijeka, Croatia

缩略语

ACE	血管紧张素转换酶	**I/D 多态性**	插入/缺失多态性
AT$_1$	血管紧张素Ⅱ受体1型	**MS**	多发性硬化症
AT$_2$	血管紧张素Ⅱ受体2型	**nAChR**	烟碱乙酯胆碱受体
AT$_4$	血管紧张素Ⅱ受体4型	**RAS**	肾素-血管紧张素系统

42.1 引言

在大脑中，星形胶质细胞合成血管紧张素原，血管紧张素原通常被肾素分解；肾素在脑组织中的浓度很低。血管紧张素转换酶（ACE）将血管紧张素Ⅰ转化为活性血管紧张素Ⅱ，血管紧张素Ⅱ再代谢为血管紧张素Ⅲ和血管紧张素Ⅳ；血管紧张素Ⅱ和血管紧张素Ⅳ可以分别转化为血管紧张素（1～7）和血管紧张素（3～7）（Guimond, Gallo-Payet, 2012; McKinley et al. 2003; Wright, Harding, 2013）（图42.1）。作为脑RAS的主要效应者，血管紧张素Ⅱ既是一种循环激素，影响心血管和电解质的稳态，又是一种神经肽，起神经递质的作用。其生物学作用主要由血管紧张素Ⅱ受体1型（AT$_1$）和2型（AT$_2$）介导。AT$_1$受体存在于大脑各处，但在多巴胺能区尤其丰富，如基底神经节和下丘脑。AT$_2$受体在大脑中的表达密度很低，仅限于特定区域（Guimond, Gallo-Payet, 2012; Marchese et al. 2016; Wright, Harding, 2013）。此外，已经证明AT$_2$受体的激活会导致与经典的AT$_1$受体介导的作用相反；因此，AT$_2$拮抗AT$_1$的许多作用（图42.1）（Guimond, Gallo-Payet, 2012; Labandeira-García et al., 2014）。此外，在大脑中还发现了其他与RAS相关的受体，包括肾素原受体、Mas受体和血管紧张素Ⅱ受体4型（AT$_4$）（Guimond, Gallo-Payet,2012;Wright, Harding, 2013）（图42.2）。

科学家们一直对大脑RAS影响中脑边缘通路中的多巴胺能信号的能力感兴趣，众所周知，中脑边缘通路在药物滥用的成瘾特性中起着关键作用。在大鼠纹状体中，血管紧张素Ⅱ刺激多巴胺的神经传递，几种ACE抑制剂（卡托普利、依那普利和培哚普利）已被证明可以调节多巴胺的周转（Jenkins, Chai, Mendelsohn, 1997; Jenkins, Mendelsohn, Chai, 1997; Obata et al. 2008）。行为学研究表明，脑RAS功能是由纹状体多巴胺能系统介导的。例如，多巴胺拮抗剂氟哌啶醇影响运动和刻板行为，几种ACE抑制剂可消除阿扑吗啡诱导的大鼠和小鼠的刻板行为；ACE抑制剂卡托普利可减少吗啡诱导的条件性位置偏好和吗啡自给药（Banks et al. 1994; Georgiev et al.

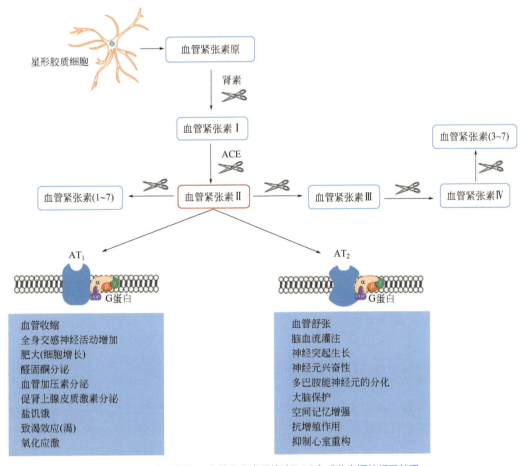

图 42.1　大脑肾素 – 血管紧张素系统（RAS）成分之间的相互关系

星形胶质细胞分泌失活的血管紧张素原，然后被血管紧张素转换酶（ACE）连续酶切（剪刀）。这导致血管紧张素Ⅱ的形成，血管紧张素Ⅱ是RAS的主要效应器。血管紧张素Ⅱ的作用主要通过血管紧张素Ⅱ受体1型（AT_1）和2型（AT_2）介导。

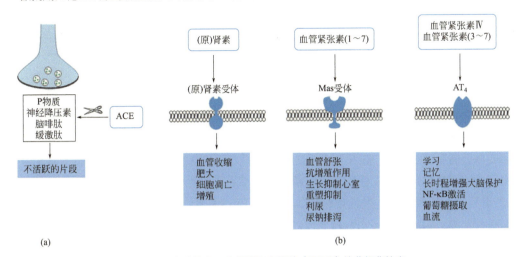

图 42.2　大脑肾素 – 血管紧张素系统（RAS）的非经典效应

（a）除了它的主要底物（血管紧张素原），血管紧张素转换酶（ACE）还可以切割（剪刀）和灭活肽类神经递质，如P物质、神经降压素、脑啡肽和缓激肽；（b）指示的RAS成分结合并激活（原）肾素受体、Mas受体和血管紧张素Ⅱ受体4型（AT_4），从而产生指示的效果。

1985; Hosseini et al.2007）。新的发现表明，RAS的成分会因药物滥用而发生显著变化。在大鼠中，饮酒降低了内侧前额叶皮质的AT_1受体密度，增加了血管紧张素原的表达（Sommer et al. 2007）；可卡因对中枢神经系统的影响被认为是额叶皮质和纹状体ACE活性和表达增加所致（Visniauskas et al. 2012）。此外，苯丙胺诱导的大鼠运动敏感化和神经认知改变与伏隔核和尾壳核中AT_1受体密度的变化有关（Marchese et al. 2016; Paz et al. 2014）。

RAS的成分是由基因决定的，基因被认为在物质滥用的脆弱性中扮演着重要的角色。然而，支持脑RAS在人群成瘾病因中的作用的数据很少；只有几项遗传学研究调查了一些RAS相关基因的多态变异（Baghai et al. 2008; Garrib, Peters, 1998; Hubacek et al. 2004; Hubacek et al. 2001; Nadalin et al. 2017; Nadalin, Ristić et al. 2017; Serý et al. 2001）。这些研究主要集中在烟碱依赖上；其中包括健康受试者和患有多种疾病/状况的个体，如抑郁症、多发性硬化症（MS）和精神分裂症。在这些疾病的背景下烟碱依赖的病因似乎很复杂；一个看似合理的潜在机制可能是一些基因变异可能导致对疾病和烟碱依赖的双重易感性（de Leon, Diaz, 2005）。因此，在疾病的背景下研究烟碱依赖的遗传学可能会为烟碱依赖提供新的见解，此外，还可以提高我们对这些疾病的发病机制的理解。在本章中，我们讨论了RAS相关基因与烟碱依赖的研究。最后，我们将把我们的视角转向未来的遗传和/或环境研究，这些研究可能揭示RAS成分和烟碱依赖之间的联系。

42.2 脑RAS基因可能与烟碱依赖有关

血管紧张素转换酶（ACE）基因（17q23）第16内含子的功能性插入/缺失（I/D）多态性（rs1799752），与ACE循环、细胞内和脑组织中的水平相关，其特征是287 bp的Alu重复序列的存在或缺失。已证实ACE-I/D多态性约占ACE水平的50%。D等位基因纯合子个体的ACE水平最高，ACE-I等位基因纯合子个体的ACE水平最低，而I和D等位基因杂合子个体的ACE水平居中（Rigat et al. 1990）。ACE-I/D多态性是研究最多的RAS相关多态变异。到目前为止，它是唯一一个与吸烟行为的病因相关的RAS相关多态性研究。大多数调查ACE-I/D多态性与吸烟行为相关性的研究都研究了健康个体（表42.1和表42.2）。Hubacek等（2001）首次推测ACE-I/D多态性可能通过影响多巴胺能神经传递而在吸烟行为中发挥作用。他们对捷克共和国的健康个体进行了两项研究；一项小规模的试点研究只包括男性受试者，另一项较大的研究包括了两种性别的个体。Baghai等（2008）假设ACE-I/D多态性可能在基因上调节吸烟行为，因此，这种多态性可能是心血管疾病和抑郁症之间高度相关的基础。他们调查了这种多态变异是否影响德国人群中抑郁症患者的吸烟习惯。为了控制抑郁状态对吸烟行为的潜在影响，他们还在研究中纳入了一小部分心理和心血管健康的对照组。在我们小组之前在克罗地亚和斯洛文尼亚人群中进行的研究中，我们研究了ACE-I/D变异与多发性硬化症和精神分裂症患者吸烟行为的潜在相关性（Nadalin et al. 2017）。有证据表明吸烟对多发性硬化症（MS）有不利影响；烟草烟雾的成分与脱髓鞘和轴突变性有关；此外，烟碱会损害血脑屏障，对T淋巴细胞有免疫调节作用（Ramanujam et al. 2015; Zhang et al. 2016）。我们推测ACE-I/D多态性可能与MS风险增加间接相关，主要是通过导致习惯性吸烟。我们还提出，ACE-I/D多态性可能通过影响中脑边缘通路（介导阳性和阴性精神分裂症症状）中的多巴胺能信号，参与精神分裂症与烟碱依赖之间的关系。据估计，精神分裂症患者的吸烟率为70%～80%，大约2/3的吸烟患者被归类为重度吸烟者［每天吸烟≥30支（1.5包）

（de Leon, Diaz, 2005）。一些研究已经报道了ACE-I/D多态性、MS和精神分裂症之间有趣的相关性，这促使我们调查这种多态变异是否可能与这些疾病患者的吸烟行为有关。如表42.3所示，在一些人群研究中，ACE-I/D多态性导致MS和精神分裂症风险增加（Crescenti et al. 2009; Kucukali et al. 2010; Lovrečić et al. 2006; Mazaheri, Saadat, 2015; Živković et al. 2016），并影响精神分裂症的严重程度，这是基于阳性和阴性综合征量表的精神病理学评估（Hui et al. 2014; Hui et al. 2015; Nadalin et al. 2012）。我们之前在克罗地亚和斯洛文尼亚人群中进行的研究也发现了其中一些积极的关联；此外，我们的数据表明，多态性的影响可能是性别特有的。研究发现ACE-I/D多态性与抑郁症呈正相关；事实上，ACE-I/D变异与疾病的发生有关（Stewart et al. 2009）。地塞米松/促肾上腺皮质激素释放激素试验结果表明，ACE-I/D变异与下丘脑-垂体肾上腺皮质系统的改变有关，这是抑郁症的主要神经内分泌异常（Baghai et al. 2002）。最后，一项荟萃分析表明，ACE-I/D多态变异对抑郁症有深远影响；事实上，在某些人群中，ACE-I/D多态性被认为是抑郁症的危险因素（Wu et al. 2012）（表42.4）。基于ACE-I/D多态性变异与烟碱依赖风险之间的联系（表42.1），我们推测ACE-I/D多态性在精神疾病（例如抑郁症和精神分裂症）中的相关性可能高于其他疾病。与精神分裂症相似，抑郁症与中脑边缘通路的变化有关，而吸烟与抑郁症之间存在高度相关性（Dichter, Damiano, Allen, 2012; Munafò, Araya, 2010）。然而，神经影像学研究表明，这两种疾病的中脑边缘信号传导不同。在抑郁症中，中脑边缘活动减弱，在精神分裂症中，中脑边缘多巴胺传递过度活跃（Brisch et al. 2014; Dichter et al. 2012）。与这些差异一致，烟碱依赖风险升高与抑郁症患者的ACE-DD基因型（暗示高ACE活性）和精神分裂症女性的ACE-ID基因型（暗示中等ACE活性）相关是合理的。ACE-DD基因型也导致健康的德国人吸烟史更长；这些发现表明，ACE-I/D多态性变异对吸烟严重程度的影响机制在健康和抑郁状态下是相似的。然而，其他关于ACE-I/D多态性与健康受试者吸烟严重程度的潜在相关性的报告不支持这种推测（表42.2）。事实上，很难评估ACE-I/D多态性在健康人群吸烟严重程度中的作用，因为对健康受试者的研究已经通过不同的方法［即每天、每周的吸烟量或吸烟史的持续时间（包年）等］进行了吸烟严重程度的评估。事实上，捷克共和国关于ACE-I/D多态性对吸烟严重程度的潜在作用的初步研究没有在更大的样本中得到重复，这可能是因为纳入标准不同。这项初步研究包括现在和过去的吸烟者，而规模更大的研究只包括现在的吸烟者。几项发现可能解释了ACE-I/D多态性与烟碱依赖之间的性别差异。其中一个因素可能是雌激素替代疗法有助于降低具有特定ACE-I/D基因型的绝经后妇女的血清或血浆ACE活性。一项研究表明，携带ACE-ID和ACE-II基因型的妇女血浆ACE活性显著降低（Sanada et al. 2001），另一项研究表明，携带ACE-ID和ACE-DD基因型的妇女血浆ACE活性降低（Sumino et al. 2003）。另一个因素可能是雌激素减少了多巴胺能神经传递。在大鼠中，雌激素治疗降低了几个脑区的多巴胺受体D2水平（Chavez et al. 2010）。

表42.1 与ACE-I/D多态性相关的烟碱依赖风险

参考文献	人群	吸烟者/非吸烟者	研究群体	主要结果
Hubacek et al.（2001）	捷克共和国人	男性：189/113	健康受试者	ACE-I/D多态性与吸烟风险无关（$P>0.05$）
Hubacek et al. (2004)	捷克共和国人	男性：707/497 女性：478/897	健康受试者	ACE-I/D多态性与吸烟风险无关（$P>0.05$）

续表

参考文献	人群	吸烟者/非吸烟者	研究群体	主要结果
Baghai et al. (2008)	德国人	总计：17/93	健康受试者	ACE-I/D多态性与吸烟风险无关（$P>0.05$）
Baghai et al. (2008)	德国人	总计：53/430	重度抑郁症患者	ACE-DD纯合子基因型导致总病例组吸烟风险增加（$\chi^2=7.0$；$P=0.03$）
Nadalin, Buretić-Tomljanović et al. (2017); Nadalin, Ristić, et al. (2017)	克罗地亚人和斯洛文尼亚人	男性：66/73 女性：150/232	多发性硬化症患者	ACE-I/D多态性与吸烟风险无关（$P>0.05$）
Nadalin, Buretić-Tomljanović et al. (2017); Nadalin, Ristić, et al. (2017)	克罗地亚人	男性：99/41 女性：77/50	精神分裂症患者	ACE-ID纯合子基因型增加了女性患者吸烟的风险（OR=2.3；95% CI = 1.1～4.7；$P=0.03$）

表42.2　ACE-I/D多态性与吸烟严重程度的关系

参考文献	研究群体	主要结果
Hubacek et al. (2001)	健康受试者（仅男性）	ACE-Ⅱ纯合子基因型导致每周吸烟量高（$P=0.005$）
Hubacek et al. (2004)	健康受试者	ACE-I/D多态性与每周吸烟量无关（$P>0.05$）
Baghai et al. (2008)	健康受试者	ACE-DD纯合子基因型导致更长的吸烟史（以包年计算）（$F=3.3$；$P=0.04$）
Baghai et al. (2008)	重度抑郁症患者	ACE-DD纯合子基因型导致每日吸烟量高（$F=3.2$；$P=0.04$）
Nadalin, Buretić-Tomljanović et al. (2017); Nadalin, Ristić et al. (2017)	多发性硬化症患者	ACE-I/D多态性与每日吸烟量和每周吸烟量均无相关性（$P>0.05$）

注：没有对精神分裂症患者进行吸烟严重程度评估。

表42.3　ACE-I/D多态性与多发性硬化症和精神分裂症的潜在相关性

参考文献	人群	患者/对照	研究群体	主要结果
Lovrečić et al. (2006)	克罗地亚人和斯洛文尼亚人	313/376	多发性硬化症患者	ACE-DD纯合子基因型导致男性患者多发性硬化症风险增加
Živković et al. (2016)	塞尔维亚人	384/395	多发性硬化症患者	ACE纯合子基因型（ACE-DD和ACE-Ⅱ）均可增加多发性硬化症的风险
Crescenti et al. (2009)	西班牙人	243/291	精神分裂症及相关障碍患者	ACE-D等位基因被认为对精神分裂症、分裂情感障碍、急性精神障碍和妄想障碍有保护作用
Kucukali et al. (2010)	土耳其人	239/210	精神分裂症患者	ACE-Ⅰ等位基因被认为对精神分裂症有保护作用
Nadalin et al. (2012)	克罗地亚人	211/187	精神分裂症患者	ACE-D等位基因导致全部患者组的阴性和总PANSS评分增加，而男性患者的PANSS评分更高
Hui et al. (2014)	中国人	212/538	首发精神分裂症患者	ACE-DD纯合子基因型和ACE-D等位基因与较高的阴性PANSS评分相关
Hui et al. (2015)	中国人	382/538	精神分裂症患者	ACE-D等位基因可增加全部患者组和男女患者组的精神分裂症的风险；ACE-DD患者的PANSS抑郁评分低于ACE-Ⅱ纯合子基因型患者
Mazaheri, Saadat (2015)	伊朗人	363/363	精神分裂症患者	ACE-Ⅱ纯合子基因型可降低女性患者的精神分裂症风险

注：PANSS为阳性和阴性综合征量表。

表42.4 ACE-I/D多态性与重度抑郁症的潜在相关性

参考文献	人群	研究样本量	主要结果
Baghai et al. (2002)	德国人	115例患者	ACE-D等位基因与地塞米松/促肾上腺皮质激素释放激素试验中较高的皮质醇刺激有关
Stewart et al. (2009)	芬兰人	119例耐药患者	ACE-I等位基因导致男性抑郁症发病较早,但在女性中,较早发病与ACE-ID杂合基因型有关
Wu et al. (2012)	亚洲人和欧洲人	2479例患者和7744例对照	ACE-DD纯合子基因型与白种人和由几个欧洲人群(德国人、英国人、比利时人、芬兰人和以色列人)和亚洲人群(日本人和中国人)组成的混合种族群体患抑郁症的风险增加有关

注:最近的一些药物遗传学研究也表明,对特定抗抑郁药物的治疗反应与ACE-I/D多态性有关(未显示)。

我们应该意识到,ACE-I/D变异在烟碱依赖中的作用的研究存在许多局限性。最重要的局限性就是只研究了一种RAS相关的多态性。此外,没有一项研究用更具体的方法来评估烟碱依赖,如烟碱依赖的Fagerstrom测试。此外,大多数研究参与者数量较少,而针对精神分裂症和多发性硬化症患者的研究缺乏对照组。最后,多发性硬化症的男女比例或精神分裂症的吸烟者/非吸烟者比例的不平衡可能会导致统计分析中的偏差。

42.3 结论和展望

尽管遗传学研究的结果可能存在争议,但他们认为ACE-I/D多态变异对吸烟习惯的调节作用较弱。此外,ACE-I/D多态性与烟碱依赖的相关性因特定疾病和/或条件的不同而不同;实际上,这种多态性可能与精神障碍患者的吸烟风险最为相关。未来的研究应研究其他功能性ACE多态性,调查其他RAS相关多态变异(如血管紧张素原和AT_1或AT_2基因的变异)的相关性,并纳入来自不同种族背景的人群。另一个需要澄清的重要问题是,除了血管紧张素Ⅱ,ACE还有其他潜在的底物,如P物质、神经降压素和脑啡肽(图42.2),这些物质也影响中脑边缘系统的多巴胺能神经传递(Binder et al. 2001; Gerfen et al. 1991)。此外,在其他疾病,特别是可能由吸烟引起的疾病(如肺癌)的背景下,研究ACE-I/D多态性与烟碱依赖的关联将是有趣的。全基因组关联研究表明,中脑边缘系统基因的许多多态变异(特别是nAChR亚基基因)与肺癌有关(Amos et al. 2008);其他研究也报道了ACE-I/D多态性与肺癌易感性相关(Wang et al. 2015)。

一些环境因素可能与RAS相关基因相互作用,从而影响特定疾病和/或条件下的吸烟行为。例如,服用单胺摄取抑制剂会降低纹状体中P物质的水平(Porcelli et al. 2011),而抗精神病药物可能会减少或增加ACE的表达/活性(Segman et al. 2002)。一个新的发现是,广泛用于MS治疗的干扰素-β干扰了某些RAS成分。例如,复发和缓解的MS患者接受干扰素-β及伴随的AT_1拮抗剂和血管紧张素转换酶抑制剂的治疗;与仅接受干扰素-β治疗的患者相比,这些患者的复发率更高。(Doerner et al. 2014)。最后,吸烟也可能影响ACE的表达/活性;烟碱及其代谢物增加了人内皮细胞的ACE的表达和活性。此外,慢性吸烟者表现出RAS激活增强和循环ACE水平升高(Ljungberg et al. 2011)。

抑郁症、精神分裂症和多发性硬化症也可能改变吸烟习惯。自我用药假说认为,精神疾病人群对烟碱的高依赖率和/或高吸烟率是由于烟碱的有益作用。吸烟通过烟碱对多巴胺能系统的中枢作用恢复多巴胺能传递；因此，吸烟被认为可以缓解抑郁和焦虑症状、阴性和阳性精神分裂症症状、抗精神病药物的锥体外系副作用以及认知缺陷（Fluharty et al. 2017; Sagud et al. 2009）。研究还表明，通过扩展的残疾状态量表进行衡量，发现吸烟的多发性硬化症患者经历了更严重的病程和更快的残疾进展（Healy et al. 2009）。因此，由于疾病，从长远来看，多发性硬化症患者可能会减少吸烟或戒烟。最后，在确定吸烟是否会增加患抑郁症的风险时，动物试验表明，长期暴露于卷烟烟雾中对抑郁症动物的下丘脑-垂体肾上腺皮质调节失调有重要作用（Fluharty et al. 2017）。

42.4 对治疗的影响

在我们看来，长期使用干扰RAS成分的药物（即ACE抑制剂或AT_1阻滞剂），安全地用于治疗高血压和心脏保护，是否可能是烟碱依赖的有效治疗方法将是一件有趣的事情。这种疗法可能对精神疾病患者特别有益，因为他们养成的吸烟习惯使他们的心血管疾病风险大大增加。与ACE-I/D多态性的功能特性相一致，同样值得阐明的是，烟碱依赖治疗的反应是否可能与特定的ACE基因型有关。此外，吸烟已被证明通过增加细胞色素家族中的酶的活性来增加许多药物的新陈代谢，包括抗抑郁药和抗精神病药（Oliveira et al. 2017; Sagud et al. 2009）。因此，根据ACE-I/D多态性导致抑郁症和精神分裂症患者吸烟行为的证据，对这些患者进行基因分型也可能为适当地调整药物治疗提供有用的信息。

术语解释
- 血管紧张素转换酶（ACE）：它是RAS中的关键酶；它将失活的十肽（血管紧张素Ⅰ）转化为有活性的八肽（血管紧张素Ⅱ）。
- 功能多态性：它们是已被证明可以改变基因表达和/或功能的基因变异。
- 基因多态性：它们是在人群中发现的单一基因的常见变异。
- 插入/缺失多态性：这是一种基因改变，包括额外序列的加入（插入）或序列的删除（缺失）。
- 重度抑郁症：这是一种精神障碍，其特征是情绪低落或在日常活动中失去兴趣和乐趣，持续两周以上。
- 中脑边缘通路：它是大脑中的一个回路，在这个回路中，多巴胺从腹侧被盖区传递到伏隔核、杏仁核、海马体和前额叶皮质。除了产生奖励刺激，它还与成瘾行为、抑郁症和精神分裂症有关。
- 多发性硬化症：这是一种慢性中枢神经系统自身免疫性疾病，以炎症、髓鞘破坏和神经元变性为特征。
- 肾素-血管紧张素系统（RAS）：它是一种肽能系统，经典地被描述为激素系统。它的主要功能是调节全身血压，维持钠和液体的动态平衡。此外，许多组织都有独立于经典RAS调节的局部RAS组分。
- 精神分裂症：它是一种慢性精神疾病，以积极症状（妄想和幻觉）、消极症状（迟钝的情绪和社交孤立）和认知缺陷为特征，包括注意力、记忆力和执行功能的损害。
- 物质滥用：它是过度使用一种潜在的上瘾物质；上瘾的特征是无法减少消耗以及社会或职业功能的损害。

- RAS的经典功能是调节全身血压，维持钠和液体的动态平衡。
- 当RAS效应在不同的人体组织中被发现，特别是在大脑中时，人们对RAS的兴趣重新燃起。
- 所有经典的RAS成分（血管紧张素原、肽酶、血管紧张素和受体蛋白）都在血脑屏障内的不同脑区被识别出来。
- 脑RAS控制着许多中枢功能，包括脑血流调节、神经元再生、记忆巩固、饮酒和应激；此外，RAS被认为在许多疾病的病因中扮演着不同的角色。
- 越来越多的证据表明，脑RAS可能通过影响中脑边缘通路中的多巴胺能信号，在物质滥用病因中起着重要的决定作用。

- 脑肾素-血管紧张素系统（RAS）可能通过影响多巴胺能信号在物质滥用的病因中发挥重要作用。
- 在人类群体中，将RAS与成瘾联系起来的数据很少；这些数据大多来自一些遗传学研究，这些研究调查了血管紧张素转换酶（ACE）基因的功能性插入/缺失（I/D）多态性是否影响吸烟行为。
- 除了健康受试者，这些研究还包括抑郁症、多发性硬化症和精神分裂症患者。
- 结果表明，ACE-I/D多态性对吸烟行为的调节作用较弱，在不同的疾病和/或条件下，这种多态性与烟碱依赖的相关性可能有所不同。
- 研究结果表明，与其他疾病和/或条件相比，ACE-I/D多态性在预测精神疾病的吸烟风险方面可能更具相关性。

参考文献

Amos, C. I.; Wu, X.; Broderick, P.; Gorlov, I. P.; Gu, J.; Eisen, T. et al. (2008). Genome-wide association scan of tag SNPs identifies a susceptibility locus for lung cancer at 15q25. 1. Nature Genetics, 40, 616-622.

Baghai, T. C.; Schule, C.; Zwanzger, P.; Minov, C.; Zill, P.; Ella, R. et al. (2002). Hypothalamic-pituitary-adrenocortical axis dysregulation in patients with major depression is influenced by the insertion/ deletion polymorphism in the angiotensin I-converting enzyme gene. Neuroscience Letters, 328, 299-303.

Baghai, T. C.; Varallo-Bedarida, G.; Born, C.; Häfner, S.; Schule, C.; Eser, D. et al. (2008). A polymorphism in the angiotensin-converting enzyme gene is associated with smoking behavior. Journal of Clinical Psychiatry, 69, 1983-1985.

Banks, R. J.; Mozley, L.; Dourish, C. T. (1994). The angiotensin converting enzyme inhibitors captopril and enalapril inhibit apomorphineinduced oral stereotypy in the rat. Neuroscience, 58, 799-805.

Binder, E. B.; Kinkead, B.; Owens, M. J.; Nemeroff, C. B. (2001). Neurotensin and dopamine interactions. Pharmacological Reviews, 53, 453-486.

Brisch, R.; Saniotis, A.; Wolf, R.; Bielau, H.; Bernstein, H. G.; Steiner, J. et al. (2014). The role of dopamine in schizophrenia from a neurobiological and evolutionary perspective: old fashioned, but still in vogue. Frontiers in Psychiatry. 5, https://doi. org/10. 3389/ fpsyt. 2014. 00047.

Chavez, C.; Hollaus, M.; Scarr, E.; Pavey, G.; Gogos, A.; van den Buuse, M. (2010). The effect of estrogen on dopamine and serotonin receptor and transporter levels in the brain: an autoradiography study. Brain Research, 1321, 51-59.

Crescenti, A.; Gassó, P.; Mas, S.; Abellana, R.; Deulofeu, R.; Parellada, E. et al. (2009). Insertion/deletion polymorphism of the angiotensinconverting enzyme gene is associated with schizophrenia in a Spanish population. Psychiatry Research, 165, 175-180.

de Leon, J.; Diaz, F. J. (2005). A meta-analysis of worldwide studies demonstrates an association between schizophrenia and tobacco smoking behaviors. Schizophrenia Research, 76, 135-157.

Dichter, G. S.; Damiano, C. A.; Allen, J. A. (2012). Reward circuitry dysfunction in psychiatric and neurodevelopmental disorders and genetic syndromes: animal models and clinical findings. Journal of Neurodevelopmental Disorders, 4, 19.

Doerner, M.; Beckmann, K.; Knappertz, V.; Kappos, L.; Hartung, H. P.; Filippi, M. et al. (2014). Effects of inhibitors of the renin-angiotensin system on the efficacy of interferon beta-1b: a post hoc analysis of the BEYOND study. European Neurology, 71, 173-179.

Fluharty, M.; Taylor, A. E.; Grabski, M.; Munafò, M. R. (2017). The association of cigarette smoking with depression and anxiety: a systematic review. Nicotine, Tobacco Research, 19, 3-13.

Garrib, A.; Peters, T. (1998). Angiotensin-converting enzyme (ACE) gene polymorphism and alcoholism. Biochemical Society Transactions, 26, S136.

Georgiev, V.; György, L.; Getova, D.; Markovska, V. (1985). Some central effects of angiotensin II. Interactions with dopaminergic transmission.

Acta physiologica et pharmacologica Bulgarica, 11, 19-26.

Gerfen, C. R.; McGinty, J. F.; Young, W. S.; 3rd. (1991). Dopamine differentially regulates dynorphin, substance P, and enkephalin expression in striatal neurons: in situ hybridization histochemical analysis. Journal of Neuroscience, 11, 1016-1031.

Guimond, M. O.; Gallo-Payet, N. (2012). The angiotensin II type 2 receptor in brain functions: an update. International Journal of Hypertension, 2012, 351758.

Healy, B. C.; Ali, E. N.; Guttmann, C. R.; Chitnis, T.; Glanz, B. I.; Buckle, G. et al. (2009). Smoking and disease progression in multiple sclerosis. Archives of Neurology, 66, 858-864.

Hosseini, M.; Sharifi, M. R.; Alaei, H.; Shafei, M. N.; Karimooy, H. A. (2007). Effects of angiotensin II and captopril on rewarding properties of morphine. Indian Journal of Experimental Biology, 45, 770-777.

Hubacek, J . A.; Adamkova, V.; Skodova, Z.; Lanska, V.; Poledne, R . (2004). No relation between angiotensin-converting enzyme gene polymorphism and smoking dependence. Scandinavian Journal of Clinical and Laboratory Investigation, 64, 575-578.

Hubacek, J. A.; Pitha, J.; Skodova, Z.; Poledne, R. (2001). Angiotensin converting enzyme gene—a candidate gene for addiction to smoking? Atherosclerosis, 159, 237-238.

Hui, L.; Wu, J. Q.; Ye, M. J.; Zheng, K.; He, J. C.; Zhang, X. et al. (2015). Association of angiotensin-converting enzyme gene polymorphism with schizophrenia and depressive symptom severity in a Chinese population. Human Psychopharmacology, 30, 100-107.

Hui, L.; Wu, J. Q.; Zhang, X.; Lv, J.; Du, W. L.; Kou, C. G. et al. (2014). Association between the angiotensin-converting enzyme gene insertion/deletion polymorphism and first-episode patients withschizophrenia in a Chinese Han population. Human Psychopharmacology, 29, 274-279.

Jenkins, T. A.; Chai, S. Y.; Mendelsohn, F. A. (1997). Effect of angiotensin II on striatal dopamine release in the spontaneous hypertensive rat. Clinical and Experimental Hypertension, 19, 645-658.

Jenkins, T. A.; Mendelsohn, F. A.; Chai, S. Y. (1997). Angiotensin converting enzyme modulates dopamine turnover in the striatum. Journal of Neurochemistry, 68, 1304-1311.

Kucukali, C. I.; Aydin, M.; Ozkok, E.; Bilge, E.; Zengin, A.; Cakir, U.; et al. (2010). Angiotensin-converting enzyme polymorphism in schizophrenia, bipolar disorders, and their first-degree relatives. Psychiatric Genetics, 20, 14-19.

Labandeira-García, J. L.; Garrido-Gil, P.; Rodriguez-Pallares, J.; Valenzuela, R.; Borrajo, A.; Rodriguez-Perez, A. I. (2014). Brain renin-angiotensin system and dopaminergic cell vulnerability. Frontiers in Neuroanatomy, 8, 67.

Ljungberg, L.; Alehagen, U.; Länne, T.; Björck, H.; De Basso, R.; Dahlström, U. et al. (2011). The association between circulating angiotensin-converting enzyme and cardiovascular risk in theelderly: a cross-sectional study. Journal of the Renin-Angiotensin-Aldosterone System, 12, 281-289.

Lovre ćić, L.; Ristić, S.; Starčević-čizmarević, N.; Jazbec, S. S.; Sepčić, J.; Kapović, M. et al. (2006). Angiotensin-converting enzyme I/D gene polymorphism and risk of multiple sclerosis. Acta Neurologica Scandinavica, 114, 374-377.

Marchese, N. A.; Artur de la Villarmois, E.; Basmadjian, O. M.; Perez, M. F.; Baiardi, G.; Bregonzio, C. (2016). Brain angiotensin II AT1 receptors are involved in the acute and long-term amphetamine-induced neurocognitive alterations. Psychopharmacology (Berlin), 233, 795-807.

Mazaheri, H.; Saadat, M. (2015). Association between insertion/deletion polymorphism in angiotension converting enzyme and susceptibility to schizophrenia. Iranian Journal of Public Health, 44, 369-373.

McKinley, M. J.; Albiston, A. L.; Allen, A. M.; Mathai, M. L.; May, C. N.; McAllen, R. M. et al. (2003). The brain renin-angiotensin system:location and physiological roles. The International Journal of Biochemistry, Cell Biology, 35, 901-918.

Munafò, M. R.; Araya, R. (2010). Cigarette smoking and depression: a question of causation. British Journal of Psychiatry, 196, 425-426.

Nadalin, S.; Buretić-Tomljanović, A.; Lavtar, P.; Starčević čizmarević, N.; Hodžić, A.; Sepčić, J. et al. (2017). The lack of association between angiotensin-converting enzyme gene insertion/deletion polymorphism and nicotine dependence in multiple sclerosis. Brain and Behavior. 7, e00600.

Nadalin, S.; Buretić-Tomljanović, A.; Rubeša, G.; Jonovska, S.; Tomljanović, D.; Ristić, S. (2012). Angiotensin-converting enzyme gene insertion/deletion polymorphism is not associated with schizophrenia in a Croatian population. Psychiatric Genetics, 22, 267-268.

Nadalin, S.; Ristić, S.; Rebić, J.; Šendula Jengić, V.; Kapović, M.; Buretić-Tomljanović, A. (2017). The insertion/deletion polymorphism in the angiotensin-converting enzyme gene and nicotine dependence in schizophrenia patients. Journal of Neural Transmission (Vienna), 124, 511-518.

Obata, T.; Takahashi, S.; Kashiwagi, Y.; Kubota, S. (2008). Protective effect of captopril and enalaprilat, angiotensin-converting enzyme inhibitors, on para-nonylphenol-induced *OH generation and dopamine efflux in rat striatum. Toxicology, 250, 96-99.

Oliveira, P.; Ribeiro, J.; Donato, H.; Madeira, N. (2017). Smoking and antidepressants pharmacokinetics: a systematic review. Annals of General Psychiatry, 16, 17.

Paz, M. C.; Marchese, N. A.; Stroppa, M. M.; Gerez de Burgos, N. M.; Imboden, H.; Baiardi, G. et al. (2014). Involvement of the brain renin-angiotensin system (RAS) in the neuroadaptive responses induced by amphetamine in a two-injection protocol. Behavioural Brain Research, 272, 314-323.

Porcelli, S.; Drago, A.; Fabbri, C.; Gibiino, S.; Calati, R.; Serretti, A. (2011). Pharmacogenetics of antidepressant response. Journal of Psychiatry and Neuroscience, 36, 8 7-113.

Ramanujam, R.; Hedström, A. K.; Manouchehrinia, A.; Alfredsson, L.; Olsson, T.; Bottai, M. et al. (2015). Effect of smoking cessation on multiple sclerosis prognosis. JAMA Neurology, 72, 1117-1123.

Rigat, B.; Hubert, C.; Alhenc-Gelas, F.; Cambien, F.; Corvol, P.; Soubrier, F. (1990). An insertion/deletion polymorphism in the angiotensin I-converting enzyme gene accounting for half the variance of serum enzyme levels. Journal of Clinical Investigation, 86, 1343-1346.

Sagud, M.; Mihaljević-Peles, A.; Mück-Seler, D.; Pivac, N.; VuksanCusa, B.; Brataljenović, T. et al. (2009). Smoking and schizophrenia. Psychiatria Danubina, 21, 371-375.

Sanada, M.; Higashi, Y.; Nakagawa, K.; Sasaki, S.; Kodama, I.; Tsuda, M. et al. (2001). Relationship between the angiotensinconverting enzyme genotype and the forearm vasodilator response to estrogen replacement therapy in postmenopausal women. Journal of the American College of Cardiology, 37, 1529-1535.

Segman, R. H.; Shapira, Y.; Modai, I.; Hamdan, A.; Zislin, J.; HerescoLevy, U. et al. (2002). Angiotensin converting enzyme gene insertion/deletion polymorphism: case-control association studies in schizophrenia, major affective disorder, and tardive dyskinesia and a family-based association study in schizophrenia. American Journal of Medical Genetics, 114, 310-314.

Serý, O.; Vojtová, V.; Zvolský, P. (2001). The association study of DRD2, ACE and AGT gene polymorphisms and metamphetamine dependence. Physiological Research, 50, 43-50.

Sommer, W. H.; Rimondini, R.; Marquitz, M.; Lidström, J.; Siems, W. E.; Bader, M. et al. (2007). Plasticity and impact of the central reninangiotensin system during development of ethanol dependence. Journal of Molecular Medicine (Berlin), 85, 1089-1097.

Stewart, J. A.; Kampman, O.; Huuhka, M.; Anttila, S.; Huuhka, K.; Lehtimäki, T. et al. (2009). ACE polymorphism and response to electroconvulsive therapy in major depression. Neuroscience Letters, 458, 122-125.

Sumino, H.; Ichikawa, S.; Ohyama, Y.; Nakamura, T.; Kanda, T.; Sakamoto, H. et al. (2003). Effects of hormone replacement therapy on serum angiotensin-converting enzyme activity and plasma bradykinin in postmenopausal women according to angiotensinconverting enzyme-genotype. Hypertension Research, 26, 53-58.

Visniauskas, B.; Perry, J. C.; Oliveira, V.; Dalio, F. M.; Andersen, M. L.; Tufik, S. et al. (2012). Cocaine administration increases angiotensin I-converting enzyme (ACE) expression and activity in the rat striatum and frontal cortex. Neuroscience Letters, 506, 84-88.

Wang, N.; Yang, D.; Ji, B.; Li, J. (2015). Angiotensin-converting enzyme insertion/deletion gene polymorphism and lung cancer risk: a meta-analysis. Journal of the Renin-Angiotensin-Aldosterone System, 16, 189-194.

Wright, J. W.; Harding, J. W. (2013). The brain renin-angiotensin system: a diversity of functions and implications for CNS diseases. Plfügers Archiv—European Journal of Physiology, 465, 133-151.

Wu, Y.; Wang, X.; Shen, X.; Tan, Z.; Yuan, Y. (2012). The I/D polymorphism of angiotensin-converting enzyme gene in major depressive disorder and therapeutic outcome: a case-control study and metaanalysis. Journal of Affective Disorders, 136, 971-978.

Zhang, P.; Wang, R.; Li, Z.; Wang, Y.; Gao, C.; Lv, X. et al. (2016). The risk of smoking on multiple sclerosis: a meta-analysis based on 20, 626 cases from case-control and cohort studies. PeerJ. 4, e1797.

Živković, M.; Kolaković, A.; Stojković, L.; Dinčić, E.; Kostić, S.; Alavantić, D. et al. (2016). Renin-angiotensin system gene polymorphisms as risk factors for multiple sclerosis. Journal of the Neurological Sciences, 15(363), 29-32.

43

烟碱依赖与 *CHRNA5/CHRNA3/CHRNB4* 烟碱受体调节组

Sung-Ha Lee[1], Elizabeth S. Barrie[2], Wolfgang Sadee[3], Ryan M. Smith[4]

1. Center for Pharmacogenomics, College of Medicine, The Ohio State University, Columbus, OH, United States
2. Institute for Genomic Medicine, Nationwide Children's Hospital, Columbus, OH, United States
3. Center for Pharmacogenomics, Department of Cancer Biology and Genetics, College of Medicine, The Ohio State University, Columbus, OH, United States
4. Division of Pharmaceutics and Translational Therapeutics, Department of Pharmaceutical Sciences and Experimental Therapeutics, College of Pharmacy, University of Iowa, Iowa City, IA, United States

缩略语

CNS	中枢神经系统	**MeQTL**	甲基化数量性状基因座
CpG	胞嘧啶磷酸鸟嘌呤	**mRNA**	信使核糖核酸
DNA	脱氧核糖核酸	**ND**	烟碱依赖
GTEx	基因型-组织表达	**RNA**	核糖核酸
GWAS	全基因组关联研究	**SNP**	单核苷酸多态性
LD	连锁不平衡	**UTR**	未翻译区
MAF	次要等位基因频率		

43.1 引言：烟碱的α5、α3、β4亚基的组织表达和功能

编码α5、α3和β4亚基的基因（*CHRNA5*、*CHRNA3*和*CHRNB4*）位于染色体15q25.1上的单基因簇中。*CHRNA5*的编码方向为5′—3′，而*CHRNA3*、*CHRNB4*和非编码核糖核酸*RP11-650L12.2*（ENST00000567141）的编码方向与之相反（3′—5′）（图43.1）。这个区域跨度约为76kb，包含紧密连锁不平衡的块（LD；图43.1）。*CHRNA5*和*CHRNA3*在它们注释的基因组序列的3′端有466个碱基对重叠，导致它们延伸的mRNA转录本之间有互补的碱基对。

成对相关性表明，*CHRNA5*、*CHRNA3*、*CHRNB4*和RP11-650L12.2 mRNA在大多数组织中共表达，这表明存在共同的调控机制（Barrie et al. 2017）。CHRNA5与其反义*RNA RP11-650L12.2*高度相关的生物学意义尚不清楚。除了PSMA4和MORF4L1（Barrie et al. 2017）外，邻近该簇的大多数蛋白质编码基因都不共表达，这表明局部"调节组"的影响可能也延伸到这两个基因。

翻译后，α3和β4亚基共同组装形成功能性α3β4*通道，有时会合并α5亚基（α3β4α5）（Vernallis, Conroy, Berg, 1993; Wang et al. 1996）。在肾上腺（Hone et al. 2015）、外周神经节（Mao et al. 2006; Vernallis et al. 1993; Yeh et al. 2001）和上皮结构中，特别是缰核和脚间核中（Frahm et al. 2011; Yeh et al. 2001; Zoli, Le Novere, Hill Jr., Changeux, 1995），可以观察到不同的受体化学计量学（图43.2）。一般而言，α3β4*通道调节神经节细胞的兴奋性，从而调节活动依赖性神经递质的释放，即自主神经节和感觉神经元兴奋时（Genzen, McGehee, 2003; Mao et al. 2006; Zhang, Albers, Gold, 2015）的去甲肾上腺素释放（Yokotani et al. 2000）。

与成瘾相关的是，α3β4*通道在缰核、垂体、反折束和脚间核等上皮结构中有较好的表达（Shih et al. 2014）。缰核及其相关结构调节负性奖励，对负性或厌恶刺激作出反应而激活。因此，α3β4*通道在成瘾后的奖励行为中起着重要作用。在内侧缰核有更多α3β4*通道表达的转基因小鼠的烟碱消耗减少（Frahm et al. 2011），因为过量的烟碱是令人厌恶的。许多上皮α3β4*通道也含有α5受体亚基。虽然这个亚基不是烟碱相关奖励或厌恶行为的表现所必需的（Jackson et al. 2013），但在α5/α3/β4调节组的背景下，这个亚基的重要性是显而易见的。

43.2 调控CHRNA5/CHRNA3/CHRNB4转录的蛋白质

背景对于确定调控CHRNA5、CHRNA3或CHRNB4表达的蛋白质至关重要，因为每个基因都有自己的启动子和相互作用的增强子，这些启动子和相互作用的增强子可以跨发育时间线以组织依赖的方式发挥作用或响应外部干扰。特异性蛋白（SP）转录因子家族调节这三个基因的表达，每个启动子都有多个SP结合位点（Bigger et al. 1996; Bigger et al. 1997; Campos-Caro et al. 1999; Fornasari et al. 1997）。与这三个亚基的组织特异性表达相比，SP转录因子的几乎无处不在的表达强烈表明，更多的蛋白质参与了亚基的表达调控。人类和啮齿动物的表达表现出组织调节特异性，在神经细胞中由Pou3f1和PHOX2A调节α3（Benfante et al. 2007; Yang et al. 1994），在神经细胞中由Sox10调节α3和β4（Liu et al. 1999），在海马细胞中由多发性内分泌癌蛋白调节α5（Getz et al. 2017）。青蒿素诱导炎症后三叉神经节和皮肤神经元内α3和β4的表达（Albers et al. 2014）。

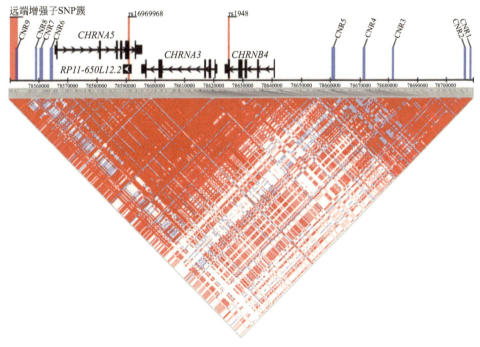

图 43.1 *CHRNA5/CHRNA3/CHRNB4* 基因座

CHRNA5/CHRNA3/CHRNB4基因座位于染色体15q25.1上。用黑色表示的是蛋白质编码基因和非编码基因。最厚的基因区域表示蛋白质编码潜力，中等厚度的区域表示非翻译区，薄的区域表示内含子，箭头方向表示转录方向。红色阴影区域表示与临床相关的功能多态性。根据Xu等（2006）的研究，蓝色阴影区域表示保守的烟碱调节区（CNR1—9）。基因图下方是一个连锁不平衡曲线图，显示出很强的连锁不平衡，用红色阴影表示，延伸到整个基因簇。

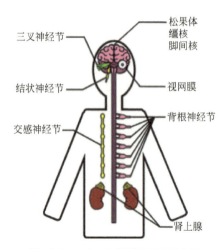

图 43.2　α3β4* 受体在体内的表达

α3β4* 受体在中枢、外周神经系统和外周组织中均有表达。在大脑内，α3β4* 受体在介导奖励的上皮结构中表达。在外周神经系统中，α3β4* 受体分布于多种类型的神经节上，这些神经节支配着大多数器官，调节兴奋性和神经递质的释放。

烟碱基因的接近形成了一个系统发育保守的簇以及不同的组织特异性共表达模式，这表明它们的表达受到共同调控元件的共同调控。Xu、Scott 和 Deneris（2006）绘制了 A5/A3/B4 簇周围的保守区域图，以确定保守的调控元件，发现 9 个区域的长度 >200bp，序列一致性 >70%（图 43.1）。α3 和 β4 在松果体和颈上神经节的表达受 β4 上游元件的共同调控（Xu et al. 2006）。总之，强有力的证据支持多种调控元件以组织依赖的方式协调所有三种烟碱基因的表达。

43.3　调控 CHRNA5/CHRNA3/CHRNB4 mRNA 表达的多态性

CHRNA5 mRNA 的表达受遗传变异的调节（Smith et al. 2011; Wang et al. 2009; Wang et al. 2009），但 A5/A3/B4 基因座上紧密的 LD（见图 43.1）使得从替代标记中分离致病功能多态性具有挑战性。利用等位基因表达来缓解 LD 的混淆，Smith 等（2011）发现了 CHRNA5 基因位点上游约 15kb 的增强子区域，这与 Xu 等（2006）发现的保守区一致（图 43.1），并由 Doyle 等（2011）以及 Ramsay 等（2015）在皮质下结构中复制。这个由 6 个 SNPs（rs1979905、rs1979906、rs1979907、rs880395、rs905740 和 rs7164030）标记的增强子区域，使前额叶皮质 CHRNA5 的表达增加了 4 倍。增强子还影响许多外周组织中的表达（GTEx Consortium, 2013; Ramsay et al. 2015）。

这个增强子区域对 CHRNA3 和 CHRNB4 表达的影响是未知的或被认为是不显著的，因为它不像 CHRNA5 那样显著。然而，使用多组学方法，Barrie 等（2017）发现远端增强子区域也影响了 CHRNA3 和反义 RP11-650L12.2 在中枢神经系统和外周神经系统的表达。这表明，这些烟碱亚基的 mRNA 表达受到临床上显著的功能多态性和远端增强子区域的共同调控，后者是该簇 mRNA 表达的主要调控因子。CHRNB4 在可供研究的 CNS 组织中的低表达排除了对基因型-组织表达（GTEx）数据的分析，以确定增强子是否调节 CHRNB4 的表达，但研究 CHRNB4 在表达较高的上皮组织中的表达可能解决这个问题（Shih et al. 2014）。

虽然远端增强子的多态性对中枢和外周组织中 CHRNA5 和 CHRNA3 的表达有结构性的调节作用，但有一个显著的例外，其与成瘾有很大的关系。在纹状体（包括尾状核、壳核和伏隔核）

中，rs1948与GTEx数据中*CHRNA3*的表达相关性最强（Barrie et al. 2017），其中次要等位基因与*CHRNA3* mRNA表达增加相关。这个大脑区域与多巴胺依赖的奖励行为密切相关，这是成瘾的基础。在非人灵长类动物的壳核中检测到的大部分活性或烟碱诱发多巴胺的释放，都是由α3亚基与α6和β2亚基共同负责的（Perez, O'Leary, Parameswaran, McIntosh, Quik, 2009）。体外模拟不同3'UTR长度的*CHRNB4*的构建中，rs1948对*CHRNB4*表达的影响是明显的（Flora et al. 2013; Gallego, Cox, Laughlin, Stitzel, Ehringer, 2013）。

43.4　调控*CHRNA5*/*CHRNA3*/*CHRNB4*的表观遗传学和环境因素

环境因素可以动态调节脱氧核糖核酸（DNA）中与胞嘧啶磷酸鸟嘌呤（CpGs）相邻的胞嘧啶核苷酸的甲基化。在暴露于逆境中的儿童中，*CHRNA5*启动子上的CpG岛被高甲基化（Zhang, Wang, Kranzler, Zhao, Gelernter, 2013）。在性别特异性基因-环境交互作用的一个例子中，rs16969968次要等位基因的男性携带者暴露于童年逆境中会增加ND的风险（Xie et al. 2012）。此外，A5/A3/B4簇中的显著甲基化数量性状基因座（meQTL）在该区域的特定CpG位点在多个组织中是明显的（Hancock et al. 2015; Ramsay et al. 2015; Volkov et al. 2016）。这些发现建立了遗传和表观遗传（包括环境）因素之间的联系。因此，人们可能认为童年的逆境和meQTL多态性的存在汇聚在一起，导致*CHRNA5*基因启动子的高甲基化，降低*CHRNA5* mRNA的表达，增加ND的风险。然而，包括同一样本的表达、甲基化和基因型的后续分析发现，甲基化和表达之间没有直接关系（Hancock et al. 2015; Ramsay et al. 2015）。除了CpG甲基化，A5/A3/B4基因簇的表观遗传调控可以通过组蛋白的化学修饰和染色质的结构变化来发生。针对A5/A3/B4基因座的研究很少，但主要调控元件的发现应该会加强进一步的努力。

43.5　与*CHRNA5*/*CHRNA3*/*CHRNB4*调节组的临床相关性

候选基因和单SNP研究确定A5/A3/B4簇是ND的易感基因座（Bierut et al. 2007; Saccone et al. 2007），后来得到了关于ND和相关临床表型的全基因组关联研究（GWAS）的证实（表43.1）（Amos et al. 2008; Saccone et al. 2010; Tobacco, Genetics Consortium, 2010）。*CHRNA5*中的一个非同义SNP rs16969968（D398N）与ND密切相关。该变异体降低了它所结合的通道的激动剂诱发活性，而不改变激动剂或拮抗剂的正构体结合（George et al. 2012; Tammimäki et al. 2012）。rs16969968抑制缰核中含有α5受体的信号，从而减少对成瘾物质的厌恶（Fowler, Lu, Johnson, Marks, Kenny, 2011; Frahm et al. 2011; Jensen et al. 2015）。

在具有不同LD结构和变异的不同种族人群中，考虑A5/A3/B4调节组与吸烟行为的关系是很有必要的。在非裔美国人中，rs16969968对吸烟行为也有类似的影响（Olfson et al. 2016）；然而，次要等位基因在非洲和亚洲人群中并不常见（1%～5%）。其他多态性，如*CHRNA3*中的rs1317286和rs8040806，在非裔美国人中显示与ND相关（Li et al. 2010），但在韩国人中，烟碱受体簇与吸烟行为的相关性很弱（Li et al. 2010）。此外，调控多态性在这些人群中没有得到很好的研究，使得知识驱动的单倍型分析更难构建和解释。

在进化选择中，由频繁的SNPs产生的具有长单倍型的同源基因簇，形成了一个局部的"调节组"（Barrie et al. 2017; Sadler et al. 2015）。由于rs16969968为ND风险提供了最切实的证据，研究人员在rs16969968的背景下衡量了更多候选SNPs的综合效应。Saccone等（2010）报道，在控制rs16969968基因型后，rs578776对吸烟的保护作用减弱但显著。*CHRNA5*和rs1948远端增强子中的SNP只有在与rs16969968一起考虑时才会传递ND的风险（Barrie et al. 2017; Smith et al. 2011）。简而言之，由rs16969968、rs880395和rs1948构建的四种主要单倍型以等位基因剂量依赖的方式传递风险（Barrie et al. 2017; 表43.2），这与它们对基因表达和配体相关信号特性的已知影响是一致的（表43.3）。在该基因位点常见SNPs的功能效应的指导下，可以构建反映调节组赋予的不同烟碱受体生物学的单倍型。

表43.1 报道的rs1051730、rs8034191、rs16969968、rs578776和rs588765与欧美人群烟碱依赖和/或相关表型的关联

SNP	位置[①]（相关基因符号）	等位基因（MAF）	功能注释	临床关联
rs8034191	15: 78513681 (HYKK)	T>C(0.37)	内含子变体	肺癌
rs588765	15: 78573083 (CHRNA5)	C>T(0.4)	内含子变体	吸烟量
rs16969968	15: 78590583 (CHRNA5)	G>A(0.36)	非同义变体 [D(Asp)->N(Asn)]	吸烟量 烟碱依赖型肺癌
rs578776	15: 78596058 (CHRNA3)	G>A (0.28)	3'-UTR	吸烟量
rs1051730	15: 78601997 (CHRNA3)	G>A (0.36)	同义变体	烟碱依赖型肺癌，吸烟量

① 基于GRCh39/hg38组件。

表43.2 关键SNPs的单倍型、对吸烟行为的影响及其在人群中的分布

rs16969968/rs880395/rs1948	对吸烟行为的影响	具有单倍型的群体的平均百分比
AGG	增加风险	35
GAA	增加中度风险	31
GGG	基线风险	20
GAG	降低风险	11

表43.3 关键SNPs对mRNA表达和吸烟行为的影响

项目	rs16969968	rs880395	rs1948
吸烟风险等位基因	A	G	A
功能影响	减少CHRNA5信号	减少CHRNA5 mRNA	增加CHRNA3 mRNA
主要等位基因	G	G	G

术语解释

- 增强子：DNA区域，它结合促进与基因启动子相互作用的蛋白质，以增加信使RNA的表达，并能以组织特异性的方式发挥作用。

- 表观遗传：可遗传的和动态的DNA修饰影响基因表达和表型呈现，包括但不限于组蛋白修饰和DNA甲基化。

- 上丘脑：邻近丘脑的脑区，包括缰核和松果体。

- 功能多态性：一种明显影响生物学的DNA变异。例如，影响配体结合的基因表达的改变或编码蛋白的改变。

- 单倍型：同一等位基因上的一组多态性。
- 连锁不平衡：同一等位基因上两个或多个多态性在群体中的非随机共存；例如，多态性能可靠地预测相同等位基因频率的其他多态性的存在。
- 非同义替换：改变蛋白质中的一种氨基酸的多态性。
- 表现型：一种可观察到的特征，由于遗传或环境，群体中不同的个体会有不同的表现。
- 启动子：DNA区域，通常位于基因上游，编码启动基因转录所需的蛋白质结合位点。
- 数量性状基因座：DNA的多态区域，与数量表型相关，如基因表达水平或甲基化水平。
- 调控元件：编码调节RNA表达的蛋白质结合位点的DNA区域。它们包括增强子和启动子。
- 调节组：调节一个或多个基因协调表达的调节因子的集合。调节组可以根据背景的不同而不同，如发育阶段或组织。

基因表达的关键事实

- 在调控元件的引导下，基因以时间和组织依赖的方式表达。
- 基因多态性可以对基因表达的方方面面产生巨大影响，包括转录、选择性剪接、运输和翻译。
- 几乎所有的多外显子基因，包括非编码RNA，在人类体内都经历了选择性剪接，以产生独特的RNA异构体，这种异构体在不同的组织中会有所不同。
- 虽然基因是在细胞核中转录的，但它们可以被运输到特定的亚细胞位置，在那里它们执行调节功能或就地翻译。
- 蛋白质编码基因只占转录基因总数的一小部分，转录基因还包括非编码RNA，如小RNA（微RNA和核仁小RNA）、长非编码RNA和调节RNA（转移RNA和核糖体RNA）。

要点总结

- CHRNA5/CHRNA3/CHRNB4基因簇位于染色体15q25.1上的紧密连锁不平衡区域。
- CHRNA5、CHRNA3和CHRNB4经常是共表达的，并在外周和与奖励加工直接相关的脑区形成功能性配体门控离子通道。
- 这种烟碱基因簇包含许多控制这些亚基协调表达的调控元件，其中一些还含有进一步调节表达的遗传变异。
- 远端增强子的多态性显著增加了CHRNA5和CHRNA3在大脑和外周的表达，其中以CHRNA5的影响最大。
- CHRNB4（rs1948）的3′非翻译区的多态性以组织特异性的方式调节了CHRNA3的表达，显著增加了纹状体的表达。
- 表观遗传因素，如CpG甲基化，与该基因簇中的单核苷酸多态性显著相关，但它们对成瘾的重要性尚未确定。
- 在烟碱成瘾的临床关联研究中，非同义多态性rs16969968驱动着最强、最具重复性的单一信号。
- 了解CHRNA5/CHRNA3/CHRNB4基因座多态性的功能效应，可以创建rs16969968的单倍型用于临床分析，揭示通过测量与单个变异的关联而没有观察到的关联。

参考文献

Albers, K. M.; Zhang, X. L.; Diges, C. M.; Schwartz, E. S.; Yang, C. I.; Davis, B. M. et al. (2014). Artemin growth factor increases nicotinic cholinergic receptor subunit expression and activity in nociceptive sensory neurons. Molecular Pain, 10, 31.

Amos, C. I.; Wu, X.; Broderick, P.; Gorlov, I. P.; Gu, J.; Eisen, T. et al. (2008). Genome-wide association scan of tag SNPs identifies a susceptibility locus for lung cancer at 15q25. 1. Nature Genetics, 40 (5), 616-622.

Barrie, E. S.; Hartmann, K.; Lee, S. H.; Frater, J. T.; Seweryn, M.; Wang, D. et al. (2017). The CHRNA5/CHRNA3/CHRNB4 nicotinic receptor regulome: genomic architecture, regulatory polymorphisms, and clinical associations. Human Mutation, 38(1), 112-119.

Benfante, R.; Flora, A.; Di Lascio, S.; Cargnin, F.; Longhi, R.; Colombo, S. et al. (2007). Transcription factor PHOX2A regulates the human alpha3 nicotinic receptor subunit gene promoter. The Journal of Biological Chemistry, 282(18), 13290-13302.

Bierut, L. J.; Madden, P. A.; Breslau, N.; Johnson, E. O.; Hatsukami, D.; Pomerleau, O. F. et al. (2007). Novel genes identified in a highdensity genome wide association study for nicotine dependence. Human Molecular Genetics, 16(1), 24-35.

Bigger, C. B.; Casanova, E. A.; Gardner, P. D. (1996). Transcriptional regulation of neuronal nicotinic acetylcholine receptor genes. Functional interactions between Sp1 and the rat beta4 subunit gene promoter. The Journal of Biological Chemistry, 272(51), 32842-32848.

Bigger, C. B.; Melnikova, I. N.; Gardner, P. D. (1997). Sp1 and Sp3 regulate expression of the neuronal nicotinic acetylcholine receptor beta4 subunit gene. The Journal of Biological Chemistry, 272(41), 25976-25982.

Campos-Caro, A.; Carrasco-Serrano, C.; Valor, L. M.; Viniegra, S.; Ballesta, J. J.; Criado, M. (1999). Multiple functional Sp1 domains in the minimal promoter region of the neuronal nicotinic receptor alpha5 subunit gene. The Journal of Biological Chemistry, 274(8), 4693-4701.

Doyle, G. A.; Wang, M. J.; Chou, A. D.; Oleynick, J. U.; Arnold, S. E.; Buono, R. J. et al. (2011). In vitro and ex vivo analysis of CHRNA3 and CHRNA5 haplotype expression. PLoS One. 6(8), e23373.

Flora, A. V.; Zambrano, C. A.; Gallego, X.; Miyamoto, J. H.; Johnson, K. A.; Cowan, K. A. et al. (2013). Functional characterization of SNPs in CHRNA3/B4 intergenic region associated with drug behaviors. Brain Research, 1529, 1-15.

Fornasari, D.; Battagliolo, E.; Flora, A.; Terzano, S.; Clementi, F. (1997). Structural and functional characterization of the human alpha3 nicotinic subunit gene promoter. Molecular Pharmacology, 51(2), 250-261.

Fowler, C. D.; Lu, Q.; Johnson, P. M.; Marks, M. J.; Kenny, P. J. (2011). Habenular alpha5 nicotinic receptor subunit signalling controls nicotine intake. Nature, 471(7340), 597-601.

Frahm, S.; Slimak, M. A.; Ferrarese, L.; Santos-Torres, J.; AntolinFontes, B.; Auer, S. et al. (2011). Aversion to nicotine is regulated by the balanced activity of beta4 and alpha5 nicotinic receptor subunits in the medial habenula. Neuron, 70(3), 522-535.

Gallego, X.; Cox, R. J.; Laughlin, J. R.; Stitzel, J. A.; Ehringer, M. A. (2013). Alternative CHRNB4 3'-UTRs mediate the allelic effects of SNP rs1948 on gene expression. PLoS One. 8(5)e63699.

Genzen, J. R.; McGehee, D. S. (2003). Short- and long-term enhancement of excitatory transmission in the spinal cord dorsal horn by nicotinic acetylcholine receptors. Proceedings of the National Academy of Sciences of the United States of America, 100(11), 6807-6812.

George, A. A.; Lucero, L. M.; Damaj, M. I.; Lukas, R. J.; Chen, X.; Whiteaker, P. (2012). Function of human alpha3beta4alpha5 nicotinic acetylcholine receptors is reduced by the alpha5(D398N) polymorphism. The Journal of Biological Chemistry, 287(30), 25151-25162.

Getz, A. M.; Xu, F.; Visser, F.; Persson, R.; Syed, N. I. (2017). Tumor suppressor menin is required for subunit-specific nAChR alpha5 transcription and nAChR-dependent presynaptic facilitation in cultured mouse hippocampal neurons. Scientific Reports, 7(1), 1768.

GTEx Consortium. (2013). The genotype-tissue expression (GTEx) project. Nature Genetics, 45(6), 580-585.

Hancock, D. B.; Wang, J. C.; Gaddis, N. C.; Levy, J. L.; Saccone, N. L.; Stitzel, J. A. et al. (2015). A multiancestry study identifies novel genetic associations with CHRNA5 methylation in human brain and risk of nicotine dependence. Human Molecular Genetics, 24(20), 5940-5954.

Hone, A. J.; McIntosh, J. M.; Azam, L.; Lindstrom, J.; Lucero, L.; Whiteaker, P. et al. (2015). Alpha-conotoxins identify the alpha3beta4* subtype as the predominant nicotinic acetylcholine receptor expressed in human adrenal chromaffin cells. Molecular Pharmacology, 88(5), 881-893.

Jackson, K. J.; Sanjakdar, S. S.; Muldoon, P. P.; McIntosh, J. M.; Damaj, M. I. (2013). The alpha3beta4* nicotinic acetylcholine receptor subtype mediates nicotine reward and physical nicotine withdrawal signs independently of the alpha5 subunit in the mouse. Neuropharmacology, 70, 228-235.

Jensen, K. P.; DeVito, E. E.; Herman, A. I.; Valentine, G. W.; Gelernter, J.; Sofuoglu, M. (2015). A CHRNA5 smoking risk polymorphism decreases the aversive effects of nicotine in humans. Neuropsychopharmacology, 40(12), 2813-2821.

Li, M. D.; Xu, Q.; Lou, X. Y.; Payne, T. J.; Niu, T.; Ma, J. Z. (2010). Association and interaction analysis of polymorphisms in CHRNA5/CHRNA3/CHRNB4 gene cluster with nicotine dependence in African and European Americans. American Journal of Medical Genetics Part B, Neuropsychiatric Genetics, 153B(3), 745-756.

Li, M. D.; Yoon, D.; Lee, J. Y.; Han, B. G.; Niu, T.; Payne, T. J. et al. (2010). Associations of polymorphisms in CHRNA5/A3/B4 gene cluster with smoking behaviors in a Korean population. PLoS One. 5(8) e12183, https://doi. org/10. 1371/journal. pone. 0012183.

Liu, Q.; Melnikova, I. N.; Hu, M.; Gardner, P. D. (1999). Cell typespecific activation of neuronal nicotinic acetylcholine receptor subunit genes by Sox10. The Journal of Neuroscience, 19(22), 9747-9755.

Mao, D.; Yasuda, R. P.; Fan, H.; Wolfe, B. B.; Kellar, K. J. (2006). Heterogeneity of nicotinic cholinergic receptors in rat superior cervical and nodose Ganglia. Molecular Pharmacology, 70(5), 1693-1699.

Olfson, E.; Saccone, N. L.; Johnson, E. O.; Chen, L. S.; Culverhouse, R.; Doheny, K. et al. (2016). Rare, low frequency and common coding polymorphisms in CHRNA5 and their contribution to nicotine dependence in European and African Americans. Molecular Psychiatry, 21(5), 601-607.

Perez, X. A.; O'Leary, K. T.; Parameswaran, N.; McIntosh, J. M.; Quik, M. (2009). Prominent role of alpha3/alpha6beta2* nAChRs in regulating evoked dopamine release in primate putamen: effect of long-term nicotine treatment. Molecular Pharmacology, 75(4), 938-946.

Ramsay, J. E.; Rhodes, C. H.; Thirtamara-Rajamani, K.; Smith, R. M. (2015). Genetic influences on nicotinic alpha5 receptor (CHRNA5) CpG methylation and mRNA expression in brain and adipose tissue. Genes Environment, 37, 14.

Saccone, N. L.; Culverhouse, R. C.; Schwantes-An, T. H.; Cannon, D. S.; Chen, X.; Cichon, S. et al. (2010). Multiple independent loci at chromosome 15q25. 1 affect smoking quantity: a meta-analysis and comparison with lung cancer and COPD. PLoS Genet. 6(8).

Saccone, S. F.; Hinrichs, A. L.; Saccone, N. L.; Chase, G. A.; Konvicka, K.; Madden, P. A. et al. (2007). Cholinergic nicotinic receptor genes implicated in a nicotine dependence association study targeting 348 candidate genes with 3713 SNPs. Human Molecular Genetics, 16 (1), 36-49.

Sadler, B.; Haller, G.; Edenberg, H.; Tischfield, J.; Brooks, A.; Kramer, J. et al. (2015). Positive selection on loci associated with drug and alcohol dependence. PLoS One. 10(8)e0134393.

Shih, P. Y.; Engle, S. E.; Oh, G.; Deshpande, P.; Puskar, N. L.; Lester, H. A. et al. (2014). Differential expression and function of nicotinic acetylcholine receptors in subdivisions of medial habenula. The Journal of Neuroscience, 34(29), 9789-9802.

Smith, R. M.; Alachkar, H.; Papp, A. C.; Wang, D.; Mash, D. C.; Wang, J. C. et al. (2011). Nicotinic alpha5 receptor subunit mRNA expression is associated with distant 5ʹupstream polymorphisms. European Journal of Human Genetics, 19(1), 76-83. https://doi.org/10.1038/ejhg.2010.120.

Tammimäki, A.; Herder, P.; Li, P.; Esch, C.; Laughlin, J. R.; Akk, G. et al. (2012). Impact of human D398N single nucleotide polymorphism on intracellular calcium response mediated by alpha3beta4alpha5 nicotinic acetylcholine receptors. Neuropharmacology, 63(6), 1002-1011.

Tobacco, Genetics Consortium (2010). Genome-wide meta-analyses identify multiple loci associated with smoking behavior. Nature Genetics, 42(5), 441-447.

Vernallis, A. B.; Conroy, W. G.; Berg, D. K. (1993). Neurons assemble acetylcholine receptors with as many as three kinds of subunits while maintaining subunit segregation among receptor subtypes. Neuron, 10(3), 451-464.

Volkov, P.; Olsson, A. H.; Gillberg, L.; Jorgensen, S. W.; Brons, C.; Eriksson, K. F. et al. (2016). A genome-wide mQTL analysis in human adipose tissue identifies genetic polymorphisms associated with DNA methylation, gene expression and metabolic traits. PLoS One. 11(6)e0157776.

Wang, F.; Gerzanich, V.; Wells, G. B.; Anand, R.; Peng, X.; Keyser, K. et al. (1996). Assembly of human neuronal nicotinic receptor alpha5 subunits with alpha3, beta2, and beta4 subunits. The Journal of Biological Chemistry, 271(30), 17656-17665.

Wang, J. C.; Cruchaga, C.; Saccone, N. L.; Bertelsen, S.; Liu, P.; Budde, J. P. et al. (2009). Risk for nicotine dependence and lung cancer is conferred by mRNA expression levels and amino acid change in CHRNA5. Human Molecular Genetics, 18(16), 3125-3135.

Wang, J. C.; Grucza, R.; Cruchaga, C.; Hinrichs, A. L.; Bertelsen, S.; Budde, J. P. et al. (2009). Genetic variation in the CHRNA5 gene affects mRNA levels and is associated with risk for alcohol dependence. Molecular Psychiatry, 14(5), 501-510.

Xie, P.; Kranzler, H. R.; Zhang, H.; Oslin, D.; Anton, R. F.; Farrer, L. A. et al. (2012). Childhood adversity increases risk for nicotine dependence and interacts with alpha5 nicotinic acetylcholine receptor genotype specifically in males. Neuropsychopharmacology, 37(3), 669-676.

Xu, X.; Scott, M. M.; Deneris, E. S. (2006). Shared long-range regulatory elements coordinate expression of a gene cluster encoding nicotinic receptor heteromeric subtypes. Molecular and Cellular Biology, 26(15), 5636-5649.

Yang, X.; McDonough, J.; Fyodorov, D.; Morris, M.; Wang, F.; Deneris, E. S. (1994). Characterization of an acetylcholine receptor alpha 3 gene promoter and its activation by the POU domain factor SCIP/Tst-1. The Journal of Biological Chemistry, 269(14), 10252-10264.

Yeh, J. J.; Yasuda, R. P.; Davila-Garcia, M. I.; Xiao, Y.; Ebert, S.; Gupta, T. et al. (2001). Neuronal nicotinic acetylcholine receptor alpha3 subunit protein in rat brain and sympathetic ganglion measured using a subunit-specific antibody: regional and ontogenic expression. Journal of Neurochemistry, 77(1), 336-346.

Yokotani, K.; Wang, M.; Okada, S.; Murakami, Y.; Hirata, M. (2000). Characterization of nicotinic acetylcholine receptor-mediated noradrenaline release from the isolated rat stomach. European Journal of Pharmacology, 402(3), 223-229.

Zhang, H.; Wang, F.; Kranzler, H. R.; Zhao, H.; Gelernter, J. (2013). Profiling of childhood adversity-associated DNA methylation changes in alcoholic patients and healthy controls. PLoS One. 8(6) e65648.

Zhang, X. L.; Albers, K. M.; Gold, M. S. (2015). Inflammation-induced increase in nicotinic acetylcholine receptor current in cutaneous nociceptive DRG neurons from the adult rat. Neuroscience, 284, 483-499.

Zoli, M.; Le Novere, N.; Hill, J. A., Jr.; Changeux, J. P. (1995). Developmental regulation of nicotinic ACh receptor subunit mRNAs in the rat central and peripheral nervous systems. The Journal of Neuroscience, 15 (3 Pt 1), 1912-1939.

44
大脑、Nrf2 和烟草：吸烟氧化应激介导的脑血管效应的机制和反馈机制

Shikha Prasad[1], Taylor Liles[2], Luca Cucullo[2]

1. Department of Neurology, Northwestern University Feinberg School of Medicine, Chicago, IL, United States
2. Department of Pharmaceutical Sciences, TTUHSC, School of Pharmacy, Amarillo, TX, United States

缩略语

ARE	抗氧化反应元件	NRF2	核因子红系 2 相关因子
BBB	血脑屏障	Nrf2	核因子红系 2 相关因子
COPD	慢性阻塞性肺疾病	OS	氧化应激
CS	卷烟烟雾	ROS	活性氧
CSE	卷烟烟雾提取物	SOD	超氧化物歧化酶
GSH	谷胱甘肽	TJ	紧密连接
MF	二甲双胍	TS	烟草烟雾
NQO-1	NAD(P)H 醌还原酶 I	ZO-1	闭合小带 -1

44.1 引言

在全球范围内，烟草使用每年造成约600万人死亡，预测报告称，按照目前的趋势，预计到2030年，每年将有800多万人死于烟草使用。目前，吸烟在美国每年造成超过48万人死亡，是美国可预防死亡的主要原因。平均而言，吸烟者比不吸烟者早10年死亡，如果青少年吸烟的比例继续保持目前的水平，预计每13名17岁或以下的美国人中就有一人会过早死亡于与吸烟有关的疾病。尽管近几年（2015年与2005年相比）吸烟率下降了约5%，但吸烟者仍占美国成年人口的15%。同样令人担忧的是，48万人中有4.1万人死于二手烟。此外，在过去的十年中，标榜是卷烟更安全替代品的电子烟的消费量有所上升，尽管这些说法没有科学证据支持（CDC, 2016b）。

对TS的成瘾主要是由烟碱引起的。然而，最近的研究也表明，烟草中的非烟碱成分，如假木贼碱、新烟草碱和降哈尔满本身就具有成瘾特性，并能进一步增强烟碱的成瘾性。烟草烟雾中含有7000多种化合物，包括63种不同的致癌物和一些氧化元素，它们可以严重影响细胞和组织功能，是引发重大健康疾病的先兆（How Tobacco Smoke Causes Disease, 2010）。

44.2 健康统计数据

在美国，每年因吸烟而死亡的人数可以统计如下：肺癌约29%，其他癌症约8%，缺血性心脏病约28%，慢性阻塞性肺疾病（COPD）约21%，中风约4%，其他疾病约10%（Surgeon General's

Report, 2015）。吸烟导致的肺癌死亡人数约占所有肺癌死亡人数的90%（不分性别）。对于每一个因吸烟而死亡的人，至少有30个人受到其影响，并患有与吸烟有关的严重疾病（CDC, 2016a）。

吸烟者患冠心病和中风的可能性是非吸烟者的2～4倍，患肺癌的可能性大约是非吸烟者的25倍。此外，吸烟还会导致糖尿病、类风湿性关节炎、肺炎、哮喘、失明、动脉硬化、生育力下降以及免疫系统受损，从而增加各种感染的风险和发展。吸烟者患糖尿病的风险比非吸烟者高30%～40%，其影响取决于吸烟量。孕期吸烟会增加异位妊娠、早产、死产、低出生体重、婴儿口裂和婴儿猝死综合征的风险（CDC, 2016b; The Health Consequences, 2014）。此外，吸烟是许多脑血管和神经疾病的前驱危险因素，包括中风（Surgeon General's Report, 2015）、阿尔茨海默病（Cataldo et al. 2010）、抑郁症（Martini et al. 2002）、认知障碍和血管性痴呆（Anstey et al. 2007）。吸烟对脑血管和神经的负面影响在很大程度上是由于烟草烟雾中高度浓缩的活性氧（ROS）（Naik et al. 2014; Sobczak et al. 2004）（另见图44.1），随之而来的炎症

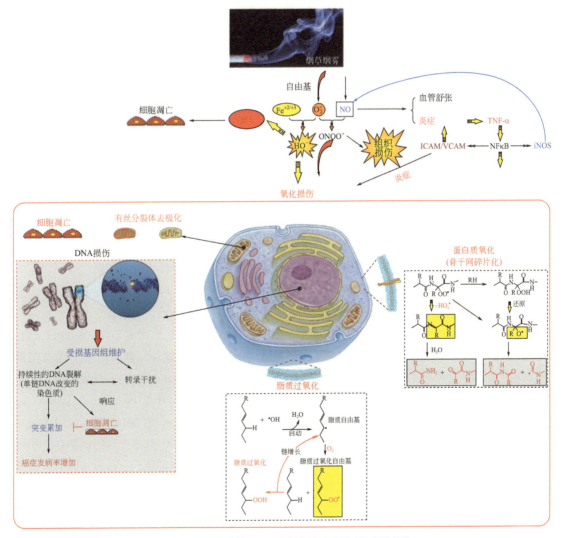

图44.1　TS衍生的ROS促进细胞炎症反应和氧化损伤

示意图描绘了主要的OS激活的途径，通过这些途径，烟草燃烧产生的ROS可以诱导脂质过氧化、蛋白质降解和DNA损伤，从而导致细胞损伤和炎症。

（Arnson, Shoenfeld, Amital, 2010）和血脑屏障（BBB）的损害（Rosenberg, 2012）。事实上，怀孕期间吸烟会影响胎儿的脑血管发育（How Tobacco Smoke Causes Disease, 2010; The Health Consequences, 2014）。

44.3 吸烟者：健康管理和当前挑战

烟草成瘾和依赖使得确保向想要戒烟的吸烟者提供有效的行为和药物戒烟治疗是很重要的（Galanti, 2008）。戒烟是恢复吸烟者健康的唯一有效途径。根据美国疾病控制与预防中心（CDC）的数据，戒烟一年可以显著降低心脏病发作和中风的风险。戒烟10年后，患肺癌的风险降低了一半（Larzelere, Williams, 2012）。Fagerström烟碱依赖测试有助于了解成瘾的严重程度。Fagerström总分越高，患者对烟碱的身体依赖就越强烈。临床上，针对烟碱成瘾的不同方面的治疗，如强化、戒断和线索相关的学习，从完全戒烟到用危害较小的产品替代，都会相应地实施。烟碱替代疗法和部分α4β2激动剂（烟碱乙酰胆碱受体配体）的药理干预被用来减少渴望（Wilkes, 2008）。在许多情况下，安非他酮被用来平息戒烟带来的负面情绪（Wilkes, 2008）。不幸的是，对于这些患者（既往吸烟者）或暴露在二手烟（SHS）环境中的人进行临床治疗，以减轻吸烟对健康的影响，目前还没有指南。美国国家科学院食品与营养委员会建议吸烟者摄入更多的维生素C（每天比不吸烟者多35mg）（ODS, 2016）；然而，这种疗法对慢性吸烟者的健康益处和整体影响仍不确定。至于其他抗氧化剂的预防性治疗，其结果相当有争议，并且高度依赖于实验设置、试剂的纯度和给药方案（Frei, 2004; Kaisar et al. 2015）。研究已经报道了一些流行的抗氧化剂和保健品的有益效果，强调它们清除ROS和/或抗炎的特性（Liu et al. 2014），如维生素、白藜芦醇、褪黑素和硫辛酸，而没有考虑它们对癌细胞生长和增殖的影响（Muller, Hengstermann, 2012）。

戒烟者戒烟的时间长短、在二手烟中的烟雾暴露水平、预先确定的健康状况和遗传学（以及长期吸烟引起的表观遗传学改变）等因素，几乎不是开始评估针对慢性吸烟者和既往吸烟者（特别是早期前吸烟者）（包括那些经常接触二手烟的人）的预防和/或治疗影响所需评估的标准。

更令人担忧的是，在过去十年中，许多替代雾化产品已经进入市场，迅速赢得了包括成年人在内的消费者，特别是青少年的喜爱（FDA, 2016）。电子烟碱传递系统或电子烟（e-cigs）已经成为抢手的产品，部分原因是人们相信它们比传统卷烟安全得多。此外，众所周知，TS与血管内皮细胞功能障碍之间的关联（Chen et al. 2004; Naik et al. 2014; Raij et al. 2001）是致因的和剂量依赖的（Gill et al. 1989），主要与TS中的活性氧（ROS）（Naik et al. 2014; Panda et al. 1999）、组织氧化应激（OS）驱动/组织氧化应激（OS）驱动的炎症（Arnson et al. 2010; Naik et al. 2014）和烟碱（Das et al., 2009; Paulson et al. 2010）有关。目前的科学观点认为OS介导的通路在这些疾病（特别是中风）的发病机制中起着重要作用（Cojocaru, Cojocaru, Sapira, Ionescu, 2013）。临床前研究还表明，烟碱（电子烟中使用的电子烟液的主要成分）也会导致OS、加重脑缺血和继发性脑损伤（Bradford et al. 2011; Li et al. 2016）。同样，最近的研究表明，长期吸食电子烟可能会导致脑血管损伤的前兆，并促进下列脑血管状况：加大中风的发生概率和加重缺血后的脑损伤（Kaisar et al. 2017; Prasad et al. 2017）。电子烟对健康的影响现在是公众和监管机构关注的一个主要问题，美国卫生局（E-Cigarette Use Among Youth and Young Adults, 2016）和美国食品药品监督管理局（FDA）最近的报告清楚地表明了这一点。

44.4 脑血管视角：吸烟、烟碱和血脑屏障

在细胞水平上，血脑屏障由血管内皮细胞衬里构成，脑微血管与星形细胞末端足突紧密相连（图44.2）（Abbott, Patabendige, Dolman, Yusof, Begley, 2010）。血脑屏障内皮细胞具有独特的跨膜运输系统的表达模式（细胞极化），以调节物质进出脑实质的运输。此外，内皮细胞间紧密连接的表达、缺乏窗口和最少的胞饮转运（这与调节和维持脑微环境的动态平衡有关）是血脑屏障内皮细胞的独特特征。相邻内皮细胞之间的紧密连接（TJ）形成扩散屏障，选择性地阻止大多数血源性物质（包括电解质和其他水溶性化合物）和外来极性物质通过细胞旁途径进入大脑（Abbott et al. 2010）。

还存在专门的外排转运机制［如P-糖蛋白、乳腺癌耐药蛋白（BCRP）和多药耐药蛋白-4（MRP-4）］，以调节两亲性和疏水性分子的通道，保护大脑免受潜在有害物质的伤害（Abbott et al. 2010）。

血脑屏障在保护大脑免受卷烟烟雾产生的氧化和炎症应激方面起着至关重要的作用。然而，烟草烟雾中含有各种ROS，如过氧化氢、环氧化物、二氧化氮和过氧亚硝酸盐（ONOO⁻），它们都具有氧化损伤作用，能够通过TJ修饰和激活促炎/抗炎途径导致血脑屏障的破坏（Naik et al. 2014; Pun, Lu, Moochhala, 2009）。在正常情况下，在细胞内超氧化物歧化酶、过氧化氢酶、谷胱甘肽过氧化物酶（Hayes, Strange, 1995）或（细胞外）抗氧化维生素如抗坏血酸（维生素C）和α-生育酚（维生素E）的作用下，ROS被清除或转化为活性较低的分子（Davitashvili et al. 2010; Gallo et al. 2010）。然而，无论是主动吸烟还是被动吸烟，其产生的ROS都超过了人体可以有效消除的水平。支持这一事实的是，几项研究表明，慢性吸烟者有抗氧化剂短缺的情况，这是因为它增加了动员来对抗由富含ROS的TS引起的系统性氧化应激（Dietrich et al. 2003; Tsuchiya et al. 2002）。此外，当补充某些抗氧化剂时，由TS在动物和细胞中诱导的氧化和炎症似乎有不同程度的减少（Hossain et al. 2011; Kaisar et al. 2015）。最近的研究表明，卷烟烟雾提取物（CSE）含有高浓度的一氧化氮和过氧化氢，这对应于细胞氧化应激（使用CellROX®Green试剂测量）的显著增加，并诱导BBB内皮功能障碍和强烈的炎症反应。这包括①TJ蛋白表达ZO-1和闭合蛋白的下调和再分布，② VE-cadherin和claudin-5的上调（可能是一种细胞保护性反调节活性），③黏附分子的表达增强，④促炎细胞因子的释放，包括白细胞介素-6（IL-6）和基质金属蛋白酶-2（MMP-2）（Naik et al. 2014）。这些事件可导致持续（慢性）CS暴露（如慢性吸烟者）对脑血管系统和血脑屏障的氧化损伤，并促进脑血管疾病的发生和发展（Hossain et al. 2009）。最近发表的数据有力地表明，慢性TS和电子烟暴露引起的大量脑血管和血脑屏障损伤在很大程度上是由于核因子红系2相关因子（Nrf2）调节的内源性抗氧化反应元件（ARE）的改变，Nrf2是一种普遍表达的氧化还原敏感转录因子，也是通过抗氧化、药物代谢、抗炎、解毒和清除自由基而参与氧化还原稳态的复杂分子系统网络的组成性或诱导性表达的主要调节者（Hayes, Dinkova-Kostova, 2014a）。相反，Nrf2的缺失或下调已证明增强了细胞对促氧化剂和炎性刺激的毒性效应的敏感性，包括细胞生物能量学的崩溃，从而导致细胞和组织损伤（Holmstrom et al. 2013; Mitsuishi et al. 2012）（见图44.3）。

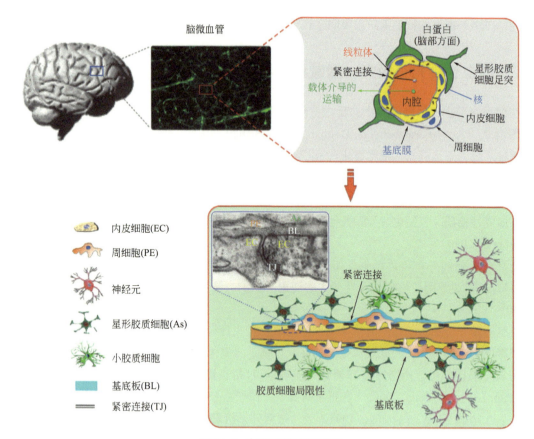

图 44.2 血脑屏障解剖示意图

脑微血管的横切面显示内皮细胞（EC）的最内腔位于基底板（BL）支撑上，周围环绕着另外一层连续的周细胞（PE）和星形胶质细胞（AS）足突，这些突起将血管与脑实质分开。紧密连接（TJ）存在于大脑内皮细胞之间，选择性地阻止极性分子通过细胞旁途径进入大脑，而主动运输系统允许营养物质和其他基本因素的通过。

44.5 Nrf2通路在TS所致的脑血管功能障碍中的作用

正常情况下，Nrf2通过kelchECH相关蛋白1（keap1）/cullin-3/Rbx-1被胞质中的26S蛋白酶体降解。然而，细胞内的稳态是通过Nrf2在细胞核中的基础积累来维持的，Nrf2介导了ARE依赖基因的正常表达。在应激条件下或在ARE诱导剂存在的情况下，多泛素化被抑制，从而导致Nrf2的激活。内源性p62（自噬的选择性底物）的增加会抑制keap1介导的Nrf2泛素化和降解，从而激活Nrf2并诱导ARE依赖基因。Nrf2还受磷酸化[通过各种蛋白激酶（如PKC和AMPK)]和乙酰化/去乙酰化过程的调节。除此之外，组蛋白磷酸化和乙酰化、CpG岛甲基化[胞嘧啶（C）碱基紧跟鸟嘌呤（G）碱基]以及特定miRNAs的合成（表观遗传机制）是细胞调节Nrf2水平的另一种手段（Hayes, Dinkova-Kostova, 2014b; Sandberg et al. 2014）。

外源Nrf2-ARE诱导剂有多种来源，从天然植物化学衍生物（如齐墩果酸、萝卜硫素、染料木素和姜黄素等）到合成产品（如对乙酰氨基酚和尼美舒利）。在某些情况下，这些药物被发现比前列腺素等内源性诱导剂更有效。到目前为止，许多诱导剂正在动物和人类身上进行严格的预防和治疗应用研究（Ma, He, 2012）。

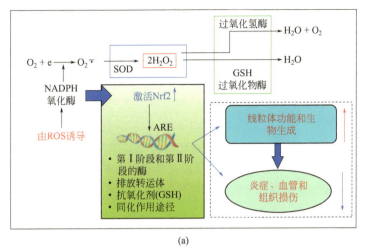

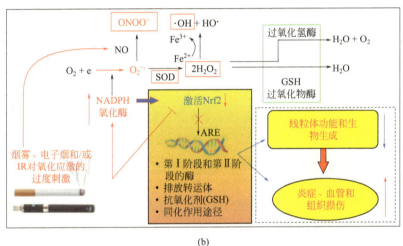

图 44.3 正常和应激条件下细胞抗氧化反应元件的激活

（a）在正常情况下，对损伤的反应是适应性的，旨在恢复动态平衡，保护细胞免受进一步的损伤。（b）在TS促进的氧化应激下，NADPH氧化酶被激活，产生过量的O_2^-，O_2^-在一氧化氮（TS中也存在丰富的NO）的存在下导致过氧亚硝酸盐（$ONOO^-$）的形成。此外，过量的H_2O_2会导致羟基自由基（$OH·$；芬顿反应）的形成。Nrf2活性的失调阻止了细胞对这些OS刺激的反应，导致线粒体功能和生物发生的损害和细胞损伤。

44.6 靶向Nrf2预防吸烟所致的脑血管功能障碍

概念验证实验表明，Nrf2缺陷小鼠在慢性CS暴露6个月后出现早期广泛的肺气肿（Rangasamy et al. 2004）。此外，合成的三萜类1[2-氰基-3,12-二氧代齐墩甲烷-1,9(11)-二烯-28-油基]咪唑（CDDO-Im），一种已知的Nrf2诱导剂，显著减少了慢性CS暴露引起的肺氧化应激、肺泡破坏和肺气肿（Sussan et al. 2009）。TS本身含有数不清的单功能和双功能Nrf2诱导剂，在急性体外实验环境中，已经证明这些诱导剂能激活许多细胞保护基因的表达。然而，体外和体内的慢性TS暴露都已证明对Nrf2水平有负面影响，从而增加了细胞和组织的氧化负担。例如，Goven等的研究表明，TS冷凝物能激活人巨噬细胞THP-1细胞中Nrf2的核定位，并在作用6h后引起HO-1表达增加，72h后Nrf2核定位和HO-1表达降低（Goven et al. 2009）。该研究小组后来还报道，与非肺气肿患者相比，肺气肿患者全肺组织和肺泡巨噬细胞（细胞质和细胞核）中的 Nrf2 蛋白水平显著降低（Goven et al. 2008）。

在这种脑微血管系统的背景下，一些研究试图确定 Nrf2 在维持血脑屏障功能完整性和防止与各种中枢神经系统病理相关的脑血管功能障碍的发生中的作用（Li et al. 2014; Zhao et al. 2007）。例如，Zhao 等之前的发现（Zhao et al. 2007）提出，脑损伤后 Nrf2 信号的药理激活可以恢复紧密连接（TJ）的丢失，防止血脑屏障的破坏。同样，Nrf2-ARE 系统的激活被认为可以防止缺血性中风后血脑屏障的破坏和神经功能障碍（Alfieri et al. 2013）。Nrf2 在血脑屏障完整性和活性方面的重要性最近在体外和体内都得到了证实，而二甲双胍诱导 Nrf2 的表达水平和激活（核转位），从而促进 TJ 蛋白的上调，而沉默 Nrf2 的表达则取消了它们的表达（Sajja, Green, Cucullo, 2015）。

总体而言，这些发现表明，靶向 Nrf2 系统可能是一个可行的治疗选择（尽管探索仍然很少），以开发新的、更有效的策略来预防神经血管功能障碍和继发性中枢神经系统损伤，不仅对 TS 和类似产品，而且对其他几种与 OS 相关的致病刺激也有反应。因此，制药行业对 Nrf2 激活剂（如萝卜硫素、姜黄素和对乙酰氨基酚）用于开发动物和人类的预防和治疗应用产生极大兴趣是不足为奇的（Crunkhorn, 2012）。最近，二甲双胍（一种成熟的抗糖尿病药物）被证明可以有效地防止 TS 损害血脑屏障功能，并促进促凝状态，从而增加中风的风险。这种作用似乎是通过 Nrf2-ARE 功能的正向调节（激活）来实现的（Ashabi et al. 2014; Kaisar et al. 2017; Prasad et al. 2017）。

总之，有必要进一步深入研究 TS 引起的血管和脑血管损伤的机制，特别是考虑到市场上推出的许多替代产品。在吸烟者、戒烟者和二手吸烟者中识别指示氧化应激水平和相关脑血管损伤的标志物，对于评估中枢神经系统疾病的发展和开始临床治疗以降低风险和戒烟将是非常有用的。这还包括确定诸如吸烟者的表观遗传突变（Nrf2 突变与癌细胞在进一步刺激下逐渐生长有关）等条件，这表明 OS 损伤的进一步易感性和/或排除在基于 Nrf2-ARE 的临床治疗之外。

术语解释

- 激动剂：一种在结合时激活受体的化学物质。
- 双官能团：具有两个高活性位点的化学结构。
- 血脑屏障：存在于脑微血管水平的高度选择性血管屏障。
- 宫外孕：胎儿在子宫外发育，大部分在输卵管内发育。
- 流出物：从一种物质中排出。
- 表观遗传：可遗传的基因表达变化。
- 单官能团：具有单一高活性位点的化学结构。
- 突变：指基因结构的改变。
- 泛素化：标记蛋白质降解的过程。
- 促炎剂：导致发炎的物质。
- 预防药：预防性的药物。
- 活性氧物种：含氧的化学反应分子。
- 死产：怀孕 24 周后胎儿死亡。
- 外源化合物：对身体来说是外来的物质。

烟草烟雾的关键事实

- 烟草是一种原产于美洲、澳大利亚、西南非洲和南太平洋的草本植物（茄科），用于生产制造卷烟的烟叶。
- 烟草烟雾中含有约7000种化学物质，其中已经确定了60种成分人体吸入癌症的风险值和38种成分非癌症吸入风险值。
- 非癌症风险包括直接鼻部损伤、呼吸影响、慢性活动性炎症和肺纤维化、神经疾病，以及对消化、肝/肾和生殖的影响。
- 烟草的主要成瘾成分是烟碱，它可以在 10~20s 内到达大脑。

烟碱的关键事实

- 烟碱是主要的烟草生物碱，在商品卷烟中的含量约为 1.5%，约占总生物碱含量的 95%。
- 烟碱本身通过呼吸道、肺泡和皮肤的小气道被很好地吸收（不是从胃吸收，但在小肠中被很好地吸收）。
- 烟碱吸收后进入血液，在 pH = 7.4 时，大约 69% 的烟碱被电离，31% 的烟碱处于未电离状态。
- 吸烟使烟碱迅速进入肺静脉循环，然后迅速进入全身动脉循环和大脑。
- 烟碱主要在肝脏中代谢，主要代谢物是可替宁，它通常被用作暴露于烟草烟雾中的生物标志物。

核因子红系2相关因子（Nrf2）的关键事实

- Nrf2是一种转录因子，它调节抗氧化蛋白的表达，保护其免受损伤和炎症引发的氧化损伤。
- Nrf2也是解毒和细胞防御基因表达的主要调节因子。
- Nrf2在大脑、肾脏、肌肉、心脏、肺和肝脏中普遍表达，浓度很高。

要点总结

- 本章重点研究吸烟对脑血管系统的影响，以及核因子红系2相关因子（Nrf2）作为对抗TS诱导的氧化应激的应对机制的作用。
- 目前的科学观点认为，OS在中风、血管性痴呆、小血管缺血性疾病和阿尔茨海默病（AD）等与TS相关的主要脑血管和神经炎性疾病的发病机制中发挥重要作用。
- 慢性TS暴露会损害脑血管水平的抗氧化反应系统，从而成为神经疾病发病的一个强有力的前驱因素。
- Nrf2是一种氧化还原敏感的转录因子，是细胞抗氧化防御的主要调节因子。
- Nrf2活性对细胞氧化还原动态平衡至关重要，Nrf2信号缺陷（如慢性TS暴露时观察到的Nrf2信号缺陷）与多种中枢神经系统疾病有关。

参考文献

Abbott, N. J.; Patabendige, A. A.; Dolman, D. E.; Yusof, S. R.; Begley, D. J. (2010). Structure and function of the blood-brain barrier. Neurobiology of Disease, 37, 13-25.

Alfieri, A.; Srivastava, S.; Siow, R. C.; Cash, D.; Modo, M.; Duchen, M. R. et al. (2013). Sulforaphane preconditioning of the Nrf2/HO-1 defense pathway protects the cerebral vasculature against blood-brain barrier disruption and neurological deficits in stroke. Free Radical Biology, Medicine, 65, 1012-1022.

Anstey, K. J.; von, S. C.; Salim, A.; O'Kearney, R. (2007). Smoking as a risk factor for dementia and cognitive decline: a meta-analysis of prospective studies. American Journal of Epidemiology, 166, 367-378.

Arnson, Y.; Shoenfeld, Y.; Amital, H. (2010). Effects of tobacco smoke on immunity, inflammation and autoimmunity . Journal of Autoimmunity, 34, J258-J265.

Ashabi, G.; Khalaj, L.; Khodagholi, F.; Goudarzvand, M.; Sarkaki, A. (2014). Pre-treatment with metformin activates Nrf2 antioxidant pathways and inhibits inflammatory responses through induction of AMPK after transient global cerebral ischemia. Metabolic Brain Disease 30(3), 747-754. (2014).

Bradford, S. T.; Stamatovic, S. M.; Dondeti, R. S.; Keep, R. F.; Andjelkovic, A. V. (2011). Nicotine aggravates the brain postischemic inflammatory response . American Journal of Physiology—Heart and Circulatory Physiology, 300, H1518-H1529.

Cataldo, J. K.; Prochaska, J. J.; Glantz, S. A. (2010). Cigarette smoking is a risk factor for Alzheimer's disease: an analysis controlling for tobacco industry affiliation. Journal of Alzheimer's Disease, 19, 465-480.

CDC (Ed.). (2016). Fast facts (12-20-2016). https://www. cdc. gov/tobacco/data_statistics/fact_sheets/fast_facts/index. htm.

CDC (Ed.). (2016). Health effects of cigarette smoking (12-1-2016). https:// www. cdc. gov/tobacco/data_statistics/fact_sheets/health_effects/ effects_cig_smoking/.

Chen, H. W.; Chien, M. L.; Chaung, Y. H.; Lii, C. K.; Wang, T. S. (2004). Extracts from cigarette smoke induce DNA damage and cell adhesion molecule expression through different pathways. ChemicoBiological Interactions, 150, 233-241.

Cojocaru, I. M.; Cojocaru, M.; Sapira, V.; Ionescu, A. (2013). Evaluation of oxidative stress in patients with acute ischemic stroke. Romanian Journal of Internal Medicine, 51, 97-106.

Crunkhorn, S. (2012). Deal watch: abbott boosts investment in NRF2 activators for reducing oxidative stress. Nature Reviews Drug Discovery, 11, 96.

Das, S.; Gautam, N.; Dey, S. K.; Maiti, T.; Roy, S. (2009). Oxidative stress in the brain of nicotine-induced toxicity: protective role of Andrographis paniculata Nees and vitamin E. Applied Physiology, Nutrition, and Metabolism, 34, 124-135.

Davitashvili, D. T.; Museridze, D. P.; Svanidze, I. K.; Pavliashvili, N. S.; Sanikidze, T. V. (2010). Correction of oxidative stress in the rat brain cortical cellular culture with vitamines E and C. Georgian Medical News, (180), 56-60.

Dietrich, M.; Block, G.; Norkus, E. P.; Hudes, M.; Traber, M. G.; Cross, C. E. et al. (2003). Smoking and exposure to environmental tobacco smoke decrease some plasma antioxidants and increase gammatocopherol in vivo after adjustment for dietary antioxidant intakes. The American Journal of Clinical Nutrition, 77, 160-166.

E-Cigarette Use Among Youth and Young Adults. (2016). A report of the surgeon general. U. S. Department of health and human services. FDA (2016). Youth tobacco use: results from the 2014 national youth tobacco survey. Frei, B. (2004). Efficacy of dietary antioxidants to prevent oxidative damage and inhibit chronic disease. Journal of Nutrition, 134, 3196S-3198S.

Galanti, L. M. (2008). Tobacco smoking cessation management: integrating varenicline in current practice. Vascular Health and Risk Management, 4, 837-845.

Gallo, C.; Renzi, P.; Loizzo, S.; Loizzo, A.; Piacente, S.; Festa, M. et al. (2010). Potential therapeutic effects of vitamin e and C on placental oxidative stress induced by nicotine: an in vitro evidence. Open Biochemistry Journal, 4, 77-82.

Gill, J. S.; Shipley, M. J.; Tsementzis, S. A.; Hornby, R.; Gill, S. K.; Hitchcock, E. R. et al. (1989). Cigarette smoking. A risk factor for hemorrhagic and nonhemorrhagic stroke. Archives of Internal Medicine, 149, 2053-2057.

Goven, D.; Boutten, A.; Lecon-Malas, V.; Boczkowski, J.; Bonay, M. (2009). Prolonged cigarette smoke exposure decreases heme oxygenase-1 and alters Nrf2 and Bach1 expression in human macrophages: roles of the MAP kinases ERK(1/2) and JNK. FEBS Letters, 583, 3508-3518.

Goven, D.; Boutten, A.; Lecon-Malas, V.; Marchal-Somme, J.; Amara, N.; Crestani, B. et al. (2008). Altered Nrf2/Keap1-Bach1 equilibrium in pulmonary emphysema. Thorax, 63, 916-924.

Hayes, J. D.; Dinkova-Kostova, A. T. (2014a). The Nrf2 regulatory network provides an interface between redox and intermediary metabolism. Trends in Biochemical Sciences, 39, 199-218.

Hayes, J. D.; Strange, R. C. (1995). Potential contribution of the glutathione S-transferase supergene family to resistance to oxidative stress. Free Radical Research, 22, 193-207.

Holmstrom, K. M.; Baird, L.; Zhang, Y.; Hargreaves, I.; Chalasani, A.; Land, J. M. et al. (2013). Nrf2 impacts cellular bioenergetics by controlling substrate availability for mitochondrial respiration. Biology Open, 2, 761-770.

Hossain, M.; Mazzone, P.; Tierney, W.; Cucullo, L. (2011). In vitro assessment of tobacco smoke toxicity at the BBB: do antioxidant supplements have a protective role? BMC Neuroscience, 12, 92.

Hossain, M.; Sathe, T.; Fazio, V.; Mazzone, P.; Weksler, B.; Janigro, D. et al. (2009). Tobacco smoke: a critical etiological factor for vascular impairment at the blood-brain barrier. Brain-Research, 1287, 192-205.

How Tobacco Smoke Causes Disease. (2010). The biology and behavioral basis for smoking-attributable disease: a report of the surgeon general. Chapter 3. Publications and Reports of the Surgeon General.

Kaisar, M. A.; Prasad, S.; Cucullo, L. (2015). Protecting the BBB endothelium against cigarette smoke-induced oxidative stress using popular antioxidants: are they really beneficial? Brain Research, 1627, 90-100.

Kaisar, M. A.; Villalba, H.; Prasad, S.; Liles, T.; Sifat, A. E.; Sajja, R. K. et al. (2017). Offsetting the impact of smoking and e-cigarette vaping on the cerebrovascular system and stroke injury: is metformin a viable countermeasure? Redox Biology, 13, 353-362.

Larzelere, M. M.; Williams, D. E. (2012). Promoting smoking cessation. American Family Physician, 85, 591-598.

Li, C.; Sun, H.; Arrick, D. M.; Mayhan, W. G. (2016). Chronic nicotine exposure exacerbates transient focal cerebral ischemia-induced brain injury. Journal of Applied Physiology, 120, 328-333.

Li, T.; Wang, H.; Ding, Y.; Zhou, M.; Zhou, X.; Zhang, X. et al. (2014). Genetic elimination of Nrf2 aggravates secondary complications except for vasospasm after experimental subarachnoid hemorrhage in mice. Brain Research, 1558, 90-99.

Liu, H.; Ren, J.; Chen, H.; Huang, Y.; Li, H.; Zhang, Z. et al. (2014). Resveratrol protects against cigarette smoke-induced oxidative damage and pulmonary inflammation. Journal of Biochemical and Molecular Toxicology, 28, 465-471.

Ma, Q.; He, X. (2012). Molecular basis of electrophilic and oxidative defense: promises and perils of Nrf2. Pharmacological Reviews, 64, 1055-1081.

Martini, S.; Wagner, F. A.; Anthony, J. C. (2002). The association of tobacco smoking and depression in adolescence: evidence from the United States. Substance Use, Misuse, 37, 1853-1867.

Mitsuishi, Y.; Taguchi, K.; Kawatani, Y.; Shibata, T.; Nukiwa, T.; Aburatani, H. et al. (2012). Nrf2 redirects glucose and glutamine into anabolic pathways in metabolic reprogramming. Cancer Cell, 22, 66-79.

Muller, T.; Hengstermann, A. (2012). Nrf2: friend and foe in preventing cigarette smoking-dependent lung disease. Chemical Research in Toxicology, 25, 1805-1824.

Naik, P.; Fofaria, N.; Prasad, S.; Sajja, R. K.; Weksler, B.; Couraud, P. O. et al. (2014). Oxidative and pro-inflammatory impact of regular and denicotinized cigarettes on blood brain barrier endothelial cells: is smoking reduced or nicotine-free products really safe? BMC Neuroscience, 15, 51.

ODS. (Ed.), (2016). Vitamin C [2-11-2016]. https://ods. od. nih. gov/ factsheets/VitaminC-HealthProfessional/#en8.

Panda, K.; Chattopadhyay, R.; Ghosh, M. K.; Chattopadhyay, D. J.; Chatterjee, I. B. (1999). Vitamin C prevents cigarette smoke induced oxidative damage of proteins and increased proteolysis. Free Radical Biology, Medicine, 27, 1064-1079.

Paulson, J. R.; Yang, T.; Selvaraj, P. K.; Mdzinarishvili, A.; Van der Schyf, C. J.; Klein, J. et al. (2010). Nicotine exacerbates brain edema during in vitro and in vivo focal ischemic conditions. Journal of Pharmacology and Experimental Therapeutics, 332, 371-379.

Prasad, S.; Sajja, R. K.; Kaisar, M. A.; Park, J. H.; Villalba, H.; Liles, T. et al. (2017). Role of Nrf2 and protective effects of metformin against tobacco smoke-induced cerebrovascular toxicity. Redox Biology, 12, 58-69.

Pun, P. B.; Lu, J.; Moochhala, S. (2009). Involvement of ROS in BBB dysfunction. Free Radical Research, 43, 348-364.

Raij, L.; Demaster, E. G.; Jaimes, E. A. (2001). Cigarette smoke-induced endothelium dysfunction: role of superoxide anion. Journal of Hypertension, 19, 891-897.

Rangasamy, T.; Cho, C. Y.; Thimmulappa, R. K.; Zhen, L.; Srisuma, S. S.; Kensler, T. W. et al. (2004). Genetic ablation of Nrf2 enhances susceptibility to cigarette smoke-induced emphysema in mice. Journal of Clinical Investigation, 114, 1248-1259.

Rosenberg, G. A. (2012). Neurological diseases in relation to the bloodbrain barrier. Journal of Cerebral Blood Flow, Metabolism, 32, 1139-1151.

Sajja, R. K.; Green, K. N.; Cucullo, L. (2015). Altered Nrf2 signaling mediates hypoglycemia-induced blood-brain barrier endothelial dysfunction in vitro. PLoS One, 10, e0122358.

Sandberg, M.; Patil, J.; D'Angelo, B.; Weber, S. G.; Mallard, C. (2014). NRF2-regulation in brain health and disease: implication of cerebral inflammation. Neuropharmacology, 79, 298-306.

Sobczak, A.; Golka, D.; Szoltysek-Boldys, I. (2004). The effects of tobacco smoke on plasma alpha- and gamma-tocopherol levels in passive and active cigarette smokers. Toxicology Letters, 151, 429-437.

Surgeon General's Report. (2015). Surgeon general's report: the health consequences of smoking—50 years of progress. .

Sussan, T. E.; Rangasamy, T.; Blake, D. J.; Malhotra, D.; El-Haddad, H.; Bedja, D. et al. (2009). Targeting Nrf2 with the triterpenoid CDDOimidazolide attenuates cigarette smoke-induced emphysema and cardiac dysfunction in mice. Proceedings of the National Academy of Sciences of the United States of America, 106, 250-255.

The Health Consequences. (2014). The health consequences of smoking-50 years of progress: a report of the surgeon general. .

Tsuchiya, M.; Asada, A.; Kasahara, E.; Sato, E. F.; Shindo, M.; Inoue, M. (2002). Smoking a single cigarette rapidly reduces combined concentrations of nitrate and nitrite and concentrations of antioxidants in plasma. Circulation, 105, 1155-1157.

Wilkes, S. (2008). The use of bupropion SR in cigarette smoking cessation. International Journal of Chronic Obstructive Pulmonary Disease, 3, 4 5-53.

Zhao, J.; Moore, A. N.; Redell, J. B.; Dash, P. K. (2007). Enhancing expression of Nrf2-driven genes protects the blood brain barrier after brain injury. The Journal of Neuroscience, 27, 10240-10248.

45
烟碱和组蛋白脱乙酰酶抑制剂对大脑的影响

Maria Paula Faillace, Ramon O. Bernabeu

Departamento de Fisiología e Instituto de Fisiología y Biofísica (IFIBIO-Houssay, UBA-CONICET), Universidad de Buenos Aires (UBA), Paraguay 2155, Buenos Aires, Argentina

缩略语

CPA	条件性位置厌恶	NaB	丁酸钠
CpG	胞嘧啶-鸟嘌呤岛	NAcc	伏隔核
CPP	条件性位置偏好	nAChR	烟碱乙酰胆碱受体
CREB	环磷酸腺苷反应元件结合蛋白	NOR	新奇物体识别
DNMT	DNA甲基转移酶	OR	物体识别
dStr	背侧纹状体	pCREB	磷酸化CREB
H3	组蛋白3	PFC	前额叶皮层
H4	组蛋白4	PhB	丁酸苯酯
HAT	组蛋白乙酰转移酶	PrL	前额叶区域
HDAC	组蛋白脱乙酰酶	TSA	曲古抑素A
HDACi	HDAC抑制剂	VTA	腹侧被盖区

45.1 引言

遗传信息存储在极长的核苷酸线性序列中，因此真核生物中的遗传物质被排列成复杂的结构，有效地将DNA包装在细胞核内（Horn, Peterson, 2002）。DNA链与核蛋白一起形成染色质。组蛋白（H）是染色质中主要的结构性和组成性调节蛋白。146个碱基对的DNA被一个八聚体的组蛋白缠绕两次。每个八聚体由每种类型的组蛋白的两个亚基组成：H2A、H2B、H3和H4。染色质的这种基本结构单位称为核小体。

表观发生涉及由大量染色质变化决定的效应，这些变化主要是由DNA甲基化和组蛋白翻译后修饰引起的（Jiang et al. 2008）。其他过程也可以通过染色质结构重塑来控制基因转录，所有的表观遗传改变都是可遗传的和可逆的。然而，在表观遗传调控过程中，DNA或蛋白质序列没有发生变化。DNA甲基化是长期表观遗传变化的核心，多年来，DNA甲基化被认为仅仅是胞嘧啶甲基化。然而，几年前，人们发现鸟嘌呤和腺嘌呤也可以甲基化（O'Brown, Greer, 2016）。此外，组蛋白的酶修饰是最常见和被研究的表观遗传改变，可以引起染色质结构的长期和短期变化。组蛋白有一条尾巴延伸出核小体的八聚体核心。氨基末端经过翻译后修饰，包括乙酰化、甲基化、磷酸化、ADP-核糖化、法尼基化、脯氨酸异构化和泛素化（Tollefsbol, 2011）。这些化学基团改变组蛋白-DNA和组蛋白-蛋白相互作用，重塑染色质，从而影响转录、DNA复制和修复（Jenuwein, Allis, 2001）。因此，基因表达可以由组蛋白的乙酰化和甲基化驱动，这改变了DNA-蛋白质的结合和染色质结构（图45.1）。染色质的松弛或浓缩形式分别有利于或减少转录。组蛋白残基的乙酰化和去甲基化诱导DNA松弛，促进转录因子和重塑蛋白的相互作用（Kouzarides, 2007; Marmorstein, Zhou, 2014）。

在这一章中，我们分析了涉及组蛋白乙酰化的表观遗传机制。此外，我们还描述了组蛋白脱乙酰酶抑制剂（HDACi）对动物行为的影响以及与烟碱奖励特性相关的蛋白质表达的研究结果。

45.2 乙酰基转移酶和脱乙酰基酶对组蛋白的乙酰化和脱乙酰化

环境中的许多因素可以激活调节组蛋白修饰的酶。组蛋白乙酰化是影响染色质结构的重要因素。组蛋白乙酰化是一个动态和可逆的过程，由一系列称为组蛋白乙酰转移酶（HAT）和组蛋白脱乙酰酶（HDAC）的酶控制。HAT将乙酰基转移到赖氨酸残基上，HDAC从这些氨基酸中去除乙酰基。1995年在酵母中发现了第一个HAT，一年后，第一个HDAC被提纯并命名为HDAC-l（Yang, Seto, 2007）。HAT和HDAC的激活为理解组蛋白乙酰化和转录是如何调控的提供了一种机制。例如，涉及A型HAT（GCN5、p300/CBP、TAFII250、P55和PCAF）的研究提供了有关核小体组蛋白乙酰化的信息，而涉及B型HAT的研究则报道了细胞质中新合成的组蛋白的乙酰化机制（Jeanteur, 2005）。

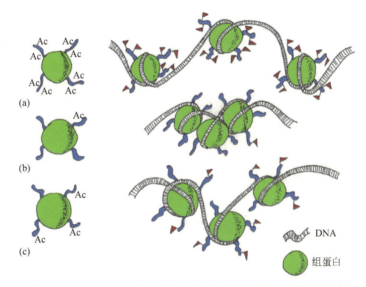

图45.1 组蛋白乙酰化和去乙酰化是表观遗传机制，会对染色质结构和基因表达产生相反的影响

卡通图说明了组蛋白3和组蛋白4（H3和H4）尾部赖氨酸残基的组蛋白乙酰化的表观遗传机制。组蛋白的乙酰化和去乙酰化分别介导松弛和浓缩染色质形式之间的转换。（a）组蛋白尾部完全乙酰化，导致染色质处于开放状态，这更容易促进转录的转录因子相互作用。组蛋白乙酰转移酶的活性促进了乙酰化状态。（b）组蛋白尾部去乙酰化使染色质浓缩，从而减少转录。从赖氨酸残基中去除乙酰基是通过组蛋白脱乙酰酶实现的。（c）中间乙酰化状态促进异质染色质结构，差异地调节转录。组蛋白脱乙酰酶抑制剂（HDACi）诱导更高程度的乙酰化，通常有利于基因表达。表观遗传调节剂(如烟碱)可以诱导染色质特定部分的乙酰化，从而差异地调节基因的表达。R. O. Bernabeu未发表的原创艺术作品。

45.2.1 组蛋白脱乙酰酶抑制剂

HDAC抑制剂维持组蛋白乙酰化，并能将平衡倾斜到染色质的"开放"构型状态，从而导致转录允许状态。以HDAC抑制剂为特征的不同药物已被用于治疗神经精神疾病和药物成瘾性疾病。例如，丙戊酸盐是一种HDAC抑制剂，已被广泛用于治疗神经精神疾病。丙戊酸盐诱导成年小鼠脑内DNA去甲基化（Dong et al. 2010）。同样，曲古抑素A（TSA）增加组蛋白乙酰化，减少DNA甲基化。然而，用DNA甲基转移酶抑制剂处理并不影响组蛋白乙酰化，这表明乙酰化可以调节甲基化，但甲基化不能调节乙酰化（Vaissière, Sawan, Herceg, 2008）。SIRT1（III类HDAC）使DNA甲基转移酶1（DNMT1）去乙酰化，因此HDAC活性抑制剂很可能通过改变关键的甲基转移酶活性来调节DNA甲基化水平（Peng et al. 2011）。此外，在适当的时间点使用HDAC抑制剂可以减轻酒精戒断时所观察到的负面烦躁情绪（Sakharkar et al. 2014）。

目前，已有40多种药物被描述为HDAC抑制剂。其中一些化合物已获得美国食品和药品监督管理局（FDA）的批准，主要用于治疗不同类型的癌症，而其他化合物正在等待临床使用的批准。在本章中，我们重点介绍了两种HDAC抑制剂：丁酸钠（NaB）和丁酸苯酯（PhB），这两种抑制剂已经在烟碱依赖的动物模型上显示了显著的生物学和行为学效应。

45.2.2 组蛋白脱乙酰酶和烟碱对神经系统的影响

45.2.2.1 烟碱模拟HDAC抑制剂的作用

滥用药物（包括烟碱）会引起奖励通路神经元中FosB的急剧增加和积聚，主要是在伏隔核（NAcc）中（Soderstrom et al. 2007）。FosB蛋白显示出一个被截断且稳定的剪接变异体，命名为δ-FosB，它的积累对成瘾行为的建立至关重要（Kowiański et al. 2018）。可卡因通过抑制HDAC诱导fosb基因表达（Nestler, 2008）。同样，研究发现烟碱抑制HDAC，并在诱导FosB表达的小鼠纹状体中的FosB启动子处产生强有力的H3和H4乙酰化（Levine et al. 2011）。

然而，烟碱对HDAC活性的抑制是否会导致组蛋白在其他基因的启动子上发生更广泛的乙酰化还有待检验。烟碱通过抑制HDAC使染色质过度乙酰化的能力可能导致短暂和稳定的长期乙酰化状态。

45.2.2.2 HDACi和烟碱对记忆的影响

烟碱乙酰胆碱受体（nAChR）在神经系统的广泛分布可能是烟碱引起多种生理效应的原因。多项研究表明，烟碱可以提高吸烟者的认知能力。也有反复报道称烟碱对学习、记忆和注意力有积极的调节作用。遗传学研究表明，多巴胺受体（DR）和nAChR都参与烟碱诱导的认知改善（Herman, Sofuoglu, 2010）。此外，据报道，烟碱调节有助于成瘾过程的突触学习机制。（Subramaniyan, Dani, 2015）。

在一项有趣的研究中，我们分析了预先接触烟碱对啮齿动物可卡因奖励的影响。他们发现，应用组蛋白脱乙酰酶抑制剂辛二酰苯胺异羟肟酸羟肟酸可以模拟烟碱对可卡因诱导的齿状回长时程增强的增强作用（Huang et al. 2014）。这些发现与先前的研究一致，表明烟碱可能作为一种促进特定基因转录的HDAC抑制因子发挥作用（Levine et al. 2011）。

一些研究证实了丁酸钠（一种HDAC抑制剂）对新奇物体识别（NOR）记忆的影响。对NOR的长期记忆对组蛋白乙酰化的修饰特别敏感。研究结果显示，HDAC抑制有利于组蛋白过度乙酰化，这是一种通常会被遗忘的认知事件，被转化为长期记忆（Stefanko, Barrett, Ly, Reolon, Wood, 2009）。因此，长期记忆需要由组蛋白乙酰化引起的结构染色质修饰，这提供了表观遗传线索，保留了与巩固记忆相关的基因表达。

研究发现，通过突变组蛋白乙酰转移酶来减少组蛋白乙酰化，会损害对物体定位的长期记忆，而通过抑制组蛋白脱乙酰酶来增强组蛋白乙酰化，则会改善对物体定位的长期记忆。此外，海马内注射非特异性HDAC抑制剂TSA或Ⅰ类HDAC选择性抑制剂MS275可增强物体定位的长期记忆，这表明抑制Ⅰ类HDAC活性对于巩固海马依赖的空间记忆非常重要（Hawk et al. 2011）。

另一方面，以斑马鱼作为实验模型，我们评估了在烟碱和HDACi PhB等影响啮齿动物注意力和记忆保持的药物存在的情况下其对物体的记忆。最初修改的物体识别任务被用来区分熟悉的物体和新的物体（Faillace et al. 2017）。我们首次证明了斑马鱼对探索一些有色物体比其他物体有先天的偏好。此外，斑马鱼更善于辨别颜色变化，而不是形状或大小的适度变化。这些发现还表明，必须事先对物体进行评估，才能了解斑马鱼对物体的先天偏好或厌恶（图45.2）。此外，烟碱显著增强了短期的先天新奇物体偏好或识别，而PhB在长期先天物体偏好或识别上表现出类似的效果。PhB处理抑制HDAC的生理后果只有在暴露于PhB几小时后才能观察到，因为它的影响是由基因转录介导的。相比之下，急性烟碱效应可以更快、更短暂地观察到。研究结果表明，烟碱和PhB可以促进斑马鱼的物体识别，这可能涉及记忆。有趣的是，当测试过程中的配对对象中有一个是自然偏好的对象，而另一个是非偏好的对象时，烟碱和PhB通常会增强，但在某些情况下会逆转自然的偏好。这些影响并不一定意味着记忆，但可能涉及感知和注意力的改善。因此，烟碱和PhB分别改变了天生的知觉敏锐度和修改了的短期和长期记忆。

45.2.2.3　HDACi对烟碱增强性能的影响

烟碱改变腹侧被盖区（VTA）多巴胺神经元的放电，从而在NAcc释放DA是导致烟碱奖励的第一步，但激活nAChR下游的细胞内信号通路可能是烟碱长期暴露的后果（包括条件性奖励）的关键（Walters et al. 2005）。这些研究还确定了VTA和NAcc是环磷酸腺苷反应元件结合蛋白（CREB）所在的大脑区域，其活性对于建立研究烟碱诱导的条件性位置偏好（CPP）至关重要。我们的研究表明，在CPP过程中，烟碱可诱导中脑边缘区CREB的磷酸化（pCREB）和Fos的表达（Pascual et al. 2009）。

烟碱诱导的CPP的获得和维持而不是烟碱诱导的条件性位置厌恶（CPA）的获得和维持增加了VTA以及NAcc、前额叶皮层（PFC）和背侧纹状体（dStr）的pCREB和Fos蛋白，这表明与特定的环境线索有关的烟碱诱导形成中脑边缘通路的不同结构的神经元活性发生了变化（Pascual et al. 2009; Walters et al.2005）。此外，美加明（一种非选择性nAChR拮抗剂）可消除pCREB的增加，表明烟碱-环境联合可诱导CREB的特异性激活。

组蛋白脱乙酰酶通过激活或停止转录来差异调节pCREB的靶基因（Fass et al. 2003）。已有研究表明，HDAC1可与pCREB和蛋白磷酸酶1（PP1）形成复合物，导致pCREB去磷酸化和乙酰基去除，抑制基因转录（Canettieri et al. 2003）。事实上，HDAC抑制剂TSA可增强cAMP对CRE报告基因的激活。因此，促进特定基因转录的pCREB活性至少在一定程度上被HDAC的招募所抑制。

HDAC对药物成瘾的影响主要是在大鼠自身注射可卡因（Kumar et al. 2005; Romieu et al. 2008）或条件性位置偏好（Raybuck et al. 2013）的实验中检验的。只有两项研究评估了HDAC抑制对大鼠烟碱奖励特性的影响（Castino et al. 2015; Pastor et al. 2011）。烟碱会引起大脑结构的长期改变，但人们对烟碱偏好的长期神经可塑性的机制知之甚少（Barik, Wonnacott, 2009）。

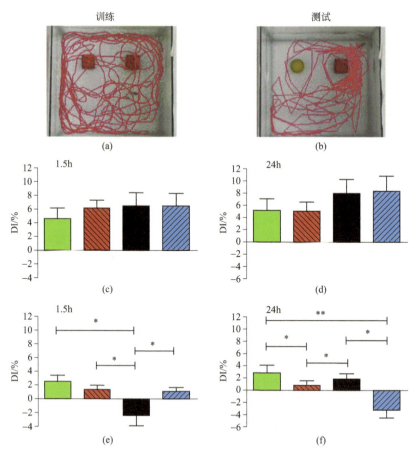

图 45.2 烟碱和丁酸苯酯对斑马鱼新物体偏好的影响

斑马鱼在训练过程中接触到两个相同的红色立方体（在本例中），然后在测试过程中接触到相同的红色立方体（a）或一个红色立方体（熟悉的物体）和一个黄色的球（新物体）（b）。斑马鱼在训练10min后立即暴露于池水、烟碱、丁酸苯酯（组蛋白脱乙酰酶抑制剂PhB）或丁酸苯酯+烟碱。在引入鱼之前，药物立即被溶解在水箱中。在训练后1.5h（c和e）或24h（d和f）进行测试。条形图描述了测试过程中的物体偏好，并在没有药物的情况下通过对比两个红色立方体（c和d）或一个红色立方体和一个黄色球体（e和f）进行评估。斑马鱼表现出对红色的自然偏好和对黄色物体的厌恶。斑马鱼能够辨别相同大小物体的颜色变化和形状的轻微变化。烟碱显著增强了短期内对新奇物体的偏好或厌恶（取决于物体的颜色），而丁酸苯酯在训练后24h表现出类似的效果。判别指数百分比（DI）计算如下：[（探索新物体的时间）－（探索熟悉的物体的时间）/（探索新物体的时间+探索熟悉的物体的时间）] ×100（Stefanko et al. 2009）。使用 DI 时，正值表示动物花更多时间探索新物体，而负值表示动物更喜欢探索熟悉的物体。该图显示，当斑马鱼暴露于烟碱、间隔1.5h后，或暴露于PhB、延迟24h后，它们探索熟悉的红色物体的时间比新发现的黄色物体的时间更长。数据用±SEM描述；每组动物数为10～12只。结果表明，当它们接触烟碱并在1.5h后进行测试，或在PhB中进行延迟24h的测试时，斑马鱼对熟悉的红色物体的探索时间比对新的黄色物体的探索时间更长。方差分析后经Newman-Keuls检验，*$P<0.05$；**$P<0.01$。

表观遗传机制是理解烟碱对大脑的生物学作用的主要候选机制之一。如上所述，组蛋白乙酰化是迄今为止研究的主要修饰，不仅因为它在控制基因表达方面起着至关重要的作用，而且因为HDAC抑制剂目前被用于癌症和神经疾病的治疗。关于成瘾，仔细研究了NaB对烟碱自给药的消退和恢复的影响。HDAC抑制剂通过增强大鼠消退记忆的巩固，促进了静脉注射烟碱自给药的消退（Castino et al. 2015）。然而，烟碱自给药和消退过程中涉及的表观遗传机制仍不清楚。

在我们的实验室中，我们使用条件性位置偏好任务作为自给药的替代测试来研究烟碱的奖励特性。通过对烟碱诱导的大鼠CPP、消退和复发的研究，我们证明了在CPP表达和复发期间，奖励通路神经元中HDAC2蛋白水平升高。相反，H3的赖氨酸9位乙酰化水平（H3-K9Ac）没有明显变化（图45.3和图45.4）。

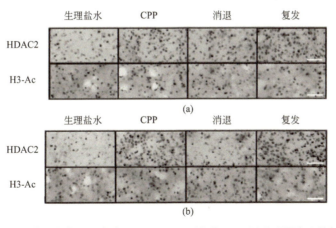

图45.3 大鼠伏隔核（Nacc）中H3-K9Ac乙酰化的HDAC2和组蛋白3的免疫反应

显微照片显示了不同实验组大鼠的Nacc、核心（a）和外壳（b）中HDAC2和H3-Ac阳性免疫染色的代表性图像：生理盐水（对照组）、CPP（烟碱条件性位置偏好组）、消退（烟碱诱导的CPP消退组）和复发（烟碱诱导的CPP恢复组）关于老鼠行为群体的详细信息见Pascual等（2009）。CPP，条件性位置偏好。比例尺，50μm。未发布的图片。

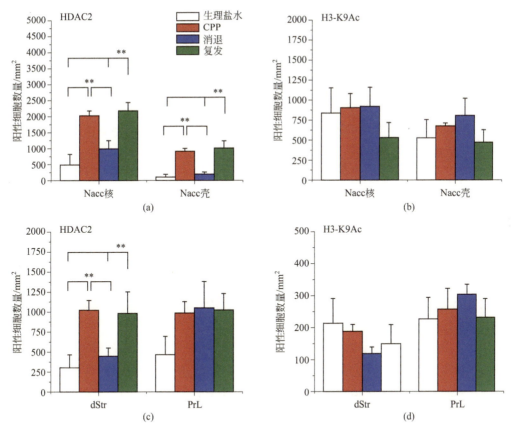

图45.4 大鼠中脑边缘通路不同结构中HDAC2和H3-Ac阳性细胞的定量分析

不同实验组大鼠的伏隔核（NAcc、核与壳）、背侧纹状体（dStr）和前额叶区域（PrL）均有HDAC2［(a)和(c)］和H3-K9Ac免疫阳性细胞［(b)和(d)］。由于每个细胞都有两种标志物，所以严格的标准被用来仅将密度大于平均值的细胞（较暗）计数为免疫阳性细胞。条形表示±SEM，每组7～9只动物。方差分析后，行为组间采用Newman-Keuls检验，**$P<0.01$。HDAC2，组蛋白脱乙酰酶2；H3-K9Ac，组蛋白3在赖氨酸9位乙酰化。

此外，我们还证明了 PhB 在 CPP 任务中显著降低了对烟碱的偏好，而不改变药物的厌恶特性（Pastor et al. 2011）。事实上，高剂量烟碱会引起场所厌恶（Le Foll, Goldberg, 2005; Pascual et al. 2009），这不受 PhB 治疗的影响。这些发现表明，烟碱偏好的潜在机制不同于对这种药物的潜在厌恶。评估 HDAC 抑制剂对烟碱自给药和烟碱诱导的 CPP 影响的实验获得的行为数据表明，HDAC 活性参与了食欲性寻药行为，而对厌恶行为没有明显影响。HDAC 活性至少在两个时间窗内相关：在无条件刺激条件性刺激关联的巩固期间（通过巴甫洛夫 CPP 观察到的）和在条件性记忆消失期间（通过烟碱自给药观察到的）。药物-线索关联行为的发展和消亡是减少使用 HDAC 抑制剂的滥用药物强化特性的适当时间窗口。

为了探讨 PhB 抑制烟碱诱导的 CPP 的可能机制，本实验室对组蛋白乙酰化水平、HDAC2 和甲基 CpG 结合蛋白 2（MeCP2）的表达以及 CREB 的磷酸化进行了分析。通过测定 H3-K9Ac 的乙酰化水平来评价 PhB 的作用。用 PhB 处理的动物的乙酰化水平提高了 2～3 倍。此外，在烟碱条件下的大鼠中脑边缘通路的不同结构中表达 pCREB 的细胞数量在 HDAC 抑制剂处理后略有减少。这些发现表明，尽管 CREB 的磷酸化是建立 CPP 所必需的（Pascual et al. 2009），但它显然在条件反射过程中 HDAC 抑制剂诱导的 CPP 的降低中起不到重要作用（Pastor et al. 2011）。有趣的是，PhB 处理后烟碱诱导 CPP 组大鼠纹状体内 HDAC2 免疫阳性细胞数显著减少，而烟碱诱导 CPA 组动物纹状体内 HDAC2 免疫阳性细胞数无明显变化。因此，HDAC2 是烟碱条件性位置偏好所必需的，当药物寻求行为减少时，HDAC2 被下调。这些发现巩固了 HDAC2 在学习中的作用（Franklin, Mansuy, 2010）。

最后，MeCP2 与 mSin3A（HDAC1/2 抑制子复合体的重要成分）形成复合体，HDAC2 与甲基化的 DNA 结合并强烈抑制基因转录（Yang, Seto, 2008）。类似于使用可卡因进行的实验（Cassel et al. 2006），烟碱诱导的 CPP 增加了大鼠 dStr 中表达 MeCP2 的细胞的数量，而不影响 Nacc 或 PFC（Pastor et al. 2011）。

综上所述，我们的研究结果表明，HDAC 抑制能够调节与烟碱奖励相关的药物寻求行为。此外，HDAC2 在建立位置条件性烟碱偏好所必需的中脑边缘通路 Nacc 和 dStr 的突触可塑性中起着重要作用。

45.3 治疗应用

人类广泛使用和滥用烟草、卷烟和卷烟中的烟碱被认为是导致成瘾的主要因素。制药公司和公共卫生项目已经开发和评估了抑制组蛋白脱乙酰酶（HDAC）活性的化合物。这些化合物是有效治疗不同类型癌症和神经精神疾病的工具。此外，科学报告表明，HDAC 抑制剂可以控制酒精和可卡因消费等成瘾行为，并可能非常有效地避免烟碱依赖和复发。此外，pCREB 和 δ-FosB 的激活负责烟碱奖励，这些分子也被认为可能是帮助结束人类烟草使用和滥用的治疗靶点。

术语解释
- **成瘾**：对动物大脑中边缘多巴胺系统中突触可塑性的终生修饰，一旦建立，就会诱导一种寻求行为，以获得特定的奖励或避免不快。动物的大脑奖励回路（中边缘通路）已经增强，并在很大程度上控制了动物的行为，几乎完全以寻求和获得奖励为导向。
- **条件性位置偏好**：巴甫洛夫式或经典的条件性测试，测试动物是否愿意更频繁地访问或在以前被认为与有效药物相关的地方待更长时间。非条件刺激是一种特定的药物，而条件刺激则代表动物接受药物的特定环境。药物-环境关联可以在动物的中性环境中建立，也可以在单纯的非偏好环境中建立，这可以进一步证明在条件建立的情况下实验者可诱导动物的药物寻求行为。

- δ-FosB和FosB：δ-FosB和FosB是转录因子和Fos家族的成员。fosb基因可以将FosB和δ-FosB作为剪接变异体表达，它们参与滥用药物的动机和奖励，并诱导神经适应，从而建立成瘾行为。在不接触药物的情况下，纹状体内过表达δ-FosB可使小鼠产生成瘾行为（McClung et al. 2004）。

- 表观遗传：永久性或长期的化学酶修饰，如DNA或核小体中的组蛋白的甲基化或乙酰化（对于组蛋白，有时在细胞质中），改变染色质结构（松弛与凝聚）和特定基因表达的可能性。这些修饰可以遗传，但不影响DNA核苷酸序列或蛋白质同一性。表观遗传机制有利于或抑制参与不同生物过程的特定基因的转录。

- 组蛋白乙酰转移酶：具有催化活性的酶，主要将乙酰基从细胞质或细胞核或适当的人工反应介质中的其他分子转移到组蛋白的赖氨酸残基上。

- 组蛋白脱乙酰酶（HDAC）：位于细胞核和细胞质中的酶，调节形成核小体的组蛋白的乙酰化程度。它们催化组蛋白中主要赖氨酸残基的脱乙酰化。高组蛋白脱乙酰酶活性导致低乙酰化程度（少量乙酰化赖氨酸残基），从而导致DNA缩合抑制基因转录（图45.1）。组蛋白脱乙酰酶2是哺乳动物脑中表达最强的HDAC。

- 甲基CpG结合蛋白2（MeCP2）：这种蛋白通过与基因组上胞嘧啶-鸟嘌呤岛（CpG）高频率区域的甲基化启动子特异性结合来抑制基因转录。MeCP2与5-甲基胞嘧啶结合，促进染色质重塑和转录抑制复合体的募集，使染色质处于浓缩状态。该蛋白在乳腺癌进展和胚胎发育过程中起着关键作用。该蛋白编码基因（MBD2）的突变可能导致Rett综合征。它也可以作为一种去甲基酶来促进转录。

- 丁酸苯酯（PhB）：一种抑制组蛋白脱乙酰酶活性的化合物。PhB可能通过使平衡向形成核小体的组蛋白的高乙酰化状态倾斜而增加基因转录的可能性（图45.1）。

- 磷酸化环磷酸腺苷反应元件结合蛋白（pCREB）：CREB被磷酸化激活，磷酸化受细胞细胞质中激酶的调节，激酶对不同的细胞信号通路作出反应。pCREB转移到细胞核，在那里它通过与基因启动子区的CRE序列结合来调节一组基因的转录。pCREB增强表明细胞的功能激活，如可兴奋细胞的去极化。

- 突触可塑性或神经适应：显著改变神经回路中突触功效或活动的任何持久的形态或分子变化。发芽、树突或突触末端回缩、脊柱形成、修剪、膜受体上调和下调、神经递质释放或摄取上调和下调、突触前和/或突触后功效修饰，如长时程增强、长时程抑制和突触促进。

关键事实

- 表观遗传学的关键事实：表观遗传机制是理解烟碱诱导的大脑突触可塑性长期变化的主要候选机制之一。

- 烟碱-环境关联和中边缘通路的关键事实：在调节任务中，烟碱与特定的环境线索相关联，导致中边缘通路不同结构的神经元活性发生变化。

- 组蛋白脱乙酰酶（HDAC）的关键事实：HDAC抑制促进大鼠静脉内烟碱自给药的消失。

- 组蛋白脱乙酰酶2（HDAC2）的关键事实：HDAC2在触发伏隔核和中脑边缘通路背侧纹状体神经元活动的变化中起着重要作用，这是建立烟碱条件性位置偏好所必需的。

- 组蛋白脱乙酰酶和磷酸化CREB的关键事实：组蛋白脱乙酰酶通过促进转录的激活或终止来差异地调节磷酸化CREB的靶基因。

- 磷酸化CREB的关键事实：CREB磷酸化是建立烟碱依赖的位置偏好所必需的，但显然在组蛋白去乙酰化酶抑制剂丁酸苯酯引起的烟碱依赖的位置偏好的减少中不起重要作用。

> - 组蛋白脱乙酰酶抑制剂的关键事实：这些抑制剂目前用于威胁生命的疾病的医学治疗，它们可以以适当的剂量用于治疗烟碱成瘾和帮助吸烟者戒烟。

要点总结
> - 我们在此描述了组蛋白脱乙酰酶抑制剂对动物行为和蛋白质表达的影响的已发表结果，这些结果与烟碱的奖励特性有关。
> - 组蛋白去乙酰化酶活性的抑制增强了消退记忆的巩固，因此减弱了烟碱的恢复。
> - 组蛋白去乙酰化酶2是烟草诱导的位置偏好调节所必需的，并且当药物寻求行为减少时，组蛋白脱乙酰酶2被下调。
> - 经验证据表明，烟碱可能作为组蛋白脱乙酰酶抑制剂，通过促进特定基因转录来调节特定脑区的突触可塑性。
> - 组蛋白去乙酰化酶活性抑制剂增加了厌恶性长期记忆，但降低了烟碱的位置偏好。
> - 烟碱导致短期改善，而组蛋白脱乙酰酶抑制导致对物体识别的物体感知和记忆的长期增强。

参考文献

Barik, J.; Wonnacott, S. (2009). Molecular and cellular mechanisms of action of nicotine in the CNS. Handbook of Experimental Pharmacology, 192, 173-207.

Canettieri, G.; Morantte, I.; Guzmán, E.; Asahara, H.; Herzig, S.; Anderson, S. D. et al. (2003). Attenuation of a phosphorylationdependent activator by an HDAC-PP1 complex. Nature Structural Biology, 10(3), 175-181.

Cassel, S.; Carouge, D.; Gensburger, C.; Anglard, P.; Burgun, C.; Dietrich, J. B. et al. (2006). Fluoxetine and cocaine induce the epigenetic factors MeCP2 and MBD1 in adult rat brain. Molecular Pharmacology, 70(2), 487-492.

Castino, M. R.; Cornish, J. L.; Clemens, K. J. (2015). Inhibition of histone deacetylases facilitates extinction and attenuates reinstatement of nicotine self-administration in rats. PLoS One, 10(4)e0124796.

Dong, E.; Chen, Y.; Gavin, D. P.; Grayson, D. R.; Guidotti, A. (2010). Valproate induces DNA demethylation in nuclear extracts from adult mouse brain. Epigenetics, 5(8), 730-735.

Faillace, M. P.; Pisera-Fuster, A.; Medrano, M. P.; Bejarano, A. C.; Bernabeu, R. O. (2017). Short- and long-term effects of nicotine and the histone deacetylase inhibitor phenylbutyrate on novel object recognition in zebrafish. Psychopharmacology, 234(6), 943-955.

Fass, D. M.; Butler, J. E.; Goodman, R. H. (2003). Deacetylase activity is required for cAMP activation of a subset of CREB target genes. The Journal of Biological Chemistry, 278(44), 43014-43019.

Franklin, T. B.; Mansuy, I. M. (2010). The prevalence of epigenetic mechanisms in the regulation of cognitive functions and behaviour. Current Opinion in Neurobiology, 20(4), 441-449.

Hawk, J. D.; Florian, C.; Abel, T. (2011). Post-training intrahippocampal inhibition of class I histone deacetylases enhances long-term object-location memory. Learning, Memory, 18(6), 367-370.

Herman, A. I.; Sofuoglu, M. (2010). Cognitive effects of nicotine: genetic moderators. Addiction Biology, 15(3), 250-265.

Horn, P. J.; Peterson, C. L. (2002). Chromatin higher order foldingwrapping up transcription. Science, 297(5588), 1824-1827.

Huang, Y. Y.; Levine, A.; Kandel, D. B.; Yin, D.; Colnaghi, L.; Drisaldi, B. et al. (2014). D1/D5 receptors and histone deacetylation mediate the Gateway. Effect of LTP in hippocampal dentate gyrus. Learning, Memory, 21(3), 153-160.

Jeanteur, P. (2005). Epigenetics and chromatin (1st ed.). Germany: Springer-Verlag.

Jenuwein, T.; Allis, C. D. (2001). Translating the histone code. Science, 293(5532), 1074-1080.

Jiang, Y.; Langley, B.; Lubin, F. D.; Renthal, W.; Wood, M. A.; Yasui, D. H. et al. (2008). Epigenetics in the nervous system. The Journal of Neuroscience, 28(46), 11753-11759.

Kouzarides, T. (2007). Chromatin modifications and their function. Cell, 128(4), 693-705.

Kowianski, P.; Lietzau, G.; Steliga, A.; Czuba, E.; Ludkiewicz, B.; Wa skow, M. et al. (2018). Nicotine-induced CREB and DeltaFosB activity is modified by caffeine in the brain reward system of the rat. Journal of Chemical Neuroanatomy, 88, 1-12.

Kumar, A.; Choi, K. H.; Renthal, W.; Tsankova, N. M.; Theobald, D. E.; Truong, H. T. et al. (2005). Chromatin remodeling is a key mechanism underlying cocaine-induced plasticity in striatum. Neuron, 48(2), 303-314.

Le Foll, B.; Goldberg, S. R. (2005). Nicotine induces conditioned place preferences over a large range of doses in rats. Psychopharmacology, 178(4), 481-492.

Levine, A.; Huang, Y.; Drisaldi, B.; Griffin, E. A Jr.; Pollak, D. D.; Xu, S.; Yin, D.; Schaffran, C.; Kandel, D. B.; Kandel, E. R. (2011). Molecular mechanism for a gateway drug: epigenetic changes initiated by nicotine prime gene expression by cocaine. Sci Transl med, 3 (107):107ra109.

Marmorstein, R.; Zhou, M. M. (2014). Writers and readers of histone acetylation: structure, mechanism, and inhibition. Cold Spring Harbor Perspectives in Biology, 6(7), a018762.

McClung, C. A.; Ulery, P. G.; Perrotti, L. I.; Zachariou, V.; Berton, O.; Nestler, E. J. (2004). DeltaFosB: a molecular switch for long-term adaptation in the brain. Brain Research. Molecular Brain Research. 132, 146-154.

Nestler, E. J. (2008). Transcriptional mechanisms of addiction: role of DeltaFosB. Review. Philosophical Transactions of the Royal Society of London. Series B, Biological Sciences, 363(1507), 3245-3255.

O'Brown, Z. K.; Greer, E. L. (2016). N6-methyladenine: a conserved and dynamic DNA mark. Advances in Experimental Medicine and Biology, 945, 213-246.

Pascual, M. M.; Pastor, V.; Bernabeu, R. O. (2009). Nicotineconditioned place preference induced CREB phosphorylation and Fos expression in the adult rat brain. Psychopharmacology, 207(1), 57-71.

Pastor, V.; Host, L.; Zwiller, J.; Bernabeu, R. O. (2011). Histone deacetylase inhibition decreases preference without affecting aversion for nicotine. Journal of Neurochemistry, 116(4), 636-645.

Peng, L.; Yuan, Z.; Ling, H.; Fukasawa, K.; Robertson, K.; Olashaw, N. et al. (2011). SIRT1 deacetylates the DNA methyltransferase 1 (DNMT1) protein and alters its activities. Molecular and Cellular Biology, 31(23), 4720-4734.

Raybuck, J. D.; McCleery, E. J.; Cunningham, C. L.; Wood, M. A.; Lattal, K. M. (2013). The histone deacetylase inhibitor sodium butyrate modulates acquisition and extinction of cocaine-induced conditioned place preference. Pharmacology, Biochemistry, and Behavior, 106, 109-116.

Romieu, P.; Host, L.; Gobaille, S.; Sandner, G.; Aunis, D.; Zwiller, J. (2008). Histone deacetylase inhibitors decrease cocaine but not sucrose self-administration in rats. The Journal of Neuroscience, 28(38), 9342-9348.

Sakharkar, A. J.; Zhang, H.; Tang, L.; Baxstrom, K.; Shi, G.; Moonat, S. et al. (2014). Effects of histone deacetylase inhibitors on amygdaloid histone acetylation and neuropeptide Y expression: a role in anxietylike and alcohol-drinking behaviours. The International Journal of Neuropsychopharmacology, 17(8), 1207-1220.

Soderstrom, K.; Qin, W.; Williams, H.; Taylor, D. A.; McMillen, B. A. (2007). Nicotine increases FosB expression within a subset of reward- and memory-related brain regions during both peri- and post-adolescence. Psychopharmacology, 191, 891-897.

Stefanko, D. P.; Barrett, R. M.; Ly, A. R.; Reolon, G. K.; Wood, M. A. (2009). Modulation of long-term memory for object recognition via HDAC inhibition. Proceedings of the National Academy of Sciences of the United States of America, 106(23), 9447-9452.

Subramaniyan, M.; Dani, J. A. (2015). Dopaminergic and cholinergic learning mechanisms in nicotine addiction. Annals of the New York Academy of Sciences, 1349, 46-63.

Tollefsbol, T. (2011). Handbook of epigenetics, the new molecular and medical genetics (1st ed.). London: Academic Press. Vaissière, T.; Sawan, C.; Herceg, Z. (2008). Epigenetic interplay between histone modifications and DNA methylation in gene silencing. Mutation Research, 659(1-2), 40-48.

Walters, C. L.; Cleck, J. N.; Kuo, Y. C.; Blendy, J. A. (2005). Mu-opioid receptor and CREB activation are required for nicotine reward. Neuron, 46(6), 933-943.

Yang, X. J.; Seto, E. (2007). HATs and HDACs: from structure, function and regulation to novel strategies for therapy and prevention. Oncogene, 26(37), 5310-5318.

Yang, X. J.; Seto, E. (2008). Lysine acetylation: codified crosstalk with other posttranslational modifications. Molecular Cell, 31(4), 449-461.

46
L型钙离子通道与烟碱

Yudan Liu[1], *Meghan Harding*[2]

1. Department of Neuroendocrine Pharmacology, School of Pharmacy, China Medical University, Shenyang, Liaoning, China
2. Family Medicine Physician Candidate, UCONN School of Medicine, Hartford, CT, United States

缩略语

AChR	乙酰胆碱受体	**DHP**	二氢吡啶
CaMKⅡ	钙/钙调蛋白依赖性蛋白激酶Ⅱ	**EPM**	高架加迷宫
CPA	条件性位置厌恶	**LTCC**	L型钙离子通道
CPP	条件性位置偏好	**NAcc**	伏隔核
DA	多巴胺	**VTA**	腹侧被盖区
DBI	地西泮结合抑制剂		

46.1 什么是L型钙离子通道?

1985年，耶鲁大学的三位科学家将L型钙离子通道（LTCC）定义为"L"，因为与具有瞬时内向电流的T型钙离子通道相比，L型钙离子通道在去极化过程中具有持久的电流（Nowycky, Fox, Tsien, 1985）。LTCC也被称为Ca_v1钙离子通道，以钙离子通道的主要亚基命名。LTCC在骨骼肌兴奋-收缩偶联等生理和病理过程中发挥重要作用。LTCC是第一批纯化的电压门控性钙离子通道，最初来源于兔骨骼肌，发现有5个亚基（图46.1）：α1（170kDa）、α2（150kDa）、β（52kDa）、δ（17～25kDa）和γ（32kDa）亚基（Takahashi, Seagar, Jones, Reber, Catterall, 1987; Tanabe et al. 1987），其中α2亚基和δ亚基通常整合成α2δ亚基。其中，α1亚基是最重要的亚基，因为它是成孔亚基，也是最重要的调节剂和药物（如1,4-二氢吡啶化合物）的结合位点。α2δ、β和γ亚基是参与调节功能的辅助亚基（Hofmann, Flockerzi, Kahl, Wegener, 2014）。事实上，LTCC与其他电压钙离子通道（如N型、P/Q型和T型钙离子通道）的区别在于其对DHP化学物质（如硝苯地平）的高度敏感性，DHP化学物质不仅是分离LTCC的基本药理工具，也是治疗心血管疾病（如高血压）的关键药物。LTCC家族关于其α1亚基有四种亚型（表46.1）：$Ca_v1.1$、$Ca_v1.2$、$Ca_v1.3$和$Ca_v1.4$。这四种亚型有相似的生理特性，如持久的内向电流，但是它们在亚基组成、组织分布和一些电生理特性上有所不同。例如，$Ca_v1.2$通道只由三个亚基组成，即α1、α2δ、β亚基，没有γ亚基（Hofmann et al.2014）。例如，$Ca_v1.1$亚型主要分布在骨骼肌中，而$Ca_v1.4$亚型主要局限于视网膜。然而，$Ca_v1.2$和$Ca_v1.3$亚型在许多组织中大量表达，如心脏和脑。在特定情况下，$Ca_v1.2$和$Ca_v1.3$处于同一位置中，如在大脑神经元的突触后树突中。在电生理特性方面，$Ca_v1.2$具有典型的LTCC特性：激活阈值较高（如-40～-20mV），去极化电流持续时间长，对DHP药物高度敏感。然而，与$Ca_v1.2$相比，$Ca_v1.3$被较低的电压（−60～−40mV）激活，对DHP药物的敏感性降低。亚型之间的分子差异意味着它们可能偶联到不同的信号通路，从而在神经元中介导不同的生理作用。例如，$Ca_v1.3$通道在通过响应小的膜去极化来调节Ca^{2+}内流的过程中起着至关重要的作用，而膜去极化对于维持神经元的自发节律性放电是必不可少的。与此一致，Liu等的结果显示，$Ca_v1.3$设定了基本基调，以维持基本的单峰放电，而$Ca_v1.2$和$Ca_v1.3$都介导了腹侧被盖区（VTA）多巴胺（DA）细胞的特定放电模式"爆发式放电"（Liu et al. 2014）。在VTA中，单峰放电维持终末区的基本DA水平，并发出预期环境刺激的信号；然而，"爆发式放电"显著增强了DA突触传递，并对意外刺激进行行为编码。出于疾病治疗和研究的目的，已经开发了各种类型的LTCC拮抗剂（表46.2），包括DHP（如硝苯地平）、苯基烷基胺（如维拉帕米）、苯并噻嗪类（如地尔硫䓬）和二苯基烷基胺（如氟桂利嗪）。

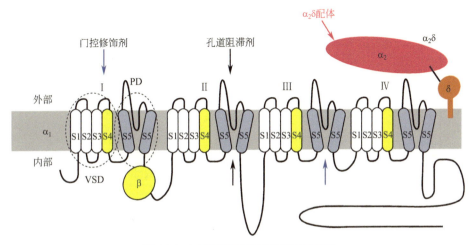

图 46.1 L型钙离子通道结构模型示意图

该图显示了L型钙离子通道中的主要药物结合位点。药物通过改变通道门控（蓝色箭头，门控修饰剂，如硝苯地平）、通过直接阻断孔道（黑色箭头，孔道阻滞剂）或通过两种机制（如苯基烷基胺阻滞剂）来阻断通道。α2δ配体（洋红色箭头）可以修改通道交易。来自 Zamponi, G. W.;Striessnig, J.;Koschak, A.;Dolphin, A. C. (2015). The physiology, pathology, and pharmacology of voltage-gated calcium channels and their future therapeutic potential. Pharmacological Reviews, 67(4), 821-870.

表46.1　不同L型钙离子通道亚型的主要性质

亚型	α1亚基	编码基因	主要分布
$Ca_v1.1$	α1S	CACNA1S	骨骼肌
$Ca_v1.2$	α1C	CACNA1C	脑、心脏、血管、肠、膀胱平滑肌、胰腺、肾上腺髓质
$Ca_v1.3$	α1D	CACNA1D	脑、听觉毛细胞、前庭毛细胞、心脏、胰腺、肾上腺
$Ca_v1.4$	α1F	CACNA1F	视网膜

注：该表介绍了L型钙离子通道的四种亚型及其主要亚基、编码基因和主要分布。

表46.2　L型钙离子通道激活剂和抑制剂的主要亚类

化合物	对LTCC的作用	典型药物
1,4-二氢吡啶	抑制剂	硝苯地平、尼莫地平、尼卡地平、氨氯地平、依拉地平
苯基烷基胺	抑制剂	维拉帕米
苯并噻嗪类	抑制剂	地尔硫䓬

续表

化合物	对LTCC的作用	典型药物
二苯基烷基胺	抑制剂	氟桂利嗪
苯甲酰基吡咯	激活剂	FPL 64176
1,4-二氢吡啶	激活剂	(S)-(−)-Bay K8644

注：该表列出了用于动物研究和临床的主要L型钙离子通道药物。

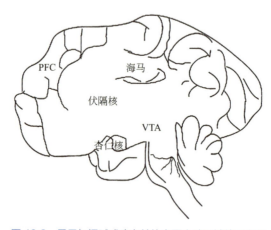

图46.2 显示与烟碱成瘾有关的主要大脑区域的示意图

涉及烟碱成瘾的主要脑区：PFC，前额叶皮质；VTA，腹侧被盖区。

46.2 LTCC与烟碱治疗的关系

烟碱滥用是一种复杂的多脑区功能障碍（图46.2）。经典理论认为，烟碱激活中脑边缘系统中的DA神经元，该神经元起源于VTA，主要位于伏隔核（NAcc）中的目标区域；破坏大脑区域，包括与奖励和学习有关的区域，如海马体和额叶皮层；然后招募与压力和焦虑有关的相互关联的大脑回路，如杏仁核。在所有这些脑区中，只有$Ca_v1.2$和$Ca_v1.3$ LTCC亚型高度分布（Chan et al. 2007; Dragicevic, Schiemann, Liss, 2015; Olson et al. 2005）。在这些脑区中，89%的LTCC包含$Ca_v1.2$亚型，而$Ca_v1.3$亚型仅占11%（Hell et al. 1993; Sinnegger-Brauns et al. 2009）。在某些领域，它们的表达比例可能会逆转；例如，Takada等（Takada, Kang, Imanishi, 2001）谈到$Ca_v1.3$ LTCC免疫组织化学定位于大多数中脑神经元，并分布于整个神经元，而$Ca_v1.2$ LTCC在中脑显示较少。不同LTCC亚型在烟碱相关脑区的密集表达暗示了LTCC与烟碱依赖之间的联系。事实上，在动物研究中，已经在行为和分子水平上分析了长期使用和滥用烟碱的影响（表46.3）。

表46.3 L型钙离子通道（LTCC）和烟碱的动物研究总结

索引	烟碱模型	动物	LTCC药物	参考文献
苯丙胺诱导的前额叶皮层多巴胺释放	5μmol/L	Sprague Dawley 大鼠	尼群地平	J Neurochem, 77 (2001) 839-848
抗伤害作用	1.5mg/kg皮下注射	癌症研究所（ICR）小鼠	尼莫地平、硝苯地平	J Pharmacol Exp Ther, 266 (1993) 1330-1338

续表

索引	烟碱模型	动物	LTCC药物	参考文献
抗伤害作用	每天6mg/kg，持续28d	Sprague Dawley大鼠	硝苯地平、维拉帕米	Life Sci, 60 (1997) 1651-1658
抗伤害作用	每天24mg/kg，持续14d	ICR小鼠	硝苯地平、维拉帕米	J Pharmacol Exp Ther 315 (2005) 959-964
抗伤害作用	每只小鼠鞘内注射20μg	C57BL/6小鼠	尼莫地平、维拉帕米	J Pharmacol Exp Ther 320 (2007) 244-249
抗伤害作用 运动	1.75mg/kg皮下注射或1.5mg/kg皮下注射	ICR小鼠	硝苯地平、尼莫地平、维拉帕米、Bay K8644	Drug Alcohol Depend 32 (1993) 73-79
抗伤害作用 运动	2mg/kg，每日2次，持续10d	ICR小鼠	Bay K8644	Eur J Pharmacol 322 (1997) 129-135
焦虑	急性，0.1mg/kg或0.5mg/kg；慢性，0.1mg/kg，持续6d	Swiss小鼠	尼莫地平、氟桂利嗪、维拉帕米、地尔硫䓬	Life Sci 79 (2006) 81-88
焦虑	0.1mg/kg s.c.；1d或6d	Swiss小鼠	尼莫地平、氟桂利嗪、维拉帕米、地尔硫䓬	Prog Neuropsychopharmacol Biol Psychiatry 32 (2008) 54-61
辨别	0.4mg/kg皮下注射	大鼠	依拉地平	Pharmacol Biochem Behav 41 (1992) 807-812
大脑皮层神经元中地西泮结合抑制剂mRNA的表达	0.1μmol/L，24h	ddY品系小鼠	脑地西泮结合抑制剂mRNA	Brain Res Mol Brain Res 80 (2000) 132-141
LTCC亚型致敏的表达	0.175mg/kg，1d或14d	C57BL/6N小鼠	$Ca_v1.2$、$Ca_v1.3$的mRNA表达 硝苯地平	Nicotine Tob Res 16 (2014) 774-785
LTCC和ERK磷酸化在原代皮层神经元中的表达	100μmol/L	C57BL/6J小鼠	硝苯地平、地尔硫䓬	J Neurochem 103(2007) 666-678
LTCC在大脑皮层神经元中的表达	0.1μmol/L，72h；1mg/kg s.c.，每日3次，持续7d	ddY品系小鼠	[^{3}H]维拉帕米结合试验 蛋白质电泳与免疫印迹	J Biol Chem 277 (2002) 7979-7988
LTCC在小鼠脑内的表达	1mg/kg，每日3次，持续7d	ddY品系小鼠	α1C、α1D、α1F、α2/δ1、β4亚基	Brain Res Mol Brain Res 135 (2005) 280-284
运动	0.4mg/kg腹腔注射	Sprague Dawley大鼠	尼莫地平	Psychopharmacology 128 (1996) 359-361
运动	0.5mg/kg腹腔注射5d	Swiss小鼠	维拉帕米、地尔硫䓬、尼莫地平	Pol J Pharmacol 56(2004)391-397
运动 位置偏好	0.5mg/kg，5d运动试验；0.5mg/kg，4dCPP试验	Wistar大鼠	尼莫地平、维拉帕米、地尔硫䓬	Pol J Pharmacol 55(2003)327-335
运动 位置偏好	0.5mg/kg	Wistar大鼠 Swiss小鼠	尼莫地平、维拉帕米、地尔硫䓬	J Pharm Pharmacol 56 (2004) 1021-1028
记忆	0.0175mg/kg皮下注射、0.035mg/kg皮下注射、0.175mg/kg皮下注射或0.35mg/kg皮下注射	Swiss小鼠	氟桂利嗪、维拉帕米、氨氯地平、尼莫地平、硝苯地平和尼卡地平	Naunyn Schmiedebergs Arch Pharmacol 386 (2013) 651-664

续表

索引	烟碱模型	动物	LTCC药物	参考文献
记忆（短期和长期）	0.05mg/kg皮下注射、0.1mg/kg皮下注射和0.5mg/kg皮下注射	Swiss小鼠	氨氯地平、尼卡地平、维拉帕米	Behav Brain Res 317 (2017) 27-36
与记忆相关的响应	0.035mg/kg、0.175mg/kg和0.35mg/kg	Swiss小鼠	尼莫地平、氟桂利嗪、维拉帕米、地尔硫䓬	Pharmacol Rep 61 (2009) 236-244
激励效应	1.168mg/kg皮下注射，每日3次，持续11d	Wistar大鼠	尼莫地平、维拉帕米和氟桂利嗪	Behav Brain Res 228 (2012) 144-150
激励效应	0.1～1mg/kg，0.5mg/kg最佳方式为皮下注射3d	C57BL/6J小鼠	硝苯地平Cav1.2 Cav1.3转基因小鼠	Prog Neuropsychopharmacol Biol Psychiatry75 (2017)176-182
神经损伤	卷烟烟雾暴露，每天20min，持续14d	白化Wistar大鼠	硝苯地平、维拉帕米	Ann Plast Surg 70 (2013) 222-226
复发	0.5mg/kg腹腔注射，持续3d	Wistar大鼠	尼莫地平、氟桂利嗪	Pharmacol Biochem Behav 89 (2008) 116-125
皮瓣坏死	卷烟烟雾暴露，每天20min，持续21d	白化Wistar大鼠	硝苯地平、维拉帕米	Plast Reconstr Surg 125 (2010) 866-871
躯体体征	2.5mg/kg皮下注射，每日4次，持续7d	Swiss小鼠	尼莫地平、维拉帕米、地尔硫䓬、氟桂利嗪	Pharmacol Res 51 (2005) 483-488
躯体体征激励信号	每天36mg/kg，使用14d或28d微型泵	C57BL/6J小鼠	尼莫地平或维拉帕米（±）Bay K8644	J Pharmacol Exp Ther 330 (2009) 152-161
电生理学	卡巴胆碱，类毒素A	Sprague Dawley大鼠	硝苯地平	J Physiol 568 (2005) 469-481
电生理学		Sprague Dawley大鼠	(S)-(−)-BAY K8644 FPL 64176 硝苯地平	J Biol Chem 282 (2007) 8594-8603
电生理学		C57BL/6J小鼠	硝苯地平 LTCC亚型	J Neurophysiol 112 (2014) 1119-1130
电生理学	卡巴胆碱	Sprague Dawley大鼠	硝苯地平	Brain Res 1245 (2008) 41-51

注：该表列出了有关L型钙离子通道和烟碱在动物体内的主要研究，并提供了详细的参考信息。

46.3 镇痛作用

在早期阶段，许多研究人员关注LTCC药物对烟碱诱导的抗伤害作用的影响。甩尾技术是一种主要的伤害感测量方法，除了尾巴以外，动物的身体都会受到约束，一束光投射到动物的尾巴上。Damaj的研究小组证明，LTCC激活剂（±）-Bay K8644可增强烟碱诱导的急性或慢性抗伤害作用，而LTCC抑制剂尼莫地平和硝苯地平则阻断烟碱单独或（±）-Bay K8644与烟碱合用的抗伤害作用（Damaj, 1997, 2005, 2007; Damaj, Martin, 1993; Damaj, Welch, Martin, 1993）。Damaj（2007）还指出，LTCC对烟碱诱导的抗伤害性感受的影响是通过脊髓中含有β2的乙酰胆碱受体介导的，这需要通过LTCC的钙内流来激活钙/钙调蛋白依赖性蛋白激酶Ⅱ（CaMKⅡ），从而产生烟碱镇痛。此外，LTCC还参与小鼠烟碱耐受的表达和发展（Damaj, 2005）。然而，大鼠研究的结果与Damaj的实验结果不同，后者显示硝苯地平（15mg/kg，腹腔注射）增强了烟碱诱导的抗伤害作用（Zbuzek, Cohen, Wu, 1997）。

46.4　运动

此外，还研究了LTCC对烟碱诱导的运动改变的影响。Damaj等的结果表明，Bay K8644（0.75 mg/kg i.p.）在烟碱注射引起的自发活动减少中产生5～10倍的增强效果（Damaj, Martin, 1993），这一作用可被硝苯地平阻断。Hart等注意到LTCC抑制剂尼莫地平（10mg/kg和20mg/kg）可以逆转急性烟碱注射后的运动增加（Hart et al. 1996）。成瘾行为的一个特征是一种称为敏化的现象：在反复、间歇使用成瘾药物治疗后，某些药物诱导的效应（如运动）逐渐增强。Biala等（Biala, 2003；Biala, Weglinska, 2004a, 2004b）和Bernardi等（Bernardi et al. 2014）表明，4种LTCC抑制剂硝苯地平、尼莫地平、维拉帕米和地尔硫䓬都可以阻断烟碱诱导的运动敏化的获得和表达；维拉帕米和地尔硫䓬可以减弱烟碱和乙醇的交叉敏化；但尼莫地平和维拉帕米可降低烟碱与吗啡或MK-801的交叉增敏作用。

46.5　依赖性

条件性位置偏好（CPP）范式是研究烟碱强化特性的一种流行而有效的方法。Biala等（2003）发现，尼莫地平、维拉帕米或地尔硫卓10μmol/L腹腔注射可阻断烟碱诱导的CPP（烟碱0.5mg/kg腹腔注射）。此外，在交叉致敏实验中，吗啡（5mg/kg）只诱导烟碱注射动物的CPP，尼莫地平、维拉帕米或地尔硫卓分别以10mg/kg和20mg/kg的剂量腹腔注射，可以剂量依赖性地阻止这种敏感化（Biala, Weglinska, 2004b）。我们的团队进一步研究了所涉及的LTCC亚型，表明$Ca_v1.2$亚型而不是$Ca_v1.3$亚型通过不表达$Ca_v1.3$（Cav1.3$^{-/-}$）的转基因小鼠模型介导了CPP的获得，或者包含$Ca_v1.2$的DHP（$Ca_v1.2DHP^{-/-}$）位点的突变（Liu, Harding, Dore, Chen, 2017）。

CPP也是研究药物恢复的有效范式。药物成瘾是一种复发性脑功能障碍，其神经生物学改变导致强迫性寻药行为。长期戒断后的高复发率是成瘾治疗中的主要问题之一。Biala等指出LTCC拮抗剂尼莫地平和氟桂利嗪的腹腔注射剂量分别为5mg/kg和10mg/kg，可减弱大麻素受体激动剂WIN55、212-2和乙醇诱导的烟碱CPP的恢复（Biala, Budzynska, 2008）。

此外，烟碱戒断症状会促进持续吸烟和戒烟后的复发。长期服用烟碱后戒断烟碱会导致以身体和情感症状为特征的戒断综合征（Biala, Weglinska, 2005）。Biala等（Biala, Weglinska, 2005）和Damaj等（Jackson, Damaj, 2009）研究发现，使用LTCC拮抗剂，如尼莫地平1mg/kg或10mg/kg腹腔注射，维拉帕米1mg/kg或10mg/kg腹腔注射，或地尔硫卓10mg/kg腹腔注射，烟碱戒断后的体征显著降低，LTCC激活剂(±)-Bay K8644在0.5mg/kg剂量下表现出更多的躯体体征，表明LTCC在烟碱戒断体征中具有重要作用。条件性位置厌恶（CPA）被用来考察戒断时的厌恶动机状态或对与戒断成对的环境刺激的条件性回避。关于LTCC和烟碱诱导的CPA的研究结果是相反而复杂的。Biala等（Budzynska et al. 2012）研究表明，LTCC拮抗剂尼莫地平、维拉帕米和氟桂利嗪的腹腔注射剂量分别为5mg/kg和10mg/kg。在给药前注射美加明可减弱烟碱CPA，但Damaj等（Jackson, Damaj, 2009）发现，在美加明给药前以腹腔注射剂量为1mg/kg

预处理尼莫地平可以增强CPA反应。因此，LTCC在烟碱戒断中的作用仍然不是很清楚，也比较复杂。

46.6　焦虑

焦虑是身体依赖和烟碱戒断综合征的常见症状。在烟碱戒断过程中焦虑水平升高，这是烟碱戒断失败的主要原因，而焦虑水平随着烟碱依赖程度的降低而降低，这就是吸烟者可能继续吸烟的原因。高架加迷宫（EPM）被用来测量焦虑，其中张开手臂的入口和进入张开手臂的时间的增加意味着焦虑的增加。Biala等（Biala, Budzynska, 2006;Biala, Kruk, 2008）发现四种LTCC抑制剂尼莫地平、氟桂利嗪、维拉帕米和地尔硫䓬（剂量为10mg/kg）在急性低剂量（0.1mg/kg）烟碱和5mg/kg剂量（尼莫地平或氟桂利嗪）或20mg/kg剂量（维拉帕米或地尔硫䓬）在0.1mg/kg烟碱给药6d后可减轻焦虑作用。但在戒断试验中，Damaj等（Jackson, Damaj, 2009）没有发现LTCC抑制剂尼莫地平和维拉帕米（1mg/kg）对烟碱戒断后的焦虑效应有影响。

46.7　认知功能

烟碱已被证明具有神经保护特性，在人类中，许多研究描述了烟碱给药后认知功能的缺陷或效率的提高。因此，Biala等研究了LTCC对烟碱诱导的记忆改变的影响，尽管他们的结果本身相互矛盾。他们揭示了LTCC抑制剂氨氯地平、尼卡地平和维拉帕米可增强烟碱诱导的短时记忆和长时记忆的改善，这可能是通过激活ERK1/2或抑制长时记忆而实现的（Michalak, Biala, 2017）。然而，他们之前的发现与之恰恰相反，急性氨氯地平、尼卡地平和维拉帕米的预处理逆转了烟碱诱导的记忆获得的改善，在维拉帕米的情况下也逆转了记忆巩固；氨氯地平和维拉帕米的慢性预处理逆转了烟碱促进的记忆获得和巩固（Biala, Kruk, 2009; Biala et al. 2013）。作者自己认为，"决定LTCC抑制剂对烟碱记忆效应影响的结果差异的因素可能包括给药途径（中枢和外周）、剂量计划表（急性和慢性）、治疗时间（训练前和训练后），以及其他与行为测试相关的条件，如使用的刺激物"（Michalak, Biala, 2017）。这一评论也可以解释不同实验室在焦虑、CPA和运动实验中存在的相反结果。

除了这些主要的行为测试，LTCC还被证明参与阻断烟碱辨别（依拉地平15mg/kg）（Schechter, Meehan, 1992），减少吸烟对周围神经缺血/再灌注损伤的影响［硝苯地平10mg/(kg·d)或维拉帕米20mg/(kg·d)］（Rinker et al. 2013），改善吸烟诱导的皮瓣坏死［硝苯地平10mg/(kg·d)或维拉帕米20mg/(kg·d)］（Rinker et al. 2010）。

46.8　LTCC的表达

LTCC在烟碱诱导的行为中确实发挥着重要作用，但其潜在的大脑区域和分子机制仍未被很好地理解。Ohkuma的研究小组讨论了在原代培养和烟碱处理的小鼠大脑皮层中LTCC与烟碱暴露的关系（Hayashida et al. 2005; Katsura et al. 2000; Katsura et al. 2002）。他们发现，24h的烟碱暴露增加了地西泮结合抑制剂（DBI）的mRNA表达，这是通过激活CaMKⅡ介导的，在nAChR激活诱导膜去极化后，CaMKⅡ通过LTCC增加了细胞内的Ca^{2+}（Katsura et al. 2000）。他们还发现，在细胞培养72h（Katsura et al. 2002）或小鼠烟碱给药7d后（Hayashida et al. 2005），小鼠大脑皮层中α1C、α1D、α1F和α2/δ1亚基以及[^{3}H]地尔硫䓬结合位点的表达显著增加。他们还研究了（Katsura et al. 2002）LTCC抑制剂硝苯地平（1μmol/L）如何抑制30mmol/L KCl诱导的Ca^{2+}内流，烟碱暴露如何增强被硝苯地平抑制的Bay K8644诱导的Ca^{2+}内流，以及尼卡地平（1μmol/L）如何降低0.1mol/L烟碱作用72h后Ba^{2+}电流峰值的增加。所有这些研究表明，烟碱暴露于nAChR可激活LTCC，诱导Ca^{2+}内流，从而改变大脑皮层的细胞内过程，这可能是烟碱依赖和戒断综合征的潜在机制。最近，Bernardi等（2014）在更广泛的脑区调查了长期烟碱暴露的LTCC亚型的个体贡献，发现$Ca_v1.2$ mRNA在单次烟碱（0.175 mg/kg）暴露后没有改变，而在包括前额叶皮层、尾壳核和伏隔核（NAcc）在内的几个大脑区域观察到$Ca_v1.3$ mRNA的强烈上调。经过14d的烟碱治疗和24h的戒断，$Ca_v1.2$ mRNA在包括前额叶皮层、尾壳核、VTA和海马腹侧亚区（CA3）在内的所有脑区都下调，而$Ca_v1.3$ mRNA没有变化。戒断7d后，$Ca_v1.2$转录上调，包括前额叶皮层、尾壳核、NAcc壳和海马腹侧亚区（CA1和CA3），而$Ca_v1.3$ mRNA基本不受影响。作者认为，$Ca_v1.2$可能参与了戒断相关症状的调节，而$Ca_v1.3$似乎主要参与了烟碱暴露的早期阶段。

46.9 放电模式

我们小组从电生理的角度讲述了这个故事（图46.3）。在VTA中，DA神经元有两种不同的放电模式，即单峰放电和爆发放电，这两种放电模式分别编码不同的行为和分子信号。烟碱的暴露被认为会增加中脑爆发放电的百分比。因此，放电模式可能与烟碱依赖的理论分子途径有关。我们的研究小组发现，普通胆碱能激动剂卡巴胆碱或α4β2 nAChR激动剂anatoxin A可以诱导VTA DA神经元的爆发放电，在使用LTCC抑制剂硝苯地平后，这种放电可以被阻断或恢复为单峰放电（Zhang, Liu, Chen, 2005）。这种爆裂也可以通过(S)-(−)-Bay K8644或FPL 64176直接激活LTCC来诱导，这种激活是由蛋白激酶C裂解产生的蛋白激酶M介导的（Liu et al. 2007）。还需要注意的是，不同亚型的LTCC调节不同的放电模式，因为只有$Ca_v1.3$调节基本的单峰放电，而$Ca_v1.2$和$Ca_v1.3$的激活都支持爆发放电（Liu et al. 2014）。以上结果表明，不同亚型的LTCC和VTA内不同的放电模式可能是烟碱依赖的根本原因，并可能承担不同的责任。

综上所述，许多关于烟碱和LTCC的动物研究表明，LTCC确实在烟碱暴露和成瘾的许多方面发挥了关键作用，包括烟碱依赖和戒断综合征，这是因为在动物中使用LTCC抑制剂后可以减轻这些症状。因此，进一步评估LTCC抑制剂在治疗烟碱依赖或戒断中的作用可能是一个很有前途的领域。然而，第一，必须记住一些重要的问题，这些治疗效果只在实验室动物中表现出来，因此还不能与人类的治疗或经验直接相关。第二，临床剂量的LTCC抑制剂不会影响人类的大脑功能，尽管已经检测到皮质脊髓的可塑性发生了一些变化（Wankerl, Weise, Gentner, Rumpf, Classen, 2010）。第三，全身应用LTCC药物可能会引起明显的心血管效应，其剂量与大多数研究在实验中使用的剂量相同，尽管对自发活动的影响尚未见报道。第四，LTCC药物对烟碱相关行为的影响可能涉及多个烟碱相关区域和信号通路；因此，仅有一种理论还不能解释整个过程。

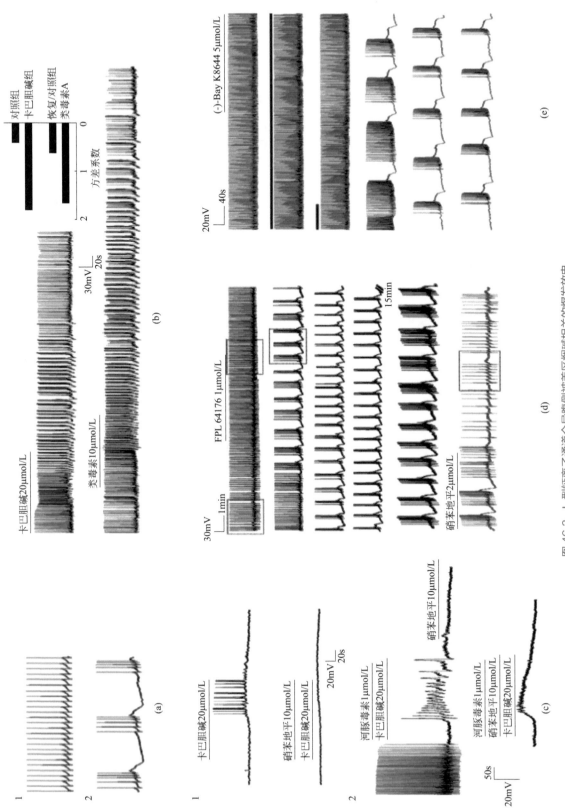

图 46.3 L 型钙离子通道介导腹侧被盖区烟碱相关的爆发放电

(a) 两种放电模式：(1) 单峰放电和 (2) 爆发放电。(b) 卡巴胆碱和 α4β2 激动剂 anatoxin A 对同一神经元均有类似的爆发放电。(c) L 型钙离子通道抑制剂硝苯地平可阻断卡巴胆碱诱发的突发性放电 (1) 和膜振荡 (2)。L 型钙离子通道激动剂 FPL 64176 (d) 和 (S)-(−)-Bay K8644 (e) 均由单次激发转变为突发性激发。(b) 和 (c) 来自 Zhang 等 (2005)，发表在 J Physiol; (a)、(d) 和 (e) 来自 Liu 等 (2007)，发表在 J Biol Chem。

| 术语解释 | - 激动剂：一种能够促进受体激活或通道开放的化学物质。
- 抑制剂：一种能够阻断受体激活或通道开放的化学物质。
- 电压门控钙离子通道：对电压变化敏感的离子通道。当它打开时，钙离子流入细胞内。
- 条件性位置偏好（CPP）：这是一种检测药物增强性能的有效方法。
- 交叉致敏作用：一种药物的致敏作用是由另一种药物引起的。
- 去极化：膜电位由低到高变化，如从 −60mV 变为 −40mV。
- 多巴胺：一种重要的神经递质，涉及生理状态（如奖励处理和运动精细调节）和疾病状态（如帕金森病、药物成瘾和精神分裂症）。
- Firing：这意味着细胞内的动作电位。放电模式是指两个动作电位之间具有不同时间间隔。
- L型钙离子通道：一种类型的钙离子通道。当它打开时，钙离子内流时间相对较长，与其他钙离子通道相比，通道失活相对较慢。
- Reinstatement：停药后恢复服药的行为。
- 敏化：一些与药物有关的作用逐渐增强，如运动。
- 腹侧被盖区：中脑的一个小区域，是大脑中多巴胺能神经元的主要来源。它的功能与奖励和疾病状态（如药物成瘾和精神分裂症）有关。
- 戒断综合征：在成瘾性戒断后，出现了复杂和多重的症状，如焦虑和颤抖增加。 |

| L型钙离子通道（LTCC）的关键事实 | - LTCC是一种在去极化过程中具有持久电流的钙离子通道。
- LTCC有四种亚型：$Ca_v1.1$、$Ca_v1.2$、$Ca_v1.3$和$Ca_v1.4$。
- LTCC是首个纯化的钙离子通道。
- LTCC抑制剂是治疗心血管疾病的常用有效临床药物。
- LTCC分布在大脑中，参与神经功能（如递质释放）、放电调节以及大脑处理（如奖励和记忆）。 |

| 要点总结 | - 本章主要介绍L型钙离子通道（LTCC）和烟碱。
- LTCC分布于脑内，主要是$Ca_v1.2$和$Ca_v1.3$亚型，它们可以位于同一神经元上，位置相同，如在树突中。
- 在动物实验中，LTCC激动剂增强烟碱相关行为，而LTCC抑制剂则抑制一些与烟碱相关的行为，如运动敏感化和条件性位置偏好。
- 烟碱的使用增加了LTCC在相关脑区的表达，如动物的皮质、伏隔核和腹侧被盖区。
- 烟碱受体激活诱导放电模式转换，参与动物LTCC的激活。
- 请记住，动物研究中使用的药物剂量可能会高于临床研究中使用的药物剂量。 |

参考文献

Bernardi, R. E.; Uhrig, S.; Spanagel, R.; Hansson, A. C. (2014). Transcriptional regulation of L-type calcium channel subtypes Cav1.2 and Cav1.3 by nicotine and their potential role in nicotine sensitization. Nicotine, Tobacco Research, 16(6), 774-785.

Biala, G. (2003). Calcium channel antagonists suppress nicotine-induced place preference and locomotor sensitization in rodents. Polish Journal of Pharmacology, 55(3), 327-335.

Biala, G.; Budzynska, B. (2006). Effects of acute and chronic nicotine on elevated plus maze in mice: involvement of calcium channels. Life Science, 79(1), 81-88.

Biala, G.; Budzynska, B. (2008). Calcium-dependent mechanisms of the reinstatement of nicotine-conditioned place preference by drug priming in rats. Pharmacology Biochemistry and Behavior, 89(1), 116-125.

Biala, G.; Kruk, M. (2008). Calcium channel antagonists suppress cross-tolerance to the anxiogenic effects of D-amphetamine and nicotine in the mouse elevated plus maze test. Progress in Neuropsychopharmacology, Biological Psychiatry, 32(1), 54-61.

Biala, G.; Kruk, M. (2009). Influence of bupropion and calcium channel antagonists on the nicotine-induced memory-related response of mice in the elevated plus maze. Pharmacological Reports, 61(2), 236-244.

Biala, G.; Kruk-Slomka, M.; Jozwiak, K. (2013). Influence of acute or chronic calcium channel antagonists on the acquisition and consolidation of memory and nicotine-induced cognitive effects in mice. Naunyn-Schmiedeberg's Archives of Pharmacology, 386(7), 651-664.

Biala, G.; Weglinska, B. (2004a). Calcium channel antagonists attenuate cross-sensitization to the locomotor effects of nicotine and ethanol in mice. Polish Journal of Pharmacology, 56(4), 391-397.

Biala, G.; Weglinska, B. (2004b). Calcium channel antagonists attenuate cross-sensitization to the rewarding and/or locomotor effects of nicotine, morphine and MK-801. Journal of Pharmacy and Pharmacology, 56(8), 1021-1028.

Biala, G.; Weglinska, B. (2005). Blockade of the expression of mecamylamine-precipitated nicotine withdrawal by calcium channel antagonists. Pharmacological Research, 51(5), 483-488.

Budzynska, B.; Polak, P.; Biala, G. (2012). Effects of calcium channel antagonists on the motivational effects of nicotine and morphine in conditioned place aversion paradigm. Behavioural Brain Research, 228(1), 144-150.

Chan, C. S.; Guzman, J. N.; Ilijic, E.; Mercer, J. N.; Rick, C.; Tkatch, T.; Surmeier, D. J. (2007). 'Rejuvenation' protects neurons in mouse models of Parkinson's disease. Nature, 447(7148), 1081-1086.

Damaj, M. I. (1997). Altered behavioral sensitivity of Ca(2+)-modulating drugs after chronic nicotine administration in mice. European Journal of Pharmacology, 322(2-3), 129-135.

Damaj, M. I. (2005). Calcium-acting drugs modulate expression and development of chronic tolerance to nicotine-induced antinociception in mice. Journal of Pharmacology and Experimental Therapeutics, 315(2), 959-964.

Damaj, M. I. (2007). Nicotinic regulation of calcium/calmodulindependent protein kinase Ⅱ activation in the spinal cord. Journal of Pharmacology and Experimental Therapeutics, 320(1), 244-249.

Damaj, M. I.; Martin, B. R. (1993). Calcium agonists and antagonists of the dihydropyridine type: effect on nicotine-induced antinociception and hypomotility. Drug and Alcohol Dependence, 32(1), 73-79.

Damaj, M. I.; Welch, S. P.; Martin, B. R. (1993). Involvement of calcium and L-type channels in nicotine-induced antinociception. Journal of Pharmacology and Experimental Therapeutics, 266(3), 1330-1338.

Dragicevic, E.; Schiemann, J.; Liss, B. (2015). Dopamine midbrain neurons in health and Parkinson's disease: emerging roles of voltagegated calcium channels and ATP-sensitive potassium channels. Neuroscience, 284, 798-814.

Hart, C.; Kisro, N. A.; Robinson, S. L.; Ksir, C. (1996). Effects of the calcium channel blocker nimodipine on nicotine-induced locomotion in rats. Psychopharmacology (Berlin), 128(4), 359-361.

Hayashida, S.; Katsura, M.; Torigoe, F.; Tsujimura, A.; Ohkuma, S. (2005). Increased expression of L-type high voltagegated calcium channel alpha1 and alpha2/delta subunits in mouse brain after chronic nicotine administration. Molecular Brain Research, 135(1-2), 280-284.

Hell, J. W.; Westenbroek, R. E.; Warner, C.; Ahlijanian, M. K.; Prystay, W.; Gilbert, M. M. et al. (1993). Identification and differential subcellular localization of the neuronal class C and class D L-type calcium channel alpha 1 subunits. Journal of Cell Biology, 123(4), 949-962.

Hofmann, F.; Flockerzi, V.; Kahl, S.; Wegener, J. W. (2014). L-type CaV1. 2 calcium channels: from in vitro findings to in vivo function. Physiological Reviews, 94(1), 303-326.

Jackson, K. J.; Damaj, M. I. (2009). L-type calcium channels and calcium/calmodulin-dependent kinase II differentially mediate behaviors associated with nicotine withdrawal in mice. Journal of Pharmacology and Experimental Therapeutics, 330(1), 152-161.

Katsura, M.; Higo, A.; Tarumi, C.; Tsujimura, A.; Takesue, M.; Mohri, Y. et al. (2000). Mechanism for increase in expression of cerebral diazepam binding inhibitor mRNA by nicotine: involvement of L-type voltage-dependent calcium channels. Molecular Brain Research, 80 (2), 132-141.

Katsura, M.; Mohri, Y.; Shuto, K.; Hai-Du, Y.; Amano, T.; Tsujimura, A. et al. (2002). Up-regulation of L-type voltage-dependent calcium channels after long term exposure to nicotine in cerebral cortical neurons. The Journal of Biological Chemistry, 277(10), 7979-7988.

Liu, Y.; Dore, J.; Chen, X. (2007). Calcium influx through L-type channels generates protein kinase M to induce burst firing of dopamine cells in the rat ventral tegmental area. The Journal of Biological Chemistry, 282(12), 8594-8603.

Liu, Y.; Harding, M.; Dore, J.; Chen, X. (2017). Cav1.2, but not Cav1.3, L-type calcium channel subtype mediates nicotine-induced conditioned place preference in miceo. Progress in Neuropsychopharmacology, Biological Psychiatry, 75, 176-182.

Liu, Y.; Harding, M.; Pittman, A.; Dore, J.; Striessnig, J.; Rajadhyaksha, A. et al. (2014). Cav1. 2 and Cav1. 3 L-type calcium channels regulate dopaminergic firing activity in the mouse ventral tegmental area. Journal of Neurophysiology, 112(5), 1119-1130.

Michalak, A.; Biala, G. (2017). Calcium homeostasis and protein kinase/phosphatase balance participate in nicotine-induced memory improvement in passive avoidance task in mice. Behavioural Brain Research, 317, 27-36.

Nowycky, M. C.; Fox, A. P.; Tsien, R. W. (1985). Three types of neuronal calcium channel with different calcium agonist sensitivity. Nature, 316(6027), 440-443.

Olson, P. A.; Tkatch, T.; Hernandez-Lopez, S.; Ulrich, S.; Ilijic, E.; Mugnaini, E. et al. (2005). G-protein-coupled receptor modulation of striatal CaV1.3 L-type Ca^{2+} channels is dependent on a Shankbinding domain. Journal of Neuroscience, 25(5), 1050-1062.

Rinker, B.; Fink, B. F.; Barry, N. G.; Fife, J. A.; Milan, M. E. (2010). The effect of calcium channel blockers on smoking-induced skin flap necrosis. Plastic and Reconstructive Surgery, 125(3), 866-871.

Rinker, B.; Fink, B. F.; Stoker, A. R.; Milan, M. E.; Nelson, P. T. (2013). Calcium channel blockers reduce the effects of cigarette smoking on peripheral nerve ischemia/reperfusion injury. Annals of Plastic Surgery, 70(2), 222-226.

Schechter, M. D.; Meehan, S. M. (1992). Further evidence for the mechanisms that may mediate nicotine discrimination. Pharmacology Biochemistry and Behavior, 41(4), 807-812.

Sinnegger-Brauns, M. J.; Huber, I. G.; Koschak, A.; Wild, C.; Obermair, G. J.; Einzinger, U. et al. (2009). Expression and 1, 4dihydropyridine-binding properties of brain L-type calcium channel isoforms. Molecular Pharmacology, 75(2), 407-414.

Takada, M.; Kang, Y.; Imanishi, M. (2001). Immunohistochemical localization of voltage-gated calcium channels in substantia nigra dopamine neurons. European Journal of Neuroscience, 13(4), 757-762.

Takahashi, M.; Seagar, M. J.; Jones, J. F.; Reber, B. F.; Catterall, W. A. (1987). Subunit structure of dihydropyridine-sensitive calcium channels from skeletal muscle. Proceedings of the National Academy of Sciences of the United States of America, 84(15), 5478-5482.

Tanabe, T.; Takeshima, H.; Mikami, A.; Flockerzi, V.; Takahashi, H.; Kangawa, K. et al. (1987). Primary structure of the receptor for calcium channel blockers from skeletal muscle. Nature, 328(6128), 313-318.

Wankerl, K.; Weise, D.; Gentner, R.; Rumpf, J. J.; Classen, J. (2010). L-type voltage-gated Ca^{2+} channels: a single molecular switch for long-term potentiation/long-term depression-like plasticity and activity-dependent metaplasticity in humans. Journal of Neuroscience, 30(18), 6197-6204.

Zbuzek, V. K.; Cohen, B.; Wu, W. (1997). Antinociceptive effect of nifedipine and verapamil tested on rats chronically exposed to nicotine and after its withdrawal. Life Science, 60(19), 1651-1658.

Zhang, L.; Liu, Y.; Chen, X. (2005). Carbachol induces burst firing of dopamine cells in the ventral tegmental area by promoting calcium entry through L-type channels in the rat. The Journal of Physiology, 568 (Pt 2), 469-481.

47

烟碱与其他物质使用和成瘾的并存：风险、机制、后果和对实践的影响，以年轻人为重点

Linda Richter

Director of Policy Research and Analysis, Center on Addiction, New York, NY, United States

47.1 引言

来自美国的国家统计数据表明，烟碱产品的使用仍然是一个严重的公共健康问题，尽管最近吸烟人数有所下降。这是因为与不再吸烟或不吸烟的人相比，许多继续吸食可燃卷烟的人在社会经济上处于更不利的地位，更容易受到烟草对健康的破坏性影响（Jamal et al. 2016）。这也反映了这样一个事实，尽管卷烟的使用率总体上有所下降，但其他烟碱产品（如电子烟和水烟）的使用率普遍上升，特别是在年轻人中（Agaku et al. 2014; Jamal et al. 2017）。虽然从公共健康的角度来看，可燃卷烟使用量的下降无疑代表着一种进步，值得称赞，但由于吸烟对发病率和死亡率造成的巨大影响，其他烟碱产品（即使是那些不含烟草的产品）使用量的增加仍然是一个令人担忧的重要因素（The National Center on Addiction and Substance Abuse, 2015; The National Center on Addiction and Substance Abuse, 2016）。

无论烟碱是通过什么设备传递的，它都不是一种无害的药物，特别是当年轻人摄入烟碱时（Klein, 2015）。烟碱会升高血压、呼吸和心率，并对神经、心血管、呼吸和生殖系统产生不利影响（Benowitz, 2009）。吸烟可能导致癌症的发展（Grando, 2014），如果口服的话可能是致命的（Mayer, 2014）。对年轻人来说，最重要的是，包括电子烟在内的所有烟碱产品都含有烟碱，这是一种高度成瘾的药物。事实上，烟碱是最容易成瘾的药物（Palmer et al. 2009），与使用其他成瘾物质的人相比，每周吸食烟碱的人成瘾的比例最高（大麻为67.3%和25.0%，酒精为15.6%）（Cougle et al. 2016）。

现今的卷烟比过去更容易成瘾，因为设计上的改变提高了烟碱的输送效率和烟草产品中的烟碱产量（Land et al. 2014）。在传统卷烟和不可燃烟碱产品中发现的添加剂和调味剂，有助于烟碱的输送，增加产品的吸引力，也可能加剧其健康后果和烟碱成瘾的风险（Alpert et al. 2016）。

47.1.1 年轻人的脆弱性

当涉及到年轻人时，烟碱的成瘾潜力尤其令人担忧。许多研究表明，首次接触某种物质的年龄越小，成瘾的风险就越高（Lanza, Vasilenko, 2015）。绝大多数对烟碱成瘾的人在青春期或成年早期就开始吸烟：84%的人在18岁之前开始吸烟，95%的人在21岁之前开始吸烟（The National

Center on Addiction and Substance Abuse, 2011)。近一半吸烟的青少年在18岁之前至少出现一种烟碱成瘾症状（Apelberg et al. 2014），1/5的人符合完整的诊断标准（Dierker et al. 2012）。对于那些从小就开始成瘾的人来说，成瘾症状可能会迅速发展，即使只是"试验性的"或偶尔使用也是如此（Dierker et al. 2012; DiFranza, 2015; McQuown et al. 2007）。使用多种烟碱产品的年轻人的成瘾风险特别高，在美国，报告使用两种或更多烟碱产品的年轻人的成瘾风险是只使用卷烟的年轻人的两倍（Apelberg et al. 2014; Lee et al. 2015）。

47.1.2 使用其他物质和成瘾的风险增加

烟碱的使用不仅与烟碱成瘾有关，还与其他形式的物质使用和成瘾的风险增加有关。Richter、Pugh、Smith和Ball（2017）发现，在报告使用任何类型烟碱产品或有烟碱成瘾的年轻人和成年人中，酒精使用、大麻使用、其他药物使用、多物质使用和物质使用障碍的概率都明显高于从未使用烟碱的人；在报告目前使用卷烟和其他烟碱产品的人中，共同发生的概率通常最高。烟碱的使用和其他物质的使用之间的关系在年轻的受访者中尤其强烈，这表明在年轻人中共同发生的潜在风险可能比年长的人更大。

对2014年全国药物使用与健康调查（Substance Abuse and Mental Health Services Administration, 2015）数据的其他分析表明，烟碱成瘾和酒精以及其他药物使用和成瘾之间存在关联。符合烟碱成瘾标准的受访者更有可能报告过去30天使用酒精（63.3%对46.2%）和过去一年的酒精使用障碍（16.5%对6.3%），以及过去30天使用其他药物（32.1%对11.2%）和过去一年的药物使用障碍（12.7%对3.0%）（见图47.1）。

更具体地说，有烟碱成瘾的人比没有烟碱成瘾的人更有可能报告过去30天使用大麻（28.2%对9.4%）和过去一年的大麻使用障碍（6.8%对2.1%），以及过去30天使用大麻以外的任何药物（11.2%对3.4%）和过去一年的药物使用障碍（7.9%对1.1%），以及过去30天滥用阿片类药物（5.9%对1.6%）和过去一年的阿片类药物使用障碍（4.2%对0.6%）。在有烟碱成瘾和没有烟碱成瘾的年轻人中，过去一年的酒精和其他药物使用障碍的发生率的差异在12～20岁的年轻人中更加明显。有烟碱成瘾的年轻人有酒精使用障碍的人数是没有烟碱成瘾的年轻人的6倍多（25.1%对4.2%），而在21岁及以上的成年受访者中的差异较小（15.4%对7.4%）。同样，有烟碱成瘾的年轻人有药物使用障碍的人数几乎是没有烟碱成瘾的年轻人的7倍（27.6%对4.0%），而成年人中的差异更小（10.8%对2.3%）（见图47.2）。

其他研究证实了青少年烟碱的使用与酒精和其他药物使用（Camenga et al. 2014; Cohen et al. 2015; Miech et al. 2016）以及酒精和其他药物使用障碍（Richter, Pugh, Ball, 2017; Richter et al. 2016）的风险之间存在着强烈的联系。

47.2 烟碱和其他物质使用和成瘾的神经生物学基础

烟碱的使用，特别是在青春期，不仅会使有害烟草产品的使用持续存在，增加烟碱成瘾的风险，而且还会增加使用其他物质的风险，并使大脑更容易受到酒精和其他药物成瘾的影响。这就是电子烟和其他非卷烟烟碱产品在年轻人中的受欢迎程度如此令人担忧的原因之一。在2016年，电子烟是美国初中生和高中生最常用的烟草产品（Jamal et al. 2017）。我们知道，年轻人使用这些产品，不仅使他们在大脑仍在发育、特别容易受到烟碱成瘾影响的时候接触到烟碱，而且还会导致或延续吸烟及其所有相关危害，即使是在那些本来没有吸烟倾向的人中也是如此（Soneji et al. 2017）。

青少年吸食任何类型的物质，包括烟碱，更容易上瘾，这似乎是由于这个年龄段的人对生物、心理和环境风险因素特别敏感（Smith et al. 2015; Yuan et al. 2015）。青春期的大脑非常敏感，在结构、功能和神经化学水平上都经历了基本的发育变化，使年轻人能够快速学习和快速适应。然而，这也意味着青少年的大脑对包括烟碱在内的成瘾物质更敏感，也更受其影响，而且这些影响，特别是与神经连接和行为调节有关的影响，可以持续到成年（Yuan et al. 2015）。

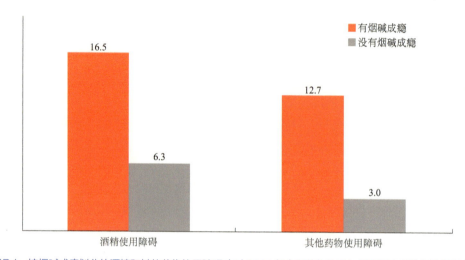

图47.1　按烟碱成瘾划分的酒精和其他药物使用障碍（对2014年全国药物使用与健康调查的数据进行了分析）

有烟碱成瘾和没有烟碱成瘾的受访者中，符合酒精或其他药物使用障碍诊断标准的百分比。基于对2014年全国药物使用与健康调查数据的分析（Substance Abuse and Mental Health Services Administration, 2015）。

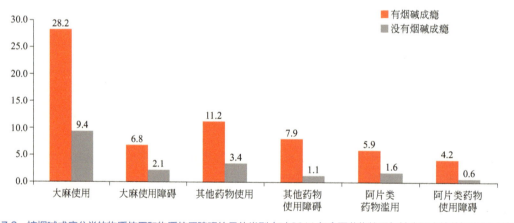

图47.2　按烟碱成瘾分类的物质使用和物质使用障碍的具体类型（对2014年全国药物使用与健康调查的数据进行了分析）

有烟碱成瘾和没有烟碱成瘾的受访者中，过去30天使用大麻、大麻以外的药物或阿片类药物滥用或过去一年有大麻使用障碍、其他药物使用障碍或阿片类药物使用障碍的受访者的百分比。基于对2014年全国药物使用与健康调查数据的分析（Substance Abuse and Mental Health Services Administration, 2015）。

烟碱乙酰胆碱受体（nAChR）是大脑中的受体蛋白，在烟碱成瘾的神经生理学中起着重要作用。它们参与神经递质系统的调节，特别是多巴胺，而多巴胺与奖励进程和成瘾物质的强化作用密切相关。它们在整个青春期的大脑成熟过程中也扮演着重要的角色（Yuan et al. 2015）。

烟碱对青少年大脑的影响比成人大脑更强烈，产生更强的奖励和更少的厌恶感。动物研究表明，与成年时期相比，青春期接触烟碱对大脑边缘系统有更深远、更不利和更长期的影响，这反过来会影响奖励进程、认知功能（如注意力减少和冲动增加）和情绪调节（与焦虑和抑郁有关）（Yuan et al. 2015）。烟碱对边缘系统的影响也使年轻人更容易使用和沉迷于其他物质（Dao et al. 2011）。在大鼠的研究中，在青春期短暂接触烟碱与更多的可卡因、甲基苯丙胺和酒精的自给药相关，这表明烟碱对大脑起作用，使其对其他成瘾物质敏感（Dao et al. 2011; Kandel, Kandel, 2014）（见表47.1）。

表47.1 影响烟碱暴露的因素

烟雾的酸碱值水平	烟雾/烟草的pH值碱性越大（无论吸入与否），越容易通过口腔黏膜被吸收，暴露程度也越大
吸入行为	吸入越多，口腔黏膜和肺部对烟碱的吸收越多，从而增加暴露
使用产品的时间/产品的消耗量	使用时间越长，烟碱暴露越多

注：烟碱的含量和浓度取决于所用产品的大小和类型、烟雾的酸碱值水平、吸入行为以及使用产品的时间/产品的消耗量。

多种形式的物质使用和物质使用障碍并存是很常见的，特别是在青少年中，可能是由于共同的遗传风险或共同的脆弱性，或者是由于神经生物学的启动或通过受体上调使大脑对成瘾物质敏感（Falk et al. 2006; Melroy-Greif et al. 2016; Palmer et al. 2009）（见表47.2）。

表47.2 按烟碱成瘾、年龄类别划分的酒精和其他药物使用障碍

项目	酒精/%	大麻/%	其他非法药物/%	处方药/%	多物质/%
共计（n=48750）	5.7	1.4	0.5	0.8	0.9
从未使用烟碱					
12～17	0.6	0.5	<0.1	0.4	0.2
18～25	3.7	0.6	<0.1	0.1	0.3
26岁及以上	1.4	<0.1	<0.1	0.2	<0.1
过去30天烟碱依赖					
12～17	25.7	25.3	7.4	9.4	16.7
18～25	23.6	12.6	6.3	7.5	12.7
26岁及以上	10.9	2.8	2.2	2.9	2.9

注：对2014年全国药物使用与健康调查数据的分析显示，与从未使用烟碱的人相比，烟碱依赖者的酒精和其他药物使用障碍更为普遍，尤其是在青少年中（Richter et al. 2017）。

47.2.1 烟碱和酒精

最常一起使用的两种成瘾物质是烟碱和酒精（Falk et al. 2006）。吸烟者比不吸烟者更有可能饮酒并患上酒精使用障碍（Richter et al. 2017）。烟碱和酒精的不良健康影响，如癌症，在同时使用这两种成瘾物质的人中会加剧（Adams, 2017; Falk et al. 2006）。烟碱和酒精同时使用的普遍现象可能是由几个因素造成的。这两种物质中的每一种物质都对另一种物质有奖励增强或增强作用，称为交叉强化，即两种物质作用于nAChR和中脑边缘多巴胺通路的相加效应。交叉强化效应的证据是：渴望增加，获得奖励的体验增加，吸烟者饮酒的动机增强，吸烟可能破坏减少饮酒的努力，饮酒可能破坏戒烟的尝试。这两种物质中的每一种物质也可以减轻或缓冲另一种物质的负面影响，即所谓的交叉耐受，如当酒精减轻烟碱的一些唤醒或刺激作用时，或烟碱减弱酒精的镇静、醉酒或抑郁作用时，否则可能会导致酒精摄入量的减少（Adams, 2017; Tolu et al. 2017）。

47.2.2 烟碱和大麻

就像酒精一样,烟碱和大麻的使用和成瘾有很高的同时发生率,其中一种物质的使用既增加了依赖另一种物质的风险,也干扰了戒烟或减少使用另一种物质的尝试(Kristman-Valente et al. 2017; Rabin, George, 2015; Richter et al. 2017)。

通常,大麻被卷进卷烟中制成大麻接头,烟草经常被添加到接头上以方便使用和降低成本,雪茄被掏空并装入大麻以制成小雪茄烟。同时使用烟草和大麻的人比只使用这两种物质中的一种的人会经历更严重的后果(Agrawal et al. 2009)。

某些神经生物学机制可以帮助解释同时使用这两种物质的吸引力。与烟碱和酒精相似,有一些证据表明大麻对烟碱有协同或增强作用,其中大脑内源性大麻素系统的启动有助于增强烟碱的奖励效应(Rabin, George, 2015)。同样,长期服用烟碱会影响大脑中大麻素受体的密度和内源性大麻素的水平,从而使烟碱增强对大麻的反应(Kristman-Valente et al. 2017)。烟碱可以提高人的觉醒和注意力,而大麻则起到相反的作用。烟碱的使用可能有助于掩盖与大麻使用相关的认知缺陷,特别是在年轻人中(Jacobsen et al. 2007)。与烟碱和酒精不同,烟碱和大麻的使用有一个共同的给药途径:吸入,这是成瘾的最有效途径;因此,使用一种物质可能会提示或激发对另一种物质的渴望(Rabin, George, 2015)。一种常见的遗传脆弱性也可能是吸食大麻的人烟碱成瘾率高的原因(Agrawal et al. 2010)。

47.2.3 烟碱和可卡因

烟碱被作为一种诱导性毒品,最常见物质是可卡因。与吸烟前使用可卡因或不经常吸烟的人相比,吸烟后开始使用可卡因的人可卡因成瘾率最高。研究发现,小鼠长期接触烟碱会使大脑变得更敏感或更容易对可卡因做出反应(Kandel, Kandel, 2014; Yuan et al. 2015)。与青少年大脑对成瘾物质的强化效应特别敏感的观点一致,在青少年中,烟碱暴露使大脑更倾向于使用可卡因的可能性很明显。暴露于烟碱(相对于生理盐水)的青春期大鼠比同样暴露的成年大鼠对可卡因(自给药可卡因)有更强的反应(McQuown et al. 2007)。

47.2.4 多种烟碱产品的使用

在使用多种烟碱产品的人群中,烟碱与其他物质的使用和成瘾并存最明显。Richter等(2017)发现,在美国全国调查中报告使用烟碱产品的受访者同时发生物质使用和物质使用障碍的发生率明显更高,尤其是那些报告使用卷烟和非卷烟烟碱产品的人。该研究还发现,报告使用任何类型的烟碱的青少年,其酒精、药物和多种物质的使用率较高,但在使用多种烟碱产品的青少年中,这种关联最为明显。

47.3 减少烟碱使用及其后果的必要条件

减少烟碱产品的使用需要持续实施全人群循证预防计划,对有风险的人进行早期干预,并对成瘾者进行及时有效的治疗,还需要仔细观察电子烟等非卷烟烟碱产品的流行。尽管电子烟和其他蒸发设备可能比烟草产品更安全,但事实上,大多数电子烟和其他蒸发设备都含有烟碱和许多其他有害物质。烟碱产品的使用一再与不良健康影响、开始吸烟、酗酒和其他吸毒成瘾有关，特别是在年轻人中（U.S. Department of Health and Human Services, 2016）。

尽管烟碱与其他形式的物质使用有相当大的共生性，但烟碱通常不会在针对酒精和其他药物的相同预防措施中得到解决。在预防规划中人为地将烟碱与其他成瘾物质分开，可能会使人们长期认为烟碱的使用与其他物质的使用和成瘾无关，而且问题可能比其他物质的使用和成瘾问题要小。为了有效防止烟碱产品的使用及其对健康的影响，并降低其他物质使用和成瘾的风险，预防方案应该解决所有烟碱产品与其他成瘾物质一起使用的问题（Richter, Foster, 2013; Richter et al. 2017）。

鉴于烟碱使用者中酒精和其他药物的共存率很高，未能在教育和医疗保健环境中筛查烟碱的使用和成瘾，可能会导致错过解决年轻人和成年人成瘾问题的机会。所有形式的烟碱使用应包括在与物质相关的筛查和评估工具中；目前，大多数此类评估工具不包括烟碱产品或仅涉及卷烟使用（Richter, Foster, 2013）。考虑到烟碱使用者，即使是那些不符合烟碱成瘾标准的人，似乎也应该关注其中那些烟碱使用较多的人，而不仅仅是成瘾者，因为烟碱使用者中发现了高水平的共生物质使用和成瘾。向使用烟碱产品的人提供或将其与循证干预联系起来，应该成为卫生保健实践的常规部分。

对治疗的启示

尽管烟碱的使用和成瘾与其他物质的使用和成瘾之间存在明显的联系，但大多数心理健康和成瘾治疗方案都没有提供戒烟服务（Knudsen et al. 2010）。一种普遍的假设认为，鼓励戒烟可能会影响人们从酒精或其他药物成瘾中成功戒烟，而事实恰恰相反。研究发现，将烟碱成瘾作为酒精和其他药物成瘾治疗的标准部分可以改善治疗结果（Lemon et al. 2004）。烟碱产品的使用干扰了药物使用障碍的恢复，并增加了复发的风险。同时治疗烟碱和共生物质使用障碍可以充分利用成功康复的心理和神经生物学机制。

术语解释
- 共现：一种以上的成瘾物质使用或物质使用障碍的存在或共病。
- 内源性大麻素：存在于大脑和全身的受体，其功能是维持动态平衡或稳定性，并允许大脑和身体内不同类型的细胞之间的交流和协调。
- 烟碱依赖/成瘾：达到过去一个月"烟碱依赖"的诊断标准，由烟碱依赖综合征量表（NDSS）衡量，NDSS是全国药物使用和健康调查中使用的成瘾衡量标准。NDSS标准一般与《精神障碍诊断与统计手册》第四版（DSM-Ⅳ）中的"烟草使用障碍"标准相同。
- 烟碱乙酰胆碱受体（nAChR）：神经递质乙酰胆碱的大脑受体，它对烟碱也有反应。
- 上调：在细胞水平上，通过增加突触后受体的数量来增加对刺激的反应。

烟碱与其他物质成瘾关系的关键事实
- 烟碱是所有药物中最容易成瘾的。每周使用烟碱产品的人中有2/3会成瘾。
- 烟碱成瘾的人使用大麻、阿片类药物和其他药物，以及患有大麻、阿片类药物或其他药物使用障碍的可能性是没有烟碱成瘾的人的3倍多。
- 烟碱成瘾的年轻人比成年人更有可能同时使用物质或患有共生物质使用障碍。
- 高共现率可能是由于共同的风险因素或烟碱对大脑的神经生物学效应。
- 与成功戒烟的人相比，继续使用烟碱的人更有可能重新患上酒精和其他药物使用障碍。

要点总结

- 本章的重点是烟碱与其他物质的使用和成瘾的共现。
- 虽然卷烟使用率一直在下降，但美国烟碱产品的总体使用率保持相对稳定，这在很大程度上是因为电子烟等非卷烟烟碱产品的使用量增加。
- 尽管不可燃烟碱产品总体上危害较小，但也不是没有风险。
- 除了烟碱使用会导致成瘾的风险外，它还与酒精和其他药物的使用和成瘾以及药物使用障碍康复患者的复发密切相关。
- 因此，预防和治疗做法应该将烟碱作为整体成瘾护理的一部分，而不是因为担心烟碱会影响酒精和其他药物使用障碍的预防或治疗而回避它。

参考文献

Adams, S. (2017). Psychopharmacology of tobacco and alcohol comorbidity: a review of current evidence. Current Addiction Reports, 4(1), 25-34.

Agaku, I. T.; King, B. A.; Husten, C. G.; Bunnell, R.; Ambrose, B. K.; Hu, S. S. et al. (2014). Tobacco product use among adults—United States, 2012-2013. Morbidity and Mortality Weekly Report, 63(25), 542-547.

Agrawal, A.; Lynskey, M. T.; Madden, P. A.; Pregedia, M. L.; Bucholz, K. K.; Heath, A. C. (2009). Simultaneous cannabis and tobacco use and cannabis-related outcomes in young women. Drug and Alcohol Dependence, 101(1-2), 8-12.

Agrawal, A.; Silberg, J. L.; Lynskey, M. T.; Maes, H. H.; Eaves, L. J. (2010). Mechanisms underlying the lifetime co-occurrence of tobacco and cannabis use in adolescent and young adult twins. Drug and Alcohol Dependence, 108(1-2), 49-55.

Alpert, H. R.; Agaku, I. T.; Connolly, G. N. (2016). A study of pyrazines in cigarettes and how additives might be used to enhance tobacco addiction. Tobacco Control, 25(4), 444-450.

Apelberg, B. J.; Corey, C. G.; Hoffman, A. C.; Schroeder, M. J.; Husten, C. G.; Caraballo, R. S. et al. (2014). Symptoms of tobacco dependence among middle and high school tobacco users: results from the 2012 National Youth Tobacco Survey. American Journal of Preventive Medicine, 47(2 Suppl 1), S4-S14.

Benowitz, N. L. (2009). Pharmacology of nicotine: addiction, smokinginduced disease, and therapeutics. Annual Review of Pharmacology and Toxicology, 49, 57-71.

Camenga, D. R.; Kong, G.; Cavallo, D. A.; Liss, A.; Hyland, A.; Delmerico, J. et al. (2014). Alternate tobacco product and drug use among adolescents who use electronic cigarettes, cigarettes only, and never smokers. Journal of Adolescent Health, 55(4), 588-591.

Cohen, A.; Villanti, A.; Richardson, A.; Rath, J. M.; Williams, V.; Stanton, C. et al. (2015). The association between alcohol, marijuana use, and new and emerging tobacco products in a young adult population. Addictive Behaviors, 48, 79-88.

Cougle, J. R.; Hakes, J. K.; Macatee, R. J.; Zvolensky, M. J.; Chavarria, J. (2016). Probability and correlates of dependence among regular users of alcohol, nicotine, cannabis, and cocaine: concurrent and prospective analyses of the National Epidemiologic Survey on alcohol and related conditions. Journal of Clinical Psychiatry, 77(4), 444-450.

Dao, J. M.; McQuown, S. C.; Loughlin, S. E.; Belluzzi, J. D.; Leslie, F. M. (2011). Nicotine alters limbic function in adolescent rat by a 5-HT1A receptor mechanism. Neuropsychopharmacology, 36(7), 1319-1331.

Dierker, L.; Swendsen, J.; Rose, J.; He, J.; Merikangas, K. (2012). Transitions to regular smoking and nicotine dependence in the Adolescent National Comorbidity Survey (NCS-A). Annals of Behavioral Medicine, 43(3), 394-401.

DiFranza, J. R. (2015). A 2015 update on the natural history and diagnosis of nicotine addiction. Current Pediatric Reviews, 11(1), 43-55.

Falk, D. E.; Yi, H. Y.; Hiller-Sturmhöfel, S. (2006). An epidemiologic analysis of co-occurring alcohol and tobacco use and disorders: findings from the National Epidemiologic Survey on Alcohol and Related Conditions. Alcohol Research, Health, 29(3), 162-171.

Grando, S. A. (2014). Connections of nicotine to cancer. Nature Reviews Cancer, 14(6), 419-429.

Jacobsen, L. K.; Pugh, K. R.; Constable, R. T.; Westerveld, M.; Mencl, W. E. (2007). Functional correlates of verbal memory deficits emerging during nicotine withdrawal in abstinent adolescent cannabis users. Biological Psychiatry, 61(1), 31-40.

Jamal, A.; Gentzke, A.; Hu, S. S.; Cullen, K. A.; Apelberg, B. J.; Homa, D. M. et al. (2017). Tobacco use among middle and high school students—United States, 2011-2016. Morbidity and Mortality Weekly Report, 66(23), 597-603.

Jamal, A.; King, B. A.; Neff, L. J.; Whitmill, J.; Babb, S. D.; Graffunder, C. M. (2016). Current cigarette smoking among adults—United States, 2005-2015. Morbidity and Mortality Weekly Report, 65, 1205-1211. (2016).

Kandel, E. R.; Kandel, D. B. (2014). A molecular basis for nicotine as a gateway drug. New England Journal of Medicine, 371(10), 932-943.

Klein, J. D. (2015). Electronic cigarettes are another route to nicotine addiction for youth. JAMA Pediatrics, 169(11), 993-994.

Knudsen, H. K.; Studts, J. L.; Boyd, S.; Roman, P. M. (2010). Structural and cultural barriers to the adoption of smoking cessation services in addiction treatment organizations. Journal of Addictive Diseases, 29(3), 294-305.

Kristman-Valente, A. N.; Hill, K. G.; Epstein, M.; Kosterman, R.; Bailey, J. A.; Steeger, C. M. et al. (2017). The relationship between marijuana and conventional cigarette smoking behavior from early adolescence to adulthood. Prevention Science, 18(4), 428-438.

Land, T.; Keithly, L.; Kane, K.; Chen, L.; Paskowsky, M.; Cullen, D. et al. (2014). Recent increases in efficiency in cigarette nicotine delivery: implications for tobacco control. Nicotine, Tobacco Research, 16(6), 753-758.

Lanza, S. T.; Vasilenko, S. A. (2015). New methods shed light on age of onset as a risk factor for nicotine dependence. Addictive Behaviors, 50, 161-164.

Lee, Y. O.; Hebert, C. J.; Nonnemaker, J. M.; Kim, A. E. (2015). Youth tobacco product use in the United States. Pediatrics, 135(3), 409-415.

Lemon, S. C.; Friedmann, P. D.; Stein, M. D. (2003). The impact of smoking cessation on drug abuse treatment outcome. Addictive Behaviors, 28(7), 1323-1331.

Mayer, B. (2014). How much nicotine kills a human? Tracing back the generally accepted lethal dose to dubious self-experiments in the nineteenth century. Archives of Toxicology, 88(1), 5-7.

McQuown, S. C.; Belluzzi, J. D.; Leslie, F. M. (2007). Low dose nicotine treatment during early adolescence increases subsequent cocaine reward. Neurotoxicology and Teratology, 29(1), 66-73.

Melroy-Greif, W. E.; Stitzel, J. A.; Ehringer, M. A. (2016). Nicotinic acetylcholine receptors: upregulation, age-related effects and associations with drug use. Genes, Brain, and Behavior, 15(1), 89-107.

Miech, R. A.; O'Malley, P. M.; Johnston, L. D.; Patrick, M. E. (2016). E-cigarettes and the drug use patterns of adolescents. Nicotine and Tobacco Research, 18(5), 654-659.

Palmer, R. H.; Young, S. E.; Hopfer, C. J.; Corley, R. P.; Stallings, M. C.; Crowley, T. J. et al. (2009). Developmental epidemiology of drug use and abuse in adolescence and young adulthood: evidence of generalized risk. Drug and Alcohol Dependence, 102(1-3), 78-87.

Prochaska, J. J.; Delucchi, K.; Hall, S. M. (2004). A meta-analysis of smoking cessation interventions with individuals in substance abuse treatment or recovery. Journal of Consulting and Clinical Psychology, 72 (6), 1144-1156.

Rabin, R. A.; George, T. P. (2015). A review of co-morbid tobacco and cannabis use disorders: possible mechanisms to explain high rates of co-use. American Journal on Addictions, 24(2), 105-116.

Richter, L.; Foster, S. E. (2013). The exclusion of nicotine: closing the gap in addiction policy and practice. American Journal of Public Health, 103, e14-e16.

Richter, L.; Pugh, B. S.; Ball, S. A. (2017). Assessing the risk of marijuana use disorder among adolescents and adults who use marijuana. American Journal of Drug and Alcohol Abuse, 43(3), 247-260.

Richter, L.; Pugh, B. S.; Peters, E.; Vaughan, R. D.; Foster, S. E. (2016). Underage drinking: prevalence and correlates of risky drinking measures among youth aged 12-20. American Journal of Drug and Alcohol Abuse, 42(4), 385-394.

Richter, L.; Pugh, B. S.; Smith, P. H.; Ball, S. A. (2017). The co-occurrence of nicotine and other substance use and addiction among youth and adults in the United States: implications for research, practice, and policy. American Journal of Drug and Alcohol Abuse, 43(2), 132-145.

Smith, R. F.; McDonald, C. G.; Bergstrom, H. C.; Ehlinger, D. G.; Brielmaier, J. M. (2015). Adolescent nicotine induces persisting changes in development of neural connectivity. Neuroscience and Biobehavioral Reviews, 55, 4 3 2-443.

Soneji, S.; Barrington-Trimis, J. L.; Wills, T. A.; Leventhal, A. M.; Unger, J. B.; Gibson, L. A. et al. (2017). Association between initial use of e-cigarettes and subsequent cigarette smoking among adolescents and young adults: a systematic review and metaanalysis. JAMA Pediatrics. https://doi. org/10. 1001/ jamapediatrics. 2017. 1488.

Substance Abuse and Mental Health Services Administration. (2015). Analysis of the National Survey on Drug Use and Health (NSDUH), 2014 [Public Use Files]. Retrieved from (2015). https://www.samhsa. gov/samhsa-data-outcomes-quality/major-datacollections/public-use-files-2014-nsduh/.

The National Center on Addiction and Substance Abuse. (2011). Adolescent substance use: America's #1 public health problem. New York: Author.

The National Center on Addiction and Substance Abuse. (2015). Understanding and addressing nicotine addiction: A science-based approach to policy and practice. New York: Author.

The National Center on Addiction and Substance Abuse. (2016). Beyond cigarettes: The risks of non-cigarette nicotine products and implications for tobacco control. New York: Author.

Tolu, S.; Marti, F.; Morel, C.; Perrier, C.; Torquet, N.; Pons, S. et al. (2017). Nicotine enhances alcohol intake and dopaminergic responses through β2* and β4* nicotinic acetylcholine receptors. Scientific Reports, 7, 4 5 1 1 6 . https://doi. org/10. 1038/ srep45116.

U. S. Department of Health and Human Services. (2016). E-cigarette use among youth and young adults: A report of the surgeon general. Atlanta, GA: Office on Smoking and Health.

Yuan, M.; Cross, S. J.; Loughlin, S. E.; Leslie, F. M. (2015). Nicotine and the adolescent brain. Journal of Physiology, 593(16), 3397-3412.

48
吸烟与赌博并存障碍：潜在机制及未来探索

Emma V. Ritchie, David C. Hodgins, Daniel S. McGrath

Department of Psychology, University of Calgary, Calgary, AB, Canada

缩略语

APA	美国精神病学协会	MAO	单胺氧化酶
AUD	酒精使用障碍	NRT	烟碱替代疗法
DGs	无序赌博/无序赌徒	SUD	物质使用障碍
DSM-5	《精神障碍诊断与统计手册》（第5版）	TUD	烟草使用障碍
GD	赌博障碍	VLT	视频彩票终端

48.1 引言

烟草使用的问题通常包括反复尝试戒烟失败、产生耐受性、戒烟症状、强烈的生理渴望；尽管烟草产品对健康、人际关系或个人安全有负面影响，但仍在继续使用（American Psychiatric Association, 2013）。这些是烟草使用障碍（TUD）的一些标准，在《精神障碍诊断与统计手册》第5版（DSM-5; APA, 2013）中，TUD被归类为物质使用障碍（SUD）。烟碱是烟草产品中含有的一种生物碱化学物质，已被确认为烟草的假定精神活性成分（Benowitz, 2008）。然而，基于证据的积累，确定了TUD中其他烟草成分的个体和协同作用（Baker et al. 2012; Fagerström, 2012），"烟草依赖"一词现已主要取代了文献中的"烟碱依赖"。烟草依赖通常不是单独发生的，而是与其他成瘾行为和精神健康障碍高度共存（Lasser et al. 2000）。不仅酒精使用障碍（AUD）与TUD有很强的关系（Falk et al. 2006），而且其他成瘾行为也经常与吸烟并存，包括赌博障碍（GD）（Lorains et al. 2011）。例如，最近的一项研究发现，与普通人群（约5%）相比，烟草依赖者的GD发病率（约14%）更高（Barnes et al. 2015）。事实上，最近的研究已经开始更专注于烟碱和烟草在维持GD和亚临床无序赌博（DG）中的作用。

最近赌博被重新归类为DSM-5中的一种成瘾行为（APA, 2013），赌博经常与其他成瘾行为同时存在，特别是烟草使用（McGrath, Barrett, 2009）。在对DG中常见的共发疾病的系统回顾中，Lorains等（2011）发现了许多心理疾病，如情绪障碍和SUD。然而，烟草使用的流行率最高，大约60%的DG者也符合TUD的标准。也有证据表明，吸烟的DG者可能代表着一种更严重的赌博病理形式。一项比较吸烟和不吸烟的DG者的研究发现，吸烟者表现出更严重的赌博症状，更可能有其他心理障碍，更可能寻求先前的治疗（Odlaug et al. 2013）（图48.1和图48.2）。

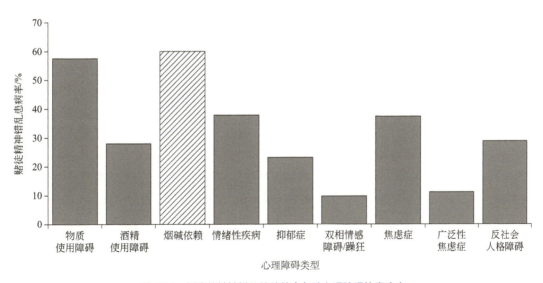

图 48.1 报告的精神错乱的赌徒中各种心理障碍的患病率

赌博障碍患者各种心理障碍的患病率（平均效应量）。数据来自Lorains等（2011）进行的荟萃分析。

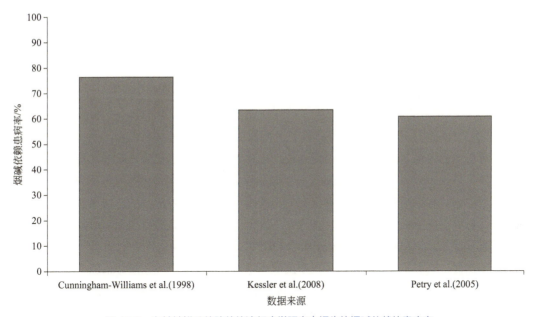

图 48.2 在精神错乱的赌徒的流行病学研究中报告的烟碱依赖的患病率

根据三项不同的研究，报告了精神错乱的赌徒样本中烟碱依赖的患病率。

48.2　吸烟和赌博共病的潜在机制

已经提出许多吸烟和赌博关系的潜在因素。例如，条件反射效应可能起到一定作用。当一个人在重复配对后学会将一种类型的刺激与另一种不同的刺激联系起来时，就会发生经典的条件反射。如果赌徒在赌博时吸烟，他们可能会将吸烟与赌博联系在一起（McGrath, Barrett, 2009）。从本质上讲，这两种行为都可以作为另一种行为的条件性提示，吸烟行为可能会引发赌博欲望，反之亦然。这种被称为交叉提示反应的现象，已经被经验证明至少部分解释了TUD和AUD的关系（如Piasecki et al. 2011），但直到最近才有与赌博和吸烟有关的研究（Wulfert et al. 2016）。

另一项研究集中在吸烟的赌徒和不吸烟的赌徒之间存在性格差异的可能性。衡量赌博严重程度的研究发现，吸烟的DG者在这些指标上得分更高（Grant et al. 2008; McGrath et al. 2012）。吸烟的DG者还倾向于表现出更多的精神症状（焦虑、抑郁和自杀倾向增加），并且更有可能患有另一种SUD（Grant et al. 2008; Pry, Oncken, 2002; Potenza et al. 2004）。此外，最近的一项研究报告称，吸烟的DGs在被称为负面紧迫感的冲动方面得分更高，即一个人在面对负面情绪或情况时会做出冲动的反应（Boothby et al. 2017）。其他人则提出，吸烟的DG者这样做可能是为了抑制他们的冲动，因为烟碱可以增强他们的认知能力（Mooney et al. 2011）。最后，吸烟者和DG者的神经质得分都较高，而责任心得分较低（Bagby et al. 2007; Terracciano, Costa Jr., 2004），尽管吸烟的DG者的人格维度得到的经验关注相对较少。

此外，烟草烟雾中的某些成分已被证明能抑制单胺氧化酶（MAO），单胺氧化酶是一种与抑郁有关的酶（Lewis et al. 2007）。有观点认为，一些人将吸烟作为一种自我治疗抑郁的方式（Benowitz, 2008）。有证据表明，DG者中血小板MAO活性也被耗尽，这与低MAO活性对5-羟色胺能系统的影响导致的冲动控制降低有关（Carrasco et al. 1994）。MAO抑制剂也被用来改善边缘型人格障碍患者的自我控制问题；DG者也有可能出现类似的过程（即他们吸烟是为了应对自己的冲动）（Carrasco et al. 1994）。

48.3 烟碱/烟草对强化行为的影响

来自动物和人类的研究结果表明，除了主要的强化作用和条件性强化特性（如吸烟提示）外，烟碱对其他行为也有强化作用。也就是说，急性服用烟碱可以增强与吸烟本身没有直接关系的奖励（参见Perkins et al. 2017）。重要的是，这些强化作用是通过将药物与可预测奖励的刺激直接配对而产生的。对这些作用的实证研究首先是在啮齿动物模型中进行的，结果显示，偶然和非偶然烟碱注射都可以增强对初级奖励（如食物）的反应；然而，这些作用似乎对视觉奖励（如视觉光和听觉音调）尤其强烈（Rupprecht et al. 2015）。烟碱增强强化作用的确切神经生物学机制尚未建立。然而，人们早就知道烟碱通过中皮质边缘通路分泌多巴胺在烟草依赖中起着关键作用（Balfour, 2015）。一些证据表明，给予选择性D_3受体拮抗剂可以特异性地增强强化作用，但不会促进烟碱的进一步自给药（Paterson, 2009）（表48.1）。

一项针对人类受试者的规模较小的研究揭示了吸烟者体内类似的烟碱强化作用。研究发现，通过卷烟急性吸食烟碱可以提高奖励视觉刺激的评级，如漂亮面孔的图片（Attwood et al. 2009; Attwood et al. 2012）。另一项研究集中在奖励形式和给药途径上。在一系列研究中，Perkins和Karelitz评估了烟碱对增强实验室操作任务表现的影响。总的来说，他们发现烟碱增强了感官奖励的强化价值，如音乐（Perkins, Karelitz, 2013a; Perkins, Karelitz, 2013b; Perkins et al. 2013）和视频（Perkins et al. 2015; Perkins, Karelitz, 2016），但不能强化金钱。与烟碱替代疗法（NRT）等纯烟碱形式相比，烟碱通过卷烟递送时，这些作用更为一致。然而，另一个研究小组的一项研究发现，急性NRT增强了由金钱强化的卡片分类任务的表现（Dawkins et al. 2009）。这些发现支持烟碱对人类感官奖励的强化作用，并可能对金钱奖励产生类似的影响。

表48.1 烟碱对人体强化作用的实验室研究摘要

参考文献	烟碱给药方法	奖励类型	结果
Attwood, Penton-Voak, Munafò (2009)	烟碱卷烟（0.60mg烟碱）与去烟碱卷烟（0.005mg烟碱）	面孔照片	吸食烟碱卷烟的参与者对吸引力的评分明显更高
Attwood, Penton-Voak, Goodwin, Munafò (2012)	烟碱卷烟（0.6mg烟碱）与去烟碱卷烟（0.005mg烟碱），在摄入酒精饮料（0.4g/kg）或安慰剂后给药	面孔和自然风光的照片	在吸食烟碱卷烟的参与者中，无论是否饮酒，他们对这两种类型照片的吸引力评分都较高；接受酒精和烟碱卷烟的参与者的吸引力评分最高
Dawkins, Powell, Pickering, Powell, West (2009)	含片（4mg烟碱）与安慰剂含片	卡片分类任务中的金钱奖励	只有重度吸烟者在含片条件下才能加强对较高任务的反应
Perkins, Karelitz (2013a)	隔夜戒断后，半支烟碱卷烟（8口）与全烟碱卷烟（16口）	音乐（偏好程度不同）和无奖励（控制）	吸食全烟碱卷烟后，增强了对高偏好音乐奖励的反应
Perkins, Karelitz (2013b)	烟碱卷烟（0.6mg烟碱）与去烟碱卷烟（<0.05mg烟碱）	金钱、音乐、停止吵闹和无奖励（控制）	吸食烟碱卷烟后，只有对音乐奖励的强化反应才会增强
Perkins, Karelitz (2014)	隔夜戒断后，烟碱卷烟（0.6mg烟碱）与去烟碱卷烟（<0.05mg烟碱）	音乐、视频、金钱和无奖励（控制）	吸食烟碱卷烟后，增强了对音乐和视频奖励的反应；吸食去烟碱卷烟与不吸烟没有区别
Perkins, Karelitz, Michael (2015)	隔夜戒断后，含有烟碱（36mg烟碱）或安慰剂（0mg烟碱）的电子烟	音乐、视频、金钱和无奖励（控制）	只有在使用含有烟碱的电子烟后，才能增强对视频奖励的反应
Perkins, Karelitz (2016)	通宵戒断与他们选择的烟碱卷烟（每次试验前抽6口烟）	音乐、视频和无奖励（控制）	吸食烟碱卷烟后，对音乐和视频奖励的反应增强；男性对视频奖励的反应更强，而女性对音乐奖励的反应更强

注：该表总结了烟碱如何增强对人类不同感官和非感官奖励的反应。

48.4 烟碱/烟草对冒险行为的影响

一项适度的研究探索了烟碱对实验室冒险任务的影响。例如，Pilarski等（2014）研究了烟碱对不吸烟者冒险行为的影响。实验任务包括手指敲击、气球模拟风险任务和红绿灯任务。将不同剂量的烟碱口香糖（2mg和4mg）与安慰剂进行了比较。与预测相反，与安慰剂相比，烟碱（4mg）实际上降低了气球模拟风险任务的风险承担。同样，接受烟碱的男性在红绿灯任务中的冒险意愿也有所下降。他们最初的假设是基于一些研究，这些研究表明烟碱对多巴胺能系统的影响应该会增加冒险行为（Sevy et al. 2006）。研究人员推测，这些相反的发现可能是由于样本中参与者的特定任务需求（如任务相关性）和个体差异（如个性）的结合。

48.5 烟碱/烟草对赌博的影响

很少有实验室研究致力于研究烟碱如何具体影响赌博。这有点令人惊讶，因为赌博提供了一个真实世界的例子，说明了与吸烟同时发生的强化行为。赌博包含感官刺激、金钱强化和冒险的因素，在之前的烟碱药物挑战实验中，每一项都被单独研究过。在一项研究中，McGrath等（2012）使用吸入器给每天吸烟的普通视频彩票终端（VLT）赌徒服用烟碱或安慰剂。他们没有发现烟碱和安慰剂在赌博欲望、赌博乐趣或赌博行为（如下注次数和每次下注金额）方面有任何不同。在一项后续研究中，McGrath等（2013）提供了烟碱和安慰剂含片，以评估烟碱对赌博欲望和吸烟的风险/紊乱赌徒行为的影响。同样，烟碱和安慰剂在赌博方面没有发现差异（表48.2）。

表48.2 烟碱对赌博和冒险任务的影响

参考文献	烟碱给药方法	任务	结果
Barrett, Collins, Stewart (2015)	烟碱卷烟（0.6mg烟碱）与去烟碱卷烟（0.05mg烟碱），这两种卷烟是在摄入酒精饮料或安慰剂后使用的	在一个旋转卷轴VLT上玩价值40美元的游戏；玩家想玩多久就玩多久（最多15min）或直到没有积分	吸食烟碱卷烟会导致更高的平均赌注；摄入酒精会增加赌博的欲望
McGrath, Barrett, Stewart, Schmid (2012)	隔夜戒烟后烟碱吸入剂（10mg烟碱）与安慰剂吸入器	在一个旋转卷轴VLT上玩价值60美元的游戏；玩家想玩多久就玩多久（最多30min）或直到没有积分	烟碱和安慰剂在赌博行为的任何衡量标准（如花费的金钱、平均赌注规模和每分钟的赌注）或赌博欲望方面没有显著差异
McGrath et al. (2013)	隔夜戒烟后烟碱含片（4mg烟碱）与安慰剂（薄荷糖）	选择在VLT上押注10美元，或将这笔钱加到他们的补偿金中	烟碱对赌博或保留金钱的决定没有影响；烟碱和安慰剂在赌博欲望方面也没有显著差异
Pilarski et al. (2014)	烟碱口香糖（2mg和4mg）与安慰剂口香糖	气球模拟风险任务	与4mg烟碱组相比，安慰剂组的冒险得分更高

注：该表总结了在受控实验室环境中烟碱对赌博行为和嗜好的影响，以及冒险任务的研究。

重要的是，上述研究通过NRT（吸入器和含片）而不是烟草卷烟进行烟碱递送。为了考察吸烟产生的烟碱可能对赌博有独特影响的可能性，Barrett等（2015）在一项VLT的研究中，向赌徒提供了烟碱卷烟、去烟碱卷烟以及酒精和安慰剂饮料。当参与者吸一支烟碱卷烟时，平均每个赌注花费的钱比他们吸一支去烟碱卷烟时要多。这一发现表明，通过烟草烟雾吸入烟碱确实对赌博行为的至少一个方面有可测量的影响。

因此，烟草烟雾中的烟碱可能具有独特和可区分的影响，吸烟和赌博的频繁并存与吸烟有关，而不是烟碱本身。这一领域的研究结果基本上是无效的，这可能是因为吸烟和赌博之间存在一种特殊的关系，而不仅仅是单独的烟碱。虽然烟碱是烟草中的主要化学物质，但吸烟还有其他明显的特征导致了它的成瘾特性。例如，吸烟被认为能将烟碱推注到大脑，而且比其他给药方法更有效（Benowitz et al. 2009）。给药后不久就会迅速产生生理效应的药物往往更容易成瘾（Samaha, Robinson, 2005）。同样，当一种奖励刺激（如吸烟的愉悦效果）在吸入后迅速呈现时，这种行为更有可能得到强化（Perkins, Karelitz, 2013b）。吸烟对烟碱的控制作用更强，这可能与烟碱对赌博等其他奖励行为的影响有直接关系。

48.6 赌博行为对烟草使用的潜在影响

虽然烟草依赖和GD明显相关，但这些障碍的时间顺序仍然不清楚。很少有人注意到赌博可能对吸烟本身起到的作用。最近，Bussu和Detotto（2015）研究了赌博和包括烟草在内的几种SUDs之间是否存在双向关系。他们在赌博场所调查了700多名赌徒，调查他们在赌博时是否饮酒、吸烟或使用其他药物，以及他们花了多少钱来赌博。有趣的是，他们没有发现赌博和烟草使用之间存在双向关系的证据；然而，更多地参与赌博似乎确实增加了个人吸烟的可能性。

最近的一项实验室研究调查了吸烟和赌博之间的交叉线索反应（Wulfert et al. 2016）。交叉线索反应描述了一种与成瘾相关的刺激的条件性线索如何引发对它经常与之配对的第二种成瘾行为的反应（如渴望）。研究人员招募了吸烟的扑克玩家、不吸烟的扑克玩家和不赌博的吸烟者。参与者暴露环境：一个装有一副纸牌的托盘（赌博提示），一个装有卷烟和打火机的托盘（吸烟提示），以及一支铅笔和一块橡皮（中性提示）。多次测量主观渴望评分和皮肤电导率。吸烟和赌博增加了吸烟的扑克牌玩家的烟草欲望，而不是纯粹的吸烟者或赌徒。有趣的是，没有发现交叉线索反应是赌欲的原因。

目前还没有研究直接评估赌博对烟碱实际自给药的影响。然而，饮酒文献中的研究表明，酒精增强了吸烟的愉悦效果，比吸烟更能增强饮酒的愉悦效果（如 Piasecki et al. 2011）。这是赌博研究领域唯一已知的关于这一主题的基于实验室的实验，Stewart 等（2002）随机分配了社区招募的 VLT 玩家（没有 AUD 的普通赌徒）进行 90min 的 VLT 游戏或观看电影（对照任务）；每个人之后都有机会用自己的钱购买酒精或非酒精饮料。对参与者可以购买的酒精饮料的数量设定了上限，以确保血液中的酒精浓度（BAC）低于 0.08%。正如预测的那样，VLT 状态下的人（15 人中的 11 人）比电影状态下（15 人中的 6 人）购买至少一种酒精饮料的人要多得多。8 名参与者达到了 BAC 的上限，无法购买任何额外的酒精饮料。这些发现表明，接触赌博会增加饮酒的可能性。可以想象，烟草管理部门也会观察到类似的模式；然而，这种可能性还没有得到经验上的探索。

48.7 需要进一步探索的领域

总而言之，吸烟和赌博的同时发生和维持仍然是一个复杂的现象，这种关系可能涉及一些潜在机制。虽然有一些证据支持烟碱对赌博行为的强化作用（如在 VLT 上的平均赌注规模），但这些影响的程度尚不确定。吸烟而不是烟碱本身导致了赌博欲望和行为，这似乎是合理的，但需要对吸烟如何影响赌博进行更多的研究。赌博结果对吸烟行为的可能影响目前正受到适度的实证关注。这种联系的方向性还远不清楚，而且共同的跨诊断对这种关系的贡献还没有具体确定。

展望未来，我们可以设想几项实验室研究，这些研究将有助于进一步阐明吸烟与赌博之间的联系。例如，大多数研究在很大程度上忽略了吸烟的娱乐性赌徒。根据研究酒精和烟草共同使用的文献，吸烟在酒精的影响下会增加，许多"社交吸烟"的人只有在酒精的影响下才会这样（McKee et al. 2004）。吸烟和娱乐性赌博之间可能存在类似的关系。另一个值得研究的领域是戒烟对赌博行为的影响，特别是纵向影响。大多数 NRT 产品都是为长时间（如数周）使用而设计的，而大多数药物挑战研究都将这些产品用于急性给药。此外，未来的研究还可以进一步研究 DGs 人群吸烟的潜在动机，因为几乎没有专门针对这一点的研究。之前的研究表明，一些 DG 者发现吸烟鼓励他们赌博，而另一些 DG 者则在试图戒赌时发现吸烟可以安抚他们。更多地了解这一群体中吸烟的动机可能会有所帮助。最后，虽然 Bussu 和 Detotto（2015）提出赌博直接影响吸烟，但没有受控的实验室研究评估不同的赌博结果（如大赢家游戏与伪装成输的胜利游戏）是否直接影响吸烟行为（表 48.3）。

表48.3　吸烟与赌博并存的关键事实

- 烟草依赖是患有另一种心理障碍的人最常见的共病之一
- 现在或过去有心理障碍的人的烟草依赖率几乎是从未被诊断出有心理障碍的人的两倍
- 据估计，赌博障碍（GD）患者的烟草依赖率在40%～60%之间
- 研究指出，烟草依赖是与GD并存的最频繁或第二频繁的成瘾
- GD最初被归类为冲动控制障碍，但最近由于研究表明，GD与物质成瘾更相似，这一点被改变了
- 在赌场吸烟曾经是一种常见的做法，直到人们对二手烟影响的担忧变得更加突出。许多赌场现在都禁止吸烟，这一禁令对博彩收入和顾客行为的影响引起了人们的极大关注

注：该表列出了烟草依赖和赌博障碍的一些关键事实，包括共病率和事实，以及每种情况的关键事实。GD，赌博障碍。

术语解释

- **双向关系**：在这一章中，这指的是吸烟和赌博之间的潜在关系，在这种关系中，吸烟和赌博都会对对方产生某种影响，即赌博鼓励人们进一步使用烟草，反之亦然。
- **经典条件反射**：无意识学习的一种类型，在两种刺激反复配对后，个体学会将一种类型的刺激与另一种不同的刺激联系起来。
- **伴随疾病**：在心理学上，这是指一个人同时经历至少两种不同的心理障碍；在本章中，它主要指个体同时患有赌博障碍和烟草使用障碍。
- **条件性强化**：这也被称为二次强化，指的是在行为之后出现的对刺激的习得性反应，以鼓励未来的行为实例。
- **交叉提示反应**：一种心理现象，其中与一种成瘾行为（如吸烟）有关的刺激引起对另一种成瘾（如赌博）的可测量的反应（如渴望），因为两者经常同时出现（如赌博时吸烟）。
- **赌博障碍**：一种行为成瘾，即一个人难以控制自己的赌博行为，当他们不能赌博时会出现戒断症状，即使反复尝试也不能戒赌，并在经济或个人受到伤害的情况下继续赌博。
- **冲动性**：一种与无序赌博和吸烟有关的心理学概念。冲动的特征是不考虑自己行为的后果而行事，也不能控制自己的行为，从而导致鲁莽或不恰当的行为。
- **主要强化**：这指的是一个自然的（非习得的）过程，在这个过程中，行为的未来实例会受到行为之后呈现的刺激的鼓励。烟碱被认为是一种主要的增强剂，因为烟碱的生理效应可以是令人愉悦的、有益的，并鼓励未来使用烟碱。
- **强化**：一种学习方式，在一种行为之后提供刺激，以鼓励该行为在未来再次发生。
- **强化增强效果**：这指的是烟碱的一种独特特性，它可以加强与吸烟无关的奖励刺激。

要点总结

- 本章重点讨论吸烟和赌博的共病，特别是有赌博障碍的人。
- 虽然许多研究已经注意到吸烟和赌博是高度共生的，但人们对为什么会发生这种情况知之甚少。
- 已经提出了一些潜在的机制来解释这种关系，包括经典条件反射的影响、潜在的心理或倾向特征，以及烟草烟雾成分对抑郁和冲动等不良心理状态的影响。
- 烟碱通过三种截然不同的方式影响强化。它是一种主要的条件性增强剂，它还能增强与吸烟和烟碱本身无关的奖励刺激的强化。
- 关于烟碱如何具体影响赌博的研究很少，尽管目前为数不多的研究表明，影响赌博行为的是吸烟，而不是烟碱本身。
- 还必须考虑赌博对吸烟行为的影响。最近的两项研究表明，赌博可能会鼓励吸烟，要么是因为赌博引发了欲望，要么是因为赌博增强了与吸烟相关的愉悦效果。
- 这仍然是一个将在未来的研究中取得丰硕成果的话题，我们已经概述了几个有助于这一领域的文献的想法。

参考文献

American Psychiatric Association. (2013). Diagnostic and statistical manual of mental disorders (5th ed.). Washington, DC: Author. Attwood, A. S.; Penton-Voak, I. S.; Goodwin, C.; Munafò, M. R. (2012). Effects of acute nicotine and alcohol on the rating of attractiveness in social smokers and alcohol drinkers. Drug and Alcohol Dependence, 125(1-2), 43-48.

Attwood, A. S.; Penton-Voak, I. S.; Munafò, M. R. (2009). Effects of acute nicotine administration on ratings of attractiveness of facial cues. Nicotine and Tobacco Research, 11(1), 44-48.

Bagby, R. M.; Vachon, D. D.; Bulmash, E. L.; Toneatto, T.; Quilty, L. C.; Costa, P. T. (2007). Pathological gambling and the five-factor model of personality. Personality and Individual Differences, 43(4), 873-880.

Baker, T. B.; Breslau, N.; Covey, L.; Shiffman, S. (2012). DSM criteria for tobacco use disorder and tobacco withdrawal: a critique and proposed revisions for DSM-5. Addiction, 107(2), 263-275.

Balfour, D. J. K. (2015). The role of mesoaccumbens dopamine in nicotine dependence. D. Balfour, M. Munafó (Eds.), Current topics in behavioural neurosciences (pp. 55-98). The neuropharmacology of nicotine dependence: Vol. 24(pp. 55-98). Basel, Switzerland: Springer International Publishing.

Barnes, G. M.; Welte, J. W.; Tidwell, M. O.; Hoffman, J. H. (2015). Gambling and substance use: co-occurrence among adults in a recent general population study in the United States. International Gambling Studies, 15(1), 55-71.

Barrett, S. P.; Collins, P.; Stewart, S. H. (2015). The acute effects of tobacco smoking and alcohol consumption on video-lottery terminal gambling. Pharmacology, Biochemistry, and Behaviour, 130, 34-39.

Benowitz, N. L. (2008). Clinical pharmacology of nicotine: Implications for understanding, preventing, and treating tobacco addiction. Clinical Pharmacology and Therapeutics, 83(4), 531-541.

Benowitz, N. L.; Hukkanen, J.; Jacob, P.; III (2009). Nicotine chemistry, metabolism, kinetics, and biomarkers. In J. E. Henningfield et al. (Ed.) Handbook of experimental pharmacology (pp. 29-60). Berlin: SpringerVerlag.

Boothby, C. A.; Kim, H. S.; Romanow, N. K.; Hodgins, D. C.; McGrath, D. S. (2017). Assessing the role of impulsivity in smoking and non-smoking disordered gamblers. Addictive Behaviours, 70, 35-41.

Bussu, A.; Detotto, C. (2015). The bidirectional relationship between gambling and addictive substances. International Gambling Studies, 15(2), 285-308.

Carrasco, J. L.; Sáiz-Ruiz, J.; Hollander, E.; César, J.; López-Ibor, J. J. (1994). Low platelet monoamine oxidase activity in pathological gambling. Acta Psychiatrica Scandinavica, 90(6), 427-431.

Dawkins, L.; Powell, J. H.; Pickering, A.; Powell, J.; West, R. (2009). Patterns of change in withdrawal symptoms, desire to smoke, reward motivation and response inhibition across 3 months of smoking abstinence. Addiction, 104(5), 850-858.

Fagerström, K. (2012). Determinants of tobacco use and renamed the FTND to the Fagerstrom test for cigarette dependence. Nicotine and Tobacco Research, 14(1), 75-78.

Falk, D. E.; Yi, H.; Hiller-Sturmhöfel, S. (2006). An epidemiologic analysis of co-occurring alcohol and tobacco use and disorders: findings from the National Epidemiologic Survey on alcohol and related conditions. Alcohol Research and Health, 29(3), 162-171.

Grant, J. E.; Kim, S. W.; Odlaug, B. L.; Potenza, M. N. (2008). Daily tobacco smoking in treatment-seeking pathological gamblers: clinical correlates and co-occurring psychiatric disorders. Journal of Addiction Medicine, 2(4), 178-184.

Kessler, R. C.; Hwang, I.; LaBrie, R.; Petukhova, M.; Sampson, N. A.; Winters, K. C. et al. (2008). DSM-IV pathological gambling in the National Comorbidity Survey Replication. Psychological Medicine, 38, 1351-1360.

Lasser, K.; Boyd, J. W.; Woolhandler, S. (2000). Smoking and mental illness: a population based prevalence study. Journal of the American Medical Association, 284(20), 2606-2610.

Lewis, A.; Miller, J. H.; Lea, R. A. (2007). Monoamine oxidase and tobacco dependence. NeuroToxciology, 28(1), 182-195.

Lorains, F. K.; Cowlishaw, S.; Thomas, S. A. (2011). Prevalence of comorbid disorders in problem and pathological gambling: systematic review and meta-analysis of population surveys. Addiction, 106, 490-498.

McGrath, D. S.; Barrett, S. P. (2009). The comorbidity of tobacco smoking and gambling: a review of the literature. Drug and Alcohol Review, 28(6), 676-681.

McGrath, D. S.; Barrett, S. P.; Stewart, S. H.; McGrath, P. R. (2012). A comparison of gambling behaviour, problem gambling indices, and reasons for gambling among smokers and nonsmokers who gamble: evidence from a provincial gambling prevalence study. Nicotine and Tobacco Research, 14(7), 833-839.

McGrath, D. S.; Barrett, S. P.; Stewart, S. H.; Schmid, E. A. (2012). The effects of acute doses of nicotine on video lottery terminal gambling in daily smokers. Psychopharmacology, 220, 155-161.

McGrath, D. S.; Dorbeck, A.; Barrett, S. P. (2013). The influence of acutely administered nicotine on cue-induced cravings for gambling in at-risk video lottery terminal gamblers who smoke. Behavioural Pharmcology, 24(2), 124-132.

McKee, S. A.; Hinson, R.; Rounsaville, D.; Petrelli, P. (2004). Survey of subjective effects of smoking while drinking among college students. Nicotine and Tobacco Research, 6(1), 111-117.

Mooney, M. E.; Odlaug, B. L.; Kim, S. W.; Grant, J. E. (2011). Cigarette smoking status in pathological gamblers: association with impulsivity and cognitive flexibility. Drug and Alcohol Dependence, 117(1), 74-77.

Odlaug, B. L.; Stinchfield, R.; Golberstein, E.; Grant, J. E. (2013). The relationship of tobacco use with gambling problem severity and gambling treatment outcome. Psychology of Addictive Behaviours, 27 (3).

Paterson, N. E. (2009). The neuropharmacological substrates of nicotine reward: reinforcing versus reinforcement-enhancing effects of nicotine.

Behavioral Pharmacology, 20(3), 211-225.

Perkins, K. A.; Karelitz, J. L. (2013a). Influence of reinforcer magnitude and nicotine amount on smoking's acute reinforcement enhancing effects. Drug and Alcohol Dependence, 133(1), 167-171.

Perkins, K. A.; Karelitz, J. L. (2013b). Reinforcement enhancing effects of nicotine via smoking. Psychopharmacology, 228(3), 479-486.

Perkins, K. A.; Karelitz, J. L. (2014). Sensory reinforcement-enhancing effects of nicotine via smoking. Experimental and Clinical Psychopharmacology, 22(6), 511-516.

Perkins, K. A.; Karelitz, J. L. (2016). Potential sex differences in the pattern of sensory reinforcers enhanced by nicotine. Experimental and Clinical Psychopharmacology, 24(3), 156-161.

Perkins, K. A.; Karelitz, J. L.; Boldry, M. C. (2017). Nicotine acutely enhances reinforcement from non-drug rewards in humans. Frontiers in Psychiatry. 8(65).

Perkins, K. A.; Karelitz, J. L.; Jao, N. C.; Stratton, E. (2013). Possible reinforcement enhancing effects of burpropion during initial smoking abstinence. Nicotine and Tobacco Research, 15, 1141-1145.

Perkins, K. A.; Karelitz, J. L.; Michael, V. C. (2015). Reinforcement enhancing effects of acute nicotine via electronic cigarettes. Drug and Alcohol Dependence, 153, 104-108.

Petry, N. M.; Oncken, C. (2002). Cigarette smoking is associated with increased severity of gambling problems in treatment-seeking gamblers. Addiction, 97(6), 745-753.

Petry, N. M.; Stinson, F. S.; Grant, B. F. (2005). Comorbidity of DSM-IV pathological gambling and other psychiatric disorders: results from the National Epidemiologic Survey on alcohol and related conditions. The Journal of Clinical Psychiatry, 66(5), 564-574.

Piasecki, T. M.; Jahng, S.; Wood, P. K.; Robertson, B. M.; Epler, A. J.; Cronk, N. J. et al. (2011). The subjective effects of alcohol-tobacco co-use: an ecological momentary assessment investigation. Journal of Abnormal Psychology, 120(3), 557-571.

Pilarski, C. R.; Skeel, R. L.; Reilly, M. P. (2014). Acute effects of nicotine on risky choice among non-smokers. The Psychological Record, 64, 151-159.

Potenza, M. N.; Steinberg, M. A.; McLaughlin, S. D.; Wu, R.; Rounsaville, B. J.; Krishnan-Sarin, S. et al. (2004). Characteristics of tobacco-smoking problem gamblers calling a gambling helpline. The American Journal on Addictions, 13(5), 471-493.

Rupprecht, L. E.; Smith, T. T.; Schassburger, R. L.; Buffalari, D. M.; Sved, A. F.; Donny, E. C. (2015). Behavioural mechanisms underlying nicotine reinforcement. In: D. Balfour, M. Munafó (Eds.), Current topics in behavioural neurosciences (pp. 19-53). The neuropharmacology of nicotine dependence: Vol. 24(pp. 19-53). Basel, Switzerland: Springer International Publishing.

Samaha, A.; Robinson, T. E. (2005). Why does the rapid delivery of drugs to the brain promote addiction?TREND in Pharmacological Sciences, 26(2), 82-87.

Sevy, S.; Hassoun, Y.; Bechara, A.; Yechiam, E.; Napolitano, B.; Burdick, K. et al. (2006). Emotion-based decision-making in healthy subjects: shortterm effects of reducing dopamine levels. Psychopharmacology, 188(2), 228-235.

Stewart, S. H.; McWilliams, L. A.; Blackburn, J. R.; Klein, R. M. (2002). A laboratory-based investigation of relations among video lottery terminal (VLT) play, negative mood, and alcohol consumption in regular VLT players. Addictive Behaviours, 27(5), 819-835.

Terracciano, A.; Costa, P. T.; Jr. (2004). Smoking and the five-factor model of personality. Addiction, 99(4), 472-481.

Wulfert, E.; Harris, K.; Broussard, J. (2016). The role of cross-cue reactivity in coexisting smoking and gambling habits. Journal of Gambling Issues, 32, 2 8-43.

49

烟草和强效可卡因使用的神经科学：新陈代谢、效果和症状学

Antonio Gomes de Castro-Neto[1], *Rossana Carla Rameh-de-Albuquerque*[2], *Pollyanna Fausta Pimentel de Medeiros*[1], *Roberta Uchôa*[3], *Beate Saegesser Santos*[1]

1. Study Group on Alcohol and other Drugs, Research Group on Biomedical Nanotechnology, Department of Pharmaceutical Sciences, Federal University of Pernambuco, Cidade Universitária, Recife, Pernambuco, Brazil
2. Study Group on Alcohol and other Drugs, Federal Institute of Education, Science and Technology of Pernambuco, Cidade Universitária, Recife, Pernambuco, Brazil
3. Department of Social Work, Federal University of Pernambuco, Economistas Avenue, Cidade Universitária, Recife, Pernambuco, Brazil

缩略语

ACTH	促肾上腺皮质激素	**LTSP**	长时程突触增强
ADHD	注意缺陷多动障碍	**MDU**	多药使用
AEME	脱水芽子碱甲酯	**mGluR2/3**	第二组代谢型谷氨酸受体
CHT	突触前高亲和力胆碱转运体	**nAChR**	烟碱乙酰胆碱受体
CPP	条件性位置偏好	**SAHA**	辛二酰苯胺异羟肟酸
DHEA	脱氢表雄（甾）酮	**US**	美国
HDAC	组蛋白去乙酰化酶	**VTA**	腹侧被盖区
KO	敲除大鼠	**WT**	野生型大鼠
LH	黄体化激素		

49.1 引言

尽管20世纪60年代末的科学报告指出了烟草（或卷烟）的有益使用，但如今众所周知，这种习惯是极其有害的。关于烟碱的事情已经确立，但烟草仍然是世界上消费最多的药物之一，具有重要的强化因素：有价值的市场（及其利润）和与其使用模式相关的许多文化方面（Pinto et al. 2017; Reitsma et al. 2017）。

另一方面，吸食强效可卡因现在是世界各地一种确定的药物滥用形式。目前，巴西是这种可卡因的最大使用者，据观察，大多数强效可卡因使用者将这种药物与烟草结合使用。

烟草和可卡因（不同形式）的结合实际上是由世界各地的使用者以不同的方式进行的。南美的一些研究报告了吸食古柯膏、烟草或大麻制成的一种名为 Pitillos 或 Papilloes 的卷烟的药物 Basuco（Jeri, 1980; Siegel, 1982）。虽然这种习惯是一个严重的健康问题，但仍只有少数定量和定性研究描述了使用者在联合使用烟草和强效可卡因时的经历，并试图理解其原因（Gonçalves, Nappo, 2015）。

在位于巴西东北部海岸的累西腓（Recife），crack 可卡因与烟草结合被称为 capeta，与大麻结合被称为中 mesclado 或 melado（图 49.1）。

使用者报告说，这些组合减少了人们的渴望，尤其是对大麻的渴望。capeta 使用者表示，与不使用 crack 可卡因的人相比，他们对 crack 可卡因的使用有更多的控制权，尽管这种控制的强度因使用者而异。以下以使用者上报的部分数据为例：

除了生物力学上的相似性，使用块状海洛因，有必要将烟灰插入管道底部或锡罐来进行燃烧。换句话说，……使用烟草吸食强效可卡因势在必行（Zeni, Araujo, 2011, p. 32）。

所有的可卡因使用者都一致认为：燃烧块状海洛因后残留在管道中的灰烬非常有价值，并被认为比块状海洛因本身具有更大的能量（Alves, 2016, p.5）。

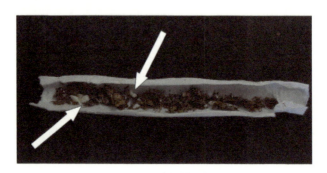

图 49.1　卡佩塔卷烟

手工制作的烟草卷烟和强效可卡因。白色箭头表示一些块状海洛因。

已经观察到，强效可卡因与烟草之间的联系是一种优先使用模式。然而，许多使用者称，他们只使用烟草灰来缓解燃烧过程：

……这样，卷烟混在块状海洛因中是不可避免的，并且人们也乐于产生了新的烟灰。并非所有人都吸烟，因为许多可卡因使用者都不吸烟。为此，卷烟被点燃，然后保持垂直燃烧，以在不吸入烟雾的情况下获得烟灰……（Alves, 2016, p.5）。

在同时使用烟草和强效可卡因时，必须提到的其他重要特征是它们的兴奋剂作用和消费方式的相似性。吸烟的烟斗 "boris" 与吸食强效可卡因的烟斗非常相似，尤其是它们的曲线形式（Jorge, Quindere, Yasui, Albuquerque, 2013）。换句话说，它们的行为方向带来了协同作用的对应关系，促进了同时使用：

卷烟对禁止吸食可卡因至关重要。这是通过 "卷烟者" 社会观察到的，他们负责在吸毒现场向可卡因使用者提供卷烟，分包装或单位销售，甚至用烟灰销售……（Alves, 2016, p. 9）。

此外，当单独使用烟草时，它会作为刺激 crack 可卡因使用的触发器。然而，当烟草与 crack 可卡因同时使用时，这种渴望就会减弱。失控是 crack 可卡因使用者最常见的问题之一；因此，应进一步研究使用烟草或大麻结合强效可卡因作为控制减少危害的策略（Acioli Neto, 2014）。

49.2　烟草作为门户

一些作者认为吸烟是通往其他毒品的门户，如大麻、可卡因和 crack 可卡因。然而，目前尚不清楚烟草的活性物质烟碱是如何促进门户机制的。门户理论是由 Kandel（1975）在观察到年轻人按阶段和顺序吸毒时提出的。她指出，在美国和其他西方社会的普通人群中，有一个明确的发展性毒品使用顺序，从合法的毒品开始，然后再发展到非法的毒品（图 49.2）。具体地说，烟草和酒精的使用导致使用大麻仅次于可卡因，然后导致使用其他非法药物（Degenhardt et al. 2010; Kandel, 2002; Kandel, Yamaguchi, Chen, 1992; Wagner, Anthony, 2002）。

除了门户理论，MDU是基于常见药物使用敏感性的概念。这意味着，使用一种以上的药物会增加发展为MDU的风险（Palmer et al., 2009; Vanyukov et al. 2012）。

流行病学和生物学研究结合表明了一个模型，即烟碱通过抑制纹状体中的HDAC对可卡因起初始作用。这种抑制诱导了伏隔核中组蛋白乙酰化的一般变化，已知在使用可卡因时，不同 *FosB* 基因的转录变化，这表明烟碱在响应可卡因时增加了 *FosB* 的转录（Kandel, Kandel, 2014; Levine et al. 2011）。这些因素创造了一个诱导基因表达的环境。当长期接触烟碱后再使用可卡因时，伏隔核的长时程增强就会被阻断，这可能减弱了VTA中多巴胺能神经元的抑制，从而导致更好的多巴胺释放。

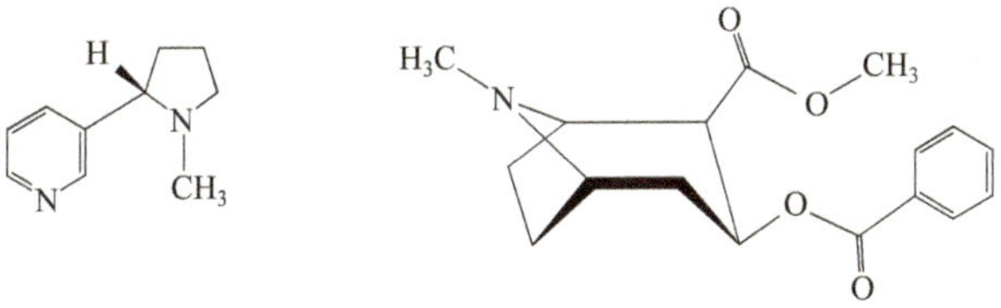

图49.2 烟碱和可卡因的化学结构

烟碱和可卡因分别是烟草和强效可卡因的主要活性物质。

采用 ^1H NMR 的代谢组学模型研究了大鼠伏隔核和纹状体的代谢谱。该模型显示，预给药烟碱显著增加了2mg/kg可卡因诱导的CPP，与单独使用高剂量（20mg/kg）可卡因诱导的CPP相似。奇怪的是，代谢谱显示这两种模型之间有相当大的重叠。这些重叠的代谢物主要包括参与能量稳态和细胞代谢的神经递质和分子。这些结果表明，烟碱强化可卡因行为反应可能与伏隔核和纹状体中某些特定代谢物的变化有关，从而创造一个有利的代谢环境，增加可卡因条件反射和奖励效应（Li et al. 2014）。

49.3 吸烟加剧了药物滥用

可卡因热解产物AEME（图49.3）是乙酰胆碱M1和M3毒蕈碱受体的部分激动剂和其他亚型的拮抗剂。与单独使用可卡因相比，可卡因和AEME联合使用显著增强了成年Wistar大鼠的可卡因作用。观察到尾壳核中多巴胺水平升高，而该脑区D1受体的蛋白水平下降。在伏隔核内发生了多巴胺水平的增加，而D_1和D_2受体的蛋白水平没有变化。这些行为和神经化学数据表明，AEME本身并不会引起行为敏感性。另一方面，当共同给药时，它显著增强可卡因效应，导致尾壳核和伏隔核的多巴胺增加，这些大脑区域的多巴胺释放是由胆碱能活动介导的（Garcia et al. 2016）。

49.4 与可卡因相关的烟碱作用机制

烟碱和可卡因通过细胞外多巴胺的增加产生正强化作用。边际强化剂量的组合可以产生一种成瘾的多巴胺增加，这可能解释了同时使用烟草和强效可卡因比单独使用这两种药物的效果更强烈。事实上，烟碱的增加可诱导可卡因在伏隔核中的细胞外多巴胺水平（Mello, Newman, 2011）。此外，药理学研究表明，一些烟碱和可卡因的作用可以被多巴胺激动剂模拟或被多巴胺拮抗剂阻断（Corrigall, Coen, 1991; Desai, Barber, Terry, 2003）。

甲胺是一种非竞争性拮抗剂烟碱受体，可以避免大鼠可卡因的增加。据临床研究报道，甲胺减少了烟碱和可卡因共同依赖的个体对可卡因的渴望（Reid et al. 1999）。

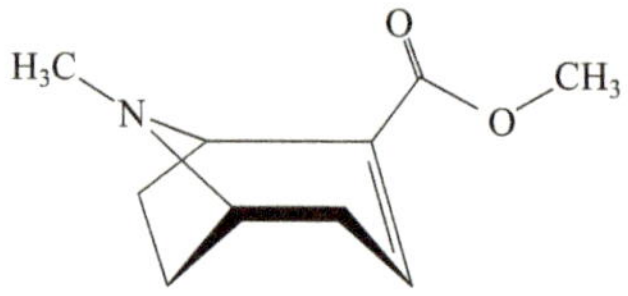

图 49.3 AEME 的化学结构

AEME 是可卡因的主要热解产物。

烟碱显著改善了可卡因诱导的纹状体突触可塑性的变化。短期（1d）和长期（7d）预先接触烟碱有助于可卡因在杏仁核中诱导 LTSP，杏仁核是参与情绪协调和药物依赖的大脑区域。LTSP 的这种效应是单向的，使用可卡因后接触烟碱是无效的。这种烟碱对可卡因的化生作用是长期存在的，尽管它是可逆的。LTSP 的促进作用可在 24d 内达到，但在烟碱停止使用后的 40d 内不能达到。与纹状体一样，用 HDAC 抑制剂 SAHA 进行预处理，可以模拟烟碱的起始效应。这些结果提供了额外的证据，表明烟碱起始效应至少部分可以通过组蛋白乙酰化抑制，这表明杏仁核似乎是大脑中处理烟碱生化效应的重要结构部分，而不是可卡因（Huang et al. 2013）。

烟碱和可卡因刺激下丘脑-垂体-肾上腺-性腺轴中的激素。越来越多的证据表明，激素环境可以调节与这些药物滥用相关的影响。烟碱和可卡因刺激 LH 和 ACTH 快速增加，随后皮质醇和 DHEA 逐渐增加。在使用烟碱或可卡因后，对积极的主观影响的估计会立即增加（Mello, 2010）。

49.5 烟碱与可卡因结合的分子机制

中边缘通路中通过 nAChR 的胆碱能信号与烟碱和可卡因等药物的滥用奖励效应有关。美加明（一种 nAChR 非选择性拮抗剂）可抑制可卡因诱导的大鼠的 CPP 和行为致敏。同时给药 nAChR 亚型选择性拮抗剂，如二氢-β-赤藓红、β2 选择性拮抗剂和甲基烟碱、α7 选择性拮抗剂，避免可卡因行为致敏（Khroyan et al. 2015）。

两种强 α3β4 nAChR 选择性配体 AT-1001 和 AT-1012，在可卡因剂量为 5～30mg/kg 的大鼠中产生强大的 CPP，而运动活动行为敏感性仅在更高剂量（20～30mg/kg）中观察到。AT-1001（1～10mg/kg）或 AT-1012（3～10mg/kg）预处理可阻断 5mg/kg 可卡因诱导的 CPP，而不能阻断 30mg/kg 可卡因诱导的 CPP。低剂量的 AT-1001（0.3mg/kg）和 AT-1012（1～3mg/kg）不会增加 5mg/kg 或 30mg/kg 可卡因诱导的运动能力。然而，在这些剂量下，AT-1001 可以阻断 30mg/kg 可卡因引起的运动敏化。这表明 α3β4 nAChR 在可卡因奖励和行为效应中发挥作用，其选择性配体可以减弱可卡因诱导的行为表达。功能性 α3β4 nAChR 拮抗剂 AT-1001 也能阻断大鼠的烟碱自给药（Khroyan et al. 2015）。

其他烟碱受体，如 α6 nAChR（及其许多亚型）在烟碱行为效应中起着重要作用。然而，关于α6 nAChR的许多亚型对烟碱奖励效应的作用知之甚少。在动物模型中，与WT相比，α6 KO表现出烟碱剂量-应答曲线的直接变化；但α4 KO对烟碱没有偏好，这表明α6α4β2 nAChR（及其亚型）参与了该药物的积极作用。此外，在伏隔核中发现的α6β2 nAChR在条件性烟碱奖励中起重要作用，伏隔内注射α-共毒素MII（α6β2选择性）可阻断烟碱CPP。与烟碱相比，α6 KO对可卡因没有条件反射，但α4 KO中的可卡因CPP被保留了下来。有趣的是，α-共毒素MII阻断了α4 KO条件下的可卡因，这意味着α6β2 nAChR（及其亚型）的可卡因奖励。值得注意的是，这些影响不能一概而论，因为α6 KO表现出对气候的厌恶，受氯化锂和可口食物CPP的制约。此外，α6 KO和WT的多巴胺吸收没有差异（Sanjakdar et al. 2015）。

中枢神经系统中的多巴胺信号通路介导了引起多种药物依赖的能力，如烟碱和可卡因。VTA中多巴胺能神经元的激活和伏隔核神经元投射的多巴胺释放受nAChR介导的胆碱能信号的密切控制。胆碱能信号传导能力由CHT Slc5a7的可用性和活性所决定。根据突触活性的不同，胆碱的再摄取又促进了乙酰胆碱的合成。在大鼠（CHT+/−）中，通过Slc5a7基因拷贝的基因消除介导的CHT结构性表达缺失，导致伏隔核基础细胞外多巴胺水平显著降低。此外，CHT杂合性导致烟碱和可卡因全身给药后多巴胺的增加减弱。这加强了乙酰胆碱能力在强直信号传导和药物调节中的关键作用。然而，他们证明了CHT施加的基因减少导致多巴胺信号的减少，以及对奖励刺激的弱回应。这些机制可能导致了与胆碱能信号通路干扰相关的紊乱（图49.4），包括抑郁症和ADHD（Dong et al. 2013）。

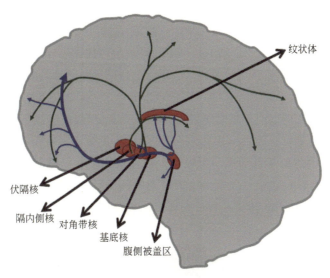

图49.4 多巴胺能和胆碱能途径
受烟碱和可卡因效应影响的主要大脑结构。蓝色箭头表示多巴胺能途径；绿色箭头表示胆碱能途径。

代谢型谷氨酸受体，主要是mGluR2/3，在药物奖励的行为介导和复发机制中起着重要作用。一项应用mGluR2/3原型激动剂LY379268的研究显示，在大鼠模型中，存在由药物搜索建议诱导的烟碱强化衰减和重新整合，以及与不同药物（可卡因、海洛因和甲基苯丙胺）滥用相关的刺激和环境诱导的重新整合。然而，在灵长类动物中，LY379268显示出与可卡因滥用效应相反的结果。在自给药模型中，这种物质阻断了烟碱，但没有阻断可卡因。在影响烟碱和食物自给药的剂量之间存在部分重叠。在戒断的灵长类动物中，LY379268阻断了mGluR2/3，这取决于烟碱的剂量，而不取决于可卡因的剂量，从而导致药物复发。对于烟碱和可卡因研究动物组，

LY379268 显著减少了对药物寻求行为的诱导调整。这些发现为 mGluR2/3 激动剂可能用于烟碱依赖治疗提供了强有力的支持，并建议将它们用于预防与药物使用相关的环境因素引起的复发（Justinova et al. 2016）。

49.6 烟碱和可卡因的依赖和渴望

在一项以安慰剂为对照的双盲交叉研究中，20名吸烟者被随机分配了单剂量的烟碱和安慰剂。用对可卡因渴望和情绪的视觉模拟量表测量了可卡因提示前后的渴望和焦虑。在可卡因提示前后记录皮肤电导率和温度。在接触了强效可卡因的提示后，所有的受试者都报告了与初始记录相关的渴望和焦虑程度的增加，而且皮肤电导率增加，皮肤温度降低。强效可卡因暗示引起的焦虑增加被烟草强烈强化。与皮肤测量相关的反应不受烟草的影响。然后得出结论，可卡因的使用是由烟碱高度诱导的。这种反应发生在没有烟草提示的情况下，这表明烟碱可能具有与可卡因欲望直接相关的精神药理学效应（Reid et al. 1998）。

烟碱和可卡因会促进运动活动的变化。可卡因预处理的大鼠出现了对可卡因运动反应的敏感性增加以及对尼古丁-交叉的运动神经元敏化。在自给药的实验中，反复服用可卡因会导致烟碱用量耐受性的增加和强迫性药物的摄入量的增加（Leão et al. 2013）。

延迟折扣是一种冲动性测量方法，它描述了强化如何在使用延迟增加时失去其值。与一般人群相比，在与MDU相关的疾病患者中可以观察到更高的延迟折扣。比较了四组延迟折扣：烟草单独依赖组、可卡因单独依赖组、烟草和可卡因依赖组以及对照组。结果显示，烟草和可卡因依赖组的延迟折扣明显高于烟草单独依赖组和对照组。与烟草单独依赖组和对照组相比，可卡因单独依赖组的延迟折扣也更高，但烟草和可卡因依赖组和可卡因单独依赖组之间没有观察到差异。延迟折扣因MDU类型而不同，而不是MDU数量（García-Rodriguez et al. 2013）。

烟草会改变对高剂量可卡因的高度主观分类和渴望以及其他主观效应。吸烟者称，使用 crack 克可卡因（可卡因的游离碱形式，可吸食）强烈增加了他们同时吸食烟碱和快克可卡因的欲望。数据表明，同时吸烟和吸食可卡因的行为增加了吸食可卡因的渴望（Brewer III et al. 2013）。图49.5描述了渴望机制的循环。

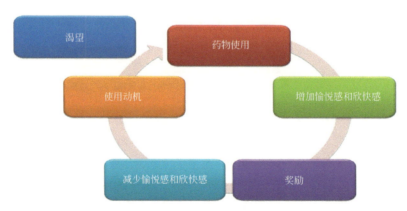

图 49.5 渴望机制

渴望是如何在个体中形成的。药物使用会增加愉悦感和欣快感，这是由奖励机制调节的。这些感觉的减少促使个体再次寻找药物。如果这种追求是不断的，那么一个人就有了渴望。

烟草使用表明，烟草和可卡因渴望的频率呈线性增加。在戒断期间，烟草显著减少了对可卡因的渴望，并且有减少早晨烟草使用的趋势（不显著）。因此，烟草的使用与强效可卡因的使用及其渴望密切相关，反之亦然。对烟草的依赖治疗应从一开始就与其他药物治疗同时提供，而不是单独治疗（Epstein et al. 2010）。

49.7 烟碱和可卡因依赖性的药物治疗

理想的治疗方法应同时减少对烟草和吸食可卡因的滥用。伐伦克林是一种临床上用于α4β2和α6β2 nAChR（及其亚型）的部分激动剂和α7 nAChR的完全激动剂。它有助于在临床研究中的戒烟，减少烟碱自给药，并在临床前研究中替代烟碱辨别性刺激。伐伦克林（图49.6）对单独烟碱或烟碱联合可卡因均有反应，且呈剂量依赖性，但对饮食模式没有显著影响。然而，伐伦克林在低剂量自给药中并没有显著减少单独烟碱、单独可卡因以及烟碱联合可卡因（分别为0.001mg/kg、0.0032mg/kg和0.01mg/kg）。因此，伐伦克林选择性地减弱了单独的烟碱强化效应，而不是可卡因效应，因为它取决于烟碱和可卡因组合的可卡因剂量（Mello et al. 2014）。

丁螺环酮（图49.6）是一种非苯二氮䓬类抗焦虑药物，可抑制血清素能和多巴胺能系统。在临床前研究中，恒河猴接受急性和慢性治疗后，可卡因自给药减少。丁螺环酮不仅对单独的烟碱剂量有剂量依赖性反应，而且对烟碱和可卡因联合剂量也有剂量依赖性反应，但对饮食模式没有显著影响。丁螺环酮在灵长类非人类自给药药物模型中选择性减弱单独的烟碱以及烟碱/可卡因的联合强化效应（Mello et al. 2013）。

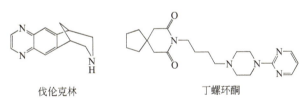

伐伦克林　　　　丁螺环酮

图49.6　烟草和可卡因药物治疗的主要药物

49.8 最终结论

MDU增强了具有这种特性的用户的更多药物使用。烟草的使用是对可卡因使用者的一种生理刺激，但与此同时，烟草减少了对可卡因的渴望，从而减少了可卡因的使用频率。这些机制是由于烟碱和可卡因在伏隔核和纹状体等多巴胺能受体和胆碱能受体中的作用。

本章显示的对烟草和可卡因滥用治疗的一些影响是，治疗不仅应关注其中一种药物，而且应同时关注这两种药物，因为一种药物可强化另一种药物。因此，由于烟草和可卡因的高度化学依赖性，应结合烟草和可卡因治疗，并支持药物治疗。最后，为了更好地了解烟草和crack可卡因联合的神经药理机制，应该开发新的治疗方法、行为疗法和药物治疗。

术语解释	- Basuco：可卡因碱与烟草或大麻的混合物。
- Boris：用来吸食强效可卡因的管道类型。
- capeta：由强效可卡因和烟草的混合物制成的卷烟。
- 条件性位置偏好：动物模型测试，反映了环境刺激的能力，最初是中性的，在反复呈现给一种具有滥用潜力的物质后，获得积极的动机特性。
- FosB：被 *FosB* 基因解码的参与药物依赖发展的细胞膜蛋白。
- 敲除大鼠：通过DNA人工成分而失活、改变或阻断现有基因的转基因大鼠。
- 长时程突触增强：两个神经元之间信号传递的长期改善，从而导致它们的刺激以同步进行。
- mesclado 或 melado：由强效可卡因和大麻的混合物制成的卷烟。
- 代谢组学：生命系统对生理病理刺激或基因修饰的动态多参数代谢反应的定量测量。
- 促代谢受体：突触后受体由结合神经递质的胞外结构域和结合蛋白的胞内结构域组成。
- pitillos 或 papilloes：Basuco 的其他名称。
- 复发：当一个人试图改变或戒掉一个有问题的行为时，在这种情况下，继续使用有问题的药物但失败了。
- Rock：描述强效可卡因的流行术语。
烟碱和可卡因滥用的关键事实	- 大多数时候，crack可卡因的使用者也是烟草使用者。
- 烟草减少了对可卡因的渴望，尽管它是使用可卡因的引子。
- crack可卡因热解产物会增强可卡因的作用。
- 烟碱和可卡因在奖励途径中起协同作用。
- 由于药物的协同作用，烟碱和可卡因依赖性的治疗必须同时进行。
要点总结	- 大多数crack可卡因吸食者使用烟草来减少渴望，也因为烟灰有助于可卡因的燃烧。
- 烟碱和可卡因在多巴胺和乙酰胆碱介导的奖励途径中起协同作用。
- 烟碱的使用促进了大脑区域的变化（主要是在伏隔核和纹状体中），有利于可卡因促进的作用。
- 烟碱和可卡因的协同作用增加了正强化效应，使依赖性的治疗更加困难。
- 强效可卡因和烟草化学依赖治疗必须同时进行，这是药物治疗这种情况最重要的策略之一。

参考文献

Acioli Neto, M. L. (2014). Os contextos de uso do crack: representac¸ões e prá- ticas sociais entre usuários. Recife: Novas Edições Acadêmicas.
Alves, Y. D. D. (2016). O uso do crack como ele é: o cachimbo, o "bloco" eo usuário. Etnográfica, 20, 495-515.
Brewer, A. J.; III, Mahoney, J. J.; Ⅲ, Nerumalla, C. S.; Newton, T. F.; Garza, R. D. L.; II. (2013). The influence of smoking cigaretteson the high and desire for cocaine among active cocaine users. Pharmacology, Biochemistry and Behavior, 106, 132-136.
Corrigall, W. A.; Coen, K. M. (1991). Selective dopamine antagonistsreduce nicotine self-administration. Psychopharmacology, 104, 171-176.
Degenhardt, L.; Dierker, L.; Chiu, W. T.; Medina-Mora, M. E.; Neumark, Y.; Sampson, N. et al. (2010). Evaluating the drug use"gateway" theory using cross-national data: consistency and associations of the order of initiation of drug use among participants in theWHO World Mental Health Surveys. Drug and Alcohol Dependence, 108, 84-97.
Desai, R. I.; Barber, D. J.; Terry, P. (2003). Dopaminergic and cholinergic involvement in the discriminative stimulus effects of nicotine and cocaine in rats. Psychopharmacology, 167, 335-343.
Dong, Y.; Dani, J. A.; Blakely, R. D. (2013). Choline transporter hemizygosity results in diminished basal extracellular dopamine levels in nucleus

accumbens and blunts dopamine elevations following cocaine or nicotine. Biochemical Pharmacology, 86, 1084-1088.

Epstein, D. H.; Marrone, G. F.; Heishman, S. J.; Schmittner, J.; Preston, K. L. (2010). Tobacco, cocaine, and heroin: craving and use during daily life. Addictive Behaviors, 35, 318-324.

Garcia, R. C. T.; Torres, L. H.; Balestrin, N. T, Andrioli, T. C.; Flório, J. C.; Oliveira, C. D.; Costa, J. L.; Yonamine, M.; Sandoval, M. R.; Camarini, R.; Marcourakis, T. (2016) Anhydroecgonine methyl ester, a cocaine pyrolysis product, may contribute to cocaine behavioral sensitization, Toxicology, 376, 44-50.

García-Rodriguez, O.; Secades-Villa, R.; Weidberg, S.; Yoon, J. H. (2013). A systematic assessment of delay discounting in relation to cocaine and nicotine dependence. Behavioural Processes, 99, 100-105.

Gonc¸alves, J. R.; Nappo, S. A. (2015). Factors that lead to the use of crack cocaine in combination with marijuana in Brazil: a qualitative study. BMC Public Health, 15, 706-713.

Huang, Y. Y.; Kandel, D. B.; Kandel, E. R.; Levine, A. (2013). Nicotine primes the effect of cocaine on the induction of LTP in the amygdala. Neuropharmacology, 74, 126-134.

Jeri, F. R. (1980). Nuevas observaciones sobre los síndromes producidos por fumar pasta de coca. In F. R. Jeri (Ed.), Cocaína 1980. Lima: Pacific Press.

Jorge, M. S. B.; Quindere, P. H. D.; Yasui, S.; Albuquerque, R. A. (2013). Ritual de consumo do crack: aspectos socioantropológicos e repercussões para a saúde dos usuários. Ciência, Saúde Coletiva, 18, 2909-2918.

Justinova, Z.; Foll, B. L.; Redhi, G. H.; Markou, A.; Goldberg, S. R. (2016). Differential effects of the metabotropic glutamate 2/3 receptor agonist LY379268 on nicotine versus cocaine self administration and relapse in squirrel monkeys. Psychopharmacology, 233, 1791-1800.

Kandel, D. B. (1975). Stages in adolescent involvement in drug use. Science, 190, 912-914.

Kandel, D. B. (2002). Stages and pathways of drug involvement: examining the gateway hypothesis. Cambridge: Cambridge University Press.

Kandel, D. B.; Yamaguchi, K.; Chen, K. (1992). Stages of progression in drug involvement from adolescence to adulthood: further evidence for the gateway theory. Journal of Studies on Alcohol and Drugs, 53, 447-457.

Kandel, E. R.; Kandel, D. B. (2014). A molecular basis for nicotine as a gateway drug. The New England Journal of Medicine, 371, 932-943.

Khroyan, T. V.; Yasuda, D.; Toll, L.; Polgar, W. E.; Zaveri, N. T. (2015). High affinity α3β4 nicotinic acetylcholine receptor ligands AT-1001 and AT-1012 attenuate cocaine-induced conditioned place preference and behavioral sensitization in mice. Biochemical Pharmacology, 97, 531-541.

Leão, R. M.; Cruz, F. C.; Carneiro-de-Oliveira, P. E.; Rossetto, D. B.; Valentini, S. R.; Zanelli, C. F. et al. (2013). Enhanced nicotine-seeking behavior following pre-exposure to repeated cocaine is accompanied by changes in BDNF in the nucleus accumbens of rats. Pharmacology, Biochemistry and Behavior, 104, 169-176.

Levine, A.; Huang, Y. Y.; Drisaldi, B.; Griffin, E. A.; Jr.; Pollak, D. D.; Xu, S. et al. (2011). Molecular mechanism for a gateway drug: epigenetic changes initiated by nicotine prime gene expression by cocaine. Science Translational Medicine, 3, 107-109.

Li, H.; Bu, Q.; Chen, B.; Shao, X.; Hu, Z.; Deng, P. et al. (2014). Mechanisms of metabonomic for a gateway drug: nicotine priming enhances behavioral response to cocaine with modification in energy metabolism and neurotransmitter level. PLoS One, 9, e87040.

Mello, N. K. (2010). Hormones, nicotine, and cocaine: clinical studies. Hormones and Behavior, 58, 57-71.

Mello, N. K.; Fivel, P. A.; Kohut, S. J. (2013). Effects of chronic Buspirone treatment on nicotine and concurrent nicotine + cocaine selfadministration. Neuropsychopharmacology, 38, 1264-1275.

Mello, N. K.; Fivel, P. A.; Kohut, S. J.; Carroll, F. I. (2014). Effects of chronic varenicline treatment on nicotine, cocaine, and concurrent nicotine + cocaine self-administration. Neuropsychopharmacology, 39, 1222-1231.

Mello, N. K.; Newman, J. L. (2011). Discriminative and reinforcing stimulus effects of nicotine, cocaine, and cocaine + nicotine combinations in rhesus monkeys. Experimental and Clinical Psychopharmacology, 19, 203-214.

Palmer, R. H. C.; Young, S. E.; Hopfer, C. J.; Corley, R. P.; Stallings, M. C.; Crowley, T. J. et al. (2009). Developmental epidemiology of drug useand abuse in adolescence and young adulthood: evidence of generalized risk. Drug and Alcohol Dependence, 102, 78-87.

Pinto, M.; Bardach, A.; Palacios, A.; Biz, A. N.; Alcaraz, A.; Rodríguez, B. et al. (2017). Carga de doenc¸a atribuível ao uso do tabaco no Brasil e potencial impacto do aumento de prec¸os por meio de impostos. Documento tecnico IECS N 21. Buenos Aires: Instituto de Efectividad Clínica y Sanitaria.

Reid, M. S.; Mickalian, J. D.; Delucchi, K. L.; Berger, S. P. (1999). A nicotine antagonist, mecamylamine, reduces cueinduced cocaine craving in cocaine-dependent subjects. Neuropsychopharmacology, 20, 297-307.

Reid, M. S.; Mickalian, J. D.; Delucchi, K. L.; Hall, S. M.; Berger, S. P. (1998). An acute dose of nicotine enhances cue-induced cocaine craving. Drug and Alcohol Dependence, 49, 95-104.

Reitsma, M. B. et al. (2017). Smoking prevalence and attributable disease burden in 195 countries and territories, 1990-2015: a systematic analysis from the global burden of disease study 2015. The Lancet, 389, 1885-1906.

Sanjakdar, S. S.; Maldoon, P. P.; Marks, M. J.; Brunzell, D. H.; Maskos, U.; McIntosh, J. M. et al. (2015). Differential roles of α6β2* and α4β2* neuronal nicotinic receptors in nicotine- and cocaine-conditioned reward in mice. Neuropsychopharmacology, 40, 350-360.

Siegel, R. K. (1982). Cocaine smoking. Journal of Psychoactive Drugs, 14, 277-559.

Vanyukov, M. M.; Tarter, R. E.; Kirillova, G. P.; Kirisci, L.; Reynolds, M. D.; Kreek, M. J. et al. (2012). Common liability to addiction and "gateway hypothesis": theoretical, empirical and evolutionary perspective. Drug and Alcohol Dependence, 123(Suppl 1), S3-S17.

Wagner, F. A.; Anthony, J. C. (2002). Into the world of illegal drug use: exposure opportunity and other mechanisms linking the use of alcohol, tobacco, marijuana, and cocaine. American Journal of Epidemiology, 155, 918-925.

Zeni, T. C.; Araujo, R. B. (2011). Relationship between craving for tobacco and craving for crack in patients hospitalized for detoxification. Brazilian Journal of Psychiatry, 60, 28-33.

50
唾液可替宁测定

M. Inês G.S. Almeida[1], Luisa Barreiros[2], Spas D. Kolev[1], Marcela A. Segundo[2]

1. School of Chemistry, The University of Melbourne, Parkville, Melbourne, VIC, Australia
2. Department of Chemical Sciences, Faculty of Pharmacy, University of Porto, Porto, Portuga

缩略语

ASAP	大气压固体分析探头	LC-MS	液相色谱-质谱联用
ELISA	酶联免疫吸附测定	LC-MS/MS	液相色谱法-串联质谱联用
ETS	环境烟草烟雾	LLE	液液萃取
GC-FID	气相色谱-火焰电离检测	MS-qTOF	四极杆飞行时间串联质谱
GC-MS	气相色谱-质谱联用	POC	医疗点技术
IgG	免疫球蛋白G	SPE	固相萃取
LC-DAD	液相色谱-二极管阵列检测		

50.1 引言

可替宁是烟草生物碱烟碱的主要代谢物（图50.1）（Hukkanen et al. 2005）。作为一种生物标记物，可替宁被选择用于监测戒烟计划的依从性（Gorber et al. 2009），也用于评估环境烟草烟雾（ETS）暴露（Avila-Tang et al. 2013），因为可替宁比其他化合物（如一氧化碳和硫氰酸盐）更可靠，且其水平不受饮食或常见污染暴露的影响（Jarvis et al. 1987），所以它更适合用作生物标志物。

唾液中的可替宁浓度被定义为区分吸烟者和非吸烟者的切点，烟碱和烟草研究协会建议血浆或唾液中的可替宁浓度为15ng/mL（SNRT,2002）。然而，最近的研究（Kim,2016）指出，两个人群（非吸烟者和吸烟者）的可替宁浓度的双峰分布可能会随着时间的推移而变化。随着公共场所对烟草的控制日益严格，非吸烟者中可替宁浓度的分布将倾向于转向较低的值，而且根据目前的分析技术，并且更多的不吸烟者可能具有当前分析技术检测不到的浓度。因此，临界点也会下调。事实上，这是在美国国家健康和营养检查调查（1999—2004）中观察到的，在此基础上提出了较低的截止值（3ng/mL）（Benowitz et al. 2009）。因此，需要合适的分析方法来检测微量可替宁浓度，近年来对开发这类方法提出了越来越大的挑战。因此，需要合适的分析方法来检测微量可替宁浓度，近年来对开发这类方法提出了越来越大的挑战。

在这种情况下，唾液比血浆更适合用于生物监测方案，因为它的收集是无创的，特别适合用于ETS暴露研究中的儿童取样。由于可替宁是一种弱碱，它通过被动扩散从血液运输到唾液中，不需要与其他分子的额外结合。此外，一些研究表明，唾液/血浆可替宁浓度比高于统一水平，而且几乎是不变的（Michalke et al. 2015）。因此，唾液可替宁可以提供一个准确的血浆水平的替代方法，避免了需要采血的不便和疼痛。然而，从分析化学的角度来看，唾液是一个具有挑战性的样本（表50.1）。唾液主要由水组成（97%～99%），但它也含有脂质、蛋白质和无机化合物，当用仪器分析方法定量可替宁时，它们会产生显著干扰。

当大分子的数量比可替宁高几个数量级时（例如，总蛋白在微克/毫升级存在，而可替宁在纳克/毫升级存在时），就会产生这些干扰。此外，一些分光光度检测系统受到吸收用于可替宁检测的相同波长辐射的物种的干扰。另一个常见的干扰原因，是离子的存在，特别是在质谱检测中，这可能导致可替宁的电离增强或抑制，从而对其准确测定造成阻碍。因此，当针对唾液中低纳克/毫升水平的可替宁时，样品必须要进行前处理。

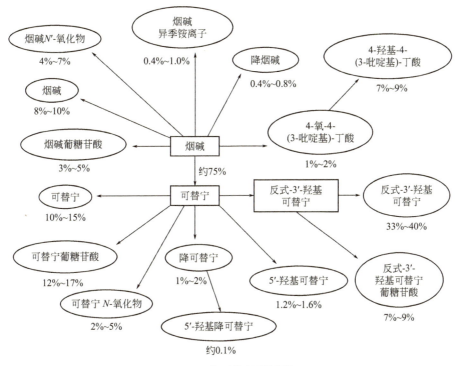

图 50.1 烟碱的主要代谢物

烟碱代谢的定量表，基于代谢物的平均排泄占总尿烟碱的百分比的估计。来自 Pharmacological Reviews, Metabolism and Disposition Kinetics of Nicotine, 57, 2005, 79, J. Hukkanen, P. Jacob, N. L. Benowitz. © 2005 ASPET, reproduced with permission from The American Society for Pharmacology and Experimental Therapeutics。

表50.1 唾液作为分析样本的关键事实

- 唾液是一个具有挑战性的样本体系，因为其复杂、动态的组成和固有的个体间和个体内的变异性
- 唾液由三对大唾液腺和舌、脸颊、嘴唇和上颚黏膜中的小唾液腺产生
- 健康的成年人每天产生 500～2500mL 的唾液，唾液流速高达6mL/min（未受刺激）或高达10mL/min（受刺激）
- 唾液主要由水（97%～99%）、脂质、蛋白质和无机化合物组成
- 唾液中的主要脂质是胆固醇和胆固醇酯、甘油三酯、游离脂肪酸和磷脂，而蛋白质主要以糖蛋白、白蛋白、代谢酶和免疫球蛋白为代表
- 唾液的无机部分含有多种电解质，包括钠、钾、钙、镁、碳酸氢盐和磷酸盐，这些电解质的水平可能受到唾液生成速率的影响
- 唾液pH值的范围为5.8～7.8，这主要取决于碳酸氢盐水平，当刺激唾液分泌时，碳酸氢盐水平会增强
- 在未受刺激的条件下，应优先收集唾液，因为pH值的增加可以改变生物标志物的电离形式的比例
- 整个唾液可以通过引流、吐痰、抽吸、冲洗或使用吸收介质来收集

注：1. 本表列出了唾液作为分析样本的关键事实，包括人类生理学、收集方法和影响其在生物标志物分析方法中使用的化学成分等方面。
2. 信息收集自 Michalke, B.; Rossbach, B.; Goen, T.; Schaferhenrich, A.; Scherer, G. (2015)。

50.2 分析方法

如上所述，唾液可替宁测定法用于评估对戒烟计划的依从性或评估特定人群中的ETS暴露情况。在这些情况下，检测要求可能会有显著差异。在第一种情况下，如果从一直吸烟的人那里收集唾液，预计就会有高水平的可替宁（>100ng/mL）（Avila-Tang et al. 2013）。因此，一种具有半定量特征来区分背景和正值的筛选方法是合适的。在第二种情况下，非暴露受试者的预期水平为<15ng/mL，最近的数据表明，临界点为3ng/mL（Benowitz et al. 2009），因此需要最先进的分析技术。

医疗点（POC）技术（表50.2）满足筛选方法的要求。有几种策略可用于直接测量唾液中的可替宁，包括NicAlert条带、安全护理生物技术条带、iScreen OFD条和Salimetrics ELISA试剂盒。所有方法都依赖于通过目测或使用酶标仪的分光光度法对可替宁进行免疫化学检测。这是Salimetrics ELISA试剂盒的情况，样品中的可替宁与可替宁-辣根过氧化物酶偶联物竞争微滴度板上的抗体结合位点，结合偶联物使用四甲基联苯胺作为比色试剂测量。定量结果的检测限为0.15ng/mL，使该试验适用于ETS暴露的筛选。尽管它作为一种分析性POC技术具有易于使用的特性，但它的主要缺点是它仍然需要实验室设备进一步分析读数。

表50.2 医疗点方法的关键事实

- 医疗点的目的是提供现场的分析结果，这意味着在医生的办公室或患者/目标个体所在的任何其他地点收集和分析样本
- POC方法适用于无创样本（唾液和尿液）或少量血液（一滴或两滴）
- 目前的设备是基于带有固定化试剂的膜基测试条，封闭在塑料外壳中或连接到传感器和电子元件
- 结果主要是半定量的，表明阳性或阴性结果（如妊娠试验）或在一定浓度范围内的结果（如尿葡萄糖条）
- 当定量结果与治疗方法的实施相关时（如用于设置胰岛素丸的血糖分析仪的结果）时，也有更精确的POC方法

注：本表包括了一些关于医疗点技术的关键事实，如样本收集、应用范围和定性或半定量的反应类型。

安全护理生物技术条带和iScreen OFD条带只能提供定性结果，阳性反应的临界值较高（>30ng/mL）。因此，这些条带适用于吸烟状况的评估，但不适用于ETS的筛查。NicAlert条带提供了一种半定量的方法，基于使用金颗粒包覆的单克隆抗体和一系列对这些抗体具有不同亲和力的分子阱，依次放置在分析条带中。因此，可替宁分子与固定在金颗粒上的抗体结合，该金颗粒携带多种抗体（40～100个受体位点）。被占据位点的数量是样品中可替宁浓度的函数。因此，含有更多未结合抗体（样品中可替宁较少）的颗粒将首先被低亲和力陷阱保留，而含有较少未结合抗体（样品中可替宁较多）的颗粒将被高亲和力陷阱保留在另一个区域内。使用这种策略，通过测定10～1000ng/mL的可替宁，可以评估吸烟状况。

最先进的分析技术可达到纳克/毫升的水平，目前只能在实验室条件下进行，如使用质谱仪（表50.3）探测器。除了ELISA格式下的免疫分析（Langone, Bjercke, 1989），液相色谱法结合串联质谱法（LC-MS/MS）被认为是该领域的金标准，可同时测定其他烟碱代谢物 [反式-3′-羟基可替宁和降可替宁（图50.1）]，（Bentley et al. 1999; Jacob et al. 2011; Shakleya, Huestis, 2009），甚至其他受控物质（Concheiro et al. 2010）。图50.2显示了在三重四极杆光谱仪中获得的可替宁的质谱（Perez-Ortuno et al., 2015）。分子离子（m/z 180.2）在正离子模式下的电喷雾电离，可以识别出两个主要的片段。m/z 80.1处较丰富的片段对应吡啶部分，已用于定量，m/z 98.1处的片段归于甲基吡咯烷酮环，已用于鉴定。为了准确定量，经常使用氘化可替宁-d_3作为内标，在m/z 80.1处

生成相同的定量片段，在 m/z 101.1 处生成相同的鉴定片段，说明了添加到结构中的三个重氢。

除了 LC-MS/MS、LC-MS（Kataoka et al. 2009）、LC-DAD（Machacek, Jiang,1986）、GC-MS（Shin et al. 2002）和 GC-FID（Feyerabend, Russell, 1980）已被提出用于符合ETS暴露评估水平的唾液中可替宁的定量。这些方法的工作范围为 0.5～5000ng/mL，检测限为 0.02～1ng/mL。为了达到如此低的检测水平，需要进行样品预处理需以除干扰，也需要预浓缩可替宁（图50.3）。

表50.3 质谱与液体界面耦合的关键事实

- 质谱基于测量气相中电离分子的质荷比，表示为 m/z
- 为了将液体界面连接到质谱分析仪，需要去除溶剂、电离目标分子和过渡到气相
- 液流和质谱分析仪之间最常见的界面基于电喷雾电离（ESI）和大气压化学电离（APCI）
- ESI 可以在正模式或负模式下进行，获得或失去一个氢原子，导致母离子的 m/z 值比目标分子的分子质量多于或少于1Da
- 有几种类型的质谱分析仪（四极杆、飞行时间、离子阱等），主要区别在于报告的 m/z 的准确性和精度
- 串联质谱是指两个或更多的质谱分析仪的串联，允许鉴定/定量由母离子产生的片段离子
- 高分辨率质谱是基于 m/z 值的精确测量，提供小数位数的值，并使元素组成的测定成为可能

注：该表包括了质谱与液体界面耦合的一些关键事实，即通过电离和转化为气相来检测分子所需的步骤、最常见的界面以及它们如何产生离子。介绍了一些类型的探测器以及高分辨率和串联质谱的特点。

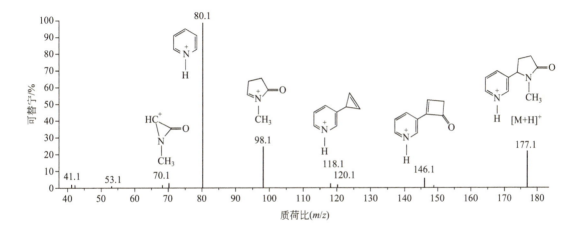

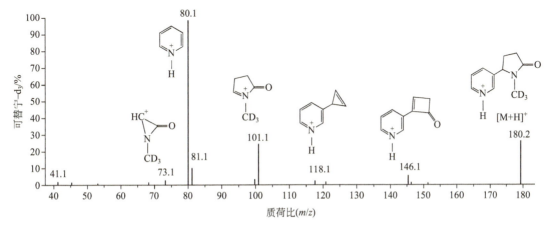

图 50.2 可替宁和可替宁 $-d_3$ 的质谱

使用三重四极杆设备（串联质谱）获得的可替宁和可替宁 -d_3 的质谱，显示了基于前体离子 [M+H]⁺ 在 m/z 177 处的断裂而获得的可替宁的产物离子质谱。内标可替宁-d_3（前体离子 [M+H]⁺ 在 m/z 180 处）的产物离子质谱也可显示。并给出了每个观测峰的化学结构。

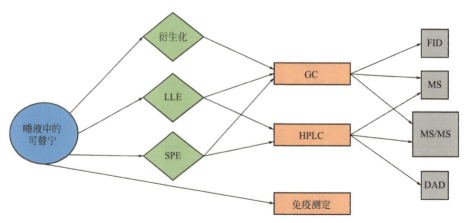

图 50.3 唾液可替宁测定的分析工作流程

在应用分析技术（以矩形和正方形放置）之前，唾液预处理（插入菱形中的操作）所采用的程序示意图。箭头表示到目前为止在文献中描述的可能的组合。

液液萃取（LLE）包括添加液体萃取溶剂（如二氯甲烷）、通过离心分离液相和萃取剂的回收，已被认为是一种简单、方便、直接的定量分离可替宁的方法，回收率>83%。固相萃取（SPE）被认为是一种更环保的样品预处理方法，也被应用于唾液中可替宁的测定。已经提出了几种类型的吸附剂，包括传统的硅-C18、亲水性亲脂性聚合物和分子印迹聚合物。

根据所选择的仪器分析方法，还需要进行其他类型的样品预处理。例如，敏感的气相色谱分析要求分离下的物种是挥发性的。因此，提出的唾液中可替宁测定的气相色谱方法需要事先使用 N-甲基-三甲基硅基-三氟乙酰胺和三甲基氯硅烷进行衍生化（da Fonseca et al. 2012），从可替宁中产生更多的挥发性化合物。

50.3 样品预处理和可替宁测定的最新进展

在过去的几年中，已经观察到关于最小化或消除样品预处理和小型化的新趋势。关于唾液预处理的自动化，最近提出了一种基于珠注射概念的自动微固相萃取方法（Ramdzan et al. 2016）。使用介观流控-阀上实验室平台（如图50.4所示），SPE的所有步骤都是通过计算机控制完成的，促进了对溶液的精确测量和对应用流速的严格控制。对几种反相聚合物吸附剂进行了测试，发现球形Oasis HLB吸附剂具有更好的充填和回收特性。可替宁洗脱使用与色谱流动相组成相同的溶液［乙腈-100mmol/L乙酸铵缓冲液，95∶5（体积比），pH = 5.8］，促进洗脱液直接引入液相色谱仪，基于亲水相互作用（HILIC）进行分离。这种操作方式特别适用于极性化合物，由于色谱流动相主要由有机溶剂组成，直接注入SPE洗脱液时不存在增带效应，因此无需通过蒸发和再悬浮切换溶剂，节省了时间。该方法适用于直接引入唾液，尽管唾液具有黏性成分，但样品在磷酸盐缓冲液中被稀释。这种稀释并不影响方法的灵敏度，因为原样品中所有可替宁都保留在固相萃取柱中，检测限和定量限分别为1.5ng/mL和3ng/mL，采样率为每小时6个样品，包括样品预处理。

为了进一步缩小规模，采用微芯片格式下的ELISA法测定可替宁（Cheng et al. 2013）。在聚二甲基硅氧烷中，采用标准软光刻技术设计和制造了最多可进行8次平行检测的微流控芯片

（图50.5）。可替宁的测定采用蛋白A包被聚苯乙烯微球固定可替宁-IgG的方法。检测方案包括：将可替宁-IgG微球固定在微芯片内，灌注稀释的示踪剂（可替宁-辣根过氧化物酶）溶液中的样品，孵育，与Amplex Red反应后进行荧光检测，荧光值越低，可替宁水平越高。12μL唾液最低检测浓度为1ng/mL，样品通量为每小时12个样品。该方法成功地应用于检测接受ETS的吸烟者和非吸烟者唾液样本中的可替宁。

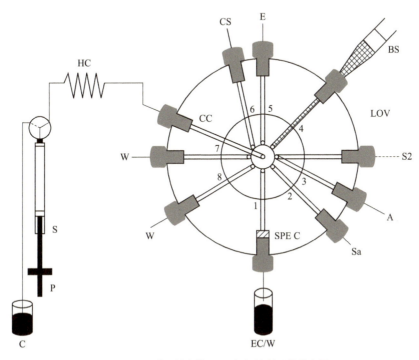

图50.4　唾液可替宁微SPE阀门注射系统的介绍

为唾液可替宁自动SPE设计的阀上实验室设备示意图。试剂和吸附剂被置在一个中央通道周围，从中吸入或输送溶液和珠状悬浮液，以执行SPE所需的所有步骤，包括柱填充和调节、样品加载和去除基质干扰、可替宁洗脱和吸附剂的处理。所有这些操作都是通过计算机控制来自动执行的。P，低压活塞泵；S，注射器；HC，固定线圈；C，载体（1.20mmol/L磷酸一钾，pH＝6.8）；E，洗脱液；SPE C，SPE柱；Sa，样品；A，空气；BS，珠悬液；CS，调节溶液［乙腈-水，50：50（体积比）］；CC，中央通道；EC，洗脱液收集；W，废物。来自Journal of Chromatography A, Determination of salivary cotinine through solid phase extraction using a bead-injection lab-on-valve approach hyphenated to hydrophilic interaction liquid chromatography, 1429, 2016, 284, A. N. Ramdzan, L. Barreiros, M. I. G. S. Almeida, S. D. Kolev, M. A. Segundo. © 2015 Elsevier B. V, 经Elsevier许可复制。

流行病学研究需要具有更高的通量和简单、直接的样本处理方法。针对这些特征，提出了一种HPLC-MS/MS方法，可应用于唾液、尿液和头发样本（Perez-Ortuno et al. 2015），每次色谱运行只需要2min来测定可替宁和烟碱。利用与LC（或GC）设备耦合的自动采样器的内置特性，可以编程针穿透瓶中的深度，直接在瓶中进行LLE，直接探测底部有机相。因此，将0.5mL唾液与碱性内标溶液和二氯甲烷直接在瓶中混合。如前所述，HILIC的实现是由于其与高水平的有机溶剂的相容性和对极性化合物的分离能力。唾液中可替宁的校准范围为0.1～2000ng/mL。

最后，微量分析的最近趋势集中在完全消除样品预处理上，例如，当分析物直接从样品转移到质谱仪的电离室时。已提出使用四极杆飞行时间串联质谱仪（MS-qTOF）耦合的大气压固体分析探头（ASAP）筛选可替宁的方法（Carrizo et al. 2016）。将玻璃毛细管浸入唾液（或尿液）样品中两次，并引入电离室，以正模式进行大气压电离。对戒烟计划下的个体样本进行分析，并

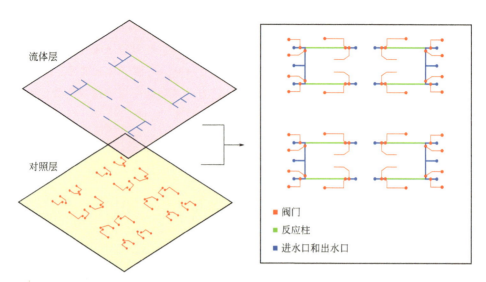

图 50.5　制备用于快速检测可替宁的微流控芯片示意图

微流控分析芯片是由聚二甲基硅氧烷构建的两个独立部件，使用光刻工艺制作的不同图案的模具制作的（方案左侧）。图右部分描述了模具中设计的图案及芯片不同部件的功能，包括用于液体通道的阀门、通过通道限制的免疫吸附剂夹带（反应柱）和溶液出入口点（入口和出口）。来自 Biomedical Microdevices, Microfluidic immunoassay for rapid detection of cotinine in saliva, 15, 2013, 951; K. P. Cheng, W. Zhao, S. X. Liu, G. D. Sui. ©Springer Science+Business Media New York 2013, 经 Springer 许可复制。

观察到白天可替宁值的相对差异，但未确定相应的确切可替宁浓度。因此，尽管这种分析方法很方便，但其应用仍然是半定量的，但它显示出在多分析物检测和综合诊断方面的巨大潜力，因为qTOF检测器可提供准确的质量测定，从而能够鉴定多种临床上感兴趣的化合物。

　　使用一种更传统的电离方法，该方法基于对纸载体上的唾液样本应用高压直流电，通过应用氘化内标实现了定量分析（Wang et al. 2013）。不需要进行样品预处理，即将5μL唾液直接浸入纸三角形（基部7mm，高度12mm）中，然后加入20μL乙腈。因此，通过将纸载体放置在质谱仪入口前，并施加高压，获得了正模式电离后的质谱特征。虽然未应用于流行病学研究，但该方法显示出定量和快速测定可替宁的潜力。

　　总之，尽管迄今为止做出了努力，但仍需要快速定量唾液中可替宁的方法，特别是那些使POC测量精度更好、检测限更低的方法。

术语解释

- **自动采样器**：目前存在于大多数色谱设备中，允许将样品自动引入色谱柱。最近的模型允许外部编程，允许在自动采样器内自动进行样品预处理。
- **注珠注射**：是一种流动分析技术，其中颗粒悬浮液被困在流动管道（通常是测量单元）内，并在分析操作完成后自动丢弃。
- **ELISA**：ELISA是酶联免疫吸附测定的缩写。它是基于目标化合物的固定化（通过与表面的特定相互作用，通过反应基团或使用特定的抗体），然后使用免疫复合物进行检测。
- **阀上实验室**：是一种中流体平台，采用聚合物材料建造，与选择阀和可逆活塞泵相结合，允许开发一种用于（生物）化学分析自动化的流量分析系统。
- **检测限**：是提供可与无分析物时获得的信号区分的分析信号的最低浓度。有几种方法可以评估检测限。其中最普遍的一种是基于信噪比，其中最低的可检测浓度对应于在没有分析物时获得的信号加上其标准差的三倍。

- 液液萃取：这是一种基于两个不可混溶液相之间传质的分离过程。
- 质谱：将电流强度（或相对丰度）表示为质荷比的函数。需要注意的是，由于可以形成不同的离子（正离子、负离子或加合物）和不同的碎片，一个给定的物质可以根据所应用的质量探测器的类型和选定的电离过程提供不同的光谱。
- 采样率：采样率也指定为样品通量，对应于在给定时间内（通常为1小时或1个工作日），给定分析技术可以处理的样品数量。
- 硅C18：这是十八烷基二氧化硅的常见名称，是反相液相色谱中最常用的固定相材料。它也经常被用于固相萃取方案。
- 固相萃取：这是一种基于从液相到固相的传质过程的分离过程。对于大多数分析过程，分析物从固相洗脱到一个新的液相，然后使用仪器分析方法进行定量。
- 吸附剂：是在固相萃取中保留分析物的固相。
- 工作范围：对于分析方法，工作范围由应用所建立的校准曲线可以确定的最低浓度和最高浓度来确定。

要点总结

- 本章重点测定唾液中可替宁作为吸烟或环境烟草烟雾暴露的生物标志物。
- 唾液是通过无创程序采集的，适用于流行病学研究。
- 医疗点方法提供了有关吸烟习惯的定性或半定量结果。
- 由于敏感性不足，目前的医疗点方法不适合评估环境烟草烟雾暴露。
- 液相色谱法结合串联质谱法是目前唾液中可替宁定量的金标准，其优点是为其他生物标记物同时提供结果。
- 分析方法倾向于使用基于纸张、微流控设备和中流控设备自动化、最小化或消除样品预处理。
- 快速定量唾液中可替宁的精度和更低的检测限仍然需要在医疗点应用。

参考文献

Avila-Tang, E.; Al-Delaimy, W. K.; Ashley, D. L.; Benowitz, N.; Bernert, J. T.; Kim, S. et al. (2013). Assessing secondhand smokeusing biological markers. Tobacco Control, 22, 164-171.

Benowitz, N. L.; Bernert, J. T.; Caraballo, R. S.; Holiday, D. B.; Wang, J. T. (2009). Optimal serum cotinine levels for distinguishing cigarettesmokers and nonsmokers within different racial/ethnic groups inthe United States between 1999 and 2004. American Journal of Epidemiology, 169, 236-248.

Bentley, M. C.; Abrar, M.; Kelk, M.; Cook, J.; Phillips, K. (1999). Validation of an assay for the determination of cotinine and3-hydroxycotinine in human saliva using automated solid-phaseextraction and liquid chromatography with tandem mass spectrometric detection. Journal of Chromatography B, 723, 185-194.

Carrizo, D.; Nerin, I.; Domeno, C.; Alfaro, P.; Nerin, C. (2016). Directscreening of tobacco indicators in urine and saliva by atmospheric pressure solid analysis probe coupled to quadrupole-time of flight mass spectrometry (ASAP-MS-Q-TOF-). Journal of Pharmaceutical and Biomedical Analysis, 124, 149-156.

Cheng, K. P.; Zhao, W.; Liu, S. X.; Sui, G. D. (2013). Microfluidic immunoassay for rapid detection of cotinine in saliva. Biomedical Microdevices, 15, 949-957.

Concheiro, M.; Gray, T. R.; Shakleya, D. M.; Huestis, M. A. (2010). High-throughput simultaneous analysis of buprenorphine, methadone, cocaine, opiates, nicotine, and metabolites in oral fluid by liquid chromatography tandem mass spectrometry. Analytical and Bioanalytical Chemistry, 398, 915-924.

da Fonseca, B. M.; Moreno, I. E. D.; Magalhaes, A. R.; Barroso, M.; Queiroz, J. A.; Ravara, S. et al. (2012). Determination of biomarkers of tobacco smoke exposure in oral fluid using solid-phase extraction and gas chromatography-tandem mass spectrometry. Journal of Chromatography B-Analytical Technologies in the Biomedical and Life Sciences, 889, 116-122.

Feyerabend, C.; Russell, M. A. H. (1980). Rapid gas-liquid?chromatographic determination of cotinine in biological-fluids. Analyst, 105, 998-1001.

Gorber, S. C.; Schofield-Hurwitz, S.; Hardt, J.; Levasseur, G.; Tremblay, M. (2009). The accuracy of self-reported smoking: a system?atic review of the relationship between self-reported and cotinine-assessed smoking status. Nicotine, Tobacco Research, 11, 12-24.

Hukkanen, J.; Jacob, P.; Benowitz, N. L. (2005). Metabolism and dis?position kinetics of nicotine. Pharmacological Reviews, 57, 79-115.

Jacob, P.; Yu, L. S.; Duan, M. J.; Ramos, L.; Yturralde, O.; Benowitz, N. L. (2011). Determination of the nicotine metabolites cotinine and trans-3′-hydroxycotinine in biologic fluids of smokers and non-smokers using liquid chromatography-tandem mass spectrom?etry: biomarkers for tobacco smoke exposure and for phenotyping cytochrome P450 2A6 activity. Journal of Chromatography B-Analytical Technologies in the Biomedical and Life Sciences, 879, 267-276.

Jarvis, M. J.; Tunstallpedoe, H.; Feyerabend, C.; Vesey, C.; Saloojee, Y. (1987). Comparison of tests used to distinguish smokers from nonsmokers. American Journal of Public Health, 77, 1435-1438.

Kataoka, H.; Inoue, R.; Yagi, K.; Saito, K. (2009). Determination of nic?otine, cotinine, and related alkaloids in human urine and saliva by automated in-tube solid-phase microextraction coupled with liquid chromatography-mass spectrometry. Journal of Pharmaceutical and Biomedical Analysis, 49, 108-114.

Kim, S. (2016). Overview of cotinine cutoff values for smoking status classification. International Journal of Environmental Research and Public Health, 13. https://dx. doi. org/10. 3390/ijerph13121236.

Langone, J. J.; Bjercke, R. J. (1989). Idiotype anti-idiotype hapten immunoassays—assay for cotinine. Analytical Biochemistry, 182, 187-192.

Machacek, D. A.; Jiang, N. S. (1986). Quantification of cotinine in plasma and saliva by liquid-chromatography. Clinical Chemistry, 32, 979-982.

Michalke, B.; Rossbach, B.; Goen, T.; Schaferhenrich, A.; Scherer, G. (2015). Saliva as a matrix for human biomonitoring in occupational and environmental medicine. International Archives of Occupational and Environmental Health, 88, 1-44.

Perez-Ortuno, R.; Martinez-Sanchez, J. M.; Fernandez, F.; Pascual, J. A. (2015). High-throughput wide dynamic range procedure for thesimultaneous quantification of nicotine and cotinine in multiple biological matrices using hydrophilic interaction liquid chromatography-tandem mass spectrometry. Analytical and Bioanalytical Chemistry, 407, 8463-8473.

Ramdzan, A. N.; Barreiros, L.; Almeida, M. I. G. S.; Kolev, S. D.; Segundo, M. A. (2016). Determination of salivary cotinine through solid phase extraction using a bead-injection lab-on-valve approach hyphenated to hydrophilic interaction liquid chromatography. Jour?nal of Chromatography A, 1429, 284-291.

Shakleya, D. M.; Huestis, M. A. (2009). Optimization and validation of a liquid chromatography-tandem mass spectrometry method for the simultaneous quantification of nicotine, cotinine, 417 REFERENCES trans-30-hydroxycotinine and norcotinine in human oral fluid. Analytical and Bioanalytical Chemistry, 395, 2349-2357.

Shin, H. S.; Kim, J. G.; Shin, Y. J.; Jee, S. H. (2002). Sensitive and simple method for the determination of nicotine and cotinine in human urine, plasma and saliva by gas chromatography-mass spectrometry. Journal of Chromatography B-Analytical Technologies in the Biomedical and Life Sciences, 769, 177-183.

Society for Research on Nicotine and Tobacco - Subcommittee on Biochemical Verification. (2002). Biochemical verification of tobacco and cessation. Nicotine, Tobacco Research, 4, 149-159.

Wang, H.; Ren, Y.; McLuckey, M. N.; Manicke, N. E.; Park, J.; Zheng, L. X. et al. (2013). Direct quantitative analysis of nicotine alkaloids from biofluid samples using paper spray mass spectrometry. Analytical Chemistry, 85, 11540-11544.

51
关于吸烟状态分类的可替宁截止值的概述

Sungroul Kim

Department of Environmental Health Sciences, SoonChunHyang University, Asan, South Korea

缩略语

IARC	国际癌症研究机构	USDHHS	美国卫生与公众服务部
NRC	国家研究委员会（美国）		

准确评估吸烟状况是至关重要的，原因有很多；其中包括它在评估全球烟草控制项目进展、记录烟草流行和估计人口吸烟风险方面的效用（IARC，2004；NRC，1986；USDHHS，2006；Warren et al. 2006）。在评估吸烟流行率和接触二手烟（SHS）时，研究人员最常用的是标准化问卷。

然而，这种方法在准确评估受试者的真实吸烟状况的能力上受到了限制。这些限制包括受试者难以回忆过去吸烟的细节和受访者偏见，其程度随着时间的推移而增加，由于社会规范的改变，烟草使用的社会接受程度降低。此外，问卷并不能完全准确地评估非吸烟者的SHS暴露情况，而且问卷在试图确定SHS暴露水平可能不同的近期前吸烟者的吸烟状况时尤其不足（Kawachi, Colditz, 1996; Wells et al. 1998）。

由于这些原因，进行流行率调查和流行病学研究的研究人员多年来一直利用烟草暴露的生物标志物来验证报告的吸烟状况（Benowitz, 1983, 1999; Coultas et al. 1987; DeLorenze et al. 2002; Eliopoulos et al. 1996; Etzel, 1990; NRC, 1986, 1989），并监测和跟踪考虑人、地点和时间的烟草暴露。这些生物标志物可以包括与烟雾相关的成分的浓度或代谢物，以及烟雾中生物物质和化学物质相互作用的产物。

烟碱及其代谢物是烟草特异性的生物标记物（Benowitz, Jacob III, 1994; Benowitz et al. 1994; Jacob, Byrd, 1999）。烟碱与活跃吸烟者吸入的烟雾中的颗粒结合，并且在SHS中只处于气相（Benner et al. 1986; Ogden et al. 1993）。肝脏主要将吸收的烟碱代谢为可替宁（Benowitz, Jacob III, 1994; Benowitz et al. 1994）；烟碱在体内的半衰期为2～3h，而可替宁的半衰期为12～20h（Benowitz, 1996; Hammond, Leaderer, 1987; Jaakkola, Jaakkola, 1997）。尿液中排出的少量可替宁（10%～15%）进一步代谢为反式-3′-羟基可替宁及其他副产物（Benowitz et al. 1994）。可替宁具有较长的半衰期，是烟草烟雾暴露的常用生物标志物，可在唾液、血清或尿液中测量。Benowitz（1999）发表了一篇关于烟草烟雾暴露生物标志物的综述，这些生物标志物的水平受到暴露后体内吸收、分布、代谢和消除的影响。

特定于烟草烟雾的生物标志物（如烟碱或可替宁）的分布应该是双峰的，并反映吸烟者和非吸烟者在这两种人群中的潜在分布。两个关键的自我报告有效性指标可以通过比较自我报告的吸烟状态和生物标志物的二分模板计算：敏感性（%）（自我报告的吸烟者被生物监测分类为吸烟者的百分比）和特异性（%）（自我报告的非吸烟者被生物监测分类为非吸烟者的百分比）。这里一个特别关键的问题是漏报，即假阴性，即那些报告为非吸烟者但生物标志物水平为阳性的人。非吸烟者通常不会自我报告为吸烟者，但由于暴露于SHS，可能具有阳性生物标志物水平，这使得特异性>100%。暴露状态的特异性越低，就越容易低估暴露与疾病发生之间的相关性（Flegal et al. 1986）。

如上所述，被动吸烟模式应反映在非吸烟者中的生物标志物分布中，而主动吸烟者中的这种分布应反映他们的吸烟情况。设置一个截止值的目的是优化敏感性和特异性，同时认识到这两者之间不可避免地存在权衡。在双峰分布中，较低的截止值通常会获得较高的敏感度，但较高的截止值将具有更大的特异性；换句话说，更多的非吸烟者将表现出超过临界值的生物标志物水平。较高的截止值比较低的截止值具有较大的特异性，但敏感性较低。

在选择一个截止值时，最好都要考虑吸烟者和非吸烟者中生物标志物的潜在分布；然而，这些分布可能会随着时间的推移而变化。对烟草的有效控制将使这些值在非吸烟者中的分布转移到较低的水平，较少的非吸烟者具有可检测水平的吸烟生物标志物。这种转变也会降低截止点。由于不同的主动吸烟模式和SHS暴露，这些生物标志物的分布在不同人群之间可能存在差异。

可替宁被广泛用于暴露状态分类的验证标准（Boyd et al. 1998; Etter, Vu, Perneger, 2000; Etzel, 1990; Hegaard et al. 2007; Jarvis et al. 1984, 1987; Luepker et al. 1989; McNeill et al. 1986; Murray et al. 1993; Pierce et al. 1987; Stookey et al. 1987）。烟碱和烟草研究学会的一个小组委员会已经评估了可替宁、一氧化碳和硫氰酸盐作为烟草使用和戒烟的生物标志物的效用，并推荐了它们在临床试验中的应用临界值（SRNT, 2002）。

本研究在1985～2014年在公共文献数据库PubMed中使用关键词"可替宁""截止"或"自我报告""吸烟状况"和"验证"（$n = 104$）。以自我报告或可替宁试验作为金标准，证明了自我报告吸烟状况与可替宁试验之间的一致性和差异，结果描述了如何确定给定的可替宁浓度的截止值。同时检索已鉴定文章的文献资料，以确定所引用的截止测定方法。本概述包括对青少年和成人研究人群的结果的比较。描述可替宁试验条或可替宁试纸法的文章被排除在外。本概述共包括32篇文章。

总结了截止值、测定方法和研究种群特征。敏感性和特异性也被总结，以区分吸烟者和非吸烟者，自我报告作为一种金标准测试，使用三种生物样本：唾液、血清和尿液。还评估了截止值随时间的变化以及它们在种群和地区方面的差异，并描述了确定截止值过程中所产生的问题。

表51.1～表51.3总结了研究人群的特征以及确定截止值的方法；唾液、血清和尿液可替宁截止值；以及自我报告吸烟和不吸烟的人数。本文回顾的大多数研究都是在20世纪80年代中期至2013年期间在北美或欧洲进行的，样本量在24～24332例之间。采用了许多方法来选择截止值。这些研究包括：（1）非吸烟者（Benowitz, 1983）、被动吸烟者（Hoffmann et al. 1984）、吸烟者（Slattery et al. 1989）的可替宁水平；（2）一个2×2表（Jarvis et al. 1987; Luepker et al. 1989; Martinez et al. 2004; Murray et al. 1993; Pierce et al. 1987）；（3）吸烟者和非吸烟者中可替宁浓度的双峰分布有一个分离点（Pirkle et al. 1996）。最近的一种选择截止值的方法是受试者工作特征（ROC）曲线，它优化了敏感性和特异性，同时以最高的比率正确分类吸烟状态（Benowitz et al. 2009; Boyd et al. 1998; Goniewicz et al. 2011; Hegaard et al. 2007; Jarvis et al. 2008）。还介绍了使用生物标本（血清、唾液和尿液）的截止值细节和测定方法。

51.1 唾液可替宁

在11项研究中，用于区分吸烟者和非吸烟者的唾液可替宁的截止值为10～到44ng/mL。敏感性和特异性的总体范围分别为69%～99%和74%～99%（图51.1）。Jarvis等（1987）研究了英国伦敦的211名成年门诊患者，报告了唾液可替宁的截止值为14.2ng/mL；这是使用2×2表选择的（表51.1）。该值的敏感性为96.4%，特异性为99.0%。Pierce等（1987）在一项针对澳大利亚975名14岁以上人口的研究中报告了以44ng/mL作为截止值。Etzel（1990）回顾了1973～1989年MEDLINE英文检索的关键词为唾液和可替宁22项研究的结果，结果报告的截止值为10ng/mL。这个截止值是通过比较唾液可替宁与吸烟状况的分布而确定的：被动吸烟者的数值不超过5ng/mL，重度被动吸烟者的数值为10ng/mL或稍高，不经常吸烟者的数值在10～100ng/mL之间，而经常主动吸烟者的数值等于或超过100ng/mL。然而，Etzel（1990）确定的10ng/mL值的敏感性和特异性尚不清楚。Jarvis等（2008）最近报道了唾液可替宁的新截止值为12ng/mL；这是根据1996～2003年英国健康调查（HSE）中16岁及以上参与者的一项研究确定的，通过ROC曲线，敏感性为96.7%，特异性为96.9%，以区分吸烟者和从不吸烟者。图51.1显示了表51.1～表51.3中总结的可替宁不同截止水平的敏感性和特异性值的分布。

表51.1 唾液可替宁截止值及其测定方法

参考文献	研究人群特征				截止值/(ng/mL)	自我报告的数量		截止值测定方法
	说明	n	年龄	女性比例/%		吸烟者	非吸烟者	
Jarvis et al.（1987）	英国伦敦圣玛丽医院的门诊病人	211	平均年龄55岁	24.6	14.2	111	100	2×2表：提供正确分类的吸烟者和非吸烟者的最高数量的截止值
McNeill et al.（1987）	英国伦敦女子综合学校的学生	508	11～16岁	100	14.7	173	335	截止值采用Jarvis等（1987）的研究结果
Pierce et al.（1987）	在澳大利亚一个社区中随机选中的居民	975	14岁或以上	49.2	44	353	622	2×2表
Stookey et al.（1987）	美国一项评估促进戒烟措施的临床试验的参与者	236	NA	NA	10	216	20	截止值采用Benowitz（1983）的研究结果："没有非吸烟者的血液可替宁值大于10ng/mL"（文献第21页）
Luepker et al.（1989）	在美国明尼苏达州明尼阿波利斯市，随机抽取高中生进行调查	263	17～21岁	NA	20	87	176	2×2表
Etzel[①]（1990）	1973～1989年期间发表的22项研究的参与者	NA	NA	NA	10	NA	NA	在1973～1989年期间发表的22篇研究论文中，通过比较唾液可替宁浓度与吸烟状况的分布，选择了截止值

续表

参考文献	研究人群特征				截止值 /(ng/mL)	自我报告的数量		截止值测定方法
	说明	n	年龄	女性比例/%		吸烟者	非吸烟者	
Murray et al. (1993)	在美国和加拿大进行的"肺健康研究"临床试验中,有证据表明接受常规护理的参与者早期存在慢性阻塞性肺疾病	1498	35～60岁（平均48.5岁）	36	20	1345	153	截止值被选择为唾液可替宁水平,提供了正确分类的吸烟状态的最高百分比
Boyd et al. (1998)	在伯明翰4家公共卫生产科诊所进行的第2次试验中的孕妇	548	平均24.6岁	100	24	441	107	受试者工作特征（ROC）曲线：提供最大百分比的截止值

① Etzel没有提供金标准信息，但本文中包含了截止值，该值是在审查了大量论文后获得的。

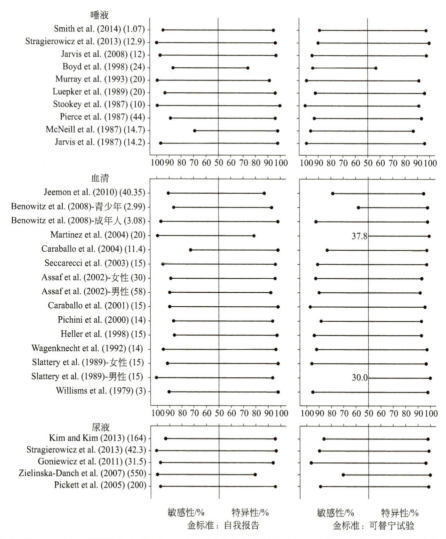

图 51.1 根据唾液或血清可替宁的截止值绘制的敏感性和特异性图（括号内的数字表示作者选择的截止值）

51.2 血清可替宁

14项研究评估的血清可替宁截止值为3.0～20ng/mL，其敏感性范围为73.2%～98.9%，特异性范围为78.7%～99.0%。其中8项研究提供了1989～2004年期间14或15ng/mL的截止值（Caraballo et al. 2001; Heller et al. 1998; Nafstad et al.1996; Pichini et al. 2000; Pirkle et al. 1996; Seccareccia et al. 2003; Slattery et al. 1989; Wagenknecht et al. 1992）（表51.2）。

Slattery等（1989）报道的截止值为15ng/mL，相当于他们的研究中吸烟者平均血清可替宁水平的6%。Pirkle等（1996）选择15ng/mL作为血清可替宁截止值，因为该值标志着美国第三次国家健康和营养检查调查报告的烟草使用者和非使用者血清可替宁水平双峰分布的分离点（NHANES Ⅲ，1988～1991）（$n=10270$，年龄≥4）。Pirkle的研究没有包括敏感性和特异性方面的信息。NHANES研究是基于相对较多的健康参与者的不同年龄和种族，其报告值15ng/mL符合ROC曲线中意大利人心血管疾病的横断面研究的截止值（MATISS项目，$n=3379$）（Seccareccia et al. 2003）。Caraballo等（2001）使用了NHANES Ⅲ数据集，但调查期延长（1988～1994年），成年参与者年龄为17岁（$n=15357$），使用Pirkle等（1996）指出的截止值验证并提出新的敏感性（89.5%）和特异性（98.5%）。他们随后报告了他们自己的11.4ng/mL的新截止值，对应的敏感性（73.2%）和特异性（98.4%）来自同一数据集（NHANES Ⅲ，1988～1994）的青少年人群（$n=2107$），这是使用ROC曲线计算的。表51.3所示的血清可替宁截止值在很大程度上具有可比性，只有少数例外（Assaf et al. 2002; Jeemon et al. 2010; Williams et al. 1979），并在8～20ng/mL范围内。然而，Benowitz等最近利用1999～2004年NHANES数据的ROC分析报道了更低的截止值，成人为3.08ng/mL，青少年为2.99ng/mL。

表51.2 血清可替宁截止值及其测定方法

参考文献	研究人群特征				截止值 /（ng/mL）	自我报告的数量		截止值测定方法
	说明	n	年龄	女性比例/%		吸烟者	非吸烟者	
Williams et al.（1979）	参加学校健康教育计划的高中生在美国随机采血	118	14～17岁	53	3.0	21	97	2×2表
Benowitz（1983）	一项评估可替宁消除半衰期的参与者。他们在研究病房停止吸烟（平均19.1h；范围为10.9～37.0h）	16	NA	NA	10	NA	NA	作者从不吸烟者的一系列浓度中选择了临界值，并报告说"没有不吸烟者的血可替宁值高于10ng/mL"
Slattery et al.（1989）	参与者在(1)一项关于饮食摄入和激素的横断面研究，(2)美国犹他州宫颈鳞状细胞癌的病例对照研究	(1) 112 (2) 547	17岁或以上	(1)仅男性 (2)仅女性	15	(1) 3 (2) 163	(1) 109 (2) 379	作者通过计算研究中吸烟者平均血清可替宁水平的6%来选择截止值
Wagenknecht et al.（1992）	美国心血管疾病研究队列中的年轻人	4984	17～30岁	NA	14	1540	3444	ROC

续表

参考文献	研究人群特征				截止值/(ng/mL)	自我报告的数量		截止值测定方法
	说明	n	年龄	女性比例/%		吸烟者	非吸烟者	
Pirkle et al.[①] (1996)	美国第三次全国健康和营养检查调查（NHANES）的参与者	10270	4岁或以上	50	15	NA	NA	作者从烟草使用者和非使用者血清可替宁双峰分布的分离点中选择了截止值
Nafstad et al.[①] (1996)	挪威奥斯陆生育院的孕妇	202	平均30岁（范围19～43岁）	100	14	42经常+24偶尔	136	传统使用的截止值（14ng/mL）是由作者自行选择的
Heller et al. (1998)	1987～1988年，在德国，世卫组织监测心血管疾病趋势和决定因素项目参与者中的追随者	3661	TBA	50.9	15	1227	2434	采用Wagenknecht等（1992）的研究结果中的截止值
Pichini et al. (2000)	西班牙巴塞罗那德尔马医院的孕妇	404	TBA	100	14	136	268	采用Nafstad等（1996）的研究结果中的截止值
Caraballo et al. (2001)	1988～1994年，美国第三次全国健康和营养检查调查中的成年人	15357	17岁或以上	53.8	15	4274	11083	采用Pirkle等（1996）的研究结果中的截止值
Assaf et al. (2002)	在Pawtucket心脏健康计划（1985～1986年）中进行可替宁试验的美国成年人	784	18～65岁	57.5	58（男性）30（女性）	131（男性）141（女性）	172（男性）279（女性）	ROC
Seccareccia et al. (2003)	意大利马蒂斯高级卫生研究所（MATISS）马蒂斯-马拉蒂心血管动脉硬化症项目参与者血清样本提供者	3379	20～79岁	39.5	15	977		ROC
Caraballo et al. (2004)	美国第三次全国青少年健康和营养检查调查(NHANES)，1988～1994年	2107	12～17岁	53.8	11.4	213	1894	ROC
Martinez et al. (2004)	美国亚利桑那州菲尼克斯市腺瘤复发饮食试验参与者	824	40～80岁	31	20	95	729	2×2表
Benowitz et al. (2008)	1999～2004年国家健康和营养检查调查（NHANES）的美国参与者	9901名成年人，5138名青少年	20岁以上、12～19岁	50.6的成年人，49.6的青少年	3.08成年人和2.99青少年	2340 515	7561 4623	ROC
Jeemon et al. (2010)	印度新德里心血管疾病监测项目参与者	426	18岁以上	TBA	40.35	142	284	ROC

① Benowitz（1983）、Pirkle等（1996）和Nafstad等（1996）未提供敏感性和特异性值，但本综述中包含了截止值，因为这些值是在审查了大量研究人群后获得的，或者截止值是参考其他研究的。

表51.3 尿液可替宁截止值及其测定方法

参考文献	研究人群特征				截止值/(ng/mL)	自我报告的数量		截止值测定方法
	说明	n	年龄	女性比例/%		吸烟者	非吸烟者	
Hoffmann et al.[①] (1984)	志愿者参加了一项关于侧流烟雾吸收的研究	NA	NA	NA	55	NA	NA	该值是从唾液烟碱水平恢复到基线水平时（即5h后）收集的尿样中获得的，研究受试者在密闭室内暴露于SHS（空气烟碱浓度为280mg/m³）1h
Riboli et al.[①] (1990)	来自10个国家的已婚不吸烟妇女	1369	年龄42～60岁	NA	50	NA	NA	选择截止值作为提供3.4%错误分类的值。它还与Hoffmann等（1984）的研究结果进行了比较
Pickett et al. 2005	1986年至1992年间在美国东波士顿社区健康中心就诊的孕妇，允许多次就诊	998	19岁或以上	NA	200	1272	3566	ROC
Zielinska-Danch (2007)	住在波兰索斯诺维茨的志愿者	327	19～60	57.2	550	111	216	作者从自我报告的吸烟者和非吸烟者的尿液可替宁双峰分布的分离点中选择了一个截止值
Goniewicz et al. (2011)	在美国旧金山和波兰西里西亚进行的三项不同研究中的吸烟者；以及在美国匹兹堡、波兰和墨西哥进行的其他三项研究中的非吸烟者	601	18岁或以上	52.7	31.5	373	228：仅被动吸烟者	ROC
Stragierowicz et al. (2013)	波兰母婴队列研究中的孕妇	69	平均26.4岁	100	53.0	17	52	ROC
Kim, Jung (2013)	2008～2010年韩国国家健康和营养检查调查（KNHANES）参与者，韩国	11629	19岁以上	55.5	164	2547	9082	ROC

① Hoffmann等（1984）和Riboli等（1990）未提供敏感性和特异性值，但本综述中包含了截止值，因为这些值是其他研究参考的少数可用值之一，或分别在审查大量研究人群后获得的值。

51.3 尿液可替宁

我们的综述仅包括少数关于尿液可替宁的研究（$n=5$），截止值在31.5～550ng/mL之间（Goniewicz et al. 2011; Hoffmann et al.1984; Pickett et al. 2005; Riboli et al. 1990; Zielinska-Danch et al. 2007）。Pickett等（2005）使用ROC曲线提供了200ng/mL的截止值，并根据美国东波士顿社区健康中心的998名孕妇的数据进行了计算。

一项波兰研究的327名受试者的截止值为550ng/mL（Zielinska-Danch et al. 2007）。这个截止值是根据自我报告的吸烟者和非吸烟者中尿液可替宁的双峰分布的一个分离点选择的。Goniewicz等（2011）通过对六项不同研究的受试者数据进行ROC分析，得出了31.5ng/mL的截止值，以区分成人主动吸烟者和被动吸烟者。Kim和Jung（2013）最近利用韩国国家健康和营养检查调查数据库（2008～2010，$n=11629$），发现尿液可替宁的截止值为164ng/mL。尿可替宁的截止值的敏感性为93.2%，特异性为95.7%。

51.4 确定截止值的问题

旨在确定截止值的唾液可替宁研究的结果因研究人群的特征而有很大差异（表51.1）。三项关于唾液可替宁的研究（Boyd et al.1998；Murray et al.1993；Stookey et al.1987）对戒烟临床试验的受试者进行了研究，而Jarvis等。（1987）对伦敦一家医院的门诊病人进行了一项研究。表51.2涵盖了血清可替宁的研究结果（Heller et al. 1998; Martinez et al. 2004; Slattery et al. 1989; Wagenknecht et al. 1992; Williams et al. 1979），参与者来自心血管疾病研究、健康教育项目和临床试验。戒烟临床试验或其他与健康相关的研究的参与者可能会低估他们的吸烟暴露水平。先前的研究也表明，社会规范压力会影响吸烟者低估自己的吸烟情况（Fendrich et al. 2005; Perez-Stable et al. 1990）。

孕妇是三项唾液研究（Boyd et al. 1998; Smith et al. 2014; Stragierowicz et al. 2013）、两项血清研究（Nafstad et al. 1996; Pichini et al. 2000）和一项尿液研究（Kim, Jung, 2013）的重点。人们普遍认为，怀孕会影响烟碱的摄取和新陈代谢（Rebagliato et al.1998）。上述研究确定，怀孕期间每支卷烟的唾液可替宁的比例（中位数为3.53ng/mL）远低于怀孕后（每支卷烟的中位数为9.87ng/mL）。这些发现表明，怀孕人群的截止值不能适用于一般人群。

表51.1中11项研究中的3种（Murray et al. 1993; Piercc et al. 1987; Smith et al. 2014）仅针对白种人进行。Wells等（1998）最近的一项研究报告称，美国少数族裔中偶尔吸烟或经常吸烟的女性的错误分类率（15.3%或2.8%）高于美国非西班牙裔白种人（6.0%或0.8%）。这种错误分类的模式在男性中很相似，但略高于女性。不同种族的特异性差异给定截止值被报道（Jarvis et al. 2008）：98.4%的白种人参与者和90.2%的南亚移民，这表明可能有必要对这些亚洲人口应用不同的截止值。在印度、巴基斯坦和孟加拉国，口服烟草制品的消费非常频繁，而妇女吸烟一度是禁忌，现在在日本、韩国和中国等一些亚洲国家急剧增加（WHO, 2008）。Benowitz等（2009）基于1999～2004年的NHANES数据（3078名吸烟者和13078名非吸烟者），报道了血清可替宁截止值因种族/民族而不同。这些值被发现，非西班牙裔黑人为5.92ng/mL，非西班牙裔白人为4.85ng/mL，墨西哥裔美国人为0.84ng/mL。尿液可替宁的估计截止值分别为15ng/mL和60ng/mL，分别由美国血清可替宁截止值（3ng/mL）和英国唾液可替宁截止值（12ng/mL）转换而成。这些值明显低于报道的韩国尿液可替宁截止值。这表明，从白种人人口中获得的值不能推广到其他种族/民族群体，应确定国家、民族和性别的截止值，并验证妇女的吸烟状况。

我们的综述表明，研究设计之间的一致性不足以便于比较。在不同的研究中，敏感性和特异性检测方法不同（即使用自我报告或可替宁检测）。当选择相同的截止值时，当在几项研究中使用可替宁检测而不是自我报告时，敏感性从90%下降到<80%（Benowitz et al. 2009; Jeemon et al. 2010; Martinez et al. 2004; Slattery et al. 1989）（图51.1）；这表明，自我报告并不是真实吸烟状况的准确指标。基于此概述，建议根据两个金标准及其对应的2×2表，提供给定截止值的敏感性和特异性，以便进行比较和验证。当特异性为95%时，也应报告敏感性，反之亦然，以比较在不同时间和/或不同人群和区域之间进行的类似研究类型。这些从基于大量人群的研究中获得的信息将非常有用。

51.5 在过去20年里截止值下降

虽然在个体研究中可替宁在唾液、血清或尿液中的水平可以用来区分吸烟者和非吸烟者，目前很难概括任何特定的研究敏感性和特异性，因其容易受种族、人群特征（如性别和位置）、烟草产品及其使用模式、SHS暴露和吸收途径的影响。因此，吸烟者和非吸烟者分类的最佳截止值可能因人口特征、地区或时间而不同。将1988～1994年和1999～2004年NHANES数据中获得的唾液可替宁截止值与Jarvis等在1987年和2008年在英国报道的两个唾液可替宁截止值进行了比较。表51.1显示这是真的。

Jarvis等（2008）最近报道的12ng/mL的截止值表明，在过去的20年里，英国人口的唾液可替宁截止值从14.2ng/mL下降到12ng/mL；然而，这比美国人口的差异相对较小。

根据1999～2004年NHANES数据（9901名成年人和5138名青少年）的ROC分析，Benowitz等（2009）最近报道的成年人的截止值（3.08ng/mL）和青少年的截止值（2.99ng/mL）远低于Caraballo等（2001）报道的早期数据和Caraballo等（2004）使用1988～1994年的NHANES数据：成年人15ng/mL（$n=15357$）和青少年11.4ng/mL（$n=2107$）（Caraballo et al. 2001, 2004）。这些研究者均采用了ROC分析。这些结果表明，美国人群的血清可替宁截止值在20年内有所下降。该较低的截止值可能是由于在过去的20年里，吸烟者吸烟数量的减少和非吸烟者暴露于SHS的减少，这是由于美国加大了烟草控制的力度，包括烟草消费税、无烟工作场所、青少年接触法和增加了控烟资金（Stoner, Foley, 2006）。

Jarvis等（2008）基于HSE数据的最新唾液可替宁截止值与Benowitz等最近报道的来自美国NHANES数据库的血清可替宁截止值进行了比较，使用了从血清可替宁到唾液可替宁截止值的转换因子（1.16）。这表明Jarvis等（2008）的结果远高于Benowitz等（2009）的结果。两国之间吸烟流行率的差异可能是造成截止值差异的原因。世界卫生组织关于全球烟草流行情况的一份报告（WHO, 2008）表明，英国和美国的年龄标准化成人吸烟流行率分别为28.4%和18.7%。非吸烟者中烟草烟雾生物标志物的分布应反映从不吸烟或被动吸烟的模式，而主动吸烟者的分布应反映他们的吸烟情况。这种分布可能会随着时间的推移而改变；随着有效的烟草控制，非吸烟者的值的分布将向左转移，更多的非吸烟者将有无法检测到的水平。这种向左的移动也可能导致截止点向左的移动，即达到一个较低的值。

本概述的局限性包括它主要使用PubMed数据库来提取文章，而忽略了其他可能也包含有用文章的数据库。然而，我们的综述中包含的文章数量更高，因为包含的文章的书目也被搜索。另一个局限性是概述通过自我报告或使用提供的2×2表的可替宁测试来计算敏感性和特异性，假设每个研究中使用的可替宁测试为100%准确。

本研究的目的是检查已报告可替宁截止值的研究，以及将这些研究报告的唾液或血清可替宁截止值应用于一般人群时存在的潜在问题。更希望为大规模人群的不同暴露类别提供特定国家或多种生物标志物截止值，即主动吸烟者与被动吸烟者以及被动与非吸烟者。这将使未来的研究人员能够为他们自己的研究进行比较和应用最相关的数据。此外，应用更多的研究来评估1999～2004年NHANES数据库中获得的新的血清截止值（3ng/mL）的效用将是有益的。

术语解释
- 敏感性（%）：通过生物监测将自我报告的吸烟者归类为吸烟者的百分比。
- 特异性（%）：生物监测将自我报告的非吸烟者分类为非吸烟者的百分比。

截止值的关键事实
- 烟草烟雾特有的生物标志物包括烟碱和可替宁；预计这是双峰的，反映了吸烟者和非吸烟者在人群中的两种基本分布。
- 两个关键的自我报告效度指标可以在二分模板中计算出来，比较自我报告的吸烟状况和生物标志物：敏感性（%）（经生物监测归类为吸烟者的自我报告吸烟者的百分比）和特异性（%）（经生物监测归类为非吸烟者的自我报告非吸烟者的百分比）。
- 设置截止值的目的是优化敏感性和特异性；然而，两者之间不可避免地会有一种权衡。
- 在双峰分布中，通常可以通过较低的截止值来实现较高的灵敏度；然而，当截止值较高时，特异性会降低。换句话说，更多的非吸烟者具有超过截止值的生物标志物水平。
- 相比之下，较高的截止值意味着较大的特异性，但敏感性较低。

要点总结
- 我们描述了如何导出截止值，并解释了在推广截止值时发生的问题。
- 我们在PubMed上对1985～2014年的英国文献进行了检索，关键词为"可替宁""截止"或"自我报告""吸烟状况"和"验证"。在总共获得的104篇文章中，有32篇提供了（1）敏感性和特异性和（2）确定所应用的截止值的方法。
- 可替宁截止值范围为10～25ng/mL（唾液可替宁）、10～20ng/mL（血清可替宁）和50～200ng/mL（尿液可替宁）。这些数据通常被用来通过2×2表或受试者的工作特征曲线来验证自我报告的吸烟状况。
- 虽然传统上被接受，但血清和唾液中的可替宁截止值分别为15ng/mL和14ng/mL；最近在美国和英国进行的大规模人群研究报告称，血清中3ng/mL值较低，唾液中12ng/mL值较低。
- 时间、地点和种族可以影响吸烟状况分类的最佳截止值。

参考文献

Assaf, A. R.; Parker, D.; Lapane, K. L.; McKenney, L.; Jr.; Carleton, R. A. (2002). Are there gender differences in self-reported smoking practices? Correlation with thiocyanate and cotinine levels insmokers and nonsmokers from the Pawtucket Heart Health Program. Journal of Women's Health, 11(10), 899-906.

Benner, C. L.; Bayona, J. M.; Caka, F. M.; Tang, H.; Kewis, L.; Crawford, J. et al. (1986). Chemical composition of environmentaltobacco smoke. 2. Particulate-phase compounds. Environmental Science, Technology, 23, 688-699.

Benowitz, N. L. (1983). The use of biologic fluid samples in assessing tobacco smoke consumption. In: NIDA research monograph, no. 48, Measurement in the analysis and treatment of smoking behavior. Rockville, MD: National Institute on Drug Abuse.

Benowitz, N. L. (1996). Cotinine as a biomarker of environmental tobacco smoke exposure. Epidemiologic Reviews, 18(2), 188-204.

Benowitz, N. L. (1999). Biomarkers of environmental tobacco smoke exposure. Environmental Health Perspectives, 107(Suppl. 2), 349-355.

Benowitz, N. L.; Bernert, J. T.; Caraballo, R. S.; Holiday, D. B.; Wang, J. (2009). Optimal serum cotinine levels for distinguishing cigarette smokers and nonsmokers within different racial/ethnic groups in the United States between 1999 and 2004. American Journal of Epidemiology, 169(2), 236-248.

Benowitz, N. L.; Jacob, P.; III (1994). Metabolism of nicotine to cotinine studied by a dual stable isotope method. Clinical Pharmacology and Therapeutics, 56(5), 483-493.

Benowitz, N. L.; Jacob, P.; III, Fong, I.; Gupta, S. (1994). Nicotine metabolic profile in man: comparison of cigarette smoking and transdermal nicotine. The Journal of Pharmacology and Experimental Therapeutics, 268(1), 296-303.

Boyd, N. R.; Windsor, R. A.; Perkins, L. L.; Lowe, J. B. (1998). Quality of measurement of smoking status by self-report and saliva cotinine among pregnant women. Maternal and Child Health Journal, 2(2), 77-83.

Caraballo, R. S.; Giovino, G. A.; Pechacek, T. F. (2004). Self-reported cigarette smoking vs. serum cotinine among U. S. adolescents. Nicotine, Tobacco Research, 6(1), 19-25.

Caraballo, R. S.; Giovino, G. A.; Pechacek, T. F.; Mowery, P. D. (2001). Factors associated with discrepancies between self-reports on cigarette smoking and measured serum cotinine levels among persons REFERENCESaged 17 years or older, Third National Health and Nutrition Examination Survey, 1988-1994. American Journal of Epidemiology, 153(8), 807-814.

Coultas, D. B.; Howard, C. A.; Peake, G. T.; Skipper, B. J.; Samet, J. M. (1987). Salivary cotinine levels and involuntary tobacco smoke exposure in children and adults in New Mexico. The American Review ofRespiratory Disease, 136(2), 305-309.

DeLorenze, G. N.; Kharrazi, M.; Kaufman, F. L.; Eskenazi, B.; Bernert, J. T. (2002). Exposure to environmental tobacco smoke in pregnant women: the association between self-report and serum cotinine. Environmental Research, 90(1), 21-32.

Eliopoulos, C.; Klein, J.; Koren, G. (1996). Validation of self-reported smoking by analysis of hair for nicotine and cotinine. Therapeutic Drug Monitoring, 18(5), 532-536.

Etter, J. F.; Vu, D. T.; Perneger, T. V. (2000). Saliva cotinine levels in smokers and nonsmokers. American Journal of Epidemiology, 151(3), 251-258.

Etzel, R. A. (1990). A review of the use of saliva cotinine as a marker of tobacco smoke exposure. Preventive Medicine, 19(2), 190-197.

Fendrich, M.; Mackesy-Amiti, M. E.; Johnson, T. P.; Hubbell, A.; Wislar, J. S. (2005). Tobacco-reporting validity in an epidemiological drug-use survey. Addictive Behaviors, 30(1), 175-181.

Flegal, K. M.; Brownie, C.; Haas, J. D. (1986). The effects of exposure misclassification on estimates of relative risk. American Journal of Epidemiology, 123, 736-751.

Goniewicz, M. L.; Eisner, M. D.; Lazcano-Ponce, E.; Zielinska-Danch, W.; Koszowski, B.; Sobczak, A. et al. (2011). Comparison of urine cotinine and the tobacco-specific nitrosamine metabolite 4-(methylnitrosamino)-1-(3-pyridyl)-1-butanol (NNAL) and their ratio to discriminate active from passive smoking. Nicotine, Tobacco Research, 13(3), 202-208.

Hammond, S. K.; Leaderer, B. P. (1987). A diffusion monitor to measure exposure to passive smoking. Environmental Science, Technology, 21(5), 494-497.

Hegaard, H. K.; Kjaergaard, H.; Moller, L. F.; Wachmann, H.; Ottesen, B. (2007). Determination of a saliva cotinine cut-off to distinguish pregnant smokers from pregnant non-smokers. Acta Obstetricia et Gynecologica Scandinavica, 86(4), 401-406.

Heller, W. D.; Scherer, G.; Sennewald, E.; Adlkofer, F. (1998). Misclassification of smoking in a follow-up population study in southern Germany. Journal of Clinical Epidemiology, 51(3), 211-218.

Hoffmann, D.; Haley, N. J.; Adams, J. D.; Brunnemann, K. D. (1984). Tobacco sidestream smoke: uptake by nonsmokers. Preventive Medicine, 13(6), 608-617.

International Agency for Research on Cancer. (2004). IARC monographs on the evaluation of carcinogenic risks to humans. Tobacco smoke and involuntary smoking: Vol. 38. Lyon: International Agency for Research on Cancer.

Jaakkola, M. S.; Jaakkola, J. J. (1997). Assessment of exposure to environmental tobacco smoke. The European Respiratory Journal, 10(10), 2384-2397.

Jacob, P. I.; Byrd, G. D. (1999). Use of gas chromatographic and mass spectrometric techniques for the determination of nicotine and its metabolites. In: J. W. Gorrod, P. I. Jacob (Eds.), Analytical determination of nicotine and related compounds and their metabolites (pp. 191-224). 1999. Amsterdam: Elsevier Science.

Jarvis, M. J.; Fidler, J.; Mindell, J.; Feyerabend, C.; West, R. (2008). Assessing smoking status in children, adolescents and adults: cotinine cut-points revisited. Addiction, 103(9), 1553-1561.

Jarvis, M.; Tunstall-Pedoe, H.; Feyerabend, C.; Vesey, C.; Salloojee, Y. (1984). Biochemical markers of smoke absorption and self reported exposure to passive smoking. Journal of Epidemiology and Community Health, 38(4), 335-339.

Jarvis, M.; Tunstall-Pedoe, H.; Feyerabend, C.; Vesey, C.; Salloojee, Y. (1987). Comparison of tests used to distinguishsmokers from nonsmokers. American Journal of Public Health, 77(11), 1435-1438.

Jeemon, P.; Agarwal, S.; Ramakrishnan, L.; Gupta, R.; Snehi, U.; Chaturvedi, V. et al. (2010). Validation of self-reported smoking status by measuring serum cotinine levels: an Indian perspective. The National Medical Journal of India, 23(3), 134-136.

Kawachi, I.; Colditz, G. A. (1996). Invited commentary: confounding, measurement error, and publication bias in studies of passive smoking. American Journal of Epidemiology, 144(10), 909-915.

Kim, S.; Jung, A. (2013). Optimum cutoff value of urinary cotinine distinguishing South Korean adult smokers from nonsmokers using data from the KNHANES (2008-2010). Nicotine, Tobacco Research, 15(9), 1608-1616.

Luepker, R. V.; Pallonen, U. E.; Murray, D. M.; Pirie, P. L. (1989). Validity of telephone surveys in assessing cigarette smoking in young adults. American Journal of Public Health, 79(2), 202-204.

Martinez, M. E.; Reid, M.; Jiang, R.; Einspahr, J.; Alberts, D. S. (2004). Accuracy of self-reported smoking status among participants in a chemoprevention trial. Preventive Medicine, 38(4), 492-497.

McNeill, A. D.; West, R. J.; Jarvis, M.; Jackson, P.; Bryant, A. (1986). Cigarette withdrawal symptoms in adolescent smokers. Psychopharmacology, 90(4), 533-536.

Murray, R. P.; Connett, J. E.; Lauger, G. G.; Voelker, H. T. (1993). Error in smoking measures: effects of intervention on relations of cotinine and carbon monoxide to self-reported smoking. The Lung Health Study Research Group. American Journal of Public Health, 83(9), 1251-1257.

Nafstad, P.; Kongerud, J.; Botten, G.; Urdal, P.; Silsand, T.; Pedersen, B. S. et al. (1996). Fetal exposure to tobacco smoke products: a comparison between self-reported maternal smoking and concentrations of cotinine and thiocyanate in cord serum. Acta Obstetricia et Gynecologica Scandinavica, 75(10), 902-907.

National Research Council. (1986). Environmental tobacco smoke: Measuring exposures and assessing health effects. Washington, DC: National Academy Press.

National Research Council. (1989). Biologic markers of pulmonary toxicology. Washington, DC: National Academy Press.

Ogden, M. W.; Maiolo, K. C.; Nelson, P. R.; Heavner, D. L.; Green, C. R. (1993). Artifacts in determining the vapor-particulate phase distribution of environmental tobacco smoke nicotine. Environmental Technology, 14, 779-785.

Perez-Stable, E. J.; Marin, B. V.; Marin, G.; Brody, D. J.; Benowitz, N. L. (1990). Apparent underreporting of cigarette consumption among Mexican American smokers. American Journal of Public Health, 80(9), 1057-1061.

Pichini, S.; Basagana, X. B.; Pacifici, R.; Garcia, O.; Puig, C.; Vall, O. et al. (2000). Cord serum cotinine as a biomarker of fetal exposure to cigarette smoke at the end of pregnancy. Environmental Health Perspectives, 108(11), 1079-1083.

Pickett, K. E.; Rathouz, P. J.; Kasza, K.; Wakschlag, L. S.; Wright, R. (2005). Self-reported smoking, cotinine levels, and patterns of smoking in pregnancy. Paediatric and Perinatal Epidemiology, 19(5), 368-376.

Pierce, J. P.; Dwyer, T.; DiGiusto, E.; Carpenter, T.; Hannam, C.; Amin, A. et al. (1987). Cotinine validation of self-reported smoking in commercially run community surveys. Journal of Chronic Diseases, 40(7), 689-695.

Pirkle, J. L.; Flegal, K. M.; Bernert, J. T.; Brody, D. J.; Etzel, R. A.; Maurer, K. R. (1996). Exposure of the US population to environmental tobacco smoke: the Third National Health and Nutrition Examination Survey, 1988 to 1991. JAMA, 275(16), 1233-1240.

Rebagliato, M.; Bolumar, F.; Florey, C. V.; Jarvis, M. J.; Perez-Hoyos, S.; Hernandez-Aguado, I. et al. (1998). Variations in cotinine levels in smokers during and after pregnancy. American Journal of Obstetrics and Gynecology, 178(3), 568-571.

Riboli, E.; Preston-Martin, S.; Saracci, R.; Haley, N. J.; Trichopoulos, D.; Becher, H. et al. (1990). Exposure of nonsmoking women to environmental tobacco smoke: a 10-country collaborative study. Cancer Causes, Control, 1(3), 243-252.

Seccareccia, F.; Zuccaro, P.; Pacifici, R.; Meli, P.; Pannozzo, F.; Freeman, K. M. et al. (2003). Serum cotinine as a marker of environmental tobacco smoke exposure in epidemiological studies: the experience of the MATISS project. European Journal of Epidemiology, 18(6), 487-492.

Slattery, M. L.; Hunt, S. C.; French, T. K.; Ford, M. H.; Williams, R. R. (1989). Validity of cigarette smoking habits in three epidemiologic studies in Utah. Preventive Medicine, 18(1), 11-19.

Smith, J. J.; Robinson, R. F.; Khan, B. A.; Sosnoff, C. S.; Dillard, D. A. (2014). Estimating cotinine associations and a saliva cotinine level to identify active cigarette smoking in Alaska native pregnant women. Maternal and Child Health Journal, 18(1), 120-128.

SRNT Subcommittee on Biochemical Verification. (2002). Biochemical verification of tobacco use and cessation. Nicotine, Tobacco Research, 4(2), 149-159.

Stoner, W. I.; Foley, B. X. (2006). Current tobacco control policy trends in the United States. Clinics in Occupational and Environmental Medicine, 5(1), 85-99. ix.

Stookey, G. K.; Katz, B. P.; Olson, B. L.; Drook, C. A.; Cohen, S. J. (1987). Evaluation of biochemical validation measures in determination of smoking status. Journal of Dental Research, 66(10), 1597-1601.

Stragierowicz, J.; Mikołajewska, K.; Zawadzka-Stolarz, M.; Polanska, K.; Ligocka, D. (2013). Estimation of cutoff values of cotinine in urine and saliva for pregnant women in Poland. Article ID 386784, 11 pages. BioMed Research International. 2013, https://dx. doi. org/ 10. 1155/2013/386784 [Epub 2013 Oct 21].

U. S. Department of Health and Human Services. (2006). The health consequences of involuntary smoking: A report of the surgeon general. Rockville, MD: Public Health Service, Centers for Disease Control, Center for Health Promotion and Education, Office on Smoking and Health.

Wagenknecht, L. E.; Burke, G. L.; Perkins, L. L.; Haley, N. J.; Friedman, G. D. (1992). Misclassification of smoking status in the CARDIA study: a comparison of self-report with serum cotinine levels. American Journal of Public Health, 82(1), 33-36.

Warren, C. W.; Jones, N. R.; Eriksen, M. P.; Asma, S. (2006). Patterns of global tobacco use in young people and implications for future chronic disease burden in adults. Lancet, 367(9512), 749-753.

Wells, A. J.; English, P. B.; Posner, S. F.; Wagenknecht, L. E.; PerezStable, E. J. (1998). Misclassification rates for current smokers misclassified as nonsmokers. American Journal of Public Health, 88(10), 1503-1509.

Williams, C. L.; Eng, A.; Botvin, G. J.; Hill, P.; Wynder, E. L. (1979). Validation of students' self-reported cigarette smoking status with plasma cotinine levels. American Journal of Public Health, 69(12), 1272-1274.

World Health Organization. (2008). WHO report on the global tobacco epidemic, 2008. In The MPOWER package, Geneva. 08.

Zielinska-Danch, W.; Wardas, W.; Sobczak, A.; SzoltysekBoldys, I. (2007). Estimation of urinary cotinine cut-off points distinguishing non-smokers, passive and active smokers. Biomarkers, 12(5), 484-496.

52
戒烟预期问卷

Lorra Garey[1], *Fiammetta Cosci*[2], *Michael J. Zvolensky*[1]

1. Department of Psychology, University of Houston, Houston, TX, United States
2. Department of Health Sciences, University of Florence, Florence, Italy

缩略语

SAEQ 戒烟预期问卷

52.1 吸烟：流行率和全球影响

烟草使用是世界上可预防的死亡和残疾的主要原因（WHO，2008），每年造成近600万人死亡（WHO，2015b）。吸烟导致死亡的人数超过结核病、艾滋病毒/艾滋病和疟疾的总和（WHO，2015b）。烟草使用也会产生严重的社会、环境和经济后果（WHO，2015b）。事实上，全球烟草使用的经济负担如此之大，据估计将超过所有低收入和中等收入国家的年度卫生支出总额（Gibson et al. 2013）。尽管造成了众所周知的健康和经济后果，但全球仍有约11亿人吸烟（WHO，2015a）。

52.2 理论和临床关系：戒烟预期和吸烟

近年来，人们对了解可能影响吸烟行为的认知过程越来越感兴趣（King et al. 1996; Schwarzer, 2008）。与吸烟有关的一组很有前途的认知过程是预期。预期被概念化为个人从其行为中预计的结果（Bandura, 1977b）。在吸烟文献中，研究人员主要关注吸烟者对吸烟使用的结果影响的预期（Brandon et al. 1999）。然而，近年来，人们对了解戒烟影响的预期越来越感兴趣（Svicher et al. 2017）。与对吸烟结果影响的预期相反，戒烟预期是对烟碱戒断的急性影响的信念；因此，它们是戒烟的短期心理和生理后果（Abrams et al. 2011）。

健康行为的几个著名理论包括反应预期理论（Kirsch, Lynn, 1999）、社会学习理论（Bandura, 1977a）、健康信念模型（Rosenstock, 1974）和预期理论（Brandon et al.1999），强调对预期结果的评估。应用于物质使用，这些理论共同假设物质使用预期影响药物的使用和效果。例如，从理论上讲，在戒烟后预期的负面后果大于积极后果的吸烟者可能不太可能尝试戒烟（Hendricks et al. 2011）。相反，那些预期主要是积极后果而很少有负面后果的人可能在戒烟方面表现出更多的成功。与理论研究一致，戒烟预期与一系列吸烟后果有关。例如，消极的戒烟预期与更严重的戒断、更严重的烟草依赖症状和更低的戒烟成功概率有关（Hendricks et al. 2011, 2014; Hendricks, Leventhal, 2013）。事实上，吸烟剥夺预期经常得到吸烟者的认可，这通常反映了他们对戒烟期间可能经历的负面后果的担忧（Svicher et al. 2017），如戒断症状。因此，短期戒烟预期在一定程度上可能是维持吸烟的一个病因（Farris et al. 2015）。然而，有证据表明，在短暂剥夺吸烟的情况下，可以操纵戒烟预期（Tate et al.1994）。从理论上讲，在戒烟尝试的背景下挑战戒烟预期可能有助于成功戒烟。

52.3 测量发展：戒烟预期问卷

戒烟预期在动态吸烟过程中的理论重要性导致了戒烟预期问卷（SAEQ; Abrams et al.2011）的发展。这项测量是在主要是白种人的成年日常吸烟者的样本中制订的。SAEQ由28个项目组成，包括四个独特的因素：消极情绪、躯体症状、有害后果和积极后果（见表52.1）。消极情绪因素是指人们认为戒烟会导致的消极情绪因素（如我的脾气会变得暴躁）。躯体症状因素评估了人们期望的因戒烟而产生的负面生理反应（如我将有胃气）。有害后果因素衡量的是戒烟所预期的心理或生理上的负面影响（如我感觉我正在失去控制）。积极后果因素评估戒烟预期的积极后果（即我会感到精力充沛）（Abrams et al. 2011）。前三个分量表代表对戒烟的消极期望，而第四个分量表代表对戒烟的积极期望。值得注意的是，躯体症状和有害后果因素通常被概念化为内感受性威胁相关的戒烟预期（Farris, Langdon et al. 2015; Farris, Paulus et al. 2015），因为它们评估（错误）对内部身体症状和感觉的解释（Spielberger, Spielberger, 1966）。SAEQ分量表的评分算法和总分见表52.2。

表52.1 戒烟预期问卷（SAEQ）

戒烟预期问卷（SAEQ）							
说明：评估如果你在一天内戒烟而不使用任何其他形式的烟碱，你认为每一种后果的可能性或不可能性							
项目	不太可能						很有可能
（1）我的喉咙会觉得干	0	1	2	3	4	5	6
（2）我会觉得很生气	0	1	2	3	4	5	6
（3）我觉得我要疯了	0	1	2	3	4	5	6
（4）我会感到精力充沛	0	1	2	3	4	5	6
（5）我的脚会感到刺痛	0	1	2	3	4	5	6
（6）我的脾气会变得暴躁	0	1	2	3	4	5	6
（7）我感觉我正在失去控制	0	1	2	3	4	5	6
（8）我会感到快乐	0	1	2	3	4	5	6
（9）我会感到呼吸急促	0	1	2	3	4	5	6
（10）我会感到沮丧	0	1	2	3	4	5	6
（11）我觉得我快死了	0	1	2	3	4	5	6
（12）我发现记住一些东西很容易	0	1	2	3	4	5	6
（13）我将有胃气	0	1	2	3	4	5	6
（14）我会感到紧张	0	1	2	3	4	5	6
（15）我会让自己在别人面前难堪	0	1	2	3	4	5	6

戒烟预期问卷（SAEQ）							
说明：评估如果你在一天内戒烟而不使用任何其他形式的烟碱，你认为每一种后果的可能性或不可能性							
项目	不太可能			很有可能			
（16）我会感到平静	0	1	2	3	4	5	6
（17）我会比平时出更多的汗	0	1	2	3	4	5	6
（18）我很难和难相处的人相处	0	1	2	3	4	5	6
（19）我周围的东西似乎不真实	0	1	2	3	4	5	6
（20）我会睡上整整一个晚上	0	1	2	3	4	5	6
（21）我会感到头晕	0	1	2	3	4	5	6
（22）我会感到焦虑	0	1	2	3	4	5	6
（23）我会恐慌	0	1	2	3	4	5	6
（24）我发现集中注意力很容易	0	1	2	3	4	5	6
（25）我的胸部会觉得紧	0	1	2	3	4	5	6
（26）我的神经会很紧张	0	1	2	3	4	5	6
（27）我将会心脏病发作	0	1	2	3	4	5	6
（28）我会感到身体很舒服	0	1	2	3	4	5	6

注：重新印自 Abrams, K.;Zvolensky, M. J.;Dorman, L.;Gonzalez, A.;Mayer, M. (2011). Development and validation of the smoking abstinence expectancies questionnaire.Nicotine, Tobacco Research, 13(12), 1296-1304, 经牛津大学出版社许可。

表52.2　SAEQ评分点

项目编号	SAEQ分量表
2, 6, 10, 14, 18, 22, 26	消极情绪
1, 5, 9, 13, 17, 21, 25	躯体症状
3, 7, 11, 15, 19, 23, 27	有害后果
4, 8, 12, 16, 20, 24, 28	积极后果

注：表中总结了加载到相应SAEQ子量表中的项目。要计算每个SAEQ子量表的得分，请将加载到子量表的项目相加。总分是对积极后果子量表中的项目进行反向评分后，所有项目的所有回答的总和。

　　Abrams等（2011）在SAEQ的发展过程中进行了初步的心理测量测试。该小组发现了这些因素之间关系的证据、不同因素的收敛和鉴别效度，并构建了阻碍或促进戒烟的理论以及重测信度。具体来说，就是带有积极结果因素的结果。在收敛效度方面，所有负预期因素与戒断严重程度和烟草依赖正相关，而正结果与这些因素负相关。消极情绪和不良后果与吸烟率呈正相关。对戒烟有害后果的预期也与过去的戒烟行为呈负相关，而对积极后果的预期则与该变量呈正相关。在鉴别效度测试中，所有的负预期因素与负性倾向正相关。积极后果与消极情绪呈负相关，与积极情绪呈正相关。随着时间的推移，所有因素都证明了可接受的测试稳定性。

　　重要的是，尽管使用该指标的工作主要集中在个人因素上，但Abrams等（2011）将SAEQ总分纳入了他们对该指标的评估中。值得注意的是，SAEQ总分代表了更多的戒烟消极预期，因为分数是在对积极后果项目进行反向编码后，将所有项目相加得出的（Abrams et al. 2011）。总分与评估吸烟恶化消极预期的因素呈正相关，与积极后果呈负相关。观察到的趋同分析和判别分析的趋势通常反映了观察到的与禁烟相关的消极预期的趋势。也就是说，总分与戒断严重程度、烟草依赖、吸烟率和负面影响呈正相关，而与戒烟史呈负相关。在某种程度上，在总分中观察到的关联模式的相似性以及与戒烟相关的消极预期是总分评分算法的直接结果。总分具有较高的重测信度。

综上所述，Abrams等（2011）的研究结果为SAEQ作为心理测量学上对戒烟积极和消极预期的有力指标提供了初步支持。在其评估的背景下，对SAEQ因素和总分的广泛结构效度证据进行了审查和综合。研究结果支持独特但相关的因素，这些因素表明与核心吸烟行为、过程以及随时间变化的稳定性的不同强度。这一信息的综合表明了研究人员的立场，这一措施可以作为一个重要的研究和临床工具，因为它有助于理解成功戒烟的动态模型和影响吸烟、治疗计划和发展的认知过程。SAEQ在吸烟行为动态过程中的启发式模型见图52.1，包括戒烟前行为、戒烟和复发（Baker et al. 2011; Hendershot et al. 2011）。

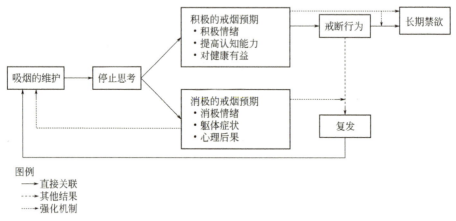

图 52.1 积极和消极的戒烟预期在动态戒烟过程中的作用的启发式模型

启发式模型代表了吸烟行为、积极和消极的戒烟预期和戒烟行为之间的关联。实线表示直接关联。短划线表示其他结果。点线表示强化机制。

性别差异：SAEQ的性别差异已经被报道过，但鉴于这些差异在不同样本之间的不一致性，这些差异的稳健性是推测性的。例如，一些研究发现，女性报告的有害后果因素得分高（Abrams et al. 2011），而其他研究却没有发现这一因素与性别之间的任何联系（Farris, Langdon et al. 2015; Farris, Paulus et al.2015; Kauffman et al. 2017; Zvolensky et al. 2017）。在躯体症状方面也有类似的混合发现，一些研究表明两者有关联（Farris, Langdon et al. 2015），而另一些研究报告没有差异或关联（Abrams et al. 2011; Farris, Paulus et al. 2015; Kauffman et al. 2017; Zvolensky et al. 2017）。事实上，消极情绪因素是唯一一个在戒烟预期方面一直与性别相关的研究（Abrams et al. 2011; Robles et al. 2017）。事实上，有一致的证据表明，女性在这方面的得分高于男性。最后，虽然Abrams等（2011）没有发现积极后果的性别差异，但这一发现并未在独立样本中进行调查。总的来说，有一些科学证据表明SAEQ可能存在性别差异，尤其是在消极情绪方面，但还需要进一步的研究。

交叉验证。几个独立的研究小组已经评估了SAEQ因素和吸烟行为之间的联系，以及被认为阻碍或促进戒烟成功的结构。为了将这项工作置于更大的吸烟文献中，SAEQ的交叉验证工作集中于与内感受性威胁相关的负面戒烟预期（即躯体症状和有害后果）（Farris, Langdon et al. 2015; Farris, Paulus et al. 2015; Kauffman et al. 2017; Zvolensky et al. 2017）。在某种程度上，该研究主要集中在这些因素上，以解决日益增长的理论和实证文献中的一个关键差距，这些文献假设使用卷烟是避免和逃避吸烟者的负面内部刺激的一种手段（Baker et al. 2004）。也就是说，在这项工作之前，我们还不清楚与内感受性威胁相关的戒烟预期如何符合这些更大的烟草使用概念模型。

在这一假设下，研究人员进行评估并发现，内感受性威胁戒烟预期因素与吸烟行为（即吸烟率和烟草依赖）相关（Farris, Paulus et al. 2015; Kauffman et al. 2017; Zvolensky et al. 2017）和维持并加剧烟草依赖的心理构建，包括焦虑症状、创伤后应激障碍症状、睡眠障碍症状、情绪失调、焦虑敏感性和负面情绪的存在（Farris, Langdon et al. 2015; Farris, Paulus et al. 2015; Kauffman et al. 2017; Zvolensky et al. 2017）。此外，内感受性威胁戒烟预期因素与吸烟动机和期望吸烟减轻负面影响、感知的戒烟障碍和之前的戒烟相关问题密切相关（Farris, Langdon et al. 2015; Farris, Paulus et al. 2015; Kauffman et al. 2017; Zvolensky et al. 2017）。重要的是，内感受性威胁戒烟预期为情感脆弱性和戒烟前认知过程之间的关系提供了一个机制功能，情感脆弱性使一个人有更大的使用问题和戒烟前的认知过程（Farris, Langdon, et al. 2015; Leventhal, Zvolensky, 2015）。

随着对内感受性威胁戒烟预期对吸烟行为和过程的影响的基础理解，研究工作已经开始评估其他SAEQ因素。在最近的一篇文章中Robles等（2017）研究人员发现，经济压力通过抑郁症状间接影响了对消极情绪后果的戒断预期。在双变量相关分析中，消极情绪与情绪过程（即消极情绪和抑郁症状）、影响调节吸烟过程（即消极情绪减少吸烟动机和感知戒烟障碍）以及教育呈正相关。有趣的是，对于消极情绪后果和抑郁症状的戒断预期只有11.6%的差异；因此，这些结构中的每一个都利用了与吸烟维持和戒烟行为相关的独特过程。

人群：已经证明了SAEQ在不同吸烟人群中适用性的普遍性。事实上，SAEQ已经被用于寻求治疗的吸烟者（Farris, Paulus et al. 2015; Zvolensky et al. 2017）和不寻求治疗的吸烟者（Abrams et al. 2011; Kauffman et al. 2017）。这些研究的比较显示，与不寻求治疗的吸烟者相比，寻求治疗的吸烟者总体上有更高的消极戒烟期望。这一观察在某种程度上挖掘了寻求治疗的吸烟者的严重性。具体来说，与不寻求治疗的药物使用者相比，寻求治疗的药物使用者往往是更严重的药物使用人群，这可以从严重的依赖性、更多的负面后果、对其使用的控制更少、更多的使用和使用频率得到证明（Ray et al. 2017）。因此，寻求治疗的吸烟者可能表现出与不寻求治疗的吸烟者不同的特征和信念。SAEQ也适用于脆弱人群，包括患有精神病的吸烟者（Farris, Paulus et al. 2015）。在这项工作中，有和没有精神病的人在有害后果和躯体症状方面的差异的统计测试支持有害后果因素的显著得分。重要的是，交叉研究比较支持一个普遍的趋势，即在有害后果和躯体症状方面，有精神病的人得分更高。然而，这些差异的统计意义还需要进一步调查。在不同的人群中，值得注意的是，SAEQ与情感脆弱性（如焦虑敏感性和消极影响）以及吸烟行为和过程之间出现了相似的关联模式。然而，这些关联的程度因人群而异。因此，有初步证据表明SAEQ可以区分吸烟者群体，并识别出那些可能更容易受到情绪困扰的人，这些情绪困扰可能会阻碍戒烟行为或成功。

临床和研究意义。临床上，SAEQ有几个重要的考虑因素。首先，SAEQ可能有助于筛查吸烟者戒烟难度的增加，从而有助于建立成功戒烟的预测模型。例如，那些期望戒烟会带来更多负面后果（如负面影响或不愉快的生理感受）的人可能不太可能成功戒烟。SAEQ提供了一种简单的、标准化的方法来评估这些维度，可用于告知治疗方案。其次，SAEQ有可能使临床医生在戒烟治疗期间靶向特定的预期。事实上，患有SAEQ的临床患者可以为临床医生提供一个机会，以更高的特异性分离和靶向特异性戒断预期。例如，如果戒烟后出现医学或精神症状的可能性是最严重的或可能干扰戒烟过程的，临床医生可能会试图改变这种不合理的信念。这种方法将允许一个更个性化的治疗计划，可能促进更大的戒烟成功。最后，继续使用SAEQ可以使研究人员和临床医生更广泛地了解影响吸烟的认知过程，包括戒烟前行为、戒烟和复发（见图52.1）。

52.4 替代措施

有两种不同的戒烟预期方法值得简要评论。首先，意大利版SAEQ目前正在流通（Svicher et al. 2017）。翻译版SAEQ在366名意大利吸烟者身上进行了测试。探索性因素分析技术与翻译措施支持一个三因素的解决方案。因此，文化方面的考虑可能会在将来引起这种措施的注意。因此，与SAEQ合作时，在对不同文化的人群进行管理时应谨慎行事。其次，Hendricks等（2011）编制了戒烟问卷。这项测量评估了短期、中期和长期的戒烟预期。尽管这项措施涉及更多的戒烟预期，但它可能会给研究参与者和临床客户带来过重的负担。具体地说，这个度量包含的条目几乎是SAEQ的两倍。此外，戒烟问卷与成人吸烟后果问卷有相当大的重叠（Copeland et al. 1995）。因此，这一措施可能不能真正评估目前在理论或经验工作中概念化的戒烟预期的潜在症结。

52.5 未来方向

构建有效性。四因素SAEQ结构尚未通过验证性因素分析技术进行评估。因此，这种结构的可复制性仍然是未知的。同样，研究也没有评估跨群体（即性别、种族/人种和年龄）或随着时间的推移的结构的稳定性。这限制了研究人员能够得出结论的程度，即观察到的差异是真实差异的结果，而不是测量偏差的人为结果（Vandenberg, Lance, 2000）。此外，SAEQ与戒烟之间的理论化的前瞻性关系尚未得到实证研究，而且在本质上仍然是理论上的。这些疏忽要求考虑对SAEQ进行额外的心理测量测试。

可塑性。未来研究的一个重要领域将是评估SAEQ对治疗反应的延展性。事实上，尽管有理论研究表明戒烟预期是一个可针对性的治疗因素，但没有研究表明参与戒烟治疗后SAEQ的变化。因此，这些变化可能如何影响戒烟尚不清楚。

发展起源。对SAEQ的科学调查产生了有希望的发现。事实上，目前对维持戒烟预期的了解是有限的。对戒烟预期感兴趣的理论工作认为，学习历史或环境压力源可能会影响它们的发展和维持。然而，对SAEQ的使用和理解，包括其组成部分和总分，仍然不发达。SAEQ在吸烟行为的负强化模型中概念化风险和保护性吸烟过程的模型中的独特作用有待继续调查（见图52.1）。

52.6 结论

戒烟预期可以阻碍或促进戒烟行为，从而实现戒烟成功。戒烟预期问卷是一个心理测量学上评估戒烟预期可靠临床相关工具。此外，解释戒烟预期问卷的性质、它在动态吸烟过程中的作用以及它与精神病理学和可能阻碍戒烟成功的过程的关系的工作继续增加。未来的工作需要进一步构建该措施的效度，揭示其对操纵的可塑性，并评估其在更大的吸烟行为和认知模型中的地位。

术语解释
- **情感脆弱性**：提高了精神病理症状，包括焦虑和/或抑郁症状，这可能会使一个人患精神障碍的风险增加。
- **焦虑敏感性**：是指一个人害怕与焦虑相关的症状和感觉的倾向。

- 内感受性：与一个人的内部状态有关，包括认知和内部生理感觉。
- 戒烟预期：相信戒烟的积极后果和消极后果。

要点总结

- 本章着重于戒烟预期和评估这些预期的常用方法，即戒烟预期问卷。
- 理论和实证工作支持戒烟预期与更有问题的吸烟和戒烟结果之间的关系。
- 戒烟预期问卷作为戒烟预期的有效测量指标，显示出强烈的心理测量特征，在几个独立样本中通过强的收敛和鉴别效度和内部一致性得到证明。
- 统计建模的最新进展为未来关于戒烟预期问卷的结构效度论证的工作提供了一个领域。
- 我们认为，戒烟预期问卷是一种心理测量学上可靠的临床相关工具，用于评估戒烟预期，并提倡将其作为临床和研究环境中的筛查工具。

参考文献

Abrams, K.; Zvolensky, M. J.; Dorman, L.; Gonzalez, A.; Mayer, M. (2011). Development and validation of the smoking abstinence expectancies questionnaire. Nicotine, Tobacco Research. 13(12), 1296-1304. https://doi. org/10. 1093/ntr/ntr184.

Baker, T. B.; Mermelstein, R.; Collins, L. M.; Piper, M. E.; Jorenby, D. E.; Smith, S. S. et al. (2011). New methods for tobacco dependence treatment research. Annals of Behavioral Medicine, 41(2), 192-207.

Baker, T. B.; Piper, M. E.; McCarthy, D. E.; Majeskie, M. R.; Fiore, M. C. (2004). Addiction motivation reformulated: an affective processing model of negative reinforcement. Psychological Review, 111(1), 33.

Bandura, A. (1977a). Self-efficacy: toward a unifying theory of behavioral change. Psychological Review, 84(2), 191.

Bandura, A. (1977b). Social learning theory. Englewood Cliffs, NJ: Prentice-Hall.

Brandon, T. H.; Juliano, L. M.; Copeland, A. L. (1999). Expectancies for tobacco smoking. In I. Kirsch (Ed.), How expectancies shape experience (pp. 263-299). Washington, DC: American Psychological Association.

Copeland, A. L.; Brandon, T. H.; Quinn, E. P. (1995). The Smoking Consequences Questionnaire-Adult: measurement of smoking outcome expectancies of experienced smokers. Psychological Assessment, 7(4), 484.

Farris, S. G.; Langdon, K. J.; DiBello, A. M.; Zvolensky, M. J. (2015). Why do anxiety sensitive smokers perceive quitting as difficult?The role of expecting "interoceptive threat" during acute abstinence. Cognitive Therapy and Research, 39(2), 236-244.

Farris, S. G.; Paulus, D. J.; Gonzalez, A.; Mahaffey, B. L.; Bromet, E. J.; Luft, B. J. et al. (2015). Anxiety sensitivity mediates the association between post-traumatic stress symptom severity and interoceptive threat-related smoking abstinence expectancies among World Trade Center disaster-exposed smokers. Addictive Behaviors, 51, 204-210.

Gibson, G. J.; Loddenkemper, R.; Lundb€ack, B.; Sibille, Y. (2013). Respiratory health and disease in Europe: The new European lung white book. European Respiratory Journal, 42(3), 559-563.

Hendershot, C. S.; Witkiewitz, K.; George, W. H.; Marlatt, G. A. (2011). Relapse prevention for addictive behaviors. Substance Abuse Treatment, Prevention, and Policy, 6(1), 17.

Hendricks, P. S.; Leventhal, A. M. (2013). Abstinence-related expectancies predict smoking withdrawal effects: Implications for possible causal mechanisms. Psychopharmacology, 230(3), 363-373.

Hendricks, P. S.; Westmaas, J. L.; Ta Park, V. M.; Thorne, C. B.; Wood, S. B.; Baker, M. R. et al. (2014). Smoking abstinence-related expectancies among American Indians, African Americans, and women: potential mechanisms of tobacco-related disparities. Psychology of Addictive Behaviors, 28(1), 193.

Hendricks, P. S.; Wood, S. B.; Baker, M. R.; Delucchi, K. L.; Hall, S. M. (2011). The Smoking Abstinence Questionnaire: measurement of smokers' abstinence-related expectancies. Addiction, 106(4), 716-728.

Kauffman, B. Y.; Farris, S. G.; Alfano, C. A.; Zvolensky, M. J. (2017). Emotion dysregulation explains the relation between insomnia symptoms and negative reinforcement smoking cognitions among daily smokers. Addictive Behaviors, 72, 33-40.

King, T. K.; Marcus, B. H.; Pinto, B. M.; Emmons, K. M.; Abrams, D. B. (1996). Cognitive-behavioral mediators of changing multiple behaviors: smoking and a sedentary lifestyle. Preventive Medicine, 25(6), 684-691.

Kirsch, I.; Lynn, S. J. (1999). Automaticity in clinical psychology. American Psychologist, 54(7), 504.

Leventhal, A. M.; Zvolensky, M. J. (2015). Anxiety, depression, and cigarette smoking: a transdiagnostic vulnerability framework to understanding emotion-smoking comorbidity. Psychological Bulletin, 141(1), 176.

Ray, L. A.; Bujarski, S.; Yardley, M. M.; Roche, D. J.; Hartwell, E. E. (2017). Differences between treatment-seeking and non-treatmentseeking participants in medication studies for alcoholism: do they matter? The American Journal of Drug and Alcohol Abuse, 1-8.

Robles, Z.; Anjum, S.; Garey, L.; Kauffman, B. Y.; Rodríguez-Cano, R.; Langdon, K. J. et al. (2017). Financial strain and cognitive-based smoking processes: the explanatory role of depressive symptoms among adult daily smokers. Addictive Behaviors, 70, 18-22.

Rosenstock, I. M. (1974). The health belief model and preventive health behavior. Health Education Monographs, 2(4), 354-386.

Schwarzer, R. (2008). Modeling health behavior change: how to predict and modify the adoption and maintenance of health behaviors. Applied Psychology, 57(1), 1-29.

Spielberger, C. D.; Spielberger, C. D. (1966). Theory and research on anxiety. Anxiety and Behavior, 1, 3-20.

Svicher, A.; Zvolensky, M. J.; Cosci, F. (2017). The Smoking Abstinence Expectancies Questionnaire—Italian version: analysis of psychometric properties. Journal of Addictive Diseases, 36(1), 80-87.

Tate, J. C.; Stanton, A. L.; Green, S. B.; Schmitz, J. M.; Le, T.; Marshall, B. (1994). Experimental analysis of the role of expectancy in nicotine withdrawal. Psychology of Addictive Behaviors, 8(3), 169.

Vandenberg, R. J.; Lance, C. E. (2000). A review and synthesis of the measurement invariance literature: suggestions, practices, and recommendations for organizational research. Organizational Research Methods, 3(1), 4-70.

World Health Organization. (2008). WHO report on the global tobacco epidemic, 2008: The MPOWER package.

World Health Organization. (2015a). Global Health Observatory (GHO) data: Prevalence of tobacco use 2015. Available from:(2015a). http:// www. who. int/gho/tobacco/use/en/. Accessed 2 November 2015.

World Health Organization. (2015b). WHO global report on trends in prevalence of tobacco smoking 2015. World Health Organization. Zvolensky, M. J.; Paulus, D. J.; Langdon, K. J.; Robles, Z.; Garey, L.; Norton, P. J. et al. (2017). Anxiety sensitivity explains associations between anxious arousal symptoms and smoking abstinence expectancies, perceived barriers to cessation, and problems experienced during past quit attempts among low-income smokers. Journal of Anxiety Disorders, 48, 70-77.

53
由药剂师主导的戒烟服务：当前和未来的展望

Chee Fai Sui[1], Long Chiau Ming[2,3]

1. Department of Pharmacy, Hospital Tapah, Perak, Malaysia
2. Faculty of Pharmacy, Quest International University Perak, Perak, Malaysia
3. Unit for Medication Outcomes Research and Education, Pharmacy, University of Tasmania, Hobart, Tasmania, Australia

缩略语

CSCSP	经认证的戒烟服务提供商	**Non-NRD**	非烟碱替代药物
E-cigarette	电子烟	**NRD**	烟碱替代药物
FDA	美国食品药品监督管理局	**SCS**	戒烟服务
FIP	国际药学联合会	**WHO**	世界卫生组织
mQuit	马来西亚戒烟在线门户网站		

53.1 引言

药店和烟碱之间的历史联系始于20世纪初，当时烟草在药店中被用于医药目的而销售。由于其高需求和其强大的效果，这种做法在十年内发展为"香烟销售药店"。随着时间的推移，在吸烟的危害和有害影响被发现和验证后，该服务转变为"戒烟药房"（Anderson, 2007）。因此，该社区的药房模式在20世纪60年代从烟草香烟销售商转变为戒烟顾问。在此期间，许多非处方药制剂在英国等国的药店中被广泛销售，以帮助慢性吸烟者戒烟。活性成分主要是亚铁盐和洛贝林盐，没有在临床上进行有效性或安全性测试（Anderson, 2007）。

随后，一种替代的烟碱传递系统被引入，作为一种使用"纯烟碱"，消除商业化香烟中发现的各种有毒化学物质。第一个烟碱替代药物（NRD），2mg烟碱口香糖，在1984年被美国食品和药物管理局（FDA）批准作为帮助戒烟的处方药。药剂师在戒烟方面的作用在咨询、监测和配药NRD方面变得更加重要。20世纪90年代初，当NRD可以作为没有处方的情况下的药剂师物品出售时，专业职责和责任增加了一倍（Callahan-Lyon, 2010）。从那时起，由于满足用户不同需求的研发，NRD产品的范围有所增长。在目前的市场上，NRD包括口香糖、贴剂、喷雾剂、吸入器、舌下注射和含片。NRD的可用性取决于每个国家的规定。除了NRD，还有一些非烟碱制剂，如瓦伦尼克林，2006年批准的烟碱阻滞剂和安非他酮，1997年批准的安抑郁药，这两种药物都可能受到处方的限制。

药房提供戒烟服务（SCS）的绝佳地点，无论他们是在社区、医院还是初级卫生诊所，因为他们经常与公众互动，公众要么寻求建议，要么得到重复的处方。药剂师和药房工作人员有许多适合戒烟活动的场合，如鼓励和激励人们开始尝试戒烟或提供一个完整的SCS，如图53.1所示。在全球范围内，对药剂师领导的SCS的支持已被纳入指导方针和方案。世界卫生组织（WHO, 1998）提名药剂师是帮助吸烟者戒烟和防止未来使用者的关键角色。2009年，国际药学联合会

（FIP）通过其出版物《遏制烟草大流行:药学的全球作用》（Brock, Taylor, Wuliji, 2009）和英国国民保健服务（NHS）通过其《基于药学的戒烟服务指南：优化调试》（NHS Employers, 2009）颁布了药剂师在SCS中的重要角色。两份指南都提供了启动药剂师主导的SCS的易于遵循的步骤，并为药剂师主导的项目的成功提供了证据。亚洲和欧洲共有14个国家实施了药剂师提供的强化SCS，并将其整合到公共资助的卫生项目中。除指南外，每个国家的药学机构在更新和向所有药学相关人员提供基于证据的关于SCS的持续药学教育方面发挥着重要作用。例如，马来西亚和新加坡的药房分会实施了在线培训项目，以认证SCS的药剂师（CSCSP, 2017; Pharmaceutical Society of Singapore, 2016）。在芬兰，药剂师反吸烟的行动（PAS）模式被用作在药房提供戒烟指南（Maguireet al. 2001）（见表53.1）。

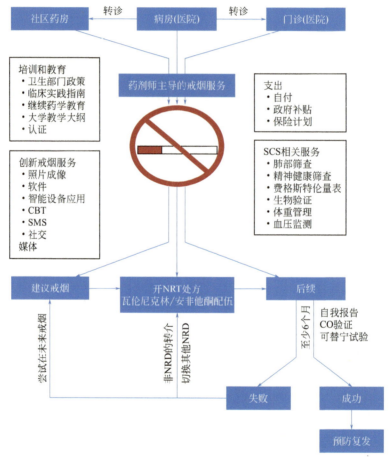

图 53.1　由药剂师主导的 SCS 的概念框架

表53.1　药剂师领导的SCS的教育、培训、指南和认证

社会/团体	年份	标题	类型	参考文献
欧洲制药论坛与世卫组织烟草或卫生股合作	1998	药剂师和烟草行动	准则	WHO（1998）
伦敦大学药学院，国际医药联合会（FIP）	2007	遏制烟草大流行：药学的全球作用	报告	Brock et al.（2009）

续表

社会/团体	年份	标题	类型	参考文献
PATH是苏格兰卫生协会、苏格兰国民保健协会和苏格兰政府之间的一项联合举措，旨在减少苏格兰烟草使用的流行率	2016	苏格兰戒烟服务的最低数据集（包括提供全国社区药房戒烟服务的药房）	准则	Partnership on tobacco Health（2016）
阿拉巴马药房协会	2014	药剂师戒烟指南	继续教育	Boutwell et al.（2014）
卫生发展局（HDA）与英国皇家制药学会和药房保健联系合作	2005	帮助吸烟者戒烟：英国药剂师的建议	准则	McRobbie McEwen（2005）
普罗维登斯健康和服务，俄勒冈州	NA	药剂师辅助戒烟班：实施指南	准则	Bentz, Grazy, Swan（2007）
不列颠哥伦比亚省药学协会	2013	药剂师主导的戒烟服务	临床服务提案	British Columbia Pharmacy Association（2013）
英国国民健康雇主协会	2009	基于药房的戒烟服务：优化调试	准则	NHS Employers（2009）
烟草管制网络	2017	通过药剂师获得戒烟药物	议定书	Tobacco Control Network（2017）
新加坡医药学会	2016	轻微疾病实践指南（PG-MA）模块5：戒烟	培训	Pharmaceutical Society of Singapore（2016）
安大略省卫生和长期护理部	2011	药房戒烟计划，药剂师在戒烟系统中的作用	准则	Ministry of Health and Long-Term Care（2011）
马来西亚药学院	2010	注册戒烟服务提供者（CSCSP）	培训	CSCSP（2017）
戒烟信托管理服务（SCTMS）	2013	戒烟服务提供者指南：美国处方药房服务	准则	Smoking Cessation Trust（2013）

53.2 由药剂师主导的SCS的不同设置

药剂师被选为美国公众眼中最值得信赖的职业（Norman，2016）。同样，波兰的药剂师被评为（Goniewicz et al. 2010）吸烟者会询问的第一个关于戒烟药物治疗的健康专业人员。社区药房很容易接触到寻求医疗保健和疾病护理的公众，而不需要预约或支付额外的诊疗费（Patwardhan et al. 2010）。许多潜在的戒烟者和家人一起到药店寻求健康建议或保健品。药剂师可以提出一系列封闭和开放性问题，引导患者自己激励戒烟（Boutwell et al. 2014），例如，通过问为自己、子女、伴侣或其他家庭成员购买咳嗽、感冒药的患者"你是否吸烟？"。通过这种方式，可以提供更多的信息给那些吸烟和有兴趣了解SCS的患者。

与社区药剂师相比，医院药剂师经常处理许多住院病人，例如，有呼吸系统、心血管疾病和并发症等特殊医疗需要的患者。因此，他们的理想位置是提供建议，并为任何吸烟者提供必要的帮助。此外，与公众患者亲属和护理人员直接接触的医院药剂师在吸引潜在戒烟者加入SCS方面也发挥了作用。与社区药剂师的同等作用相比，在医院环境中，药剂师在提供SCS方面的作用在文献中没有很好的记载。Freund等（2008）对1994～2005年期间医院吸烟护理流行情况的回顾表明，只有13%的卫生专业人员提供了烟碱替代疗法（NRT）或建议使用，39%提供了转诊或随访。类似地，澳大利亚一项由药剂师主导的在医院环境下戒烟的研究招募了102名吸烟者，并随机分为三组：最小干预组（没有NRT贴片）、医院组和社区组。6个月的随访后，在医院（戒烟率为38%）和社区药房（戒烟率为24%）之间没有发现显著差异，但戒烟率优于最小干预组（戒烟率为4.6%）（Vial et al. 2002）。

由药剂师领导的戒烟诊所大多包括一个综合团队，如医务人员、护士和医疗助理，并由一个国家卫生基金提供补贴。许多国家为有兴趣戒烟的患者提供选定设施的免费治疗，例如英国国民保健服务（Dobbie et al. 2015）、美国信托计划（Smoking Cessation Trust, 2013）和马来西亚卫生部（Fai et al. 2016）。有兴趣的患者可以选择离他们最近的设施，并决定是使用私人或公共资助的设施（专科诊所、医院或社区药房）来帮助他们戒烟。药剂师领导的SCS的成功并不仅仅依赖于药物治疗。创新方法和附加保健服务在增加某人在特定时期内成功戒烟的机会方面发挥了重要作用。

53.3 导致药剂师主导的SCS成功的促成因素

戒烟药物的开发渠道是有限的。只有少数制药公司愿意花费数百万美元研发旨在戒烟的新药，尽管全球有多达10亿人吸烟（WHO, 2017）。最近的一项系统综述证实，仅依靠毅力本身可以产生大约3%～5%的戒烟率，但尼古丁替代疗法可以将成功率提高50%～70%（Stead et al. 2012）。已有基于证据的研究评估了药剂师主导的戒烟服务（SCS），文献中大多数药剂师主导的SCS的禁欲率超过10%，但Hoving等（2010）的一项研究，成功率仅为0.8%。这表明，药剂师主导的SCS的有效性可能取决于具体的计划和方法。总体而言，继续投资于戒烟药物的研究和开发，并探索有效的方法非常重要，如药剂师主导的SCS以帮助个人戒烟。

不同药剂师主导的SCS所采用的策略（图53.2）在借助药理学治疗提高成功率方面发挥着至关重要的作用。由于烟碱的戒断症状和使人上瘾的成分，戒烟的尝试不能保证成功。Stead等（2012）证实，短信系统（SMS）短信、小册子、电话和网站提供的52周戒烟率分别约为9%、5%、8%和8%。交互式智能手机应用程序是SCS的最新创新，药剂师领导的SCS应该纳入这一策略，以吸引更多潜在的戒烟者。Bricker等的一项随机研究中，在智能手机戒烟应用程序上的试点报告显示，智能手机提供的戒烟应用程序（SmartQuit）的接受和承诺疗法的成功率为13%，国家癌症研究所的戒烟应用程序（QuitGuide）的成功率为8%。一个创新方法的例子是2016年在马来西亚推出的名为mQuit的公共资助诊所和社区药房联合网站，该网站为SCS提供了多个地点的选择。感兴趣的用户可以选择一个SCS位置，决定他们想要私人或公共资助，并通过网站注册（mQuit, 2016）。

许多吸烟者可能需要多次尝试才能完全戒烟，而另一些人可能会在戒烟期间偶尔复发。这种慢性复发的过程不仅需要药理学和行为支持，还需要多种方法。二线药物可能不如一线治疗有效，它们可能有更多的副作用，每次治疗会产生更高的成本。药剂师应在所有医疗保险或公共卫生计划的价值包范围内提供戒烟策略，以促进所有寻求戒烟帮助的潜在戒烟者获得这些干预措施。

表53.2 关于药剂师领导的SCS的证据

参考文献	环境	设计	样本量	干预/战略	药物疗法	成功率/%	随访期/月	验证成功
Sinclair et al. (1998)	社区药房	RCT	492	药剂师支持计划	是	26 (12.0)	9	自我报告
Maguire et al. (2001)	社区药房	RCT	484	药剂师行动计划	是	38 (14.3)	12	带有可替宁检测的自我报告

续表

参考文献	环境	设计	样本量	干预/战略	药物疗法	成功率/%	随访期/月	验证成功
Kennedy, Giles, Chang, Small, Edwards (2002)	社区药房	单组非盲目	48	戒烟培训手册	是	12 (25.0)	12	问卷
Vial et al. (2002)	从医院到社区药房	群体	102	咨询研究药剂师	是	8 (24.0)	12	使用CO-Level进行自我报告
McEwen, West, McRobbie (2006)	社区初级保健	准实验	1501	一对一基础药剂师/护士	是	285 (19.0)	4	未知
Dent, Harris, Noonan (2009)	社区诊所	RCT	101	药剂师团队组织的三场面对面小组活动	是	28 (28.0)	12	带有可替宁验证的自我报告
Bauld, Chesterman, Ferguson, Judge (2009)	社区药房	观察性实验	1785	药房提供一对一支持	是	256 (18.6)	4	使用CO-Level进行自我报告
Philbrick, Newkirk, Farris, McDanel, Horner (2009)	大学诊所	潜在的、单一群体	21	结构化团体咨询	是	11 (52.4)	6	自我报告
Hoving et al. (2010)	社区药房	RCT	545	计算机生成的定制建议	未提及	2 (0.8)	12	未提及
Bock, Hudmon, Christian, Graham, Bock (2010)	社区药房	未提及	200	使用ExperQuit软件进行药剂师咨询	是	28 (28.0)	6	未提及
Costello et al. (2011)	未提及	RCT	6987	药剂师主导的行为干预	是	612 (17.5%) 604 (18.0%)	1周 5周	自我报告
Taskila et al. (2012)	社区药房	随机析因试验	160	行为支持	支持	尚未公布	34周	使用CO-Level进行自我报告
Burford, Jiwa, Carter, Parsons, Hendrie (2013)	社区药房	RCT	160	使用基于互联网的人脸老化（年龄进展）软件APRIL对吸烟者和非吸烟者进行数字照相	带建议的标准护理	11 (13.8)	6	使用CO-Level进行自我报告
Fai et al. (2016)	公共卫生诊所	典型	176	药房主导的综合服务	是	75 (42.6)	6	使用CO-Level进行自我报告
Augustine, Taylor, Pelger, Schiefer, Warholak (2016)	药品管理中心	回溯性审查	238	药剂师提供电话戒烟咨询服务	是	24 (55.0)	13	自我报告
El Hajj et al. (2017)	流动药房	RCT	314	药剂师提供戒烟计划	是	40 (23.9)	12	使用CO-Level进行自我报告

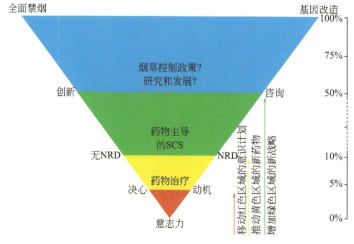

图 53.2　SCS 成功金字塔

红色，意志力区；黄色，药物治疗区；绿色，SCS 区战略；蓝色，烟草控制政策或研发。

53.4　由药剂师主导的SCS的未来发展

戒烟虽然被证明是预防非传染性疾病的一种经济和有效的方法，但仍需要药剂师反复加强，以确保其成功。在冠状动脉事件发生后，戒烟仍然比口服药物或手术干预更具成本效益；然而，仍需要给予持续的 SCS 来说服患者戒烟。2013 年，澳大利亚启动了一项多中心随机对照试验（给予），以评估药剂师主导的医院戒烟的有效性（Thomas et al. 2013）。结果显示，在 6 个月时，药剂师主导的 SCS 组和常规护理组的持续戒烟率没有显著差异 [11.6% (34/294) 对 12.6% (37/294)；优势比 (OR) = 0.91, 95% 置信区间 (CI) 0.55～1.50] 和 12 个月 [11.6% (34/292) 对 11.2% (33/294)；OR = 1.04, 95% CI = 0.63～1.73]（Thomas et al. 2016）。

Thomas 等的研究结果（2016）表明以医院药剂师为主导的 SCS 并不优于常规护理，这对使用临床试验证实其意义提出了挑战。在他们的研究中，常规护理组也接受了组织良好的 SCS，这也得到了药学团队的部分或全部支持。例如，常规护理组的患者还可以要求病房药剂师和护士启动和建议使用 NRD 和非 NRD 药物作为常规 SCS 的一部分（Thomas et al. 2016）。在这种情况下，使用聚类随机试验和交叉研究设计将更适合于减少最小化治疗组污染和霍桑效应。本研究的主要教训是，药剂师应定期随访其全科医生和社区药剂师，以加强吸烟者的动机。

从新的药物疗法的角度来看，有三个可能治疗烟碱成瘾患者的新的关键进展：①电子烟，不含吸食普通香烟的有害副产品（Rahman et al. 2015）；②针对烟碱受体的疫苗；③马钱子碱，在金合欢和新西兰合欢树等植物中发现的天然产物胞苷。

NRDs 和非 NRDs 已被证明可以提高戒烟率，伐伦克林显示出最大的益处。然而，这些产品并没有香烟的爆裂感和热感，对消费者的吸引力和产品满意度。与此同时，虽然电子烟既有吸引力又令人满意，但目前还没有关于其声称在成分方面更安全的长期数据（Mukhtar et al. 2016）。电子烟被误用于娱乐目的，而不是作为帮助戒烟。许多不吸烟者和青少年为了装酷而吸电子烟，而传统吸烟者正在成为双重吸烟者（Rahman et al. 2015）。需要进一步的研究和监管来澄清公众对戒烟的实际意义的困惑，而不仅仅是从香烟转向电子烟。与此同时，针对烟碱受体的疫苗尚未问世，目前正在临床试验中。研究人员乐观地认为，这种疫苗将防止未来烟碱成瘾的发展，同时治疗已经上瘾的患者。同样，一种名为马钱子碱的天然物质，以Tabex的名义销售，在一些欧洲国家已经作为一种传统的戒烟药物被使用了几十年。马钱子碱的结构和作用机制类似于烟碱，但其危害要小得多。然而，关于马钱子碱有效性的出版物并不多（Etter，2006）。Walker等（2014）的一项研究报道了马钱子碱在1周、2个月和6个月的禁断率方面优于NRDs。

除了开发新药外，还需要采取打破传统的创新的战略，以使该方案对公众更具吸引力和接受，认为其在预防心血管疾病和癌症等非传染性疾病方面具有重要的治疗意义。

53.5 治疗的影响

社区药房、医院药房和保健诊所药房参与了SCS，使戒烟更加有效，减少了等待时间和多个地点可供选择。药剂师可以根据患者的需要和负担性考虑个性化治疗计划。SCS药剂师应提供短期或长期的戒烟干预，以帮助戒烟的过程。他们还应该走出社区药房或医院冒险进入学校和大学，以帮助年轻吸烟者戒烟。

术语解释	■ 戒除：不吸烟的一段时间。不同的设施或国家可能会有不同的定义。 ■ 成瘾：对每天持续吸食香烟的依赖。 ■ 行为支持：一项战略计划，以一种知情的方式让吸烟者通过强化动机从吸烟者转变为戒烟者。 ■ 生化验证：一种通过测量尿液中的可替宁或呼出的空气或血液中的一氧化碳水平来确认是否吸烟的方法。 ■ 电子烟：一种由电池驱动的装置，当使用者从嘴部吸入时，它会释放出蒸汽。它模仿了吸烟的感觉，但有害成分更少。 ■ 药物治疗：使用药物（例如NRD、安非他酮和伐伦克林）对烟瘾进行管理。 ■ 戒烟指南/戒烟计划结构方案：包括戒烟日期的设定、药物治疗方式的选择、签署戒烟誓约、戒烟技巧及戒断症状的克服、副作用的管理等。 ■ 复吸：在戒烟期间吸烟或成功戒烟后重新开始吸烟。 ■ 智能手机应用程序：在移动设备上运行的用于戒烟的移动软件应用程序。"app"是"soft application"的缩写。 ■ 戒烟服务：是一个复杂的系统，在招募吸烟者和停止吸烟习惯的过程中，对吸烟上瘾的人使用药物治疗和行为支持。 ■ 戒断症状：在不吸烟期间，人类的行为和生理反应的变化，如强烈的渴望、疲劳、食欲增加、易怒和难以集中注意力。症状可以在最后一剂香烟内开始，最长可达几个月。
药剂师领导的SCS的关键事实	■ 药剂师领导的SCS的核心是指导和建议吸烟者戒烟，摆脱各种形式的烟碱成瘾。 ■ 药学专业的参与将SCS的覆盖范围扩大到社区、初级卫生环境和医院环境。 ■ 不同强度的SCS项目，从低强度到高强度，都是基于随访的次数和每次随访的时间。 ■ 药剂师接受过培训，可以为任何需要药物的患者开具、分发、监测和建议使用NRD和非NRD。

- NRD的类型会根据患者的适合性而量身定制，患者可以选择通过面对面、电话、短信或社交媒体进行随访。
- 药剂师主导的SCS在社区环境中的优势是节省成本、易于获得和药物的可用性。
- 在药物治疗和行为支持下，药剂师主导的SCS的成功率高达50%。

要点总结
- 根除吸烟和烟碱成瘾已成为一项重要的药学服务。
- 药剂师领导的SCS的成功，除了吸烟者自己的决定外，还取决于联合药物治疗和行为支持的方式。
- 对药学机构的培训、教育和认证对于提高SCS中药剂师和药学相关工作人员的技能和更新知识至关重要。
- 药剂师可以帮助传播正确的信息，以防止年轻一代中的吸烟习惯。当地政府和药房机构对药剂师领导的SCS的支持已被证明可以减少吸烟习惯。

参考文献

Anderson, S. (2007). Community pharmacists and tobacco in Great Britain: from selling cigarettes to smoking cessation services. Addiction, 102(5), 704-712.

Augustine, J. M.; Taylor, A. M.; Pelger, M.; Schiefer, D.; Warholak, T. L. (2016). Smoking quit rates among patients receiving pharmacist-447 REFERENCES provided pharmacotherapy and telephonic smoking cessation counseling. Journal of the American Pharmaceutical Association, 56(2), 129-136.

Bauld, L.; Chesterman, J.; Ferguson, J.; Judge, K. (2009). A comparison of the effectiveness of group-based and pharmacyled smoking cessation treatment in Glasgow. Addiction, 104(2), 308-316.

Bentz, C. J.; Gray, M.; Swan, C. (2007). Pharmacist-assisted smoking cessation class: a guide to implementation. Available from: https://smokingcessationleadership.ucsf.edu/sites/smokingcessationleadership.ucsf.edu/files/Downloads/Toolkits/HospGuide.pdf. Accessed 1 September 2017.

Bock, B. C.; Hudmon, K. S.; Christian, J.; Graham, A. L.; Bock, F. R. (2010). A tailored intervention to support pharmacy-basedcounseling for smoking cessation. Nicotine, Tobacco Research, 12(3), 217-225.

Boutwell, L.; Cook, L.; Norman, K.; Lindsey, W. T. (2014). A pharmacist's guide for smoking cessation. Available from: http://c.ymcdn.com/sites/www.aparx.org/resource/resmgr/imported/CE_Winter%20Smoking%20Cessation.pdf/. Accessed 1 September 2017.

Bricker, J. B.; Mull, K. E.; Kientz, J. A.; Vilardaga, R.; Mercer, L. D.; Akioka, K. J. et al. (2014). Randomized, controlled pilot trial of asmartphone app for smoking cessation using acceptance and commitment therapy. Drug and Alcohol Dependence, 143, 87-93.

British Columbia Pharmacy Association (2013). British Columbia Pharmacy Association, clinical service proposal pharmacist-led smoking cessation services. Available from: https://www.bcpharmacy.ca/uploads/Smoking%20Cessation.pdf. Accessed 1 September 2017.

Brock, T.; Taylor, D.; Wuliji, T. (2009). Curbing the tobacco pandemic: The global role for pharmacy. London: International Pharmaceutical Federation.

Burford, O.; Jiwa, M.; Carter, O.; Parsons, R.; Hendrie, D. (2013). Internet-based photoaging within Australian pharmacies to promote smoking cessation: randomized controlled trial. Journal of Medical Internet Research, 15(3), e64.

Callahan-Lyon, P. (2010). Nicotine replacement therapy: the CDER experience. Available from: http://www.fda.gov/downloads/AdvisoryCommittees/Commi-tteesMeetingMaterials/TobaccoProductsScientificAdvisoryCommittee/UCM288284.pdf. Accessed 1 June 2017.

Costello, M. J.; Sproule, B.; Victor, J. C.; Leatherdale, S. T.; Zawertailo, L.; Selby, P. (2011). Effectiveness of pharmacist counseling combined with nicotine replacement therapy: a pragmatic randomized trial with 6,987 smokers. Cancer Causes & Control, 22(2), 167-180.

CSCSP. (2017). Certified Smoking Cessation Service Provider, Malaysia Academy of Pharmacy. Available from:(2017). http://www.acadpharm.org.my/index.cfm?&menuid=2. Accessed 1 September 2017.

Dent, L. A.; Harris, K. J.; Noonan, C. W. (2009). Randomized trial assessing the effectiveness of a pharmacist-delivered program for smoking cessation. The Annals of Pharmacotherapy, 43(2), 194-201.

Dobbie, F.; Hiscock, R.; Leonardi-Bee, J.; Murray, S.; Shahab, L.; Aveyard, P. et al. (2015). Evaluating long-term outcomes of NHS stop smoking services (ELONS): A prospective cohort study. Health Techndogy Assessment, 19(95), 1-56.

EI Hajj, M.S.; Kheir, N.; Al Mull, A.M. Shami, R.; Fanous, N.; Mahfoud, Z. R. (2017). Effectiveness of a pharmacist-delivered smoking cessation program in the State of Qatar: a randomized controlledtrial. BMC Public Health, 17(1), 215.

Etter, J. F. (2006). Cytisine for smoking cessation: a literature review and a meta-analysis. Archives of Internal Medicine, 166(15), 1553-1559.

Fai, S. C.; Yen, G. K.; Malik, N. (2016). Quit rates at 6 months in a pharmacist-led smoking cessation service in Malaysia. Canadian Pharmaceutical Journal, 149(5), 303-312.

Freund, M.; Campbell, E.; Paul, C.; McElduff, P.; Walsh, R. A.; Sakrouge, R. et al. (2008). Smoking care provision in hospitals: a review of prevalence. Nicotine, Tobacco Research, 10(5), 757-774.

Goniewicz, M. L.; Lingas, E. O.; Czogala, J.; Koszowski, B.; Zielinska-Danch, W.; Sobczak, A. (2010). The role of pharmacists in smoking cessation in Poland. Evaluation, the Health Professions, 33(1), 81-95.

Hoving, C.; Mudde, A. N.; Dijk, F.; Vries, H. d. (2010). Effectiveness of a smoking cessation intervention in Dutch pharmacies and general practices. Health Education, 110(1), 17-29.

Kennedy, D. T.; Giles, J. T.; Chang, Z. G.; Small, R. E.; Edwards, J. H. (2002). Results of a smoking cessation clinic in community pharmacy practice. Journal of the American Pharmaceutical Association, 42(1), 51-56.

Maguire, T. A.; McElnay, J. C.; Drummond, A. (2001). A randomized controlled trial of a smoking cessation intervention based in community pharmacies. Addiction, 96(2), 325-331.

McEwen, A.; West, R.; McRobbie, H. (2006). Effectiveness of specialist group treatment for smoking cessation vs. one-to-one treatment in primary care. Addictive Behaviors, 31(9), 1650-1660.

McRobbie, H.; McEwen, A. (2005). Helping smokers to stop: advice for pharmacists in England. National Institute for Health and Clinical Excellence, 14-15.

Ministry of Health and Long-Term Care (2011). Pharmacy Smoking Cessation Program, the pharmacist's role in a smoking cessation system. Available from:(2011). http://www. health. gov. on. ca/en/pro/programs/drugs/ smoking/. Accessed 1 September 2017.

mQuit. (2016). Malaysia Quit Smoking Service (mQuit). Available from: (2016). http://jomquit. moh. gov. my/mquitcenters. Accessed 1 September 2017.

Mukhtar, M.; Khan, T. M.; Long, C. M. (2016). E-cigarette: more harm than good? Proceedings of Singapore Healthcare, 25(2), 115-116.

NHS Employers. (2009). Pharmacy-based stop smoking services: optimising commissioning. Available from:(2009). http://archive. psnc. org. uk/data/files/smoking_cessation_guidance. pdf. Accessed 1 September 2017.

Norman, J. (2016). Americans rate healthcare providers high on honesty, ethics. Gallup.

Partnership on Tobacco and Health. (2016). The minimum dataset for Scottish smoking cessation services (including pharmacies offering the national community pharmacy smoking cessation service).

Patwardhan, P. D.; Chewning, B. A. (2010). Tobacco users' perceptions of a brief tobacco cessation intervention in community pharmacies. Journal of the American Pharmaceutical Association, 50(5), 568-574.

Pharmaceutical Society of Singapore. (2016). Module 5: Smoking cessation, practice guides for minor ailments. Available from:(2016). https://www. pss. org. sg/product/pss-pgma-module-5-smoking-cessation. Accessed 1 September 2017.

Philbrick, A. M.; Newkirk, E. N.; Farris, K. B.; McDanel, D. L.; Horner, K. E. (2009). Effect of a pharmacist managed smoking cessation clinic on quit rates. Pharmacy Practice (Granada), 7(3), 150-156.

Rahman, M. A.; Hann, N.; Wilson, A.; Mnatzaganian, G.; Worrall-Carter, L. (2015). E-cigarettes and smoking cessation: evidence from a systematic review and meta-analysis. PLoS ONE, 10(3) e0122544.

Sinclair, H. K.; Bond, C. M.; Lennox, A. S.; Silcock, J.; Winfield, A. J.; Donnan, P. T. (1998). Training pharmacists and pharmacy assistants in the stage-of-change model of smoking cessation: a randomised controlled trial in Scotland. Tobacco Control, 7(3), 253-261.

Smoking Cessation Trust. (2013). Smoking cessation provider guide: US script pharmacy services. (2013). https://www. smokingcessationtrust. org/AvailableServices. aspx#. Wdwu2GiCzIU.

Stead, L. F.; Perera, R.; Bullen, C.; Mant, D.; Hartmann-Boyce, J.; Cahill, K. et al. (2012). Nicotine replacement therapy for smoking cessation. Cochrane Database of Systematic Reviews, 11, CD000146.

Taskila, T.; Macaskill, S.; Coleman, T.; Etter, J. F.; Patel, M.; Clarke, S. et al. (2012). A randomised trial of nicotine assisted reduction to stop in pharmacies - The RedPharm study. BMC Public Health, 12, 182.

Thomas, D.; Abramson, M. J.; Bonevski, B.; Taylor, S.; Poole, S. G.; Paul, E. et al. (2016). Integrating smoking cessation into routine care in hospitals—a randomized controlled trial. Addiction, 111(4), 714-723.

Thomas, D.; Abramson, M. J.; Bonevski, B.; Taylor, S.; Poole, S.; Weeks, G. R. et al. (2013). A pharmacist-led system-change smoking cessation intervention for smokers admitted to Australian public hospitals (GIVE UP FOR GOOD): study protocol for a randomised controlled trial. Trials, 14(1), 148.

Tobacco Control Network. (2017). Access to tobacco cessation medication through pharmacists. Tobacco Control Network. Availablefrom: http://www. astho. org/Prevention/Tobacco/Tobacco-CessationVia-Pharmacists/ (Accessed 1 September 2017).

Vial, R. J.; Jones, T. E.; Ruffin, R. E.; Gilbert, A. L. (2002). Smoking cessation program using nicotine patches linking hospital to the community. Journal of Pharmacy Practice and Research, 32(1), 57-62.

Walker, N.; Howe, C.; Glover, M.; McRobbie, H.; Barnes, J.; Nosa, V. et al. (2014). Cytisine versus nicotine for smoking cessation. The New England Journal of Medicine, 371(25), 2353-2362.

World Health Organization. (1998). Pharmacists and action on tobacco. Available from:(1998). http://apps. who. int/iris/bitstream/10665/108128/ 1/ E61288. pdf. Accessed 1 September 2017.

World Health Organization. (2017). WHO report on the global tobacco epidemic 2017 (Monitoring tobacco use and prevention policies). Available from:(2017). http://www. who. int/tobacco/global_report/2017/en/. Accessed 12 September 2017.

54
青少年的烟碱使用和体重控制：预防和早期干预的意义

Adrian B. Kelly[1], *Rebekah Thomas*[2], *Gary C.K. Chan*[3]

1. School of Psychology and Counselling, Institute for Health and Biomedical Innovation, Queensland University of Technology, Brisbane, QLD, Australia
2. School of Psychology, University of Queensland, Brisbane, QLD, Australia
3. Centre for Youth Substance Abuse Research, University of Queensland, Brisbane, QLD, Australia

缩略语

BMI	体重指数	**ATT**	损耗
NR	全国代表性	**prev**	患病率

人们普遍认为，吸烟可以通过抑制食欲来促进体重控制，这对公共健康构成了重大挑战。西方社会的超重率很高，这可能会增加担心体重的人吸烟的风险。在英国，16～24岁的年轻人中有36%超重或肥胖（Baker, 2017; Public Health England, 2015），而在美国，12～19岁的青少年中大约有20.5%的人肥胖（Ogden et al. 2015）。在澳大利亚，近30%的14～17岁青少年超重或肥胖（AIHW, 2017）。开始吸烟通常发生在青少年时期，这是一个对体重高度关注的发展期。戒烟尝试的成功可能也会在青少年中受到影响，因为他们对体重的担忧通常很严重。长期来看，吸烟还会损害健康和锻炼习惯，从而增加增重的风险。

在本章中，我们提供了一个关于吸烟与体重、超重和体重的关系的实证文献的更新。我们首先概述了烟草使用与体重和体重控制之间联系的理论解释；然后，我们回顾了过去15年里这两个因素之间关联的实证文献。我们关注过去15年的流行烟草使用，超重和肥胖的变化趋势（OECD, 2017; WHO, 2015）。根据过去15年的数据，我们寻求回答的核心研究问题如下：

（1）超重或担心超重是否会增加青春期吸烟的风险？
（2）如果体重因素增加了吸烟的风险，那么这种影响在女性中是否比男性更强呢？
（3）这些发现对预防项目有什么影响？

54.1 将体重问题和体重减轻与烟草使用之间的联系的机制

体重和吸烟之间联系的关键理论解释围绕着代谢过程、社会发展机制和社会生态驱动因素。代谢机制试图通过研究吸烟是否对食欲有明显的影响来解释这种关联。社会认知机制强调个人对吸烟和体重控制的信念。社会生态驱动因素包括关于健康风险行为的家庭和媒体信息。

54.1.1 代谢驱动程序

一个长期和普遍的看法是，吸烟可能通过提高心率促进新陈代谢，从而消耗更多的卡路里

（Wack et al. 1982）。文献综述表明，摄入烟碱增加热量消耗，并可能通过减少热量吸收而降低食欲（Chiolero et al. 2008; Wehby et al. 2012）。例如，吸烟已被证明在吸烟后30分钟内使热量消耗增加3%（Dallosso et al. 1984）。虽然近端效应已经被证明，但关于吸烟对热量消耗的慢性影响的发现是复杂的。根据大规模的研究，可以观察到吸烟开始的影响和自相关影响可以控制，证据的平衡表明，吸烟并没有在长期限制体重增加（Robertson, McGee, Hancox, 2014）体重增加是一种普遍趋势，而不是戒烟的结果。有对照的大型纵向研究也表明，非吸烟者的体重增加比吸烟的人少，或者其影响是不一致的，因文化背景而异（Chiolero et al. 2008）。这些发现表明，近端效应可能在最初是有益的，因此是早期巩固吸烟的重要驱动因素，但吸烟侵蚀锻炼机制，因此可能导致长期体重增加（Nagaya et al. 2007；见图54.1）。

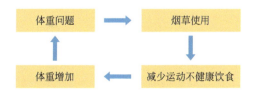

图 54.1　吸烟对体重的短期和长期新陈代谢的影响

54.1.2　社会认知驱动因素

对药物使用的社会认知方法的一个关键原则是，个人对某种行为（期望）的个人后果产生了信念，这种行为会导致健康风险行为。这些期望被认为是源于个人的学习历史（例如，父母/同伴/媒体信息和个人经验）。就吸烟而言，认为吸烟可以抑制体重增加的信念会促使人们吸烟，尤其是对那些关心自己体重的人（见图54.2）。在青少年中，驱使吸烟的期望主要与控制负面情绪和体重管理有关。例如，消极影响缓解预期可以预测吸烟结果和吸烟行为和烟碱依赖的增加（Heinz et al. 2010）。对于女性和男性来说，体重控制、无聊缓解和消极影响管理的预期可以预测当前和未来的吸烟（Wahl et al. 2005）。这些吸烟和体重控制的社会驱动因素与认知研究相吻合，这些研究表明，吸烟可以缓解负面情绪，并有证据表明，对体重的担忧是青少年痛苦、抑郁和焦虑的主要来源。

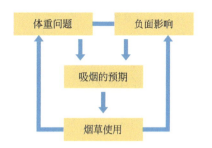

图 54.2　一种关于吸烟和体重控制的社会认知模型

54.1.3　社会生态框架

社会生态方法（Bronfenbrenner, 1989; Ennett et al. 2008）关注家庭、同伴、社区和媒体对青少年健康风险行为的嵌套影响（Mehus et al. 2018; Smith et al. 2014）（见图54.3）。吸烟最可能开始于对同伴影响的敏感性最高的时候（Monahan et al. 2009）和青少年适应主要转变，包括青春期和高中。父母、兄长和同伴吸烟是青少年烟草使用的最强有力的预测因素（Kelly et al. 2011），而家庭管理（冲突、监督和监测）是烟草使用的预测因素（Kelly et al. 2011; Mehus et al. 2018）和正在出现的体重控制关注（Hinchliff et al. 2016; Thomas et al. 2018）。系统和持续地曝光媒体信息，促进瘦的理想（Dittmar et al. 2009; Harrison, 2000）可能会增加抑郁/焦虑，增加吸烟的可能性以限制体重和/或管理负面影响（Dittmar et al. 2009; Thomas et al. 2018）。生活在社会经济条件不利的社区的青少年可能有更大的开始吸烟的风险，因为吸烟和超重的流行率往往高于社会经济条件有利的社区。

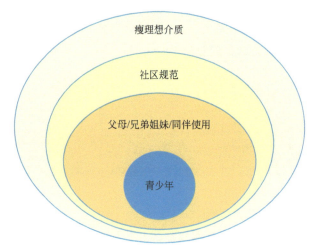

图 54.3　影响脆弱青少年吸烟的社会生态系统

54.1.4　总结和集成

青少年的体重问题和烟草使用之间的联系可以通过关注代谢过程、社会认知过程和社会生态/学习方法来理解。吸烟可能对食欲有近端影响，但从长期来看，吸烟实际上可能通过增加久坐生活方式和减少定期锻炼而导致体重问题（Nagaya et al. 2007）。青少年的吸烟预期往往与负面影响和体重管理有关，这些可能导致早期吸烟。关于瘦理想的媒体信息可能会增加吸烟的风险，特别是女孩，而青少年通过家庭和同龄人网络接触吸烟时吸烟的风险很高。来自低社会经济地位社区的青少年面临着吸烟和超重的高风险。

54.2　最近的实证文献告诉了我们什么？

为了收集关于该关联的实证研究，我们搜索了心理信息、PubMed、谷歌学者和纳入论文的参考文献列表。搜索词包括少年、年轻人、青少年、吸烟、烟草、体重和体重控制。要纳入研究，研究必须关注少年（年龄<18岁），至少有一种吸烟、BMI和/或感知体重和烟草预期的测量方法，并在2004年或以后的同行评议期刊上发表。

54.2.1　跨部门研究

表54.1概述了研究特征（原产国、样本量、测量方法和结果）。关于体重问题/控制与吸烟之间关系的研究结果是复杂的。14项研究中的6项发现，女性对吸烟对体重影响的看法和/或对体

重的担忧与吸烟状况有关。特别是，女性吸烟者报告说，她们更担心戒烟后体重会增加（Cavallo et al. 2006; Seo et al. 2009）；更多的女性吸烟者比男性吸烟者使用烟草控制体重（Cawley et al. 2016; Xie et al. 2006）。

表54.1 烟草吸烟与体重关注/控制之间的交叉研究

参考文献	试样量	样本特征	主要吸烟措施	关键发现
Cavallo（2006）	N=103	吸烟者，年龄14~18岁，美国	三十天吸烟；相信雪茄有助于控制体重；如果戒烟，要担心体重	与男性相比，女性更担心体重增加
Cawley et al.（2016）	N=10442	14~16岁，美国	目前吸烟状况（不吸烟，任何吸烟/周）	46%的女性，30%的男性吸烟来控制体重。当发现超重时，吸烟减肥更常见
Chung（2014）	N=93911	韩国/美国学生（9~11年级）	最近30天吸烟天数（>1支雪茄，吸烟者；0，不吸烟者）	体重感知/控制→↑目前吸烟情况
Cook, MacPherson, Langille（2007）	N=1133	10~12年级女生，四所学校，加拿大	最近30天吸烟天数（签注月份内所有天数）	与感知体重无关
Delk et al.（2017）	N=2733	7~11年级，美国	卷烟和电子烟的终生吸烟率、30天吸烟率	男性：与健康体重相比，肥胖→30天吸烟增加。女性：无关联
Johnson, Eaton, Pederson, Lowry（2009）	N=13917	9~12年级，美国	最近30天吸烟天数（>1支雪茄，吸烟者；0，不吸烟者）	努力减肥与吸烟有关。没有性别影响
Kendzor（2007）	N=727	2~6年级，预防试验，5所学校，美国	终生吸烟（是/否）	吸烟→节食增加，与不吸烟的人相比，体重问题上升。性别差异不显著
Lange et al.（2015）	N=15425	9~12年级，美国	终生吸烟，根/天，吸烟天数/最近30天（>1支，吸烟者；0，非吸烟者）	感知体重预测终生吸烟；BMI预测所有吸烟指标；感知体重和BMI预测女性吸烟，而不是男性
Leatherdale（2008）	N=25060	9~12年级，76所学校，加拿大	吸烟易感性（三项）	吸烟的易感性与超重有关
Pénzes（2012）	N=2208	6~9年级，78所学校，匈牙利	30天前；雪茄数量/最后30天。对体重控制和吸烟的看法	BMI→吸烟；认为吸烟控制体重是这种联系的中介。不因减肥/增重动机而有所不同。女性：比男性有更强的信念
Seo（2009）	N=13~15000/调查	9~12年级，美国	吸烟/30天（>1支雪茄，吸烟者；0，不吸烟者）	感知体重和BMI→目前正在吸烟。女性：感知超重→吸烟者。男性：不显著
Thomas（2018）	N=10273	7~11年级，澳大利亚	吸烟30天（是/否）	在控制人口统计、焦虑/抑郁、青春期、同龄人使用和吸烟之后！控制女性体重，但不控制男性体重
Weiss（2007）	N=3515	8~9年级学生，美国	吸烟/30天（是，即使是几口/否）	体重问题→吸烟的风险增加了40%。没有检查性别-体重的相互作用
Xie（2006）	N=6863	中学生/高中生，中国	吸烟/30天（是，即使是几口/否）	体重不满→吸烟增多；对女孩来说很重要，而不是男孩

在女性中，BMI与吸烟有关（Pénzes et al. 2012; Seo et al.2009），吸烟控制体重介导这种关联（Pénzes et al. 2012），饮食和减肥态度与吸烟有关（Thomas et al. 2018）。Lange等（2014）发现，女性的感知吸烟和BMI与吸烟有关，但只有BMI与男性吸烟有关。只有一项研究发现了相反的影响（Delk et al. 2017），但值得注意的是，对男孩的显著影响仅限于肥胖范围内的男孩。由于统计力量有限，确定的吸烟者人数非常少（例如，42名30天吸烟者；Delk et al. 2017）。其他研究要么没有发现体重交互作用的性别证据，要么没有测试这种交互作用（性别通常被视为控制/调整变量）。体重认知/体重控制与吸烟之间存在非性别特异性的关联（Chung, Joung, 2014; Kendzor et al. 2007; Leatherdale et al. 2008; Weiss et al. 2007）。

54.2.2 纵向研究

纵向研究为评估体重/体重控制对吸烟的影响方向提供了可能性。如果体重/体重控制增加了吸烟的风险，在考虑了潜在的混淆因素后，我们应该看到纵向关联。当然，影响这种纵向研究有效性的一个关键因素是，流失率可以很低。流失率超过25%是有问题的，因为有多重问题的青少年通常在那些退出纵向研究的人中占了过多的比例（Gustavson et al. 2012; Western et al. 2016）。为了减少对内部和外部有效性的威胁，对于3年或更长时间的调查研究，建议流失率小于25%（Hansen et al. 1990; Nemes et al. 2002）。因此，我们关注的是损耗小于25%的纵向研究，研究特征总结见表54.2。在具有全国代表性的研究（基于全国青年纵向调查的美国研究，增加健康研究）中，研究结果相对一致。据估计，15岁女孩中因感觉超重而开始吸烟的比例接近20%（Caria et al. 2009）。在人口流失率最低的研究中，超重或试图减肥的女性比男性更有可能开始吸烟（Cawley et al. 2004）。其他的研究已经发现，吸烟与人们认为的而不是实际的体重有关（Harakeh et al. 2010; Koval et al. 2008）。Koval等（2008）发现女性认为自己超重会增加吸烟的可能性，但对于男性来说，BMI（而不是体重）与吸烟有关，这表明身体形象很重要，而且对女孩来说比男孩更重要。Kaufman和Augustson（2008）也发现，在吸烟的简单模型中，感知体重和试图减肥预测一年后吸烟，但一旦自尊在多变量分析中被考虑，这些影响就变得不显著了。这些研究结果强调了自尊作为吸烟决定因素的重要性，并指出关注体重可能是低自尊的标志。5年的纵向研究结果表明，对身体的不满与女性中一些不健康的体重控制策略有关，包括频繁节食和使用食物替代品，但女性中吸烟没有显著影响（Neumark-Sztainer et al. 2006）。相反，这项研究发现了男性对身体不满和吸烟之间的联系。有可能两次评估之间的长时间间隔（5年）削弱了对女孩的影响（对女孩的影响在单变量分析中是显著的），并且存在差异摩擦，也可能削弱了影响。作者指出，大约10%的女性和5%的男性称吸烟是为了减肥。

表54.2 吸烟与体重关注/控制关系的纵向研究

参考文献	样本量	样品特征	方法/调查	关键措施	主要发现
Caria (2009)	$N=2922$	11.6岁，瑞典	7年f/u, ATT=18%	终生吸烟、终生烟支数量、常规使用	女性：超重/自认为超重→吸烟
Cawley, Markowitz, Tauras (2004)	$N=9022$	12～16岁，NR	四轮，ATT=4%～9%	开始吸烟	女性：高BMI/报告试图减肥/报告超重→开始吸烟增加，与其他女性相比

续表

参考文献	样本量	样品特征	方法/调查	关键措施	主要发现
Harakeh (2010)	$N=428$ 个家族	完好无损的家庭，荷兰，NR	两轮，ATT=3%	体重控制动机、BMI、吸烟频率	控制体重的动机→开始吸烟增多，一般体重测量没有。没有性别差异
Hong, Rice, Johnson (2011)	$N=921$	9年级的女性，美国，不是NR	f/u 12年级，ATT=34.5%	吸烟天数/30天(>1支)	对超重和低吸烟风险的看法→吸烟增多
Kaufman (2008)	$N=6956$	仅限女性，7~12年级	一轮和两轮，增加健康，ATT=11.4%	经常吸烟(30天内每天吸烟1支以上)	在多变量模型中，感知体重不能预测吸烟
Koval (2008)	$N=1598$	6年级学生，107所学校，加拿大，不是NR	四轮到22岁，ATT(最后一次f/u)=21.5%	寿命/30天预测	女性：对超重的看法(8/11年级)→最近的吸烟者增多 男性：BMI(8/11年级)
Neumark-Sztainer et al. (2006)	$N=2516$	初中/高年级，31所学校，美国，不是NR	两轮，5年间隔，ATT=22.6%	过去一年的吸烟频率、BMI、身体满意度、节食/体重控制	女性：身体满意度降低→节食危害健康的行为增多，但不吸烟 男性：身体满意度降低→日吸烟量增加
Rees, Sabia (2010)	$N=$ 大约15000	11~23岁，美国，NR	增加健康：132所学校，5年 f/u ATT=11.4%~22.6%	吸烟天数/30天，吸烟>1/4包，烟>1/2包	超重→开始吸烟增多
Tanner-Smith (2010)	$N=5591$	10~15岁女孩，美国	三轮，ATT=15.4%（第二轮）	终生吸烟	体重指数调节青春期早期与物质使用的关系

54.2.3 总结和集成

在过去的15年里，大约23项实证研究调查了关注体重/控制与青少年吸烟之间的联系。有相反结果的研究很少。纵向研究大多在美国进行，损耗相对较低，且具有全国代表性的样本。总的来说，经验证据表明，有与体重相关的担忧（真实的或可感知到的）会增加吸烟的风险，而且这种效应对女性比男性更强。这篇综述的发现表明，相对于2004年的一项研究支持是混合的回顾发现，在过去的15年里，围绕研究问题的证据变得更加有力、更加一致（Potter et al. 2004）。在这项包括8项纵向研究的早期综述中，3项研究发现了支持我们发现的证据，2项没有发现关系，3项有相互矛盾的发现。这些发现对预防和早期干预具有紧迫的意义，因为尽管青少年吸烟率正在下降，但低社会经济地位社区的下降要慢得多，而且与吸烟相关的政策和项目在这些社区的影响范围似乎有限（AHPRA, 2013）。此外，在社会经济地位较低的地区，超重和肥胖率要高得多，因此这些社区的青少年会同时接触到成人吸烟和不令人满意的饮食/锻炼。本综述强调了体重关注/控制与相关的抑郁和焦虑在开始维持和解决吸烟方面的潜在重要性。根据本研究的结果，我们对预防方案提出了三个建议（见表54.3）。

表54.3 关于预防和早期干预的几点建议

早期发现	根据BMI、感知超重和与吸烟相关的信念/预期筛查高危青少年： · 体重担忧可能比实际体重/BMI更能预测吸烟风险 · 评估人们对烟草使用的预期体重和负面影响。这些可能预示着吸烟或复发的风险
普遍预防	将上述发现纳入吸烟预防计划： · 互动讨论"瘦理想"媒介、吸烟预期、体重、抑郁/焦虑和烟草使用之间的联系

续表

普遍预防	・挑战吸烟的期望值。预期挑战策略（交互式而不是基于信息的）在酒精文献中被证明是有效的（Darkes & Goldman, 1993） ・讨论吸烟对体重的短期影响和长期影响 ・提供有关减肥的健康替代品的互动教育 ・讨论与父母/兄弟姐妹/同伴吸烟有关的压力，特别是对担心自己体重的青少年
接触易受伤害社区的青少年	・来自低社会经济地位社区的青少年吸烟/超重的风险增加，但他们是最难接触到的 ・基于社区的联盟方法对于建立可持续的方法和向社区利益攸关方传授预防技能非常重要（Rowland et al. 2013, 2018） ・以社区为基础的联盟方法导致青少年烟草使用的大幅减少（Hawkins et al. 2009）

术语解释
- 体重指数（BMI）：通过体重单位为公斤除以身高，单位为平方米计算。
- 吸烟预期：对吸烟的个人后果的信念。
- 社会生态系统：青少年是社会系统中接近青少年的成员，通常嵌套（例如，社区内学校内的同龄人）。
- 瘦理想媒介：端口、厚度最理想，超重最不理想。
- 体重控制：通过饮食和体重管理策略对体重和体重管理的持续和侵入性的关注。

关于吸烟、饮食和减肥控制的关键事实
- 吸烟最常开始于青春期早期到中期。
- 青春期是一个极易受到"瘦的理想"（媒介信息是瘦的理想或完美的身材）影响的时期。
- 在脆弱的青少年中，理想体重和实际体重之间的差异与抑郁和焦虑有关。
- 烟草的使用被广泛认为有助于控制体重和管理负面影响。
- 吸烟预防计划应该强调与体重相关的吸烟预期的效用。

要点总结
- 担心自己体重的青少年开始吸烟的风险会升高。
- 预防吸烟的计划应该纳入解决体重问题、抑郁情绪和吸烟之间联系的策略。
- 弱势青少年可能居住在社会经济地位低、成人吸烟率高的社区。
- 传统的反吸烟政策和项目在高风险社区的"影响范围"可能较小。
- 授权当地社区联盟实施有效预防计划可能会加强对高危青少年的预防方案。

参考文献

AHPRA. (2013). Smoking and disadvantage: Evidence brief. Canberra: Commonwealth of Australia.
AIHW. (2017). Overweight and obesity in Australia: A birth cohort analysis. Canberra: Commonwealth of Australia.
Baker, C. (2017). Obesity statistics: Briefing paper number 3336. London: House of Commons.
Bronfenbrenner, U. (1989). Ecological systems theory. In R. Vasta (Ed.), Annals of child development. Six theories of child development: Revised formulations and current issues (pp. 1-103). Greenwich: JAI.
Caria, M. P.; Bellocco, R.; Zambon, A.; Horton, N. J.; Galanti, M. R. (2009). Overweight and perception of overweight as predictors of smokeless tobacco use and of cigarette smoking in a cohort of Swedish adolescents. Addiction, 104(4), 661-668.
Cavallo, D. A.; Duhig, A. M.; McKee, S.; Krishnan-Sarin, S. (2006). Gender and weight concerns in adolescent smokers. Addictive Behaviors, 31(11), 2140-2146.
Cawley, J.; Dragone, D.; Von Hinke Kessler Scholder, S. (2016). The demand for cigarettes as derived from the demand for weight loss: A theoretical and empirical investigation. Health Economics, 25, 8-23.

Cawley, J.; Markowitz, S.; Tauras, J. (2004). Lighting up and slimming down: The effects of body weight and cigarette prices on adolescent smoking initiation. Journal of Health Economics, 23, 293-311.

Chiolero, A.; Faeh, D.; Paccaud, F.; Cornuz, J. (2008). Consequences of smoking for body weight, body fat distribution, and insulin resistance. The American Journal of Clinical Nutrition, 87(4), 801-809. https://doi.org/10.1093/ajcn/87.4.801.

Chung, S. S.; Joung, K. H. (2014). Risk factors for current smoking among American and south Korean adolescents, 2005-2011. Journal of Nursing Scholarship, 46(6), 408-415.

Cook, S. J.; MacPherson, K.; Langille, D. B. (2007). Weight perception, weight control, and associated risky behavior of adolescent girls in Nova Scotia. Canadian Family Physician, 63, 679-684.

Dallosso, H. M.; James, W. P. (1984). The role of smoking in the regulation of energy balance. International Journal of Obesity, 8, 365-375.

Darkes, J.; Goldman, M. S. (1993). Expectancy challenge and drinking reduction: experimental evidence for a mediational process. Journal of Consulting and Clinical Psychology, 61(2), 344-353.

Delk, J.; Creamer, M. R.; Perry, C. L.; Harrell, M. B. (2017). Weight status and cigarette and electronic cigarette use in adolescents. American Journal of Preventive Medicine, 54(1), e31-e35.

Dittmar, H.; Halliwell, E.; Stirling, E. (2009). Understanding the impact of thin media models on women's body-focused affect: the roles of thin-ideal internalization and weight-related self-discrepancy activation in experimental exposure effects. Journal of Social and Clinical Psychology, 28(1), 43-72.

Ennett, S. T.; Foshee, V. A.; Bauman, K. E.; Hussong, A. M.; Cai, L.; Luz, H. et al. (2008). The social ecology of adolescent alcohol misuse. Child Development, 79, 1777-1791.

Gustavson, K.; von Soest, T.; Karevold, E.; Røysamb, E. (2012). Attrition and generalizability in longitudinal studies: findings from a 15-year population-based study and a Monte Carlo simulation study. BMC Public Health, 12, 918.

Hansen, W. B.; Tobler, N. S.; Graham, J. W. (1990). Attrition in substance-abuse prevention research - a metaanalysis of 85 longitudinally followed cohorts. Evaluation Review, 14(6), 677-685.

Harakeh, Z.; Engels, R. C. M. E.; Monshouwer, K.; Hanssen, P. F. (2010). Adolescent's weight concerns and the onset of smoking. Substance Use, Misuse, 45(12), 1847-1860.

Harrison, K. (2000). The body electric: thin-ideal media and eating disorders in adolescents. Journal of Communication, 50(3), 119-143.

Hawkins, J. D.; Oesterle, S.; Brown, E. C.; Arthur, M. W.; Abbott, R. D.; Fagan, A. A. et al. (2009). Results of a type 2 translational research trial to prevent adolescent drug use and delinquency. Archives of Pediatrics and Adolescent Medicine, 163(9), 789-798.

Heinz, A. J.; Kassel, J. D.; Berbaum, M.; Mermelstein, R. (2010). Adolescents' expectancies for smoking to regulate affect predict smoking behavior and nicotine dependence over time. Drug and Alcohol Dependence, 111(1-2), 128-135.

Hinchliff, G. L. M.; Kelly, A. B.; Chan, G. C. K.; Toumbourou, J. W.; Patton, G. C.; Williams, J. (2016). Risky dieting behaviors amongst adolescent girls: associations with family relationship problems and depressed mood. Eating Behaviors, 22, 222-224. https://doi.org/10.1016/j.eatbeh.2016.06.001.

Hong, T.; Rice, J.; Johnson, C. (2011). Social environmental and individual factors associated with smoking among a panel of adolescent girls. Women and Health, 51, 187-203.

Johnson, J. L.; Eaton, D. K.; Pederson, L. L.; Lowry, R. (2009). Associations of trying to lose weight, weight control behaviors, and currentcigarette use among US high schoolstudents. Journal of School Health, 79, 355-360.

Kaufman, A. R.; Augustson, E. M. (2008). Predictors of regular cigarette smoking among adolescent females: does body image matter? Nicotine, Tobacco Research, 10(8), 1301-1309.

Kelly, A. B.; O'Flaherty, M.; Connor, J. P.; Homel, R.; Toumbourou, J. W.; Patton, G. C. et al. (2011). The influence of parents, siblings and peers on pre- and early-teen smoking: a multilevel model. Drug and Alcohol Review, 30, 381-387.

Kendzor, D. E.; Copeland, A. L.; Stewart, T. M.; Businelle, M. S.; Williamson, D. A. (2007). Weight-related concerns associated with smoking in young children. Addictive Behaviors, 32(3), 598-607.

Koval, J. J.; Pederson, L. L.; Zhang, X.; Mowery, P.; McKenna, M. (2008). Can young adult smok status be predicted from concern about body weight and self-reported BMI among adolescents? Results from a ten-year cohort study. Nicotine, Tobacco Research, 10(9), 1449-1455.

Lange, K.; Thamotharan, S.; Racine, M.; Hirko, C.; Fields, S. (2015). The relationship between weight and smoking in a national sample of adolescents: role of gender. Journal of Health Psychology, 20(12), 1558-1567.

Leatherdale, S. T.; Wong, S. L.; Manske, S. R.; Colditz, G. A. (2008). Susceptibility to smoking and its association with physical activity, BMI, and weight concerns among youth. Nicotine, Tobacco Research, 10(3), 499-505.

Mehus, C.; Doty, J.; Chan, G. C. K.; Kelly, A. B.; Hemphill, S.; Toumbourou, J. W. et al. (2018). Testing the social interaction learning model's applicability to adolescent substance misuse in an Australian context. Substance Use and Misuse. https://doi.org/10.1080/10826084.2018.1441307.

Monahan, K. C.; Steinberg, L.; Cauffman, E. (2009). Affiliation with antisocial peers, susceptibility to peer influence, and antisocial behavior during the transition to adulthood. Developmental Psychology, 45(6), 1520-1530.

Nagaya, T.; Yoshida, H.; Takahashi, H.; Kawai, M. (2007). Cigarette smoking weakens exercise habits in healthy men. Nicotine, Tobacco Research, 9(10), 1027-1032.

Nemes, S.; Wish, E.; Wraight, B.; Messina, N. (2002). Correlates of treatment follow-up difficulty. Substance Use, Misuse, 37(1), 19-45.

Neumark-Sztainer, D.; Paxton, S. J.; Hannan, P. J.; Haines, J.; Story, M. (2006). Does body satisfaction matter? Five year longitudinal associations between body satisfaction and health behaviors in adolescent females and males. Journal of Adolescent Health, 39, 244-251.

OECD. (2017). Obesity update 2017. Organisation for Economic Co-operation and Development. Retrieved from:(2017). www. oecd. org. Accessed 21 March 2018.

Ogden, C. L.; Carroll, M. D.; Fryar, C. D.; Flegal, K. M. (2015). Prevalence of obesity among adults and youth: United States, 2011-2014.

Pénzes, M.; Czeglédi, E.; Balázs, P.; Foley, K. L. (2012). Factors associated with tobacco smoking and the belief about weight control effects of smoking among Hungarian adolescents. Central European Journal of Public Health, 20(1), 11-17.

Potter, B. K.; Pederson, L. L.; Chan, S. S. H.; Aubut, J. -A. L.; Koval, J. J. (2004). Does a relationship exist between body weight, concerns about weight, and smoking among adolescents? An integration of theliteraturewith an emphasis on gender. Nicotine, TobaccoResearch, 6(3), 397-425. https://doi. org/10. 1080/14622200410001696529.

Public Health England. Childhood Obesity: Applying All our health, 2015, Retrieved 27/08/2018 from www.gov.uk/government/publications/childhood-obesity-applying-all-our-health.

Rees, D. I.; Sabia, J. J. (2010). Body weight and smoking initiation: Evidence from Add Health. Journal of Health Economics, 29, 774-777.

Robertson, L.; McGee, R.; Hancox, R. J. (2014). Smoking cessation and subsequent weight change. Nicotine, Tobacco Research, 16(6), 867-871.

Rowland, B.; Toumbourou, J. W.; Osborn, A.; Smith, R.; Hall, J. K.; Kremer, P. et al. (2013). A clustered randomised trial examining the effect of social marketing and community mobilisation on the age of uptake and levels of alcohol consumption by Australian adolescents: study protocol. British Medical Journal Open. 3, e002423https://doi. org/10. 1136/bmjopen-2012-002423.

Rowland, B. C.; Williams, J.; Smith, R.; Hall, J. K.; Osborn, A.; Kremer, P. et al. (2018). Social marketing and community mobilisation to reduce underage alcohol consumption in Australia: a cluster randomised community trial. Preventive Medicine. https://doi. org/10. 1016/j. ypmed. 2018. 02. 032.

Seo, D.; Jiang, N.; Kolbe, L. J. (2009). Association of smoking with body weight in US high school students, 1999-2005. American Journal of Health Behavior, 33(2), 202-212.

Smith, D.; Kelly, A. B.; Chan, G. C. K.; Toumbourou, J. W.; Patton, G. C.; Williams, J. (2014). Beyond the primary influences of parents and peers on very young adolescent alcohol use: evidence of independent neighbourhood effects. Journal of Early Adolescence, 34(5), 568-583.

Tanner-Smith, E. E. (2010). Negotiating the early developing body: Pubertal timing, body weight, and adolescent girls' substance use. Journal of Youth and Adolescence, 39, 1402-1416.

Thomas, R.; Kelly, A. B.; Chan, G. C. K.; Hides, L. M.; Quinn, C. A.; Kavanagh, D. J. et al. (2018). An examination of gender differences in the association of eating and weight loss attitudes. Substance Use, Misuse 53, 2125-2131. https://doi. org/ 10. 1080/10826084. 2018. 1455703.

Wack, J. T.; Rodin, J. (1982). Smoking and its effects on body weight and the systems of caloric regulation. The American Journal of Clinical Nutrition, 35(2), 366-380.

Wahl, S. K.; Turner, L. R.; Mermelstein, R. J.; Flay, B. R. (2005). Adolescents' smoking expectancies: psychometric properties and prediction of behavior change. Nicotine, Tobacco Research, 7(4), 613-623. https://doi. org/10. 1080/14622200500185579.

Wehby, G. L.; Murray, J. C.; Wilcox, A.; Lie, R. T. (2012). Smoking and body weight: evidence using genetic instruments. Economics and Human Biology, 10(2), 113-126.

Weiss, J. W.; Merrill, V.; Gritz, E. R. (2007). Ethnic variation in the association between weight concern and adolescent smoking. Addictive Behaviors, 32(10), 2311-2316. https://doi. org/10. 1016/j. addbeh. 2007. 01. 020.

Western, B.; Braga, A.; Hureau, D.; Sirois, C. (2016). Study retention as bias reduction in a hard-to-reach population. Proceedings of the National Academy of Sciences, 113(20), 5477.

WHO. (2015). WHO global report on trends in prevalence of tobacco smoking 2015. Geneva: World Health Organization.

Xie, B.; Chou, C. -P.; Spruijt-Metz, D.; Reynolds, K.; Clark, F.; Palmer, P. H. et al. (2006). Weight perception and weight-related sociocultural and behavioral factors in Chinese adolescents. Preventive Medicine, 42(3), 229-234. https://doi. org/10. 1016/j. ypmed. 2005.12.013.

55
锻炼是一种戒烟的辅助手段

Scott Rollo, Wuyou Sui, Harry Prapavessis

Faculty of Health Sciences, School of Kinesiology, The University of Western Ontario, London, ON, Canada

缩略语

CBT	认知行为疗法	**PA**	体育活动
NRT	烟碱替代疗法	**RCT**	随机对照试验

55.1 引言

吸烟是全球可预防死亡的主要原因,每年有600多万人死于烟草使用(WHO, 2017)。人们已经证实,吸烟对健康有害,也是许多慢性疾病的一个重要的可改变的风险因素(USDHHS, 2010)。尽管在全球范围内呈下降,但全球吸烟率仍超过11亿人(WHO, 2017)。任何年龄的戒烟都有许多健康益处和降低患吸烟相关疾病的风险,如肺癌、心脏病发作、中风和慢性肺部疾病(USDHHS,1990)。

不幸的是,戒烟是很困难的。尽管已知的健康后果,许多吸烟者发现挑战戒烟,而且失败率一直很高。在未接受正式治疗的情况下戒烟的成年吸烟者中,只有3%～5%的人在尝试戒烟1年后成功戒烟(Hughes et al. 2004)。低戒烟率可以用许多因素来解释,包括烟碱的高度成瘾特性(Hirschhorn, WHO, 2009)、强烈的渴望和戒断症状(Allen et al. 2008)、体重增加与戒烟(Klesges et al. 1988),以及吸烟的学习和强化行为(CADTH, 2014)。

许多药理学治疗[如烟碱替代疗法(NRT)、烟碱口香糖、吸入器、鼻喷雾剂、透皮贴片和含片;见图55.1和图55.2]和行为戒烟治疗[例如,认知行为疗法(CBT)]可以帮助戒烟过

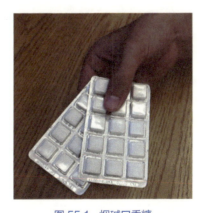

图 55.1 烟碱口香糖

一种常见的烟碱替代疗法(NRT)的例子。

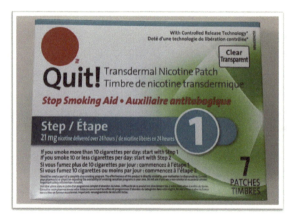

图 55.2 一个经皮烟碱贴片

NRT 的一种常见形式的说明。

程，促进戒烟维持，并预防吸烟复发（Collins et al. 2010）。虽然上述干预措施的结合可以提高戒烟成功率，但这些成功率仍然适中（即 1 年戒烟率在 8%～23%；CADTH, 2014; Lancaster, Stead, 2017）。因此，有必要探索可能有助于改善的替代治疗和/或辅助治疗方案，以改善现有的戒烟治疗和维持方法。

55.2 为什么锻炼可能是一种有效的戒烟治疗选择

来自许多大型横断面调查的证据表明，体育活动水平（PA）与吸烟率呈负相关（Picavet et al. 2011）。此外，更高水平的 PA 与开始戒烟尝试（Gauthier et al. 2012）、保持戒烟的信心（King et al. 1996）以及成功戒烟（Abrantes et al.2009）呈正相关。来自两个荟萃分析的证据表明，与对照条件相比，急性运动可以降低暂时戒烟后吸烟的冲动（Haasova et al. 2013; Roberts et al. 2012）。戒烟过程中的许多烟碱戒断症状也被证明可以通过锻炼得到改善（Ussher, Taylor, Faulkner, 2014）。此外，有研究证据表明，从长远来看，锻炼可能会减少戒烟后的体重增加（Farley, Hajek, Lycett, Aveyard, 2012）。最后，运动已被证明对其他可能防止吸烟复发的因素有积极的影响，包括抑郁（Williams, 2008）、一般疲劳和睡眠障碍（Hatsukami et al. 1984）、自尊（Spence, McGannon, Poon, 2005），以及感知的应对能力（Tritter, Fitzgeorge, Prapavessis, 2015）。综上所述，有证据支持锻炼作为烟草依赖治疗的一个组成部分的好处。

55.3 运动作为戒烟的辅助手段

许多研究已经调查了运动单独或结合传统的戒烟方法（即行为疗法和/或药物治疗）对戒烟结果的影响。当评论迄今为止的试验时，持续戒烟将作为两者都被报告的主要结果衡量指标。这可以证明，因为持续戒酒是一种更严格的戒烟措施，并更直接地与健康结果有关（Marcus et al.1999）。

（1）Cochrane 综述（Cochrane Collaboration 发布的系统性综述，通常被视为权威的医学证据）Ussher 等（2014）进行了一项系统的回顾，以确定基于运动的干预单独或联合戒烟计划是否比单独的戒烟干预更有效。在这篇综述中，确定了20项随机对照试验（RCT；$n=5870$）的运动辅助干预。在20项试验中，只有4项显示，在治疗结束时，运动辅助组的戒欲率显著高于对照组（Bock et al. 2012; Marcus et al. 1999; Marcus, Albrecht, Niaura, Abrams, Thompson, 1991; Martin et al. 1997），而只有一项研究在1年的随访中显示了运动的边缘显著益处（Marcus et al. 1999；见图55.3）。此外，只有四项研究考察了运动与NRT结合的有效性（Hill et al. 1993; Kinnunen et al. 2008; Martin et al. 1997; Prapavessis et al. 2007）。其中一项研究显示，在治疗结束和12个月的随访中，运动加贴片组的戒烟率明显高于单纯运动组（Prapavessis et al. 2007）。可以提供许多解释来解释大多数研究没有发现结果。第一，只有一项研究发现在所有领域存在低偏倚风险，只有七项研究有足够大的样本量来检测治疗和对照条件之间的显著差异。第二，研究发现戒烟和运动项目的时间和强度各不相同。第三，不同研究的戒烟结果各不相同，8个研究评估了持续禁欲，2个评估了长期戒烟，8个评估了点流行戒烟；两位没有具体说明。第四，许多试验包括干预措施，这些干预措施的强度可能不足以产生所需的运动水平变化。总之，这篇综述提供了进一步研究锻炼作为戒烟辅助作用的证据。在接下来的几页中，读者将详细了解自Ussher等（2014）Cochrane综述以来发表的运动辅助戒烟文献的状况。

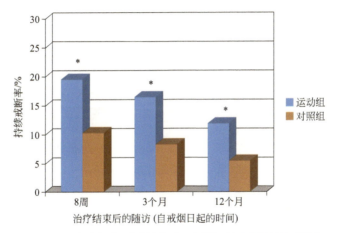

图55.3　治疗结束时、治疗结束后3个月和12个月的持续戒烟率

条形图表示在戒烟后一天的随访中，运动组相对于对照组的戒烟率。星号表示显著性（$P<0.05$）。数据来自Marcus等（1999）。

（2）强化运动辅助治疗

Abrantes等（2014）认为，在以前的运动干预试验中，固有的一些方法局限性（如干预强度不足、缺乏增加依从性的努力以及缺乏接触控制条件）可能会降低其作为戒烟辅助工具的有效性。为了解决这些限制，Abrantes和同事进行了一项为期12周的随机对照试验，以检验对吸烟者的行为运动干预（$n=61$）的有效性。在有氧运动（AE）条件下的参与者接受了有监督的锻炼课程（每周一次；见图55.4），进行家庭中等强度运动（每周2～4次），每周认知行为小组咨询课程，以及基于治疗依从性的经济激励成分。健康教育接触控制（HEC）的参与者被要求参加每周一小时的健康教育课程。所有参与者都接受了为期8周（从第5周开始）的戒烟方案，包括每周20分钟的电话咨询和NRT治疗（即透皮贴剂）。在基线、3个月（治疗结束）、6个月和12个月随访时进行评估。两组的治疗依从性都相当高（即75%）。AE组的参与者表现出更高的持续戒烟率（EOT：30%与25.8%，OR 1.23；6个月随访：23.3%与9.7%，OR 2.83；12个月随访：13.3%与

3.2%，OR 4.64）与HEC组相比；然而，这些差异并没有达到统计学意义（见图55.5）。研究还发现，AE条件下的参与者在戒烟后的PA水平显著升高（$b = 1.37$，$SE = 0.43$，$P < 0.01$）。这种干预包括一些显著的特征来促进运动坚持包括监督下的中强度有氧运动，在戒烟前1个月开始运动的顺序方法，监督加在家锻炼的结合，基于竞争的经济激励成分，认知行为锻炼咨询。总之，这项初步试验提供了有希望的证据，表明与单纯的标准治疗相比，行为锻炼干预可能是一种有用的辅助手段，可以改善戒烟结果。

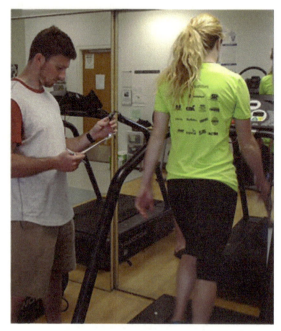

图55.4　有监督的戒烟运动训练

这张图说明了在运动辅助戒烟计划中现场组织有氧运动的例子。

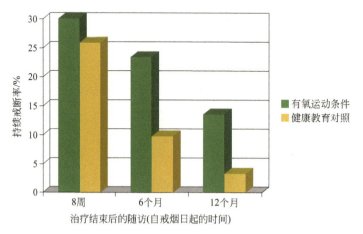

图55.5　治疗结束时、治疗结束后6个月和12个月的持续戒断率

条形图显示有氧运动条件与健康教育接触对照条件下的戒断率（%）。改编自Abrantes等的数据（2014）。

（3）特殊人群

运动作为一种戒烟辅助手段也对高危人群进行了调查。例如，Ussher等（2015）实施了一项大规模、多中心随机对照试验，以确定PA干预作为怀孕吸烟者戒烟辅助工具（$n=789$）的有效性。参与者被随机接受6周单独的个人行为戒烟支持（对照）或行为戒烟支持加上PA干预，包括PA咨询和14次监督的中等强度运动（第1～6周每周两次，第6～8周每周一次）。在目标戒烟日期前一周开始进行干预。从戒烟日期到怀孕结束之间进行了生物化学验证的持续戒断评估。研究结果表明，在怀孕末期，两组之间的戒烟率没有显著差异。PA组和对照组的持续戒断率分别为8%和6%（OR 1.21, 95% CI: 0.70～2.10）。然而，与对照组相比，在戒烟后的第1、4和6周，PA组每周自我报告的PA分钟显著增加了33%（95% CI: 14%～56%）、28%（95% CI: 7%～52%）和36%（95% CI: 12%～65%）。这些发现表明，与单独的行为支持相比，PA干预结合行为戒烟支持并不能显著提高怀孕吸烟者的戒烟率。尽管在PA组出席率低（只有29%的依从性），PA咨询部分可能仍然有助于增加PA水平。作者认为，也许要求同时改变两种健康行为（即吸烟和PA），同时应对怀孕是一项太困难的任务。未来怀孕期间戒烟的干预措施应该在预期戒烟日期之前就开始锻炼，以减轻那些试图戒烟的人的负担，并最大限度地利用锻炼来帮助戒烟。

经济上处于不利地位的不打算戒烟的吸烟者可能受益于旨在减少他们吸烟的治疗。通过一项实验性RCT，Thompson等（2016）评估了与常规护理相比，运动辅助减少然后戒烟干预对16周吸烟和PA结果的影响。那些希望减少吸烟但不戒烟的弱势吸烟者（$n=99$）被随机分配到接受常规护理或常规护理加上运动辅助的减少然后戒烟干预。干预包括多达12周的以参与者为中心的个人激励支持会议，以促进减少吸烟和增加PA。与对照组相比，干预组的参与者更有可能尝试戒烟（35.5%与9.7%; OR 5.05, 95% CI: 1.10～23.15），更大比例的参与者在16周吸烟至少减少了50%（分别为63.3%与32.3%; OR 4.21, 95%置信区间:1.32～13.39）。此外，在4周的随访中，组间在戒烟后的戒烟方面发现了有希望的差异（23%与6%; OR 4.91, 95% CI: 0.80～30.24）。不幸的是，没有发现干预对PA有影响，而且参与支持会议的比例（52.5%）在干预吸烟者中可能更高。这项研究是第一个检验行为干预对PA的有效性的研究之一，以促进最初不想戒烟的吸烟者减少吸烟。研究结果表明，在减少吸烟方面，运动辅助的行为咨询干预似乎比单纯的常规护理更有效。

在最近的一项研究中，Smits等（2016）进行了一项随机对照试验，以检测高焦虑敏感性、久坐不动的日常成年吸烟者中，高强度运动辅助戒烟的有效性。所有参与者（$n=136$）接受了15周的标准戒烟治疗（ST; 也就是说，7周的认知行为治疗以及从第6周开始的NRT贴片），并被要求在第6周尝试戒烟。此外，参与者被随机分配到15周有监督的锻炼计划（ST+EX）或15周健康教育接触控制条件（ST+CTRL），每组每周3次，每次35分钟。在目标戒烟日期后10周（治疗结束）、16周（即4个月）和24周（即6个月）进行评估。结果显示，参与者平均参加了45次运动或健康教育治疗中的24次（即53%）。在戒烟方面，研究结果表明，在焦虑敏感性高的人群中，在每个评估期，ST+EX条件下的持续戒烟率显著高于ST+CTRL条件下的持续戒烟率［持续戒烟: $b=-0.98$, $SE=0.346$, $t(132)=-2.84$, $P=0.005$］，但在低焦虑敏感性人群中不存在。在那些焦虑敏感性高的患者中，ST+EX组和ST+CTRL组在治疗结束、戒烟4个月后和戒烟6个月后的持续戒烟率分别为25.9%和11.6%、24.8%和11.0%、23.3%和10.2%。因此，在焦虑敏感性高的成年吸烟者中，与单独的标准护理相比，结合运动和标准护理可能增加戒烟成功的概率。

（4）锻炼和戒烟

Prapavessis等（2016）进行了一项名为Getting Physical on Cigarettes的RCT，以检查一个运

动辅助的NRT戒烟干预计划的有效性，该计划内置了运动和戒烟维持成分，对干预后14周、26周和56周的持续戒烟进行了测试。Prapavessis和他的同事认识到坚持锻炼辅助戒烟计划成功的重要性，他们也试图确定整个计划的坚持是否对吸烟状态有影响。希望戒烟的女性吸烟者（$n = 413$）被招募参加一个为期14周的监督锻炼和NRT（即透皮贴片）戒烟计划，随后被随机分为四种情况之一：运动维护加戒烟维护、运动维护加接触控制、戒烟维护加接触控制、接触控制。为第四周设定了一个目标戒烟日期。运动维持组在第8周和第14周期间接受了5次基于组的CBT治疗以促进运动坚持，在第26周和第52周期间接受了电话咨询以保持运动行为。戒烟加接触控制组和接触控制组在第8周、14周接受了5次健康教育，在第26周、第52周接受了关于女性健康问题的电话咨询。在第14周，戒烟维持小组收到了针对戒烟和复发预防的信息小册子。有监督的运动阶段（66%）、NRT方案（68.81%）和CBT运动维持组（54%）的依从率显著高于干预后电话运动维持组（38%）。研究发现，与吸烟者相比，戒烟者有更高的治疗依从率，并得到更多的维持。在第14周（57%与43%）、第26周（27%与21%）和第56周（26%与23.5%），运动组和等量接触非运动维持组之间的持续吸烟戒断率存在差异（见图55.6）。尽管存在这些有临床意义的差异，但只有第14周吸烟状况的差异接近显著性（$\chi^2[1, n = 409] = 2.36$和$P = 0.08$）。这些发现表明，需要考虑在终止由运动辅助的NRT戒烟计划后提供其他运动维持的方法。

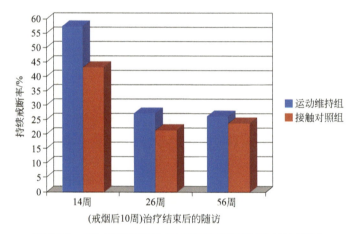

图55.6　在治疗结束时以及26周和56周随访时的持续戒断率

条形图表示运动维持但与同等接触的非运动维持组的戒断率。数据来自Prapavessis等（2016）。

55.4 未来方向

关于锻炼作为戒烟辅助手段的作用，可以提出一些未来的建议。为了确定运动对戒烟的影响，需要进行更大样本的试验，至少适度运动强度的结构化现场运动干预，同等的接触控制条件，以生物化学方法验证的持续戒烟作为主要结果，以及至少6个月的随访期。在干预设计方面，有人认为要求同时改变两种健康行为可能太困难了（例如，Prapavessis et al. 2007, 2016; Ussher et al. 2015）。因此，建议在吸烟者开始尝试戒烟之前开始锻炼计划，从而使个人在被要求显著改变吸烟行为之前专注于变得更积极（Ussher et al. 2014）。基于本文报告的研究结果，也建议未来的试验包括药理或行为疗法作为戒烟治疗的基础。有证据表明，结合锻炼和NRT或行为咨询的方法可以提高戒烟率，并增加任何一种单独治疗方法成功戒烟的可能性。

未来研究的一个关键重点是找到新颖和创新的方法，以最大限度地坚持这些戒烟计划。在Prapavessis等（2016）的研究中，提高运动辅助戒烟计划的坚持率的一个可能的解决方案是关注运动和戒烟的维持阶段。所有的戒烟计划（包括运动辅助戒烟计划）都显示出早期的希望，在治疗和随访结束时出现复发效果。因此，至关重要的是，这些类型的计划将初始戒烟和运动维持的组成部分结合到他们的设计中，以防止这两种行为的复发。到目前为止，那些让吸烟者从监督下的锻炼中戒掉的项目并没有成功地促进参与者在项目终止后的独立锻炼。未来的工作需要研究更有效的方法来维持长期的戒烟和锻炼。有可能面对面的技术和应用与实时反馈可能提供可行的选择，以改善运动维护和减少吸烟复发（Free et al. 2011）。为了准确地评估治疗依从性，建议未来的研究包括对治疗依从性的客观测量和随访。进一步的研究也需要测试不同形式的运动处方，并确定最有效的时间、强度和运动方式。在现实世界的设置中，演习辅助戒烟方案的设计和实施也保证允许这种方法作为一种戒烟援助的未来传播。最后，还需要进行更多的研究，以调查运动在种族更多样化的人群、风险人群（如心血管疾病患者）和不同年龄组（如青年吸烟者）中对戒烟的作用。

55.5 结论

运动和戒烟都对健康是独立有益的。因此，将运动与现有的戒烟治疗方案相结合，可能被证明是促进和维持戒烟的最佳方法。基于迄今为止的研究结果，有一些研究证据支持运动作为行为咨询和药物治疗（即NRT）治疗选择的辅助手段在戒烟方面的有效性。有证据表明，与传统的戒烟治疗相比，运动有可能提高持续的戒断率；然而，坚持锻炼是一个一致的问题，特别是在项目终止后。这是不幸的，因为坚持运动和戒烟结果之间有明显的联系。未来的试验需要探索如何提高运动治疗的依从性，并在锻炼辅助戒烟计划终止后保持锻炼，以便对戒烟和与健康相关的结果产生最大的影响。

术语解释

- **有氧运动**：是一种主要挑战心肺系统的运动。它包括步行、骑自行车、跑步和游泳等活动。
- **行为咨询**：是一种疗法，包括动机支持、强化非吸烟行为、放松训练、应对技能训练、应急管理、自我控制和认知行为疗法。行为治疗方法的强度和传递形式各不相同。
- **持续戒断**：指自戒烟日期以来吸烟不超过5支。
- **锻炼体育活动**：有计划、有组织和重复的活动，侧重于改善或维持身体健康和/或心理健康的措施。有目的的运动通常在中等强度进行，并以>10min的周期累积。
- **中等强度的运动**：需要适度的努力，并显著加速心率（即最大心率的50%～70%）。例如，快走、跳舞和骑自行车。
- **烟碱替代疗法**：NRT例如，口香糖、透皮贴片、吸入器、鼻喷雾剂和含片替代血液中烟草衍生的烟碱，并减少消除吸烟者时与烟碱相关的渴望和戒断症状。
- **身体活动**：由骨骼肌产生的任何身体运动，导致超过休息水平的能量消耗。
- **戒烟尝试**：吸烟者戒烟的一段时间；定义为至少24小时的戒断时间。
- **7天流行点戒断**：在过去7天内不吸一支烟。

	■ 戒烟：停止吸烟的过程；通常是指一个人达到戒烟的程度。
	■ 吸烟复发：是指吸烟者在戒烟事件后继续吸烟。
	■ 剧烈运动：需要大量的努力，并导致快速呼吸和心率显著增加（即最大心率的70%～85%）的运动。例如，跑步和快速游泳。
运动作为一种戒烟辅助手段的关键事实	■ 运动可以减少戒烟期间与烟碱相关的渴望和戒断症状。 ■ 运动可以减少戒烟后的体重增加。 ■ 运动在许多健康方面都有好处。 ■ 在工业国家，只有15%的成年人定期进行体育活动。 ■ 生活中的早期身体活动模式可以强烈地预测生活后期的身体活动模式。
要 点 总 结	■ 本章着重介绍了运动的有效性，无论是单独的，或与传统的戒烟治疗相结合，作为一种戒烟援助。 ■ 尽管有现有的治疗方案，但只有8%～23%的人在尝试戒烟1年后仍成功戒烟。 ■ 最近，运动被提议作为戒烟的一种帮助手段，因为它被证明可以减少与烟碱相关的渴望和戒断症状。 ■ 有一些证据表明，与单纯的传统戒烟治疗相比，运动辅助戒烟计划有可能提高持续的戒烟率；然而，坚持运动是一个一致的问题，特别是在项目终止后。 ■ 需要新的和创新的方法来改善运动治疗的坚持，并在运动辅助戒烟计划终止后维持锻炼。

参考文献

Abrantes, A. M.; Bloom, E. L.; Strong, D. R.; Riebe, D.; Marcus, B. H.; Desaulniers, J. et al. (2014). A preliminary randomized controlled trial of a behavioral exercise intervention for smoking cessation. Nicotine, Tobacco Research, 16(8), 1094-1103.

Abrantes, A. M.; Strong, D. R.; Lloyd-Richardson, E. E.; Niaura, R.; Kahler, C. W.; Brown, R. A. (2009). Regular exercise as a protectivefactor in relapse following smoking cessation treatment. American Journal on Addictions, 18(1), 100-101.

Allen, S. S.; Bade, T.; Hatsukami, D.; Center, B. (2008). Craving, withdrawal, and smoking urges on days immediately prior to smoking relapse. Nicotine, Tobacco Research, 10(1), 35-45.

Bock, B. C.; Fava, J. L.; Gaskins, R.; Morrow, K. M.; Williams, D. M.; Jennings, E. et al. (2012). Yoga as a complementary treatment forsmoking cessation in women. Journal of Women's Health, 21(2), 240-248.

Canadian Agency for Drugs and Technologies in Health. (2014). Nicotine replacement therapy for smoking cessation or reduction: a review of the clinical evidence. Ottawa, ON: CADTH.

Collins, S. E.; Witkiewitz, K.; Kirouac, M.; Marlatt, G. A. (2010). Preventing relapse following smoking cessation. Current Cardiovascular Risk Reports, 4(6), 421-428.

Farley, A. C.; Hajek, P.; Lycett, D.; Aveyard, P. (2012). Interventions for preventing weight gain after smoking cessation. Cochrane Database of Systematic Reviews, 1.

Free, C.; Knight, R.; Robertson, S.; Whittaker, R.; Edwards, P.; Zhou, W. et al. (2011). Smoking cessation support delivered via mobile phone text messaging (txt2stop): a single-blind, randomised trial. Lancet, 378(9785), 49-55.

Gauthier, A. P.; Snelling, S. J.; King, M. (2012). "Thinking outside the pack": examining physically active smokers and implications for practice among Ontario residents. Health Promotion Practice, 13(3), 395-403.

Haasova, M.; Warren, F. C.; Ussher, M.; Janse Van Rensburg, K.; Faulkner, G.; Cropley, M. et al. (2013). The acute effects of physical activity on cigarette cravings: systematic review and meta-analysis with individual participant data. Addiction, 108(1), 26-37.

Hatsukami, D. K.; Hughes, J. R.; Pickens, R. W.; Suilis, D. (1984). Tobacco withdrawal symptoms: an experimental analysis. Psychopharmacology, 84, 231-236.

Hill, R. D.; Rigdon, M.; Johnson, S. (1993). Behavioral smoking cessation treatment for older chronic smokers. Behavior Therapy, 24(2), 321-329.

Hirschhorn, N.; World Health Organization. (2009). Evolution of the tobacco industry positions on addiction to nicotine: A report prepared for the Tobacco Free Initiative. World Health Organization. WHO Tobacco Control Papers (NLM No. HD 9149).

Hughes, J. R.; Keely, J.; Naud, S. (2004). Shape of the relapse curve and long-term abstinence among untreated smokers. Addiction, 99, 29-38.

King, T. K.; Marcus, B. H.; Pinto, B. M.; Emmons, K. M.; Abrams, D. B. (1996). Cognitive-behavioral mediators of changing multiple behaviors: smoking and a sedentary lifestyle. Preventive Medicine, 25(6), 684-691.

Kinnunen, T.; Leeman, R. F.; Korhonen, T.; Quiles, Z. N.; Terwal, D. M.; Garvey, A. J. et al. (2008). Exercise as an adjunct to nicotine gum in treating tobacco dependence among women. Nicotine, Tobacco Research, 10(4), 689-703.

Klesges, R. C.; Brown, K.; Pascale, R. W.; Murphy, M.; Williams, E.; Cigrang, J. A. (1988). Factors associated with participation, attrition, and outcome in a smoking cessation program at the workplace. Health Psychology, 7(6), 575-589.

Lancaster, T.; Stead, L. F. (2017). Individual behavioural counselling for smoking cessation. Cochrane Database of Systematic Reviews, 3.

Marcus, B. H.; Albrecht, A. E.; King, T. K.; Parisi, A. F.; Pinto, B. M.; Roberts, M. et al. (1999). The efficacy of exercise as an aid for smoking cessation in women: a randomized controlled trial. Archives of Internal Medicine, 159(11), 1229-1234.

Marcus, B. H.; Albrecht, A. E.; Niaura, R. S.; Abrams, D. B.; Thompson, P. D. (1991). Usefulness of physical exercise for maintaining smoking cessation in women. The American Journal of Cardiology, 68(4), 406-407.

Martin, J. E.; Calfas, K. J.; Patten, C. A.; Polarek, M.; Hofstetter, C. R.; Noto, J. et al. (1997). Prospective evaluation of three smoking interventions in 205 recovering alcoholics: one-year results of Project SCRAP-Tobacco. Journal of Consulting and Clinical Psychology, 65(1), 190-194.

Picavet, H. S. J.; Wendel-vos, G. W.; Vreeken, H. L.; Schuit, A. J.; Verschuren, W. M. M. (2011). How stable are physical activity habits among adults? The Doetinchem Cohort Study. Medicine, Science in Sports, Exercise, 43(1), 74-79.

Prapavessis, H.; Cameron, L.; Baldi, J. C.; Robinson, S.; Borrie, K.; Harper, T. et al. (2007). The effects of exercise and nicotine replacement therapy on smoking rates in women. Addictive Behaviors, 32(7), 1416-1432.

Prapavessis, H.; De Jesus, S.; Fitzgeorge, L.; Faulkner, G.; Maddison, R.; Batten, S. (2016). Exercise to enhance smoking cessation: the getting physical on cigarette randomized control trial. Annals of Behavioral Medicine, 50(3), 358-369.

Roberts, V.; Maddison, R.; Simpson, C.; Bullen, C.; Prapavessis, H. (2012). The acute effects of exercise on cigarette cravings, withdrawal symptoms, affect, and smoking behaviour: systematic review update and meta-analysis. Psychopharmacology, 222(1), 1-15.

Smits, J. A.; Zvolensky, M. J.; Davis, M. L.; Rosenfield, D.; Marcus, B. H.; Church, T. S. et al. (2016). The efficacy of vigorous-intensity exercise as an aid to smoking cessation in adults with high anxiety sensitivity: a randomized controlled trial. Psychosomatic Medicine, 78(3), 354-364.

Spence, J. C.; McGannon, K. R.; Poon, P. (2005). The effect of exercise on global self-esteem: a quantitative review. Journal of Sport and Exercise Psychology, 27(3), 311-334.

Thompson, T. P.; Greaves, C. J.; Ayres, R.; Aveyard, P.; Warren, F. C.; Byng, R. et al. (2016). An exploratory analysis of the smoking and physical activity outcomes from a pilot randomized controlled trial of an exercise assisted reduction to stop smoking intervention in disadvantaged groups. Nicotine, Tobacco Research, 18(3), 289-297.

Tritter, A.; Fitzgeorge, L.; Prapavessis, H. (2015). The effect of acute exercise on cigarette cravings while using a nicotine lozenge. Psychopharmacology, 232(14), 2531-2539.

U. S. Department of Health, Human Services. (1990). The health benefits of smoking cessation: A report of the surgeon general. Atlanta, GA: U. S. Department of Health and Human Services, Public Health Service, Centers for Disease Control, Center for Chronic Disease Prevention and Health Promotion, Office on Smoking and Health.

U. S. Department of Health, Human Services. (2010). How tobacco smoke causes disease: The biology and behavioral basis for smoking-attributable disease: A report of the surgeon general. Atlanta, GA: U. S. Department of Health, Human Services, Centers for Disease Control and Prevention, National Center for Chronic Disease Prevention and Health Promotion, Office on Smoking and Health.

Ussher, M.; Lewis, S.; Aveyard, P.; Manyonda, I.; West, R.; Lewis, B. et al. (2015). Physical activity for smoking cessation in pregnancy: randomized controlled trial. BMJ, 350, h2145.

Ussher, M. H.; Taylor, A. H.; Faulkner, G. E. (2014). Exercise interventions for smoking cessation. The Cochrane Library, 8.

WHO. (2017). WHO report on the global tobacco epidemic, 2017: Monitoring tobacco use and prevention policies. Geneva: World Health Organization. Licence: CC BY-NC-SA 3. 0 IGO.

Williams, D. M. (2008). Increasing fitness is associated with fewer depressive symptoms during successful smoking abstinence among women. International Journal of Fitness, 4(1), 39-44.

56
伐伦克林：治疗吸烟成瘾和精神分裂症

Do-Un Jung, Sung-Jin Kim

Department of Psychiatry, Busan Paik Hospital, Inje University College of Medicine, Busan, Republic of Korea

缩略语

CBT	认知行为疗法	mCEQ	改良卷烟评价问卷
CDSS	卡尔加里精神分裂症抑郁量表	nAChR	烟碱乙酰胆碱受体
EAGLES study	全球戒烟研究中评估不良事件	NRT	烟碱替代疗法
HIV	人类免疫缺陷病毒		

56.1 慢性精神疾病：精神分裂症

精神分裂症是一种严重的慢性精神疾病，在普通人群中发病率约为1%（McGrath et al. 2008）。精神分裂症的临床症状可分为阳性症状、阴性症状和认知性症状。阳性症状，包括幻觉、妄想、言语混乱和行为紊乱，是患者在疾病急性期寻求治疗的主要原因。阴性症状，包括情感淡化、冷漠和心碎，导致许多患者在重返社会时遇到困难（Crow, 1985）。认知性症状曾经被归类为阳性症状或阴性症状，但最近被划分为一个独立的症状域（Green, Harvey, 2014）。尽管已经尝试了不同的治疗方法来改善认知症状，但这些治疗方法对阳性和阴性症状的效果不如那些（Goff et al. 2011）。如本文所示，精神分裂症表现出多种症状，不仅会影响患者的日常功能，还会影响患者的社会和职业功能（Dickinson et al. 2007）。即使在治疗后，相当数量的精神分裂症患者仍会出现残留症状，并报告生活质量较低（Huber et al. 1980）。

56.2 精神分裂症人群中的物质相关障碍

精神分裂症患者有较高的物质相关障碍共病。据悉，精神分裂症患者表现出更高的物质滥用水平，这是因为海马体和额叶皮质的发育变化。这些改变可能会增加多巴胺的释放，从而促进药物奖赏途径的积极强化效应，这会进一步促进药物寻找行为（Chambers et al. 2001）。大约40%～50%的精神分裂症患者经历终生物质使用障碍，这会对精神分裂症的治疗和愈后产生负面影响（Blanchard et al. 2000）。事实上，物质使用障碍与治疗依从性降低、精神病症状、暴力行为、无家可归和总体治疗费用增加有关（Dixon, 1999）。此外，物质使用障碍还会导致其他医疗问题，并对精神分裂症患者此类问题的治疗产生负面影响（Dickey et al. 2000）。

56.3 精神分裂症患者吸烟成瘾情况调查

烟草是一种使人上瘾的物质,可能导致物质使用障碍,并在停止使用后导致戒断症状。最近,由于多方面的努力,日常吸烟的流行率一直在下降,例如许多国家的政府实施了禁烟政策,但随着人口的增加,吸烟者的数量仍在逐渐增加(Ng et al. 2014)。吸烟是众所周知的重大全球健康问题,据报道与许多其他医学疾病相关,包括心血管疾病和癌症(Ambrose, Barua, 2004; Gandini et al. 2008)。Lasser等(2000)报告,与普通人群相比,患有精神疾病的人吸烟的可能性大约是普通人的两倍。此外,de Leon和Diaz(2005)进行的荟萃分析发现,尤其是精神分裂症患者的吸烟率大约是普通人群的5.9倍(男性的优势比为7.2,女性的优势比为3.3)。几项研究报告称,精神分裂症患者的患病率从50%~90%不等。据报道,在精神分裂症患者中,重度吸烟和高度烟碱依赖的患病率高于普通人群,而戒烟率则较低。吸烟是一种可预防的死亡原因,精神分裂症患者的内科疾病死亡率和吸烟率高于健康人。因此,在精神分裂症人群中戒烟似乎对于个人、社会和经济上都有很大的好处(Saha et al. 2007)。

56.4 吸烟成瘾与精神分裂症的假说

有几个假设试图解释精神分裂症人群中的高吸烟成瘾率。首先,吸烟会增加几种抗精神病药物的代谢,因此患者可能会通过吸烟来减少这些药物的副作用(Desai et al. 2001)。Goff等(1992)评估了78名精神分裂症患者的药物副作用和吸烟之间的关系,发现精神分裂症吸烟者比不吸烟者表现出较低的帕金森症水平和较高的抗精神病药物使用量。此外,Barnes等(2006)报告了吸烟与低水平不安定症状(一种药物副作用,常见于抗精神药使用者,表现为无法忍受的内部不安和运动不适,导致患者无法停止移动或静止不动)之间的联系。

第二种假设是精神分裂症患者使用烟碱(一种精神活性物质)来治疗自身的症状(Potvin et al. 2003)。烟碱增加伏隔核和前额叶皮质的中层双皮质多巴胺能活动,这似乎可以减轻精神分裂症的症状(Lyon,1999)。Sacco和他的同事(Sacco et al. 2005)报告,患有精神分裂症的吸烟者戒烟后在视觉空间工作记忆测试和持续表现测试中得分降低。此外,经皮烟碱可提高精神分裂症非吸烟者的注意力表现并改善冲动反应抑制(Barr et al. 2008)。另一项研究还表明,精神分裂症非吸烟者在接受烟碱激动剂治疗时,阴性症状显著改善(Freedman et al. 2008)。

关于吸烟成瘾和精神分裂症的第三个假说是,精神分裂症患者吸烟可以用心理社会因素来解释。由于症状的严重性,相当多的精神分裂症患者的社会和职业功能下降,避免与社会关系,并且通常倾向于不活跃。在这种情况下,吸烟可以成为消除无聊的工具(Hughes et al. 1986)。此外,吸烟可以减轻精神分裂症引起的焦虑、抑郁和压力,这与精神分裂症的精神病理症状无关。因此,吸烟最终可以改善社会关系(Lyon,1999)。为了支持这一假设,Smith等(2001)报道,无论卷烟中含有多少烟碱,吸烟都可以改善精神分裂症患者的负面症状。虽然卷烟可能会起到自我治疗的作用,但这些结果突出了吸烟在心理社会方面的意义。

56.5 伐伦克林是治疗精神分裂症吸烟成瘾的有吸引力的选择

吸烟成瘾的治疗方法可以分为心理社会疗法和药物疗法,根据患者的情况,这两种疗法可以单独使用，也可以联合使用。心理社会治疗涉及多种方法，从简单的建议或基础教育到动机增强疗法、认知行为疗法（CBT）、正念疗法或其他方法（Brewer et al. 2013;Grimshaw, Stanton,2006;Lancaster, Stead,2004）。药理治疗主要包括烟碱替代疗法（NRT）、安非他酮或伐伦克林（Cahill et al. 2013）。

伐伦克林是目前最广为人知的治疗吸烟成瘾的药物。该药是α4β2烟碱乙酰胆碱受体（nAChR）的部分激动剂，也是α7 nAChR的完全激动剂（Mihalak et al. 2006）。因此，它以一种持续和适度的水平刺激多巴胺的分泌来减少烟碱奖励和减轻戒烟过程中出现的戒断症状和渴望来帮助患者戒烟（Coe et al. 2005; Rollema et al. 2007）。

全球戒烟研究中评估不良事件（EAGLES）包括8144名参与者（精神病队列中4116人，非精神病队列中4028人），并评估了伐伦克林、安非他酮和烟碱贴片的安全性和有效性。该研究报告称，与烟碱贴片或安慰剂相比，伐伦克林显示出最高的疗效水平，并且没有显著增加精神不良事件（Anthenelli et al. 2016）。此外，Stapleton等（2008）比较了NRT和伐伦克林对参加每周小组支持会议的烟草依赖型精神疾病患者的有效性和安全性，发现伐伦克林组在开始戒烟后4周的短期戒烟率高于NRT组，安全性结果与无精神疾病的参与者的结果相似。因此，伐伦克林不仅在普通人群中，而且在精神病患者中，都被认为是治疗烟瘾的有效药物。从成本效益的角度来看，伐伦克林已被发现比安非他酮、NRT、去甲替林和无辅助戒烟更有利（Hoogendoorn, Welsing, Rutten-van Molken, 2008）。

对精神分裂症患者的尸检研究发现，包括海马体和扣带回在内的几个大脑区域的α7 nAChR显著减少。这一下降可能不仅与精神分裂症症状有关，还与吸烟模式有关（Brunzell, McIntosh, 2012）。Tidey等（2014）比较了吸烟者、精神分裂症吸烟者和非精神疾病吸烟者在72小时戒烟期后的几种症状，发现精神分裂症吸烟者表现出更严重的烟瘾和戒烟症状、更高的烟碱偏好、更早恢复吸烟。基于上述研究结果，人们认为伐伦克林是治疗精神分裂症患者吸烟成瘾的一种有吸引力的治疗选择。

Jeon等（2016）进行了一项随机、双盲、安慰剂对照试验，包括60名吸烟的精神分裂症患者，发现伐伦克林在减少吸烟方面有显著疗效。研究人员观察到，在为期8周的研究期间，时间和组之间的相互作用与卷烟数量、呼出的一氧化碳水平和改良卷烟评价问卷（mCEQ）的结果显著相关。此外，Smith等（2016）进行的一项研究旨在检查精神分裂症吸烟者的吸烟减少情况，该研究还报告了在连续8周每天服用2mg伐伦克林的患者中，卷烟数量、呼出的一氧化碳水平、血浆可替宁和吸烟欲望显著降低。对于在不容易戒烟的精神分裂症患者中，减少吸烟是否是一个合适的治疗和研究目标存在争议。然而，大量减少吸烟最终可以通过降低烟碱依赖的严重程度和增加戒烟的动机来降低吸烟的可能性（Tidey, Miller, 2015）。

目前已有几项关于伐伦克林戒烟效果的研究。Williams等（2012）对128名精神分裂症和分裂情感患者进行了一项随机、双盲、安慰剂对照试验，并报告称，经过12周的治疗期后，伐伦克林治疗组患者对戒烟满意的比例明显高于安慰剂组（19.0%与4.7%）。此外，伐伦克林组在24周时的戒烟率高于安慰剂组（11.9%与2.3%），但这种差异没有统计学意义。此外，Pachas等（2012）进行了一项研究，其中112名精神分裂症吸烟者服用了伐伦克林并每周进行CBT治疗，为期12周。治疗完成后，14天连续戒烟率为47.3%，28天连续戒烟率为34%。

精神分裂症患者长期服用伐伦克林似乎与持续的高戒烟率有关。在一项包括87名精神分裂症患者（77名）和双相情感障碍患者（10名）的研究中，Evins等（2014）在12周的开放标签期内将伐伦克林与CBT联合应用于患者，之后他们进行了一项双盲、安慰剂对照试验。在试验中，参与者被分为伐伦克林组和安慰剂组，从第12周到第52周服用安慰剂或伐伦克林和CBT，并从第52周到第76周进行无治疗的随访。伐伦克林组在第52周的点患病率戒断率（60%）明显高于安慰剂组（19%），伐伦克林组在第12～64周和第12～76周的持续戒断率也较高（分别为45%与15%和30%与11%）。表56.1总结了伐伦克林对吸烟治疗效果的研究。

几项研究调查了精神分裂症患者伐伦克林的阳性反应预测因子。当精神分裂症患者服用伐伦克林和CBT 12周时，Dutra等（2012）报告，戒烟率增加，情感扁平化减少。Schuster等（2017）对精神分裂症（$n=130$）和双相情感障碍（$n=23$）患者进行了一项研究，并报告称，戒断与较少的戒断症状、较少的吸烟、更好的注意力表现、酒精依赖史和较少的他人支持预期呈正相关。DRD4变异，已知与烟碱奖励效应相关，也可能是一种生物学预测因子，尽管尚未对其与伐伦克林的直接联系进行研究（Harrell et al. 2016; Jeon et al. 2016）。

表56.1 关于伐伦克林对精神分裂症患者吸烟治疗效果的研究总结

参考文献	目的	方法	N（MA+SD; M/F）	评价方法	结果
Jeon et al. (2016)	研究伐伦克林的戒烟效果	双盲，随机对照试验，门诊患者，精神分裂症，8周	Va=29（41.10±8.86; 26/3）Pla=30（41.53±8.83; 29/1）	mNWs、QSU-Brief、mCEQ、呼出的CO、卷烟数量	Va在呼出CO（$P=0.046$）、mCEQ（$P=0.002$）和卷烟数量（$P=0.007$）中有显著的时间×基团交互作用
Smith et al. (2016)	评价伐伦克林的减少吸烟效果和其他方面（认知、精神症状和副作用）	随机双盲对照试验，门诊和住院患者，精神分裂症，分裂情感性精神病，8周	Va=42（46.6±8.9; 35/7）Pla=45（43.6±10.6; 39/6）	QSU-Brief，呼出的CO，卷烟数量，血浆烟碱和可替宁水平，CDS	Va在呼出的CO（$P=0.035$）和可替宁水平（$P<0.001$）中有显著的时间-基团交互作用
Williams et al. (2012)	评价伐伦克林的戒烟效果	随机双盲对照试验，门诊患者，精神分裂症，分裂情感性精神病，24周	Va=84（40.2±11.9; 65/19）Pla=43（43.0±10.2; 33/10）	戒烟定义为7天内不吸烟，并通过一氧化碳水平进行验证	治疗12周时，Va组戒烟效果优于Pla组（Va组19.0%, Pla组4.7%）（$P=0.046$）。24周时，Va为11.9%, Pla为2.3%（$P=0.090$）
Pachas et al. (2012)	评价伐伦克林戒烟的疗效和安全性（联合每周一次CBT）	开放式研究，门诊患者，精神分裂症，分裂情感性精神病，12周	N=112（47.2±10; 68/44）	持续戒烟的定义是经过生化验证的连续几周的连续7天的点流行戒烟	在12周时，14天的持续戒烟率为47.3%，28天的持续戒烟率为34%
Evins et al. (2014)	评价瓦伦尼克林的戒烟维持效果（联合CBT至52周和52～76周为无治疗随访期）	随机双盲对照试验，门诊患者，精神分裂症，双相情感障碍，分裂情感性精神病，76周	Va=40（51.4±9.6; 24/16）Pla=47（45.7±10.3; 31/16）	12～64周的持续戒烟率是基于经过生化验证的戒烟情况，而12～76周的持续戒烟率是基于自我报告的吸烟行为	52周时，Va组和Pla组的点戒断率分别为60%和19%（$P<0.001$）。12～64周，Va组持续戒烟率为64.45%, Pla组为15%（$P=0.004$）。在12～76周，Va为30%; Pla为11%（$P=0.03$）

注：CDS，卷烟依赖量表；CO，一氧化碳；MA±SD，参与者的平均年龄和标准差；M/F，男女比例；mCEQ，改良卷烟评价问卷；mNWs，明尼苏达烟碱戒断量表；N，参与者人数；Pla，安慰剂组；QSU-Brief，吸烟冲动简明问卷；RCT，随机对照试验；Va，伐伦克林组。

56.6 精神分裂症患者使用伐伦克林的其他方面

在戒烟期间，精神分裂症患者通常会由于烟碱戒断症状而表现出额外的认知障碍，如注意力下降。伐伦克林不仅对精神分裂症患者的吸烟成瘾有好处，而且还能改善认知功能。这些作用与伐伦克林对nAChR的活性有关，对精神分裂症患者戒烟有重要意义。

Shim等（2012）在一组120名精神分裂症患者中研究了伐伦克林与认知功能的关系。治疗组服用2mg的瓦伦尼克林，与对照组相比，在数字符号替换测试中表现更好，在威斯康星卡片分类测试中犯的非持久性错误更少。此外，服用伐伦克林的精神分裂症吸烟者连续表现测试中的击中反应时间更短，而不吸烟者对Stroop测验的干扰减少。研究表明，伐伦克林还可以显著改善精神分裂症吸烟者的言语学习和记忆（Smith et al. 2009），并与戒烟后认知和情感恶化的严重程度降低（Liu et al. 2011）。Roh等（2014）在施用美加明（nAChR拮抗剂）、伐伦克林（nAChR激动剂）或者给不吸烟的精神分裂症患者的安慰剂后，评估认知功能，并且发现，与服用伐伦克林或安慰剂的人相比，服用美加明的人注意力下降。Hong等（2011）进行了一项包括69名精神分裂症患者的研究，以检验伐伦克林与神经生物学生物标志物之间的相关性。在他们的研究中，发现几个神经生物学生物标志物与伐伦克林相关，包括P50门控、惊吓反应和抗惊吓错误率。表56.2提供了一些在服用伐伦克林的精神分裂症患者中测量认知的研究总结。

也有报道称伐伦克林可以改善精神分裂症患者的抑郁症状。Cather等（2017）发现，在接受12周CBT和伐伦克林治疗的精神分裂症患者中，抑郁症状（使用CDSS卡尔加里精神分裂症抑郁量表评估）的减少与戒烟的效果无关。

表56.2 服用伐伦克林的精神分裂症患者认知能力测量研究总结

参考文献	目的	方法	N（MA±SD; M/F）	评价方法	结果
Shim et al.(2012)	评价伐伦克林对认知功能的影响	双盲RCT，门诊病人，精神分裂症，8周	Va=59（39.9±8.6, 38/21）Pla 58（39.9±9.9, 45/13）	CPT, SCWT, WCST, DSST, DST, VST	Va在DSST（$P=0.013$）和WCST（$P=0.043$）上的表现明显好于Pla。在吸烟者中，Va在CPT-HRT（$P=0.008$）和SI（$P=0.004$）方面优于Pla
Hong et al.(2011)	探讨伐伦克林对神经生物学和认知生物标志物的影响	双盲RCT，门诊病人，精神分裂症、分裂情感性精神病，8周	Va=32（44.03±1.82; 20/12）Pla=32（41.57±1.93; 22/10）	PPI, P50门控，SPEM, ASER, DSST, CPT	在Va组，惊恐反应性降低（$P=0.015$）；ASER降低（$P=0.034$）；吸烟者Va组P50门控缺陷减少（$P=0.006$）
Smith et al.(2016)	评价伐伦克林对认知和其他方面（吸烟、精神症状和副作用）的影响	双盲RCT，门诊和住院患者，精神分裂症、分裂情感性精神病，8周	Va=42（46.6±8.9; 35/7）Pla=45（43.6±10.6; 39/6）	无社会认知模块的MCCB	Va组认知功能未见明显改善

注：ASER，防扫视错误率；CPT，连续操作测试；DSST，数字符号替代测试；DST，数字跨度测试；HRT，命中反应时间；MA±SD，参与者的平均年龄和标准差；M/F，男女比例；MCCB，Matrics共识认知成套测验；N，参与者数量；Pla，安慰剂组；PPI，脉冲前抑制；RCT，随机对照试验；SCWT，Stroop颜色词测试；SI，Stroop干扰；SPEM，流畅的眼球运动；Va，伐伦克林组；VST，视觉跨度测试；WCST，威斯康星卡片分类测验。

56.7 不良事件和伐伦克林在精神分裂症患者中的使用

据报道,服用伐伦克林的患者经常抱怨恶心和头痛等身体不良事件。然而,即使是最常见的不良反应,如恶心,通常也只是轻微的,并且随着时间的推移会有所改善;因此,这通常不是停止治疗的原因(Cahill et al. 2016)。与这些轻微副作用相比,伐伦克林与严重心血管事件之间的关系存在很大争议。然而,最近的一项系统综述和元分析(Sterling et al. 2016)并未发现伐伦克林与严重心血管事件之间存在显著相关性。

许多研究表明,与安慰剂或其他烟碱成瘾治疗(如NRT)相比,伐伦克林不会显著增加精神不良事件(Anthenelli et al. 2016; Molero et al. 2015)。然而,不断有报道称,用伐伦克林的患者出现神经精神不良事件,包括情绪抑郁、失眠、自杀意念和攻击行为(Ahmed et al. 2013)。Williams等(2012)报道服用伐伦克林的精神分裂症和分裂情感患者经历了多种神经精神不良事件,包括异常梦境(7.1%)、焦虑(4.8%)、抑郁(4.8%)、失眠(9.5%)和自杀意念(6.0%)。然而,所有患者都有吸烟史,而伐伦克林组和安慰剂组在不良事件方面没有显著差异。因此,尚不清楚上述症状是由伐伦克林引起的还是与戒烟症状有关。总而言之,当伐伦克林用于精神分裂症等有不同精神症状的患者时,需要非常密切地监测潜在的副作用(Yousefi et al. 2011)(表56.3)。

表56.3 精神分裂症患者使用伐伦克林时需要考虑的潜在不良事件

神经精神病学	身体	神经精神病学	身体
不正常的梦	头晕	失眠	呕吐
焦虑	疲劳	兴奋	
激动	头痛	易怒	
抑郁	恶心	自杀想法	

术语解释

- 成瘾:一种强迫性的状态,在这种状态下,尽管知道某些活动会影响健康和社会生活时,但还是进行这些活动。
- 安非他酮:安非他酮作为去甲肾上腺素-多巴胺再摄取抑制剂和烟碱拮抗剂,用于治疗抑郁症和戒烟。
- 认知行为疗法:通过改变思想和行为来影响情绪和身体感觉的精神治疗方法。
- 烟碱替代疗法:通过皮肤或口腔黏膜以低吸收效率提供少量烟碱,从而缓解戒断症状而不引起烟碱成瘾的治疗方法。
- 精神分裂症:一种精神疾病,在思想、情感、感知和行为的各个方面引起广泛的临床问题。
- 物质使用障碍:物质依赖和物质滥用都可能涉及。物质依赖的特征是耐受、戒断和强迫使用,但物质滥用不是。

精神分裂症患者吸烟成瘾的关键因素

- 精神分裂症患者的吸烟率大约是普通人群的5.9倍。
- 精神分裂症患者的吸烟率为50%~90%不等。
- 存在与精神分裂症患者吸烟成瘾和药物代谢、自我药物治疗和心理社会方面之间的关联相关的假设。

- 可向精神分裂症患者和普通人群提供针对烟瘾的心理和药物治疗。
- 特别是，伐伦克林似乎是精神分裂症患者吸烟成瘾的有效药物治疗选择。

要点总结

- 在本章中，我们讨论精神分裂症患者的烟瘾以及伐伦克林作为药物的应用。
- 精神分裂症是一种主要的精神疾病，有阳性、阴性和认知症状。
- 40%～50%的精神分裂症患者患有终生物质障碍，这会影响疾病预后、健康和生活质量。
- 吸烟成瘾是精神分裂症患者中常见的物质使用问题，其在精神分裂症患者中的患病率比一般人群高（约5.9倍）。
- 药物代谢、自我治疗和心理社会方面可能与精神分裂症患者吸烟成瘾的高患病率有关。
- 伐伦克林是一种众所周知的用于治疗烟瘾的药剂，具有出色的疗效和成本效益。
- 在精神分裂症患者中，伐伦克林被发现在减少吸烟、戒烟和预防复发方面有效。
- 伐伦克林还可能影响其他精神病理学，如精神分裂症患者的认知功能。
- 因为与伐伦克林相关的神经精神副作用不断被报道，所以对有精神症状的精神分裂症患者应给予密切关注。

参考文献

Ahmed, A. I.; Ali, A. N.; Kramers, C.; Harmark, L. V.; Burger, D. M.; Verhoeven, W. M. (2013). Neuropsychiatric adverse events of varenicline: A systematic review of published reports. Journal of Clinical Psychopharmacology, 33(1), 55-62.

Ambrose, J. A.; Barua, R. S. (2004). The pathophysiology of cigarette smoking and cardiovascular disease: an update. Journal of the American College of Cardiology, 43(10), 1731-1737.

Anthenelli, R. M.; Benowitz, N. L.; West, R.; St Aubin, L.; McRae, T.; Lawrence, D. et al. (2016). Neuropsychiatric safety and efficacy of varenicline, bupropion, and nicotine patch in smokers with and without psychiatric disorders (EAGLES): A double-blind, randomised, placebo-controlled clinical trial. Lancet, 387(10037), 2507-2520.

Barnes, M.; Lawford, B. R.; Burton, S. C.; Heslop, K. R.; Noble, E. P.; Hausdorf, K. et al. (2006). Smoking and schizophrenia: is symptom profile related to smoking and which antipsychotic medication is of benefit in reducing cigarette use? The Australian and New Zealand Journal of Psychiatry, 40(6-7), 575-580.

Barr, R. S.; Culhane, M. A.; Jubelt, L. E.; Mufti, R. S.; Dyer, M. A.; Weiss, A. P. et al. (2008). The effects of transdermal nicotine on cognition in nonsmokers with schizophrenia and nonpsychiatric controls. Neuropsychopharmacology, 33(3), 480-490.

Blanchard, J. J.; Brown, S. A.; Horan, W. P.; Sherwood, A. R. (2000). Substance use disorders in schizophrenia: review, integration, and a proposed model. Clinical Psycho-logy Review, 20(2), 207-234.

Brewer, J. A.; Elwafi, H. M.; Davis, J. H. (2013). Craving to quit: psychological models and neurobiological mechanisms of mindfulness training as treatment for addictions. Psy-chology of Addictive Behaviors, 27(2), 366-379.

Brunzell, D. H.; McIntosh, J. M. (2012). Alpha7 nicotinic acetylcholine receptors mod-ulate motivation to self-administer nicotine: implications for smoking and schizophrenia. Neuropsychopharmacology, 37(5), 1134-1143.

Cahill, K.; Lindson-Hawley, N.; Thomas, K. H.; Fanshawe, T. R.; Lancaster, T. (2016). Nicotine receptor partial agonists for smoking cessation. Cochrane Database of Systema-tic Reviews, 5, CD006103.

Cahill, K.; Stevens, S.; Perera, R.; Lancaster, T. (2013). Pharmacological interventions for smoking cessation: an overview and network metaanalysis. Cochrane Database of Sy-stematic Reviews, 5, CD009329.

Cather, C.; Hoeppner, S.; Pachas, G.; Pratt, S.; Achtyes, E.; Cieslak, K. M. et al. (2017). Improved depressive symptoms in adults with schizophrenia during a smoking cessation attempt with Varenicline and behavioral therapy. Journal of Dual Diagnosis, 1-11.

Chambers, R. A.; Krystal, J. H.; Self, D. W. (2001). A neurobiological basis for subs-tance abuse comorbidity in schizophrenia. Biological Psychiatry, 50(2), 71-83.

Coe, J. W.; Brooks, P. R.; Vetelino, M. G.; Wirtz, M. C.; Arnold, E. P.; Huang, J. et al(2005). varenicline: an alpha4beta2 nicotinic receptor partial agonist for smoking cessation. Journal of Medicinal Chemistry, 48(10), 3474-3477.

Crow, T. J. (1985). The two-syndrome concept: origins and current status. Schizophrenia Bulletin, 11(3), 471-486.

de Leon, J.; Diaz, F. J. (2005). A meta-analysis of worldwide studies demonstrates an association between schizophrenia and tobacco smoking behaviors. Schizophrenia Resea-rch, 76(2-3), 135-157.

Desai, H. D.; Seabolt, J.; Jann, M. W. (2001). Smoking in patients receiving psychotro-pic medications: a pharmacokinetic perspective. CNS Drugs,

15(6), 469-494.
Dickey, B.; Azeni, H.; Weiss, R.; Sederer, L. (2000). Schizophrenia, substance use dis-orders and medical co-morbidity. The Journal of Mental Health Policy and Economics, 3(1), 27-33.
Dickinson, D.; Bellack, A. S.; Gold, J. M. (2007). Social/communication skills, cogni-tion, and vocational functioning in schizophrenia. Schizophrenia Bulletin, 33(5), 1213-1220.
Dixon, L. (1999). Dual diagnosis of substance abuse in schizophrenia: prevalence and impact on outcomes. Schizophrenia Research, 35(Suppl), S93-100.
Dutra, S. J.; Stoeckel, L. E.; Carlini, S. V.; Pizzagalli, D. A.; Evins, A. E. (2012). Var-enicline as a smoking cessation aid in schizophrenia: effects on smoking behavior and reward sensitivity. Psychopharmacology, 219(1), 25-34.
Evins, A. E.; Cather, C.; Pratt, S. A.; Pachas, G. N.; Hoeppner, S. S.; Goff, D. C. et al. (2014). Maintenance treatment with varenicline for smoking cessation in patients with schizophrenia and bipolar disorder: a randomized clinical trial. JAMA, 311(2), 145-154.
Freedman, R.; Olincy, A.; Buchanan, R. W.; Harris, J. G.; Gold, J. M.; Johnson, L. et al. (2008). Initial phase 2 trial of a nicotinic agonist in schizophrenia. The American Journal of Psychiatry, 165(8), 1040-1047.
Gandini, S.; Botteri, E.; Iodice, S.; Boniol, M.; Lowenfels, A. B.; Maisonneuve, P. et al. (2008). Tobacco smoking and cancer: a meta-analysis. International Journal of Cancer, 122(1), 155-164.
Goff, D. C.; Henderson, D. C.; Amico, E. (1992). Cigarette smoking in schizophrenia: relationship to psychopathology and medication side effects. The American Journal of Psych-iatry, 149(9), 1189-1194.
Goff, D. C.; Hill, M.; Barch, D. (2011). The treatment of cognitive impairment in sch-izophrenia. Pharmacology, Biochemistry, and Behavior, 99(2), 245-253.
Green, M. F.; Harvey, P. D. (2014). Cognition in schizophrenia: past, present, and fu-ture. Schizophrenia Research: Cognition, 1(1), e1-e9.
Grimshaw, G. M.; Stanton, A. (2006). Tobacco cessation interventions for young people. Cochrane Database of Systematic Reviews, 4, CD003289.
Harrell, P. T.; Lin, H. Y.; Park, J. Y.; Blank, M. D.; Drobes, D. J.; Evans, D. E. (2016). Dopaminergic genetic variation moderates the effect of nicotine on cigarette reward. Psycho-pharmacology, 233(2), 351-360.
Hong, L. E.; Thaker, G. K.; McMahon, R. P.; Summerfelt, A.; Rachbeisel, J.; Fuller, R. L. et al. (2011). Effects of moderate-dose treatment with varenicline on neurobiological and cognitive biomarkers in smokers and nonsmokers with schizophrenia or schizoaff-ective disorder. Archives of General Psychiatry, 68(12), 1195-1206.
Hoogendoorn, M.; Welsing, P.; Rutten-van Molken, M. P. (2008). Cost-effectiveness of varenicline compared with bupropion, NRT, and nortriptyline for smoking cessation in the Netherlands. Current Medical Research and Opinion, 24(1), 51-61.
Huber, G.; Gross, G.; Schuttler, R.; Linz, M. (1980). Longitudinal studies of schizo-phrenic patients. Schizophrenia Bulletin, 6(4), 592-605.
Hughes, J. R.; Hatsukami, D. K.; Mitchell, J. E.; Dahlgren, L. A. (1986). Prevalence of smoking among psychiatric outpatients. The American Journal of Psychiatry, 143(8), 993-997.
Jeon, D. W.; Shim, J. C.; Kong, B. G.; Moon, J. J. Seo, Y. S.; Kim, S. J. et al. (2016). Adjunctive varenicline treatment for smoking reduction in patients with schizophrenia: A randomized double-blind placebo-controlled trial. Schizophrenia Research, 176(2-3), 206-211.
Lancaster, T.; Stead, L. (2004). Physician advice for smoking cessation. Cochrane Data-base of Systematic Reviews, 4, CD000165.
Lasser, K.; Boyd, J. W.; Woolhandler, S.; Himmelstein, D. U.; McCormick, D.; Bor, D. H. (2000). Smoking and mental illness:a population-based prevalence study. JAMA, 284(20), 2606-2610.
Liu, M. E.; Tsai, S. J.; Jeang, S. Y.; Peng, S. L.; Wu, S. L.; Chen, M. C. et al. (2011). varenicline prevents affective and cognitive exacerbation during smoking abstinence in male patients with schizophrenia.
Psychiatry Research, 190(1), 79-84.
Lyon, E. R. (1999). A review of the effects of nicotine on schizophrenia and antipsychotic medications. Psychiatric Services, 50(10), 1346-1350.
McGrath, J.; Saha, S.; Chant, D.; Welham, J. (2008). Schizophrenia: a concise overview of incidence, prevalence, and mortality. Epidemiologic Reviews, 30, 67-76.
Mihalak, K. B.; Carroll, F. I.; Luetje, C. W. (2006). varenicline is a partial agonist at alpha4beta2 and a full agonist at alpha7 neuronal nicotinic receptors. Molecular Pharmaco-logy, 70(3), 801-805.
Molero, Y.; Lichtenstein, P.; Zetterqvist, J.; Gumpert, C. H.; Fazel, S. (2015). Varenicline and risk of psychiatric conditions, suicidal behaviour, criminal offending, and transport accidents and offences: population based cohort study. BMJ, 350, h2388.
Ng, M.; Freeman, M. K.; Fleming, T. D.; Robinson, M.; DwyerLindgren, L.; Thomson, B. et al. (2014). Smoking prevalence and cigarette consumption in 187 countries, 1980-2012. JAMA, 311(2), 183-192.
Pachas, G. N.; Cather, C.; Pratt, S. A.; Hoeppner, B.; Nino, J.; Carlini, S. V. et al. (2012). varenicline for smoking cessation in schizophrenia: safety and effectiveness in a 12-week, open-label trial. Journal of Dual Diagnosis, 8(2), 117-125.
Potvin, S.; Stip, E.; Roy, J. Y. (2003). Schizophrenia and addiction: an evaluation of the self-medication hypothesis. Encephale, 29(3 Pt 1), 193-203.
Roh, S.; Hoeppner, S. S.; Schoenfeld, D.; Fullerton, C. A.; Stoeckel, L. E.; Evins, A. E. (2014). Acute effects of mecamylamine and varenicline on cognitive performance in non-smokers with and without schizophrenia. Psychopharmacology, 231(4), 765-775.
Rollema, H.; Chambers, L. K.; Coe, J. W.; Glowa, J.; Hurst, R. S.; Lebel, L. A. et al. (2007). Pharmacological profile of the alpha4beta2 nicotinic acetylcholine receptor partial agonist Varenicline, an effective smoking cessation aid. Neuropharmacology, 52(3), 985-994.
Sacco, K. A.; Termine, A.; Seyal, A.; Dudas, M. M.; Vessicchio, J. C.; Krishnan-Sarin, S. et al. (2005). Effects of cigarette smoking on spatial working memory and attentional deficits in schizophrenia:involvement of nicotinic receptor mechanisms. Archives of GeneralPsychiatry, 62(6), 649-659.
Saha, S.; Chant, D.; McGrath, J. (2007). A systematic review of mortality in schizophrenia: is the differential mortality gap worsening over time? Archives of General Psychiatry, 64(10), 1123-1131.

Schuster, R. M.; Cather, C.; Pachas, G. N.; Zhang, H.; Cieslak, K. M.; Hoeppner, S. S. et al. (2017). Predictors of tobacco abstinence in outpatient smokers with schizophrenia or bipolar disorder treated with varenicline and cognitive behavioral smoking cessation therapy. Addictive Behaviors, 71, 89-95.

Shim, J. C.; Jung, D. U.; Jung, S. S.; Seo, Y. S.; Cho, D. M.; Lee, J. H. et al. (2012). Adjunctive varenicline treatment with antipsychotic medications for cognitive impairments in people with schizophrenia: a randomized double-blind placebo-controlled trial. Neuropsychopharmacology, 37(3), 660-668.

Smith, R. C.; Amiaz, R.; Si, T. M.; Maayan, L.; Jin, H.; Boules, S. et al. (2016). varenicline effects on smoking, cognition, and psychiatric symptoms in schizophrenia: a double-blind randomized trial. PLoS ONE, 11(1):e0143490.

Smith, R. C.; Infante, M.; Ali, A.; Nigam, S.; Kotsaftis, A. (2001). Effects of cigarette smoking on psychopathology scores in patients with schizophrenia: an experimental study. Substance Abuse, 22(3), 175-186.

Smith, R. C.; Lindenmayer, J. P.; Davis, J. M.; Cornwell, J.; Noth, K.; Gupta, S. et al. (2009). Cognitive and antismoking effects of varenicline in patients with schizophrenia or schizoaffective disorder. Schizophrenia Research, 110(1-3), 149-155.

Stapleton, J. A.; Watson, L.; Spirling, L. I.; Smith, R.; Milbrandt, A.; Ratcliffe, M. et al. (2008). varenicline in the routine treatment of tobacco dependence: a pre-post comparison with nicotine replacement therapy and an evaluation in those with mental illness. Addiction, 103(1), 146-154.

Sterling, L. H.; Windle, S. B.; Filion, K. B.; Touma, L.; Eisenberg, M. J. (2016). varenicline and adverse cardiovascular events: a systematic review and meta-analysis of randomized controlled trials. Journal of the American Heart Association, 5(2).

Tidey, J. W.; Colby, S. M.; Xavier, E. M. (2014). Effects of smoking abstinence on cigarette craving, nicotine withdrawal, and nicotine reinforcement in smokers with and without schizophrenia. Nicotine, Tobacco Research, 16(3), 326-334.

Tidey, J. W.; Miller, M. E. (2015). Smoking cessation and reduction in people with chronic mental illness. BMJ, 351, h4065.

Williams, J. M.; Anthenelli, R. M.; Morris, C. D.; Treadow, J.; Thompson, J. R.; Yunis, C. et al. (2012). A randomized, double-blind, placebo-controlled study evaluating the safety and efficacy of varenicline for smoking cessation in patients with schizophrenia or schizoaffective disorder. The Journal of Clinical Psychiatry, 73(5), 654-660.

Yousefi, M. K.; Folsom, T. D.; Fatemi, S. H. (2011). A review of varenicline's efficacy and tolerability in smoking cessation studies in subjects with schizophrenia. Journal of Addiction Research and Therapy, S4(1).

57

烟碱疫苗：过去、现在和未来

Yun Hu[a], Zongmin Zhao[a], Kyle Saylor[a], Chenming Zhang

Department of Biological Systems Engineering, Virginia Tech, Blacksburg, VA, United States

缩略语

nAChR	烟碱乙酰胆碱受体	PBPK	基于生理的药代动力学
NTR	烟碱替代疗法	TLR	toll样受体

57.1 简介：发展烟碱疫苗的需要

目前，世界上大约有11亿的吸烟者（Munoz et al. 2016）。近年来，吸烟一直是可预防的主要死亡原因，其对健康的损害影响是惊人的（Hu et al. 2014）。吸烟会极大地增加患多种疾病的风险，包括心血管疾病、中风和肺癌（Pope III et al. 2011; Strong et al. 2007）。在世界范围内，烟草使用每年导致500多万人死亡，研究表明，如果大流行得不到控制，到2030年，烟草使用每年将导致1000多万人死亡（Fagerstrom, 2002）。此外，世界卫生组织（WHO）估计，吸烟每年在全球造成超过5000亿美元的经济损失（Ekpu, Brown, 2015）。

由于吸烟造成的巨大死亡率、发病率和经济损失，遏制吸烟的流行至关重要。然而据报道，80%试图自行戒烟的吸烟者在一个月内重新吸烟，而每年只有3%的吸烟者成功戒烟（Benowitz,2010）。由于在无辅助戒烟方面的挑战，许多药物疗法已经被开发出来，包括烟碱替代疗法（NRT）、基于伐伦克林的疗法和基于安非他酮的疗法（Raupach, van Schayck,2011）。这些疗法通过不同的机制起作用。例如，吸烟者可以从NRT中获得烟碱，并减少他们对烟草的渴望（Schnoll et al. 2015）；伐伦克林是nAChR的部分激动剂，通过部分刺激受体和阻断烟碱的受体通路，从而减少烟碱的奖励效应（Crunelle et al. 2010）；安非他酮是nAChRs的拮抗剂，也是去甲肾上腺素-多巴胺再摄取的抑制剂，被认为是通过抑制神经元对儿茶酚胺的接触和阻止烟碱与nAChR的结合而起到辅助戒烟作用（Roddy, 2004）。这些疗法提高了戒烟成功率，但也有一定的局限性。第一，这些药物的总体戒断率约为20%（Patel et al. 2010）。第二，治疗时间可能需要长达几个月，可能会给患者的日常生活和工作带来不便（Jiloha, 2014）。第三，在某些情况下，这些疗法可能会导致严重的不良反应（Cahill et al. 2013）。第四，低收入使用者可能负担不起这些治疗的高昂费用（Muilenburg et al. 2015）。因此，开发新的烟碱成瘾治疗方法是必要和迫切的。

人们普遍认为，烟碱是烟草产品中的主要成瘾成分，它会导致长期成瘾，尽管其结果显然是有害的（Dani, De Biasi, 2001）。烟碱通过与nAChRs结合来启动其作用，nAChR随后打开离子通道，允许钠离子或钙离子进入神经细胞，导致神经递质（如多巴胺）的释放（Paterson, Nordberg, 2000）。多巴胺可以引起欣快感，并负责烟碱的强化作用（Benowitz, 2008; Nestler, 2005）。因此，吸烟成瘾在很大程度上是烟碱成瘾的问题。

57.2 过去：第一代烟碱疫苗

烟碱疫苗可以诱导免疫系统产生针对烟碱的高度特异性抗体，被认为是一种很有前途的戒烟疗法（Hall 2002; Zhao, Hu, Hoerle et al. 2017; Zhao, Powers et al. 2017; Zheng et al. 2015）。烟碱疫苗产生的抗体可以将烟碱保留在血液中，限制烟碱在大脑中的分布，从而减少烟碱的许多生理和行为影响（Pentel, Malin,2002）。与传统的药物疗法相比，烟碱疫苗有几个主要优势。第一，不需要频繁给药，血液中抗体的持久性可以确保长期疗效（Hoogsteder et al. 2014）。第二，疫苗的各项副作用都极小（Hu et al. 2016）。第三，烟碱疫苗的低成本使低收入患者能够负担得起（Goniewicz, Delijewski,2013）。

由于烟碱分子量小、结构简单，它本身不能引发免疫反应（Hu et al. 2016）。在传统的烟碱疫苗设计中，烟碱类似物与载体蛋白共价连接，以激发免疫系统的识别（图57.1）。到目前为止，已经有几种烟碱-蛋白质结合疫苗（表57.1），包括NicVAX、TA-NIC、NIC002（也称为NicQb）和Nicctine，在临床试验中进行了评估（Caponnetto et al. 2012）。根据烟碱-蛋白质结合设计，这些疫苗可归类为第一代烟碱疫苗（Pentel, LeSage,2014）。

表57.1 第一代烟碱–蛋白质结合疫苗

疫苗	公司	结构	临床试验状况	参考文献
NicVAX	Nabi 生物制药公司	3'-氨甲基烟碱铜绿假单胞菌外膜蛋白A结合疫苗	第三阶段失败	Fahim et al. (2013)
TA-NIC	Xenova/Celtic 制药公司	烟碱半抗原霍乱毒素结合物的B亚基结合疫苗	第二阶段暂停	Zalewska-Kaszubska (2015)
Nicctine	独立制药公司	烟碱半抗原破伤风类毒素结合疫苗	第二阶段暂停	Pentel, LeSage (2014)
NIC002	Cytos 生物技术公司	烟碱半抗原病毒样颗粒结合疫苗	第二阶段失败	Shen et al. (2012)

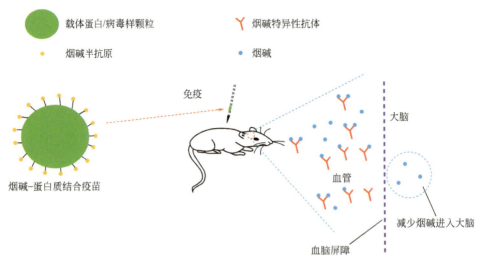

图 57.1 烟碱–蛋白质结合疫苗引起的抗体反应示意图

接种烟碱疫苗的动物或人类可以在血液中产生烟碱特异性抗体。这些抗体可以与烟碱分子结合，限制它们进入大脑，从而降低烟碱的奖励效应。

尽管第一代烟碱疫苗显示出良好的安全性和在人类中引发强烈免疫反应的能力，但由于治疗效果低于预期，它们最终在临床试验中失败（Fahim et al. 2013; Sheni et al. 2012; Zalewska-Kaszubska, 2015）。人们普遍认为，这些传统疫苗的失败可能是由于抗体浓度不足、抗体亲和力低和特异性差（Hu et al. 2016; Pentel, LeSage, 2014）。因此，需要一种能够增强这些参数的烟碱疫苗来改善治疗结果。

57.3　目前：基于纳米颗粒的烟碱疫苗

第一代烟碱结合疫苗存在一些先天缺陷，这些缺陷在很大程度上限制了它们的免疫效力，如免疫细胞识别和内化能力差、生物利用度低、难以与分子佐剂结合、免疫持久性差（Zhao, Hu, Hoerle et al. 2017）。近几十年来，纳米颗粒作为药物、蛋白质和疫苗的载体被广泛研究。纳米颗粒具有许多优势，如高效载荷能力、可控制的有效载荷释放和可调节的物理化学性质，有可能克服烟碱结合疫苗的许多缺点，因此可以作为开发能够诱导更强免疫反应的下一代烟碱疫苗的基础（Ilyinskii, Johnston, 2016）。

有希望的是，与第一代烟碱结合疫苗相比，下一代基于纳米颗粒的烟碱疫苗（图57.2）具有以下特点：①颗粒可以模仿自然存在的病原体（如细菌和病毒）的几何形状，从而使免疫细胞能够更有效地识别。②其物理化学性质（如大小和表面电荷）可以很容易地调节，以实现抗原提呈细胞的捕获和提呈。③分子佐剂可以以可控的方式容易地并入、有效地输送和高效地释放，以最大限度地提高免疫应答的幅度，同时将全身毒性降至最低（Ilyinskii, Johnston, 2016; Zhao, Powers et al. 2017）。在过去的十年中，几种基于纳米颗粒的烟碱疫苗（表57.2）一直在开发中，作为一种有效的下一代戒烟免疫治疗策略。

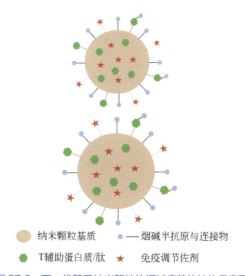

图57.2　下一代基于纳米颗粒的烟碱疫苗的结构示意图

纳米颗粒被用作颗粒载体，以有效地运送疫苗成分。T辅助蛋白/肽和免疫调节佐剂可以包裹在纳米颗粒表面或附着在纳米颗粒表面。烟碱半抗原可以通过连接物连接到纳米颗粒表面或T辅助蛋白/肽上。

表57.2　下一代纳米颗粒烟碱疫苗实例

疫苗	开发者	纳米颗粒平台	开发状况	参考文献
SEL-068	Selecta生物科学	可生物降解的聚合物颗粒	第一阶段正在进行	Pittet et al. (2012)
DNA支架烟碱疫苗	亚利桑那州立大学	自组装DNA支架	临床前	Liu et al. (2016)
脂质体烟碱疫苗	斯克里普斯学院和弗吉尼亚理工大学	脂质体	临床前	Hu et al. (2014), Lockner et al. (2013)
纳米复合烟碱疫苗（NanoNicVac）	弗吉尼亚理工大学	脂质-聚合物杂化纳米颗粒	临床前	Hu et al. (2016), Zhao, Hu, Hoerle et al. (2017)

注：表中列出了目前正在开发的所有基于纳米颗粒的烟碱纳米疫苗。

SEL-068是一种全人工合成、自组装的纳米颗粒烟碱疫苗，它是基于生物可降解和生物相容性的（聚乳酸-聚乙醇酸或聚乳酸）基质构建的。疫苗的基本成分与纳米颗粒结合或包装在纳米颗粒内。具体地说，烟碱半抗原被共价连接到纳米颗粒表面，而一种新颖的通用T细胞辅助肽和toll样受体（TLR）激动剂被包裹在纳米颗粒中。临床前研究表明，SEL-068可以在小鼠和非人类灵长类动物中诱导出对烟碱具有高亲和力的烟碱特异性抗体，并呈剂量依赖性地诱导高水平的烟碱特异性抗体（Fraser et al. 2014; Ilyinskii, Johnston, 2016; Pittet et al. 2012）。SEL-068已进入Ⅰ期临床试验，但结果尚未公布。目前，SEL-068正在通过使用双纳米颗粒策略进行重新配制，以优化人类烟碱抗体的反应。

利用自组装的DNA纳米结构作为烟碱疫苗的颗粒载体，研制了一种DNA支架烟碱疫苗。DNA支架烟碱疫苗是通过将烟碱-链霉亲和素结合物连接到由生物素化的DNA链、含CpG的寡核苷酸和其他链自组装而成的DNA四面体上构建的。临床前研究表明，使用DNA支架烟碱疫苗作为启动剂可以诱导高滴度的烟碱特异性抗体，并显著阻止烟碱进入小鼠的大脑（Liu et al. 2012; Liu et al. 2016）。这种以DNA为骨架的烟碱疫苗目前正在优化中，以进一步提高免疫效力。

脂质体已被用于开发下一代基于纳米颗粒的烟碱疫苗（Hu et al. 2014; Lockner et al. 2013）。然而，基于脂质体的烟碱纳米疫苗有一个显著的缺陷，即不稳定性，这在很大程度上限制了它们的进一步发展。通过发挥脂质体和聚合物纳米颗粒的优势并克服它们的不足，基于脂质-聚合物杂化纳米颗粒的烟碱纳米疫苗（NanoNicVac）正在开发中，这种疫苗可以共同传递烟碱半抗原、T细胞表位和分子佐剂（Hu et al. 2016; Zhao, Hu, Hoerle et al. 2017）。临床前研究表明，NanoNicVac的免疫效力可以通过多种途径来优化，包括调节颗粒大小（Zhao, Hu, Hoerle et al. 2017）、调节半抗原密度（Zhao, Powers et al. 2017）、调节半抗原定位（Zhao, Hu, Harmon et al. 2017）、筛选载体蛋白（Zhao, Hu et al. 2018）、加入分子佐剂（Zhao, Harris et al. 2018）和调节佐剂。NanoNicVac显示出更好的识别和内化、增强的免疫原性和更好的药代动力学效果（图57.3）。这种基于纳米颗粒的烟碱混合疫苗正在进一步优化，有望进入临床试验。

由于所有临床测试的烟碱结合疫苗都失败了，因此有令人信服的理由认为，有必要利用全新的范式来开发新的烟碱疫苗。使用纳米颗粒而不是蛋白质作为载体就是这样一种新的范式。尽管下一代基于纳米颗粒的烟碱疫苗仍处于早期开发阶段，但它已显示出进一步开发用于人体临床试验的巨大前景。

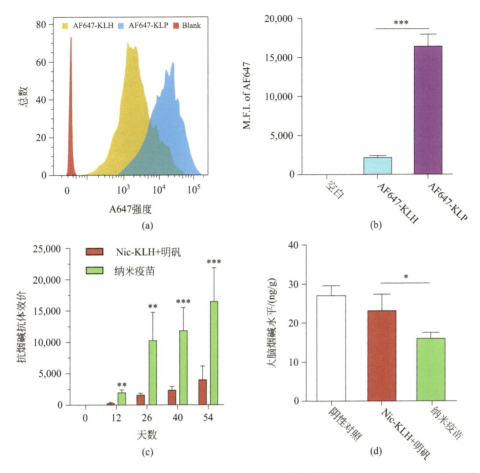

图 57.3 基于混合纳米颗粒的烟碱纳米疫苗（NanoNicVac）的功效（zhao，Powers et al. 2017）

（a）和（b）游离钥孔戚血蓝蛋白（KLH）（AF647-KLH）或混合纳米颗粒递送的 KLH（AF647-KLP）在树突细胞中的细胞摄取效率。KLH 被 Alexa Fluor 647（AF647）标记。MFI 代表平均荧光强度。显著不同：*** $P<0.001$。数据表示为平均值±标准差（$n=3$）。（c）由 Nic-KLH 结合疫苗与明矾或纳米疫苗诱导的抗烟碱抗体效价。与 Nic-KLH＋明矾相比有显著差异：** $P<0.05$，*** $P<0.001$。数据表示为平均值±标准差（$n=8$）。（d）用 0.03mg/kg 烟碱给药后，小鼠大脑中的烟碱水平。显著不同：* $P<0.05$。数据以平均值±标准差（$n=4$）表示。数据经 Elsevier 许可转载。

57.4　未来：结合以前的成功并研究新概念

过去的研究已经建立了许多可用于未来疫苗制剂的最佳方法。更具体地说，半抗原设计、半抗原定位、免疫原选择、免疫原支架、佐剂选择、疫苗接种途径和疫苗效价的影响都是经过充分研究的主题（Pentel, LeSage, 2014）。然而，当前的烟碱疫苗研究通常集中在新变量的研究上，而不是在最佳候选疫苗的评估上。这很可能是由于现有的大量专利限制了成功技术的可获得性，以及商业化是主要终点之一这一事实。如果我们希望在不久的将来看到成功的人类疫苗，请谨慎考虑过去研究的结果，并提出实施任何和所有先前积极发现的协作疫苗策略。

展望未来，用于评估疫苗效力的动物模型和基准应标准化。在过去，这些因素在测试组之间并不一致。小鼠、大鼠和兔子都已用作动物模型，主流的疗效基准在抗体效价、抗体浓度和脑中烟碱浓度降低百分比之间交替（Raupach et al. 2012）。采用与人类对烟碱疫苗的免疫反应密切相关的动物模型，将使未来的研究受益。此外，疗效基准的标准化将使独立研究之间能够更好地进行比较。

烟碱疫苗与传统疫苗的区别非常大，因为它们的功效通常仅由抗体结合动力学和抗体浓度两个因素决定，而这些参数的提高一直是过去和现在烟碱疫苗研究的重点。如果人们假设这些参数的优化将持续到将来，则有可能推测出未来烟碱疫苗研究可能采取的途径。未来研究的一些可能方向包括改进下一代基于纳米颗粒的烟碱疫苗技术，评估烟碱特异性分泌抗体对烟碱生物利用度的影响，为增强烟碱疫苗功效而对半抗原设计进行的持续研究，以及使用计算机模拟来利用动物研究数据对人类疫苗的功效做出预测。

为了提高下一代基于纳米颗粒的烟碱疫苗的免疫原性，还需要进行进一步的合理设计，例如，合理设计疫苗纳米颗粒的结构，精确控制疫苗颗粒的理化性质以及精确操作成分密度和化学计量。总体而言，开发下一代基于纳米颗粒的烟碱疫苗将有可能为治疗烟碱成瘾提供一种新颖的免疫疗法。

过去和现在的大多数烟碱疫苗研究都是非肠道注射疫苗，并且在很大程度上未能靶向黏膜免疫反应。这是不利的，因为黏膜免疫以IgA的分泌为特征，IgA是一种主要的抗体同种型，可以作为吸入的烟碱和大脑之间的另一道屏障（Neutra, Kozlowski, 2006）。在一项研究中已经看到了有希望的结果，与对照组相比，通过心脏注射放射性标记烟碱似乎使大脑中的烟碱浓度降低了75%（Fraleigh et al. 2016）。另外，在另一项研究中采用初免-加强策略时，黏膜抗体升高，全身抗体效价可与使用非肠道疫苗引起的效价相当（Cerny et al. 2002）。但是，这些研究没有研究分泌型IgA对吸入型烟碱生物利用度的影响。就易用性而言，黏膜免疫还具有无须使用针头即可在家中加强免疫力的优势。由于这些原因，在未来的烟碱疫苗制剂中应用初免-加强黏膜免疫可能是明智的。此外，使用多价烟碱疫苗可以提高烟碱特异性抗体的效价，并减少可以到达大脑的全身性烟碱的含量（de Villiers et al. 2013）。因此，使用多价、多途径疫苗接种方法也可能被证明是未来烟碱疫苗的另一种有效策略。

不幸的是，过去的烟碱疫苗的功效在最初的动物研究和后来的临床试验之间并没有很好地转化。由于这个原因，已经提出了一种新的疫苗设计方法，其中将数学模型与动物研究结合使用，以便在临床试验之前更好地预测疫苗的有效性。为此目的开发的第一个模型是简单的基于生理的药代动力学（PBPK）模型，当应用抗烟碱抗体的作用时，该模型能够有效预测大鼠血清和大脑中的烟碱浓度（Saylor, Zhang, 2016）。通过将人类特定的生理参数叠加到大鼠模型上，并使用文献中发现的时程血清烟碱浓度数据进行校准，该小组也开发了人类模型（图57.4）。如果使用在人类研究中建立的脑烟碱减少与戒烟率之间的相关性（Esterlis et al. 2013），则数学建模可以提供一种可靠的手段，从而可以在进行昂贵的临床试验之前使用动物数据来预测人类的疫苗效力。这些模型也可以用于建立疫苗功效阈值（即必需的抗体浓度、抗体亲和力和抗体选择性），从而进一步简化从动物研究到临床试验的过程。

当人们考虑过去几十年来烟碱疫苗研究的稳步发展时，很难想象没有将成功的疫苗推向市场的未来。每一项专注于实施新思想和新技术的新研究都可以进一步提高有效疫苗在人体中所需的功效。实际上，可能已经有足够的技术将有效的烟碱疫苗推向市场。但是，如前所述，由于许可问题，许多技术的传播正在放缓。此外，即使没有专利，大多数烟碱疫苗项目的特殊性质也可能会阻止各团体采用彼此的技术。最终，烟碱疫苗概念的成功似乎将归因于时间、该领域研究小组之间的合作程度以及全球资助机构的持续支持。

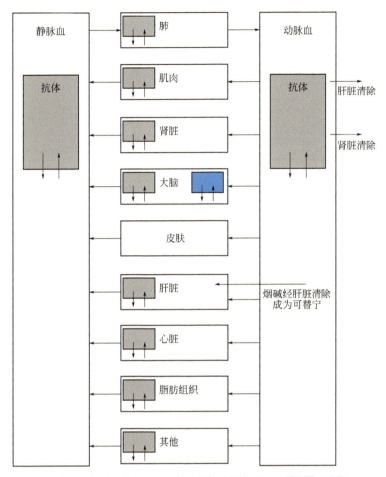

图 57.4　Saylor 和 Zhang（2016）开发的 PBPK 模型的示意图

灰色框代表结合烟碱和/或可替宁的抗体，蓝色框代表烟碱的组织保留，箭头表示烟碱和可替宁的质量作用动力学或新陈代谢。

| 术语解释 | ■ 佐剂：疫苗配方中的一种物质，能促进疫苗诱导的免疫反应。
■ 抗体的亲和力：给定抗体的结合位点与其表位之间的相互作用强度。
■ 结合疫苗：通过合适的接头将半抗原连接到基于蛋白质的载体上制成的疫苗。
■ 半抗原：一种小分子，其本身没有免疫原性，但当附着在大载体上时会具有免疫原性。
■ 免疫原性：疫苗/抗原诱导免疫反应的能力。
■ 计算机建模：一种基于计算机模拟的技术，用于模拟生理或药理过程。
■ 多价疫苗接种：一种免疫策略，其中同时向受试者施用两种或多种免疫原。
■ 纳米颗粒运载工具：使用能够携带药物化合物的纳米颗粒，将它们有效地输送到人类或动物的特定部位。
■ PBPK 模型：一种数学模型，用于预测一种物质在动物模型或人体中的吸收、分布、代谢和排泄。
■ 戒烟的药物疗法：一种通过应用药理学原理来帮助戒烟的治疗策略，包括烟碱替代疗法、基于安非他酮的疗法和基于伐伦克林的疗法。 |
|---|---|

烟碱疫苗的关键事实	■ 在全球范围内，在过去的几十年中，吸烟已经造成了巨大的死亡率、发病率和经济损失。
	■ 每年，只有3%的吸烟者自行成功戒烟。
	■ 传统的药物疗法，包括烟碱替代疗法、基于伐伦克林的疗法和基于安非他酮的疗法，被证明能有效帮助戒烟。
	■ 药物疗法面临诸多挑战，包括戒断率低、治疗时间长和副作用。
	■ 烟碱疫苗被认为是治疗烟瘾的有效疗法。
	■ 第一代烟碱疫苗是烟碱-蛋白质结合物，由于其免疫原性和特异性较低，在临床试验中显示出有限的治疗效果。
	■ 下一代烟碱疫苗是基于纳米颗粒的疫苗，可以获得比传统烟碱-蛋白质结合疫苗更好的治疗效果。

要点总结	■ 本章重点介绍烟碱疫苗，这是烟碱成瘾的潜在疗法。
	■ 烟草成瘾主要是烟碱成瘾。
	■ 烟碱疫苗可以诱导烟碱特异性抗体的产生，这种抗体可以与烟碱结合，防止其穿过血脑屏障，从而降低吸烟的奖励效应。
	■ 传统烟碱疫苗是通过将烟碱类似物与载体蛋白结合而构建的，在临床试验中显示出促进戒烟的有限功效。
	■ 下一代烟碱疫苗是基于纳米颗粒的烟碱疫苗，开发这种疫苗是为了避免传统烟碱-蛋白质结合疫苗的缺点，如低免疫原性、低特异性和短效力。
	■ 基于纳米颗粒的烟碱疫苗在临床前和临床试验中表现出很强的治疗烟碱成瘾的能力。
	■ 通过合理设计疫苗结构，优化疫苗颗粒的物理化学性质，并加入适当的分子佐剂，可以进一步提高目前基于纳米颗粒的烟碱疫苗的性能。

参考文献

Benowitz, N. L. (2008). Neurobiology of nicotine addiction: implications for smoking cessation treatment. The American Journal of Medicine, 121(4 Suppl. 1), S3-10.

Benowitz, N. L. (2010). Nicotine addiction. The New England Journal of Medicine, 362(24), 2295-2303.

Cahill, K.; Stevens, S.; Perera, R.; Lancaster, T. (2013). Pharmacological interventions for smoking cessation: an overview and network meta-analysis. Cochrane Database of Systematic Reviews, 5, CD009329.

Caponnetto, P.; Russo, C.; Polosa, R. (2012). Smoking cessation: present status and future perspectives. Current Opinion in Pharmacology, 12(3), 229-237.

Cerny, E. H.; Levy, R.; Mauel, J.; Mpandi, M.; Mutter, M.; Henzelin-Nkubana, C. et al. (2002). Preclinical development of a vaccine'against smoking'. Onkologie, 25(5), 406-411.

Crunelle, C. L.; Miller, M. L.; Booij, J.; van den Brink, W. (2010). The nicotinic acetylcholine receptor partial agonist varenicline and the treatment of drug dependence: A review. European Neuropsychopharmacology, 20(2), 69-79.

Dani, J. A.; De Biasi, M. (2001). Cellular mechanisms of nicotine addiction. Pharmacology, Biochemistry, and Behavior, 70(4), 439-446.

de Villiers, S. H.; Cornish, K. E.; Troska, A. J.; Pravetoni, M.; Pentel, P. R. (2013). Increased efficacy of a trivalent nicotine vaccine compared to a dose-matched monovalent vaccine when formulated with alum. Vaccine, 31(52), 6185-6193.

Ekpu, V. U.; Brown, A. K. (2015). The economic impact of smoking and of reducing smoking prevalence: review of evidence. Tobacco Use Insights, 8, 1-35.

Esterlis, I.; Hannestad, J. O.; Perkins, E.; Bois, F.; D'Souza, D. C.; Tyndale, R. F. et al. (2013). Effect of a nicotine vaccine on nicotine binding to beta2*-nicotinic acetylcholine receptors in vivo in human tobacco smokers. The American Journal of Psychiatry, 170(4), 399-407.

Fagerstrom, K. (2002). The epidemiology of smoking: health consequences and benefits of cessation. Drugs, 62(Suppl. 2), 1-9.

Fahim, R. E.; Kessler, P. D.; Kalnik, M. W. (2013). Therapeutic vaccines against tobacco addiction. Expert Review of Vaccines, 12(3), 333-342.

Fraleigh, N. L.; Boudreau, J.; Bhardwaj, N.; Eng, N. F.; Murad, Y.; Lafrenie, R. et al. (2016). Evaluating the immunogenicity of an intranasal vaccine against nicotine in mice using the adjuvant Finlay proteoliposome (AFPL1). Heliyon, 2(8):e00147.

Fraser, C. C.; Altreuter, D. H.; Ilyinskii, P.; Pittet, L.; LaMothe, R. A.; Keegan, M. et al. (2014). Generation of a universal CD4 memory T cell recall peptide effective in humans, mice and non-human primates. Vaccine, 32(24), 2896-2903.

Goniewicz, M. L.; Delijewski, M. (2013). Nicotine vaccines to treat tobacco dependence. Human Vaccines, Immunotherapeutics, 9(1), 13-25.

Hall, W. (2002). The prospects for immunotherapy in smoking cessation. Lancet, 360(9339), 1089-1091.

Hoogsteder, P. H.; Kotz, D.; van Spiegel, P. I.; Viechtbauer, W.; van Schayck, O. C. (2014). Efficacy of the nicotine vaccine 3′-AmNic-rEPA (NicVAX) co-administered with varenicline and counselling for smoking cessation: a randomized placebo-controlled trial. Addiction, 109(8), 1252-1259.

Hu, Y.; Smith, D.; Frazier, E.; Hoerle, R.; Ehrich, M.; Zhang, C. M. (2016). The next-generation nicotine vaccine: a novel and potent hybrid nanoparticle-based nicotine vaccine. Biomaterials, 106, 228-239.

Hu, Y.; Zheng, H.; Huang, W.; Zhang, C. M. (2014). A novel and efficient nicotine vaccine using nano-lipoplex as a delivery vehicle. Human Vaccines, Immunotherapeutics, 10(1), 64-72.

Ilyinskii, P. O.; Johnston, L. P. M. (2016). Nanoparticle-based nicotine vaccine. In I. D. Montoya (Ed.), Biologics to treat substance use disorders: vaccines, monoclonal antibodies, and enzymes (pp. 249-279): Basel, Switzerland: Springer.

Jiloha, R. C. (2014). Pharmacotherapy of smoking cessation. Indian Journal of Psychiatry, 56(1), 87-95.

Liu, X.; Hecht, S. M.; Yan, H.; Pentel, P. R.; Chang, Y. (2016). Exploration of DNA nanostructures for rational design of vaccines. In I. D. Montoya (Ed.), Biologics to treat substance use disorders: Vaccines, monoclonal antibodies, and enzymes (pp. 279-293): Basel, Switzerland: Springer.

Liu, X. W.; Xu, Y.; Yu, T.; Clifford, C.; Liu, Y.; Yan, H. et al. (2012). A DNA nanostructure platform for directed assembly of synthetic vaccines. Nano Letters, 12(8), 4254-4259.

Lockner, J. W.; Ho, S. O.; McCague, K. C.; Chiang, S. M.; Do, T. Q.; Fujii, G. et al. (2013). Enhancing nicotine vaccine immunogenicity with liposomes. Bioorganic, Medicinal Chemistry Letters, 23(4), 975-978.

Muilenburg, J. L.; Laschober, T. C.; Eby, L. T. (2015). Relationship between low-income patient census and substance use disorder treatment programs' availability of tobacco cessation services. Journal of Drug Issues, 45(1), 69-79.

Munoz, R. F.; Bunge, E. L.; Barrera, A. Z.; Wickham, R. E.; Lee, J. (2016). Using behavioral intervention technologies to help low-income and Latino smokers quit: protocol of a randomized controlled trial. JMIR Research Protocols, 5(2):e127.

Nestler, E. J. (2005). Is there a common molecular pathway for addiction? Nature Neuroscience, 8(11), 1445-1449.

Neutra, M. R.; Kozlowski, P. A. (2006). Mucosal vaccines: the promise and the challenge. Nature Reviews Immunology, 6(2), 148-158.

Patel, D. R.; Feucht, C.; Reid, L.; Patel, N. D. (2010). Pharmacologic agents for smoking cessation: a clinical review. Clinical Pharmacology, 2, 17-29.

Paterson, D.; Nordberg, A. (2000). Neuronal nicotinic receptors in the human brain. Progress in Neurobiology, 61(1), 75-111.

Pentel, P. R.; LeSage, M. G. (2014). New directions in nicotine vaccine design and use. Advances in Pharmacology, 69, 553-580.

Pentel, P.; Malin, D. (2002). A vaccine for nicotine dependence: targeting the drug rather than the brain. Respiration, 69(3), 193-197.

Pittet, L.; Altreuter, D.; Ilyinskii, P.; Fraser, C.; Gao, Y.; Baldwin, S. et al. (2012). Development and preclinical evaluation of SEL-068, a novel targeted synthetic vaccine particle (tSVP (TM)) for smoking cessation and relapse prevention that generates high titers of antibodies against nicotine. Journal of Immunology, 188.

Pope, C. A.; Ⅲ, Burnett, R. T.; Turner, M. C.; Cohen, A.; Krewski, D.; Jerrett, M. et al. (2011). Lung cancer and cardiovascular disease mortality associated with ambient air pollution and cigarette smoke:shape of the exposure-response relationships. Environmental Health Perspectives, 119(11), 1616-1621.

Raupach, T.; Hoogsteder, P. H.; Onno van Schayck, C. P. (2012). Nicotine vaccines to assist with smoking cessation: current status of research. Drugs, 72(4), e1-16.

Raupach, T.; van Schayck, C. P. (2011). Pharmacotherapy for smoking cessation: current advances and research topics. CNS Drugs, 25(5), 371-382.

Roddy, E. (2004). Bupropion and other non-nicotine pharmacotherapies. BMJ, 328(7438), 509-511.

Saylor, K.; Zhang, C. (2016). A simple physiologically based pharmacokinetic model evaluating the effect of anti-nicotine antibodies on nicotine disposition in the brains of rats and humans. Toxicology and Applied Pharmacology, 307, 150-164.

Schnoll, R. A.; Goelz, P. M.; Veluz-Wilkins, A.; Blazekovic, S.; Powers, L.; Leone, F. T. et al. (2015). Long-term nicotine replacement therapy: a randomized clinical trial. JAMA Internal Medicine, 175(4), 504-511.

Shen, X. Y.; Orson, F. M.; Kosten, T. R. (2012). Vaccines against drug abuse. Clinical Pharmacology and Therapeutics, 91(1), 60-70.

Strong, K.; Mathers, C.; Bonita, R. (2007). Preventing stroke: saving lives around the world. Lancet Neurology, 6(2), 182-187.

Zalewska-Kaszubska, J. (2015). Is immunotherapy an opportunity for effective treatment of drug addiction? Vaccine, 33(48), 6545-6551.

Zhao, Z.; Harris, B.; Hu, Y.; Harmon, T.; Pentel, P. R.; Ehrich, M. et al. (2018). Rational incorporation of molecular adjuvants into a hybrid nanoparticle-based nicotine vaccine for immunotherapy against nicotine addiction. Biomaterials, 155, 165-175.

Zhao, Z.; Hu, Y.; Harmon, T.; Pentel, P.; Ehrich, M.; Zhang, C. (2017). Rationalization of a nanoparticle-based nicotine nanovaccine as an effective next-generation nicotine vaccine: a focus on hapten localization. Biomaterials, 138, 46-56.

Zhao, Z.; Hu, Y.; Harmon, T.; Pentel, P. R.; Ehrich, M.; Zhang, C. (2018). Hybrid nanoparticle-based nicotine nanovaccines: Boosting the immunological efficacy by conjugation of potent carrier proteins. Nanomedicine, 14(5), 1655-1665.

Zhao, Z.; Hu, Y.; Hoerle, R.; Devine, M.; Raleigh, M.; Pentel, P. et al. (2017). A nanoparticle-based nicotine vaccine and the influence of particle size on its immunogenicity and efficacy. Nanomedicine, 13(2), 443-454.

Zhao, Z.; Powers, K.; Hu, Y.; Raleigh, M.; Pentel, P.; Zhang, C. M. (2017). Engineering of a hybrid nanoparticle-based nicotine nanovaccine as a next-generation immunotherapeutic strategy against nicotine addiction: a focus on hapten density. Biomaterials, 123, 107-117.

Zheng, H.; Hu, Y.; Huang, W.; de Villiers, S.; Pentel, P.; Zhang, J. et al. (2015). Negatively charged carbon nanohorn supported cationic liposome nanoparticles: a novel delivery vehicle for anti-nicotine vaccine. Journal of Biomedical Nanotechnology, 11(12), 2197-2210.

58
在精神病医院治疗烟碱依赖

Emily A. Stockings

National Drug and Alcohol Research Centre（NDARC），UNSW Sydney, Randwick, NSW, Australia

缩略语

CMS	医疗保险和医疗补助服务中心	NRT	烟碱替代疗法

58.1 引言

吸烟仍然是全球发病率和死亡率的主要原因。与普通人群相比，患有精神障碍的人吸烟率更高，更依赖烟碱，戒烟的可能性更小，死于吸烟相关疾病的可能性更大。鉴于吸烟率和烟碱依赖率在患有最严重精神障碍（包括精神分裂症和精神病）的人群中最高，精神病医院可能被证明是向这一弱势群体提供有效烟碱依赖治疗的关键场所。

在精神病医院治疗烟碱依赖一直是一个有争议的问题。一方面，考虑到广泛实施禁烟令并同时提供药物和行为戒烟支持，在精神病医院可能被视为解决高度依赖和弱势吸烟者群体吸烟问题的一个机会。另一方面，禁烟令和烟碱依赖治疗可能被视为对患者基本权利和个人自由的侵犯，因为精神病医院是患者的临时住所。精神病医院内也有一种长期的吸烟文化，历史上提供卷烟是为了奖励顺从的病人行为，并促进病人和临床工作人员之间的社会联系。尽管存在这种根深蒂固的吸烟文化，一个新的证据表明，在精神病医院治疗烟碱依赖是可能的，也是潜在有效的。

本章探讨精神病医院作为治疗烟碱依赖的环境。它涵盖了精神障碍患者吸烟的普遍程度、精神病医院内吸烟文化的概述、无烟政策的引入及其在精神病医院实施的障碍、烟碱依赖治疗的普遍程度、改善护理提供的建议方法以及出院后继续护理的考虑因素。

58.2 精神障碍患者吸烟

58.2.1 吸烟率和健康负担

基于人群的吸烟率研究估计，精神障碍患者的吸烟率至少是普通人群的两倍（Lawrence et al. 2013），吸烟率随着终生精神障碍的数量和严重程度的增加而增加（Lasser et al. 2000）；参见图58.1。

吸烟率因诊断和环境而异，焦虑症和人格障碍患者的吸烟率在36%～39%（Lineberry et al. 2009），抑郁症和情绪障碍患者的吸烟率在36%～49%（Lasser et al. 2000; Lineberry et al. 2009），精神病（包括精神分裂症和分裂情感障碍）患者的吸烟率在70%～88%。一些报告的最高吸烟率在精神病医院就诊者中已被确定，该组中吸烟率高达80%（McManus et al. 2010）；参见图58.2。除了吸烟率增加之外，患有精神障碍的吸烟者也比普通人群中的吸烟者吸烟更多，对烟碱的依赖性更强（Diaz et al. 2006）。由于这一群体的吸烟率不成比例，据估计，与普通人群相比，患有精神障碍的人的预期寿命缩短了12～15年，大多数超额死亡归因于心血管疾病和癌症（Lawrence et al. 2013）。

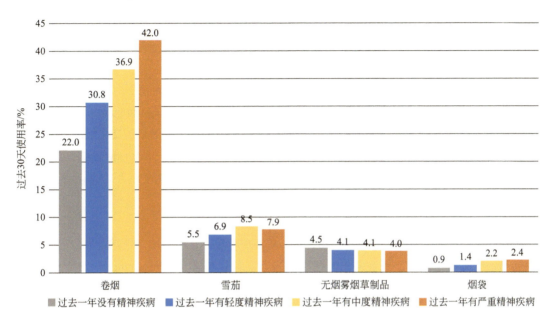

图58.1 过去30天使用特定烟草产品的成年人中，34580人过去一年没有精神疾病，4434人过去一年有轻度精神疾病，2371人过去一年有中度精神疾病，2176人过去一年有严重精神疾病

吸烟率随着精神疾病严重程度的增加而增加。过去一年患有严重精神疾病的人的吸烟率最高，大约是过去一年没有精神疾病的人的吸烟率的两倍。使用美国卫生与公众服务部2015年全国药物使用与健康调查数据绘制的图表。数据涉及18岁及以上的成年人。

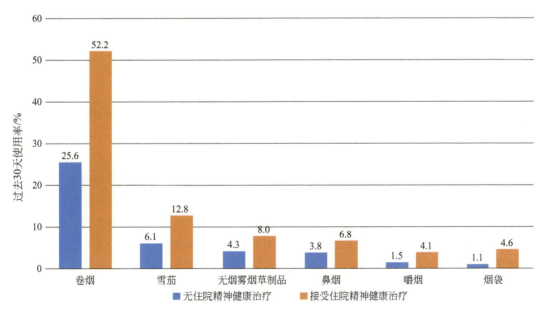

图58.2 报告过去一年接受住院精神健康治疗的成年人（n=429）与报告过去一年没有接受住院精神健康治疗的成年人（n=41115）过去30天使用特定烟草制品（%）的比较

在所有形式的烟草产品中，接受住院精神健康治疗的人的吸烟率远远高于未接受精神健康治疗的人。特别是其吸烟率（52%）大约是一般人口的估计吸烟率（26%）的两倍。使用美国卫生与公众服务部2014年全国药物使用与健康调查数据绘制的图表。数据涉及18岁及以上的成年人。

58.2.2 精神障碍患者吸烟率升高的相关因素

生物、社会和心理因素导致精神障碍患者的吸烟率高得不成比例。一些研究人员认为，与没有精神障碍的吸烟者相比，患有精神障碍的人可能具有更高的烟碱效应的遗传脆弱性，并体验到更多的奖励或愉悦感（Williams, Ziedonis, 2004）。患有精神障碍的人也可能开始吸烟，试图自我治疗（Hall, Prochaska, 2009）。还有一些证据表明烟碱可以改善精神分裂症患者的认知功能，包括持续的注意力和改善听觉信息的过滤（Depatie et al. 2002）。

造成精神障碍患者吸烟率不成比例的潜在社会因素可能包括贫困和经济压力、失业、无家可归、教育水平较低、获得医疗服务和社会支持网络的机会以及同龄人的压力（Australian Institute of Health and Welfare, 2012）。精神障碍患者也更有可能在家里和工作场所接触到吸烟的文化规范（Hiscock et al. 2012）。重要的是，患有精神障碍的吸烟者获得戒烟资源的机会减少（Williams et al. 2013），在接触卫生保健服务，特别是在住精神病医院时，也不太可能得到烟碱依赖的支持（Wye et al. 2010）。

58.2.3 吸烟的"文化"

长期以来，精神病医院中存在着吸烟文化。从历史上看，众所周知，治疗人员会定期向患者提供卷烟，在某些情况下，还会为无法这样做的患者购买卷烟（Lawn, Campion, 2013）。甚至在最近，卷烟也被用作一种行为矫正手段，例如，用来避免被感知到的攻击性或暴力行为，或奖励积极的行为，如服药依从性（Lawn, 2010）。吸烟也被发现是精神病医院患者和工作人员的一种常见的社会活动（Williams, Ziedonis, 2004），从而加强了精神病医院内吸烟的"文化"。

58.3 精神病医院的无烟政策

58.3.1 精神病医院实施无烟政策困难重重

全球大多数国家都对公共场所和工作场所（包括精神病医院）实施了吸烟限制（Callinan et al. 2010）。然而，这种禁烟令在精神病医院的实施一直存在问题。直到最近，许多精神病医院（特别是那些收容非自愿患者的精神病医院）经常被免除禁烟令（Ratschen et al. 2008）。在精神病医院引入禁烟令往往会遭到工作人员（McNally et al. 2006）和患者（Willemsen et al. 2004）的抵制，因此，据报道，禁烟令的执行和遵守情况很差（Stockings et al. 2015）。

在精神病医院有效实施禁烟和提供烟碱依赖治疗的障碍可能包括工作人员的误解，他们认为禁烟会扰乱病房的治疗环境，消极的精神症状，特别是攻击性和激动症，会随着吸烟的限制而加剧（Lawn, Campion, 2013）。然而，最近的证据表明，随着全面无烟政策的实施，发生身体暴力事件的比率实际上可能会下降（Robson et al. 2017）。在这些环境中成功实施无烟政策的另一个潜在障碍是，精神卫生工作人员普遍认为，他们的病人没有戒烟的动机、不愿意或不能够戒烟（Lawn, 2004）。与这一观点相反，精神病医院的许多吸烟者都有戒烟的动机，并经常做出几次实质性的尝试（Stockings et al. 2013）。

58.3.2 精神病医院烟碱依赖治疗的普及率

临床实践指南建议在美国、英国和澳大利亚等发达国家的精神病医院为患者提供烟碱依赖治疗（Fiore et al. 2008; New South Wales Department of Health, 2002; Ratschenet al. 2009）。这些指南要求治疗人员为所有入院时被确认为吸烟者的患者提供药理学和行为戒烟支持，如简短的戒烟建议和烟碱替代疗法（NRT）。全球卫生保健机构在不同程度上提供了这种戒烟支持，其费用通常由政府补贴。对美国和澳大利亚精神病医院提供这种烟碱依赖治疗的医疗记录审计表明，烟碱依赖治疗的记录很少（如果有的话），提供烟碱依赖治疗的情况可以忽略不计（Prochaska et al. 2004; Wye et al. 2010）。在丹麦（Willemsen et al. 2004）、美国（Bronaugh, Frances,1990）、英国（Ratschen et al. 2010）和澳大利亚（Wye et al. 2014）进行的研究也报道，偷偷吸烟继续发生在"无烟"精神病医院，使工作人员、病人和来访者暴露于环境烟草烟雾的有害影响。尽管有临床实践指南，但烟碱依赖的治疗率很低，而且违反了无烟政策，这表明需要制订策略，改善精神病医院对烟碱依赖的治疗。

58.4 改善精神病医院烟碱依赖的治疗

58.4.1 系统改变的方法

有人建议采取系统变革办法，以改善保健机构（包括精神病医院）对烟碱依赖提供及时和有效的治疗（Bonevski, 2014; Fiore et al. 2007）。表58.1总结了采用这种关键系统改变方法的策略，其中包括入院时对患者吸烟状况的系统评估、员工教育、促进支持提供烟碱依赖治疗的政策、对获得这种护理的患者提供补贴以及向工作人员补偿护理提供的费用（Fiore et al. 2007）。研究表明，与没有采取系统改变方法的医院相比，采取这种方法可以使在普通医院接受咨询或协助戒烟的患者数量增加17%（Freund et al. 2009）。

表58.1 在包括精神病医院在内的保健机构的治疗中，改善烟碱依赖治疗的提供情况的策略

序号	策略
1	实施系统，以识别和记录患者入院时的吸烟状况和烟碱依赖情况
2	为员工提供教育、资源和开发沟通渠道，以实现反馈和评估
3	指派工作人员为烟碱依赖提供治疗并评估其使用情况
4	促进支持烟碱依赖治疗的政策
5	免费或补贴提供烟碱依赖治疗
6	补偿临床医生对烟碱依赖的有效治疗，并将这种治疗纳入临床医生的规定职责

注：有许多策略可用于改善精神病医院烟碱依赖治疗的系统交付。这些策略既包括系统层面的策略，如引入具有评估烟草使用情况项目的新入院表格，也包括个人层面的策略，如提供足够的工作人员培训和反馈（Fiore et al. 2007）。

58.4.2 增加精神病医院烟碱依赖治疗的干预措施

虽然关于在精神病医院增加烟碱依赖治疗的干预措施的有效性的证据有限，但越来越多的证据表明，在普通医院环境中使用的临床实践和系统改变干预措施可能也同样有效。

2015年，在美国，医疗保险和医疗补助服务中心（CMS）引入了关于接受医疗保险基金的精神病医院烟碱依赖治疗的新报告要求。这些报告要求包括系统筛查烟草使用情况，提供烟草使

用治疗（包括咨询或戒烟药物）。未报告这些措施的设施面临2%的年度资金罚款。对一家医院在引入此类措施前后的分析发现，烟草使用筛查增加到接近100%的入院人数，转诊到戒烟咨询的人数增加了18倍，转诊到戒烟药物治疗的人数也大幅增加（Carrillo et al. 2017）。这项研究提供了很好的证据，表明基于表现的惩罚可能会改善精神病医院对烟碱依赖的治疗。

另一种在精神病医院增加烟碱依赖治疗的方法是采用多种策略，解决提供此类护理的关键障碍。例如，多策略临床实践系统-变革干预，包括领导和共识（例如，与高级工作人员协商）和使能系统和程序（例如，修改带有评估烟草使用项目的入院表格）、工作人员培训和教育、资源提供（例如，易于获取的临床实践指南副本）、审计和反馈发现，两家精神病医院的烟碱依赖治疗的所有五项指标都有所增加（Wye et al. 2017）；参见图58.3。在引入干预措施后的6个月内，在记录吸烟状况和评估烟碱依赖、提供戒烟建议、开NRT处方和提供烟碱依赖出院治疗等方面，均发现有不良反应。

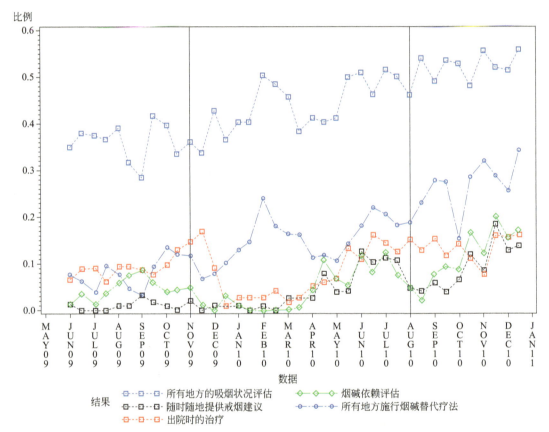

图58.3 在实施临床实践改变干预之前、期间和之后，澳大利亚精神病住院患者的审计病历中记录的烟草依赖五种治疗要素的比例变化（%）

在澳大利亚一家精神病医院引入临床实践改变干预措施，增加了对患者烟碱依赖治疗的五项关键措施的记录，这是使用审计病历进行测量的。最初由Wye等（2017）在《英国医学中心精神病学》上发表，并且该数据在此处根据知识共享署名4.0国际许可转载。

58.5 出院后继续烟碱依赖治疗

入院是解决吸烟问题的好时机；然而，如果出院后不提供持续护理，烟碱依赖住院治疗的有效性是有限的（Bowman, Stockings, 2013）。有人认为，由于住院病人和社区精神卫生服务之间缺乏协调，住院精神病患者的无烟政策对长期戒烟几乎没有影响（Campion et al. 2008）。因此，为了提高戒烟率，在从无烟医院出院后，应向患者提供长达一个月的烟碱依赖持续治疗（Rigotti et al. 2012）。在澳大利亚（Metse et al. 2017; Stockings et al. 2014）和美国（Prochaska et al. 2014）进行的随机对照试验表明，从精神病医院出院后长达4个月的烟碱依赖持续治疗可在出院后18个月内提高戒烟率。

术语解释

- 行为戒烟支持：任何包括有助于改变吸烟行为的支持性因素的戒烟方法，如支持性咨询、认知行为疗法和戒烟的简短建议。这种支持可以以多人或个人面对面的方式、在线、通过电话（如"戒烟热线"）或通过移动电话应用程序提供。
- 烟碱依赖临床实践指南：一套规则，要求临床工作人员提供烟碱依赖治疗，以管理烟碱戒断症状，并在实施无烟政策或禁烟令的环境中促进戒烟。这可能包括药物戒烟支持和行为戒烟支持。
- 精神病：也被称为"精神疾病"或"精神障碍"，是指对健康和日常生活造成损害的任何行为或精神模式。常见的精神障碍包括抑郁和焦虑，不太常见但更严重的精神障碍包括双相情感障碍、饮食障碍和精神分裂症。这些疾病由训练有素的精神健康专业人员根据诊断标准进行诊断；然而，人们可能会在不符合全部诊断标准的情况下出现精神障碍症状。如果精神障碍在过去12个月内一直存在，则通常被描述为"当前的"。
- 烟碱依赖：一种对烟碱的依赖状态，通常包括经常大量吸烟，同时伴有烟瘾或吸烟渴望以及当不使用烟碱时令人不快的戒断症状。
- 烟碱替代疗法（NRT）：允许在无烟草存在的情况下以医学上安全的方式将烟碱输送到血液中的产品。输送途径包括鼻子或口腔（如口香糖、含片和鼻喷雾剂）和皮肤（如烟碱贴片）。
- 药理学戒烟支持：任何用于治疗烟碱依赖的药物。这包括使用不构成健康风险的更安全的给药系统来替代烟碱的药物（即烟碱替代疗法）、模拟烟碱对大脑烟碱受体作用的药物（即烟碱受体部分激动剂，如伐伦克林）和抑制烟碱受体作用的药物（即烟碱拮抗剂，如安非他酮）。
- 精神病医院：为患有急性精神障碍症状的人提供治疗的医院、病房或专门的医疗服务机构。医疗机构可以在住院或门诊的基础上提供短期或长期的精神病治疗。病人可以在自愿或非自愿的基础上入院，后者通常是对可能对自己或他人造成伤害的人的法律程序。
- 无烟政策：也被称为"禁烟令"，是一套要求人们戒烟的指导方针，以保护人们免受二手烟的伤害。此类政策的范围可以从禁止在建筑物和场地内吸烟的全面禁令到可能禁止在某些区域吸烟但允许在其他区域（如指定的吸烟室）吸烟的部分禁令。

精神病医院治疗烟碱依赖的关键事实

- 人格障碍、焦虑和抑郁患者的吸烟率在36%～50%之间，包括精神分裂症和分裂情感障碍在内的精神障碍患者的吸烟率在70%～88%之间。
- 精神障碍患者的预期寿命减少了12～15年，这主要是由于与烟草有关的疾病，如心血管疾病和癌症。
- 尽管人们有普遍的看法，但患有精神障碍的吸烟者有戒烟的动机，而且许多人经常做出几次实质性的尝试。
- 精神病医院的吸烟"文化"由来已久，直到最近，许多医院才获得禁烟令的豁免。
- 在这些环境下，禁烟令的引入一直很困难，烟碱依赖治疗的接受率也很低。

- 许多普通员工对引入禁烟令的看法往往是不正确的；例如，引入全面的无烟政策实际上与减少患者的身体暴力和攻击性有关。
- 临床实践改变干预涉及整个医院的多项策略，以增加工作人员的支持，并向患者提供烟碱依赖治疗。
- 迄今为止，精神病医院的临床实践改变干预措施已导致烟草使用筛查、烟碱依赖治疗和戒烟支持的增加。
- 然而，只有在继续进行戒烟治疗的情况下，住在无烟精神病医院可能会增加吸烟者出院后戒烟的机会。

要点总结

- 本章重点介绍精神病医院的烟碱依赖治疗。
- 精神病住院患者的吸烟率最高（高达80%）；然而，接受戒烟治疗的人很少。
- 发达国家的大多数精神病医院都实行了禁烟令，以系统的方式向所有吸烟者提供烟碱依赖治疗的机会。
- 然而，精神病医院的工作人员和患者历来对禁烟令持负面看法，禁烟令经常被违反，烟碱依赖治疗的提供也很少。
- 有几种策略可用于改善精神病医院烟碱依赖治疗的系统提供，包括临床实践改变干预。
- 关于临床实践改变干预措施在精神病医院增加烟碱依赖治疗的有效性的证据仍在出现，但迄今为止的结果是令人振奋的。
- 在无烟精神病医院住院期间接受烟碱依赖治疗也可能导致出院后戒烟率增加；然而，只有在出院后继续治疗至少一个月的情况下才会发生这种情况。
- 需要将住院烟碱依赖治疗与正在进行的社区戒烟支持联系起来，以降低精神障碍患者吸烟和吸烟相关疾病的发病率升高。

参考文献

Australian Institute of Health and Welfare. (2012). Australia's health 2012. Canberra:AIHW.

Bonevski, B. (2014). System-centred tobacco management: from 'wholeperson' to 'whole-system' change. Drug and Alcohol Review, 33(1), 99-101. https://doi.org/10.1111/dar.12086.

Bowman, J.; Stockings, E. A. (2013). Smoking cessation for hospitalised patients: intensive behavioural counselling started in hospital and continued after discharge increases quit rates; with additional benefit from adding nicotine replacement therapy. Evidence-Based Nursing, 16(1), 21-22. https://doi.org/10.1136/eb-2012-100890.

Bronaugh, T. A.; Frances, R. J. (1990). Establishing a smoke-free inpatient unit: is it feasible? Hospital, Community Psychiatry, 41(12), 1303-1305.

Callinan, J. E.; Clarke, A.; Doherty, K.; Kelleher, C. (2010). Legislative smoking bans for reducing secondhand smoke exposure, smoking prevalence and tobacco consumption. Cochrane Data-base of Systematic Reviews, 4: CD005992. https://doi.org/10.1002/14651858.CD005992.pub2.

Campion, J.; Checinski, K.; Nurse, J. (2008). Review of smoking cessation treatments for people with mental illness. Advances in Psychiatric Treatment, 14, 208-216.

Carrillo, S.; Nazir, N.; Howser, E.; Shenkman, L.; Laxson, M.; Scheuermann, T. S. et al. (2017). Impact of the 2015 CMS inpatient psychiatric facility quality reporting rule on tobacco treatment. Nicotine, Tobacco Research, 19(8), 976-982. https://doi.org/10.1093/ntr/ntw386.

Depatie, L.; O'Driscoll, G. A.; Holahan, A. L.; Atkinson, V.; Thavundayil, J. X.; Kin, N. N. et al. (2002). Nicotine andbehavioral markers of risk for schizophrenia: a double-blind, placebo-controlled, cross-over study. Neuropsychopharmacology, 27(6), 1056-1070. https://doi.org/10.1016/s0893-133x(02)00372-x.

Diaz, F.; Rendon, D.; Velasquez, D.; Susce, M.; de Leon, J. (2006). Datapoints: smoking and smoking cessation among persons with severe mental illnesses. Psychiatric Services, 57(4), 462. https://doi.org/10.1176/appi.ps.57.4.462.

Fiore, M.; Jaen, C.; Baker, T. (2008). Treating tobacco use and dependence: 2008 update: Clinical practice guideline. Rockville, MD: US Department of Health and Human Services, Public Health Service.

Fiore, M. C.; Keller, P. A.; Curry, S. J. (2007). Health system changes to facilitate the delivery of tobacco-dependence treatment. American Journal of Preventive Medicine, 33 (6 Suppl), S349-S356. https:/ /doi. org/10. 1016/j. amepre. 2007. 09. 001.

Freund, M.; Campbell, E.; Paul, C.; Sakrouge, R.; McElduff, P.; Walsh, R. A. et al. (2009). Increasing smoking cessation care provision in hos-pitals: a meta-analysis of intervention effect. Nicotine, TobaccoResearch, 11(6), 650-662. https:/ /doi. org/10. 1093/ntr/ntp056.

Hall, S. M.; Prochaska, J. J. (2009). Treatment of smokers with co-occurring disorders: emphasis on integration in mental healthand addiction treatment settings. Annual Review of Clinical Psychol-ogy, 5, 409-431.

Hiscock, R.; Bauld, L.; Amos, A.; Fidler, J. A.; Munafò, M. (2012). Socioeconomic status and smoking: a review. Annals of the New YorkAcademy of Sciences, (1248), 107-123. https:/ /doi. org/10. 1111/j. 17496632. 2011. 06202. x.

Lasser, K.; Boyd, J. W.; Woolhandler, S.; Himmelstein, D. U.; McCormick, D.; Bor, D. H. (2000). Smoking and mental illness:a population based prevalence study. Journal of the AmericanMedical Association, 284(20), 2606-2610. https:/ /doi. org/10. 1001/jama. 284. 20. 2606.

Lawn, S. J. (2004). Systemic barriers to quitting smoking among institu-tionalised public mental health service populations: a comparison of two Australian sites. International Journal of Social Psychiatry, 50(3), 204-215. https:/ /doi. org/10. 1177/0020764004043129.

Lawn, S. (2010). The culture of smoking in mental health service populations. Berlin: Lambert Academic Publishing.

Lawn, S.; Campion, J. (2013). Achieving smoke-free mental healthservices: lessons from the past decade of implementation research. International Journal of Environmental Research and Public Health, 10(9), 4224-4244. https:/ /doi. org/10. 3390/ijerph10094224.

Lawrence, D.; Hafekost, J.; Hull, P.; Mitrou, F.; Zubrick, S. R. (2013). Smoking, mental illness and socioeconomic disadvantage: analysisof the Australian National Survey of Mental Health and Wellbeing. BMC Public Health, 13, 462. https:/ /doi. org/10. 1186/1471-2458-13-462.

Lawrence, D.; Hancock, K. J.; Kisely, S. (2013). The gap in life expec-tancy from preventable physical illness in psychiatric patients inWestern Australia: retrospective analysis of population basedregisters. British Medical Journal, 346.

Lineberry, T. W.; Allen, J. D.; Nash, J.; Galardy, C. W. (2009). Population-based prevalence of smoking in psychiatric inpatients:a focus on acute suicide risk and major diagnostic groups. Comprehensive Psychiatry, 50(6), 526-532. https:/ /doi. org/10. 1016/j. comppsych. 2009. 01. 004.

McManus, S.; Meltzer, H.; Campion, J. (2010). Cigarette smoking andmental health in England: Data from the Adult Psychiatric MorbiditySurvey 2007. London: National Centre for Social Research.

McNally, L.; Oyefeso, A.; Annan, J.; Perryman, K.; Bloor, R.; Freeman, S.; et al. (2006). A survey of staff attitudes to smoking-related policyand intervention in psychiatric and general health care settings. Journal of Public Health, 28(3), 192-196. https:/ /doi. org/10. 1093/pubmed/fdl029.

Metse, A. P.; Wiggers, J.; Wye, P.; Wolfenden, L.; Freund, M.; Clancy, R.; et al. (2017). Efficacy of a universal smoking cessation intervention initiated in inpatient psychiatry and continued post-discharge: arandomised controlled trial. The Australian and New Zealand Journal of Psychiatry, 51(4), 366-381. https:/ /doi. org/10. 1177/0004867417692424.

New South Wales Department of Health. (2002). Guide for the manage-ment of nicotine dependent inpatients. Sydney: State Government of New South Wales.

Prochaska, J. J.; Gill, P.; Hall, S. M. (2004). Treatment of tobaccouse in an inpatient psychiatric setting. Psychiatric Services, 55(11), 1265-1270. https://doi. org/10. 1176/appi. ps. 55. 11. 1265.

Prochaska, J. J.; Hall, S. E.; Delucchi, K.; Hall, S. M. (2014). Efficacy of initiating tobacco dependence treatment in inpatient psychiatry: a randomized controlled trial. American Journal of Public Health, 104(8), 1557-1565. https://doi. org/10. 2105/ajph. 2013. 301403.

Ratschen, E.; Britton, J.; Doody, G.; McNeill, A. (2010). Smoking attitudes, behaviour, and nicotine dependence among mental health acute inpatients: an exploratory study. International Journal of Social Psychiatry, 56(2), 107-118. https:/ /doi. org/10. 1177/0020764008101855.

Ratschen, E.; Britton, J.; McNeill, A. (2008). Smoke-free hospitals - the English experience: results from a survey, interviews and site visits. BMC Health Services Research, 8(1), 41. https://doi. org/10. 1186/1472-6963-8-41.

Ratschen, E.; Britton, J.; McNeill, A. (2009). Implementation of smoke-free policies in mental health in-patient settings in England. The British Journal of Psychiatry, 194(6), 547-551. https://doi. org/ 10. 1192/bjp. bp. 108. 051052.

Rigotti, N.; Clair, C.; Munafò, M.; Stead, L. (2012). Interventions for smoking cessation in hospitalised patients. Cochrane Database of Systematic Reviews. (5), CD001837. https://doi. org/10. 1002/14651858. CD001837. pub3.

Robson, D.; Spaducci, G.; McNeill, A.; Stewart, D.; Craig, T. J. K.; Yates, M. et al. (2017). Effect of implementation of a smoke-free policy on physical violence in a psychiatric inpatient setting: an interrupted time series analysis. Lancet Psychiatry, 4(7), 540-546. https://doi. org/10. 1016/s2215-0366(17)30209-2.

Stockings, E. A.; Bowman, J. A.; Baker, A. L.; Terry, M.; Clancy, R.; Wye, P. M. et al. (2014). Impact of a postdischarge smoking cessation Intervention for smokers admitted to an inpatient psychiatric facility: a randomized controlled trial. Nicotine, Tobacco Research, 16(11), 1417-1428. https://doi. org/10. 1093/ntr/ntu097.

Stockings, E. A.; Bowman, J. A.; Bartlem, K. M.; McElwaine, K. M.; Baker, A. L.; Terry, M. et al. (2015). Implementation of a smoke-free policy in an inpatient psychiatric facility: patient-reported adher-ence, support, andreceiptofnicotine-dependencetreatment. International Journal of Mental Health Nursing, 24(4), 342-349. https://doi. org/10. 1111/inm. 12128.

Stockings, E.; Bowman, J.; McElwaine, K.; Baker, A.; Terry, M.; Clancy, R. et al. (2013). Readiness to quit smoking and quit attempts among Australian mental health inpatients. Nicotine, Tobacco Research, 15(5), 942-949. https://doi. org/10. 1093/ntr/nts206.

Willemsen, M. C.; G€ orts, C. A.; Soelen, P. V.; Jonkers, R.; Hilberink, S. R. (2004). Exposure to environmental tobacco smoke (ETS) and determinants of support for complete smoking bans in psychiatric settings. Tobacco Control, 13, 180-185. https://doi. org/10. 1136/ tc. 2003. 004804.

Williams, J. M.; Steinberg, M. L.; Griffiths, K. G.; Cooperman, N. (2013). Smokers with behavioral health comorbidity should be designated a tobacco use disparity group. American Journal of Public Health, 103(9), 1549-1555. https://doi. org/10. 2105/ajph. 2013. 301232.

Williams, J. M.; Ziedonis, D. (2004). Addressing tobacco among individuals with a mental illness or an addiction. Addictive Behaviors, 29, 1067-

1083. https://doi.org/10.1016/j.addbeh.2004.03.009.

Wye, P.; Bowman, J.; Wiggers, J.; Baker, A.; Carr, V.; Terry, M. et al. (2010). An audit of the prevalence of recorded nicotine dependence treatment in an Australian psychiatric hospital. Australian and New Zealand Journal of Public Health, 34(3), 298-303. https://doi.org/10.1111/j.1753-6405.2010.00530.x.

Wye, P.; Gow, L. B.; Constable, J.; Bowman, J.; Lawn, S.; Wiggers, J. (2014). Observation of the extent of smoking in a mental health inpatient facility with a smoke-free policy. BMCP sychiatry, 14, 94. https://doi.org/10.1186/1471-244x-14-94.

Wye, P. M.; Stockings, E. A.; Bowman, J. A.; Oldmeadow, C.; Wiggers, J. H. (2017). Effectiveness of a clinical practice change intervention in increasing the provision of nicotine dependence treatment in inpatient psychiatric facilities: an implementation trial. BMC Psychiatry, 17, 56. https://doi.org/10.1186/s12888-017-1220-7.

59

口服18-甲氧基冠醚（18-MC）降低大鼠烟碱自给药

Amir H. Rezvani[1], *Stanley D. Glick*[2], *Edward D. Levin*[1]

1. Department of Psychiatry and Behavioral Sciences, Duke University Medical Center, Durham, NC, United States
2. Department of Neuroscience and Experimental Therapeutics, Albany Medical College, Albany, New York, United States

59.1 引言

烟碱成瘾是一个主要的健康问题，在全世界造成了严重的健康和经济后果。仅在美国，每年就有超过43万人死于吸烟，全世界每年报告的与吸烟有关的死亡人数超过300万。据预测，如果这种疾病得不到适当控制，它将成为最大的健康问题，在未来20～30年内带来毁灭性的健康和社会经济后果，每年导致全球800多万人死亡。几种药物，包括烟碱贴片、安非他酮和伐伦克林，已被批准用于治疗烟碱成瘾。但是，与其他成瘾行为类似，烟碱成瘾是一种异质性的复杂障碍；尽管有这些药理学工具，但这些药物的疗效相对较小，并且它们有一些不希望的副作用，导致高复发率。因此，开发更合适的无副作用或副作用更少的药物来覆盖更多的亚群仍然是成瘾领域的一个具有挑战性的目标。此外，可能需要更多样的有效治疗方法，至少部分根据个体的需要和基因组成进行调整。其中一种有前途的治疗剂是18-MC（18-methoxycoronaridine）（图59.1）。

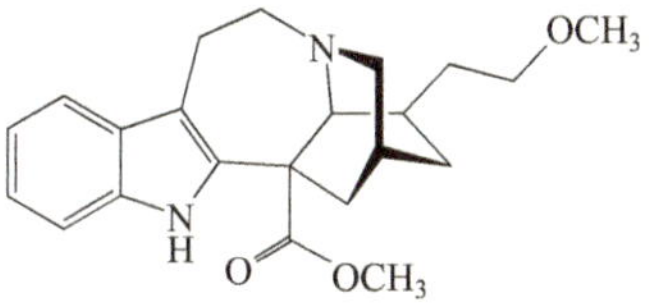

图59.1 18-MC的化学结构

18-MC是一种无毒的合成伊波加生物碱同系物，来源于伊波加因，伊波加因是一种在非洲中西部灌木伊波加（夹竹桃科）根皮中发现的吲哚生物碱（Bandarage et al. 1999）。高剂量的伊波加因本身的粗提取物会引起混乱感，有时还会产生幻觉。伊波加因本身及其主要代谢物降伊波加因通过影响大脑中的多巴胺能和5-羟色胺能系统（Glick et al. 1991），可以有效减少大鼠对烟碱、酒精、吗啡、海洛因和可卡因等成瘾性药物的自给药（Glick et al. 1996; Glick, Maisonneuve, 1998; Glick et al. 1991; Mash et al. 1998; Rezvani et al. 1995; Rezvani et al. 2003; Rezvani et al. 1997）。

伊波加因本身在高剂量下会引起严重的不良副作用（Molinari et al. 1996），这可能会妨碍其使用；因此，设计了一种合成的伊波加因类似物18-MC，它没有毒性，但对药物自给药有相同的抑制作用。

18-MC已被证明可抑制几种成瘾性药物的自给药，包括酒精（Rezvani et al. 1997）、吗啡、可卡因、甲基苯丙胺和烟碱（Glick et al. 1998;Maisonneuve, Glick,1999）。中枢多巴胺能系统已被证明与大多数滥用药物的增强特性有关，因此认为18-MC也通过调节大脑中的多巴胺能系统来发挥其作用。

为了帮助进一步确定18-MC的可能临床用途，重要的是观察它是否也能有效减少口服后的药物自给药管理。最近，进行了一项旨在确定口服18-MC对减少大鼠烟碱自给药的功效的研究。

59.2 方法

使用标准操作箱，首先对大鼠进行为期几天的静脉注射烟碱自给药训练。然后，每隔一周，大鼠通过口服18-MC（10mg/kg、20mg/kg和40mg/kg）或对照组给药，遵循重复测量平衡设计（Levin et al. 2011; Rezvani et al. 2013）。

59.3 结果

结果表明，口服18-MC可显著（$P<0.05$）降低烟碱的自给药。烟碱自给药在剂量范围内呈线性下降趋势，差异显著（$P<0.005$）。如图59.2所示，40mg/kg剂量导致烟碱自给药显著减少（$P<0.05$）。根据基线测试期间烟碱自给药的中值水平对数据进行分析时，发现低反应组大鼠平均每次烟碱注射次数为2.82±0.48，较高反应组大鼠平均每次烟碱注射次数为8.20±0.86，两组之间存在显著差异（$P<0.005$）。有趣的是，高烟碱自给药组和低烟碱自给药组在食物颗粒自给药方面没有显著差异。如图59.3所示，基线表现较低的大鼠在口服18-MC后烟碱自给药显著减少（$P<0.01$），而基线表现较高的大鼠没有表现出18-MC的显著影响。

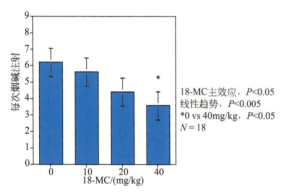

图 59.2 雌性大鼠急性口服18-MC对烟碱自给药的影响（平均值 ±SEM）

数据表示平均值±SEM（Rezvani et al. 2006）。

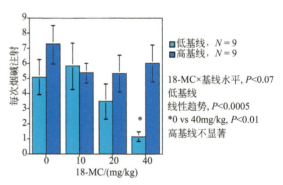

图 59.3 在低基线组（$n=9$）和高基线组（$n=9$）中，急性口服18-MC对烟碱自给药的影响

数据表示平均值±SEM（Rezvani et al. 2016）。

59.4 讨论

18-MC的全身用药已被证明能减少包括烟碱在内的几种成瘾性药物的自给药。关于18-MC的开发及其可能的临床应用，证明其口服疗效非常重要。先前的研究表明，口服18-MC可以减少大鼠的吗啡（Maisonneuve, Glick,1999）、可卡因（Glick et al. 1996）、甲基苯丙胺（Glick et al. 2000）和酒精（Rezvani et al. 1997）的自给药。目前的研究是第一个评估口服18-MC对大鼠烟碱自给药的功效的研究。

目前的研究结果表明，口服18-MC也可以显著减少静脉注射（IV）烟碱的自给药。这些发现重复和扩展了早期的发现，即急性全身注射18-MC显著减少了大鼠静脉注射烟碱的自给药（Glick et al. 2000）。有趣的是，这些发现表明，与基线表现较高的大鼠相比，口服18-MC对基线表现较低的大鼠更有效。高剂量18-MC（40mg/kg）对烟碱自给药有明显的抑制作用，而基线表现较高的大鼠没有表现出18-MC的显著影响。值得一提的是，高烟碱自给药组和低烟碱自给药组在食物颗粒自给药上没有显著差异，且颗粒自给药次数与烟碱输入量不相关，说明烟碱自给药不依赖于食物强化。

口服18-MC治疗在基线表现较低的大鼠中更有效，但在基线表现较高的大鼠中则不是，这一事实可能是由于以下几个原因。高表现者的烟碱自给药的亲和力更高，这可能为治疗提供了更困难的目标，需要比这项研究测试的更高的剂量。另一种情况是，烟碱自给药水平较高的大鼠的神经行为底物与低反应者有足够的不同，从而消除了18-MC的治疗效果。这可能是由于自给药更多烟碱的大鼠之间先前存在的差异，或者是自给药更多烟碱所产生的持久影响或这两者的结合。这些数据强化了我们的发现，即18-MC在减少烟碱自给药方面非常有效，尤其是对较少使用烟碱的人。

大多数滥用药物的增强特性部分与它们与中脑边缘多巴胺能系统的相互作用有关（Koob et al. 1994）。烟碱诱导的大鼠伏隔核中的多巴胺释放已经被一些研究者发现（Di Chiara, Imperato, 1988; Grenhoff et al. 1986; Imperato et al. 1986; Tizabi et al. 2002）。有趣的是，18-MC给药已被证明可以减少烟碱诱导的大鼠伏隔核中多巴胺的释放（Glick et al. 1998）。因此，我们认为18-MC对包括烟碱在内的成瘾药物的增强作用是通过减弱它们对中脑边缘多巴胺能系统的作用，从而降低它们的奖励效应，从而导致摄入量的减少而起作用的。

我们之前证明了大脑中的烟碱受体在烟碱和酒精增强效应中起着重要作用（Levin et al. 2010; Rezvani et al. 2010）。事实上，已经证明烟碱型α3β4受体被18-MC阻断（Glick et al. 2002）。因此，正如先前的研究证明的那样，18-MC可能通过阻断内侧缰核的这些受体来发挥作用（Glick et al. 2008; Glick et al. 2011; Taraschenko et al. 2008）。

另一个可能的机制是18-MC与脑内内源性阿片系统的相互作用。据报道，伊波加因同系物对阿片受体有亲和力。已经证明伊波加因与κ-阿片受体相互作用（Deecher et al. 1992）。因此，与伊波加因类似，其类似物18-MC有可能通过改变内源性阿片系统发挥抑制作用。还应考虑其他机制。其中包括18-MC与N-甲基-D-天冬氨酸（NMDA）受体偶联阳离子通道的相互作用（Popik et al. 1994），以及与GABA能系统的相互作用，这些都与药物成瘾有关。

59.5 结论

综上所述，这些发现表明，急性口服18-MC可以显著减少大鼠的烟碱自给药，特别是在基线烟碱摄入量较低的动物中。虽然其确切的作用机制尚不完全清楚，但它可能通过抑制或降低中脑边缘系统的多巴胺能活性和/或与其他与烟碱成瘾有关的神经系统相互作用而降低其增强作用，从而对烟碱的摄取产生抑制作用。

术语解释
- 18-MC：18-甲氧基冠醚。
- IV：静脉注射。
- 伏隔核：伏隔核是基底前脑中的一个区域，与下丘脑的视前区相对。伏隔核是奖励系统的重要组成部分。
- 操作箱：操作调节室，也被称为斯金纳箱（Skinner box），是一种封闭的装置，包含两个杠杆，动物可以按下活动杠杆，以获得食物、水或进入静脉的特定药物。
- 腹侧被盖区：腹侧被盖区（VTA）是一群位于中脑底中线附近的多巴胺能神经元。它与大脑的自然奖励回路有关。VTA中的神经元投射到大脑的许多区域，包括伏隔核和前额叶皮层。刺激VTA会导致这些结构中的多巴胺释放。

关键事实
- 急性口服18-MC可显著减少大鼠烟碱自给药。
- 18-MC对烟碱摄入量较低的大鼠更有效。
- 18-MC通过减弱烟碱引起的伏隔核多巴胺释放发挥作用。

要点总结
- 口服18-MC可显著减少大鼠烟碱自给药。
- 口服18-MC对烟碱摄入量较低的动物更有效。
- 烟碱摄入量与食物强化无关。
- 提示18-MC通过减弱烟碱诱导的中脑边缘系统多巴胺释放而影响烟碱自给药。
- 随着更全面的研究，应该考虑开发18-MC作为一种可能的对抗吸烟成瘾的新疗法。

参考文献

Bandarage, U. K.; Kuehne, M. E.; Glick, S. D. (1999). Total syntheses of racemic albifloranine and its anti-addictive congeners, including 18-methoxycoronaridine. Tetrahedron, 55, 9405-9424.

Deecher, D. C.; Teitler, M.; Soderlund, D. M.; Bornmann, W. G.; Kuehne, M. E.; Glick, S. D. (1992). Mechanisms of action of ibogaine and harmaline congeners based on radioligand binding studies. Brain Research, 571(2), 242-247.

Di Chiara, G.; Imperato, A. (1988). Drugs abused by humans preferentially increase synaptic dopamine concentrations in the mesolimbic system of freely moving rats. Proceedings of the National Academy of Sciences of the United States of America, 85, 5274-5278.

Glick, S. D.; Kuehne, M. E.; Maisonneuve, I. M.; Bandarage, U. K.; Molinari, H. H. (1996). 18-Methoxycoronaridine, a non-toxic iboga alkaloid congener: effects on morphine and cocaine self-administration and on mesolimbic dopamine release in rats. Brain Research, 719(1-2), 29-35.

Glick, S. D.; Maisonneuve, I. M. (1998). Mechanisms of antiaddictive actions of ibogaine. Annals of the New York Academy of Sciences, 844, 214-226.

Glick, S. D.; Maisonneuve, I. M.; Dickinson, H. A. (2000). 18-MC reduce methamphetamine and nicotine self-administration in rats. NeuroReport, 11, 2013-2015.

Glick, S. D.; Maisonneuve, I. M.; Kitchen, B. A. (2002). Modulation of nicotine self-administration in rats by combination therapy with agents blocking alpha3beta4 nicotinic receptors. European Journal of Pharmacology, 448(2-3), 185-191.

Glick, S. D.; Maisonneuve, I. M.; Visker, K. E.; Fritz, K. A.; Bandarage, U. K.; Kuehne, M. E. (1998). 18-Methoxycoronardine attenuates nicotine-induced dopamine release and nicotine preferences in rats. Psychopharmacology, 139, 274-280.

Glick, S. D.; Rossman, K.; Steindorf, S.; Maisonneuve, I. M.; Carlson, J. N. (1991). Effects and aftereffects of ibogaine on morphine self-administration in rats. European Journal of Pharmacology, 195(3), 341-345.

Glick, S. D.; Sell, E. M.; Maisonneuve, I. M. (2008). Brain regions mediating alpha3beta4 nicotinic antagonist effects of 18-MC on methamphetamine and sucrose self-administration. European Journal of Pharmacology, 599(1-3), 91-95.

Glick, S. D.; Sell, E. M.; McCallum, S. E.; Maisonneuve, I. M. (2011). Brain regions mediating α3β4 nicotinic antagonist effects of 18-MC on nicotine self-administration. European Journal of Pharmacology, 669(1-3), 71-75.

Grenhoff, J.; Aston-Jones, G.; Svensson, T. H. (1986). Nicotinic effects on the firing pattern of midbrain dopamine neurons. Acta Physiologica Scandinavica, 128, 151-158.

Imperato, A.; Mulas, A.; Di Chiara, G. (1986). Nicotine preferentially stimulates dopamine release in the limbic system of freely moving rats. European Journal of Pharmacology, 132, 337-338.

Koob, G. F.; Rassnick, S.; Heinrichs, S.; Weiss, F. (1994). Alcohol, the reward system and dependence. EXS, 71, 103-114.

Levin, E. D.; Rezvani, A. H.; Xiao, Y.; Slade, S.; Cauley, M.; Wells, C. et al. (2010). Sazetidine-A, a selective alpha4beta2 nicotinic receptor desensitizing agent and partial agonist, reduces nicotine self-administration in rats. The Journal of Pharmacology and Experimental Therapeutics, 332(3), 933-939.

Levin, E. D.; Slade, S.; Wells, C.; Petro, A.; Rose, J. E. (2011). D-Cycloserine selectively decreases nicotine self-administration in rats with low baseline levels of response. Pharmacology, Biochemistry, and Behavior, 98, 210-214.

Maisonneuve, I. M.; Glick, S. D. (1999). Attenuation of the reinforcing efficacy of morphine by 18-methoxycoronaridine. European Journal of Pharmacology, 383, 15-21.

Mash, D. C.; Kovera, C. A.; Buck, B. E.; Norenberg, M. D.; Shapshak, P.; Hearn, W. L. et al. (1998). Medication development of ibogaine as a pharmacotherapy for drug dependence. Annals of the New York Academy of Sciences, 844, 274-292 [Review].

Molinari, H. H.; Maisonneuve, I. M.; Glick, S. D. (1996). Ibogaine neurotoxicity: a re-evaluation. Brain Research, 737, 255-262.

Popik, P.; Layer, R. T.; Skolnick, P. (1994). The putative anti-addictive drug ibogaine is a competitive inhibitor of [^{3}H]MK-801 binding to the NMDA receptor complex. Psychopharmacology (Berl), 114(4), 672-674.

Rezvani, A. H.; Cauley, M. C.; Slade, S.; Glick, S.; Rose, J. E.; Levin, E. D. (2016). Acute oral 18-methoxycoronaridine (18-MC) decreases both alcohol intake and IV nicotine self-administration in rats. Pharmacology, Biochemistry, and Behavior, 150-151, 153-157.

Rezvani, A. H.; Overstreet, D. H.; Lee, Y. W. (1995). Attenuation of alcohol intake by ibogaine in three strains of alcohol-preferring rats. Pharmacology, Biochemistry, and Behavior, 52(3), 615-620.

Rezvani, A. H.; Overstreet, D. H.; Perfumi, M.; Massi, M. (2003). Plant derivatives in the treatment of alcohol dependency. Pharmacology, Biochemistry, and Behavior, 75(3), 593-606 [Review].

Rezvani, A. H.; Overstreet, D. H.; Yang, Y.; Maisonneuve, I. M.; Bandarage, U. K.; Kuehne, M. E. et al. (1997). Attenuation of alcohol consumption by a novel nontoxic ibogaine analogue (18-methoxycoronaridine) in alcohol-preferring rats. Pharmacology, Bio-chemistry, and Behavior, 58(2), 615-619.

Rezvani, A. H.; Sexton, H. G.; Johnson, J.; Wells, C.; Gordon, K.; Levin, E. D. (2013). Effects of caffeine on alcohol consumption and nicotine self-administration in rats. Alcoholism: Clinical and Experimental Research, 37, 1609-1617.

Rezvani, A. H.; Slade, S.; Wells, C.; Petro, A.; Lumeng, L.; Li, T. K. et al. (2010). Effects of Sazetidine-A, a selective alpha4beta2 nicotinic acetylcholine receptor desensitizing agent on alcohol and nicotine self-administration in selectively bred alcohol-preferring (P) rats. Psychopharmacology, 211, 161-174.

Taraschenko, O. D.; Rubbinaccio, H. Y.; Maisonneuve, I. M.; Glick, S. D. (2008). 18-Methoxycoronaridine: a potential new treatment for obesity in rats? Psychopharmacology, 201, 339-350.

Tizabi, Y.; Copeland, R. J.; Louis, V. A.; Taylor, R. E. (2002). Effects of combined systemic alcohol and central nicotine administration into ventral tegmental area on dopamine release in the nucleus accumbens. Alcoholism: Clinical and Experimental Research, 26, 394-399.

60
药物遗传学与戒烟

Taraneh Taghavi[1], *Rachel F. Tyndale*[2,3]

1. Departments of Pharmacology and Toxicology, and Psychiatry, University of Toronto, Toronto, ON, Canada
2. Campbell Family Mental Health Research Institute and Addictions Division, Centre for Addiction and Mental Health, Toronto, ON, Canada
3. Department of Psychiatry, Campbell Family Mental Health Research Institute and Addictions Division, University of Toronto, Centre for Addiction and Mental Health, Toronto, ON, Canada

缩略语

AGES	加性遗传效率得分	DRD_4	多巴胺 D_4 受体
COMT	儿茶酚-*O*-甲基转移酶	nAChR	烟碱乙酰胆碱受体
CYP2A6	细胞色素 P450 2A6	NMR	烟碱代谢物比率
CYP2B6	细胞色素 P450 2B6	OCT2	有机阳离子转运体2
CYP2C19	细胞色素 P450 2C19	UTR	非翻译区
DAT	多巴胺转运体	VTNR	可变数目串联重复序列
DRD_2	多巴胺 D_2 受体		

60.1 引言

尽管有三种药物疗法可用,即烟碱替代疗法、安非他酮疗法和伐伦克林疗法,但吸烟仍然存在。50%~60%的戒烟能力是可遗传的(Broms et al. 2006)。影响戒烟结果的遗传因素包括烟碱药理和戒烟药物。在没有和存在药物治疗的情况下,已经研究了单基因和多基因对戒烟的影响,本章简要总结了它们的结果(表60.1)。

表60.1 戒烟相关基因概述

基因型	基因名	类别	底物/配体
CYP2A6	细胞色素 P450,ⅡA 亚家族,多肽6	代谢型	NIC/NRT
CYP2B6	细胞色素 P450,ⅡB 亚家族,多肽6	代谢型	NIC/NRT,BUP
CHRNA5	胆碱能受体,神经元烟碱,α多肽5	靶向型	NIC/NRT,BUP,Var
DRD_2	多巴胺 D_2 受体	靶向型	神经传导物质
COMT	儿茶酚-*O*-甲基转移酶	代谢型	神经传导物质
DRD_4	多巴胺 D_4 受体	靶向型	神经传导物质
SLC6A3 (DAT)	溶质载体家族6(多巴胺转运体),成员3	转运型	神经传导物质

注:BUP,安非他酮;NIC,烟碱;NRT,烟碱替代疗法;Var,伐伦克林。

60.2 利用药物代谢酶遗传学戒烟

60.2.1 烟碱代谢物比率

烟碱从体内清除的速度会影响戒烟的能力。从卷烟烟雾中吸入的烟碱中,约有80%主要由肝酶CYP2A6代谢失活为可替宁（约90%）（Nakajima et al. 1996a, 1996b），CYP2B6的贡献很小（Al Koudsi, Tyndale, 2010）。然后可替宁进一步代谢为3'-羟基可替宁，反应完全由CYP2A6介导（Nakajima et al. 1996a,1996b）（图60.1）。这两种代谢物（3'-羟基可替宁和可替宁）的比率被称为烟碱代谢物比率（NMR），是日常吸烟者中CYP2A6活性的表型生物标志物，因此更快的CYP2A6被反映为更高的NMR（Dempsey et al. 2004）。

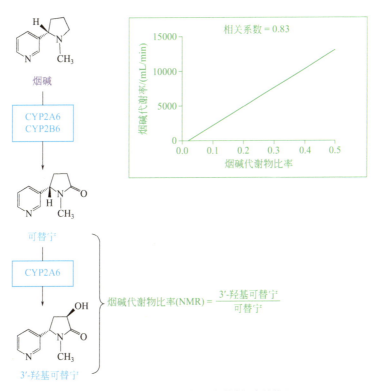

图60.1 CYP2A6在烟碱代谢途径中的作用

该图改编自Dempsey等（2004）。

60.2.2 CYP2A6与戒烟

*CYP2A6*基因具有高度多态性，有许多变异改变了CYP2A6的活性。个体可以根据其*CYP2A6*基因型对烟碱清除的预测影响，对这些变异进行基因分型，并将其分组为CYP2A6活性组（如快代谢者和慢代谢者）（Benowitz et al. 2006）。同样，基于烟碱代谢物比率，吸烟者可以分为快代谢者和慢代谢者。目前还没有单一的最佳NMR切点用来区分CYP2A6慢代谢者和快代谢者以优化戒烟；慢代谢者通常代表NMR分布的最低水平（25%～40%）（Lerman et al. 2010; Lerman et al. 2015; Lerman et al. 2006; Schnoll et al. 2009; Schnoll et al. 2013）。由*CYP2A6*基因型或NMR确定的慢烟碱代谢者具有较低的卷烟消耗量（Schoedel et al. 2004）、烟碱依赖性（Wassenaar et al. 2011）以及对吸烟线索的大脑反应（Falcone et al. 2016）。

NMR的变化与积极药物治疗的戒烟效果有关。在随机接受烟碱贴片的吸烟者中，慢烟碱代谢者（即NMR最低的1/4的人）的戒烟率高于快代谢者（Lerman et al. 2006; Schnoll et al. 2009）。比较标准烟碱贴片治疗（8周）和延长烟碱贴片治疗（6个月），基因型（基于*CYP2A6*基因型）

和表型（基于NMR）的慢烟碱代谢者在延长烟碱贴片治疗中的戒烟率高于标准烟碱贴片治疗。相比之下，快烟碱代谢者并没有从延长治疗中受益（Lerman et al. 2010）。在另一项关于快烟碱代谢者的小型试验（基于NMR）中，有一种趋势是剂量越大戒烟率越高（42mg和21mg烟碱贴片）（Schnoll et al. 2013）。因此，烟碱替代疗法对于慢烟碱代谢者比快烟碱代谢者更有效；在快速代谢者中，高剂量可能比低剂量更有效。

基于NMR随机接受治疗的吸烟者中，在快代谢者中伐伦克林比烟碱贴片更有效。在慢代谢者中，戒烟没有因治疗而有所不同（Lerman et al. 2015）[图60.2（a）]。在慢代谢者中，贴片和伐伦克林需要治疗的数量（NNT）分别为10和8。在快代谢者中，贴片和伐伦克林的NNT分别为26和5，进一步表明与安慰剂相比，使用烟碱贴片治疗的快烟碱代谢者的戒烟率更低 [图60.2（b）]。此外，与快代谢者相比，在慢代谢者中，伐伦克林与更严重的副作用有关。相比之下，两组人对烟碱贴片的耐受性都很好。这些发现表明，伐伦克林更适合用于快代谢者，而贴片更适合用于慢代谢者。

在没有药物治疗的情况下，NMR的变化也与戒烟结果有关。NMR显示，与快烟碱代谢者相比，慢烟碱代谢者在没有药物治疗的情况下（即在临床试验的安慰剂组）有更高的戒烟率（Patterson et al. 2008）。同样，在随机服用安慰剂的吸烟者中，通过替代CYP2A6活性测量（而不是NMR）测得的慢烟碱代谢者与快代谢者相比，复发风险更低（Chen et al. 2014）。

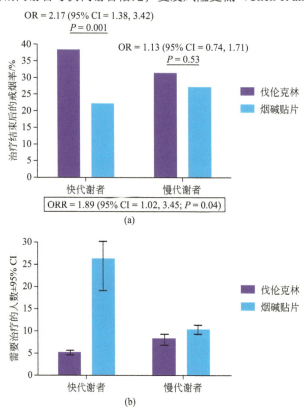

图60.2　烟碱代谢物比率（NMR）影响烟碱贴片与伐伦克林的戒烟效果

治疗结束时的戒烟率与NMR有显著的相互作用：在（a）中，OR（ORR）＝1.89（95% CI（置信区间）＝1.02, 3.45；$P=0.04$）；在（b）中，烟碱贴片和伐伦克林需要治疗的人数在慢代谢者中分别为10和8，在快代谢者中分别为26和5。该图改编自Lerman等（2015）。

60.2.3 CYP2B6 与戒烟

和CYP2A6一样，CYP2B6也是高度多态的。一种常见的CYP2B6单倍型CYP2B6*6，包括CYP2B6*4和CYP2B6*9变异体，与肝脏较低的CYP2B*6蛋白表达有关（Al Koudsi, Tyndale, 2010）。CYP2B6代谢烟碱，尽管其代谢程度比CYP2A6小（约10%与约90%）。在随机接受烟碱贴片的吸烟者中，由 *CYP2B6*6* 基因型决定的CYP2B6代谢物状态不会改变戒烟率（Lee et al. 2007a, 2007b），这与CYP2B6酶对烟碱代谢的微小贡献一致，这表明CYP2B6基因可能不是优化烟碱替代疗法辅助戒烟的理想候选者。

CYP2B6还将安非他酮代谢为羟基安非他酮（Hesse et al. 2000; Zanger et al. 2007; Zhu et al. 2012）。与安非他酮相比，羟基安非他酮在体外对nAChR的抑制作用更强（Damaj et al. 2004; Damaj et al. 2010），并且其游离血浆浓度比安非他酮高10倍（Hsyu et al. 1997; Johnston et al. 2002）。CYP2B6活性的可变性改变了羟基安非他酮的水平，这可能会影响安非他酮辅助戒烟的结果。

在接受安非他酮治疗的非裔美国吸烟者中，Zhu等研究表明CYP2B6慢性代谢者（包括那些具有CYP2B6*6单倍型的代谢者）与正常代谢者相比，羟基安非他酮水平较低，且较低的羟基安非他酮水平与较差的安非他酮辅助戒烟相关（Zhu et al. 2012）。然而，无论是高加索吸烟者（Lee et al. 2007a, 2007bb）还是非裔美国吸烟者（Zhu et al. 2012），CYP2B6*6基因型并不直接改变他们对安非他酮的反应。*CYP2B6* 基因型与戒烟结果之间缺乏直接联系可能归因于较低的效率或不完全的基因型，这表明在一项充分考虑遗传效应的较大研究中，CYP2B6缓慢基因型可能与较低的安非他酮辅助戒烟有关。

临床试验中对 *CYP2B6* 基因在安慰剂方面的潜在影响的研究发现，具有CYP2B6*6单倍型（相对于野生型）的吸烟者复吸安慰剂的可能性更高（Lee et al. 2007a, 2007b; Lerman et al. 2002），这表明与CYP2B6正常代谢者相比，CYP2B6慢代谢者戒烟的可能性较小。

60.3 利用中枢神经系统的目标基因进行戒烟

中枢神经系统奖励回路中烟碱靶点的遗传变异，包括烟碱乙酰胆碱受体和多巴胺能通路的成分（即多巴胺受体和转运体），可能有助于戒烟治疗的优化。

60.3.1 nAChR和戒烟

尽管含α4β2的nAChR是烟碱和戒烟药物的靶点，但α4β2亚基的变异与吸烟或戒烟结果无关。含α4β2的nAChR显示出高度的进化保守性，几乎没有变异（Albuquerque et al. 2009），这可能解释了缺乏相关报道的原因。

然而，已经广泛研究了位于染色体15q25上的CHRNA5-CHRNA3-CHRNB4簇的变异与戒烟成功的关系。*CHRNA5* rs16969968 A 等位基因与较高的卷烟消费量有关（Munafo et al. 2012），并会导致烟碱对nAChR反应的最大值降低（Bierut et al. 2008）。然而，最近对接受烟碱替代治疗的高加索吸烟者进行的荟萃分析显示，rs16969968与戒烟率之间没有关联（Leung et al. 2015）（图60.3）。同样，在接受伐伦克林治疗的吸烟者中，*CHRNA5* rs16969968与戒烟结果无关（Chen et al. 2015）。在高加索吸烟者中，未观察到rs16969968、rs588765和rs578776（CHRNA 5-CHRNA 3 CHRNB 4簇中的另外两个SNPs标记位点，以前与吸烟有关）与烟碱贴片或伐伦克林的戒烟结果相关（Tyndale et al. 2015）。同样，在非裔美国吸烟者中，rs16969968和rs578776均与烟碱口香糖或安非他酮治疗的戒烟结果无关（Zhu et al. 2014a, 2014b）。

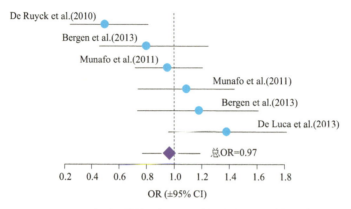

图60.3 rs16969968烟碱受体基因变异不影响烟碱替代疗法（NRT）的戒烟结果

该图改编自Leung等（2015）。

在对24项针对非吸烟高加索人的研究进行的荟萃分析中，*CHRNA5* rs16969968 AA风险基因型的吸烟者与GG吸烟者相比，戒烟的平均时间为4年（Chen, Hung et al. 2015），这表明CHRNA5活性降低会降低自发戒烟。同样，*CHRNA5* rs16969968高危基因型的吸烟者在接受安慰剂治疗时戒烟的可能性也较小（Chen et al. 2012）。然而，rs16969968对安慰剂戒烟的效果并不一致。最近的两项试验发现，在接受安慰剂治疗的高加索或非裔美国吸烟者中，CHRNA5 rs16969968与戒烟无关（Tyndale et al. 2015; Zhu et al. 2014a, 2014b）。总之，尽管有强有力的证据表明nAChR基因变异与重度吸烟和烟碱依赖有关，但缺乏nAChR基因变异和戒烟结果的重复发现，降低了该区域在优化戒烟治疗中有用的可能性。

60.3.2 多巴胺能途径和戒烟

导致多巴胺能活性降低的功能多态性被认为有助于降低戒烟成功率，并已被调查为戒烟率可变性的潜在来源（David et al. 2008）。

60.3.2.1 DRD_2

与戒烟有关的多巴胺D_2受体（DRD_2）中研究最广泛的遗传变异是Taq1A多态性（Neville et al. 2004）。Taq1A变异体可能改变DRD2基因的功能，A1等位基因与较低的纹状体D_2受体密度有关（Blum et al. 1990; Jonsson et al. 1999）。

在随机接受烟碱贴片治疗的吸烟者中，与A2/A2基因型相比，DRD_2 A1/A1或A1/A2基因型与较高的戒烟率相关（Johnstone et al. 2004）。与烟碱贴片的发现相反，在随机接受安非他酮治疗的吸烟者中，与A2/A2基因型相比，DRD_2 A1/A1或A1/A2基因型与较低的戒烟率相关（David et al. 2007）。值得注意的是，在DRD_2 A2/A2基因型的患者中，安非他酮的较高戒烟率仅限于*CYP2B6* rs3211371 TT或CT基因型的患者（David et al. 2007），这突出了评估多基因和基因-基因相互作用以确定更有可能从某种治疗中受益的吸烟者亚组的潜在重要性。同样，Lerman和他的同事报告，一种遗传变异体（DRD2-141Cdel）导致DRD_2基因（类似于Taq1A A1等位基因）的低表达与更高的烟碱替代疗法疗效相关，而高活性变体（-141Cins）与更高的安非他酮疗效相关（Lerman et al. 2006）。因此出现了一种模式，即与D_2受体密度降低相关的基因型预测烟碱替代治疗的更好结果，而与正常受体表达或功能相关的基因型预测对安非他酮的更好反应。总之，这些数据表明，对安非他酮可能没有反应的个体，部分是因为他们的DRD_2 Taq1A基因型，可能从烟碱替代疗法的使用中获得更高的疗效。

60.3.2.2　COMT

儿茶酚-O-甲基转移酶（COMT）是一种参与多巴胺代谢失活的酶，这表明COMT基因是戒烟药物遗传学研究的合理候选基因。COMT rs4680将Val高活性等位基因转化为Met低活性等位基因，导致脑酶水平和活性降低（Chen et al. 2004; Shield et al. 2004）。在随机接受烟碱替代疗法的女性中，Met等位基因与较高的戒烟率相关（Colilla et al. 2005）。Johnstone及其同事的第二项研究发现，与Met/Val或Val/Val组相比，COMT Met/Met基因型组使用烟碱替代疗法的戒烟率更高（Johnstone et al. 2007）。类似地，在随机接受安非他酮治疗的吸烟者中，两个单核苷酸多态性的COMT单倍型（包括Val/Met）与安非他酮辅助戒烟相关，尽管在男性和女性之间没有观察到这种相关性的差异（Breitling et al. 2009）。因此，COMT变异可能有助于优化烟碱替代疗法和安非他酮辅助戒烟。可能需要特别注意性别对COMT优化戒烟结果的潜在调节作用。

60.3.2.3　DRD4

与戒烟有关的多巴胺D_4受体（DRD_4）中研究最广泛的遗传变异是位于基因外显子3的可变数目串联重复序列（VNTR）多态性。大多数研究集中在VNTR的7重复（长）等位基因的存在或缺失的影响上，与6重复或更少的（短）等位基因相比，该等位基因与体外配体结合和基因表达减少有关（Van Tol et al. 1992）。与安慰剂相比，长等位基因与烟碱替代疗法的总体较低的戒烟率相关（David et al. 2008）。相比之下，相对于安慰剂，长等位基因与安非他酮的总体戒断无关（Leventhal et al. 2012）。然而，在具有长等位基因的吸烟者中，观察到基因型与治疗的相互作用，安非他酮相对于安慰剂加强戒烟；具有两个短等位基因拷贝的吸烟者没有从安非他酮中获益（Leventhal et al. 2012）。因此，安非他酮可能是更适合长等位基因吸烟者的治疗方法。考虑到安非他酮减少了线索诱发的渴望（Brody et al. 2004），它可能会缓冲那些长等位基因和D_4密度或活性较低的人在线索暴露后复发。

60.3.2.4　DAT

在编码多巴胺转运体（DAT）的基因SLC6A3中，与戒烟相关的研究最广泛的遗传变异是位于该基因的3'-非翻译区（3'-UTR）的VNTR多态性，主要关注VNTR 9-重复等位基因的效果。9-重复和10-重复等位基因与神经元表面多巴胺转运体的增加有关（Heinz, Goldman, 2000）。在最近对随机接受安非他酮或安慰剂治疗的高加索吸烟者的八项研究的荟萃分析中，9-重复等位基因与总体戒断无关（Duck, Gyoon, 2016）。因此，DAT代表了一个生物学上有希望的基因的例子，该基因可能无助于戒烟治疗的优化（图60.4）。

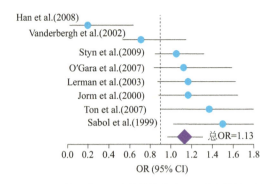

图 60.4　SLC6A3 基因（DAT）的遗传变异不影响安非他酮的戒烟效果

该图改编自 Duck 和 Gyoon（2016）。

60.4　使用多重遗传预测因子戒烟

60.4.1　CYP2A6 和 nAChR 综合遗传风险评分

在高加索吸烟者中，Chen 和他的同事根据 CYP2A6 和 CHRNA5 基因型得出的遗传风险评分（Chen et al. 2014）表明，根据风险评分，烟碱替代疗法（而非安非他酮）的戒烟结果有所不同。在最高风险组（即 CYP2A6 快速代谢加 CHRNA5 高风险 rs16969968-rs680244 基因型组合）中，烟碱替代疗法与安慰剂相比具有最大的治疗效果，而最低风险组（即 CYP2A6 慢速代谢加 CHRNA5 低风险 rs16969968-rs680244 基因型组合）的个体未从烟碱替代疗法中获益。然而，这些发现在几个方面受到了限制。当分析多个遗传标记和处理条件时，某些条件下的样本量非常小。因此，检查多基因（如多种基因变异）对戒烟结果影响的研究，包括本研究，通常力度不够，因此应谨慎解释。

60.4.2　加性遗传效率得分

在白种人吸烟者中，David 和他的同事基于假设的促进安非他酮和安慰剂戒烟的等位基因数量，计算了一个加性遗传效率得分（AGES）（David et al. 2013）。如前所述，根据与戒烟的关系选择的四个变量包括 DRD2 Taq1A、COMT rs4680、DRD4 外显子 3 VNTR 和 SLC6A3 3′ VNTR。在随机接受安非他酮治疗的吸烟者中，AGES 与首次复发或戒断的时间无关（图 60.5）；然而，在

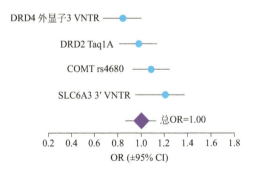

图 60.5　加性遗传效率得分（AGES）不影响安非他酮的戒烟结果

该图改编自 David 等（2013）。

随机接受安慰剂治疗的吸烟者中，较高的年龄与增加的复发风险相关。目前的遗传风险评分模型需要进一步完善，才能用于优化戒烟治疗。未来的改进可以在相关的生物途径中引入额外的基因和变异体，排除不起作用的基因和/或变异体，并确定加性与显性模型是否最适合每个基因座。

术语解释

- 安非他酮：安非他酮（商品名为Wellbutrin和Zyban）是一种去甲肾上腺素-多巴胺再摄取抑制剂和烟碱乙酰胆碱受体拮抗剂，用作抗抑郁剂和戒烟助剂。
- 烟碱代谢物比率：烟碱的两种主要代谢物，即3′-羟基可替宁和可替宁的比率；在经常吸烟的人中，它被用作衡量CYP2A6活性和烟碱代谢率的指标。
- 需要治疗的数量（NNT）：与临床试验中的对照组相比，为了让一个人从药物治疗中获得成效（如成功戒烟）而需要接受治疗的患者数量。
- 遗传药理学：研究病人的基因特征如何改变他们对药物的反应，包括副作用的研究。
- 多基因影响：多个基因位点变异的相加效应，这里用来检查对治疗药物的反应或副作用的发展。
- 伐伦克林：伐伦克林（商标名是Chantix和Champix）是烟碱乙酰胆碱受体的部分激动剂，用于戒烟。

药物遗传学的关键事实

- 药物代谢的快慢以及患者对药物的反应在一定程度上取决于他们的基因。
- 人类共有约99.5%的基因组，但个体之间0.5%的差异会影响他们对药物的反应和对副作用的敏感性。
- 了解遗传变异如何影响对药物的反应可能有助于更准确地确定哪种药物和哪种剂量最适合单个患者。
- 人类基因组中常见的两种变异包括单核苷酸多态性（SNPs）和结构变异。
- 单核苷酸多态性指的是单核苷酸碱基（A、C、T、G）的变化。
- 结构变异是指较大片段的DNA的变化，包括那些可以改变染色体结构的变化。例如包括拷贝数变化以及碱基对删除、插入和复制。

要点总结

- 根据CYP2A6基因型或表型（NMR），烟碱缓慢代谢者（相对于快速代谢者）在烟碱替代透皮贴剂和缺乏药物治疗的情况下戒烟率较高。
- NMR显示，烟碱快速代谢者（相对于缓慢代谢者）在伐伦克林上的戒烟率高于烟碱贴片；烟碱缓慢代谢者（相对于快速代谢者）对伐伦克林的副作用更大。
- 根据CYP2B6基因型，CYP2B6缓慢代谢者（相对于快速代谢者）在安非他酮和没有治疗的情况下戒烟率较低。
- 烟碱中枢神经系统靶点（如烟碱乙酰胆碱受体和多巴胺受体及转运体）的遗传变异与戒烟有关，尽管这并不一致。
- 需要考虑多基因影响和基因-基因相互作用，以便在有或没有药物治疗的情况下更准确地阐明基因对戒烟结果的影响。

参考文献

Al Koudsi, N.; Tyndale, R. F. (2010). Hepatic CYP2B6 is altered by genetic, physiologic, and environmental factors but plays little role in nicotine metabolism. Xenobiotica, 40(6), 381-392.

Albuquerque, E. X.; Pereira, E. F. et al. (2009). Mammalian nicotinic acetylcholine receptors: from structure to function. Physiological Reviews, 89(1), 73-120.

Benowitz, N. L.; Swan, G. E. et al. (2006). CYP2A6 genotype and the metabolism and disposition kinetics of nicotine. Clinical Pharmacology, Therapeutics, 80(5), 457-467.

Bergen, A. W. et al. (2013). Nicotinic acetylcholine receptor variation and response to smoking cessation therapies. Pharmacogenetics and Genomics, 23(2), 94-103.

Bierut, L. J.; Stitzel, J. A. et al. (2008). Variants in nicotinic receptors and risk for nicotine dependence. The American Journal of Psychiatry, 165(9), 1163-1171.

Blum, K.; Noble, E. P. et al. (1990). Allelic association of human dopamine D2 receptor gene in alcoholism. JAMA, 263(15), 2055-2060.

Breitling, L. P.; Dahmen, N. et al. (2009). Variants in COMT and spontaneous smoking cessation: retrospective cohort analysis of 925 cessation events. Pharmacogenetics and Genomics, 19(8), 657-659.

Brody, A. L.; Mandelkern, M. A. et al. (2004). Attenuation of cueinduced cigarette craving and anterior cingulate cortex activation in bupropion-treated smokers: a preliminary study. Psychiatry Research, 130(3), 269-281.

Broms, U.; Silventoinen, K. et al. (2006). Genetic architecture of smoking behavior: a study of Finnish adult twins. Twin Research and Human Genetics, 9(1), 64-72.

Chen, L. S.; Baker, T. B. et al. (2012). Interplay of genetic risk factors(CHRNA5-CHRNA3-CHRNB4) and cessation treatments in smoking cessation success. The American Journal of Psychiatry, 169(7), 735-742.

Chen, L. S.; Baker, T. B. et al. (2015). Genetic variation (CHRNA5), medication (combination nicotine replacement therapy vs. Varenicline), and smoking cessation. Drug and Alcohol Dependence, 154, 278-282.

Chen, L. S.; Bloom, A. J. et al. (2014). Pharmacotherapy effects on smoking cessation vary with nicotine metabolism gene (CYP2A6). Addiction, 109(1), 128-137.

Chen, L. S.; Hung, R. J. et al. (2015). CHRNA5 risk variant predicts delayed smoking cessation and earlier lung cancer diagnosis-a meta-analysis. Journal of the National Cancer Institute, 107(5).

Chen, J.; Lipska, B. K. et al. (2004). Functional analysis of genetic variation in catechol-O-methyltransferase (COMT): effects on mRNA, protein, and enzyme activity in postmortem human brain. American Journal of Human Genetics, 75(5), 807-821.

Colilla, S.; Lerman, C. et al. (2005). Association of catechol-Omethyltransferase with smoking cessation in two independent studies of women. Pharmacogenetics and Genomics, 15(6), 393-398.

Damaj, M. I.; Carroll, F. I. et al. (2004). Enantioselective effects of hydroxy metabolites of bupropion on behavior and on function of monoamine transporters and nicotinic receptors. Molecular Pharmacology, 66(3), 675-682.

Damaj, M. I.; Grabus, S. D. et al. (2010). Effects of hydroxymetabolites of bupropion on nicotine dependence behavior in mice. The Journal of Pharmacology and Experimental Therapeutics, 334(3), 1087-1095.

David, S. P.; Brown, R. A. et al. (2007). Pharmacogenetic clinical trial of sustained-release bupropion for smoking cessation. Nicotine, Tobacco Research, 9(8), 821-833.

David, S. P.; Munafo, M. R. et al. (2008). Genetic variation in the dopamine D4 receptor (DRD4) gene and smoking cessation: follow-up of a randomised clinical trial of transdermal nicotine patch. The Pharmacogenomics Journal, 8(2), 122-128.

David, S. P.; Strong, D. R. et al. (2013). Influence of a dopamine pathway additive genetic efficacy score on smoking cessation: results from two randomized clinical trials of bupropion. Addiction, 108(12), 2202-2211.

De Luca, V. et al. (2013). Analysis of nicotinic receptor genes in nicotine replacement treatment. European Psychiatry, 28(2), 113-118.

Dempsey, D.; Tutka, P. et al. (2004). Nicotine metabolite ratio as an index of cytochrome P450 2A6 metabolic activity. Clinical Pharmacology and Therapeutics, 76(1), 64-72.

De Ruyck, K. et al. (2010). Genetic variation in three candidate genes and nicotine dependence, withdrawal and smoking cessation in hospitalized patients. Pharmacogenomics, 11(8), 1053-1063.

Duck, C. H.; Gyoon, S. W. (2016). Meta-analysis update of association between dopamine transporter SLC6A3 gene polymorphism and smoking cessation. Journal of Health Psychology, 23(9), 1250-1257.

Falcone, M.; Cao, W. et al. (2016). Brain responses to smoking cues differ based on nicotine metabolism rate. Biological Psychiatry, 80(3), 190-197.

Han, D. H.; Joe, K. H.; Na, C. et al. (2008). Effect of genetic polymorphisms on smoking cessation: A trial of bupropion in Korean male smokers. Psychiatric Genetics, 18, 11-16.

Heinz, A.; Goldman, D. (2000). Genotype effects on neurodegeneration and neuroadaptation in monoaminergic neurotransmitter systems. Neurochemistry International, 37(5-6), 425-432.

Hesse, L. M.; Venkatakrishnan, K. et al. (2000). CYP2B6 mediates the in vitro hydroxylation of bupropion: potential drug interactions with other antidepressants. Drug Metabolism and Disposition, 28(10), 1176-1183.

Hsyu, P. H.; Singh, A. et al. (1997). Pharmacokinetics of bupropion and its metabolites in cigarette smokers versus nonsmokers. Journal of Clinical Pharmacology, 37(8), 737-743.

Johnston, A. J.; Ascher, J. et al. (2002). Pharmacokinetic optimization of sustained-release bupropion for smoking cessation. Drugs, 2, 11-24.

Johnstone, E. C.; Elliot, K. M. et al. (2007). Association of COMT Val108/158Met genotype with smoking cessation in a nicotine replacement therapy randomized trial. Cancer Epidemiology, Biomarkers, Prevention, 16(6), 1065-1069.

Johnstone, E. C.; Yudkin, P. L. et al. (2004). Genetic variation in dopaminergic pathways and short-term effectiveness of the nicotine patch. Pharmacogenetics, 14(2), 83-90.

Jonsson, E. G.; Nothen, M. M. et al. (1999). Polymorphisms in the dopamine D2 receptor gene and their relationships to striatal dopamine receptor density of healthy volunteers. Molecular Psychiatry, 4(3), 290-296.

Jorm, A. F.; Henderson, A. S.; Jacomb, P. A. et al. (2000). Association of smoking and personality with a polymorphism of the dopamine transporter gene: Results from a community survey. American Journal of Medical Genetics, 96, 331-334.

Lee, A. M.; Jepson, C. et al. (2007a). CYP2B6 genotype alters abstinence rates in a bupropion smoking cessation trial. Biological Psychiatry, 62(6), 635-641.

Lee, A. M.; Jepson, C. et al. (2007b). CYP2B6 genotype does not alter nicotine metabolism, plasma levels, or abstinence with nicotine replacement therapy. Cancer Epidemiology, Biomarkers, Prevention, 16(6), 1312-1314.

Lerman, C.; Jepson, C. et al. (2006). Role of functional genetic variation in the dopamine D2 receptor (DRD2) in response to bupropion and nicotine replacement therapy for tobacco dependence: results of two randomized clinical trials. Neuropsychopharmacology, 31(1), 231-242.

Lerman, C.; Jepson, C. et al. (2010). Genetic variation in nicotine metabolism predicts the efficacy of extended-duration transdermal nicotine therapy. Clinical Pharmacology and Therapeutics, 87(5), 553-557.

Lerman, C.; Schnoll, R. A. et al. (2015). Use of the nicotine metabolite ratio as a genetically informed biomarker of response to nicotine patch or varenicline for smoking cessation: a randomised, double-blind placebo-controlled trial. The Lancet Respiratory Medicine, 3(2), 131-138.

Lerman, C.; Shields, P. G. et al. (2002). Pharmacogenetic investigation of smoking cessation treatment. Pharmacogenetics, 12(8), 627-634.

Lerman, C.; Shields, P. G.; Wileyto, E. P. et al. (2003). Effects of dopamine transporter and receptor polymorphisms on smoking cessation in a bupropion clinical trial. Health Psychology, 22, 541-548.

Lerman, C.; Tyndale, R. et al. (2006). Nicotine metabolite ratio predicts efficacy of transdermal nicotine for smoking cessation. Clinical Pharmacology and Therapeutics, 79(6), 600-608.

Leung, T.; Bergen, A. et al. (2015). Effect of the rs1051730-rs16969968 variant and smoking cessation treatment: a meta-analysis. Pharmacogenomics, 16(7), 713-720.

Leventhal, A. M.; David, S. P. et al. (2012). Dopamine D4 receptor gene variation moderates the efficacy of bupropion for smoking cessation. The Pharmacogenomics Journal, 12(1), 86-92.

Munafo, M. R. et al. (2011). CHRNA3 rs1051730 genotype and short-term smoking cessation. Nicotine, Tobacco Research, 13(10), 982-988.

Munafo, M. R.; Timofeeva, M. N. et al. (2012). Association between genetic variants on chromosome 15q25 locus and objective measures of tobacco exposure. Journal of the National Cancer Institute, 104(10), 740-748.

Nakajima, M.; Yamamoto, T. et al. (1996a). Characterization of CYP2A6 involved in 30-hydroxylation of cotinine in human liver microsomes. The Journal of Pharmacology and Experimental Therapeutics, 277(2), 1010-1015.

Nakajima, M.; Yamamoto, T. et al. (1996b). Role of human cytochrome P4502A6 in C-oxidation of nicotine. Drug Metabolism and Disposition, 24(11), 1212-1217.

Neville, M. J.; Johnstone, E. C. et al. (2004). Identification and characterization of ANKK1: a novel kinase gene closely linked to DRD2 on chromosome band 11q23. 1. Human Mutation, 23(6), 540-545.

O'Gara, C.; Stapleton, J.; Sutherland, G. et al. (2007). Dopamine transporter polymorphisms are associated with short-term response to smoking cessation treatment. Pharmacogenetics and Genomics, 17, 61-67.

Patterson, F.; Schnoll, R. A. et al. (2008). Toward personalized therapy for smoking cessation: a randomized placebo-controlled trial of bupropion. Clinical Pharmacology and Therapeutics, 84(3), 320-325.

Sabol, S. Z.; Nelson, M. L.; Fisher, C. et al. (1999). A genetic association for cigarette smoking behavior. Health Psychology, 18, 7-13.

Schnoll, R. A.; Patterson, F. et al. (2009). Nicotine metabolic rate predicts successful smoking cessation with transdermal nicotine: a validation study. Pharmacology, Biochemistry, and Behavior, 92(1), 6-11.

Schnoll, R. A.; Wileyto, E. P. et al. (2013). High dose transdermal nicotine for fast metabolizers of nicotine: a proof of concept placebo-controlled trial. Nicotine, Tobacco Research, 15(2), 348-354.

Schoedel, K. A.; Hoffmann, E. B. et al. (2004). Ethnic variation in CYP2A6 and association of genetically slow nicotine metabolism and smoking in adult Caucasians. Pharmacogenetics, 14(9), 615-626.

Shield, A. J.; Thomae, B. A. et al. (2004). Human catechol O-methyltransferase genetic variation: gene resequencing and functional characterization of variant allozymes. Molecular Psychiatry, 9(2), 151-160.

Styn, M. A.; Nukui, T.; Romkes, M. et al. (2009). The impact of genetic variation in DRD2 and SLC6A3 on smoking cessation in a cohort of participants 1 year after enrollment in a lung cancer screening study. American Journal of Medical Genetics Part B: Neuropsychiatric Genetics, 150, 254-261.

Ton, T. G.; Rossing, M. A.; Bowen, D. J. et al. (2007). Genetic polymorphisms in dopamine-related genes and smoking cessation in women: A prospective cohort study. Behavioral and Brain Functions, 23, 3-22.

Tyndale, R. F.; Zhu, A. Z. et al. (2015). Lack of associations of CHRNA5-A3-B4 genetic variants with smoking cessation treatment outcomes in Caucasian smokers despite associations with baseline smoking. PLoS ONE, 10(5).

Vandenbergh, D. J.; Persico, A. M.; Hawkins, A. L. et al. (1992). Human dopamine transporter gene (DAT1) maps to chromosome 5p15. 3 and displays a VNTR. Genomics, 14, 1104-1106.

Van Tol, H. H.; Wu, C. M. et al. (1992). Multiple dopamine D4 receptor variants in the human population. Nature, 358(6382), 149-152.

Wassenaar, C. A.; Dong, Q. et al. (2011). Relationship between CYP2A6 and CHRNA5-CHRNA3-CHRNB4 variation and smoking behaviors and lung cancer risk. Journal of the National Cancer Institute, 103(17), 1342-1346.

Zanger, U. M.; Klein, K. et al. (2007). Polymorphic CYP2B6: molecular mechanisms and emerging clinical significance. Pharmacogenomics, 8(7), 743-759.

Zhu, A. Z.; Cox, L. S. et al. (2012). CYP2B6 and bupropion's smoking-cessation pharmacology: the role of hydroxybupropion. Clinical Pharmacology and Therapeutics, 92(6), 771-777.

Zhu, A. Z.; Zhou, Q. et al. (2014a). Gene variants in CYP2C19 are associated with altered in vivo bupropion pharmacokinetics but not bupropion-assisted smoking cessation outcomes. Drug Metabolism and Disposition, 42(11), 1971-1977.

Zhu, A. Z.; Zhou, Q. et al. (2014b). Association of CHRNA5-A3-B4 SNP rs2036527 with smoking cessation therapy response in African-American smokers. Clinical Pharmacology and Therapeutics, 96(2), 256-265.

61
促食欲素系统与烟碱成瘾：临床前观察

Shaun Yon-Seng Khoo[1], *Gavan P. McNally*[2], *Kelly J. Clemens*[2]

1. Center for Studies in Behavioral Neurobiology, Department of Psychology, Concordia University, Montreal, QC, Canada
2. School of Psychology, University of New South Wales, Sydney, NSW, Australia

缩略语

Acb	伏隔核	**OX-A**	促食欲素-A
DMH	背内侧下丘脑	**OX-B**	促食欲素-B
FRn	n个响应的固定比率	**PeF**	穹隆周围下丘脑
GPCR	G蛋白偶联受体	**PFC**	前额叶皮层
LH	外侧下丘脑	**PR**	累进比率
nAChR	烟碱乙酰胆碱受体	**VTA**	腹侧被盖区

目前吸烟的药物疗法的疗效很有限，失败率高达90%（Cahill et al., 2016）。促食欲素/下丘脑分泌素系统被认为是一种潜在的治疗靶点，目前正在进行可卡因的临床试验（The University of Texas Health Science Center, 2016）。在此，我们将促食欲素作为烟碱的潜在治疗靶点进行综述，因为有证据表明急性和慢性烟碱/促食欲素相互作用，也有初步证据表明基于促食欲素的药物可能有效减少吸烟。然而，虽然有希望，但有一些相互矛盾的临床前结果，只有人类研究的相关结果可用。

促食欲素/下丘脑分泌素系统是一种参与觉醒、食欲和奖励的神经肽系统。促食欲素神经元仅起源于外侧下丘脑（LH）、穹窿周围下丘脑（PeF）和背内侧下丘脑（DMH；Baldo et al. 2003; Elias et al. 1998; Peyron et al. 1998）。促食欲素纤维投射到关键的中皮质边缘奖赏区（图61.1），如腹侧被盖区（VTA）、伏隔核（NAcc）和前额叶皮层（PFC；Baldo et al. 2003; Peyron et al. 1998），那里有丰富的烟碱乙酰胆碱受体（nAChR; Lerman et al. 2007）。

促食欲素系统由两个肽[促食欲素-A和促食欲素-B（分别为OX-A和OX-B）]和两个GPCRs（OX_1和OX_2）组成（图61.2；Sakura et al. 1998）。下丘脑分泌素（人促食欲素，*HCRT*；大鼠/小鼠促食欲素，*Hcrt*）mRNA编码前促食欲素前体肽，该肽被切割形成OX-A肽和OX-B肽（Sakurai et al. 1999）。OX-A非选择性地结合两种受体，而OX-B对OX_2受体表现出一定的选择性。OX_1和OX_2都是兴奋性的，并产生升高的Ca^{2+}，提示$G\alpha_q$介导的信号传导（de Lecea et al. 1998; Sakurai et al. 1998），但它们也可以与多个第二信使途径相互作用（Kukkonen, Leonard, 2014）。促食欲素受体也形成复合物，可能是同型二聚体（Xu et al. 2011）、OX_1和OX_2异构体和CB_1或CRF受体复合物（Ellis et al. 2006; Jäntti et al. 2014; Navarro et al. 2015）。因此，促食欲素信号被认为是兴奋性的，具有$G\alpha_q$介导的信号级联，但具有与共递质和异聚受体复合物相互作用的潜力。

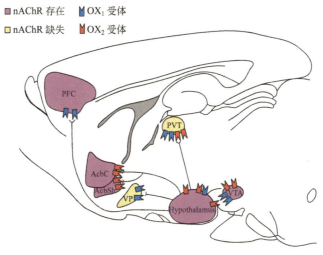

图 61.1 促食欲素系统和烟碱乙酰胆碱受体之间的解剖重叠

促食欲素受体以不同的密度存在于参与奖励的大脑关键区域。烟碱乙酰胆碱受体存在于所有这些区域,除了腹侧苍白球(VP)和丘脑室旁核(PVT)。

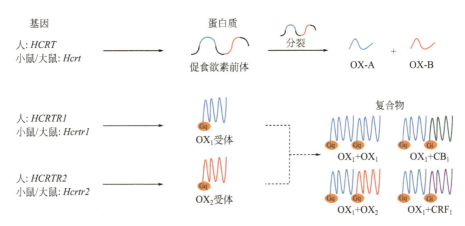

图 61.2 促食欲素信号分子示意图

这两种促食欲素肽从单一前体分裂下来,并与促食欲素受体结合,促食欲素受体可能以相互复合物的形式存在,即 CB_1 或 CRF_1 受体。

61.1 神经解剖学和分子相互作用

61.1.1 急性烟碱和促食欲素

因为胆碱能系统和促食欲素系统之间的神经解剖学和分子相互作用,促食欲素系统已被认为是一个潜在的治疗靶点。急性和慢性烟碱给药后都会发生相互作用。胆碱能神经元被 OX-A 应用激活(Fadel et al. 2005),并且促食欲素神经元被急性全身烟碱给药激活(图 61.3;Pasumarthi et al. 2006)。重要的是,通过 c-Fos 免疫组织化学测定,在下丘脑中这种激活似乎对促食欲素神经元具有特异性,表明促食欲素在烟碱介导的效应中起着关键作用。虽然这种作用被非选择性的 nAChR 拮抗剂美加明和 α4β2 nAChR 拮抗剂 DHβE 阻断,但 DHβE 单独增加了下丘脑内侧促食欲素神经元的激活，但阻断了烟碱诱导的激活（Pasumarthi et al. 2006），表明促食欲素系统存在内源性胆碱能调节。烟碱诱导的促食欲素神经元的激活似乎对基底前脑和室旁丘脑的下丘脑投射是特异性的（Pasumarthi, Fadel, 2008）。除了全身性烟碱给药，促食欲素神经元也可以通过局部烟碱应用于下丘脑而被激活，这在下丘脑中产生增加的ACh和谷氨酸流出（Pasumarthi, Fadel, 2010）。这些结果证明了激活胆碱能神经元的促食欲素之间的相互作用，烟碱系统地或直接作用于激活促食欲素神经元的下丘脑。

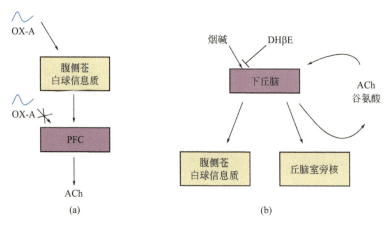

图 61.3　急性促食欲素 / 烟碱相互作用

（a）急性促食欲素可激活胆碱能神经元，（b）急性烟碱可激活促食欲素输出，导致局部谷氨酸和乙酰胆碱释放。

61.1.2　慢性烟碱和促食欲素

对慢性烟碱给药的研究表明，下丘脑分泌素基因表达和促食欲素肽的调节发生了变化（图61.4）。慢性烟碱给药（14d）增加了编码前促食欲素肽和促食欲素受体的mRNA水平（Kane et al. 2000）。烟碱暴露大鼠阻断nAChR可降低促食欲素神经元激活（Simmons et al. 2016）。对蛋白质的测量表明，在DMH中，慢性烟碱会增加OX-A和OX-B，而在室旁核中OX-B会增加（Kane et al. 2000）。然而，慢性烟碱也会减少OX-A的下丘脑结合位点（Kane et al. 2001）。这种脱敏似

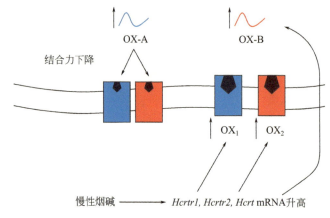

图 61.4　慢性烟碱对促食欲素调节的影响

慢性烟碱上调促食欲素肽和受体的表达，但降低了OX-A结合位点的可用性，而没有受体内化。

乎是通过模糊结合位点而发生的，但没有内化，因为OX-A继续结合但亲和力较低（Kane et al. 2001）。虽然文献中从未报道过烟碱诱导结合位点减少的确切机制的更直接的证明，但这些结果表明慢性烟碱给药对下丘脑分泌素基因表达和促食欲素肽水平都有调节作用。

61.2 促食欲素作为烟碱依赖的治疗靶点

61.2.1 烟碱自给药

促食欲素作为烟碱成瘾潜在治疗靶点的临床前研究发现，选择性和非选择性（双重）促食欲素受体拮抗剂都有效果（表61.1）。促食欲素在烟碱寻求行为中的作用的第一个直接证明涉及OX_1受体拮抗剂SB-334867的全身给药和进入岛叶皮层（Hollander et al. 2008）。OX_1受体拮抗剂选择性地抑制固定比率5（FR5）和累进比率（PR）方案中获得的烟碱输注数量，而不影响获得的食物颗粒数量。类似地，岛内给药SB-334867减少了FR5烟碱输注，但没有减少获得的食物颗粒的数量（Hollander et al. 2008）。这些结果已经用SB-334867和双重促食欲素受体拮抗剂阿莫伦特进行了复制（LeSage et al. 2010）。OX_1受体拮抗剂SB-334867和双重促食欲素受体拮抗剂阿莫伦特在FR5方案中减少了获得的烟碱输注量。然而，在这项研究中，虽然SB-334867也没有影响所获得的食物颗粒的数量，但最高剂量的阿莫伦特减少了获得的颗粒。LeSage等（2010）进一步扩展了Hollander等（2008）的发现，通过检查Hcrtr1和Hcrtr2的基因表达，发现Hcrtr1在烟碱自给药后立即在外侧LH中减少，但在自给药后5h内没有减少，而弓状核在自给药后5h内增加了Hcrtr1的mRNA，但没有立即增加。来自不同组的这些一致结果提供了强烈的迹象，表明促食欲素可能是治疗烟碱成瘾的潜在靶点。

61.2.2 恢复烟碱寻求行为

除了调节烟碱的自给药外，也有研究表明促食欲素信号在烟碱寻求的恢复中起作用，但结果并不一致。脑室给药OX-A可以恢复小鼠已消失的寻求烟碱的行为，这种作用可以被OX_1受体拮抗剂SB-334867阻断（Plaza-Zabala et al. 2010）。虽然OX_1受体拮抗剂减少了由急性烟碱注射引起的升高迷宫中的焦虑样行为，表明促食欲素参与了急性烟碱的焦虑效应，但OX_1受体拮抗剂并不影响足底电击诱发的恢复，表明这些行为是由不同的过程介导的（Plaza-Zabala et al. 2010）。在线索诱导的小鼠烟碱寻求的恢复过程中，根据c-Fos的测量，PeF和LH中的促食欲素神经元的百分比增加，显示出激活的迹象（Plaza-Zabala et al. 2013）。使用SB-334867的选择性OX_1受体拮抗剂可以减弱这种线索诱导的恢复，而不是使用TCS-OX2-29的选择性OX_2受体拮抗剂（Plaza-Zabala et al. 2013）。然而，研究表明，另一种选择性OX_2受体拮抗剂（SORA-18）能够减少线索诱导的大鼠恢复，但不能减少烟碱诱导的恢复或PR自给药（Uslaner et al. 2014）。这些研究表明，促食欲素信号在恢复行为中的作用是不一致的，可能取决于恢复的近端原因或使用的行为模式。在大鼠和小鼠中，使用促食欲素受体拮抗剂都可以减少线索诱导的恢复，但还不清楚OX_2受体是否参与其中。虽然这些结果暗示了促食欲素在线索诱导的烟碱恢复中的作用，但相对较少的研究和训练方案的差异（表61.1）使得很难得出强有力的结论。

表61.1 烟碱自给药和恢复烟碱行为研究的比较

动物	食物限制	预训练	训练	测量	药物	结果	参考文献
成对居住的雄性Wistars大鼠	到体重的85%	食物FR 5～20直到稳定	杠杆，7～14d	FR 5～20	SB-334867（腹腔注射）	↓	Hollander et al (2008)
				PR	SB-334867（腹腔注射）	↓	
				FR 5～20	SB-334867（内脑岛）	↓	
独居雄性Long-Evans大鼠	18g/d	食物至100粒/h	杠杆，(40±4.5) d	FR 5～60	SB-334867（腹腔注射）	↓	LeSage et al (2010)
			(66±8.1) d	FR 5～60	阿莫伦特（腹腔注射）	↓	
独居雄性C57BL/6J小鼠	充足	无	每日优质烟碱，鼻戳，10d	OX-A诱导恢复（脑室注射）足底电击恢复	SB-334867（腹腔注射）	↓	Plaza-Zabala et al (2010)
					SB-334867（腹腔注射）	无影响	
独居雄性C57BL/6J小鼠	充足	无	每日优质烟碱，鼻戳，10d	提示恢复	SB-334867（腹腔注射）	↓	Plaza-Zabala et al (2013)
					TCS-OX$_2$-29（腹腔注射）	无影响	
独居雄性Long-Evans大鼠	25g/d	食物FR1	杠杆，FR1×5d, FR2×2d, FR5×6d	PR	2-SORA 18（口服）	无影响	Uslaner et al (2014)
			动物再训练FR×3d	提示恢复	2-SORA 18（口服）	↓	
				烟碱恢复	2-SORA 18（口服）	无影响	
群居Sprague-Dawley大鼠	20g/d	无	鼻戳，10d 动物接受再训(共29d自我管理)	FR 1～24	TCS1102（脑室注射）	无影响	Khoo et al (2017)
				提示恢复	TCS1102（脑室注射）	无影响	
				烟碱恢复	TCS1102（脑室注射）	无影响	
				复合恢复	TCS1102（脑室注射）	无影响	

61.2.3 戒断和激活

临床前研究也证实了促食欲素信号在其他烟碱相关行为中的作用。对Hcrt$^{-/-}$小鼠或给予OX$_1$受体拮抗剂SB-334867小鼠中持续渗透微泵注射25mg/(kg·d)烟碱14d，发现甲胺沉淀戒断反应减弱，显示出促食欲素介导戒断症状（Plaza-Zabala et al. 2012），这表明促食欲素介导了戒断症状的发生。下丘脑室旁核中的促食欲素信号尤其受牵连，因为靶向微量注射SB-334867减弱了烟碱戒断的行为迹象。尽管Plaza-Zabala等（2012）没有发现OX$_2$受体拮抗剂TCS-OX$_2$-29的作用，但这可能是因为他们没有使用足够高的剂量。他们的5～10mg/kg的TCS-OX$_2$-29剂量（Plaza-Zabala et al. 2012, 2013）低于Smith等（2009）使用的10～30mg/kg的剂量，尽管后者剂量对可卡因也没有结果。之前的一项研究报道了OX$_2$受体的积极影响，使用了15mg/kg剂量的SORA-18，其效力比TCS-OX$_2$-29更强（Hirose et al. 2003；Uslaner et al. 2014）。双重促食欲素受体拮抗剂TCS 1102也减弱了烟碱增强的PR反应和烟碱诱导的蔗糖粒恢复（Winrow et al. 2010）。这些结果还支持促食欲素受体拮抗剂在治疗烟碱成瘾方面的潜在用途，因为它们可能会减轻戒断症状或减少其他与奖励相关的烟碱反应。

61.2.4 不同的发现

然而最近发现，双重促食欲素受体拮抗剂TCS 1102对烟碱自给药、线索诱导的恢复和烟碱诱导的恢复没有影响，只有在长期给予烟碱后，才对线索和烟碱诱导的恢复有微小的短暂影响

（Khoo et al. 2017）。尽管TCS 1102先前已被证明在减少烟碱的行为反应方面是有效的（Winrow et al. 2010），我们发现侧脑室内TCS 1102可以减弱OX-A诱导的摄食行为的增加，但我们没有发现任何双重促食欲素受体拮抗剂可能具有临床意义的证据。我们怀疑，我们的研究和之前的发现之间的差异可能是由于方案上的一些不同。例如，我们的大鼠接受了FR1训练，而之前的研究通常使用FR5强化和食物前训练方案（Hollander et al. 2008; LeSage et al. 2010; Uslaner et al. 2014）。在我们的研究中，大鼠被训练在整个训练期间对烟碱进行鼻触，而对食物没有反应（Khoo et al. 2017）。这可能导致我们的动物的动机水平相对较低。以前有人认为烟碱的主要强化特性相对较弱，但可能会增强其他强化剂和条件性刺激的激励特性（Chaudhri et al. 2006）。如果是这样的话，在之前的烟碱寻求或自给药的促食欲素能调节演示中使用的食物预训练方案可能增强了条件增强剂和最终与烟碱配对的反应的动机特性。此前已有研究表明，食物预训练能增强习得能力（Bongiovanni, See, 2008; Clemens et al. 2010; Garcia et al. 2014）。例如，蔗糖预训练可以促进被训练鼻触的大鼠在稍后线索诱导的烟碱寻求的恢复（Clemens et al. 2010），但食物预训练似乎不影响被训练去按下杠杆的大鼠后来的恢复测试（Garcia et al. 2014）。预训练方案的不同也可以解释为什么在我们的试验中，在FR5强化计划下自给药的大鼠相对较少（未发表的观察结果）。

这些负面结果敦促人们在寻求将促食欲素拮抗剂转化到临床时要谨慎，但他们并不一定排除以促食欲素为基础的烟碱疗法。在人类中，烟碱经常与其他药物联合使用（Cross et al. 2017）。例如，烟碱增加了男性的饮酒量（Acheson et al. 2006; Barrett et al. 2006）和醉酒的主观感觉（Kouri et al. 2004），这些结果在动物模型中得到了重复（Kalejaiye et al. 2013; Lě, et al.）烟碱的使用还与使用或依赖大麻（Taylor et al. 2017）、可卡因（Budney et al. 1993; Gorelick et al. 1997）和甲基苯丙胺（Grant et al. 2007）有关。使用多种药物可能会增加动机显著性，并使烟碱受制于促食欲素能调节。其他滥用药物也有更有力的证据证明促食欲素能调节，目前有一项使用双重促食欲素受体拮抗剂（苏沃雷生）治疗可卡因依赖的临床试验（The University of Texas Health Science Center, 2016）。然而，需要在使用多种药物的动物模型中进行进一步的临床前研究，以确定情况是否如此。

61.3 人类研究

对人类的一些研究发现了促食欲素系统和烟碱之间的联系（表61.2）。人类研究报告了促食欲素血浆浓度与自我报告的烟碱渴望之间的负相关关系（von der Goltz et al. 2010），以及与非吸烟者相比，吸烟者血液样本中Hcrt mRNA表达的降低（Rotter et al. 2012）。虽然这些研究是一致的，但它们受到外周测量促食欲素肽或Hcrt mRNA的限制。虽然OX-A肽可以扩散穿过血脑屏障，但OX-B的亲脂性低，代谢迅速（Kastin, Akerstrom, 1999）。全基因组关联研究发现，在日本样本中，HCRTR2基因的单核苷酸多态性与吸烟风险增加相关（Nishizawa et al. 2015）。然而，这些研究的结果应谨慎解释，因为有人认为，全基因组关联研究在检查复杂性状时产生的有用数据很少（Boyle et al. 2017），尽管以前的研究已经得出了生物学相关靶点或当前治疗的靶点之间的关联（Visscher et al. 2012）。而Nishizawa等（2015）发现HCRTR2多态性与吸烟、甲基苯丙胺和分裂型特征得分有关，他们还发现与甲状腺肿、主动脉瘤和骨髓瘤有关。目前对促食欲素系统和烟碱的少量人类研究表明，可能存在某种联系，但这是相关的，需要在动物和人类中进行进一步的研究，以更好地确定促食欲素系统是否真的与烟碱寻求有关。

表 61.2 人类相关研究

参与者	测量	结果	参考文献
60名吸烟者，64名非吸烟者	全血-血浆促食欲素；吸烟欲望问卷；Fagerström烟碱依赖测试	吸烟欲望与血浆促食欲素呈负相关	von der Goltz et al.（2010）
36名大麻依赖者，20名吸烟者，21名不吸烟的学生朋友	外周血淋巴细胞中全血-HCRT和OX-A的检测	吸烟者的OX-A水平较低；对HCRT启动子甲基化无影响	Rotter et al.（2012）
最初的148名GWAS患者	Fagerström烟碱依赖测试	HCRTR2单核苷酸多态性（Val308Ile）与吸烟有关	Nishizawa et al.（2015）
随访：112例腹部手术患者、203例甲基苯丙胺依赖患者、311例健康志愿者	烟草依赖筛查		
2305例尸检病例	尸检结果		

61.4　对治疗的影响

目前没有足够的证据推荐以促食欲素为基础的吸烟治疗。虽然有一些有希望的临床前研究结果和在人类中发现的相关证据，但在临床前文献中也有一些不一致的发现需要解决。需要进行进一步的研究来检验动物的训练史和烟碱寻求的促食欲素能调节之间的关系。

61.5　结论

促食欲素系统因其对各种疾病的治疗潜力而引起了极大的兴奋和兴趣。最近，随着苏沃雷生治疗失眠的批准（Coleman et al. 2017），这一潜力已经实现，并可能在可卡因成瘾方面实现（The University of Texas Health Science Center, 2016）。动物研究表明，急性烟碱刺激促食欲素神经元，慢性烟碱可以影响促食欲素系统的调节。与其他滥用药物相比，在药物自给药和寻求的临床前动物模型中，促食欲素拮抗剂对烟碱的测试频率低于其他滥用药物的测试频率，但在相对少量的研究中，关于促食欲素拮抗剂对烟碱自给药和恢复的有效性，有积极和消极的发现。对人类参与者的研究发现，促食欲素下调和烟碱使用之间存在一些一致的关联，单核苷酸HCRTR2多态性和吸烟之间存在遗传关联，但这些结果是相关的。对于烟碱和促食欲素，目前没有足够的证据表明促食欲素是烟碱成瘾的有效治疗靶点，但还需要进一步的研究来检查临床前研究中不同结果背后的原因，并跟进在人类研究中发现的关联。

术语解释
- 阿莫伦特：一种已进入临床试验的双重促食欲素受体拮抗剂。
- 双促食欲素受体拮抗剂：一种对两种促食欲素受体都有拮抗作用的化合物。
- 固定比率自给药：在临床前动物模型中使用的操作强化计划，其中通过固定数量的操作反应获得奖励。

- 下丘脑分泌素：促食欲素/下丘脑分泌素系统的命名基于其下丘脑分布和与胰岛素家族激素的相似性。指的是编码这两种多肽的基因HCRT/Hcrt，以及编码这两种受体的HCRTR1/Hcrtr1和HCRTR2/Hcrtr2。
- 促食欲素：促食欲素/下丘脑分泌素系统是根据其在食欲行为中的作用命名的。指的是与OX_1和OX_2受体结合的两种多肽，即促食欲素-A和促食欲素-B。
- 累进比率：在临床前动物模型中使用的操作强化计划，其中获得每个后续奖励所需的反应数量增加。
- 复吸：一种类似故态复萌的行为模式，它涉及以前消失的行为的回归。可能是由药物引发、奖励相关线索、背景或压力引起的。
- SB-334867：一种选择性OX_1受体拮抗剂。
- SORA-18：一种选择性OX_2受体拮抗剂。
- TCS 110：一种双重促食欲素受体拮抗剂。
- TCS-OX_2-29：一种选择性OX_2受体拮抗剂。

促食欲素系统的关键事实

- 1998年被两个小组同时发现。
- 由下丘脑泌素基因编码的两个肽，即促食欲素-A和促食欲素-B，与兴奋性G蛋白偶联受体OX_1和OX_2结合。
- 与人类发作性睡病有关的促食欲素神经元丢失。
- 刺激促食欲素系统会促进食欲行为。
- 动物研究已经证明了促食欲素在多种药物滥用中的作用。
- 苏沃雷生（Belsomra®）是第一种基于促食欲素的药物，并于2014年被批准用于治疗失眠。

要点总结

- 本章重点介绍促食欲素系统，一种涉及唤醒、食欲和奖励的神经肽系统，以及它作为烟碱成瘾治疗靶点的潜力。
- 促食欲素系统激活胆碱能神经元，并通过烟碱注射激活，慢性烟碱导致下丘脑泌素基因和促食欲素肽的表达发生变化。
- 少数临床前动物研究已经表明了各种促食欲素受体拮抗剂在自给药或恢复范例中的作用。
- 然而，不同的研究在方法上存在很大差异，一些研究还没有发现促食欲素拮抗的作用。
- 在动物和人类中进行的有限数量的研究表明，以促食欲素系统为靶点可能会有一些希望，但在临床试验之前，需要更多的研究来了解它在烟碱寻求过程中的作用。

参考文献

Acheson, A.; Mahler, S. V.; Chi, H.; de Wit, H. (2006). Differential effects of nicotine on alcohol consumption in men and women. Psychopharmacology, 186, 54.

Baldo, B. A.; Daniel, R. A.; Berridge, C. W.; Kelley, A. E. (2003). Over-lapping distribu-tions of orexin/hypocretin- and dopamine-β-hydroxylase immunoreactive fibers in rat brain regions mediatingarousal, motivation, and stress. The Journal of Comparative Neurology, 464, 220-237.

Barrett, S. P.; Tichauer, M.; Leyton, M.; Pihl, R. O. (2006). Nicotine increases alcohol self-administration in non-dependent male smokers. Drug and Alcohol Dependence, 81, 197-204.

Bongiovanni, M.; See, R. E. (2008). A comparison of the effects of different operant training experiences and dietary restriction on the reinstatement of cocaine-seeking in rats. Pharmacology, Biochemistry, and Behavior, 89, 227-233.

Boyle, E. A.; Li, Y. I.; Pritchard, J. K. (2017). An expanded view of complex traits: from polygenic to omnigenic. Cell, 169, 1177-1186.

Budney, A. J.; Higgins, S. T.; Hughes, J. R.; Bickel, W. K. (1993). Nicotine and caffeine use in cocaine-dependent individuals. Journal of Substance Abuse, 5, 117-130.

Cahill, K.; Lindson-Hawley, N.; Thomas, K. H.; Fanshawe, T. R.; Lancaster, T. (2016). Nicotine receptor partial agonists for smoking cessation. Cochrane Database of Systematic Reviews. 5, CD006103.

Chaudhri, N.; Caggiula, A. R.; Donny, E. C.; Booth, S.; Gharib, M.; Craven, L. et al. (2006). Operant responding for conditioned and unconditioned reinforcers in rats is differentially enhanced by the primary reinforcing and reinforcement-enhancing effects of nicotine. Psychopharmacology, 189, 27-36.

Clemens, K. J.; Caille, S.; Cador, M. (2010). The effects of response operandum and prior food training on intravenous nicotine self-administration in rats. Psychopharmacology, 211, 43-54.

Coleman, P. J.; Gotter, A. L.; Herring, W. J.; Winrow, C. J.; Renger, J. J. (2017). The discovery of suvorexant, the first orexin receptor drug for insomnia. Annual Review of Pharmacology and Toxicology, 57, 509-533.

Cross, S. J.; Lotfipour, S.; Leslie, F. M. (2017). Mechanisms and genetic factors underlying co-use of nicotine and alcohol or other drugs of abuse. The American Journal of Drug and Alcohol Abuse, 43, 171-185.

de Lecea, L.; Kilduff, T. S.; Peyron, C.; Gao, X. -B.; Foye, P. E.; Danielson, P. E. et al. (1998). The hypocretins: hypothalamus-specific peptides with neuroexcitatory activity. Proceedings of the National Academy of Sciences, 95, 322-327.

Elias, C. F.; Saper, C. B.; Maratos-Flier, E.; Tritos, N A.; Lee, C.; Kelly, J.; et al. (1998). Chemically defined projections linking the mediobasal hypothalamus and the lateral hypothalamic area. The Journal of Comparative Neurology, 402, 442-459.

Ellis, J.; Pediani, J. D.; Canals, M.; Milasta, S.; Milligan, G. (2006). Orexin-1 receptor-cannabinoid CB1 receptor heterodimerization results in both ligand-dependent and -independent coordinated alterations of receptor localization and function. Journal of Biological Chemistry, 281, 38812-38824.

Fadel, J.; Pasumarthi, R.; Reznikov, L. R. (2005). Stimulation of cortical acetylcholine release by orexin A. Neuroscience, 130, 541-547.

Garcia, K. L. P.; Lê, A. D.; Tyndale, R. F. (2014). Effect of food training and training dose on nicotine self-administration in rats. Behavioural Brain Research, 274, 10-18.

Gorelick, D. A.; Simmons, M. S.; Carriero, N.; Tashkin, D. P. (1997). Characteristics of smoked drug use among cocaine smokers. The American Journal on Addictions, 6, 237-245.

Grant, K. M.; Kelley, S. S.; Agrawal, S.; Meza, J. L.; Meyer, J. R.; Romberger, D. J. (2007). Methamphetamine use in rural midwesterners. The American Journal on Addictions, 16, 79-84.

Hirose, M.; Egashira, S. -i.; Goto, Y.; Hashihayata, T.; Ohtake, N.; Iwaasa, H. et al. (2003). N-Acyl 6,7-dimethoxy-1,2,3,4-tetrahydroiso-quinoline: the first orexin-2 receptor selective non-peptidic antagonist. Bioorganic, Medicinal Chemistry Letters, 13, 4497-4499.

Hollander, J. A.; Lu, Q.; Cameron, M. D.; Kamenecka, T. M.; Kenny, P. J. (2008). Insular hypocretin transmission regulates nicotine reward. Proceedings of the National Academy of Sciences, 105, 19480-19485.

Jäntti, M. H.; Mandrika, I.; Kukkonen, J. P. (2014). Human orexin/hypocretin receptors form constitutive homo- and heteromeric complexes with each other and with human CB1 cannabinoid receptors. Biochemical and Biophysical Research Communications, 445, 486-490.

Kalejaiye, O.; Bhatti, B. H.; Taylor, R. E.; Tizabi, Y. (2013). Nicotine blocks the depressogenic effects of alcohol: implications for drinking-smoking co-morbidity. Journal of Drug and Alcohol Research, 2, 235709.

Kane, J. K.; Parker, S. L.; Li, M. D. (2001). Hypothalamic orexin-A binding sites are downregulated by chronic nicotine treatment in the rat. Neuroscience Letters, 298, 1-4.

Kane, J. K.; Parker, S. L.; Matta, S. G.; Fu, Y.; Sharp, B. M.; Li, M. D. (2000). Nicotine up-regulates expression of orexin and its receptors in rat brain. Endocrinology, 141, 3623-3629.

Kastin, A. J.; Akerstrom, V. (1999). Orexin A but not orexin B rapidly enters brain from blood by simple diffusion. Journal of Pharmacology and Experimental Therapeutics, 289, 219-223.

Khoo, S. Y. -S.; McNally, G. P.; Clemens, K. J. (2017). The dual orexin receptor antagonist TCS1102 does not affect reinstatement of nicotine-seeking. PLoS ONE, 12, e0173967.

Kouri, E. M.; McCarthy, E. M.; Faust, A. H.; Lukas, S. E. (2004). Pretreatment with transdermal nicotine enhances some of ethanol's acute effects in men. Drug and Alcohol Dependence, 75, 55-65.

Kukkonen, J. P.; Leonard, C. S. (2014). Orexin/hypocretin receptor signalling cascades. British Journal of Pharmacology, 171, 314-331.

Le, A. D.; Funk, D.; Lo, S.; Coen, K. (2014). Operant self-administration of alcohol and nicotine in a preclinical model of co-abuse. Psychopharmacology, 231, 4019-4029.

Lerman, C.; LeSage, M. G.; Perkins, K. A.; O'Malley, S. S.; Siegel, S. J.; Benowitz, N. L. et al. (2007). Translational research in medication development for nicotine dependence. Nature Reviews Drug Discovery, 6, 746-762.

LeSage, M. G.; Perry, J. L.; Kotz, C. M.; Shelley, D.; Corrigall, W. A. (2010). Nicotine self-administration in the rat: effects of hypocretin antagonists and changes in hypocretin mRNA. Psychopharmacology, 209, 203-212.

Navarro, G.; Quiroz, C.; Moreno-Delgado, D.; Sierakowiak, A.; McDowell, K.; Moreno, E. et al. (2015). Orexin-corticotropin-releasing factor receptor heteromers in the ventral tegmental area as targets for cocaine. The Journal of Neuroscience, 35, 6639-6653.

Nishizawa, D.; Kasai, S.; Hasegawa, J.; Sato, N.; Yamada, H.; Tanioka, F.; et al. (2015). Associations between the orexin (hypocretin) receptor 2 gene polymorphism Val308Ile and nicotine dependence in genome-wide and subsequent association studies. Molecular Brain, 8, 50.

Pasumarthi, R. K.; Fadel, J. (2008). Activation of orexin/hypocretin projections to basal forebrain and paraventricular thalamus by acute nicotine. Brain Research Bulletin, 77, 367-373.

Pasumarthi, R. K.; Fadel, J. (2010). Stimulation of lateral hypothalamic glutamate and acetylcholine efflux by nicotine: implications for mechanisms of nicotine-induced activation of orexin neurons. Journal of Neurochemistry, 113, 1023-1035.

Pasumarthi, R. K.; Reznikov, L. R.; Fadel, J. (2006). Activation of orexin neurons by acute nicotine. European Journal of Pharmacology, 535, 172-176.

Peyron, C.; Tighe, D. K.; van den Pol, A. N.; de Lecea, L.; Heller, H. C.; Sutcliffe, J. G. et al. (1998). Neurons containing hypocretin (orexin)project to multiple neuronal systems. The Journal of Neuroscience, 18, 9996-10015.

Plaza-Zabala, A.; Flores, Á.; Maldonado, R.; Berrendero, F. (2012). Hypocretin/orexin signaling in the hypothalamic paraventricular nucleus is essential for the expression of nicotine withdrawal. Biological Psychiatry, 71, 214-223.

Plaza-Zabala, A.; Flores, A.; Martin-Garcia, E.; Saravia, R.; Maldonado, R.; Berrendero, F. (2013). A role for hypocretin/orexin receptor-1 in cue-induced reinstatement of nicotine-seeking behavior. Neuropsychopharmacology, 38, 1724-1736.

Plaza-Zabala, A.; Martín-García, E.; de Lecea, L.; Maldonado, R.; Berrendero, F. (2010). Hypocretins regulate the anxiogenic-like effects of nicotine and induce reinstatement of nicotine-seeking behavior. The Journal of Neuroscience, 30, 2300-2310.

Rotter, A.; Bayerlein, K.; Hansbauer, M.; Weiland, J.; Sperling, W.; Kornhuber, J. et al. (2012). Orexin A expression and promoter methylation in patients with cannabis dependence in comparison to nicotine-dependent cigarette smokers and nonsmokers. Neuropsycho-biology, 66, 126-133.

Sakurai, T.; Amemiya, A.; Ishii, M.; Matsuzaki, I.; Chemelli, R. M.; Tanaka, H. et al. (1998). Orexins and orexin receptors: a family of hypothalamic neuropeptides and G protein-coupled receptors that regulate feeding behavior. Cell, 92, 573-585.

Sakurai, T.; Moriguchi, T.; Furuya, K.; Kajiwara, N.; Nakamura, T.; Yanagisawa, M. et al. (1999). Structure and function of human prepro-orexin gene. Journal of Biological Chemistry, 274, 17771-17776.

Simmons, S. J.; Gentile, T. A.; Mo, L.; Tran, F. H.; Ma, S.; Muschamp, J. W. (2016). Nicotinic receptor blockade decreases fos immunoreactivity within orexin/hypocretin-expressing neurons of nicotine-exposed rats. Behavioural Brain Research, 314, 226-233. https://doi. org/ 10. 1016/j. bbr. 2016. 07. 053.

Smith, R. J.; See, R. E.; Aston-Jones, G. (2009). Orexin/hypocretin signaling at the orexin 1 receptor regulates cue-elicited cocaine-seeking. European Journal of Neuroscience, 30, 493-503. https://doi. org/10. 1111/j. 1460-9568. 2009. 06844. x.

Taylor, M.; Collin, S. M.; Munafò, M. R.; MacLeod, J.; Hickman, M.; Heron, J. (2017). Patterns of cannabis use during adolescence and their association with harmful substance use behaviour: findings from a UK birth cohort. Journal of Epidemiology and Community Health, https://doi. org/10. 1136/jech-2016-208503.

The University of Texas Health Science Center. (2016). Role of the orexin receptor system in stress, sleep and cocaine use. Retrieved from:(2016). clinicaltrials. gov/show/NCT02785406.

Uslaner, J. M.; Winrow, C. J.; Gotter, A. L.; Roecker, A. J.; Coleman, P. J.; Hutson, P. H. et al. (2014). Selective orexin 2 receptor antagonism blocks cue-induced reinstatement, but not nicotine self-administration or nicotine-induced reinstatement. Behavioural Brain Research, 269, 6 1-65.

Visscher, P. M.; Brown, M. A.; McCarthy, M. I.; Yang, J. (2012). Five years of GWAS discovery. The American Journal of Human Genetics, 90, 7-24.

von der Goltz, C.; Koopmann, A.; Dinter, C.; Richter, A.; Rockenbach, C.; Grosshans, M. et al. (2010). Orexin and leptin are associated with nicotine craving: a link between smoking, appetite and reward. Psychoneuroendocrinology, 35, 570-577.

Winrow, C. J.; Tanis, K. Q.; Reiss, D. R.; Rigby, A. M.; Uslaner, J. M.; Uebele, V. N. et al. (2010). Orexin receptor antagonism prevents transcriptional and behavioral plasticity resulting from stimulant exposure. Neuropharmacology, 58, 185-194.

Xu, T. R.; Ward, R. J.; Pediani, J. D.; Milligan, G. (2011). The orexin OX_1 receptor exists predominantly as a homodimer in the basal state:potential regulation of receptor organization by both agonist and antagonist ligands. Biochemical Journal, 439, 171-183.

62
烟草控制政策和吸烟者的反应

Philip DeCicca[1,2], *Erik Nesson*[1]

1. Department of Economics, Ball State University, Muncie, IN, United States
2. NBER, Cambridge, MA, United States

缩略语

CPS-TUS	目前的人口调查-烟草使用补充剂	**ETS**	环境烟草烟雾
NHANES	全国健康和营养检查调查	**SFA 法**	无烟空气法

62.1 引言

旨在减少吸烟的公共政策，特别是卷烟消费税和SFA法，已经成为公共卫生政策工具。在美国，卷烟消费税分州和联邦两级征收。它们提高了消费者购买卷烟的价格，因此应该会阻止吸烟。此外，美国许多州已经通过了SFA法，即限制吸烟场所的法律，影响了在餐馆和酒吧、私人工作场所、政府办公楼和教育设施等场所的吸烟。

美国不同州的吸烟率和烟草控制政策有很大差异。例如，2015年，最低的州和联邦消费税之和是1.18美元，最高的是5.36美元。大多数州已经在私人工作场所、餐馆和酒吧采用了SFA法，但各州之间SFA法的限制性差异很大。另外，成人和青少年吸烟率在各州之间也有很大差异，通常南部和阿巴契亚各州的吸烟率最高。

烟草控制政策和吸烟率也存在时间差异。图62.1和图62.2显示了这些趋势。图62.1描绘了

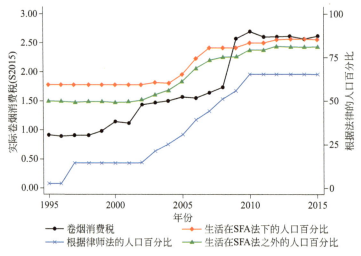

图62.1 1995～2015年烟草控制政策的趋势

来自疾病预防控制中心国家系统和烟经核算体系人口的数据。卷烟消费税代表平均州和联邦消费税，以2015年实际美元的州人口加权。生活在SFA法下的人口百分比也用州人口加权。

1995～2015年期间，经通货膨胀调整后的平均州和联邦卷烟消费税，以及根据室内清洁空气法生活在餐馆、酒吧和私人工作场所的美国人口百分比。图62.2描绘了同一时期成人和青少年参与吸烟的趋势。平均州加联邦卷烟消费税从1995年的不到1.00美元增加到2015年的近2.50美元，生活在SFA法下的美国人的百分比从1995年的略高于60%增加到2015年的近90%。在同一时期，成人和青少年吸烟的比例明显下降。

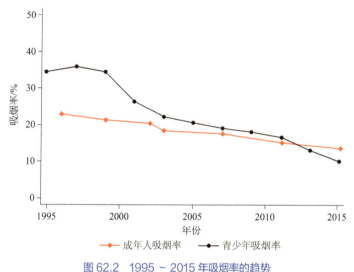

图62.2　1995～2015年吸烟率的趋势

来自疾病预防控制中心国家系统和环经核算体系人口的数据。成人吸烟率来自当前人口调查烟草使用补充问题："你现在是每天吸烟、某几天吸烟还是根本不吸烟？"青少年吸烟率来自青少年风险行为监测系统的询问："在过去的30天中，你吸烟了多少天？"

这些相关性表明，烟草控制政策可能是同时减少吸烟的主要原因，但在烟草控制政策和吸烟结果之间建立因果关系需要解决一些统计挑战。也许，最大的挑战是缺乏一个反事实的世界，在这个世界里，研究人员可以在没有烟草控制政策的情况下观察到与吸烟相关的结果。这就产生了一种可能性，即尽管烟草控制政策与减少吸烟结果相关，但这种关系不是因果关系。对烟草控制政策的经济研究主要是围绕着"差异中的差异"方法进行的，利用了这些政策在不同时期在各州的交错实施。大多数研究使用从大型调查中收集的个人层面的数据，并将个人的地理位置与该位置和时间的烟草控制政策联系起来。实施烟草控制政策的地方与没有实施烟草控制政策的地方相比，研究个人吸烟结果的变化，创造了一种反事实的环境或准实验。在一定程度上，没有实施政策的地点代表了在实施政策的地点会发生的情况，烟草控制政策和吸烟结果之间的相关性表明了因果关系。

另一个挑战是衡量吸烟的结果。直到最近，数据限制限制了研究人员根据自我报告的吸烟参与和每天吸烟的数量来衡量吸烟结果。如果烟草控制政策诱导吸烟者改变品牌，改变他们吸烟的方式，或者错误地报告他们的吸烟行为，烟草控制政策对吸烟数量的影响的估计可能不能准确地代表吸烟的变化。

下面，我们总结了烟草控制政策影响评估研究的最新进展。我们主要关注美国和最常研究的烟草控制政策、卷烟消费税和SFA法。我们研究了三个主要的与吸烟相关的结果：（1）自身的吸烟行为、（2）ETS暴露和（3）吸烟暴露对健康的影响。我们描述了每组结果的挑战和创新，并以未来研究的潜在领域结束。

62.2　成人吸烟行为

在税收和价格方面，早期的研究确定了卷烟的负价格弹性需求约为-0.4，这意味着卷烟价格每上涨10%，吸烟率就会减少4%（Chaloupka, Warner, 2000）。早期的研究普遍发现，SFA法也减少了吸烟（Chaloupka, 1992; Chaloupka, Saffer, 1992; Evans et al. 1999; Farrelly et al. 1999; Tauras, 2006）。

这些早期的研究面临着统计和数据方面的挑战。首先，很大程度上由于数据的限制，早期的研究使用自我报告的吸烟参与和每天吸烟的数量来测量吸烟行为。如上所述，误报的吸烟行为可能会使烟草控制政策对吸烟的估计影响产生偏差。与之相关的是，由于卷烟税是按每支卷烟征收的，吸烟者可能会通过改变他们吸烟的方式或改变吸烟的类型来从每支卷烟中摄取更多的烟碱。因此，卷烟消费量的减少并不意味着烟碱摄入量的减少或接触有害化学物质的减少（Harris, 1980）。Evans和Farrelly（1998）、Farrelly等（2004）首次实证检验了这个问题，他们使用了卷烟购买与焦油、烟碱和一氧化碳含量相匹配的数据集。他们都发现，尽管吸烟者减少了他们吸烟的数量以应对卷烟消费税的增加，但购买的卷烟中焦油和烟碱含量的增加抵消了这些减少。Adda和Cornaglia（2006）利用NHANES的数据推进了这一文献，这些数据包含自我报告的卷烟消费量和血清可替宁水平，可替宁是最近烟碱暴露的生物标志物。与Evans和Farrelly（1998）和Farrelly等（2004）相似，Adda和Cornaglia（2006）发现，虽然吸烟者由于卷烟消费税的增加而减少了卷烟消费，但血清可替宁水平没有相应降低，这表明吸烟者要么改变卷烟品牌，要么改变他们吸烟的强度。

然而，最近的研究发现补偿行为的证据较少。Abrevaya和Puzzello（2012）发现Adda和Cornaglia（2006）的结果是由于使用了NHANES数据的公开可用的子样本。Nesson（2017a）进一步扩展了NHANES的数据，也没有发现什么补偿行为的证据。最后，Cotti等（2016）使用家庭扫描仪数据跟踪家庭长期购买情况，并将卷烟购买与焦油、烟碱和一氧化碳含量进行匹配。他们发现焦油、烟碱和一氧化碳含量的小幅增加与卷烟购买量的减少相比微不足道。

最近的另一项创新涉及避税。Chiou和Muchlegger（2008）使用了2003年的CPS-TUS浪潮，其中包含吸烟者在哪里购买卷烟的信息。他们发现，重度吸烟者更有可能越过州边界，在低税场所购买卷烟。DeCicca等（2013a, 2013b）也使用CPS-TUS来进一步研究这个问题。DeCicca等（2013a）发现，税收较少转移到寻求较低价格的消费者身上，即购买纸盒包装卷烟而不是单独包装卷烟的吸烟者和跨州购买卷烟的吸烟者。DeCicca等（2013b）发现，这种价格搜索的影响表明，最佳卷烟消费税比当前税率低约20%，联邦卷烟税可能更有效。最后，Harding等（2012）使用家庭扫描仪数据来检查卷烟消费税对价格的影响，并发现离低税收州更近的家庭更有可能越过该州边界购买卷烟。

62.3　青少年吸烟行为

除了评估成人对烟草控制政策的反应，研究还探讨了低于法定吸烟年龄的青少年是否对烟草控制政策有反应。早期的研究表明，卷烟价格和税收影响青少年吸烟，但没有得出关于SFA法的一致结论（Chaloupka, 1991; Chaloupka, Grossman, 1996; Chaloupka, Wechsler, 1997）。然而，最近的研究得出了关于消费税的复杂结论。最近的一些研究利用了小组数据集，并经常发现较高的卷烟税导致吸烟量的微弱减少（例如，DeCicca et al. 2002; Douglas, 1998; Douglas, Hariharan, 1994; Nonnemaker, Farrelly, 2011）。另一方面，Lillard等（2013）认为，这些微弱的税收影响可能是由于有限的政策变化或这些研究检查吸烟决策的年龄。

最近的其他研究表明，政策内生性，即特定州的反吸烟情绪可能会推动烟草控制政策和减少青少年吸烟，可能会偏离青少年吸烟研究的结果。DeCicca等（2008）利用CPS-TUS对各种吸烟问题的看法，得出了一种反吸烟情绪的方法。他们发现，考虑反吸烟情绪会降低青少年对卷烟价格的反应。Carpenter和Cook（2008）使用了一个更大的重复横截面数据集，并发现一旦禁烟，卷烟税仍然会减少青少年吸烟，尽管Hansen等（2017）表明卷烟税对青少年吸烟的影响近年来有所减弱。

最后，青少年吸烟者自我报告的吸烟量和烟碱摄入量之间可能存在差异。像成年吸烟者一样，青少年吸烟者可以通过更换品牌或增加吸烟强度来补偿更高的卷烟消费税。此外，青少年可能害怕因披露吸烟行为和少报吸烟而遭到报复。如果少报的倾向与烟草控制政策有关，那么随着烟草控制政策的增加而减少吸烟可能只是反映了误报的增加。Kenkel等（2004）使用了包含同时期吸烟测量和回顾性吸烟测量的纵向数据。他们发现，在评估烟草控制政策的影响时，对误报的吸烟做出解释可能很重要。

研究人员最近在这个问题上引入了吸烟生物标志物。Edoka（2017）使用了来自英国健康调查的数据，其中包含自我报告的吸烟率和血清可替宁水平。她发现，自我报告的吸烟率低估了使用血清可替宁水平测量的吸烟率，并且这种偏差在估计吸烟决定因素的影响时减弱了边际效应。Nesson（2017b）使用来自NHANES的数据，并通过自我报告和血清可替宁水平来研究烟草控制政策对青少年吸烟的影响。虽然他发现卷烟消费税的增加降低了吸烟的参与度，这是通过自我报告和血清可替宁水平来衡量的，但他注意到了强化边际的差异。最后，Nesson（2017b）发现证据表明，针对青少年持有、使用或购买卷烟的卷烟消费税和公共政策增加了青少年中被误报的吸烟状况。

62.4　ETS暴露

直到最近，数据限制限制了烟草控制政策对特定地理位置ETS暴露的影响的研究。这项研究设计引起了人们的担忧，即与烟草控制政策相关的ETS暴露的减少实际上可能并不是由这些政策造成的。例如，Farrelly等（2005）发现，2003年纽约州的一项酒吧和餐厅SFA法减少了餐厅和酒吧员工对ETS的暴露，而CDC的一份报告发现，该法律减少了普通人群对ETS的暴露（CDC, 2007）。对马萨诸塞州、华盛顿特区、苏格兰、爱尔兰、瑞典和挪威的SFA法进行的其他研究也得出了类似的结果（Ellingsen et al. 2006; Larsson et al. 2008; Menzies et al. 2006; Mulcahy et al. 2005; Pearson et al. 2009; Siegel et al. 2004）。

随着大型调查开始询问有关ETS暴露的问题，有关ETS暴露的经济学文献不断增加。Bitler等（2010）使用CPS-TUS研究了12个特定场所的SFA法对吸烟行为和工作场所合规性的影响。他们发现，尽管酒吧SFA法导致调酒师报告增加了吸烟限制，但其他SFA法并不影响工人报告的吸烟限制。利用CPS-TUS最近的浪潮，Cheng等（2017）对Bitler等（2010）进行了扩展，同时也检查了ETS的暴露情况。他们发现，清洁室内空气法规将非吸烟者暴露于ETS的风险降低了

28%。然而，Adda和Cornaglia（2010）使用了NHANES和血清可替宁浓度的数据，几乎没有发现SFA法减少个体接触ETS的证据。事实上，他们发现的证据表明，SFA法增加了吸烟家庭儿童中ETS的暴露，因为法律促使成年吸烟者在家里吸烟更多，在餐馆和酒吧待的时间更少。也就是说，他们确实发现卷烟消费税降低了ETS暴露。

经济学家还利用了加拿大丰富的数据。Carpenter（2009）研究了加拿大安大略省1997～2004年的地方工作场所吸烟限制，发现这些限制使蓝领接触ETS的机会减少了28%～33%。然而，这些地方禁令对白领接触ETS的影响微乎其微。Carpenter等（2011）发现，SFA法减少了非吸烟者在各种公共场所接触ETS，几乎没有证据表明家庭和汽车内的迁移。同样，Nguyen（2013）研究了加拿大的汽车SFA法，发现它们在没有证据表明可以替代在家吸烟的情况下，减少了汽车中的ETS暴露。Sims等（2012）研究了2007年禁止在英国几乎所有室内公共场所和工作场所吸烟的法律是否影响非吸烟者接触ETS。作者使用了来自英国健康调查的数据，其中包含血清可替宁水平。他们发现，这项法律既降低了个体体内可替宁水平达到可测量水平的可能性，又降低了可替宁水平。作者发现，这种影响最集中在社会经济地位较高的家庭和没有吸烟者的家庭中。

62.5 与吸烟相关的健康结果

另一个较新的进展涉及烟草控制政策对吸烟相关健康结果的影响，特别是成人死亡率、怀孕和儿童健康、肥胖，以及烟草立法带来的意想不到的健康结果。

在一项早期研究中，Moore（1996）利用1954～1988年的数据研究了卷烟消费税与死亡率之间的关系，这段时期的税收增加相对较少且幅度较小。他的发现表明，卷烟消费税增加10%，每年将挽救约6000人的生命。最近的研究利用了可能提供更可信研究设计的自然试验，尽管估计这种影响的研究仍然很少。例如，Bedard和Deschenes（2006）发现由于应征服兵役而获得廉价卷烟会增加过早死亡率。最近，Darden等（2015）表明，在尝试对吸烟进行非随机分类后，吸烟对死亡率的因果影响大约是吸烟者和非吸烟者之间观察到的平均寿命差异的一半。

最近的工作还调查了SFA法对健康结果的影响。例如，Pell等（2008）发现苏格兰的一项SFA法减少了与冠状动脉相关的住院，尽管Shetty等（2011）和Barr等（2012）的研究表明没有这样的健康影响。总而言之，从研究设计的角度估计吸烟对成人死亡率和健康结果的因果影响是非常困难的。

评估烟草控制政策与婴幼儿健康之间的关系提供了更可信的研究设计。虽然最近卷烟税变化的影响似乎较小，而且集中在社会经济地位较低的妇女和婴儿中（Adams et al. 2012; Colman et al. 2003; Evans, Ringel, 1999），但在婴儿在子宫内时，卷烟税增加的影响似乎较小，并改善了分娩结果（Markowitz et al. 2013）。此外，当婴儿在子宫内时，卷烟税的增加可能会对儿童产生更晚的影响，减少在上学去看医生的病假（Simon, 2016）。也有证据表明，在儿童早期增加卷烟税可以减少婴儿猝死综合征和哮喘的发生（King et al. 2015; Markowitz, 2008; Sabia, 2008）。

除了与吸烟直接相关的健康影响外，经济学家还估计了烟草控制政策对健康的一些间接影响，既有积极的，也有消极的。积极的一面是，有证据表明，卷烟税可能通过间接影响锻炼和食物消费来降低肥胖率。此外，体重指数高的个体的肥胖率降幅最大（Courtemanche, 2009;

Wehby, Courtemanche, 2012）。最后，研究表明，酒吧SFA法的通过促使吸烟者改用无烟烟草，并驱车更远地前往仍允许吸烟的酒吧，从而增加了与酒精相关的交通死亡（Adams, Cotti, 2008; Adams et al. 2013）。

62.6 未来研究方向

鉴于我们的限制，我们忽略了吸烟经济学中的几个领域。我们相信，在讨论的领域中的研究将保持强劲，对我们确定的较新领域的兴趣将继续增长。当然，这些文献将朝着新的方向扩展，如对电子烟等新技术的评估，以及对最近政府对吸烟的监管的评估，包括美国食品和药物管理局（FDA）最近提出的关于卷烟烟碱含量的监管规定。此外，更好地解决吸烟测量问题的研究将是重要的贡献。随着具有更客观的生物标志物信息的数据变得更加广泛，将有可能更好地估计我们讨论的大多数关系，并获得相应行为的更广泛的图景。总而言之，这些将为政策制定者提供更好的信息，并推动和改进未来的吸烟经济学的研究。

术语解释
- 烟草控制政策：政府制定的政策，如卷烟税或无烟空气法，旨在降低吸烟率或吸烟可能产生的负面外部影响。
- 卷烟消费税：对卷烟在生产时征收的税，而不是在销售时征收的税。
- 无烟空气法：在地方或州级通过的法律，限制在某些场所吸烟，如私人工作场所、餐馆或酒吧。
- 吸烟率：某一特定人口目前吸烟的百分比。
- 环境烟草烟雾：由卷烟（或其他烟草产品）产生的烟雾，而不是个人吸烟行为的结果。

关键事实
- 在过去的20年中，美国成人和青少年的吸烟率都有所下降。
- 截至2015年，约14%的成人和11%的青少年报告自己是烟民。
- 经济计量问题使得确定烟草控制政策与吸烟相关结果之间的关系变得困难。
- 卷烟税的增加减少了成人吸烟，改善了儿童和婴儿的健康。
- 增加卷烟税对青少年吸烟的影响还不太清楚。

要点总结
- 卷烟消费税和SFA法减少了成人的吸烟参与和卷烟消费。
- 成年吸烟者通过更换卷烟品牌和更猛烈地吸烟来补偿更高的卷烟消费税，尽管最好的证据表明，这种行为并不能完全抵消卷烟消费量的减少。
- 关于卷烟消费税在减少青少年吸烟方面的有效性，有一场持续不断的辩论。
- 估计烟草控制政策对成人死亡率和发病率的影响是具有挑战性的，尽管有令人信服的证据表明，卷烟税改善了各种婴儿健康结果和长期儿童结果。

参考文献

Abrevaya, J.; Puzzello, L. (2012). Taxes, cigarette consumption, and smoking intensity: comment. American Economic Review, 102(4), 1751-1763.
Adams, S.; Cotti, C. (2008). Drunk driving after the passage of smoking bans in bars. Journal of Public Economics, 92(5-6), 1288-1305.

Adams, S.; Cotti, C.; Fuhrmann, D. (2013). Smokeless tobacco use following smoking bans in bars. Southern Economic Journal, 80(1), 147-161.

Adams, E. K.; Markowitz, S.; Kannan, V.; Dietz, P. M.; Tong, V. T.; Malarcher, A. M. (2012). Reducing prenatal smoking: the role of state policies. American Journal of Preventive Medicine, 43(1), 34-40.

Adda, J.; Cornaglia, F. (2006). Taxes, cigarette consumption, and smoking intensity. American Economic Review, 96(4), 1013.

Adda, J.; Cornaglia, F. (2010). The effect of bans and taxes on passive smoking. American Economic Journal: Applied Economics, 2(1), 1-32.

Barr, C. D.; Diez, D. M.; Wang, Y.; Dominici, F.; Samet, J. M. (2012). Comprehensive smoking bans and acute myocardial infarction among Medicare enrollees in 387 US counties: 1999-2008. American Journal of Epidemiology, 176(7), 642.

Bedard, K.; Desch^enes, O. (2006). The long-term impact of military service on health: evidence from World War II and Korean War veterans. The American Economic Review, 96(1), 176-194.

Bitler, M. P.; Carpenter, C. S.; Zavodny, M. (2010). Effects of venue-specific state clean indoor air laws on smoking-related outcomes. Health Economics, 19(12), 1425-1440.

Carpenter, C. (2009). The effects of local workplace smoking laws on smoking restrictions and exposure to smoke at work. Journal of Human Resources, 44(4), 1023-1046.

Carpenter, C.; Cook, P. (2008). Cigarette taxes and youth smoking: new evidence from national, state, and local youth risk behavior surveys. Journal of Health Economics, 27(2), 287-299.

Carpenter, C.; Postolek, S.; Warman, C. (2011). Public-place smoking laws and exposure to environmental tobacco smoke(ETS) in public places. American Economic Journal: Economic Policy, 3(3), 35-61.

Centers for Disease Control and Prevention. (2007). Reduced second-hand smoke exposure after implementation of a comprehensive statewide smoking ban-New York, June 26, 2003-June 30, 2004. Morbidity and Mortality Weekly Report, 56(28), 705-708.

Chaloupka, F. (1991). Rational addictive behavior and cigarette smoking. Journal of Political Economy, 99(4), 722-742.

Chaloupka, F. J. (1992). Clean indoor air laws, addiction and cigarette smoking. Applied Economics, 24(2), 193-205.

Chaloupka, F.; Grossman, M. (1996). Price, tobacco control policies and youth smoking. NBER working paper no. 5740.

Chaloupka, F. J.; Saffer, H. (1992). Clean indoor air laws and the demand for cigarettes. Contemporary Policy Issues, 10(2), 72-83.

Chaloupka, F.; Warner, K. (2000). The economics of smoking. In: A. J. Culyer, J. P. Newhouse (Eds.), Handbook of health economics(pp. 1539-1627). Vol. 1B(pp. 1539-1627). New York: North-Holland, Elsevier Science B. V.

Chaloupka, F.; Wechsler, H. (1997). Price, tobacco control policies and smoking among young adults. Journal of Health Economics, 16(3), 359-373.

Cheng, K. -W.; Liu, F.; Gonzalez, M. E.; Glantz, S. (2017). The effects of workplace clean indoor air law coverage on workers' smoking-related outcomes. Health Economics, 2(26), 226-242.

Chiou, L.; Muehlegger, E. (2008). Crossing the line: direct estimation of cross-border cigarette sales and the effect on tax revenue. B. E. Journal of Economic Analysis and Policy: Contributions to Economic Analysis and Policy, 8(1).

Colman, G.; Grossman, M.; Joyce, T. (2003). The effect of cigarette excise taxes on smoking before, during and after pregnancy. Journal of Health Economics, 22(6), 1053.

Cotti, C.; Nesson, E.; Tefft, N. (2016). The effects of tobacco control policies on tobacco products, tar, and nicotine consumption: evidence from household panel data. American Economic Journal: Economic Policy, 8(4), 103-123.

Courtemanche, C. (2009). Rising cigarette prices and rising obesity: coincidence or unintended consequence? Journal of Health Economics, 28(4), 781-798.

Darden, M.; Gilleskie, D. B.; Strumpf, K. (2015). Smoking and mortality:new evidence from a long panel. Working paper.

DeCicca, P.; Kenkel, D.; Liu, F. (2013a). Who pays cigarette taxes? Theimpact of consumer price search. The Review of Economics and Statistics, 95(2), 516-529. https://doi. org/10. 1162/REST_a_00303.

DeCicca, P.; Kenkel, D. S.; Liu, F. (2013b). Excise tax avoidance: the case of state cigarette taxes. Journal of Health Economics 32(6), 1130-1141.

DeCicca, P.; Kenkel, D.; Mathios, A. (2002). Putting out the fires: will higher taxes reduce the onset of youth smoking? Journal of Political Economy, 110(1), 144-169.

DeCicca, P.; Kenkel, D.; Mathios, A.; Shin, Y. -J.; Lim, J. -Y. (2008). Youth smoking, cigarette prices, and anti-smoking sentiment. Health Economics, 17(6), 733-749.

Douglas, S. (1998). The duration of the smoking habit. Economic Inquiry, 36(1), 49-64.

Douglas, S.; Hariharan, G. (1994). The hazard of starting smoking: estimates from a split population duration model. Journal of Health Economics, 13(2), 213-230.

Edoka, I. (2017). Implications of misclassification errors in empirical studies of adolescent smoking behaviours. Health Economics, 26(4), 486-499.

Ellingsen, D. G.; Fladseth, G.; Daae, H. L.; Gjolstad, M.; Kjaerheim, K.; Skogstad, M. et al. (2006). Airborne exposure and biological monitoring of bar and restaurant workers before and after the introduction of a smoking ban. Journal of Environmental Monitoring, 8(3), 362-368. https://doi. org/10. 1039/b600050a.

Evans, W. N.; Farrelly, M. C. (1998). The compensating behavior of smokers: taxes, tar, and nicotine. RAND Journal of Economics, 29(3), 578-595.

Evans, W. N.; Farrelly, M. C.; Montgomery, E. (1999). Do workplace smoking bans reduce smoking? American Economic Review, 89(4), 728-747.

Evans, W. N.; Ringel, J. S. (1999). Can higher cigarette taxes improve birth outcomes? Journal of Public Economics, 72, 135-154.

Farrelly, M. C.; Evans, W. N.; Sfekas, A. E. (1999). The impact of work-place smoking bans: results from a national survey. Tobacco Control, 8(3), 272-277.

Farrelly, M. C.; Nimsch, C. T.; Hyland, A.; Cummings, M. (2004). The effects of higher cigarette prices on tar and nicotine consumption in a cohort of adult smokers. Health Economics, 13(1), 49-58.

Farrelly, M. C. et al. (2005). Changes in hospitality workers' exposure to secondhand smoke following the implementation of New York's smoke-free law. Tobacco Control, 14(4), 236-241.

Hansen, B.; Sabia, J. J.; Rees, D. I. (2017). Have cigarette taxes lost their bite? New estimates of the relationship between cigarette taxes and youth smoking. American Journal of Health Economics, 3(1), 60-75.

Harding, M.; Leibtag, E.; Lovenheim, M. F. (2012). The heterogeneous geographic and socioeconomic incidence of cigarette taxes: evidence from Nielsen Homescan data. American Economic Journal: Economic Policy, 4(4), 169-198.

Harris, J. E. (1980). Taxing tar and nicotine. American Economic Review, 70(3), 300-311.

Kenkel, D.; Lillard, D. R.; Mathios, A. (2004). Accounting for misclassification error in retrospective smoking data. Health Economics, 13(10), 1031-1044.

King, C.; Markowitz, S.; Ross, H. (2015). Tobacco control policies and sudden infant death syndrome in developed nations. Health Economics, 24(8), 1042-1048.

Larsson, M.; Boethius, G.; Axelsson, S.; Montgomery, S. M. (2008). Exposure to environmental tobacco smoke and health effects among hospitality workers in Sweden-before and after the implementation of a smoke-free law. Scandinavian Journal of Work, Environment, Health, 34(4), 267-277.

Lillard, D.; Molloy, E.; Sfekas, A. (2013). Smoking initiation and the Iron law of demand. Journal of Health Economics, 32(1), 114-127.

Markowitz, S. (2008). The effectiveness of cigarette regulations in reducing cases of sudden infant death syndrome. Journal of Health Economics, 27(1), 106-133.

Markowitz, S.; Kathleen Adams, E.; Dietz, P. M.; Tong, V. T.; Kannan, V. (2013). Tobacco control policies, birth outcomes, and maternal human capital. Journal of Human Capital, 7(2), 130-160.

Menzies, D.; Nair, A.; Williamson, P. A.; Schembri, S.; Al-Khairalla, M. Z.; Barnes, M. et al. (2006). Respiratory symptoms, pulmonary function, and markers of inflammation among bar workers before and after a legislative ban on smoking in public places. JAMA, 296(14), 1742-1748. https://doi.org/10.1001/jama.296.14.1742.

Moore, M. J. (1996). Death and tobacco taxes. RAND Journal of Economics, 27(2), 415-428.

Mulcahy, M.; Evans, D. S.; Hammond, S. K.; Repace, J. L.; Byrne, M. (2005). Secondhand smoke exposure and risk following the Irish smoking ban: an assessment of salivary cotinine concentrations in hotel workers and air nicotine levels in bars. Tobacco Control, 14(6), 384-388. https://doi.org/10.1136/tc.2005.011635.

Nesson, E. (2017a). Heterogeneity in smokers' responses to tobacco control policies. Health Economics, 26(2), 206-225.

Nesson, E. (2017b). The impact of tobacco control policies on adolescent smoking: comparing self-reports and biomarkers. American Journal of Health Economics, 3(4), 507-527.

Nguyen, H. V. (2013). Do smoke-free car laws work? Evidence from a quasi-experiment. Journal of Health Economics, 32(1), 138-148.

Nonnemaker, J. M.; Farrelly, M. C. (2011). Smoking initiation among youth: the role of cigarette excise taxes and prices by race/ethnicity and gender. Journal of Health Economics, 30(3), 560-567.

Pearson, J.; Windsor, R.; El-Mohandes, A.; Perry, D. C. (2009). Evaluation of the immediate impact of the Washington, D. C.; smoke-free indoor air policy on bar employee environmental tobacco smoke exposure. Public Health Reports, 124(Suppl. 1), 134-142.

Pell, J. P.; Haw, S.; Cobbe, S.; Newby, D. E.; Pell, A. C. H.; Fischbacher, C. et al. (2008). Smoke-free legislation and hospitalizations for acute coronary syndrome. New England Journal of Medicine, 359(5), 482-491.

Sabia, J. J. (2008). Every breath you take: the effect of postpartum maternal smoking on childhood asthma. Southern Economic Journal, 128-158.

Shetty, K. D.; DeLeire, T.; White, C.; Bhattacharya, J. (2011). Changes in US hospitalization and mortality rates following smoking bans. Journal of Policy Analysis and Management, 30(1), 6-28.

Siegel, M.; Albers, A. B.; Cheng, D. M.; Biener, L.; Rigotti, N. A. (2004). Effect of local restaurant smoking regulations on environmental tobacco smoke exposure among youths. American Journal of Public Health, 94(2), 321-325.

Simon, D. (2016). Does early life exposure to cigarette smoke permanently harm childhood welfare? Evidence from cigarette tax hikes. American Economic Journal: Applied Economics, 8(4), 128-159.

Sims, M.; Mindell, J. S.; Jarvis, M. J.; Feyerabend, C.; Wardle, H.; Gilmore, A. (2012). Did smokefree legislation in England reduce exposure to secondhand smoke among nonsmoking adults? Cotinine analysis from the health survey for England. Environmental HealthPerspectives, 120(3), 425-430. https://doi.org/10.1289/ehp.1103680.

Tauras, J. A. (2006). Smoke-free air Laws, cigarette prices, and adult cigarette demand. Economic Inquiry, 44(2), 333-342.

Wehby, G.; Courtemanche, C. (2012). The heterogeneity of the cigarette price effect on body mass index. Journal of Health Economics, 31(5), 719-729.

63
烟碱神经科学资源

Rajkumar Rajendram[1,2], Victor R. Preedy[1]

1. Department of Medicine, King Abdulaziz Medical City, Ministry of National Guard Health Affairs, Riyadh, Saudi Arabia
2. Diabetes and Nutritional Sciences Research Division, Faculty of Life Science and Medicine, King's College London, London, United Kingdom

缩略语

HIV	人类免疫缺陷病毒	USA	美国
AIDS	获得性免疫缺陷综合征	WHO	世界卫生组织
UK	英国		

烟碱是最常用的娱乐性药物之一,"吸烟"的俗语是指通过吸入烟草燃烧产生的烟雾来消耗烟碱。烟草也可以咀嚼或吮吸。目前,有超过10亿人使用与烟草相关的产品(WHO,2017)。

烟碱被用作兴奋剂已有数千年的历史(Dani, Balfour, 2011)。烟碱有过多的神经活性作用,并且极易上瘾(Dani, Balfour, 2011)。烟碱的使用自古以来就存在。然而,在烟碱研究的整体时间范围内,对烟碱的神经效应的相关机制及其治疗的了解是相对较新的发现。

到20世纪初,烟碱已经被合成出来,Langley开始研究烟碱的作用(Dani, Balfour, 2011; Langley, 1905; Maehle, 2004)。在20世纪初,他们的研究导致了Langley所说的"接受性物质"的发现(Langley, 1905)。这最终被发现是烟碱乙酰胆碱受体(Dani, Balfour,2011)。

然而,由于对烟碱上瘾,人们也会接触到烟草和相关产品中的有害成分。世界卫生组织报告称,烟草使用每年导致700万人死亡(WHO, 2017)。这大约是死亡人数的1/10,超过了艾滋病毒/艾滋病、疟疾和结核病死亡人数的总和(WHO, 2017)。

自1905年人们认识到烟碱能激活受体以来,人们对烟碱神经科学的认识和理解出现了爆炸性增长。现在即使是有经验的科学家也很难跟上时代潮流。对于那些刚进入该领域的人来说,很难知道在无数可用的来源中哪些是可靠的。为了帮助有兴趣了解更多烟碱神经科学的同事,我们在本章制作了包含可靠的、最新的资源的表格。仅有40多名专家协助编制了这些资源表,并在下文中得到确认。

表63.1~表63.4列出了与烟碱神经科学循证方法相关的监管机构和专业协会(表63.1)、烟碱神经科学期刊(表63.2)和书籍(表63.3)以及在线资源(表63.4)的最新信息。

表63.1 监管机构、专业协会和组织

名称	网址
吸烟与健康行动	www.ash.org.uk
成瘾中心	www.addictioncenter.com/nicotine
非裔美国人烟草控制领导委员会	www.savingblacklives.org

续表

名称	网址
医疗保健研究与质量局	www.ahrq.gov
酒精和药物基金会	adf.org.au
美国癌症研究协会	www.aacr.org/Pages/Home.aspx
美国癌症协会	www.cancer.org
美国神经精神药理学学院	acnp.org
美国心脏协会	www.heart.org/hearorg
美国肺脏协会	www.lung.org
美国护士协会	www.ncsbn.org
美国精神病学协会	www.psychiatry.org
美国卫生经济学会	www.ashecon.org
美国成瘾医学会	www.asam.org
美国胸科学会	www.thoracic.org
成瘾专业人员协会	www.naadac.org
澳大利亚国家健康和医学研究委员会	www.nhmrc.gov.au
澳大利亚统计局	www.abs.gov.au
澳大利亚政府现在退出	www.quitnow.gov.au
无烟儿童运动	www.tobaccofreekids.org
加拿大药物使用和成瘾中心	www.ccdus.ca
澳大利亚癌症委员会	www.cancer.org.au
澳大利亚首都地区癌症委员会	www.actcancer.org
新南威尔士州癌症研究所	www.icanquit.com.au
西澳大利亚癌症委员会	www.cancerwa.asn.au
成瘾与心理健康中心	www.camh.ca
中国控制吸烟协会	www.catcprc.org.cn
药物依赖问题学院	www.cpdd.org
杜克大学戒烟中心	www.dukesmoking.com
癫痫中心	epilepsycentre.org.au
癫痫基金会	www.epilepsy.com
癫痫学会	www.epilepsysociety.org.uk
食品和药物管理局（美国）	www.fda.gov
食品和药物管理局（美国）烟草产品中心	www.fda.gov/aboutfda/centersoffices/officeofmedicalproductsandtobacco/aboutthecenterfortobaccoproducts/default.htm

续表

名称	网址
无烟美国基金会	www.anti-smoking.org
无烟世界基金会	www.smokefreeworld.org
国际卫生经济协会	www.healtheconomics.org
马来西亚药学会，注册戒烟服务提供商	www.acadpharm.org.my/index.cfm?, menuid=2
梅奥诊所（现更名为：妙佑医疗国际）	www.mayoclinic.org
全国戒烟协作组	www.tobacco-cessation.org
全国酗酒和药物滥用顾问协会	www.naadac.org
国家成瘾和药物滥用中心	www.centeronaddiction.org
国民保健制度	www.nhs.uk
国家药物滥用研究所	www.drugabuse.gov
烟碱匿名	nicotine-anonymous.org
昆士兰癌症委员会	www.cancerqld.org.au
戒烟助手	www.quitassist.com
戒烟	www.quitcoach.org.au
戒网	quitnet.meyouhealth.com
Quit South Australia	www.quitsa.org.au
Quit Victoria	www.quit.org.au
无烟	www.nhs.uk/smokefree
无烟行动联盟	www.smokefreeaction.org.uk
神经科学学会	www.sfn.org
烟碱和烟草研究学会	www.srnt.org
成瘾研究学会	www.addiction-ssa.org
西班牙戒烟专家协会	www.sedet.org
药物滥用和精神健康服务管理局	www.samhsa.gov
循环	theloop.ucsf.edu
烟草管制科学中心	prevention.nih.gov/tobacco-regulatory-science-program/research-portfolio/centers
真相倡议	truthinitiative.org
美国卫生与人类服务部	betobaccofree.hhs.gov/health-effects/nicotine-health/index.html
佛蒙特州成瘾专业协会	vapavt.org
世界银行	www.worldbank.org
世界卫生组织	www.who.int

注：该表列出了与烟草、烟碱和成瘾有关的监管机构、专业协会和组织。其中一些网站非常全面，因为它们提供了有关烟碱及其用途的建议、资源和其他信息。虽然有些网站是特定于国家的，但这些网站中包含的一些信息对其他国家很有用。表63.4还列出了一些资源。同样重要的是要指出，烟碱的精神或神经影响不应单独考虑，因为烟草使用会导致多种疾病，如心血管疾病和癌症。事实上，也发现了一些与癌症相关的位点。请注意，网站或网址有时会更改。

表63.2 烟碱神经科学相关期刊

Nicotine and Tobacco Research	BMC Public Health
Addictive Behaviors	Neuropharmacology
Psychopharmacology	Journal of Pharmacology and Experimental Therapeutics
Drug and Alcohol Dependence	European Journal of Pharmacology
PLOS One	Journal of Neuroscience
Addiction	American Journal of Public Health
Preventive Medicine	Substance Use and Misuse
Pharmacology Biochemistry and Behavior	Journal of Adolescent Health
Tobacco Control	American Journal of Preventive Medicine
Brain Research	Neuropsychopharmacology

注：发表与神经科学和治疗相关的烟碱和烟草相关产品的原创性研究和评论文章的期刊。这份榜单包括在过去5年中发表论文数量最多的前20种期刊。作者还推荐了Nature Medicine、PLOS One 和 The New England Journal of Medicine（尽管只有PLOS One出现在这份榜单上）。

表63.3 烟碱神经科学相关书籍

Addiction Biology. Simonnet A, Cador M and Caillé S. Wiley, 2013, UK
Cigarettes, Nicotine and Health. A Biobehavioral Approach. Kozlowski LT, Henningfield JE, Brigham J. SAGE Publications, 2001, UK
Clearing the Smoke: Assessing the Science Base for Tobacco Harm Reduction. Stratton K, Shetty P, Wallace R et al.(Editors). Institute of Medicine(USA) Committee to Assess the Science Base for Tobacco Harm Reduction, National Academies Press (USA) 2001, USA
Ending the Tobacco Problem: A Blueprint for the Nation. Institute of Medicine. The National Academies Press, 2007, USA
Golden Holocaust: Origins of the Cigarette Catastrophe and the Case for Abolition. Proctor RN. University of California Press, 2012, USA
Handbook of Health Economics, Vol. 1. Culyer A, Newhouse J. Elsevier, 2000, UK
Handbook of Health Economics, Vol. 2. Pauly M, Mcguire T, Parros P. Elsevier, 2011, UK
Helping the Hard-Core Smoker: A Clinician's Guide. Seidman DF, Covey LS. Lawrence Erlbaum Associates, 1999, USA
Individual Decisions for Health. Lindgren B. Routledge, 2002, UK
Methods in Molecular Biology. Caillé S, Clemens K, Stinus L, Cador M. Springer, 2012, Germany
Negative Affective States and Cognitive Impairments in Nicotine Dependence. Hall FS, Young JW, Der-Avakian A. Academic Press, 2017, UK
Neuronal Nicotinic Receptors. Clementi F, Fornasari D, Gotti C. Springer, 2000, Germany
Neuropathology of Drug Addiction and Substance Misuse Volume 1: Foundations of Understanding, Tobacco, Alcohol, Cannabinoids and Opioids. Preedy VR (Editor). Academic Press, 2016, UK
Neuropharmacology. Simonnet A, Zamberletti E, Cador M, Rubino T, Caillé S. Elsevier 2017, The Netherlands
Nicotine. Hens G, Self W, Calleja J. Other Press, 2017, USA
Nicotine Addiction: Prevention, Health Effects and Treatment Options. Di Giovanni G. Nova Science Publishers, 2012, USA

Nicotine Addiction: Principles and Management. Orleans CT, Slade JD. Oxford University Press, UK
Nicotine and Other Tobacco Compounds in Neurodegenerative and Psychiatric Diseases. Xia W, Phillips B, Wong ET, Ho J, Oviedo A, Hoeng J, Peitsch M. Academic Press, 2018, UK
Nicotine in Psychiatry: Psychopathology and Emerging Therapeutics. Piasecki M, Newhouse PA. American Psychiatric Publishing, 2000, USA
Nicotine Psychopharmacology. Henningfield JE, Calvento E, Pogun S. Springer-Verlag, 2009, Germany
Nicotinic Acetylcholine Receptor Technologies. Li M (Editor), Springer, 2016, USA
Nicotinic receptors. Lester RAJ, Humana Press, 2014, USA
Nicotinic Receptors in the Nervous System. Levin ED (Editor). CRC Press, 2001, USA
Preventing Tobacco Use Among Youth and Young Adults: A Report of the Surgeon General. National Center for Chronic Disease Prevention and Health Promotion (USA) Office on Smoking and Health. Centers for Disease Control and Prevention (USA), 2012, USA
Progress in Respiratory Research. Caillé S, Baker AL, Todd J, Turner A, Dayas CV. Karger, 2015, Europe
Psychopharmacology. Clemens KJ, Caillé S, Cador M. European Behavioural Pharmacology Society, 2010, Europe
Public Health Implications of Raising the Minimum Age of Legal Access to Tobacco Products. Committee on the Public Health Implications of Raising the Minimum Age for Purchasing Tobacco Products; Board on Population Health and Public Health Practice; Institute of Medicine; BonnieRJ, Stratton K, Kwan LY (Editors). National Academies Press (USA), 2015, USA
Research Report Series: Tobacco Addiction. National Institute on Drug Abuse, US Department of Health and Human Services, National Institutes of Health, 2012, USA
Smoking Cessation. Lewis KE. Oxford University Press, 2010, UK
Smoking: Risk, Perception, and Policy. Slovic P. SAGE, 2001, USA
The Addicted Brain: Why We Abuse Drugs, Alcohol, and Nicotine. Kuhar M. Pearson FT Press, 2012, USA
The Cigarette Book: The History and Culture of Smoking. Harrald C, Watkins F. Skyhorse Publishing, 2010, USA
The Cigarette Century: The Rise, Fall, and Deadly Persistence of the Product that Defined America. Brandt A. Basic Books, 2009, USA
The Clinical Management of Nicotine Dependence. Cocores JA. Springer-Verlag, 1991, USA
The Economics of Tobacco and Tobacco Control. US National Cancer Institute (NHU) and WHO. WHO, 2017, Switzerland
The Health Consequences of Smoking—50 Years of Progress: A Report of the Surgeon General. National Center for Chronic Disease Prevention and Health Promotion (USA) Office on Smoking and Health. Centers for Disease Control and Prevention (USA), 2014, USA
The Molecular Basis of Drug Addiction, Volume 137. Rahman S. Elsevier, 2016, USA
The Motivational Impact of Nicotine and its Role in Tobacco Use. Bevins RA, Caggiula AR. Springer-Verlag, 2009, USA
The Neurobiology and Genetics of Nicotine and Tobacco. Balfour D, Munafo M. Springer International Publishing, 2015, Switzerland
The Neuropharmacology of Nicotine Dependence. Balfour DJK, Munafo MR. Springer, 2015, Switzerland
The science of addiction: From neurobiology to treatment. Erickson CK. WW Norton, Company, 2007, USA

续表

This is Nicotine (Addiction). Farrington K. Sanctuary Publishing, 2002, UK	
Tobacco: A Cultural History of How an Exotic Plant Seduced Civilization. Gately I. Grove Press, 2002, USA	
Treating Nicotine Dependence with Nitrous Oxide/Oxygen (PAN): A manual for Health Professionals. Gillman M. Cerebrum Publishers, 2010, South Africa	
Women and Smoking: A Report of the Surgeon General. Office on Smoking and Health (USA). Centers for Disease Control and Prevention (USA), 2001, USA	

注：该表列出了烟碱神经科学方面的书籍。

表63.4　关于新兴技术的相关在线资源和信息

医疗研究和质量机构：妊娠资源	www.ahrq.gov/professionals/prevention-chronic-care/healthier-pregnancy/preventive/tobacco.html
美国癌症协会：戒烟资源	www.cancer.org/healthy/stay-away-from-tobacco/guide-quitting-smokinghtml?from=fast
美国肺脏协会：戒烟资源	www.lung.org/stop-smoking
美国成瘾医学会：烟碱和烟草资源	www.asam.org/advocacy/find-a-policy-statement/view-policy-statement/public-policy-statements/2011/12/15/nicotine-addiction-and-tobacco
烟灰缸博客	www.ecigarettedirect.co.uk/ashtray-blog/2016/10/nicotine-overdose-vaping.html
疾病控制和预防中心：概况介绍——戒烟——吸烟和烟草使用	www.cdc.gov/tobacco/data_statistics/fact_sheets/health_effects/effects_cig_smoking/index.htm
疾病控制和预防中心：烟草资源	www.cdc.gov/tobacco/campaign/tips/partners/health/hcp/index.html
食品和药物管理局：公共卫生资源	www.fda.gov/TobaccoProducts/PublicHealthScienceResearch/default.htm
激光射线	www.laserrayli.com
Luyang Health Clinic 安卓应用 mQuit	play.google.com/store/apps/details?id = appinventor.ai_h2ocfh2ocf.JomQuitTRIAL,hl=en
梅奥诊所：烟碱依赖资源	www.mayoclinic.org/diseases-conditions/nicotine-dependence/symptoms-causes/syc-20351584
Medscape	www.medscape.com
国家成瘾和药物滥用中心：电子烟资源	www.centeronaddiction.org/e-cigarettes
国家卫生局通报：戒烟资源	www.nhsinform.scot/healthy-living/stopping-smoking/reasons-to-stop/tobacco
办公室倡导戒烟行为健康事实	www.aafp.org/patient-care/public-health/tobacco-nicotine/office-champions/behavioral-health.html
澳大利亚全科医学戒烟指南	www.health.gov.au/internet/main/publishing.nsf/Content/health-pubhlth-publicat-document-smoking_cessation-cnt.htm
烟草经济学	tobacconomics.org
烟草相关疾病研究计划	www.trdrp.org
WebMD	www.webmd.com
世界卫生组织：烟草	www.who.int/mediacentre/factsheets/fs339/en

注：该表列出了一些与烟碱神经科学和烟碱成瘾治疗相关的互联网资源和其他相关材料。表63.1中也列出了其中一些网站。请注意，网站或网址偶尔会发生变化。

术语解释
- 吸烟：通过吸入燃烧烟草的烟雾来消耗烟碱。
- 乙酰胆碱：乙酰胆碱是一种有机化学物质，是一种神经递质。胆碱能受体主要有：烟碱受体和毒蕈碱受体两种类型。
- 烟碱乙酰胆碱受体：这些跨膜蛋白受体被乙酰胆碱激活。它们也会被烟碱激活。

关键事实
- 烟碱被用作兴奋剂已有数千年的历史。
- 对烟碱作用及其治疗相关机制的理解是烟碱研究中相对较新的发现。
- 自1905年人们认识到烟碱会激活受体以来，人们对烟碱神经科学的认识和理解出现了爆炸性的增长。
- 为了帮助对了解烟碱的神经科学感兴趣的同事，我们在本章中制作了包含可靠的、最新资源的表格。

要点总结
- 烟碱是最常用的娱乐性药物之一。
- 有超过10亿烟草使用者。
- 烟碱包含在可以咀嚼、吸吮或吸食的烟草产品中。最近，通过电子烟中的液体来获取烟碱变得流行起来。
- 烟碱有许多神经活性作用，而且很容易上瘾。
- 烟碱的神经效应及其治疗机制是烟草使用时间尺度上相对较新的发现。
- 本章列出了监管和专业机构、期刊、书籍和网站上与烟碱神经科学循证方法相关的资源。

致谢（按字母顺序）

我们要感谢以下作者为这一资源的开发做出的贡献。

Alkam T, Bagdas D, Beeler J, Budzynska B, Hahn B, Michalak A, Caille S, Chukwueke C, Chylinska-Wrzos P, Cole R, Corsini S, DeCicca P, Nesson E, Ferretti F, Gipson C, Henderson B, Hritcu L, Ibañez-Tallon I, Jodłowska-Jędrych B, Khoo S, Lis-Sochocka M, McNally G, Clemens K, Kumari V, Liu Y, Macedo D, McCallum S, Nabeshima T, Eggan B, McGrath D, Morales A, Nadalin S, Jakovac H, Nistri A, Richter L, Saad S, Chen H, Schmidt H, Siraj MA, Sudweeks S, Sui CF, and WawrykGawda E.

参考文献

Dani, J. A.; Balfour, D. J. (2011). Historical and current perspective on tobacco use and nicotine addiction. Trends in Neurosciences, 34, 383-392.

Langley, J. N. (1905). On the reaction of cells and of nerve-endings to certain poisons, chiefly as regards the reaction of striated muscle to nicotine and to curari. The Journal of Physiology, 33, 374-413.

Maehle, A. H. (2004). "Receptive substances": John Newport Langley(1852-1925) and his path to a receptor theory of drug action. Medical History, 48, 153-174.

WHO (2017). Who report on the global tobacco epidemic. Geneva: World Health Organization.